CT and MRI Anatomy
guided by 3D images

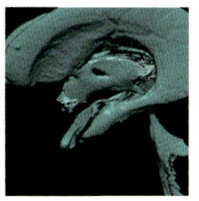
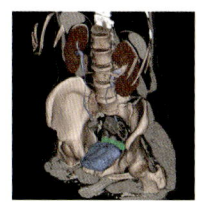
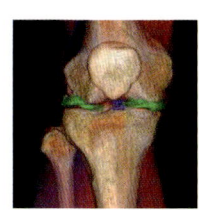
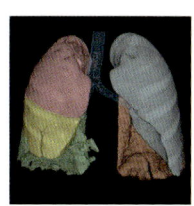
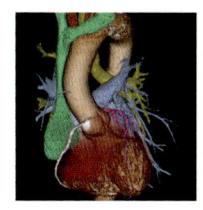

3次元画像から学ぶ
CT・MRI断層解剖

編著 ● 似鳥俊明　杏林大学医学部 放射線医学教室 教授

メディカル・サイエンス・インターナショナル

CT and MRI Anatomy guided by 3D images
First Edition
by Toshiaki Nitatori, M.D., Ph.D.

©2014 by Medical Sciences International, Ltd., Tokyo
All rights reserved.
ISBN 978-4-89592-768-0

Printed and Bound in Japan

執筆者一覧

編 集

似鳥 俊明　　杏林大学医学部 放射線医学教室 教授

編集主幹

小林 邦典　　杏林大学保健学部 診療放射線技術学科 特任教授

執 筆(五十音順)

大原 有紗　　杏林大学医学部 放射線医学教室
黒木 一典　　杏林大学保健学部 診療放射線技術学科 教授
小林 邦典　　杏林大学保健学部 診療放射線技術学科 特任教授
五明 美穂　　杏林大学医学部 放射線医学教室
小柳 正道　　杏林大学医学部付属病院 放射線部
坂本 岳士　　杏林大学保健学部 診療放射線技術学科
清水 裕太　　杏林大学医学部付属病院 放射線部
鈴木 満　　　杏林大学医学部付属病院 放射線部
髙橋 沙奈江　杏林大学医学部付属病院 放射線部
土屋 一洋　　東京逓信病院 放射線科 部長
似鳥 徹　　　岩手県立大学看護学部 解剖学 准教授
似鳥 俊明　　杏林大学医学部 放射線医学教室 教授
福島 啓太　　杏林大学医学部付属病院 放射線部
本谷 啓太　　杏林大学保健学部 診療放射線技術学科 講師
水野 将人　　杏林大学医学部付属病院 放射線部
山村 恒　　　杏林大学医学部付属病院 放射線部
横山 健一　　杏林大学医学部 放射線医学教室 准教授
吉岡 達也　　杏林大学医学部付属病院 放射線部
吉田 真衣子　杏林大学医学部 放射線医学教室

執筆協力

円城寺 正行　杏林大学医学部付属病院 放射線部
榑沼 かずみ　杏林大学医学部付属病院 放射線部
髙橋 正勝　　杏林大学医学部付属病院 放射線部
坂倉 智紀　　杏林大学医学部付属病院 放射線部
武内 啓志　　杏林大学医学部付属病院 放射線部
蓮沼 政子　　杏林大学医学部付属病院 放射線部

畦元 将吾　　株式会社 AZE 代表取締役社長
阪本 剛　　　株式会社 AZE 開発部 製品企画グループ

序

　解剖学は古くから今日まで医学の基本であり続け，CT・MRIを主とした画像診断は現代医療の要となっている．解体新書，ダ・ヴィンチ，ミケランジェロの解剖図譜の例を待つまでもなく，人体深層の実態把握のために困難な探究が行われてきたが，科学技術の進歩はこの分野でも大きく様相を変化させた．メスの力を用いずに，人体内部の形状が光の下に照らしだされ，"個人ごとの解剖図"が実用のため容易に作成される．

　CT・MRIの元データからワークステーションによりつくられる3次元立体画像は，初期の患者への説明，手術シミュレーションへの応用から，最近の飛躍的な精度向上により適応範囲が広がり，診断にすら用いられるようになっている．全体像把握には最適な観察法である．しかし，現在の撮影室，読影室，診療室で診断の際に圧倒的に多く行われる行為はモニター上での体軸横断面スクロールである．冠状断面，矢状断面も解剖構造によってしばしば使われる．まず割って見て，病態を直接的に観察できる断層面を子細に見，そしてそれを立ち止まりながら連続的に観察する．立体構造を無意識下に想像してなされる高度の作業である．

　本書の最大の目的は，各臓器構造そして臓器間の関連が理解しやすい3次元画像から，この診断に最も有用な断層面をよりやさしく深く理解し学ぶことにある．実際に元画となった2次元画像と，これよりつくられた3次元画像との相互関係を通してである．

　CT・MRIとその断層面は，機械的配置を避け，それぞれの部位で診断に適するものを柔軟に選択掲載した．また解剖学的構造と生理学的役割，そして重要な病理学的事項の略解も理解の補助のため随所にNOTEとし配した．さらに解剖学的用語の語源も可能なかぎり挿入し，解剖学という古い学問への尊敬と，医用画像を通じて想像する世界を，今いる閉ざされた病院内の小部屋を超え拡げてほしいとの願いも込めた．

　本書は杏林大学医学部と保健学部の教員，医師，技師を中心としてつくられたものだが，株式会社AZEと東芝メディカルシステムズ株式会社，そしてメディカル・サイエンス・インターナショナル編集部の正路修氏，後藤亮弘氏の多大な協力なしでは上梓できなかった．医療は直接患者に接する病院職員にとどまらず，薬品，機器，教育出版関係者など多業種にわたる医療人のチームワークで成り立つ．その基本となる画像解剖にかかわる人々の世界は広くて深い．本書が，近い将来仲間となる学生を含めたすべての医療人へ，この魅力尽きない画像解剖学を広く深く学ぶ手掛かりをお示しできればこの上ない幸いである．

2014年1月

杏林大学医学部 放射線医学教室 教授
似鳥　俊明

目 次

序 ……………………………………………………………………………… [似鳥俊明]　v

I 章　脳　Brain　[吉岡達也・五明美穂・土屋一洋]　1

頭蓋骨 …………………………………………………………………………………… 2
　・頭蓋骨 ……………………………………………………………………………… 2
　・下顎骨 ……………………………………………………………………………… 5
大脳の表面解剖 ………………………………………………………………………… 6
運動野・感覚野と神経線維 …………………………………………………………… 8
脳血管 …………………………………………………………………………………… 9
　・動　脈 ……………………………………………………………………………… 9
　・Willis 動脈輪 …………………………………………………………………… 12
　・静　脈 …………………………………………………………………………… 13
脳動脈の支配領域 …………………………………………………………………… 14
脳室・脳脊髄液 ……………………………………………………………………… 17
海馬および線条体近辺 ……………………………………………………………… 18
脳の断層解剖 ………………………………………………………………………… 19
　・横断像（MRI, T1 強調像）　1-31 〜 1-45 ………………………………… 19
　・矢状断像（MRI, T1 強調像）　1-46 〜 1-57 ……………………………… 27
　・冠状断像（MRI, T1 強調像）　1-58 〜 1-78 ……………………………… 33
脳神経 ………………………………………………………………………………… 44
　・脳神経 …………………………………………………………………………… 44
　・脳神経の分類 …………………………………………………………………… 44
脳神経の断層解剖 …………………………………………………………………… 45
　・横・矢状断像（MRI, 白黒反転 heavy T2 強調像） ………………………… 45
脳幹部の断層解剖 …………………………………………………………………… 50
　・横断像（MRI, 白黒反転 heavy T2 強調像）　1-91 〜 1-112 …………… 50
　・矢状断像（MRI, 白黒反転 heavy T2 強調像）　1-113 〜 1-122 ……… 61
　・冠状断像（MRI, 白黒反転 heavy T2 強調像）　1-123 〜 1-133 ……… 65

II章　頭頸部　Head and Neck

[吉岡達也・大原有紗]　69

- 頭頸部 70
  - ・副鼻腔・唾液腺・甲状腺 70
  - ・副鼻腔・咽喉頭 71
  - ・舌骨・甲状軟骨・輪状軟骨 71
- 頭頸部の断層解剖 72
  - ・横断像（造影CT）　2-5 〜 2-37 72
  - ・矢状断像（造影CT）　2-38 〜 2-51 89
  - ・冠状断像（造影CT）　2-52 〜 2-73 96
- 頸部リンパ節のレベルシステム 107
- 耳小骨・三半規管 109
- 側頭骨の断層解剖 110
  - ・横断像（CT）　2-81 〜 2-94 110
  - ・冠状断像（CT）　2-95 〜 2-102 115
  - ・矢状断像（CT）　2-103 〜 2-111 118

III章　脊椎　Spine

[鈴木　満・清水裕太・小柳正道・坂本岳志・五明美穂]　121

- 脊柱 122
  - ・脊柱の外観 122
- 頸椎 123
- 頸椎の断層解剖 127
  - ・横断像（CT）　3-11 〜 3-14 127
  - ・冠状断像（CT, MPR像）　3-15, 3-16 129
  - ・矢状断像（CT, MPR像）　3-17, 3-18 130
  - ・横断像（MRI, T1強調像）　3-19 〜 3-23 131
  - ・横断像（MRI, T2強調像）　3-24 133
  - ・冠状断像（MRI, T1強調像）　3-25 〜 3-27 134
  - ・矢状断像（MRI, T1強調像）　3-28, 3-29 136
  - ・矢状断像（MRI, T2強調像）　3-30 137
- 胸椎 138
- 胸椎の断層解剖 140
  - ・横断像（CT）　3-35 〜 3-37 140
  - ・冠状断像（CT, MPR像）　3-38 〜 3-40 142

- ・矢状断像(CT, MPR 像) 3-41 ～ 3-43 ……………………………… 144
- ・横断像(MRI, T2 強調像) 3-44 ～ 3-46 ……………………………… 146
- ・横断像(MRI, T1 強調像) 3-47 ……………………………………… 147
- ・冠状断像(MRI, T1 強調像) 3-48, 3-49 …………………………… 148
- ・矢状断像(MRI, T1 強調像) 3-50 ～ 3-52 …………………………… 149
- ・矢状断像(MRI, T2 強調像) 3-53 …………………………………… 150

腰 椎 ……………………………………………………………………… 151

腰椎の断層解剖 ………………………………………………………… 153
- ・横断像(CT) 3-59, 3-60 ……………………………………………… 153
- ・冠状断像(CT, MPR 像) 3-61 ～ 3-63 ……………………………… 154
- ・矢状断像(CT, MPR 像) 3-64 ～ 3-66 ……………………………… 156
- ・横断像(MRI, T2 強調像) 3-67 ～ 3-69 ……………………………… 158
- ・横断像(MRI, T1 強調像) 3-70 ……………………………………… 159
- ・冠状断像(MRI, T1 強調像) 3-71, 3-72 …………………………… 160
- ・冠状断像(MRI, T2 強調像) 3-73 …………………………………… 161
- ・矢状断像(MRI, T1 強調像) 3-74, 3-75 …………………………… 162
- ・矢状断像(MRI, T2 強調像) 3-76 …………………………………… 163

仙 椎 ……………………………………………………………………… 164

仙椎の断層解剖 ………………………………………………………… 165
- ・横断像(CT) 3-79 …………………………………………………… 165
- ・斜冠状断像(CT, MPR 像) 3-80 …………………………………… 165
- ・矢状断像(CT, MPR 像) 3-81 ……………………………………… 166
- ・横断像(MRI, T1 強調像) 3-82, 3-83 ……………………………… 167
- ・冠状断像(MRI, T1 強調像) 3-84, 3-85 …………………………… 168

IV章 胸 部 Chest
[鈴木 満・髙橋沙奈江・福島啓太・小柳正道・横山健一]　169

胸 郭 ……………………………………………………………………… 170

胸郭の断層解剖 ………………………………………………………… 175
- ・横断像(CT) 4-12 ～ 4-15 …………………………………………… 175
- ・冠状断像(CT) 4-16 ～ 4-18 ………………………………………… 177
- ・矢状断像(CT) 4-19, 4-20 …………………………………………… 179

肺 ………………………………………………………………………… 180
- ・肺区域 ………………………………………………………………… 180

気管・血管 ……………………………………………………………… 182
- ・胸部の血管 …………………………………………………………… 182
- ・区域気管支 …………………………………………………………… 183

・気管支と肺動静脈の関係	183
・気管支と肺動静脈の関係	184
縦隔の断層解剖	185
・横断像(造影CT, 縦隔条件) 4-30 ～ 4-38	185
・冠状断像(造影CT, 縦隔条件) 4-39 ～ 4-44	188
・矢状断像(造影CT, 縦隔条件) 4-45 ～ 4-52	191
肺の断層解剖	195
・横断像(造影CT, 肺野条件) 4-53 ～ 4-61	195
・冠状断像(造影CT, 肺野条件) 4-62 ～ 4-67	198
・矢状断像(造影CT, 肺野条件) 4-68 ～ 4-75	201
心　臓	205
・心臓の外観	205
・左心室短軸像	206
・左心室長軸像	206
・四腔断像	207
・三腔断像	207
冠動脈	208
冠動脈のAHA分類	211
心臓の断層解剖	213
・横断像(造影CT) 4-92 ～ 4-101	213
・矢状断像(造影CT) 4-102 ～ 4-110	218
・冠状断像(造影CT) 4-111 ～ 4-118	221
・左心室短軸像(造影CT) 4-119 ～ 4-121	224
・左心室長軸像(造影CT) 4-122	225
・四腔断像(造影CT) 4-123	226
・三腔断像(造影CT) 4-124	226

V章　腹　部　Abdomen

[小林邦典・水野将人・本谷啓太・黒木一典]　227

腹部の体表解剖	228
・体表解剖と腹部臓器	228
・腹部の9領域と腹部臓器	228
骨格と腹部臓器	229
腹部臓器(消化管を除く)	230
肝臓・脾臓と横断面	232
胆嚢・膵臓と横断面	233
腎臓・副腎と横断面	234

消化管	235
消化管のバリエーション(S状結腸過長症)	237
消化管の走行と冠状断面	238
上腹部の血管系	239
上腹部の動脈	240
上腹部の静脈	241
上腹部の動脈と横断面	242
上腹部の静脈と横断面	244
肝区域	246
・Couinaud分類	246
・肝臓の静脈・門脈	246
・血管系とCouinaud分類	246
・造影CT門脈相，静脈相，VR像(肝臓解析ソフトを使用)	247
肝区域の横断面	248
腹部の断層解剖	249
・横断像(造影CT平衡相) 5-53〜5-66	249
・冠状断像(造影CT平衡相) 5-67〜5-78	254
・矢状断像(造影CT平衡相) 5-79〜5-91	260

VI章 骨盤部 Pelvis

[小林邦典・坂本岳士・吉田真衣子] 267

男性骨盤部の体表と骨格・泌尿器	268
男性骨盤部の骨格・泌尿器・生殖器	269
男性骨盤部	270
・冠状断像(3次元画像＋造影CT)	270
・矢状断像(3次元画像＋造影CT)	272
男性骨盤部の動脈(CTA3次元表示)	273
女性骨盤部の体表と骨格・泌尿器・生殖器	274
女性骨盤部の骨格・泌尿器・生殖器	275
女性骨盤部	276
・冠状断像(3次元画像＋造影CT)	276
・矢状断像(3次元画像＋造影CT)	278
女性骨盤部の動脈(CTA3次元表示)	279
男性骨盤部の断層解剖	280
・横断像(造影CT) 6-25〜6-36	280
・冠状断像(造影CT) 6-37〜6-44	284
・矢状断像(造影CT) 6-45〜6-50	288

女性骨盤部の断層解剖 291
　・横断像（造影CT）　6-51 ～ 6-58 291
　・冠状断像（造影CT）　6-59 ～ 6-68 294
　・矢状断像（造影CT）　6-69 ～ 6-77 299

Ⅶ章　四　肢　Extremities
［山村　恒・坂本岳士・小林邦典・本谷啓太］　305

上肢の主な動脈 306
上肢の主な静脈 307
肩関節 308
　・肩関節の体表解剖 308
　・肩関節の筋 309
　・肩関節の骨 310
肩関節の断層解剖 312
　・横断像（MRI，プロトン密度強調像）　7-10 ～ 7-15 312
　・冠状断像（MRI，プロトン密度強調像）　7-16 ～ 7-21 315
　・矢状断像（MRI，プロトン密度強調像）　7-22 ～ 7-30 318
肘関節 323
　・肘関節の体表解剖 323
　・肘関節の筋 323
　・肘関節の骨 324
肘関節の断層解剖 325
　・横断像（MRI，プロトン密度強調像）　7-39 ～ 7-47 325
　・冠状断像（MRI，プロトン密度強調像）　7-48 ～ 7-56 330
　・矢状断像（MRI，プロトン密度強調像）　7-57 ～ 7-65 335
手関節と手 340
　・手関節と手の体表解剖 340
　・手関節と手の骨・腱 341
　・手関節と手の骨 342
手関節と手の断層解剖 343
　・横断像（MRI，プロトン密度強調像）　7-72 ～ 7-79 343
　・横断像：第3指（MRI，プロトン密度強調像）　7-80 ～ 7-83 ... 347
　・冠状断像（MRI，プロトン密度強調像）　7-84 ～ 7-86 349
　・矢状断像：第3指（MRI，プロトン密度強調像）　7-87 ～ 7-89 ... 351
下肢の主な動脈 353
下肢の主な静脈 354
股関節 355

- ・下肢の筋 …………………………………………………………………………………… 355
- ・骨盤の筋 …………………………………………………………………………………… 355
- ・骨盤の骨 …………………………………………………………………………………… 356
- ・右大腿骨頭 ………………………………………………………………………………… 359

股関節の断層解剖 …………………………………………………………………………… 360
- ・横断像（MRI, プロトン密度強調像） 7-102 〜 7-107 ………………………………… 360
- ・冠状断像（MRI, プロトン密度強調像） 7-108 〜 7-113 ………………………………… 363
- ・矢状断像（MRI, プロトン密度強調像） 7-114 〜 7-119 ………………………………… 366

膝関節 ………………………………………………………………………………………… 369
- ・膝部の体表解剖 …………………………………………………………………………… 369
- ・膝関節の筋 ………………………………………………………………………………… 370
- ・膝関節の筋・靱帯 ………………………………………………………………………… 371
- ・外側側副靱帯 ……………………………………………………………………………… 371
- ・内側側副靱帯 ……………………………………………………………………………… 372
- ・靱帯・半月板 ……………………………………………………………………………… 372
- ［半月板］ …………………………………………………………………………………… 373
  - ・半月板 …………………………………………………………………………………… 373
  - ・矢状断 …………………………………………………………………………………… 374
  - ・冠状断 …………………………………………………………………………………… 374
- ・膝関節の骨 ………………………………………………………………………………… 375

膝関節の断層解剖 …………………………………………………………………………… 376
- ・横断像（MRI, プロトン密度強調像） 7-136 〜 7-144 ………………………………… 376
- ・冠状断像（MRI, プロトン密度強調像） 7-145 〜 7-153 ………………………………… 381
- ・矢状断像（MRI, プロトン密度強調像） 7-154 〜 7-166 ………………………………… 386

足関節と足 …………………………………………………………………………………… 393
- ・足関節部の外観 …………………………………………………………………………… 393
- ・足関節と足の筋・腱 ……………………………………………………………………… 393
- ・足関節と足の骨 …………………………………………………………………………… 394

足関節と足の断層解剖 ……………………………………………………………………… 396
- ・横断像（MRI, プロトン密度強調像） 7-174 〜 7-185 ………………………………… 396
- ・冠状断像（MRI, プロトン密度強調像） 7-186 〜 7-200 ………………………………… 402
- ・矢状断像（MRI, プロトン密度強調像） 7-201 〜 7-213 ………………………………… 409

和文索引 ………………………………………………………………………………………… 417
欧文索引 ………………………………………………………………………………………… 428

Green NOTEs

皮質 Cortex	……………………………………	24
延髄 Medulla oblongata	………………………	26
洞 Sinus	…………………………………………	29
サンスクリットと医学用語	…………………	30
淡蒼球 Globus pallidus	………………………	38
橋 Pons	……………………………………………	40
中脳水道 Aqueduct	……………………………	52
脳室 Ventricle	…………………………………	54
白質 White matter と灰白質 Grey matter	………	61
小脳虫部 Cerebellar vermis	…………………	68
頬骨 Zygoma	……………………………………	76
頚動脈 Carotid artery	………………………	83
頚静脈 Jugular vein	…………………………	84
僧帽筋 Trapezius (muscle)	……………………	86
伴行静脈 Accompanying vein, Companion vein	…	88
耳管 Eustachian tube	………………………	117
環椎 Atlas	………………………………………	124
脊椎 Spine	………………………………………	128
椎骨 Vertebra	…………………………………	135
矢状 Sagittal	……………………………………	144
上・下椎切痕 Superior/Inferior vertebral notch		
	………………………………………………	157
黄色靱帯 Yellow ligament	……………………	159
奇静脈 Azygos vein	…………………………	191
僧帽弁 Mitral valve	……………………………	223
門脈 Portal vein	………………………………	249
横隔膜 Diaphragm	……………………………	254
副腎 Adrenal gland	…………………………	259
横隔膜脚 Crus of diaphragm	………………	261
解剖 Anatomy	…………………………………	266
卵巣 Ovary	………………………………………	298
肩峰 Acromion	…………………………………	316
尺骨 Ulna と橈骨 Radius	……………………	334
短内転筋 Adductor brevis muscle	……………	365
ハムストリング Hamstring	…………………	366
内側広筋 Vastus medialis muscle	……………	376
十字靱帯 Cruciate ligament	…………………	384
アキレス腱 Achilles tendon	…………………	412

＊緑色の NOTE は編著者が解剖用語の語源を中心に執筆した．
＊水色の NOTE は各章担当者が執筆した．

＊本書に使用した CT は東芝メディカルシステムズ社製の Aquilion™ ONE ViSION, Aquilion™ PRIME, Aquilion™ 64, MRI は同社の Vantage Titan™ 3T・1.5T, EXCELART Vantage™ powered by Atlas1.5T である．

＊3 次元画像作成は AZE 社製の AZE VirtualPlace/AZE Phoenix による．

＊解剖学用語の英語名は日本解剖学会監修，解剖学用語委員会編集の『解剖学用語』(改訂13版, 2007年)に従い，1字目は大文字表記としたが，杏林大学医学部解剖学教室の松村讓兒先生のご指導を得た．

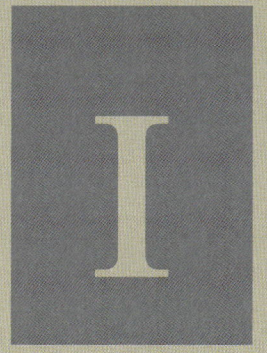

脳
Brain

頭蓋骨（CT, VR像）

1-1 頭蓋骨（正面）

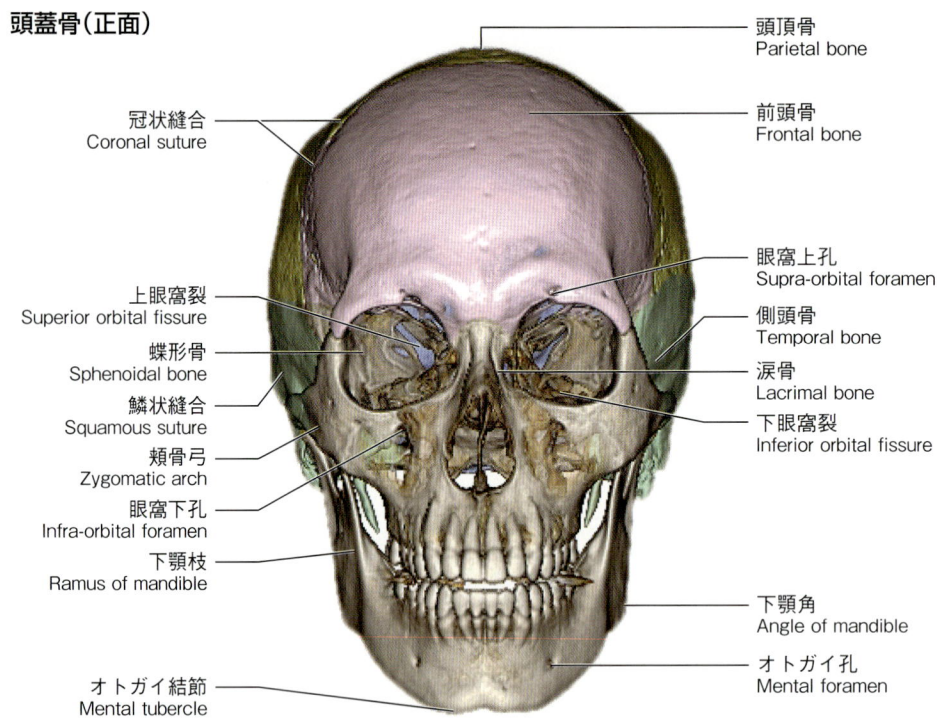

1-2 頭蓋骨（側面）

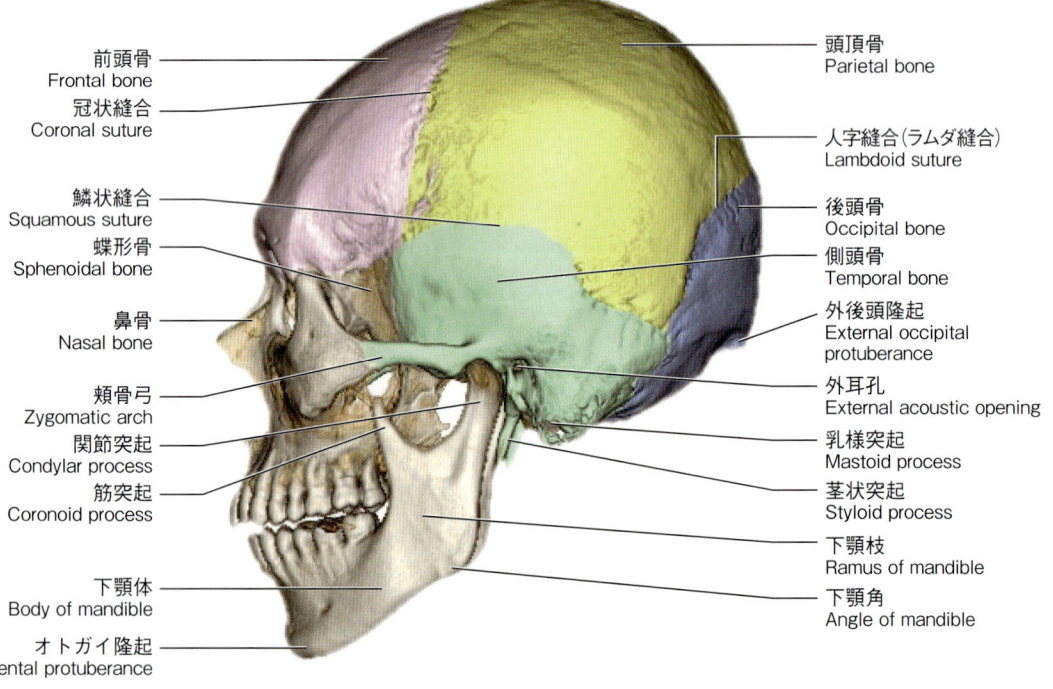

> **NOTE** 縫合の閉鎖と離開：文献によって差異があるが，主な泉門や縫合はおおむね2歳までに閉鎖する（ただし，縫合の完全な骨化は30歳以降）．単一あるいは複数の縫合が異常に早く融合すると"頭蓋縫合早期癒合症"と称される変形をきたす．逆に小児では，頭蓋内圧亢進で縫合が離開することがある．

頭蓋骨（CT, VR像） 3

1-3 頭蓋骨（後面）

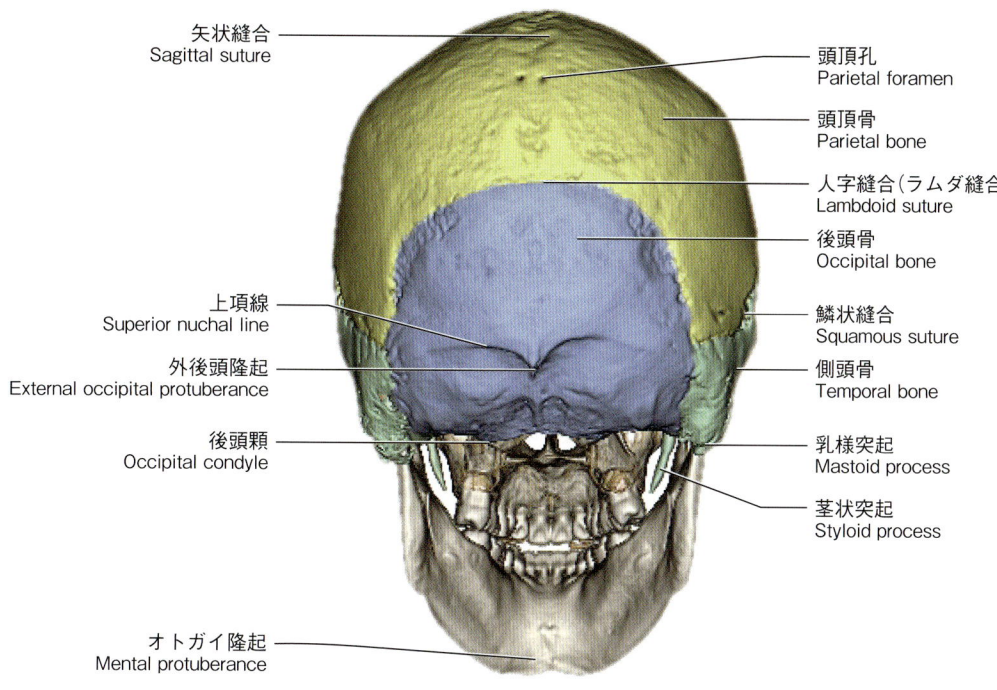

1-4 頭蓋骨（頭頂）

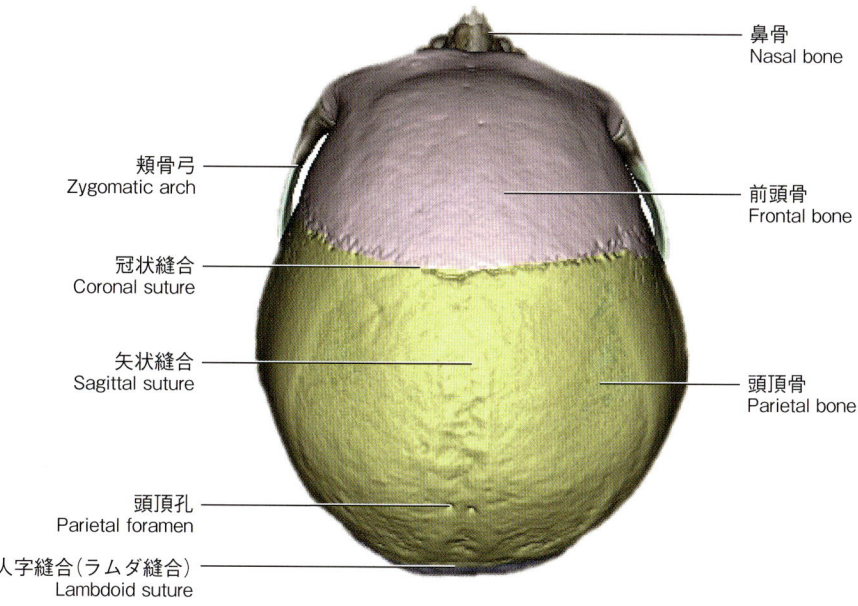

NOTE しばしばみられる縫合のバリエーション
前頭縫合：前頭骨を形成する左右の原基が完全に癒合していないもの．
縫合骨：縫合線内の独立した骨．頭頂間骨（インカ骨）はそのひとつともいうべきもので，人字（ラムダ）縫合の頂点部の後頭骨鱗部上部にみられる．

頭蓋骨

1-5 頭蓋底（CT, VR 像）

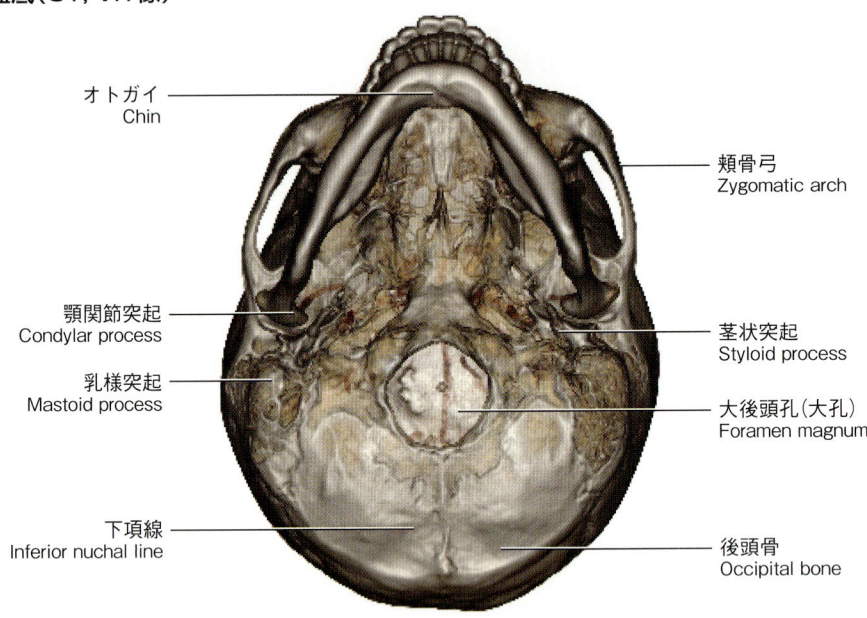

1-6 頭蓋底（標本）

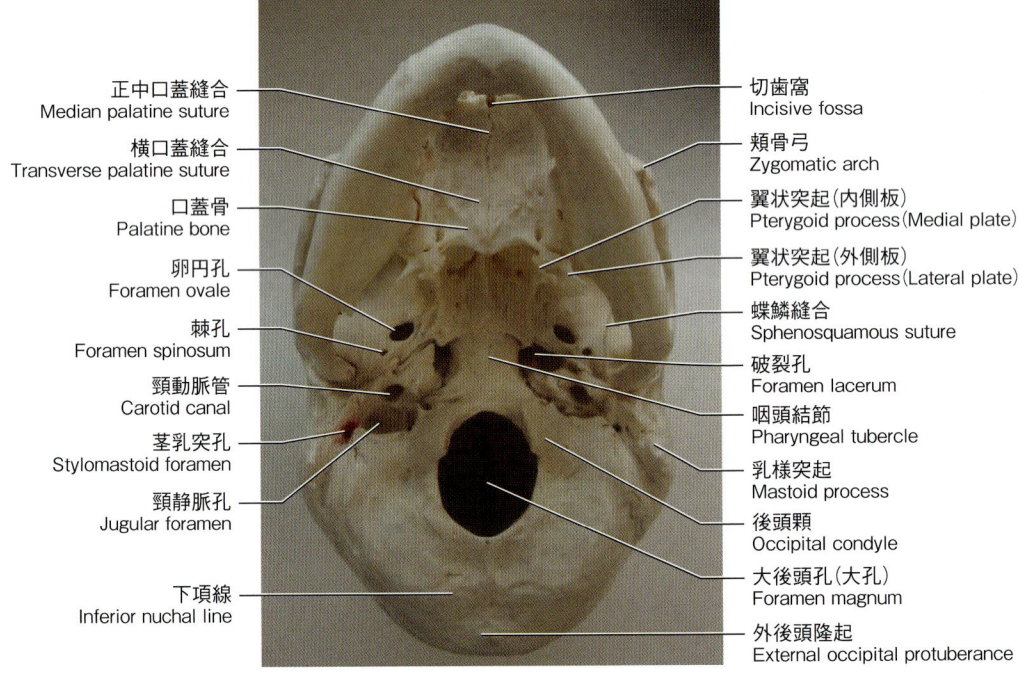

NOTE 頭蓋底の孔については，それを出入りする血管や神経を把握しておく必要がある．

下顎骨

1-7 下顎骨斜位（CT, VR像）

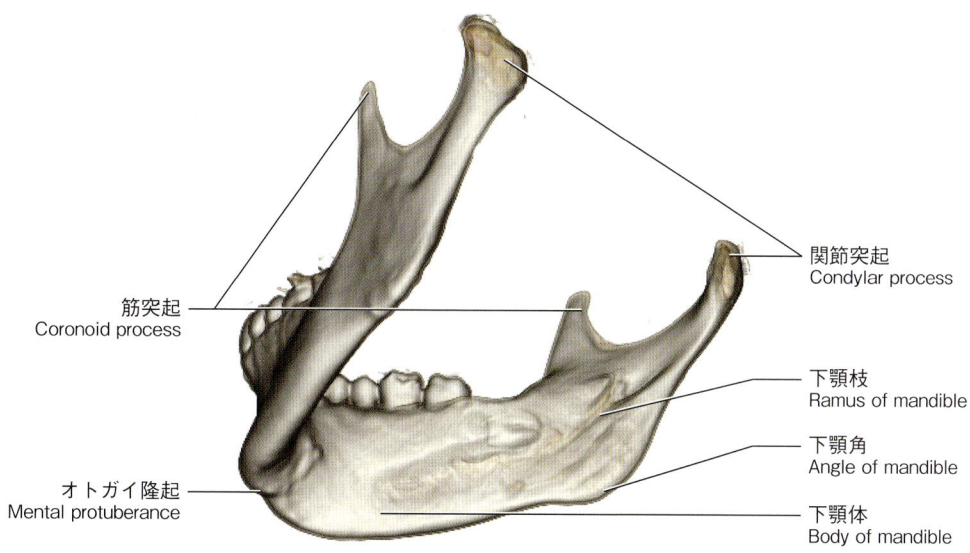

1-8 歯列（CT, CPR像）

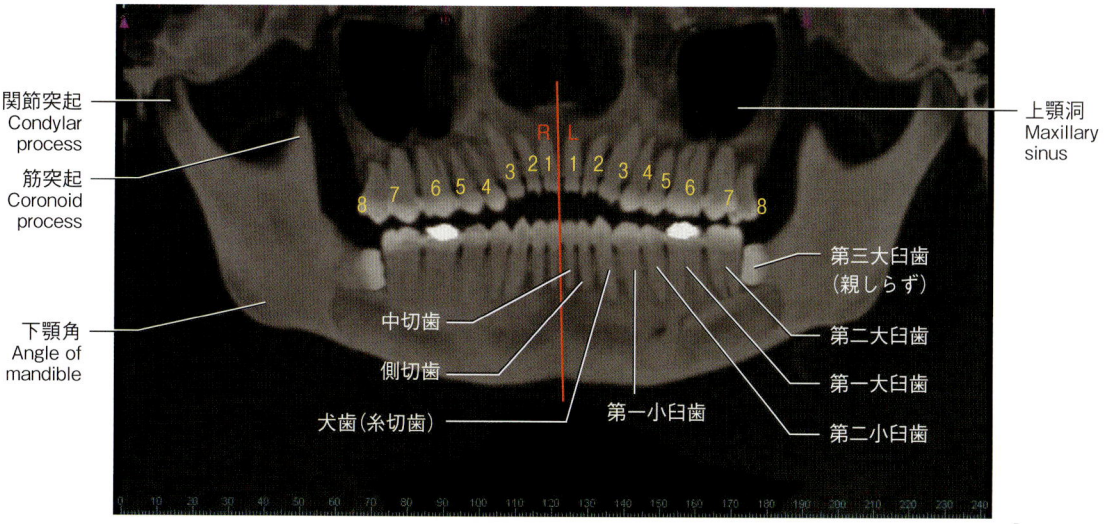

大脳の表面解剖 (MRI, 3D FLAIR 像から頭蓋や頭皮を除去)

1-9 脳葉

1-10 脳溝

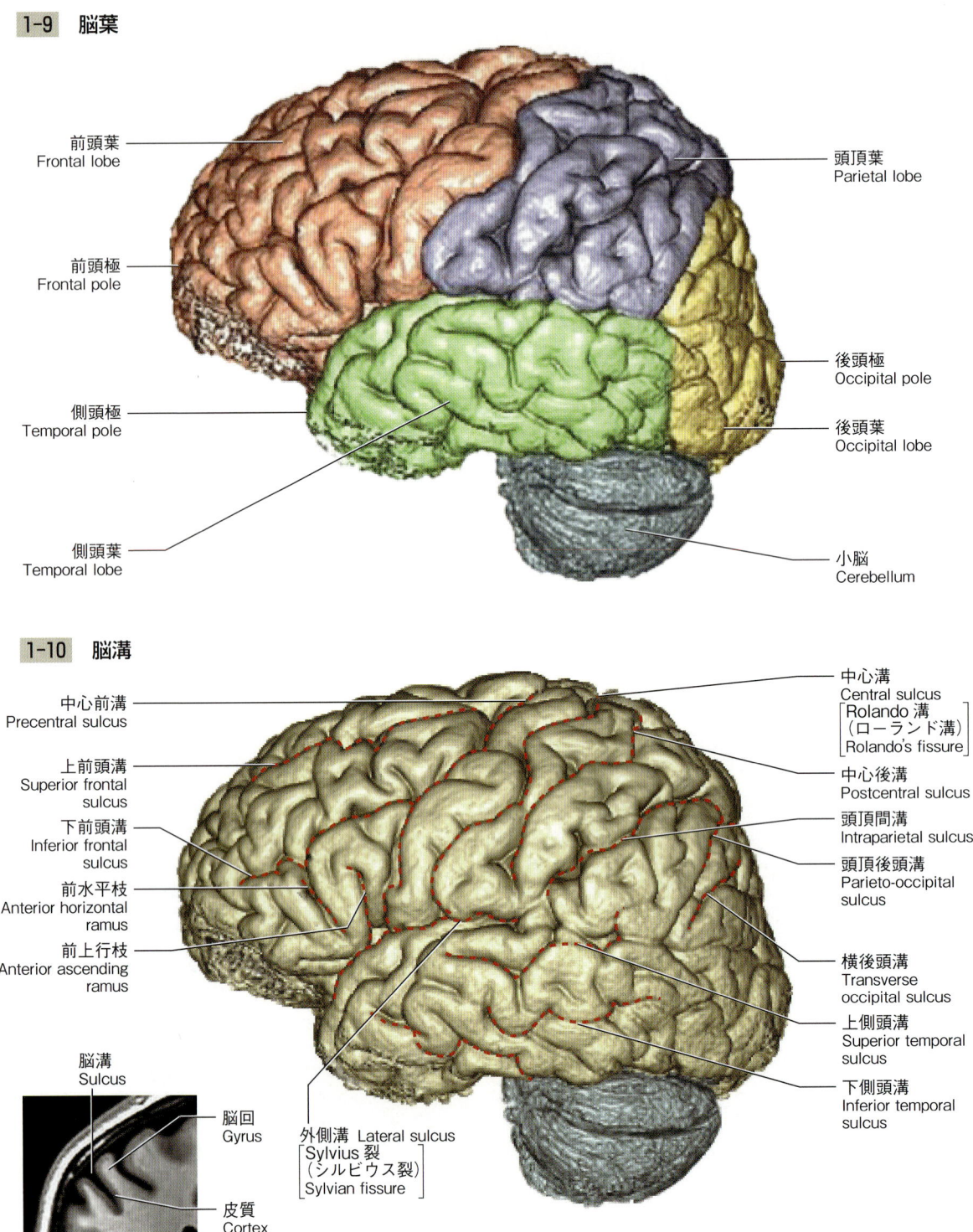

NOTE 1-9〜12の画像は，3DのFLAIR像のデータから頭蓋や頭皮をワークステーション上で除去して表示したものである．脳回などの脳表構造の良好なコントラストが得られている．

大脳の表面解剖（MRI, 3D FLAIR 像から頭蓋や頭皮を除去）

1-11 脳回

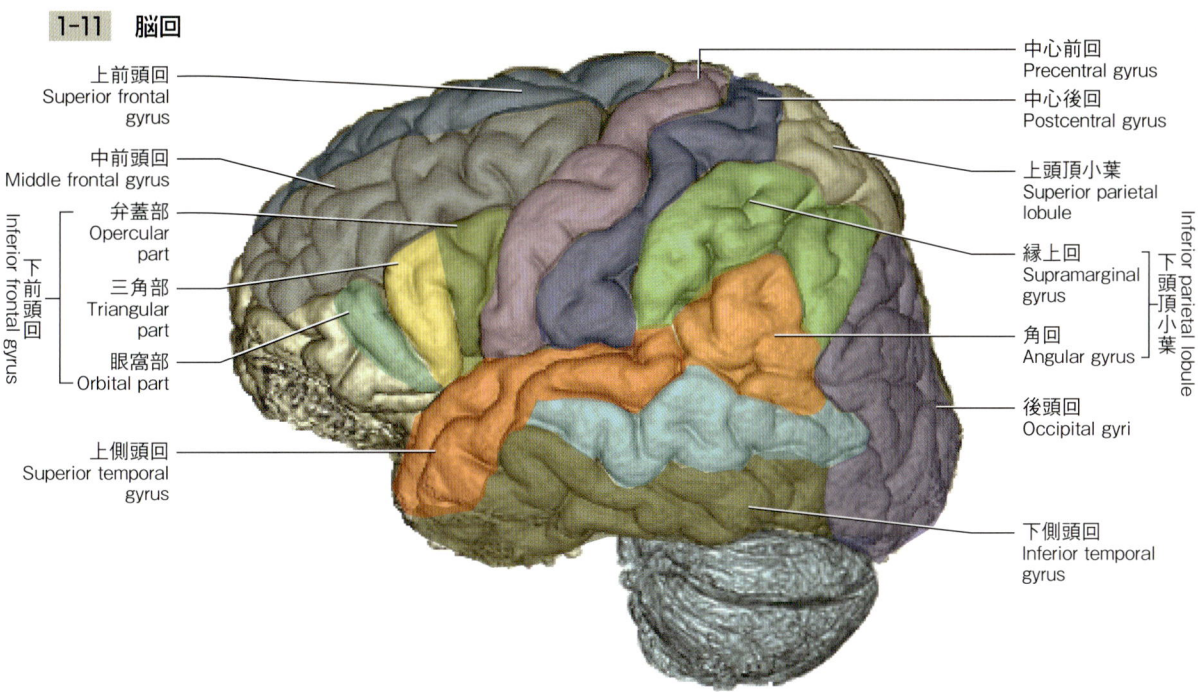

1-12 支配野

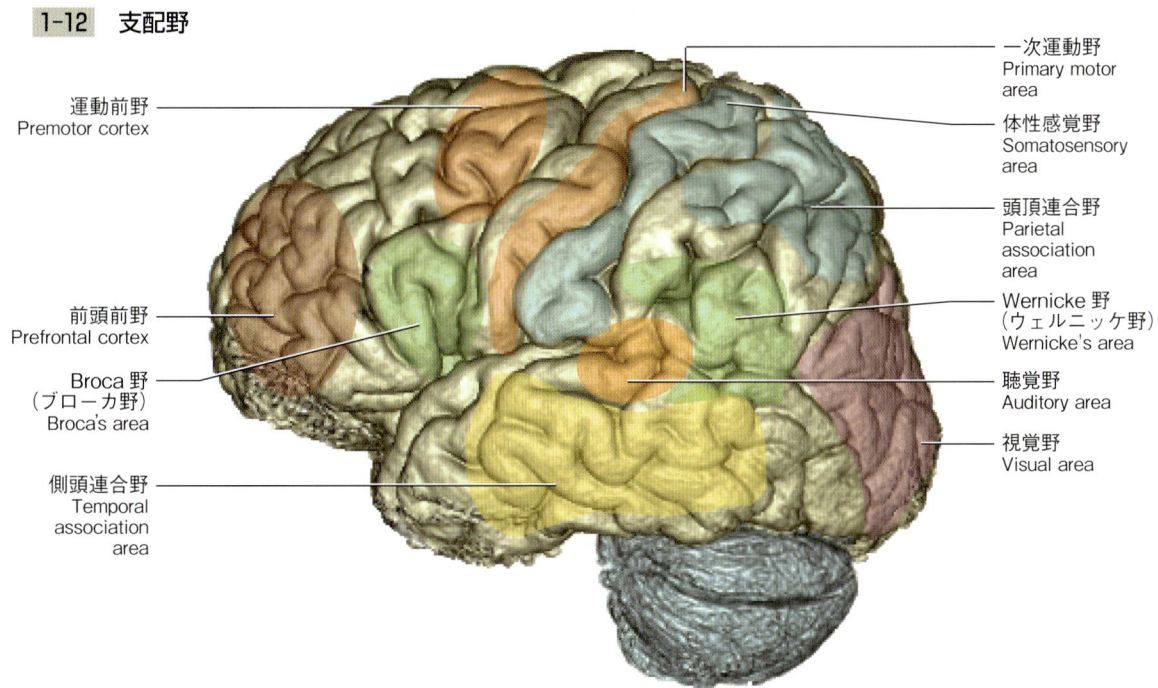

> **NOTE** 言語に関する中枢：優位半球（多くの場合は左側）のBroca（ブローカ）野は運動性言語中枢，Wernicke（ウェルニッケ）野は感覚性言語中枢である．それぞれの障害で運動失語（正しい言葉を発せられない），感覚失語（言葉を正しく理解できない）が起こる．

運動野・感覚野と神経線維

1-13 ホムンクルス

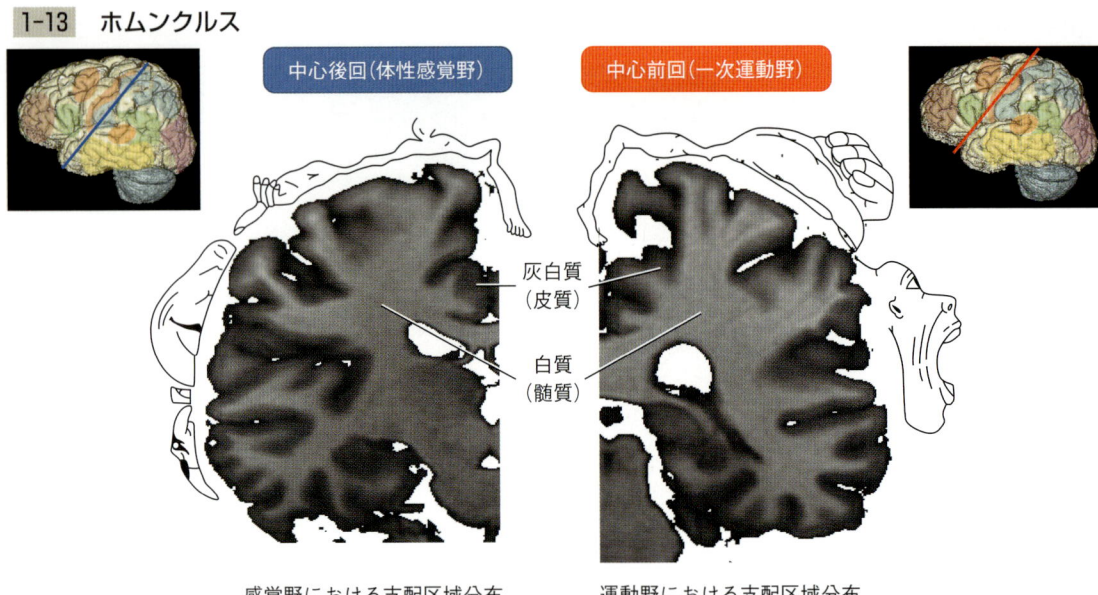

（Penfield W, Rasmussen T : The cerebral cortex of man: a clinical study of localization of function. New York : Macmillan, 1950. をもとに作成）

1-14 白質部の線維網（MR tractography）

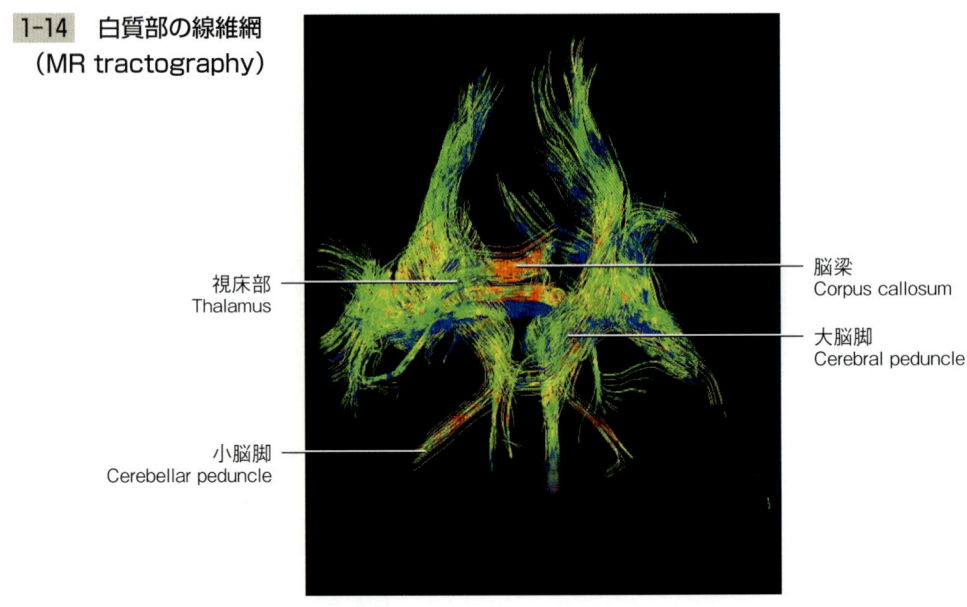

> **NOTE** 中心溝の前方が一次運動野，後方が体性感覚野である（1-13）．それぞれ絵で示された体の部位を大脳皮質のどの部位がつかさどっているのかを表している．
> 　6軸以上の拡散強調画像を解析すること（テンソル解析）で，神経線維を擬似的に描出することができる（1-14）．皮質の神経細胞と髄質の神経線維によって複雑なネットワークが構築されている．

脳血管（動脈）　(MRA, 3D-TOF 法, VR 像)

1-15　脳動脈（尾頭方向）

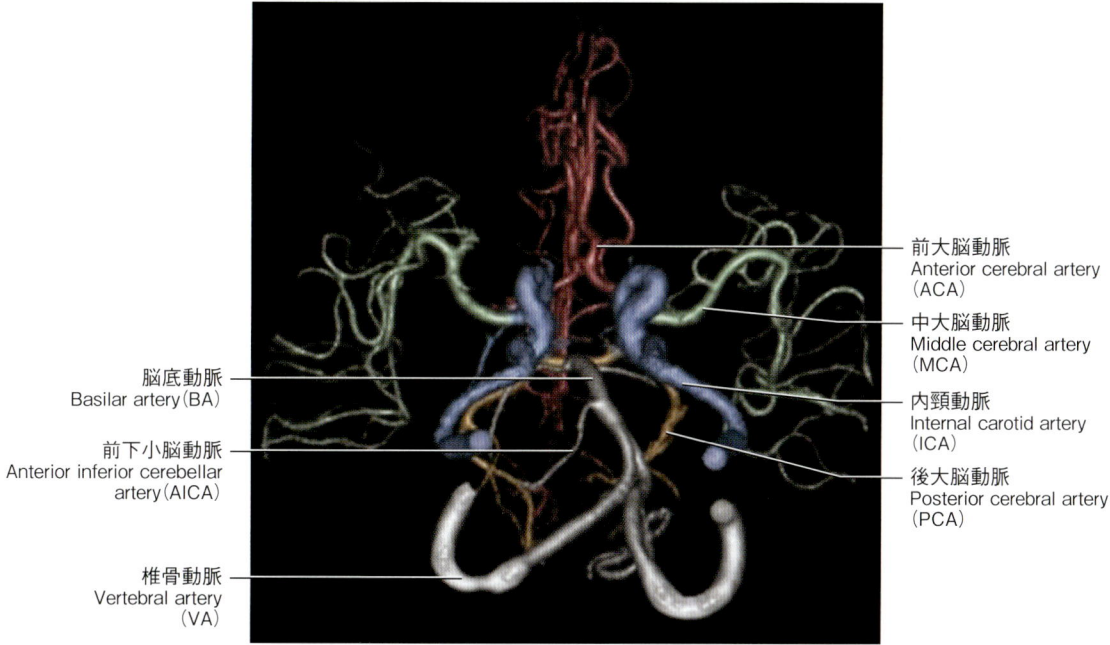

1-16　脳動脈（正面）

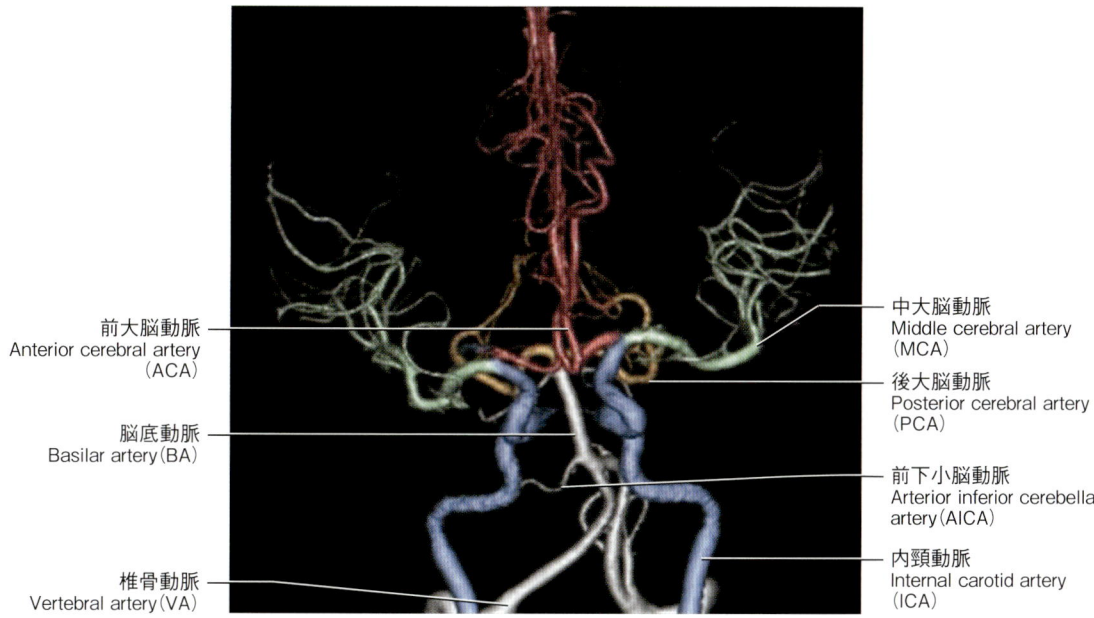

> **NOTE**　3T（テスラ）装置での 3D-TOF 法の MRA では，末梢まで信号の強い画像が得られ，1-15〜1-21 に示すような VR 法での 3 次元表示も高画質になっている．

脳血管（動脈）（MRA, 3D-TOF 法, VR 像）

1-17 脳動脈（側面）

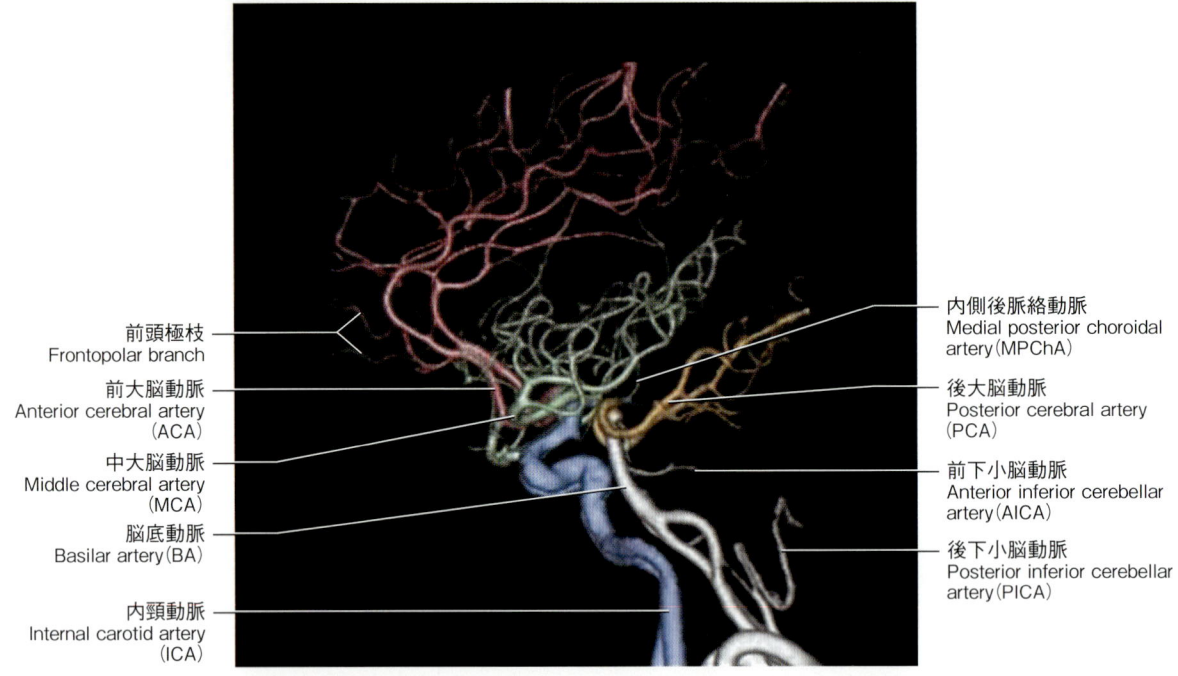

- 前頭極枝 Frontopolar branch
- 前大脳動脈 Anterior cerebral artery (ACA)
- 中大脳動脈 Middle cerebral artery (MCA)
- 脳底動脈 Basilar artery (BA)
- 内頸動脈 Internal carotid artery (ICA)
- 内側後脈絡動脈 Medial posterior choroidal artery (MPChA)
- 後大脳動脈 Posterior cerebral artery (PCA)
- 前下小脳動脈 Anterior inferior cerebellar artery (AICA)
- 後下小脳動脈 Posterior inferior cerebellar artery (PICA)

1-18 中大脳動脈の領域区分（1-16 の拡大像）

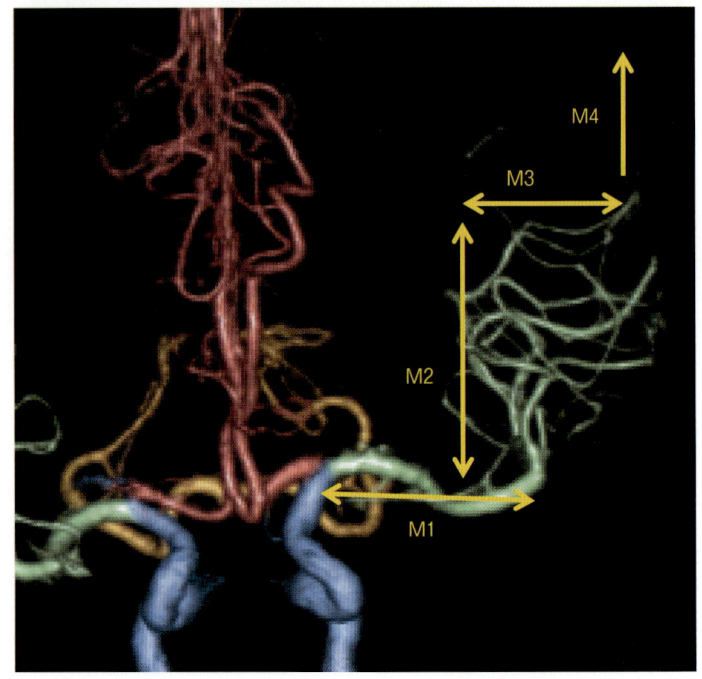

M1：水平部
M2：島部
M3：弁蓋部
M4：皮質部

脳血管（動脈）（MRA, 3D-TOF 法, VR 像）

1-19 前大脳動脈の領域区分（1-17 の拡大像）

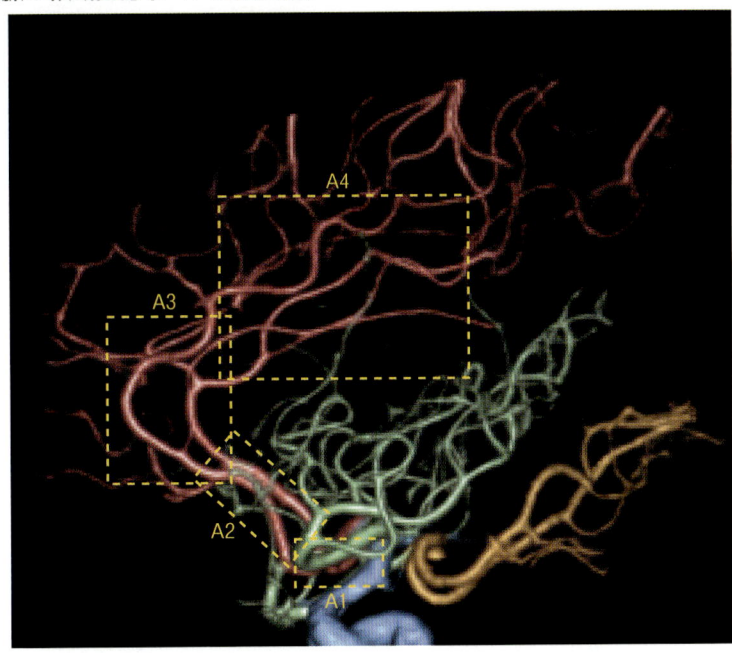

A1：水平部
A2：脳梁下部
A3：脳梁前部
A4：脳梁上部

1-20 後大脳動脈の領域区分（1-17 の拡大像）

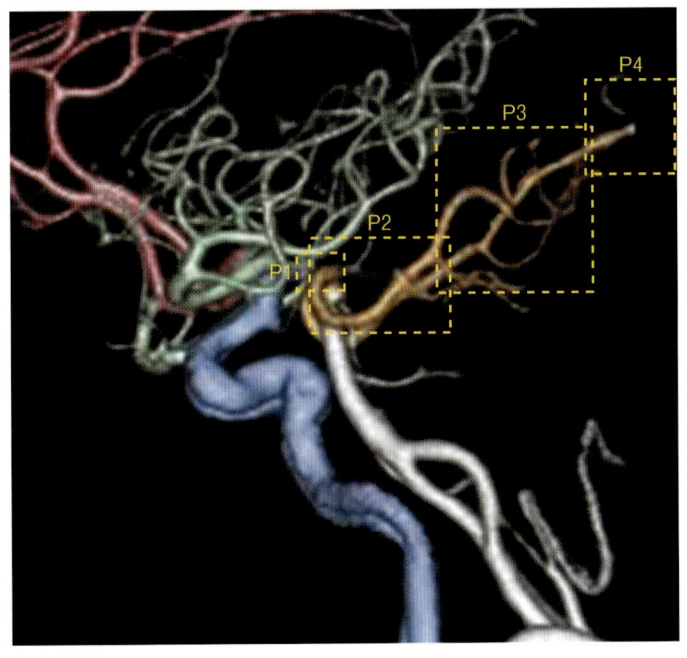

P1：交通前部
P2：脚部
P3：四丘体部
P4：皮質部

NOTE 前大脳動脈と後大脳動脈の走行区分を血管像のみで示すことは難しい．1-19, 20 では，おおよその区分を点線で記した．
【前大脳動脈】A1：内頸動脈分岐から前交通動脈分岐まで，A2：A1 より遠位で脳梁膝部に向けて前上方に向かう部分，A3：脳梁膝部の前方を回り込んで後上方に向かう部分，A4：脳梁体部の上を後方に向かって走行する部分．
【後大脳動脈】P1：後大脳動脈起始部から後交通動脈との合流点まで，P2(P2A)-脚部：P1 より遠位で脚槽を走行して大脳脚後縁まで，P2(P2P)-迂回槽部：迂回槽内を走行する部分，P3：四丘体槽を走行して鳥距溝前縁まで，P4：さらに後方の皮質枝部分．

Willis 動脈輪

1-21 Willis 動脈輪の MRA, 3D-TOF 法, VR 像

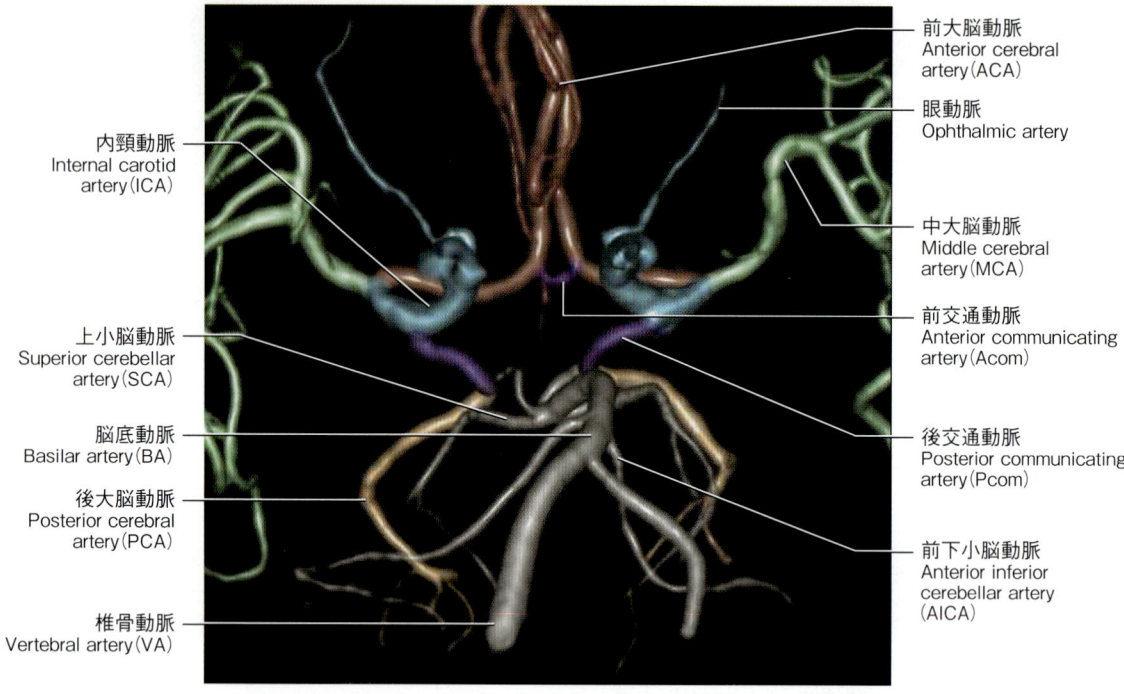

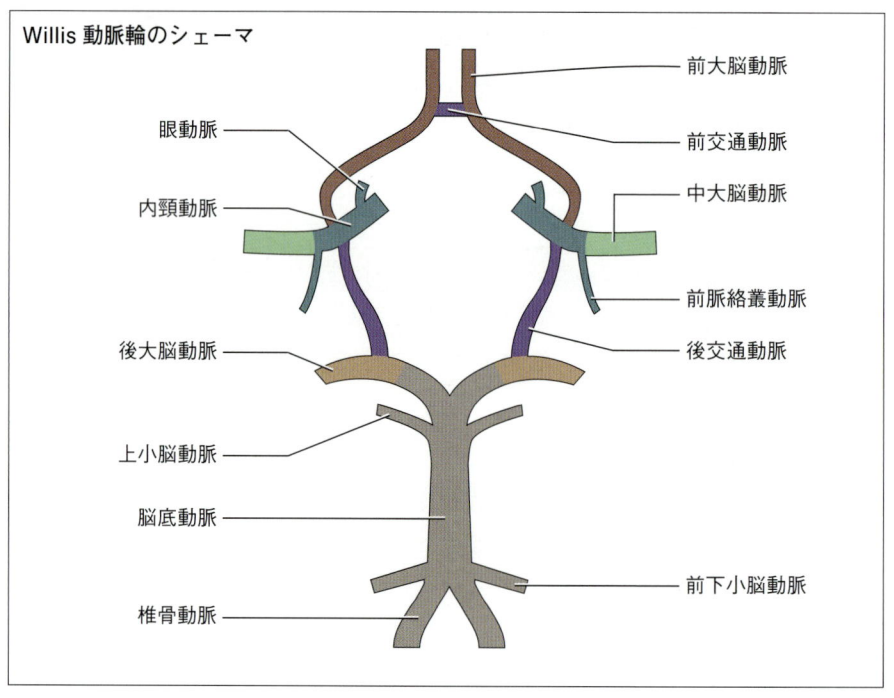

> **NOTE** MRA の施行目的のひとつとして動脈瘤の検索がある．脳動脈瘤は Willis（ウィリス）動脈輪近傍に多く，中大脳動脈の分岐部（M1-M2 移行部），内頸動脈-後交通動脈分岐部，前交通動脈で 80％ 以上を占める．

脳血管（静脈） （MRA, 3D-PC 法, VR 像）

1-22 脳静脈（尾頭方向）

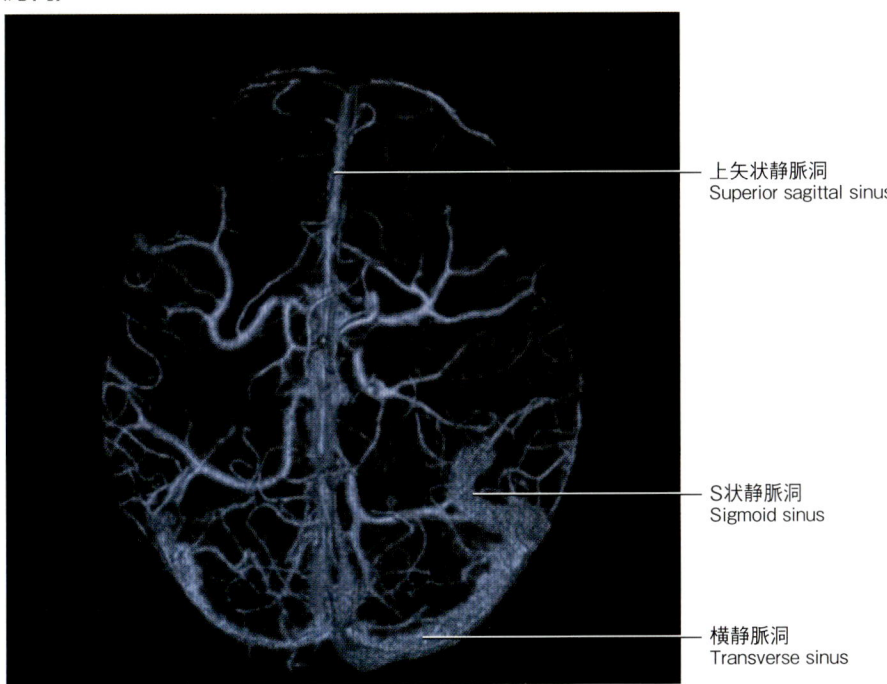

- 上矢状静脈洞 Superior sagittal sinus
- S状静脈洞 Sigmoid sinus
- 横静脈洞 Transverse sinus

1-23 脳静脈（側面方向）

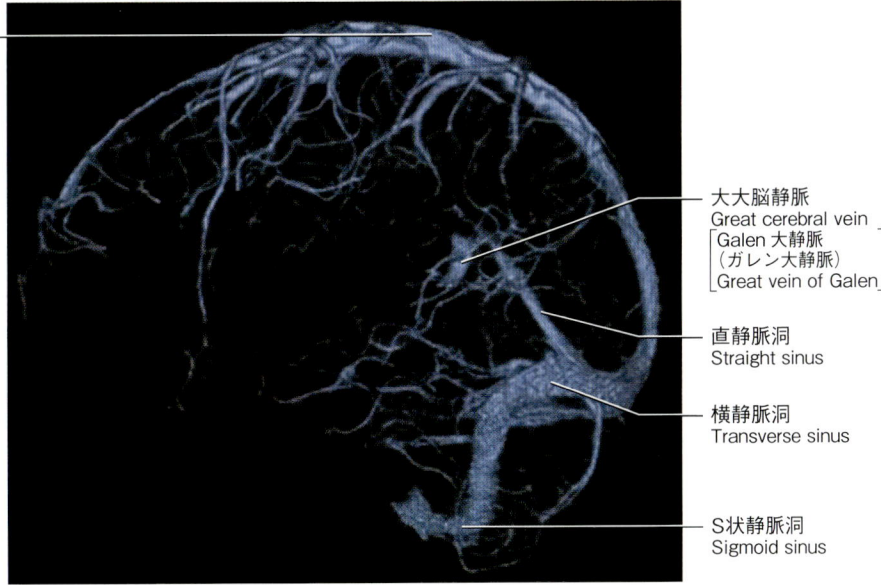

- 上矢状静脈洞 Superior sagittal sinus
- 大大脳静脈 Great cerebral vein [Galen 大静脈（ガレン大静脈）Great vein of Galen]
- 直静脈洞 Straight sinus
- 横静脈洞 Transverse sinus
- S状静脈洞 Sigmoid sinus

NOTE 血流速度の遅い静脈の描出には PC（phase contrast）法が適している．ここでは比較的血流量の多い，硬膜静脈洞（上矢状静脈洞，直静脈洞，横静脈洞，S状静脈洞）が描出されている．

脳動脈の支配領域 (MRI, T1強調像)

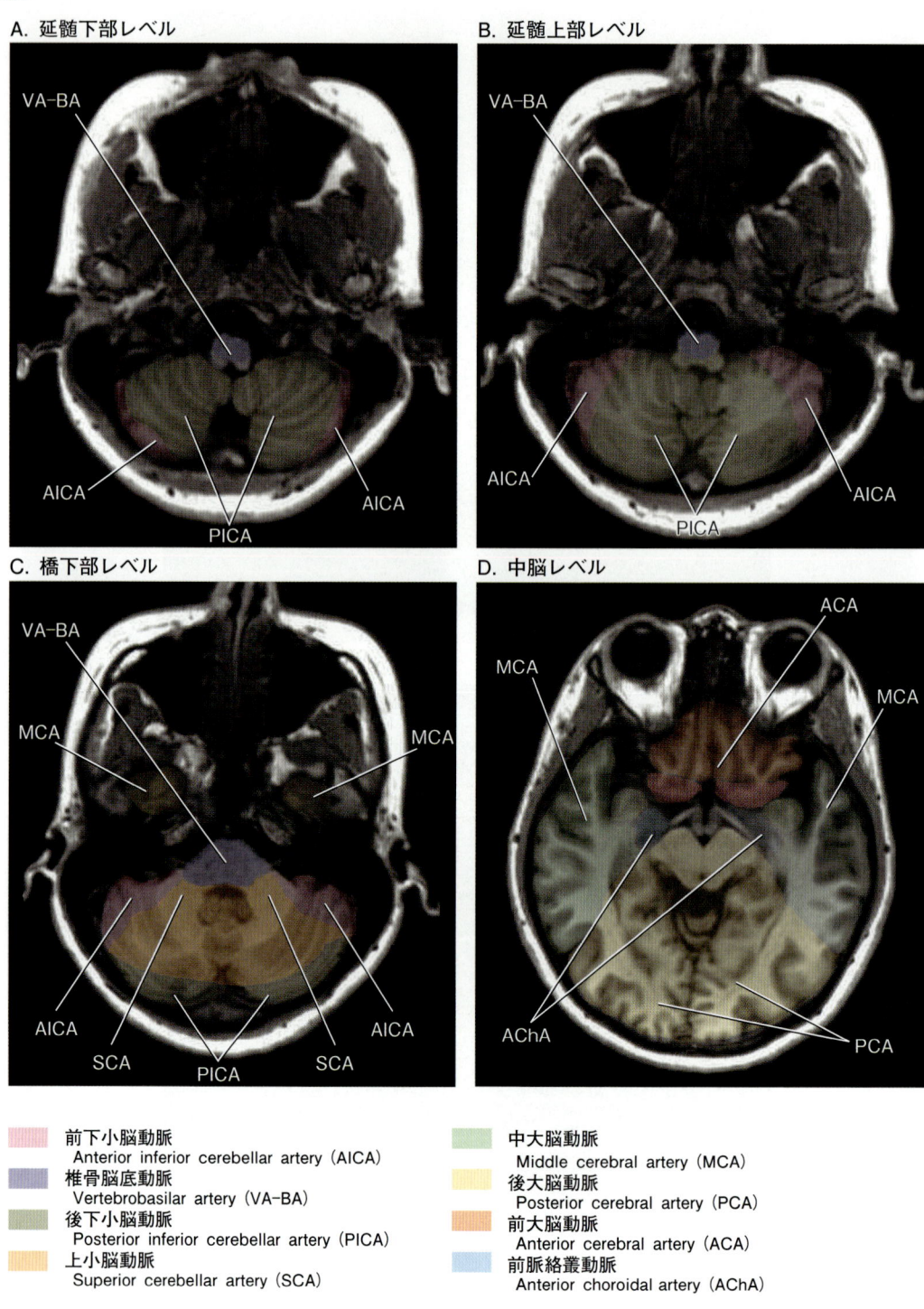

NOTE 脳動脈の支配領域は，脳梗塞の責任血管を判断するうえで重要である．ただし，後頭蓋窩（特に小脳）の動脈の支配領域は個体差が大きい．

脳動脈の支配領域（MRI, T1 強調像）

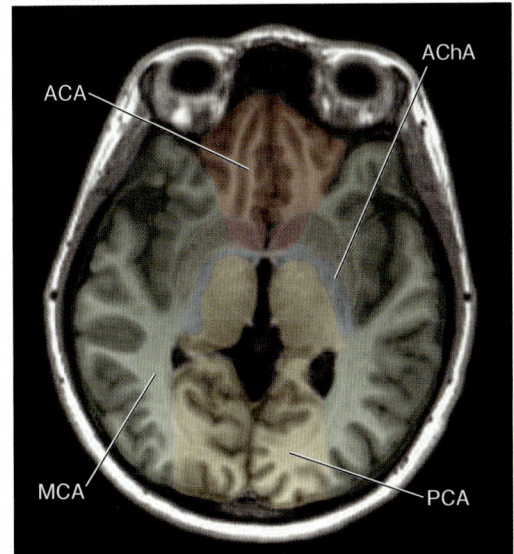

E. 基底核・視床の下部レベル

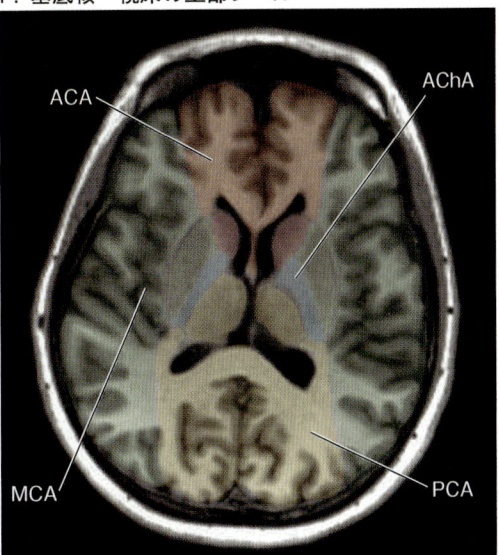

F. 基底核・視床の上部レベル

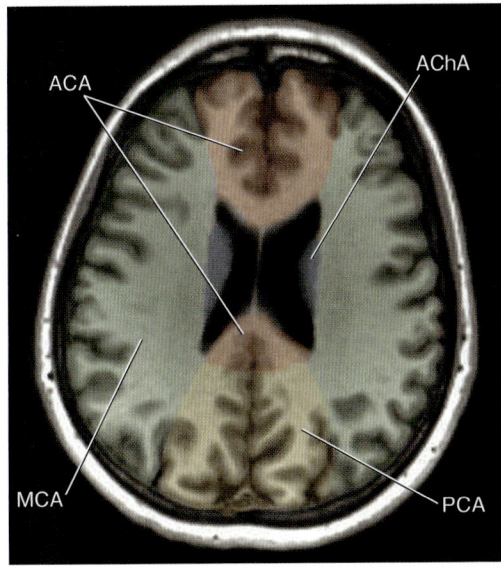

G. 放線冠レベル

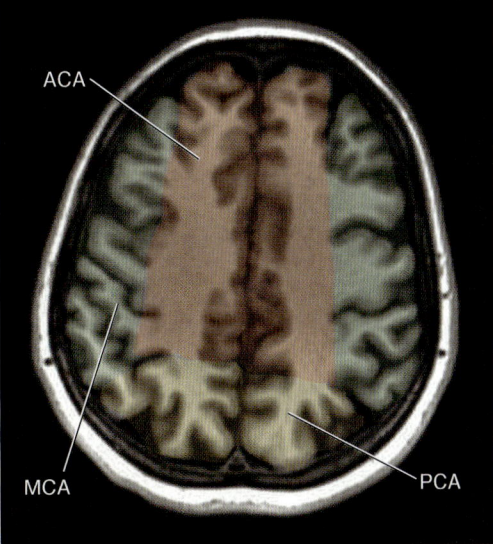

H. 半卵円中心レベル

- 中大脳動脈 Middle cerebral artery (MCA)
- 後大脳動脈 Posterior cerebral artery (PCA)
- 前大脳動脈 Anterior cerebral artery (ACA)
- 前脈絡叢動脈 Anterior choroidal artery (AChA)

脳動脈の支配領域（MRA, 3D-TOF 法, VR 像）

1-25 視床・線条体支配血管（穿通枝）

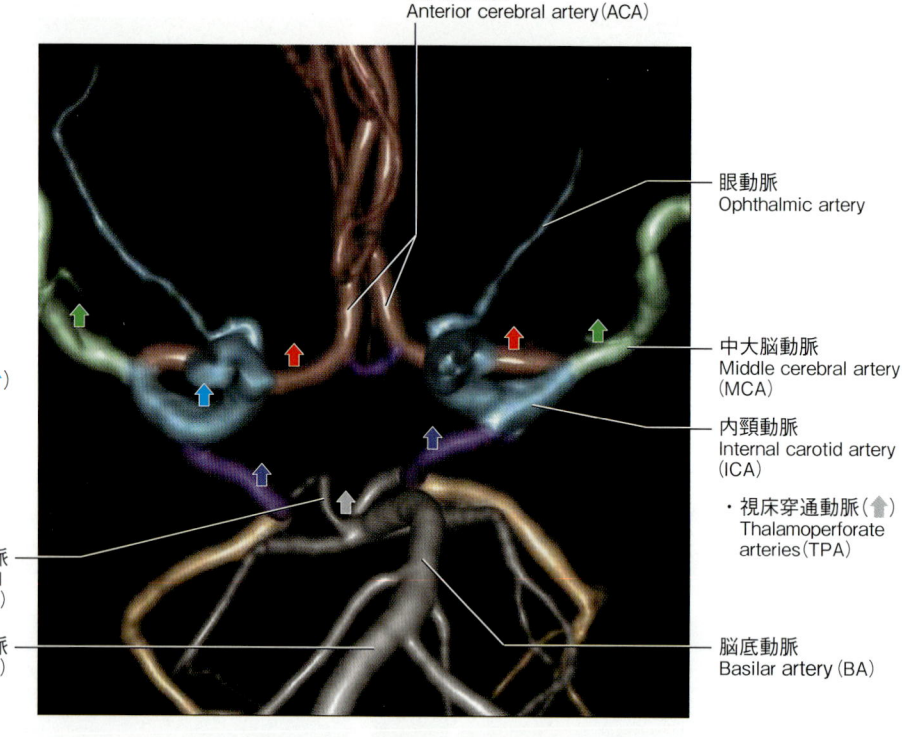

1-26 視床・線条体部

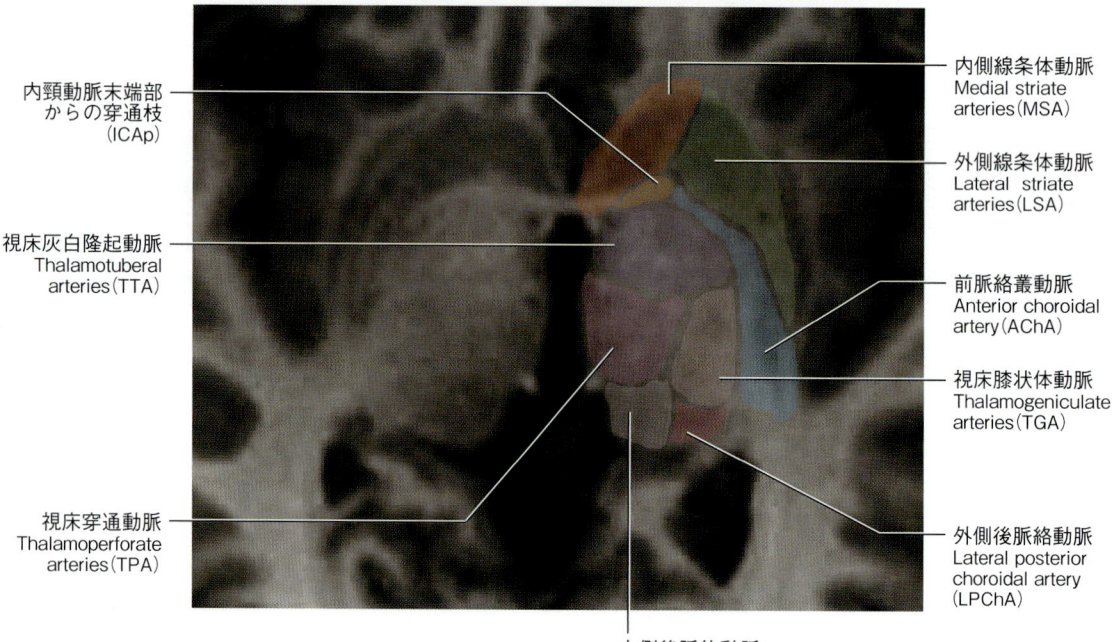

> **NOTE** 中大脳動脈や後大脳動脈に由来する穿通枝の分布領域は，梗塞や出血などの脳血管障害の好発部位として臨床的に重要である．（※1-25 の矢印は，それぞれの穿通枝の分枝部を示す．）

脳室・脳脊髄液（MRI, heavy T2 強調像, VR 像）

1-27 脳脊髄液（側面方向）

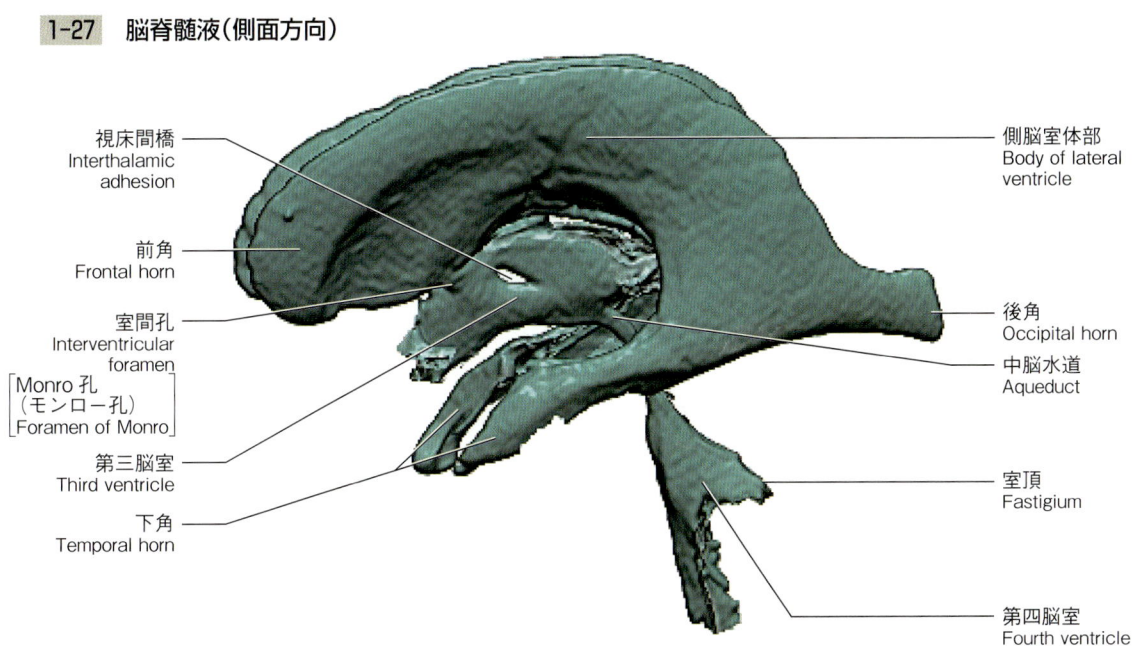

1-28 脳脊髄液（左前斜方向）

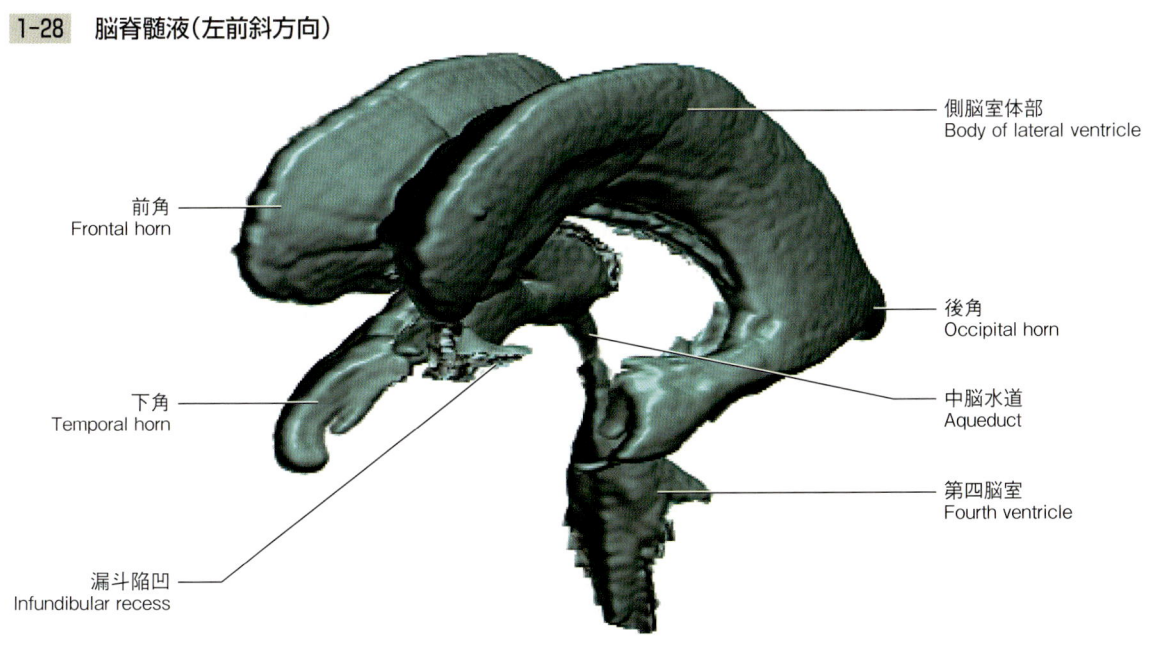

> **NOTE** 3D の heavy T2 強調像から構築した脳室系の VR 像である．側脳室内の脈絡叢で生産された脳脊髄液は Monro（モンロー）孔→第三脳室→中脳水道→第四脳室の順に追加されながら移動する．

18 海馬および線条体近辺(MRI, FLAIR＋T1 強調像の fusion 像)

1-29　海馬・視床・尾状核(側面方向)

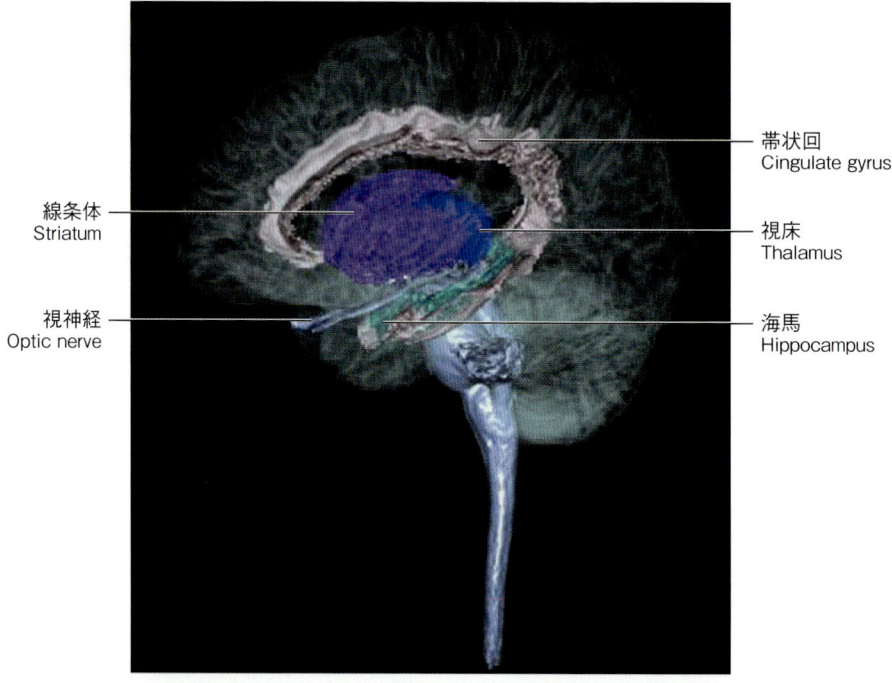

1-30　海馬・線条体(前後方向)

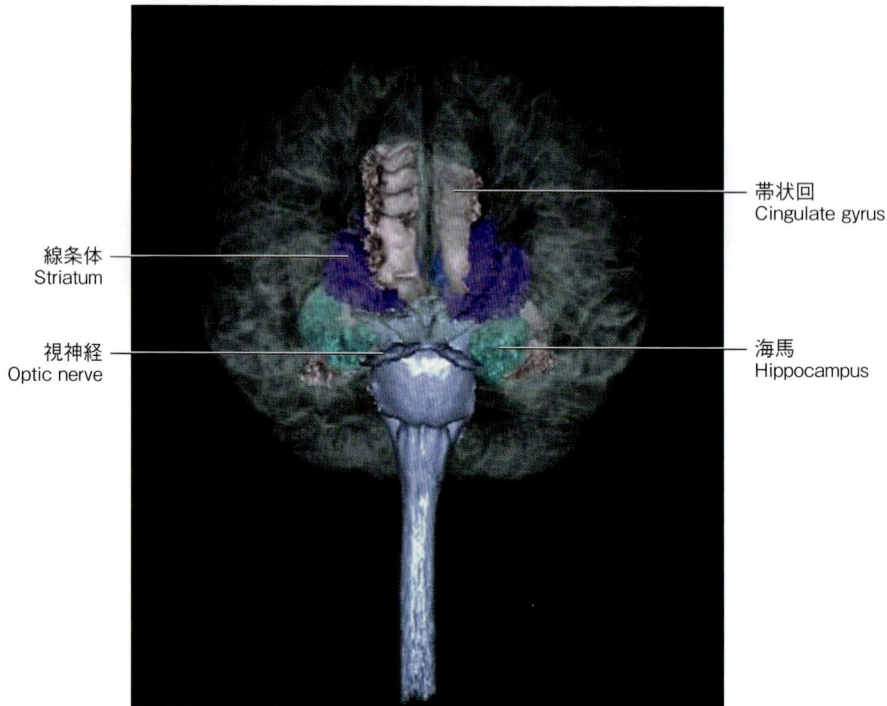

NOTE 海馬−脳弓−乳頭体−視床前核−帯状回−海馬傍回−海馬という閉鎖回路を"Papez(パペッツ)の回路"という．ヒトの記憶に大きく関与する．

脳の断層解剖 ［横断像（MRI, T1 強調像）］

1-31

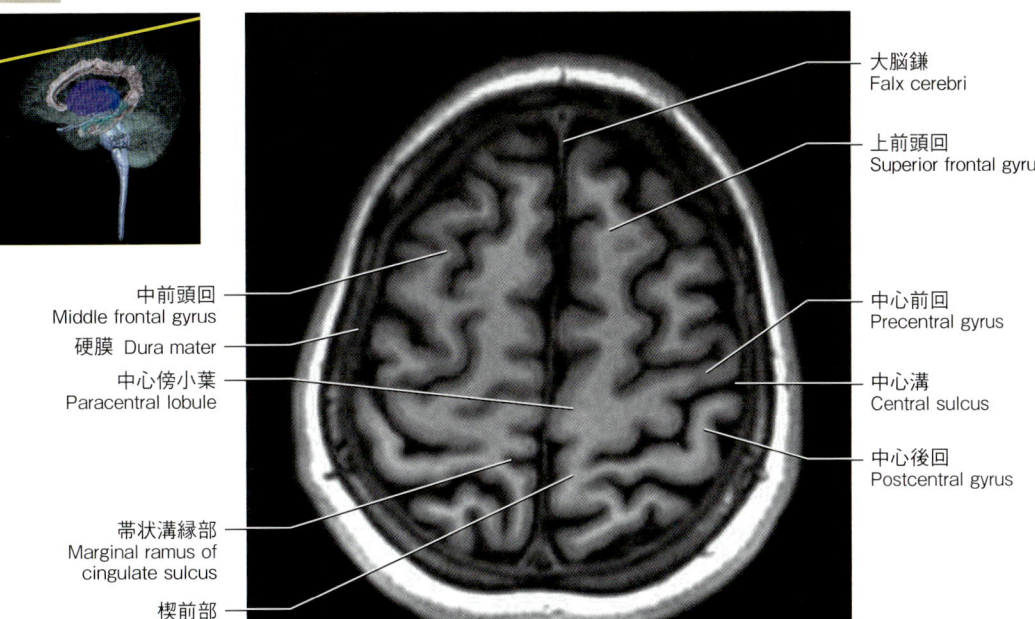

- 大脳鎌 Falx cerebri
- 上前頭回 Superior frontal gyrus
- 中前頭回 Middle frontal gyrus
- 硬膜 Dura mater
- 中心傍小葉 Paracentral lobule
- 中心前回 Precentral gyrus
- 中心溝 Central sulcus
- 中心後回 Postcentral gyrus
- 帯状溝縁部 Marginal ramus of cingulate sulcus
- 楔前部 Precuneus

1-32

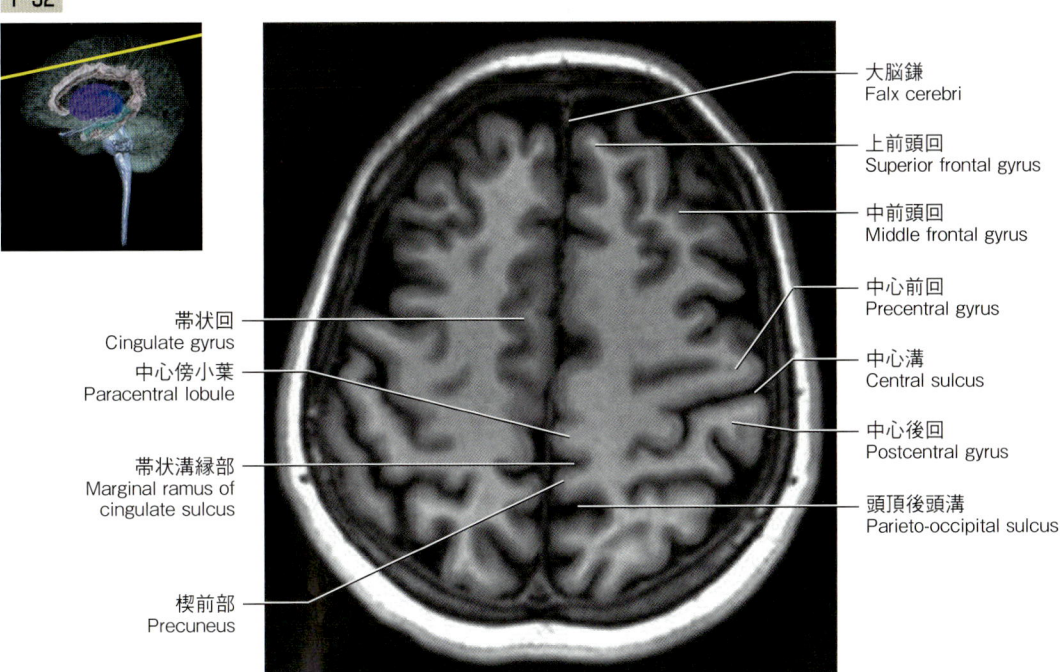

- 大脳鎌 Falx cerebri
- 上前頭回 Superior frontal gyrus
- 中前頭回 Middle frontal gyrus
- 帯状回 Cingulate gyrus
- 中心傍小葉 Paracentral lobule
- 帯状溝縁部 Marginal ramus of cingulate sulcus
- 中心前回 Precentral gyrus
- 中心溝 Central sulcus
- 中心後回 Postcentral gyrus
- 頭頂後頭溝 Parieto-occipital sulcus
- 楔前部 Precuneus

> **NOTE** 中心前回は腹側を中心前溝，背側を中心溝，尾側を Sylvius 裂に隔てられ，正中側は中心傍小葉に連続する脳回である．同脳回には一次運動野が存在し，正中側から外側に向かい下肢，体幹，上肢，顔面といった体性局在が存在するため，局在診断において重要である（1-13 を参照）．特に手指の運動野は背側に凸の形態を呈しており，"Precentral knob" とよばれる．

脳の断層解剖 ［横断像（MRI, T1 強調像）］

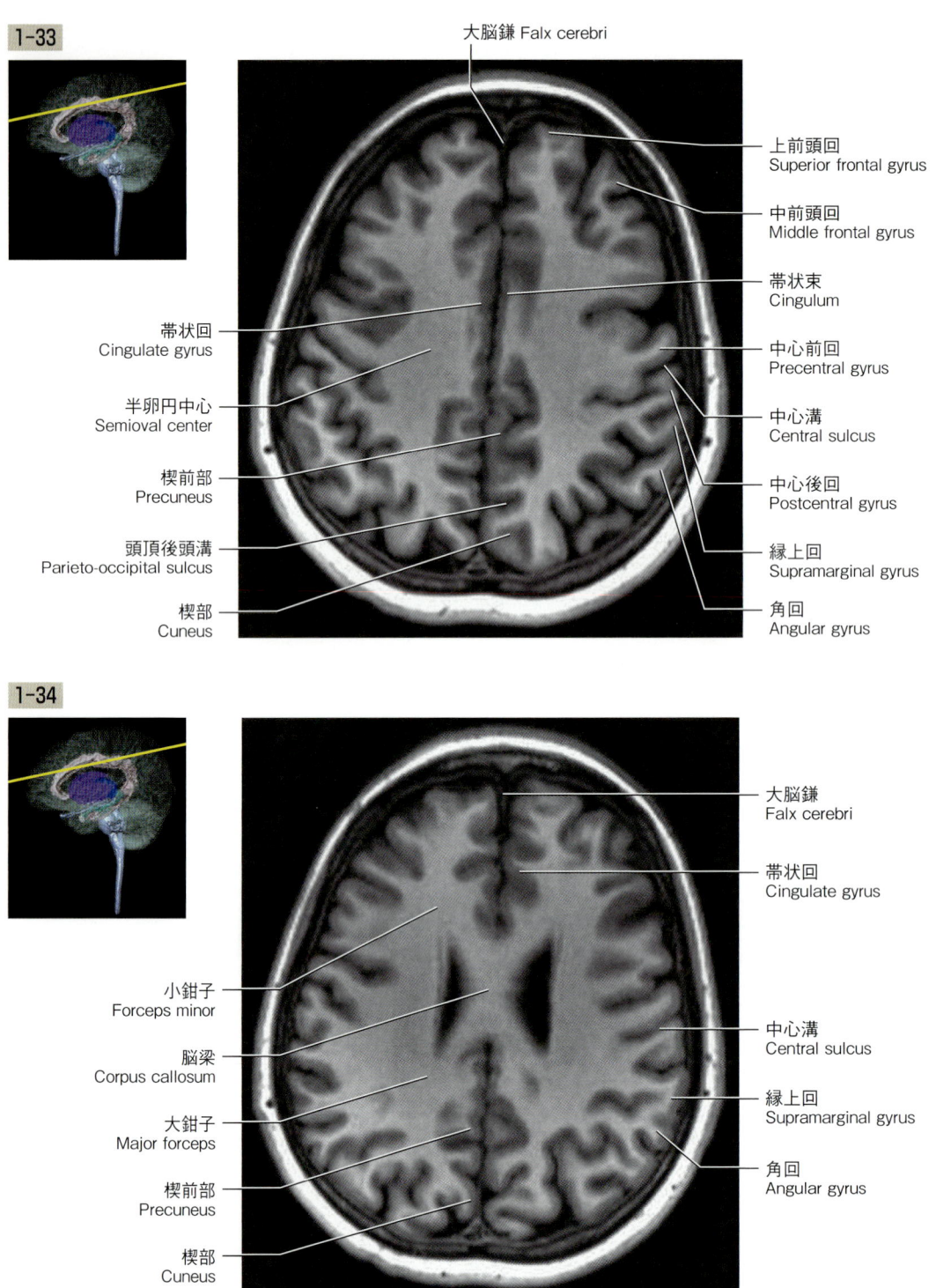

1-33

- 大脳鎌 Falx cerebri
- 上前頭回 Superior frontal gyrus
- 中前頭回 Middle frontal gyrus
- 帯状束 Cingulum
- 帯状回 Cingulate gyrus
- 半卵円中心 Semioval center
- 楔前部 Precuneus
- 頭頂後頭溝 Parieto-occipital sulcus
- 楔部 Cuneus
- 中心前回 Precentral gyrus
- 中心溝 Central sulcus
- 中心後回 Postcentral gyrus
- 縁上回 Supramarginal gyrus
- 角回 Angular gyrus

1-34

- 大脳鎌 Falx cerebri
- 帯状回 Cingulate gyrus
- 小鉗子 Forceps minor
- 脳梁 Corpus callosum
- 大鉗子 Major forceps
- 楔前部 Precuneus
- 楔部 Cuneus
- 中心溝 Central sulcus
- 縁上回 Supramarginal gyrus
- 角回 Angular gyrus

NOTE 側脳室よりも上方で，横断像にて左右の白質が向かい合わせたような半円形の形状となっている領域を半卵円中心とよぶ．この部分の傍正中には連合線維と投射線維，交連線維が混在している．通常の画像ではこれら線維束を識別することはできないが，拡散テンソル画像を用いた tractography にてこれら線維束の描出が可能となる（1-14 を参照）．

脳の断層解剖　[横断像（MRI, T1強調像）]

1-35

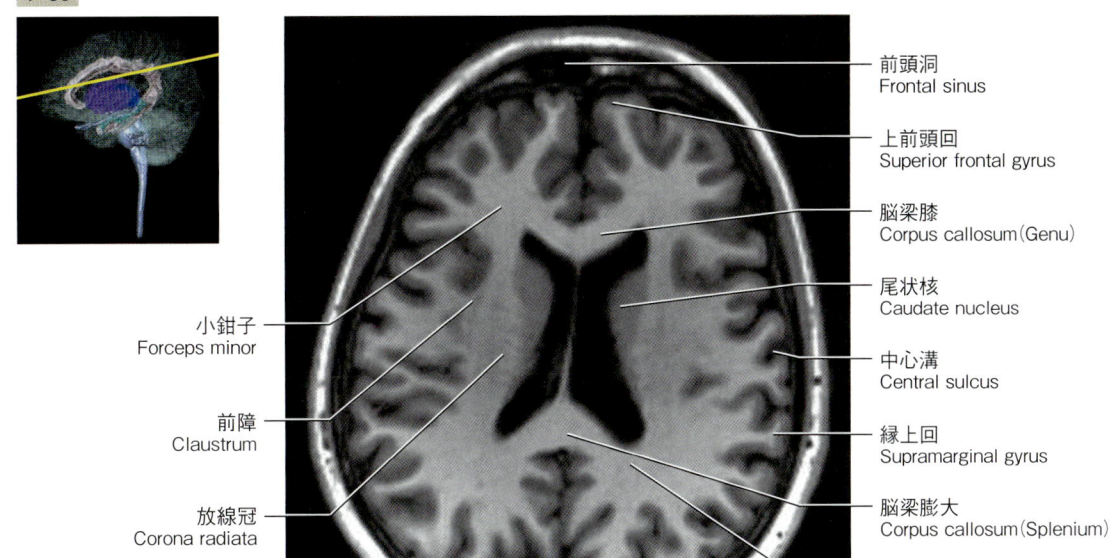

- 前頭洞 Frontal sinus
- 上前頭回 Superior frontal gyrus
- 脳梁膝 Corpus callosum (Genu)
- 尾状核 Caudate nucleus
- 中心溝 Central sulcus
- 縁上回 Supramarginal gyrus
- 脳梁膨大 Corpus callosum (Splenium)
- 大鉗子 Major forceps
- 小鉗子 Forceps minor
- 前障 Claustrum
- 放線冠 Corona radiata
- 一次視覚皮質 Primary visual cortex

1-36

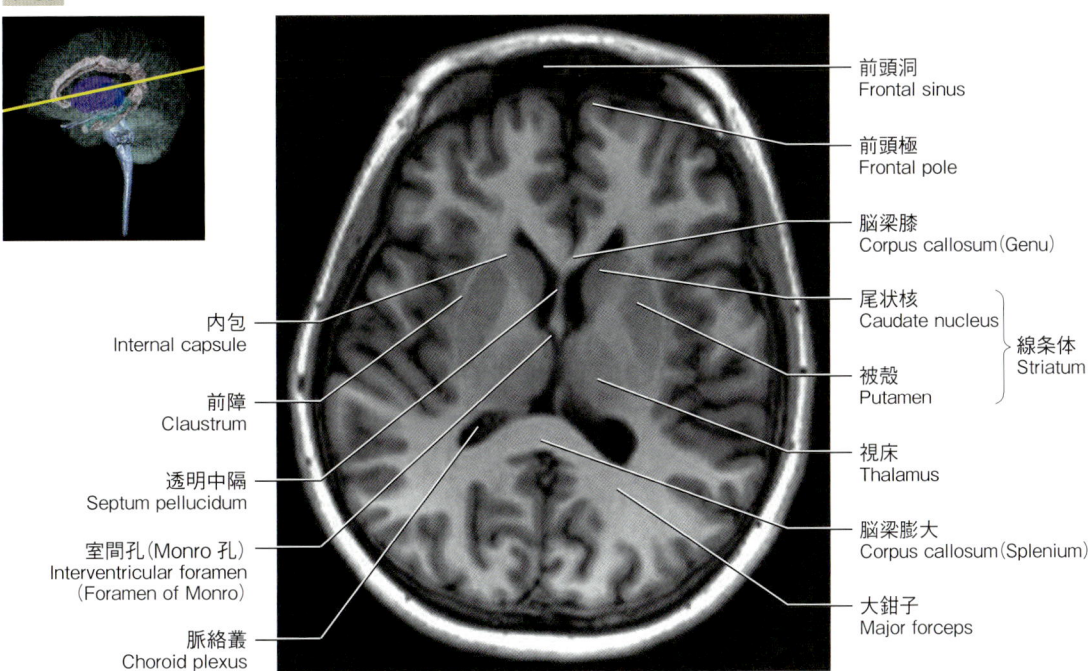

- 前頭洞 Frontal sinus
- 前頭極 Frontal pole
- 脳梁膝 Corpus callosum (Genu)
- 尾状核 Caudate nucleus ┐ 線条体 Striatum
- 被殻 Putamen ┘
- 視床 Thalamus
- 脳梁膨大 Corpus callosum (Splenium)
- 大鉗子 Major forceps
- 内包 Internal capsule
- 前障 Claustrum
- 透明中隔 Septum pellucidum
- 室間孔（Monro孔） Interventricular foramen (Foramen of Monro)
- 脈絡叢 Choroid plexus

NOTE 放線冠は投射線維のうち内包を通過する線維群が存在する領域を指す．

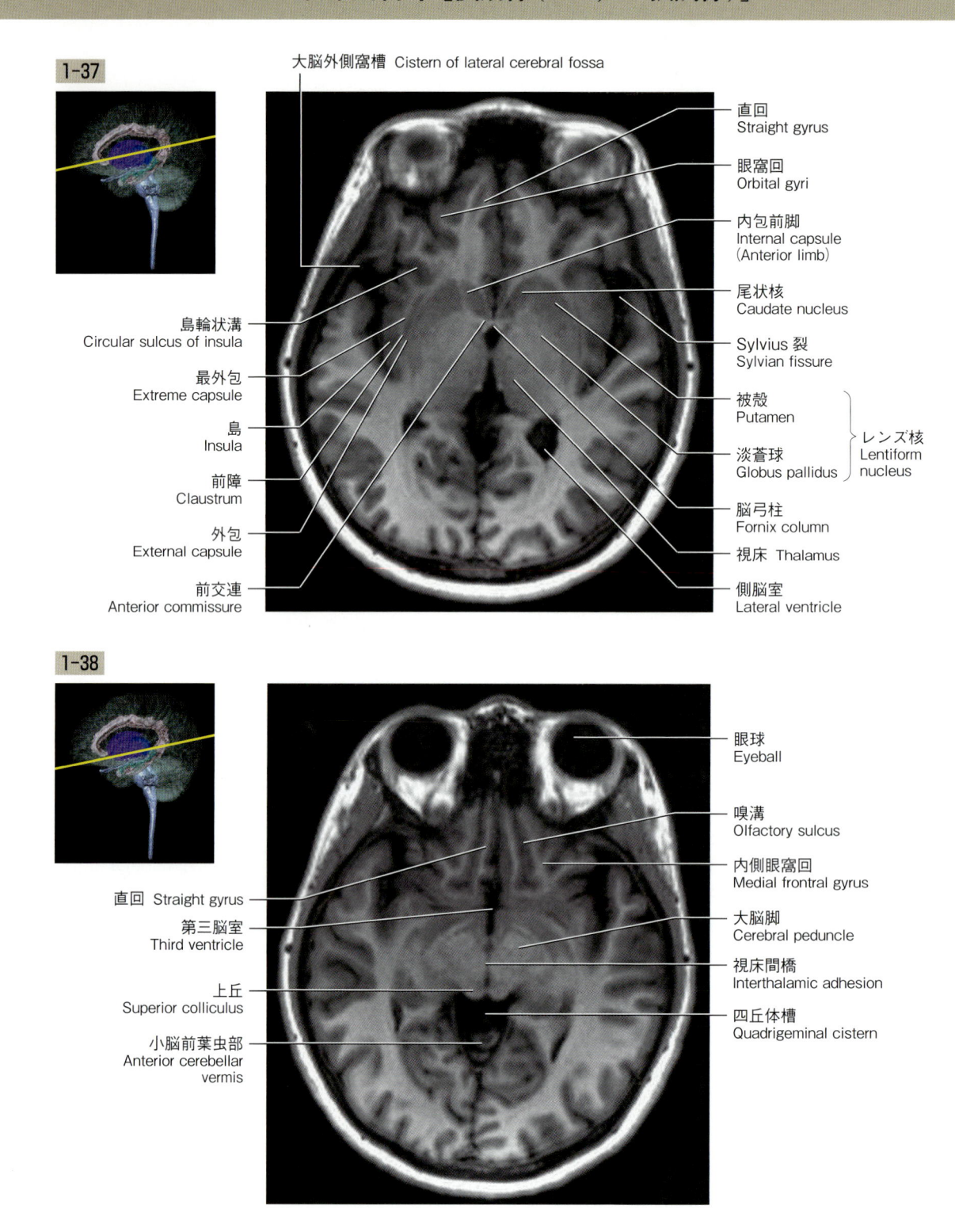

脳の断層解剖　[横断像（MRI, T1強調像）]

1-37

- 大脳外側窩槽　Cistern of lateral cerebral fossa
- 直回　Straight gyrus
- 眼窩回　Orbital gyri
- 内包前脚　Internal capsule (Anterior limb)
- 尾状核　Caudate nucleus
- Sylvius裂　Sylvian fissure
- 被殻　Putamen ⎫ レンズ核
- 淡蒼球　Globus pallidus ⎭ Lentiform nucleus
- 脳弓柱　Fornix column
- 視床　Thalamus
- 側脳室　Lateral ventricle
- 島輪状溝　Circular sulcus of insula
- 最外包　Extreme capsule
- 島　Insula
- 前障　Claustrum
- 外包　External capsule
- 前交連　Anterior commissure

1-38

- 眼球　Eyeball
- 嗅溝　Olfactory sulcus
- 内側眼窩回　Medial frontal gyrus
- 大脳脚　Cerebral peduncle
- 視床間橋　Interthalamic adhesion
- 四丘体槽　Quadrigeminal cistern
- 直回　Straight gyrus
- 第三脳室　Third ventricle
- 上丘　Superior colliculus
- 小脳前葉虫部　Anterior cerebellar vermis

NOTE　島はSylvius（シルビウス）裂の最も深部に位置する．中大脳動脈の支配領域であり（1-24のEFを参照），超急性期脳梗塞の際のCTでの島皮質の不明瞭化は"insular ribbonの消失"とよばれ，重要なサインとなる．
　内包はレンズ核と尾状核・視床間の"く"の字型の白質であり，投射線維の大部分がここを通過する．一方，被殻の外側に存在する外包は主に連合線維から構成される．

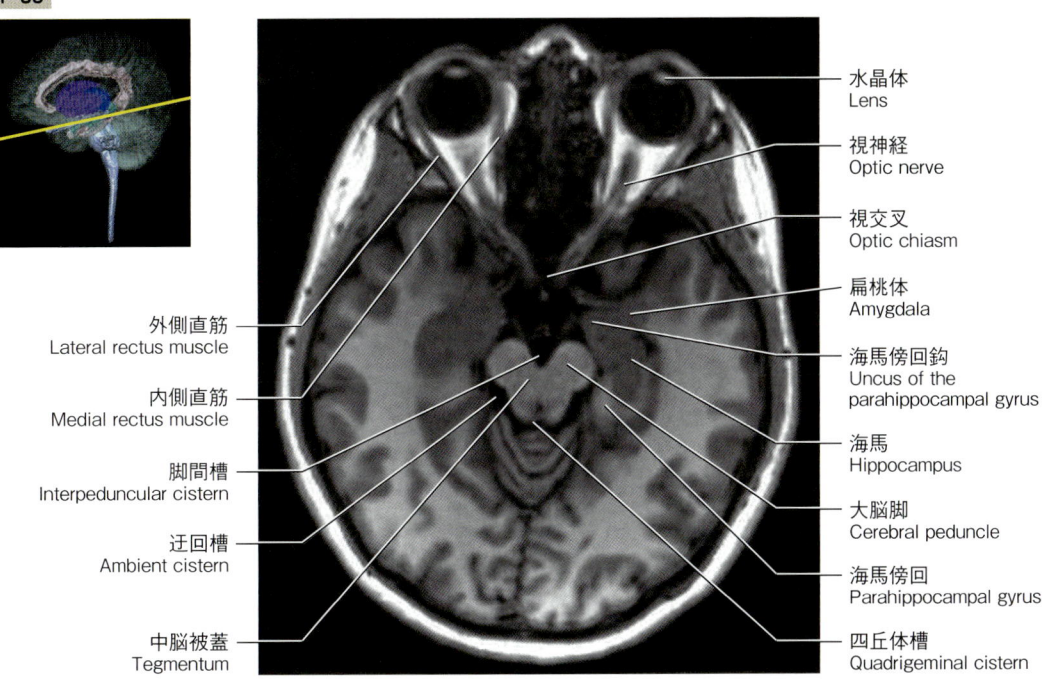

脳の断層解剖［横断像（MRI，T1 強調像）］

1-39

- 水晶体 Lens
- 視神経 Optic nerve
- 視交叉 Optic chiasm
- 扁桃体 Amygdala
- 海馬傍回鈎 Uncus of the parahippocampal gyrus
- 海馬 Hippocampus
- 大脳脚 Cerebral peduncle
- 海馬傍回 Parahippocampal gyrus
- 四丘体槽 Quadrigeminal cistern
- 外側直筋 Lateral rectus muscle
- 内側直筋 Medial rectus muscle
- 脚間槽 Interpeduncular cistern
- 迂回槽 Ambient cistern
- 中脳被蓋 Tegmentum

1-40

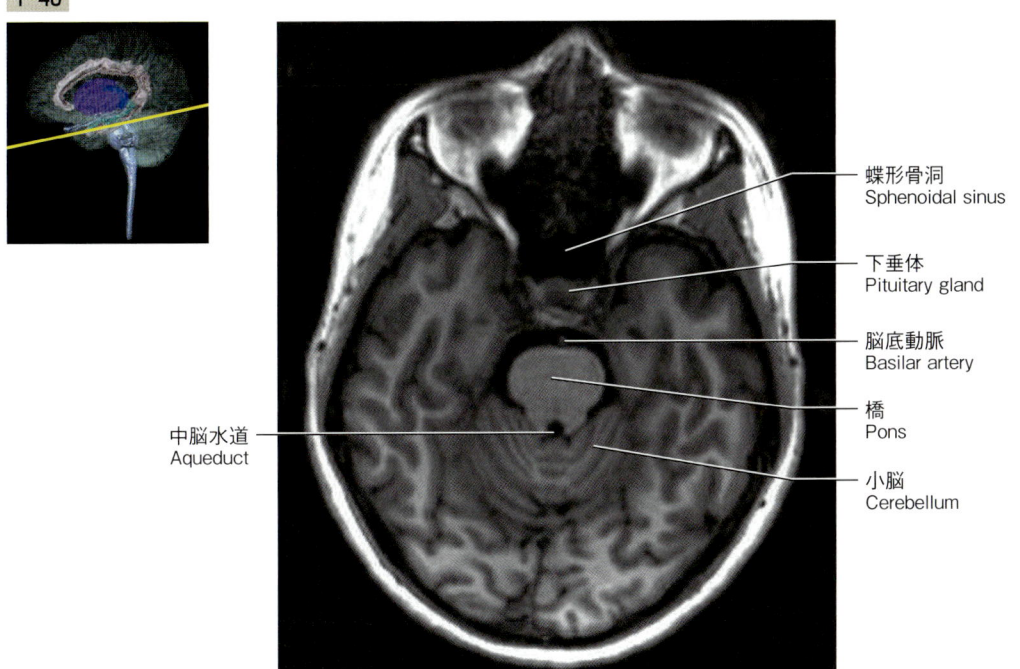

- 蝶形骨洞 Sphenoidal sinus
- 下垂体 Pituitary gland
- 脳底動脈 Basilar artery
- 橋 Pons
- 小脳 Cerebellum
- 中脳水道 Aqueduct

NOTE 脳は灰白質と白質により構成されている．灰白質は神経細胞体の集合であり，特に脳表面の灰白質を"皮質"とよぶ．一方，白質は神経細胞体から連続する神経線維よりなり，神経線維は大脳皮質と下位の脳や脊髄を連絡する投射線維，左右の大脳半球の皮質間を連絡する交連線維，同側大脳半球の皮質間を連絡する連合線維からなる．連合線維のうち隣り合う脳回の皮質間を連絡するものを"弓状線維"とよび，断面で皮質直下にU字型を呈することから"U-fiber"ともよばれる．

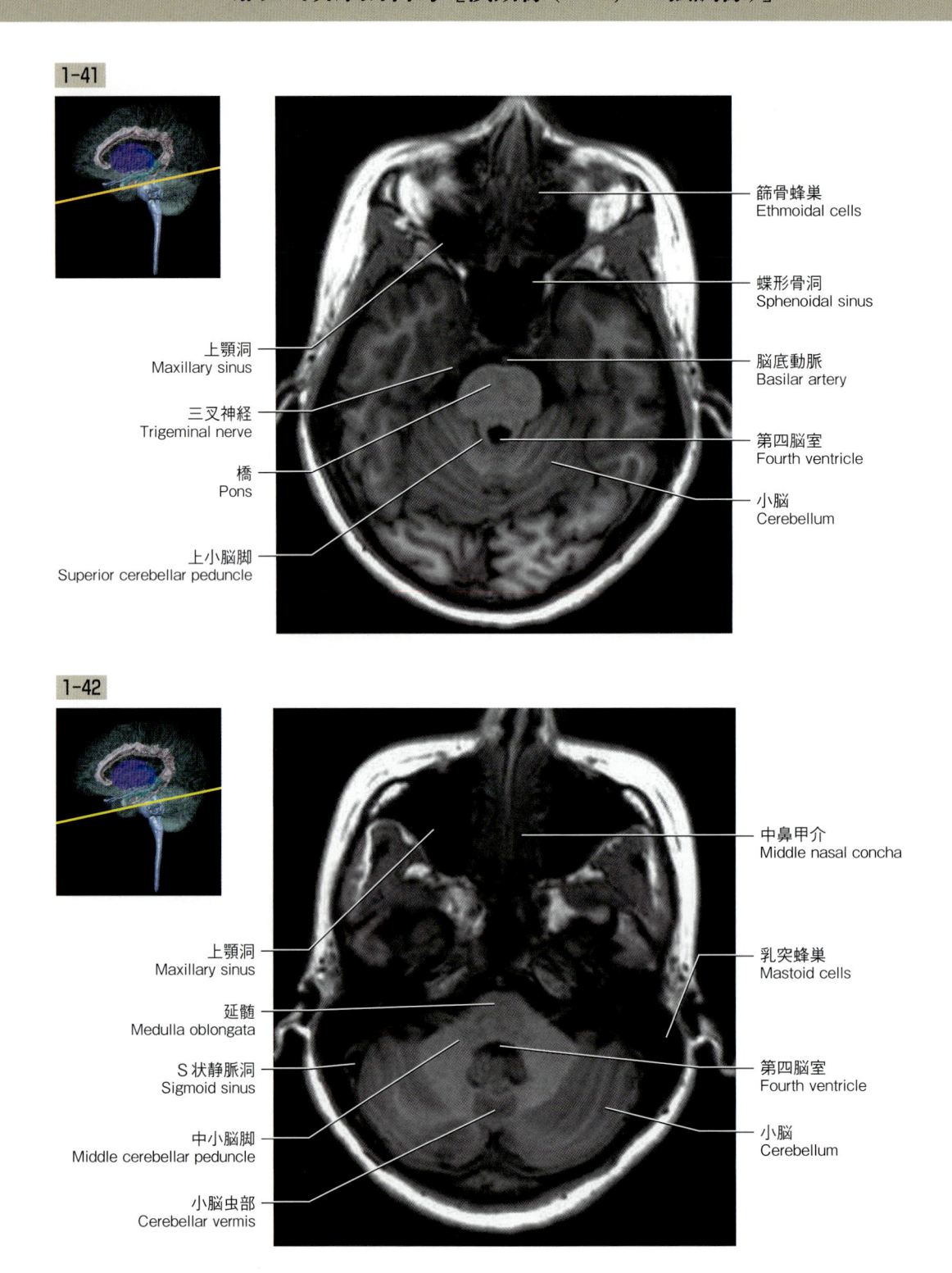

脳の断層解剖　[横断像（MRI，T1強調像）]

1-41

- 篩骨蜂巣 Ethmoidal cells
- 蝶形骨洞 Sphenoidal sinus
- 上顎洞 Maxillary sinus
- 脳底動脈 Basilar artery
- 三叉神経 Trigeminal nerve
- 第四脳室 Fourth ventricle
- 橋 Pons
- 小脳 Cerebellum
- 上小脳脚 Superior cerebellar peduncle

1-42

- 中鼻甲介 Middle nasal concha
- 上顎洞 Maxillary sinus
- 乳突蜂巣 Mastoid cells
- 延髄 Medulla oblongata
- S状静脈洞 Sigmoid sinus
- 第四脳室 Fourth ventricle
- 中小脳脚 Middle cerebellar peduncle
- 小脳 Cerebellum
- 小脳虫部 Cerebellar vermis

> **NOTE　皮質 Cortex**
> Cortexは，皮（果実・野菜・樹木），外皮の意味で，サンスクリットのkrit，kart（裂く）に由来するとされる．解剖学では骨や実質臓器の表層部を指す．その深部はMedulla（26頁のNOTEを参照）である．

脳の断層解剖　[横断像（MRI, T1 強調像）]

1-43

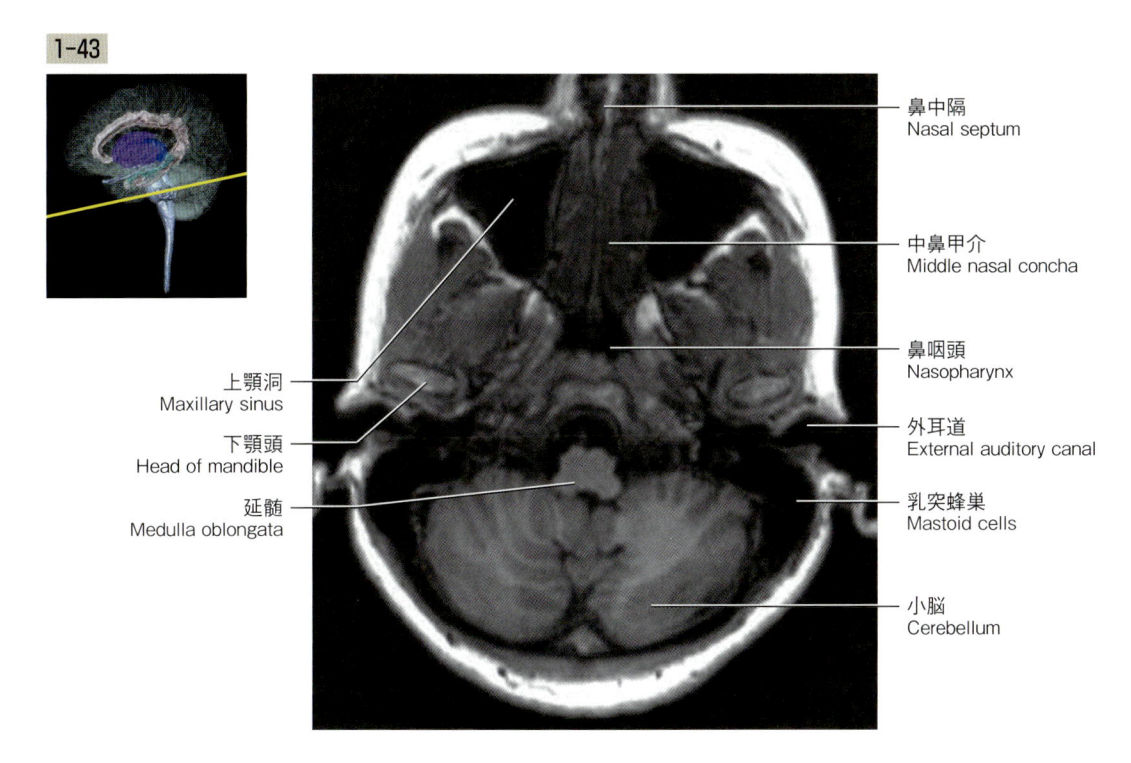

- 鼻中隔 Nasal septum
- 中鼻甲介 Middle nasal concha
- 鼻咽頭 Nasopharynx
- 外耳道 External auditory canal
- 乳突蜂巣 Mastoid cells
- 小脳 Cerebellum
- 上顎洞 Maxillary sinus
- 下顎頭 Head of mandible
- 延髄 Medulla oblongata

1-44

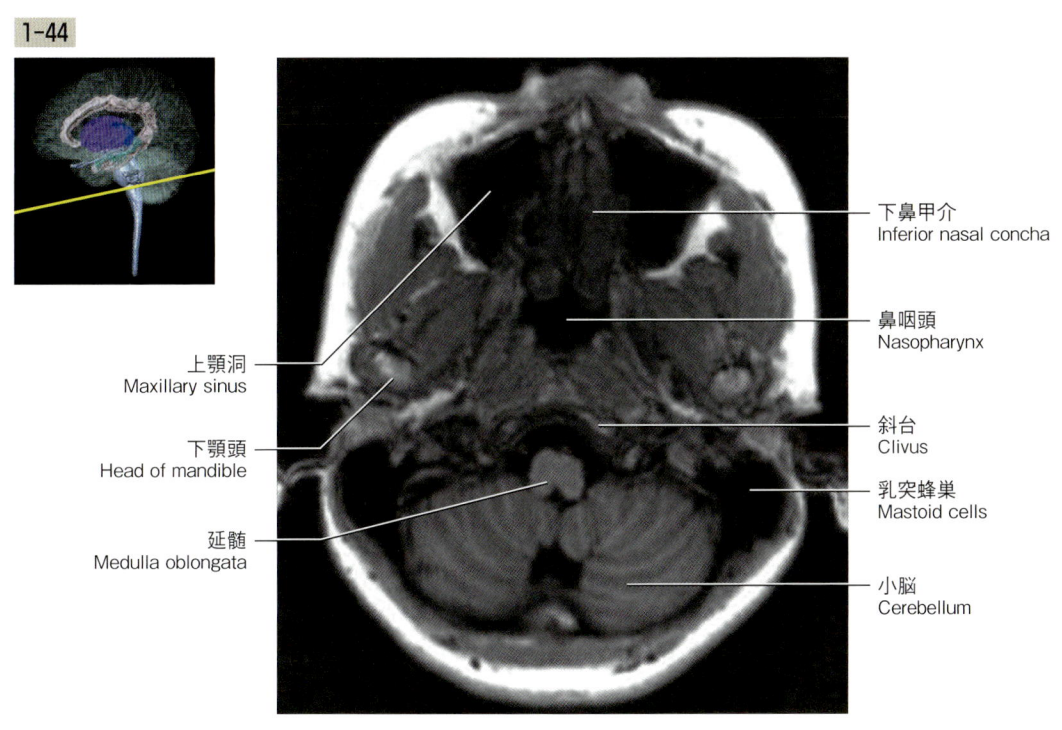

- 下鼻甲介 Inferior nasal concha
- 鼻咽頭 Nasopharynx
- 斜台 Clivus
- 乳突蜂巣 Mastoid cells
- 小脳 Cerebellum
- 上顎洞 Maxillary sinus
- 下顎頭 Head of mandible
- 延髄 Medulla oblongata

> **NOTE**　後頭蓋窩は中脳・橋・延髄からなる脳幹と小脳が占めている．
> 　小脳は両側の小脳半球と，この間でこれらを結合する虫部からなり，上小脳脚・中小脳脚・下小脳脚の3つの小脳脚によって脳幹と結合している．

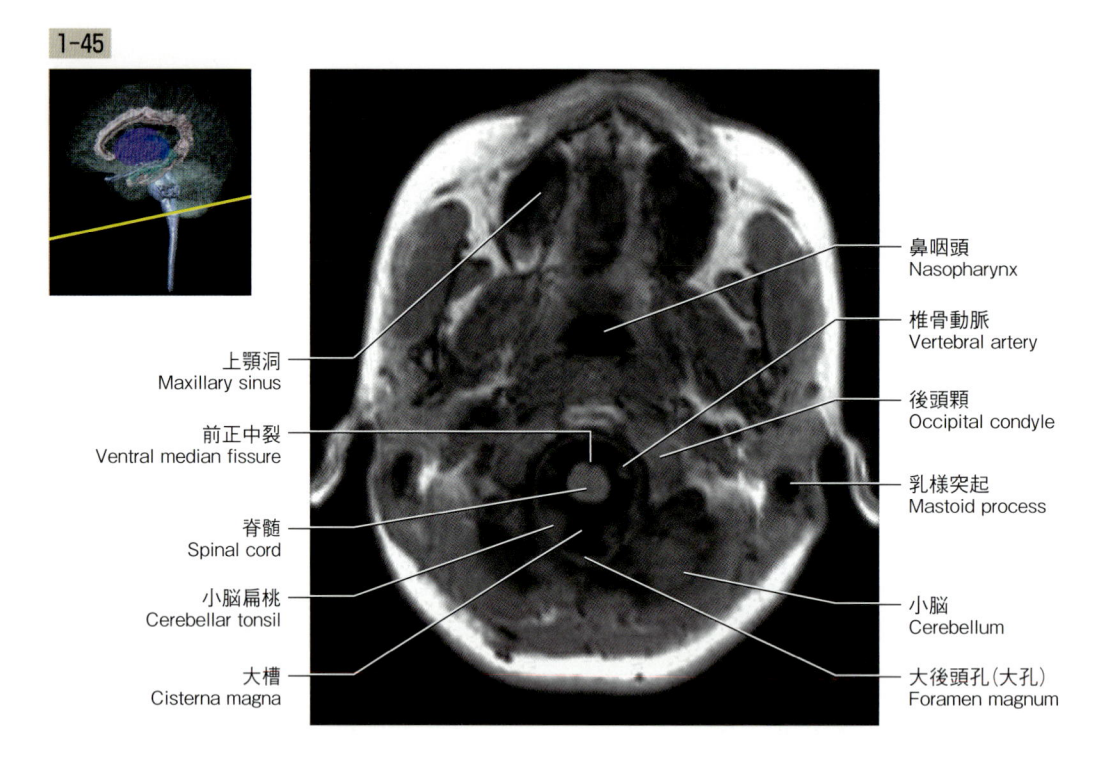

脳の断層解剖 ［横断像（MRI, T1強調像）］

1-45

- 上顎洞 Maxillary sinus
- 前正中裂 Ventral median fissure
- 脊髄 Spinal cord
- 小脳扁桃 Cerebellar tonsil
- 大槽 Cisterna magna
- 鼻咽頭 Nasopharynx
- 椎骨動脈 Vertebral artery
- 後頭顆 Occipital condyle
- 乳様突起 Mastoid process
- 小脳 Cerebellum
- 大後頭孔（大孔） Foramen magnum

> **NOTE** 延髄 Medulla oblongata
> Medullaは，medius（中央の）から由来する．近代解剖学の父 Vesalius（ヴェサリウス）（16世紀）は骨の中心，脊柱の中心などに用い，今日，骨髄（Medulla ossium），延髄（Medulla oblongata），副腎髄質（Adrenal medulla）などに残る．サンスクリットの"medhara"とも関係があるとされる．

脳の断層解剖　[矢状断像（MRI, T1 強調像）]

1-46

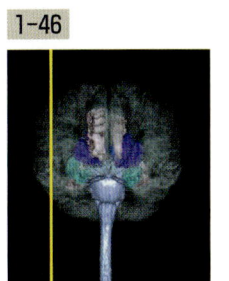

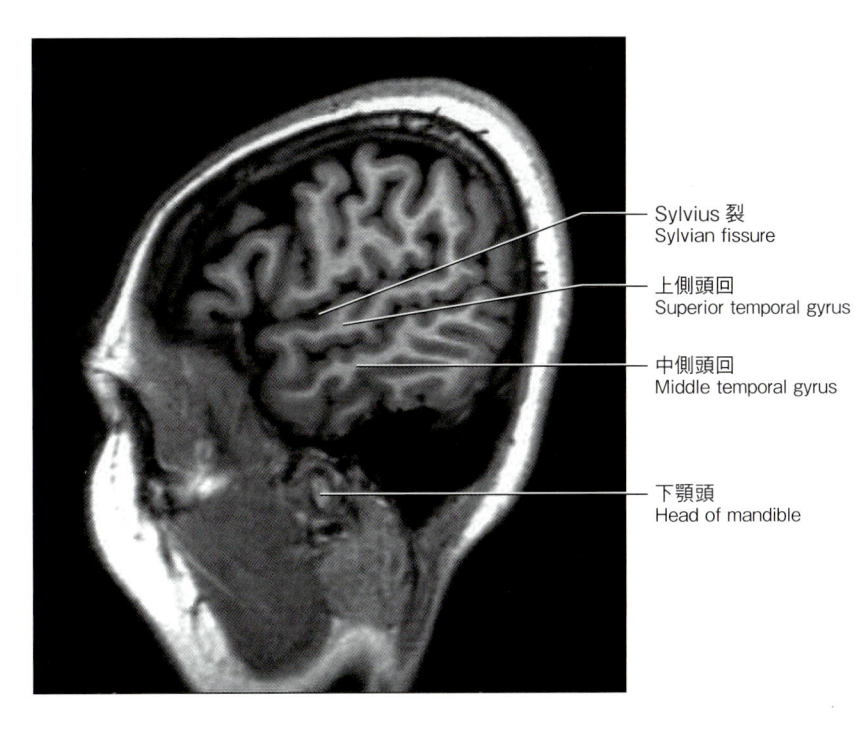

- Sylvius 裂　Sylvian fissure
- 上側頭回　Superior temporal gyrus
- 中側頭回　Middle temporal gyrus
- 下顎頭　Head of mandible

1-47

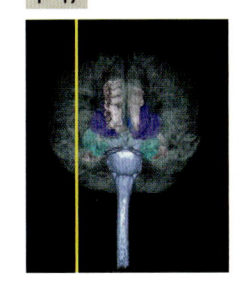

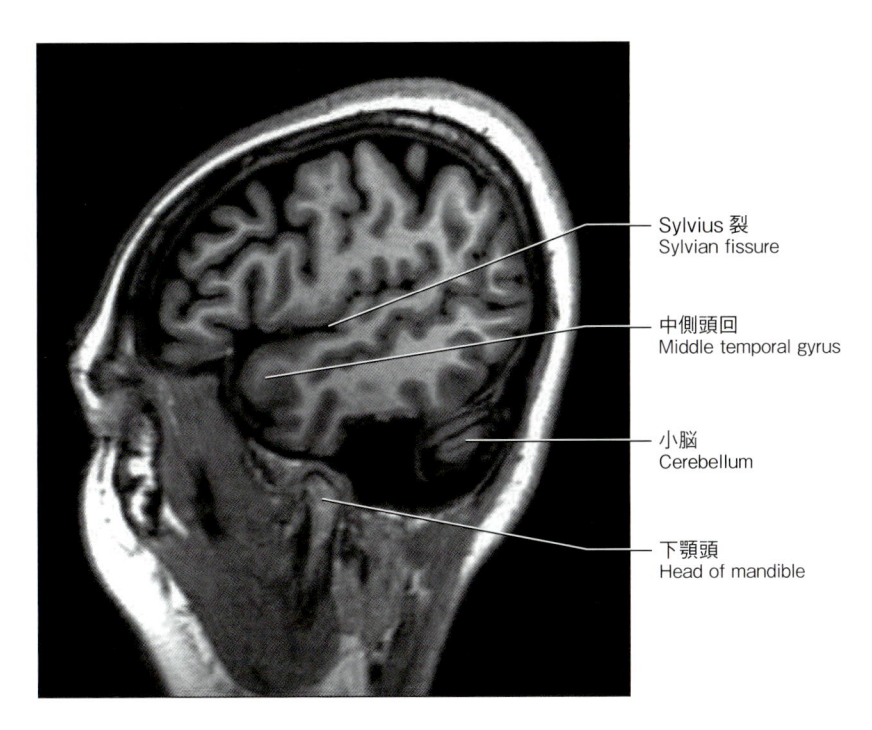

- Sylvius 裂　Sylvian fissure
- 中側頭回　Middle temporal gyrus
- 小脳　Cerebellum
- 下顎頭　Head of mandible

NOTE Sylvius 裂は大脳半球外側の深い脳溝であり，前頭葉と側頭葉とを分けている．側頭葉外側面は上・下側頭溝によって上・中・下の3つの側頭回に分けられる（1-66を参照）．通常，左側の上側頭回後部から角回にかけ感覚性言語野（Wernicke's area）が存在する（1-11, 12を参照）．

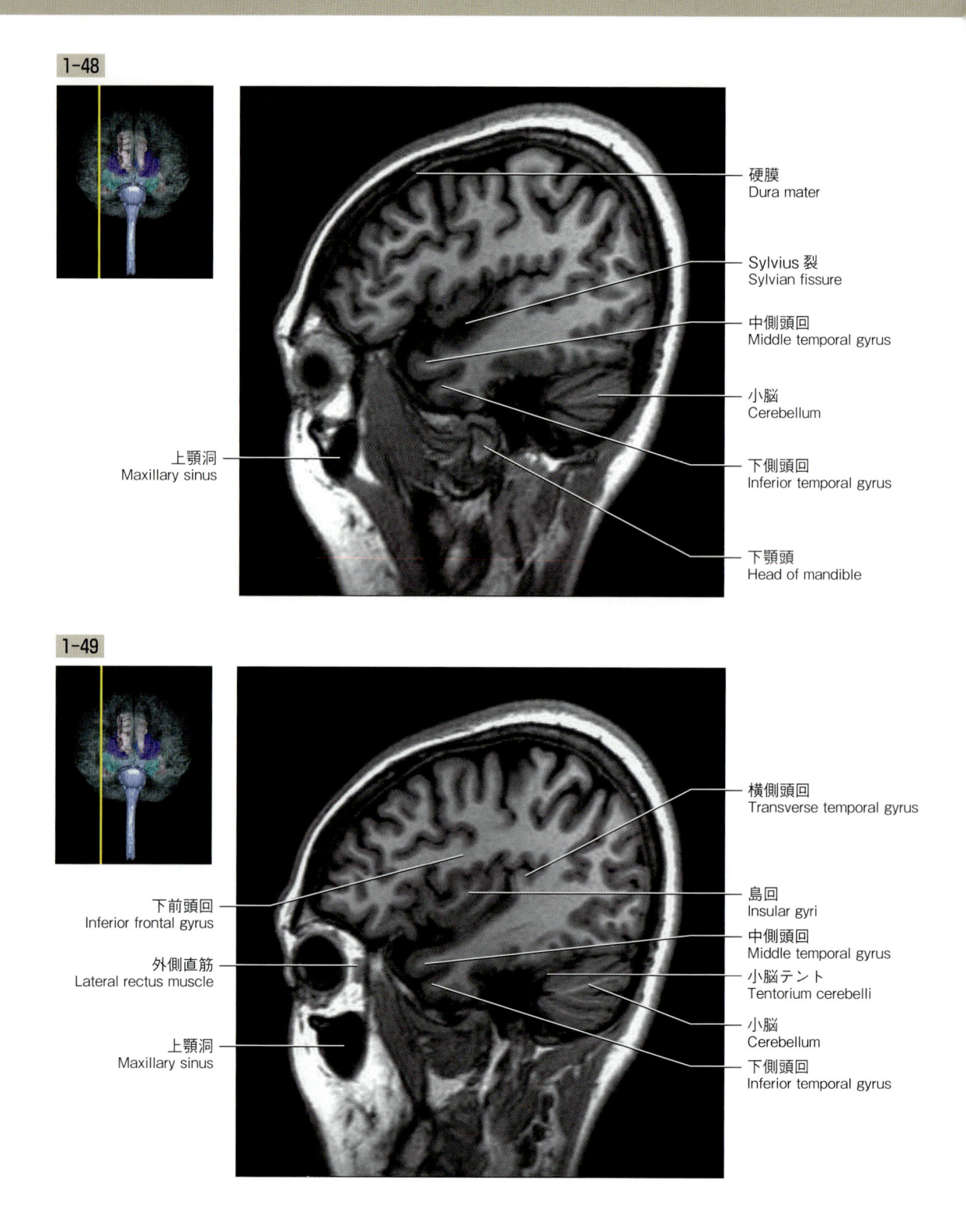

脳の断層解剖　[矢状断像（MRI, T1 強調像）]

1-48

- 硬膜 Dura mater
- Sylvius 裂 Sylvian fissure
- 中側頭回 Middle temporal gyrus
- 小脳 Cerebellum
- 下側頭回 Inferior temporal gyrus
- 下顎頭 Head of mandible
- 上顎洞 Maxillary sinus

1-49

- 横側頭回 Transverse temporal gyrus
- 島回 Insular gyri
- 中側頭回 Middle temporal gyrus
- 小脳テント Tentorium cerebelli
- 小脳 Cerebellum
- 下側頭回 Inferior temporal gyrus
- 下前頭回 Inferior frontal gyrus
- 外側直筋 Lateral rectus muscle
- 上顎洞 Maxillary sinus

NOTE 横側頭回は側頭葉上面に位置し，上方へ凸のΩ状の形状を呈する脳回である（1-72を参照）．同脳回には聴覚皮質が存在し，内側膝状体からの聴放線を受ける．

脳の断層解剖　[矢状断像（MRI, T1強調像）]

1-50

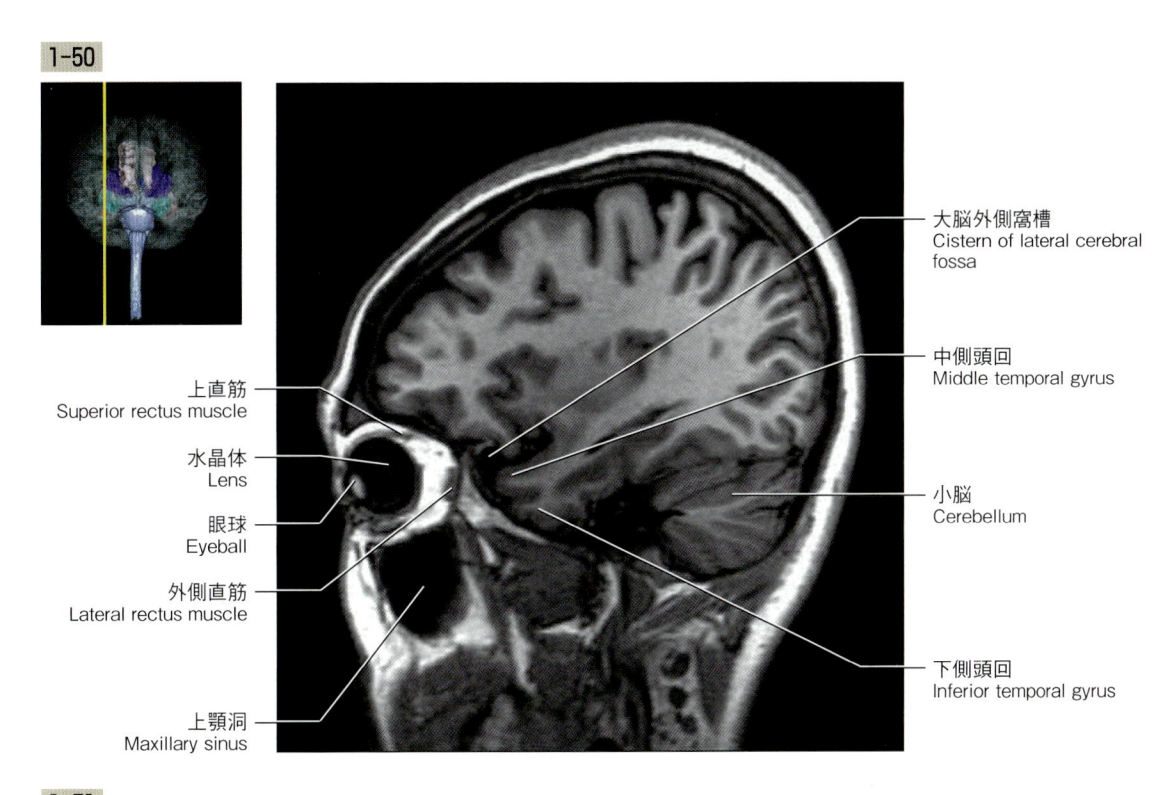

- 大脳外側窩槽　Cistern of lateral cerebral fossa
- 中側頭回　Middle temporal gyrus
- 小脳　Cerebellum
- 下側頭回　Inferior temporal gyrus
- 上直筋　Superior rectus muscle
- 水晶体　Lens
- 眼球　Eyeball
- 外側直筋　Lateral rectus muscle
- 上顎洞　Maxillary sinus

1-51

- 被殻　Putamen
- 扁桃体　Amygdala
- 海馬　Hippocampus
- 小脳　Cerebellum
- 上眼瞼挙筋　Levator palpebrae superioris muscle
- 前頭洞　Frontal sinus
- 上直筋　Superior rectus muscle
- 下直筋　Inferior rectus muscle
- 上顎洞　Maxillary sinus

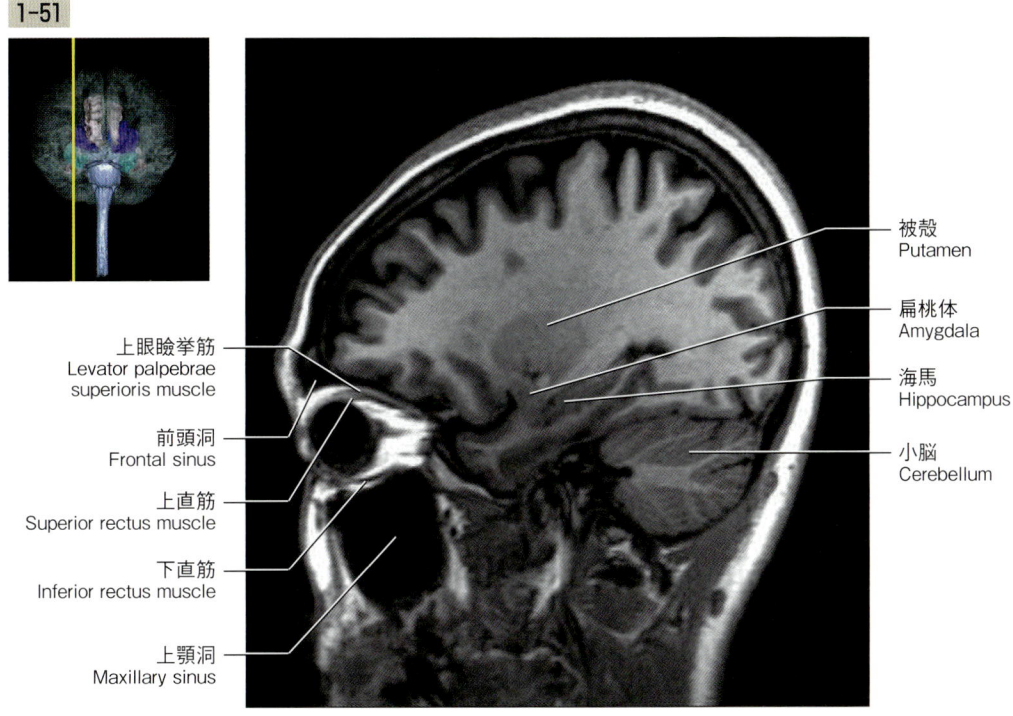

NOTE　洞　Sinus

Sinusは，船の帆を膨らました状態を意味する語．くぼみの原因であり，副鼻腔とか大動脈弁などの半月弁のポケット状の腔に用いる言葉．硬膜静脈洞（Dural sinuses）や心臓の冠状静脈洞（Coronary sinus）は，静脈血が流れていても管らしくなく，周りの組織の間隙のようにみえるために用いられるとの説がある．サンスクリットのjiva（弧の弦を意味する語）がもともとの語源とされる．

脳の断層解剖 ［矢状断像（MRI, T1 強調像）］

1-52

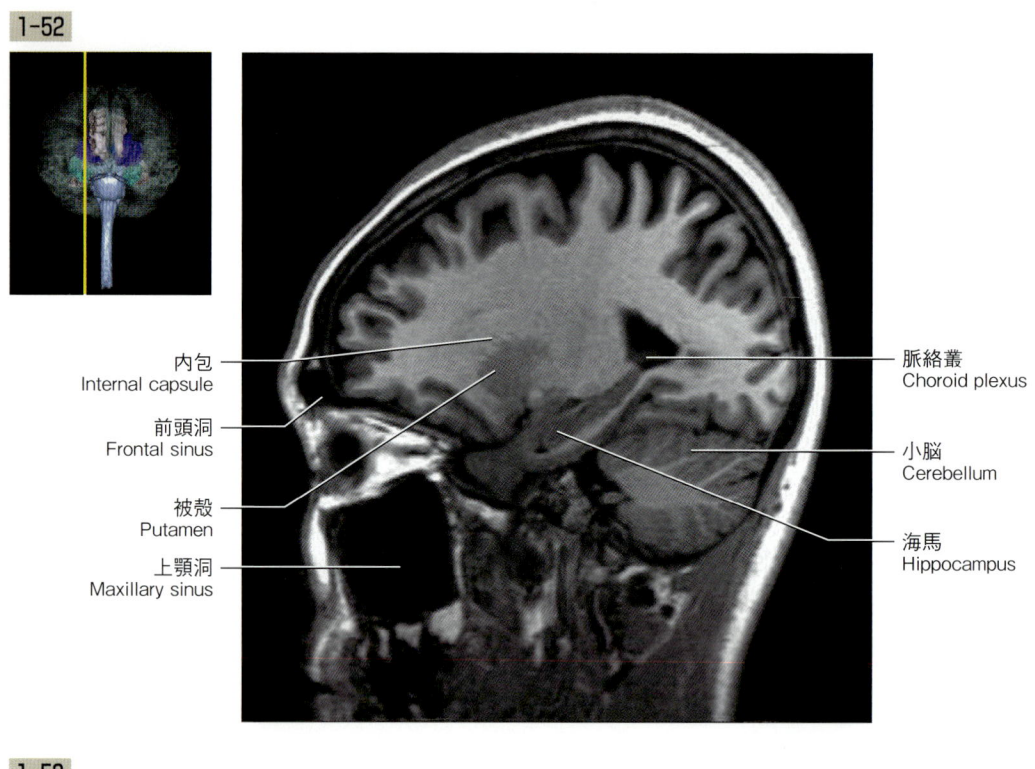

- 内包 Internal capsule
- 前頭洞 Frontal sinus
- 被殻 Putamen
- 上顎洞 Maxillary sinus
- 脈絡叢 Choroid plexus
- 小脳 Cerebellum
- 海馬 Hippocampus

1-53

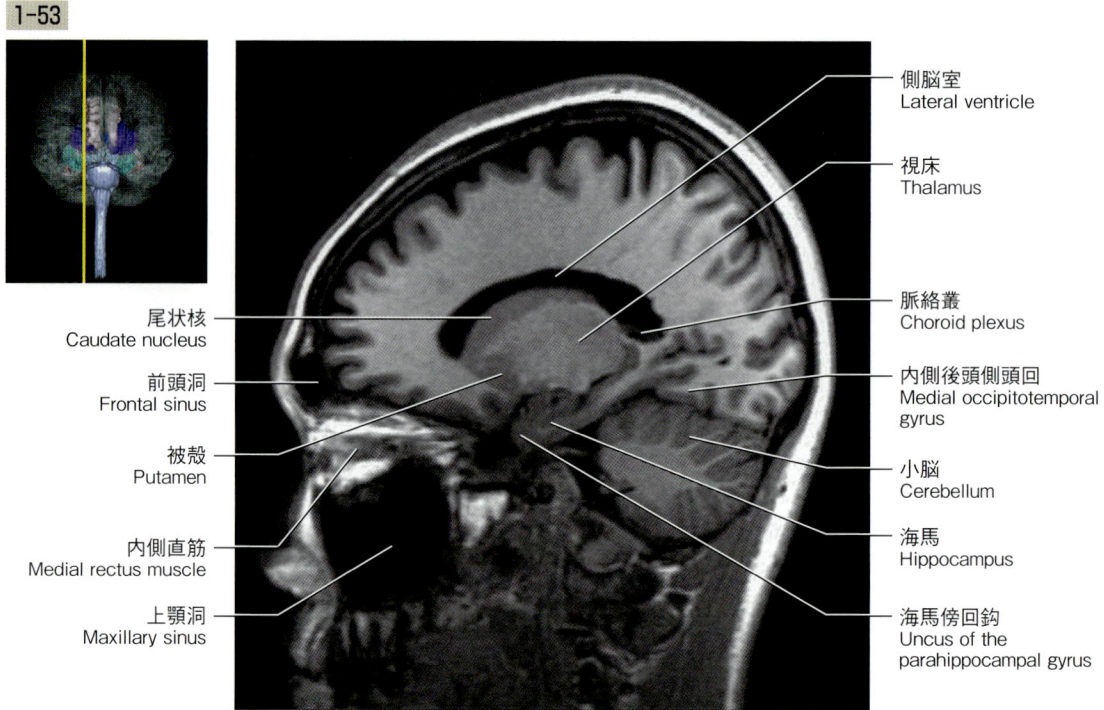

- 尾状核 Caudate nucleus
- 前頭洞 Frontal sinus
- 被殻 Putamen
- 内側直筋 Medial rectus muscle
- 上顎洞 Maxillary sinus
- 側脳室 Lateral ventricle
- 視床 Thalamus
- 脈絡叢 Choroid plexus
- 内側後頭側頭回 Medial occipitotemporal gyrus
- 小脳 Cerebellum
- 海馬 Hippocampus
- 海馬傍回鈎 Uncus of the parahippocampal gyrus

> **NOTE** サンスクリットと医学用語
> Medulla, Sinus のごとく，ギリシャ語，ラテン語の解剖名のいくつかが古代インド語 サンスクリットに由来するが，零(zero)もまた，もともと"空虚な"という意味のśūnya(シューニャ)が古代インド数字の零となり，アラビアに入って sifr，イタリアに渡り zeifro となったとされる．印欧語(インド・ヨーロッパ語)という単語のもつ意味は深い．

脳の断層解剖　[矢状断像(MRI, T1強調像)]

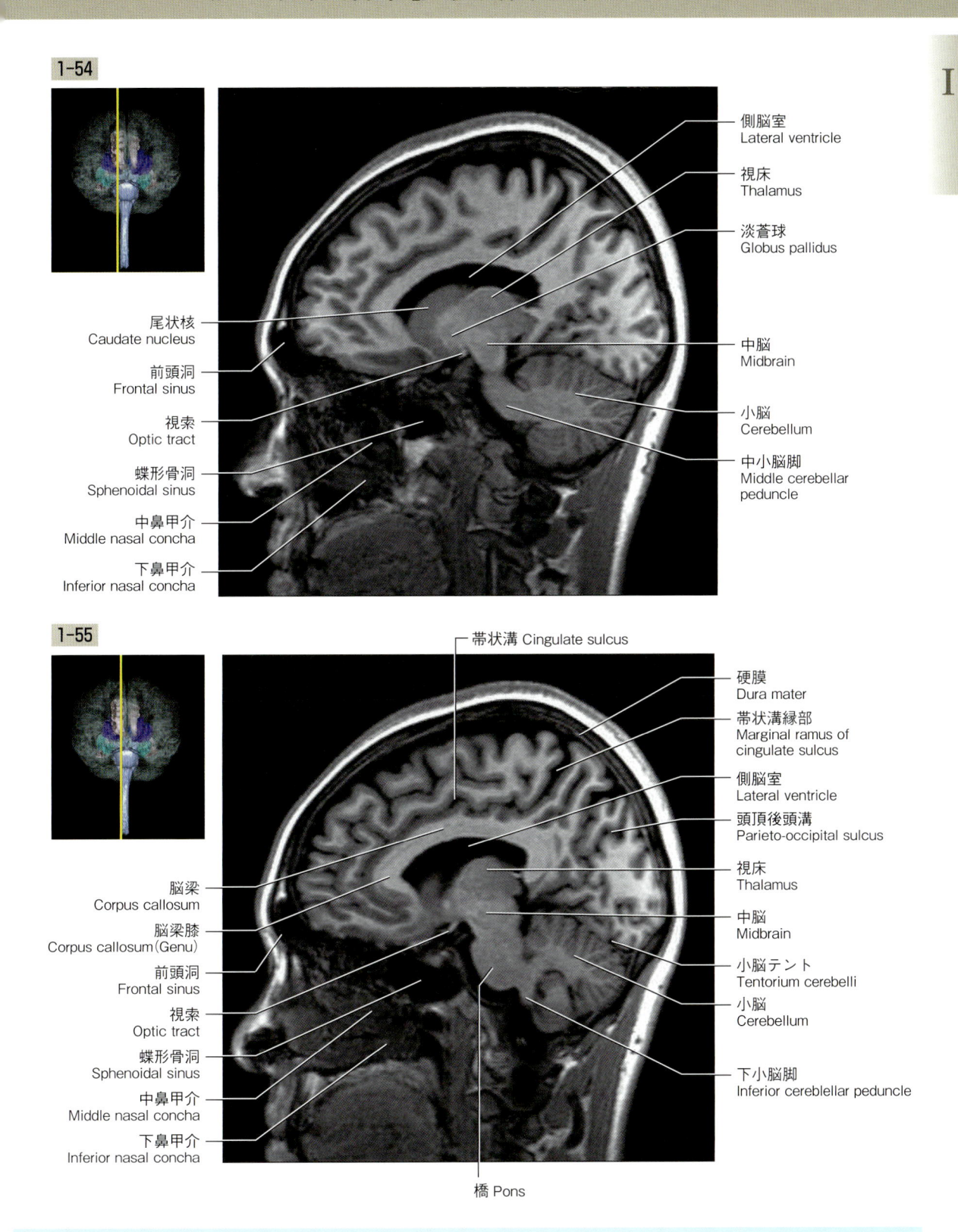

1-54

- 側脳室 Lateral ventricle
- 視床 Thalamus
- 淡蒼球 Globus pallidus
- 中脳 Midbrain
- 小脳 Cerebellum
- 中小脳脚 Middle cerebellar peduncle
- 尾状核 Caudate nucleus
- 前頭洞 Frontal sinus
- 視索 Optic tract
- 蝶形骨洞 Sphenoidal sinus
- 中鼻甲介 Middle nasal concha
- 下鼻甲介 Inferior nasal concha

1-55

- 帯状溝 Cingulate sulcus
- 硬膜 Dura mater
- 帯状溝縁部 Marginal ramus of cingulate sulcus
- 側脳室 Lateral ventricle
- 頭頂後頭溝 Parieto-occipital sulcus
- 視床 Thalamus
- 中脳 Midbrain
- 小脳テント Tentorium cerebelli
- 小脳 Cerebellum
- 下小脳脚 Inferior cerebellar peduncle
- 脳梁 Corpus callosum
- 脳梁膝 Corpus callosum (Genu)
- 前頭洞 Frontal sinus
- 視索 Optic tract
- 蝶形骨洞 Sphenoidal sinus
- 中鼻甲介 Middle nasal concha
- 下鼻甲介 Inferior nasal concha
- 橋 Pons

NOTE 帯状溝は脳梁直上の帯状回直上の脳溝である．矢状断像で前後方向に走行し，背側で上行し帯状溝縁となる．帯状溝縁の1つ前の脳溝が中心溝であるため，帯状溝の同定は中心溝を同定するうえで有用である．また，頭頂後頭溝は後上方から前下方へ走る脳溝であり，これにより頭頂葉と後頭葉が分けられる．

脳の断層解剖　［矢状断像（MRI, T1強調像）］

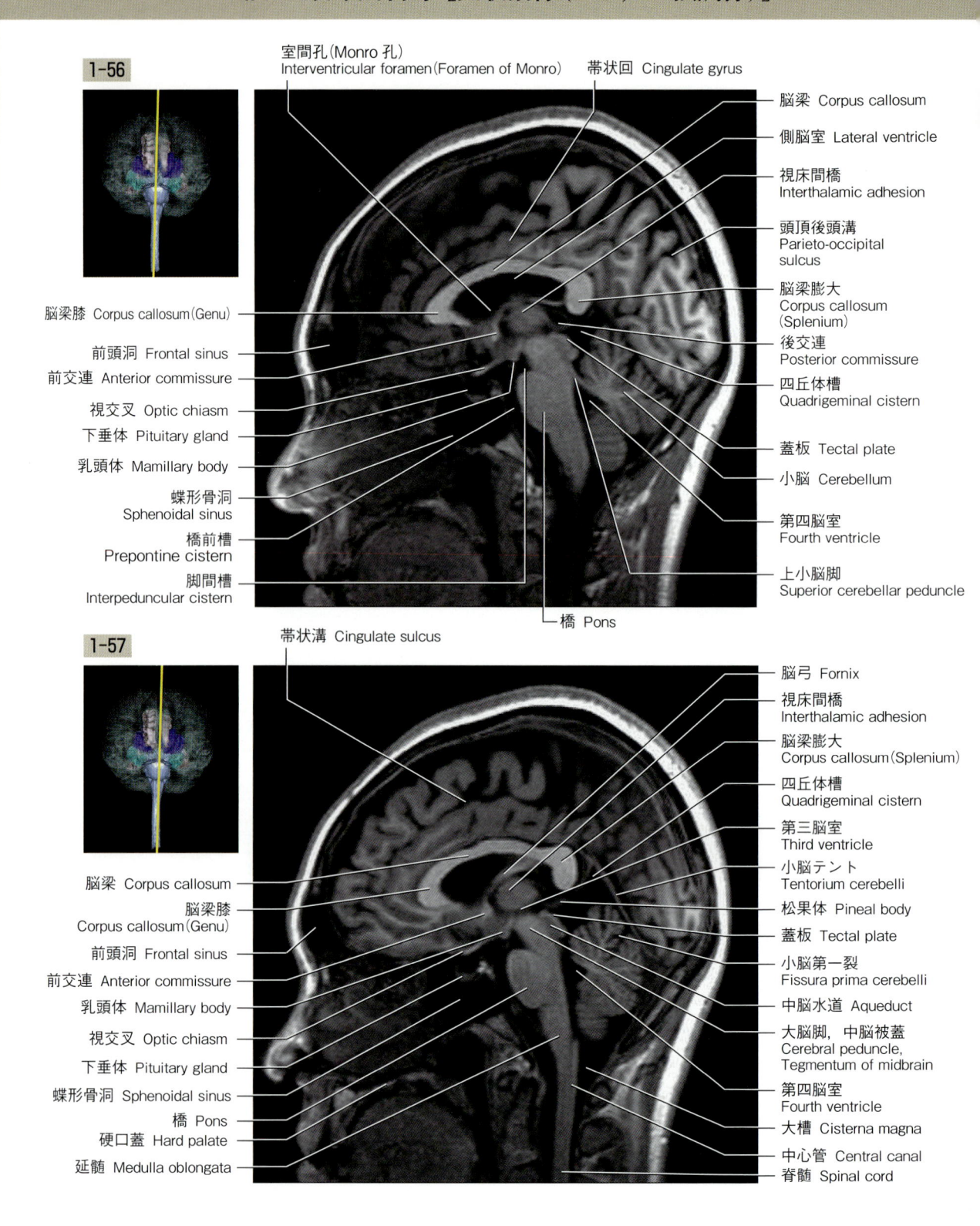

1-56

ラベル：
- 室間孔（Monro 孔） Interventricular foramen (Foramen of Monro)
- 帯状回 Cingulate gyrus
- 脳梁 Corpus callosum
- 側脳室 Lateral ventricle
- 視床間橋 Interthalamic adhesion
- 頭頂後頭溝 Parieto-occipital sulcus
- 脳梁膨大 Corpus callosum (Splenium)
- 後交連 Posterior commissure
- 四丘体槽 Quadrigeminal cistern
- 蓋板 Tectal plate
- 小脳 Cerebellum
- 第四脳室 Fourth ventricle
- 上小脳脚 Superior cerebellar peduncle
- 脳梁膝 Corpus callosum (Genu)
- 前頭洞 Frontal sinus
- 前交連 Anterior commissure
- 視交叉 Optic chiasm
- 下垂体 Pituitary gland
- 乳頭体 Mamillary body
- 蝶形骨洞 Sphenoidal sinus
- 橋前槽 Prepontine cistern
- 脚間槽 Interpeduncular cistern
- 橋 Pons

1-57

ラベル：
- 帯状溝 Cingulate sulcus
- 脳弓 Fornix
- 視床間橋 Interthalamic adhesion
- 脳梁膨大 Corpus callosum (Splenium)
- 四丘体槽 Quadrigeminal cistern
- 第三脳室 Third ventricle
- 小脳テント Tentorium cerebelli
- 松果体 Pineal body
- 蓋板 Tectal plate
- 小脳第一裂 Fissura prima cerebelli
- 中脳水道 Aqueduct
- 大脳脚, 中脳被蓋 Cerebral peduncle, Tegmentum of midbrain
- 第四脳室 Fourth ventricle
- 大槽 Cisterna magna
- 中心管 Central canal
- 脊髄 Spinal cord
- 脳梁 Corpus callosum
- 脳梁膝 Corpus callosum (Genu)
- 前頭洞 Frontal sinus
- 前交連 Anterior commissure
- 乳頭体 Mamillary body
- 視交叉 Optic chiasm
- 下垂体 Pituitary gland
- 蝶形骨洞 Sphenoidal sinus
- 橋 Pons
- 硬口蓋 Hard palate
- 延髄 Medulla oblongata

> **NOTE**　脳梁は最大の交連線維であり，大脳半球間の知覚情報の統合を行う．小脳は上小脳脚によって中脳と，中小脳脚によって橋と，下小脳脚によって延髄とそれぞれ結合している．
> 　1-57 に示されている正中矢状断には重要な構造物が多く，十分な理解が必要である．

脳の断層解剖 ［冠状断像（MRI, T1 強調像）］

1-58

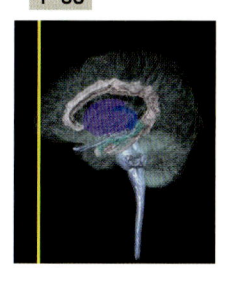

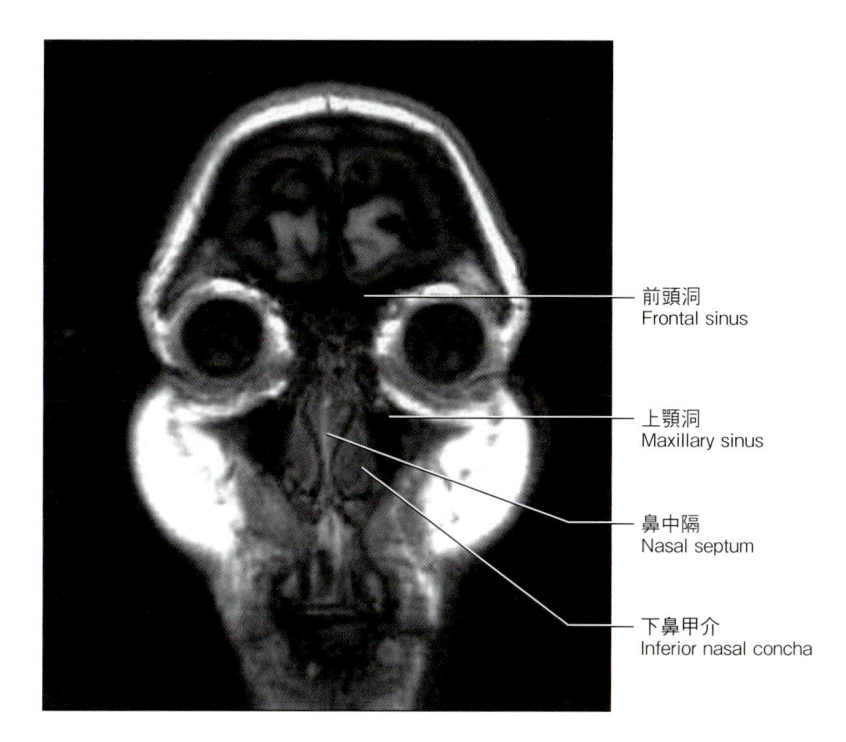

- 前頭洞 Frontal sinus
- 上顎洞 Maxillary sinus
- 鼻中隔 Nasal septum
- 下鼻甲介 Inferior nasal concha

1-59

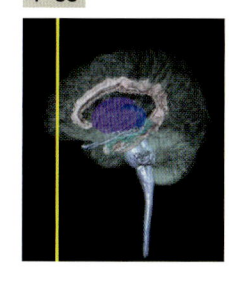

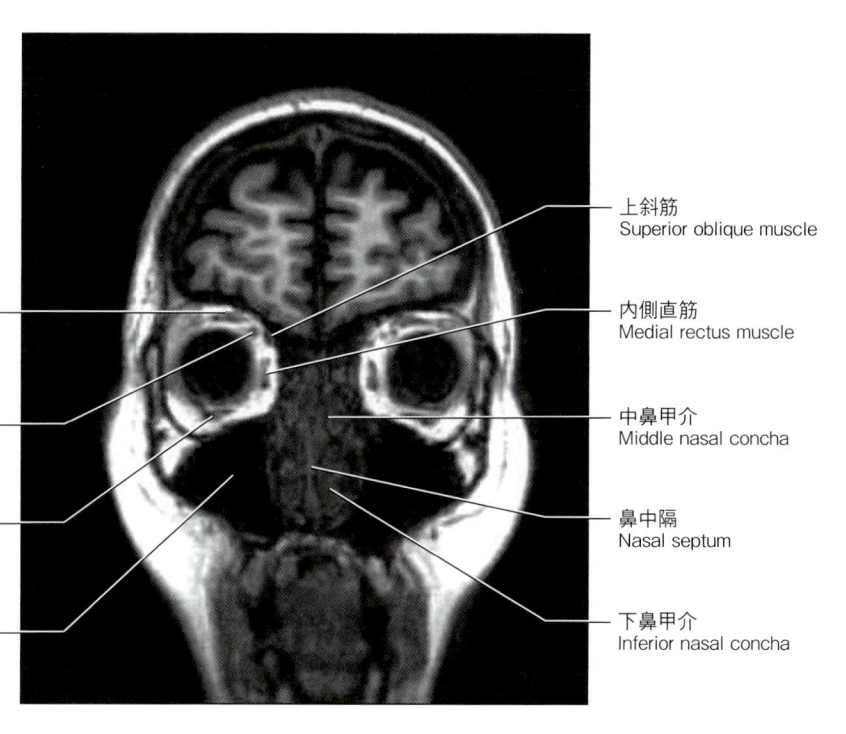

- 上直筋 Superior rectus muscle
- 上眼瞼挙筋 Levator palpebrae superioris muscle
- 下直筋 Inferior rectus muscle
- 上顎洞 Maxillary sinus
- 上斜筋 Superior oblique muscle
- 内側直筋 Medial rectus muscle
- 中鼻甲介 Middle nasal concha
- 鼻中隔 Nasal septum
- 下鼻甲介 Inferior nasal concha

脳の断層解剖 ［冠状断像（MRI, T1 強調像）］

1-60

- 半球間槽 Interhemisphaerica cisterm
- 上眼瞼挙筋 Levator palpebrae superioris muscle
- 上斜筋 Superior oblique muscle
- 内側直筋 Medial rectus muscle
- 中鼻甲介 Middle nasal concha
- 下鼻甲介 Inferior nasal concha
- 上直筋 Superior rectus muscle
- 外側直筋 Lateral rectus muscle
- 下直筋 Inferior rectus muscle
- 上顎洞 Maxillary sinus

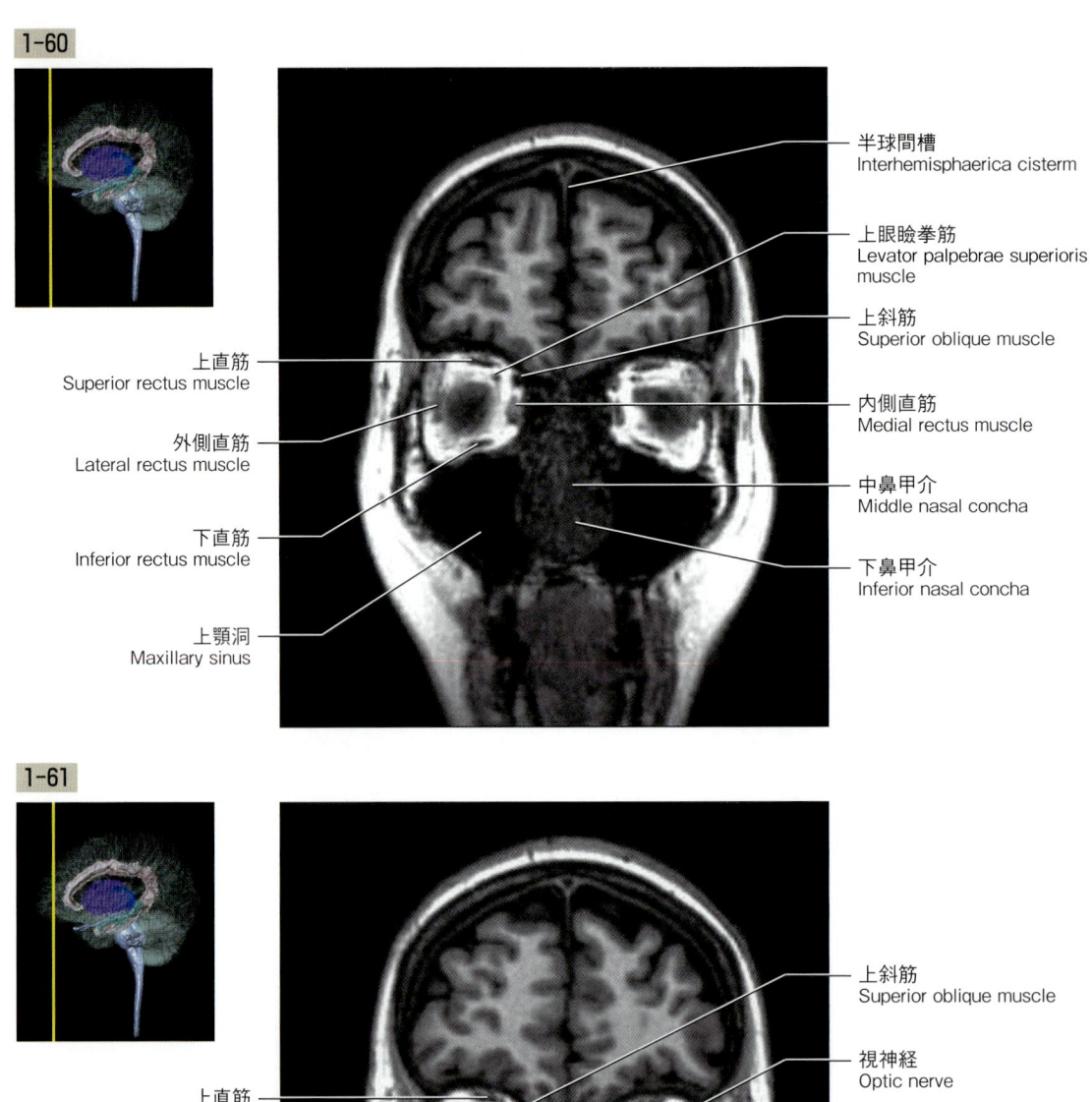

1-61

- 上斜筋 Superior oblique muscle
- 視神経 Optic nerve
- 内側直筋 Medial rectus muscle
- 中鼻甲介 Middle nasal concha
- 下鼻甲介 Inferior nasal concha
- 上直筋 Superior rectus muscle
- 外側直筋 Lateral rectus muscle
- 下直筋 Inferior rectus muscle
- 上顎洞 Maxillary sinus

脳の断層解剖　[冠状断像（MRI, T1強調像）]

1-62

- 上直筋 Superior rectus muscle
- 外側直筋 Lateral rectus muscle
- 上顎洞 Maxillary sinus
- 直回 Straight gyrus
- 視神経 Optic nerve
- 中鼻甲介 Middle nasal concha
- 下鼻甲介 Inferior nasal concha

1-63

- 側頭極 Temporal pole
- 上顎洞 Maxillary sinus
- 直回 Straight gyrus
- 下前頭回 Inferior frontal gyrus
- 眼窩回 Orbital gyri
- 視神経 Optic nerve
- 中鼻甲介 Middle nasal concha

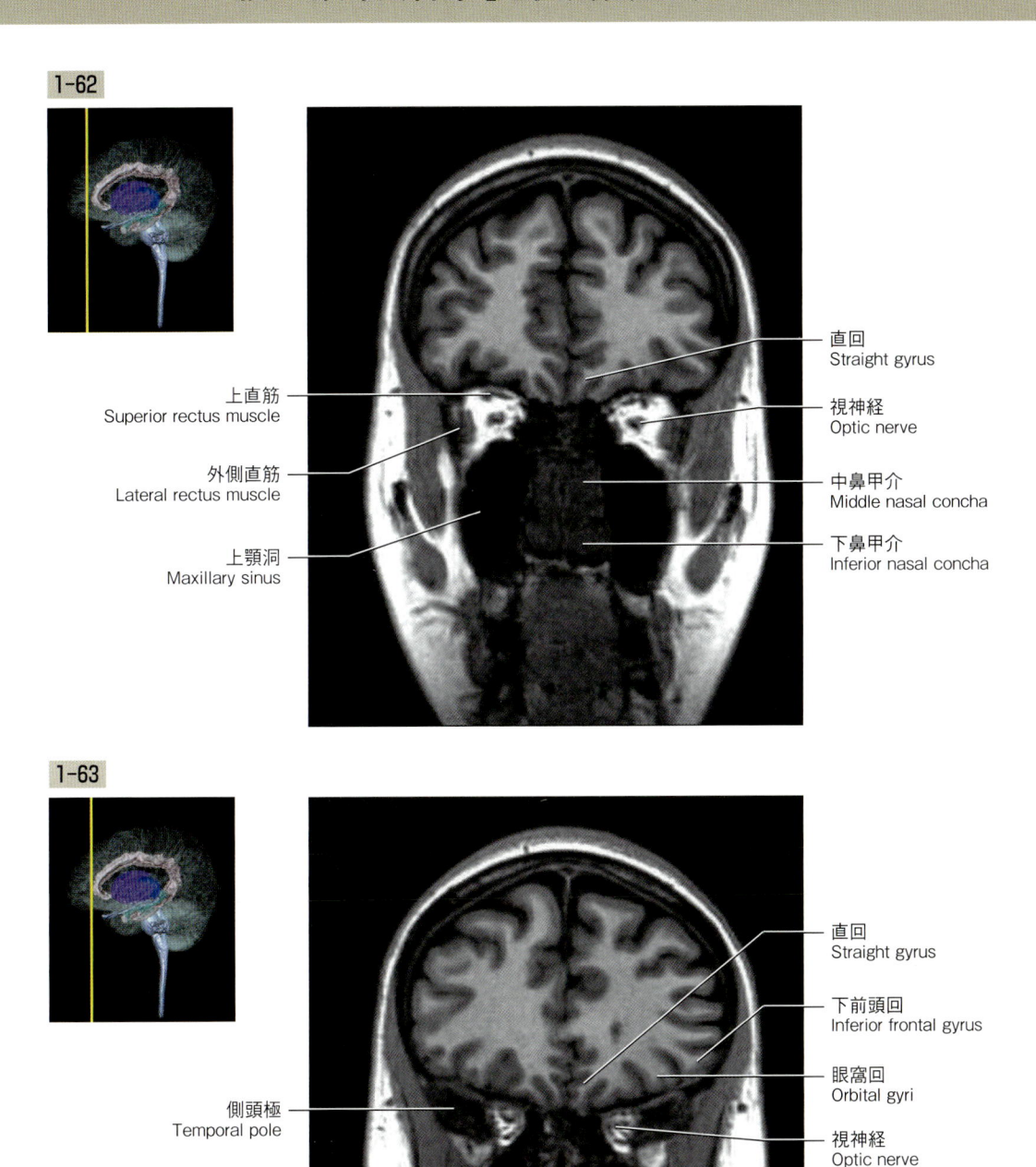

NOTE 直回は前頭葉底部腹内側に位置し，外側の眼窩回との間には嗅溝が存在する（1-38を参照）．直下の嗅球から連続する嗅索が嗅溝を走行する．

脳の断層解剖 ［冠状断像（MRI, T1強調像）］

1-64

- 側脳室前角 Lateral ventricle (Frontal horn)
- 側頭極 Temporal pole
- 蝶形骨洞 Sphenoidal sinus
- 帯状回 Cingulate gyrus
- 脳梁膝 Corpus callosum (Genu)
- 視神経 Optic nerve
- 中鼻甲介 Middle nasal concha
- 上顎洞 Maxillary sinus

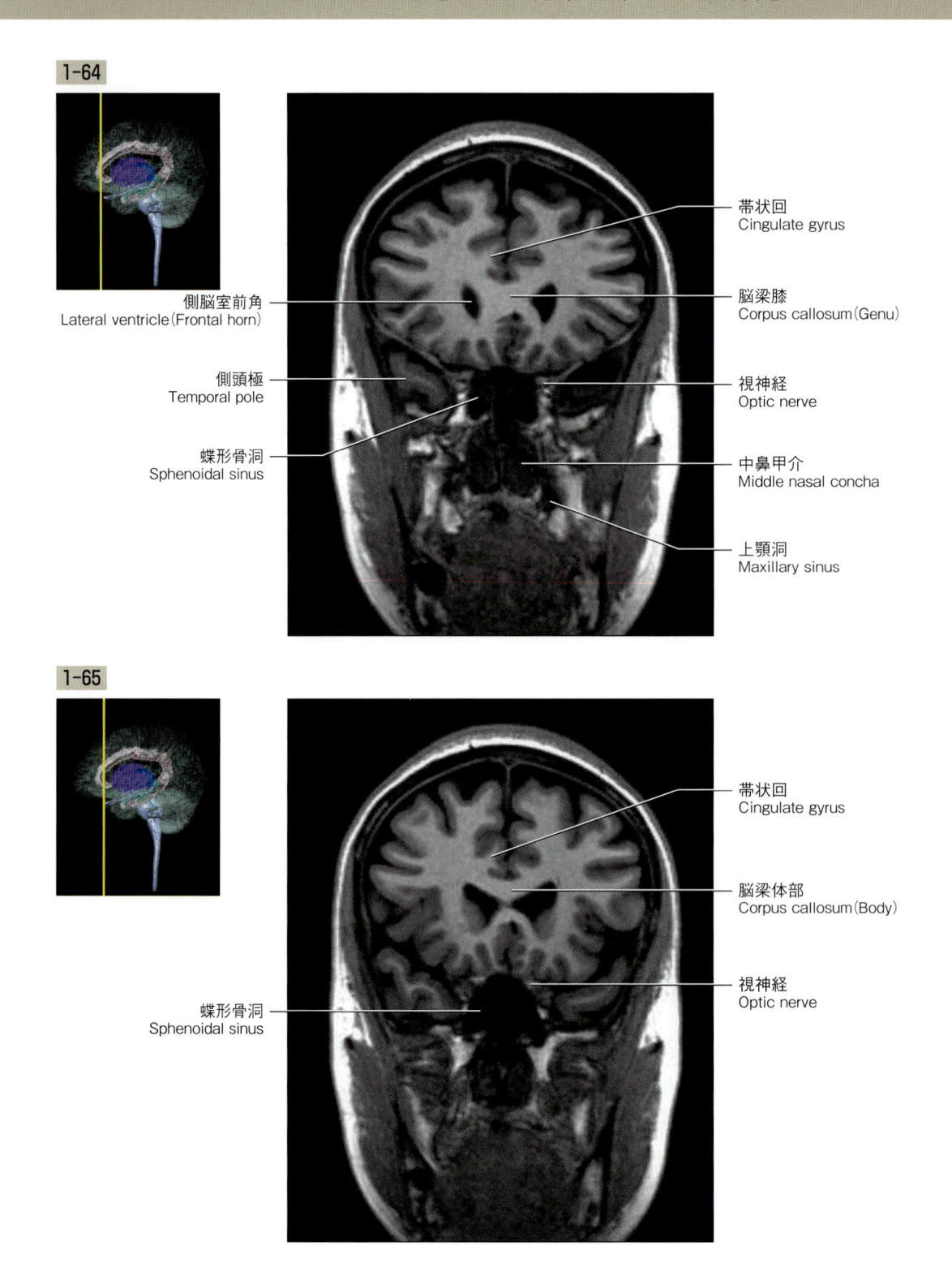

1-65

- 蝶形骨洞 Sphenoidal sinus
- 帯状回 Cingulate gyrus
- 脳梁体部 Corpus callosum (Body)
- 視神経 Optic nerve

NOTE 前頭洞や蝶形骨洞など副鼻腔と頭蓋内は頭蓋底部で隣接しており，副鼻腔炎からの炎症が直接波及し髄膜炎を生じることがある．髄膜炎の画像診断の際には副鼻腔炎の有無を確認することも大切である．

脳の断層解剖［冠状断像（MRI, T1強調像）］

1-66

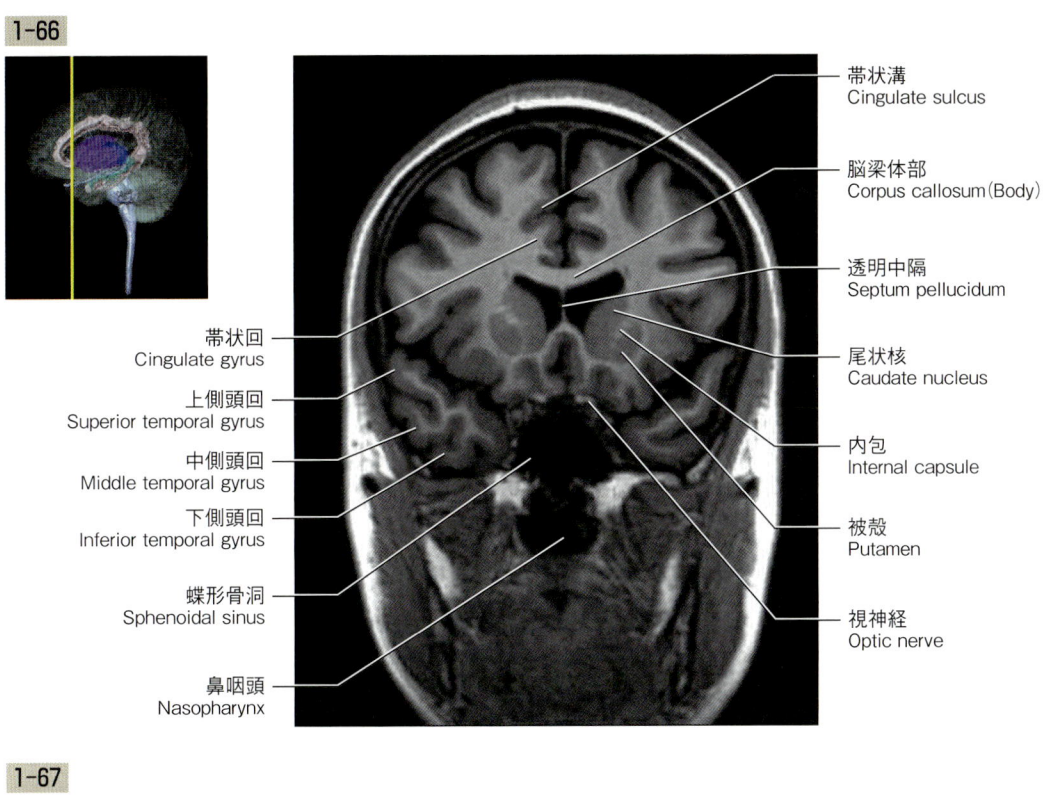

- 帯状溝 Cingulate sulcus
- 脳梁体部 Corpus callosum（Body）
- 透明中隔 Septum pellucidum
- 尾状核 Caudate nucleus
- 内包 Internal capsule
- 被殻 Putamen
- 視神経 Optic nerve
- 帯状回 Cingulate gyrus
- 上側頭回 Superior temporal gyrus
- 中側頭回 Middle temporal gyrus
- 下側頭回 Inferior temporal gyrus
- 蝶形骨洞 Sphenoidal sinus
- 鼻咽頭 Nasopharynx

1-67

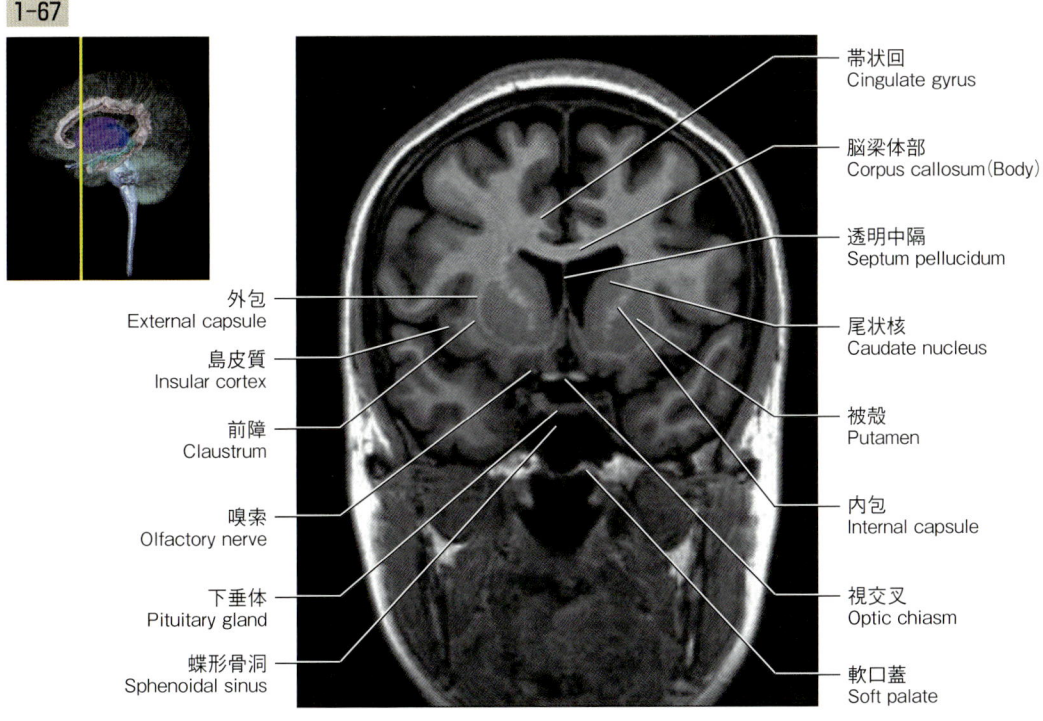

- 帯状回 Cingulate gyrus
- 脳梁体部 Corpus callosum（Body）
- 透明中隔 Septum pellucidum
- 尾状核 Caudate nucleus
- 被殻 Putamen
- 内包 Internal capsule
- 視交叉 Optic chiasm
- 軟口蓋 Soft palate
- 外包 External capsule
- 島皮質 Insular cortex
- 前障 Claustrum
- 嗅索 Olfactory nerve
- 下垂体 Pituitary gland
- 蝶形骨洞 Sphenoidal sinus

NOTE 下垂体の直上には視交叉が存在する．このため上方へ進展する下垂体腫瘍や鞍上部腫瘍の際には視交叉が圧排され視野障害が生じることになる．

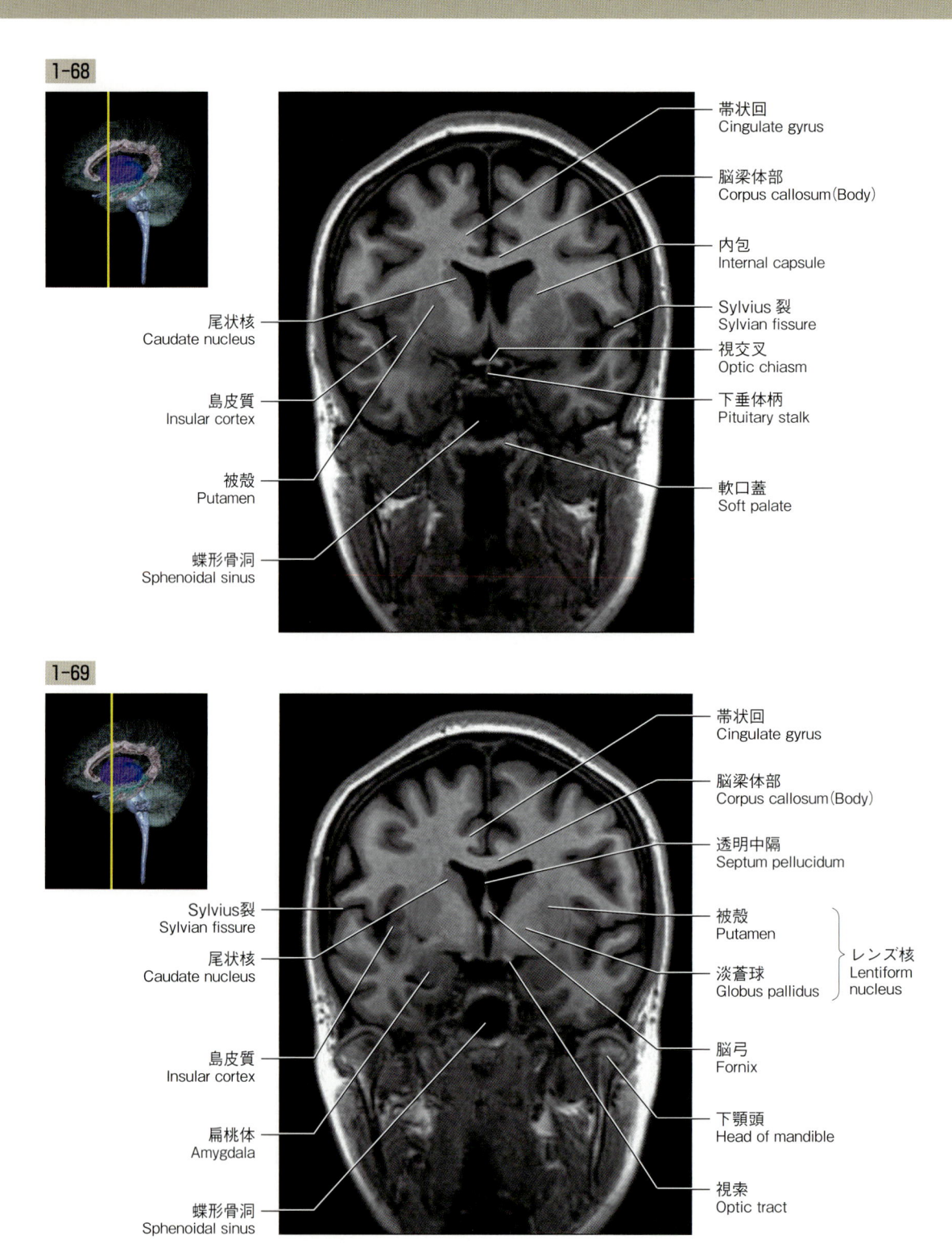

脳の断層解剖［冠状断像（MRI, T1 強調像）］

1-68

- 帯状回 Cingulate gyrus
- 脳梁体部 Corpus callosum (Body)
- 内包 Internal capsule
- Sylvius 裂 Sylvian fissure
- 視交叉 Optic chiasm
- 下垂体柄 Pituitary stalk
- 軟口蓋 Soft palate
- 尾状核 Caudate nucleus
- 島皮質 Insular cortex
- 被殻 Putamen
- 蝶形骨洞 Sphenoidal sinus

1-69

- 帯状回 Cingulate gyrus
- 脳梁体部 Corpus callosum (Body)
- 透明中隔 Septum pellucidum
- 被殻 Putamen
- 淡蒼球 Globus pallidus
- レンズ核 Lentiform nucleus
- 脳弓 Fornix
- 下顎頭 Head of mandible
- 視索 Optic tract
- Sylvius 裂 Sylvian fissure
- 尾状核 Caudate nucleus
- 島皮質 Insular cortex
- 扁桃体 Amygdala
- 蝶形骨洞 Sphenoidal sinus

> **NOTE** 淡蒼球 Globus pallidus
> pallidus は青白いの意，英語の pale の語源である．

脳の断層解剖 ［冠状断像（MRI, T1 強調像）］

1-70

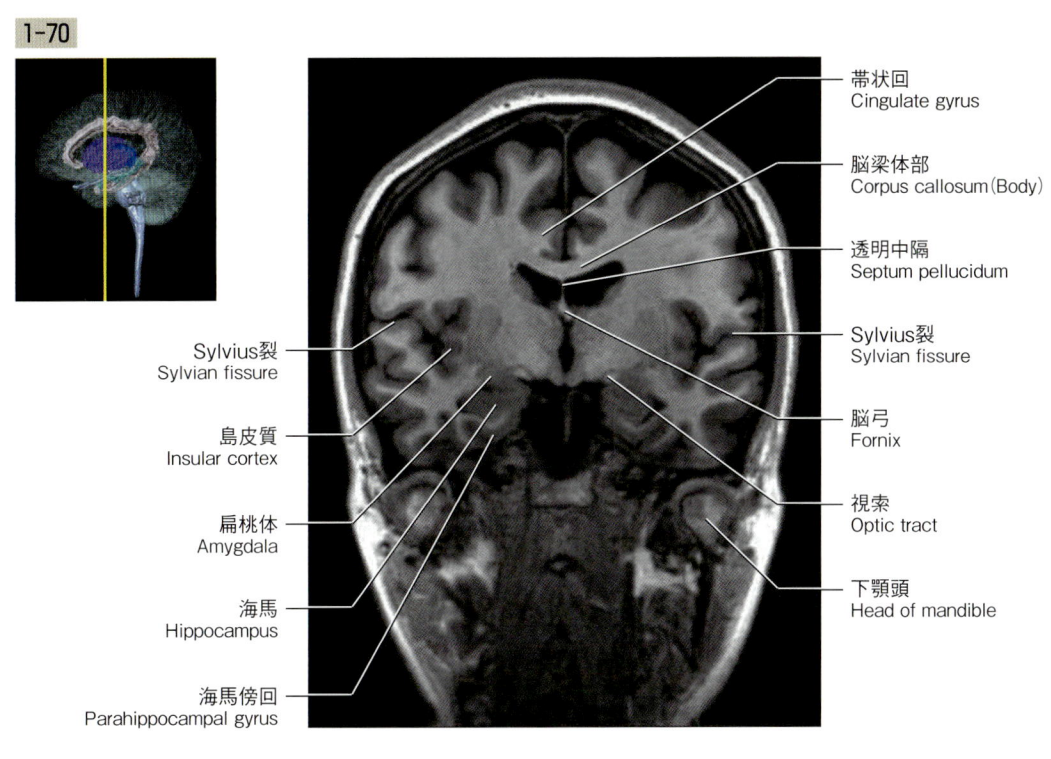

- 帯状回 Cingulate gyrus
- 脳梁体部 Corpus callosum (Body)
- 透明中隔 Septum pellucidum
- Sylvius裂 Sylvian fissure
- 脳弓 Fornix
- 視索 Optic tract
- 下顎頭 Head of mandible
- Sylvius裂 Sylvian fissure
- 島皮質 Insular cortex
- 扁桃体 Amygdala
- 海馬 Hippocampus
- 海馬傍回 Parahippocampal gyrus

1-71

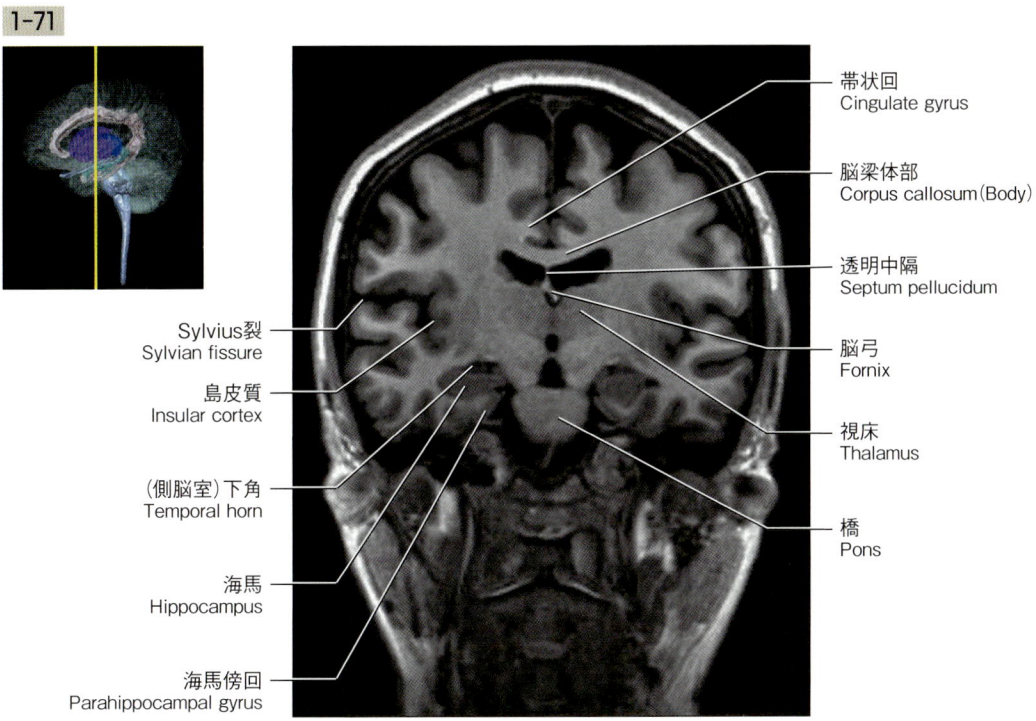

- 帯状回 Cingulate gyrus
- 脳梁体部 Corpus callosum (Body)
- 透明中隔 Septum pellucidum
- 脳弓 Fornix
- 視床 Thalamus
- 橋 Pons
- Sylvius裂 Sylvian fissure
- 島皮質 Insular cortex
- （側脳室）下角 Temporal horn
- 海馬 Hippocampus
- 海馬傍回 Parahippocampal gyrus

NOTE 海馬やその近傍の構造物は Alzheimer（アルツハイマー）病でしばしば異常所見がみられる．正常の構造や信号を把握しておく必要がある．

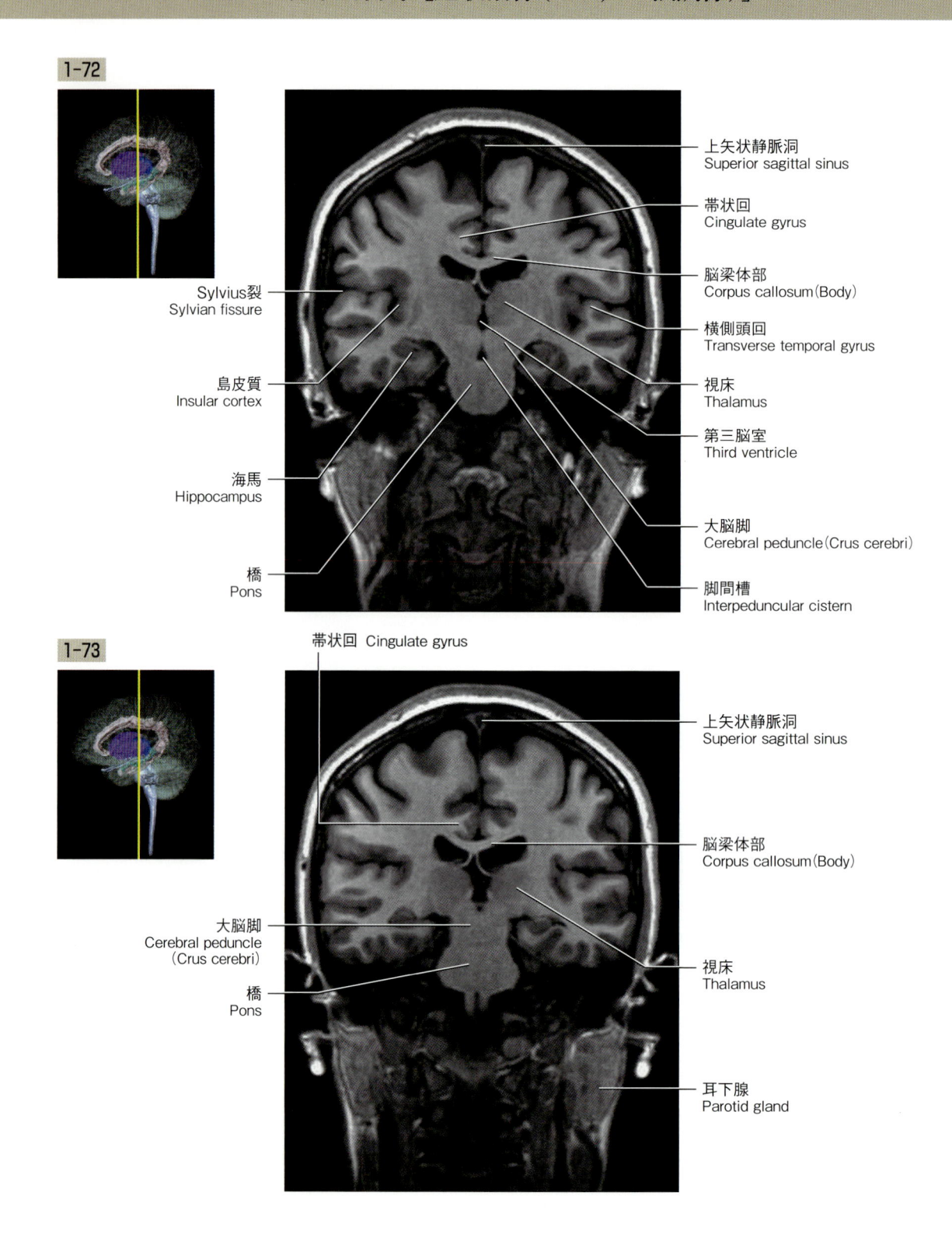

脳の断層解剖 ［冠状断像（MRI, T1強調像）］

1-72

- 上矢状静脈洞 Superior sagittal sinus
- 帯状回 Cingulate gyrus
- 脳梁体部 Corpus callosum (Body)
- 横側頭回 Transverse temporal gyrus
- 視床 Thalamus
- 第三脳室 Third ventricle
- 大脳脚 Cerebral peduncle (Crus cerebri)
- 脚間槽 Interpeduncular cistern
- Sylvius裂 Sylvian fissure
- 島皮質 Insular cortex
- 海馬 Hippocampus
- 橋 Pons

1-73

- 帯状回 Cingulate gyrus
- 上矢状静脈洞 Superior sagittal sinus
- 脳梁体部 Corpus callosum (Body)
- 視床 Thalamus
- 耳下腺 Parotid gland
- 大脳脚 Cerebral peduncle (Crus cerebri)
- 橋 Pons

NOTE　橋 Pons

Pons とはラテン語の橋の意味そのままで，小脳から出た線維束（中小脳脚）が脳幹を乗り越え盛り上がってみえることからこの名がついた．フランス最大の古代ローマの水道橋は，Pont du Gard（ポン・デュ・ガール）である．

脳の断層解剖 ［冠状断像（MRI, T1 強調像）］

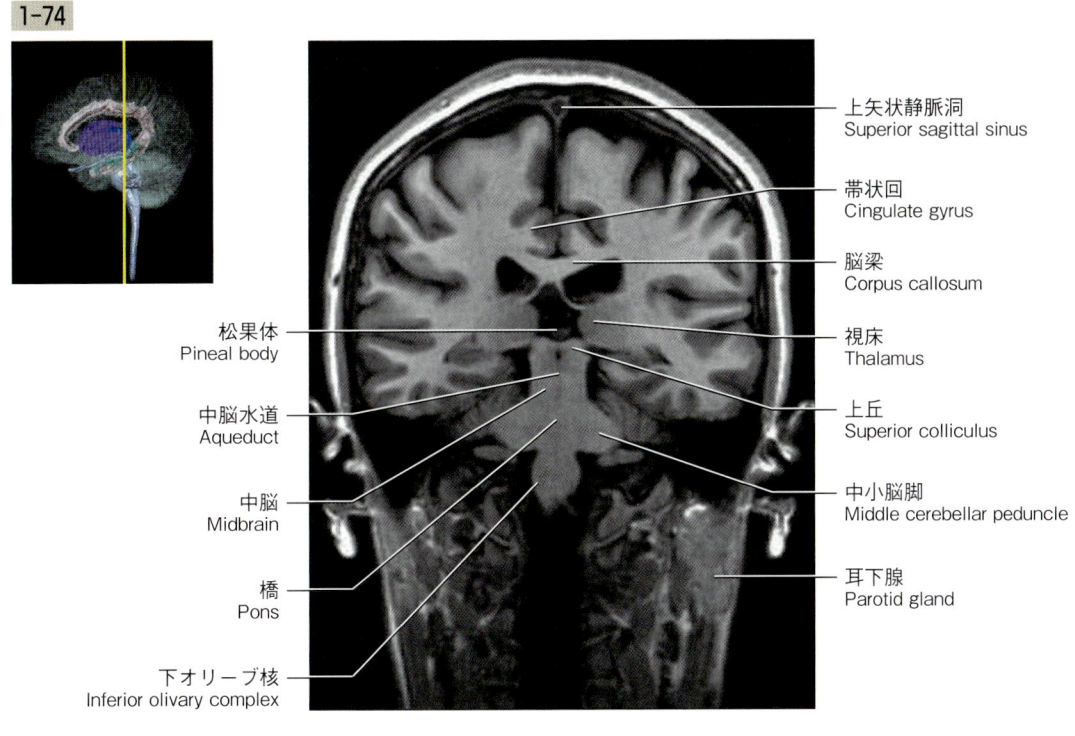

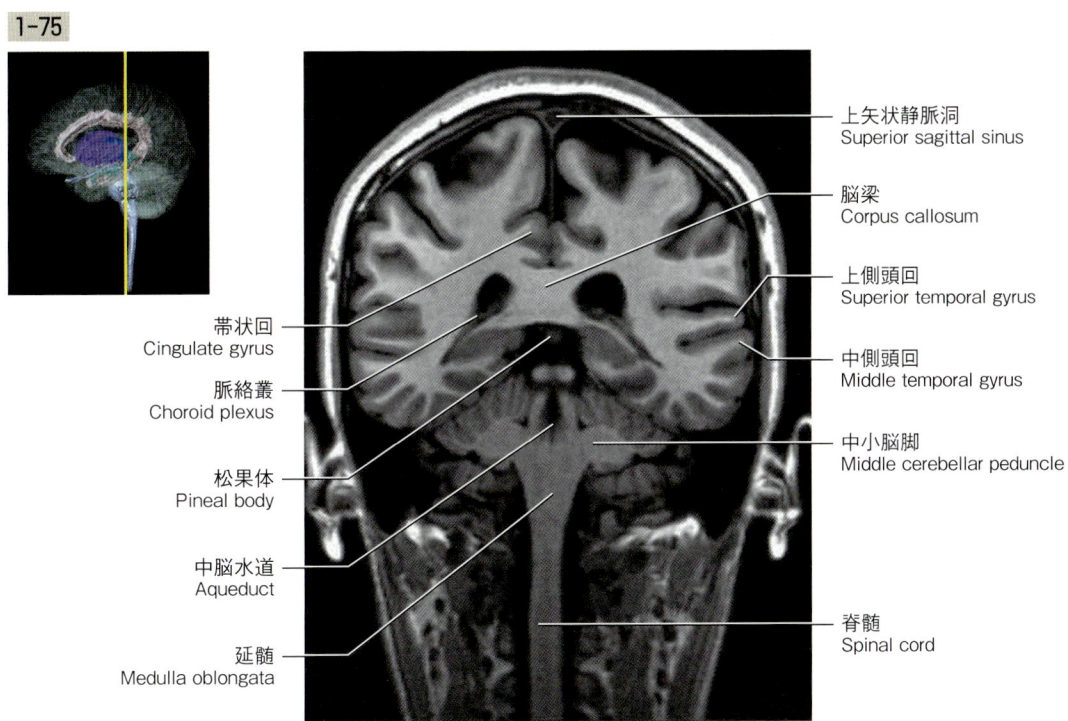

1-74

- 松果体 Pineal body
- 中脳水道 Aqueduct
- 中脳 Midbrain
- 橋 Pons
- 下オリーブ核 Inferior olivary complex
- 上矢状静脈洞 Superior sagittal sinus
- 帯状回 Cingulate gyrus
- 脳梁 Corpus callosum
- 視床 Thalamus
- 上丘 Superior colliculus
- 中小脳脚 Middle cerebellar peduncle
- 耳下腺 Parotid gland

1-75

- 帯状回 Cingulate gyrus
- 脈絡叢 Choroid plexus
- 松果体 Pineal body
- 中脳水道 Aqueduct
- 延髄 Medulla oblongata
- 上矢状静脈洞 Superior sagittal sinus
- 脳梁 Corpus callosum
- 上側頭回 Superior temporal gyrus
- 中側頭回 Middle temporal gyrus
- 中小脳脚 Middle cerebellar peduncle
- 脊髄 Spinal cord

脳の断層解剖［冠状断像（MRI, T1強調像）］

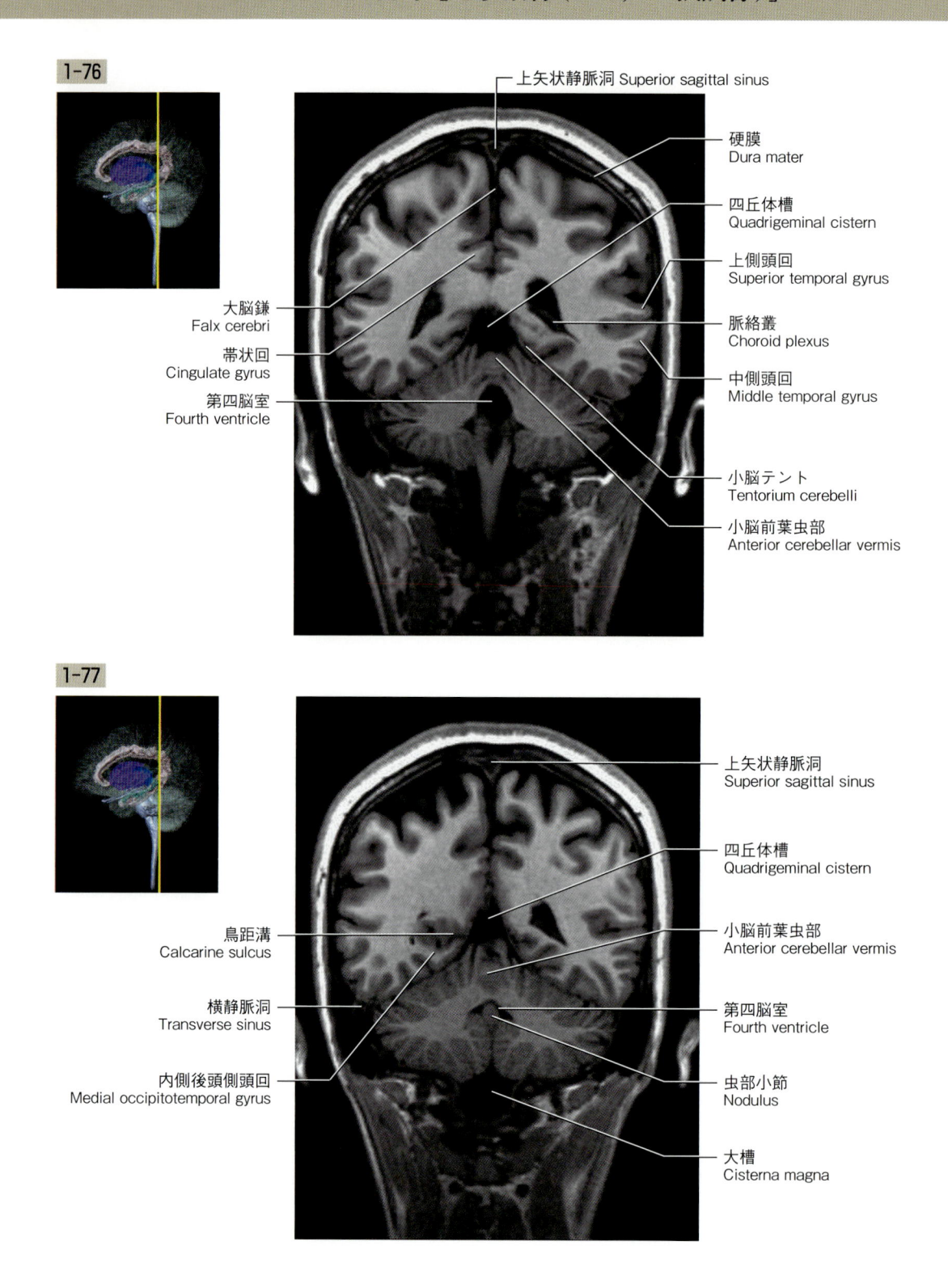

1-76

- 上矢状静脈洞 Superior sagittal sinus
- 硬膜 Dura mater
- 四丘体槽 Quadrigeminal cistern
- 上側頭回 Superior temporal gyrus
- 脈絡叢 Choroid plexus
- 中側頭回 Middle temporal gyrus
- 小脳テント Tentorium cerebelli
- 小脳前葉虫部 Anterior cerebellar vermis
- 大脳鎌 Falx cerebri
- 帯状回 Cingulate gyrus
- 第四脳室 Fourth ventricle

1-77

- 上矢状静脈洞 Superior sagittal sinus
- 四丘体槽 Quadrigeminal cistern
- 小脳前葉虫部 Anterior cerebellar vermis
- 第四脳室 Fourth ventricle
- 虫部小節 Nodulus
- 大槽 Cisterna magna
- 鳥距溝 Calcarine sulcus
- 横静脈洞 Transverse sinus
- 内側後頭側頭回 Medial occipitotemporal gyrus

NOTE 脳は髄膜とよばれる3層の膜によって包まれている．髄膜は外側から順に硬膜，くも膜と，脳表面に密着した軟膜からなる．硬膜とくも膜との間は潜在腔であり，血腫や水腫がない限り同定は困難である．くも膜下腔は脳脊髄液で満たされており，脳実質は髄液内に浮いた状態で存在している．

脳の断層解剖　[冠状断像（MRI, T1 強調像）]

1-78

- 上矢状静脈洞　Superior sagittal sinus
- 大脳鎌　Falx cerebri
- 楔部　Cuneus
- 鳥距溝　Calcarine sulcus
- 外側後頭側頭回　Lateral occipitotemporal gyrus
- 内側後頭側頭回　Medial occipitotemporal gyrus
- 小脳虫部　Cerebellar vermis
- 縁上回　Supramarginal gyrus
- 楔前部　Precuneus
- 横静脈洞　Transverse sinus
- 直静脈洞　Straight sinus

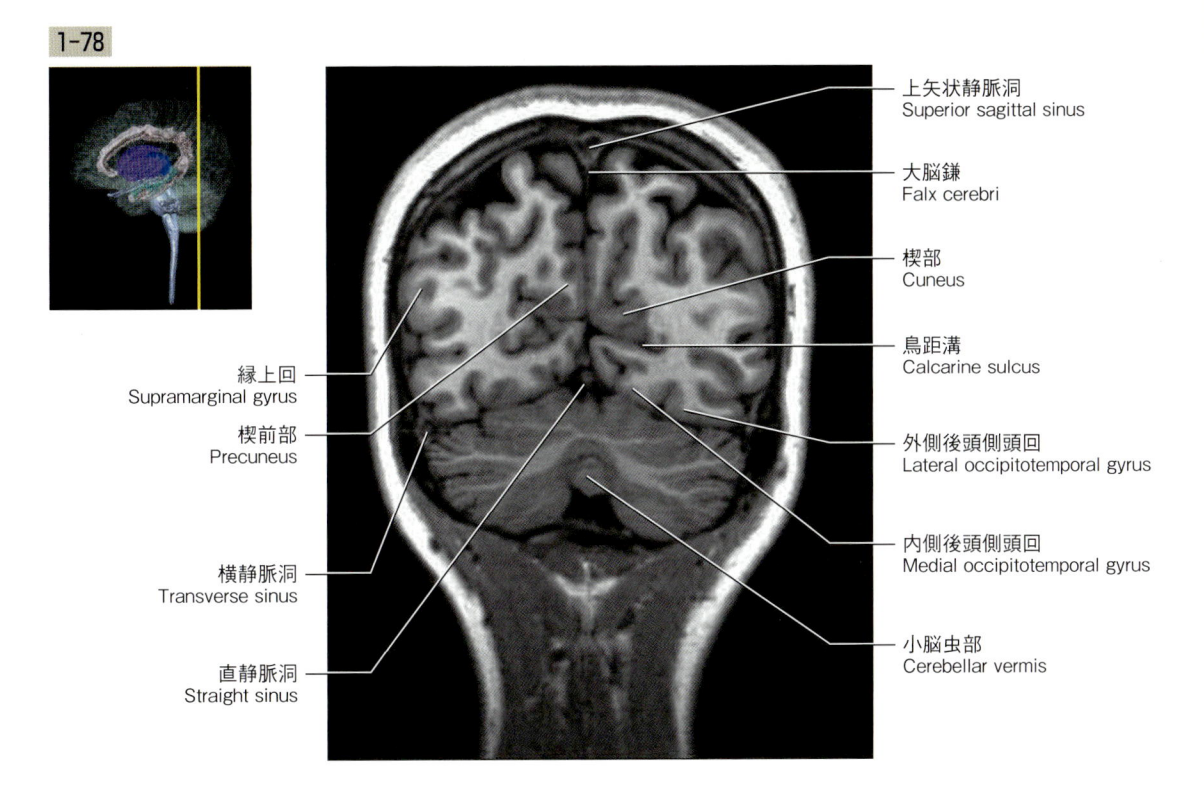

NOTE　硬膜（1-76 を参照）は正中部では大脳鎌を，後頭蓋窩では小脳テントを形成し，前者は左右の大脳半球間，後者は大脳と小脳間の仕切りとなっている．

脳神経

1-79 脳神経（MRI, T1強調像, VR像）

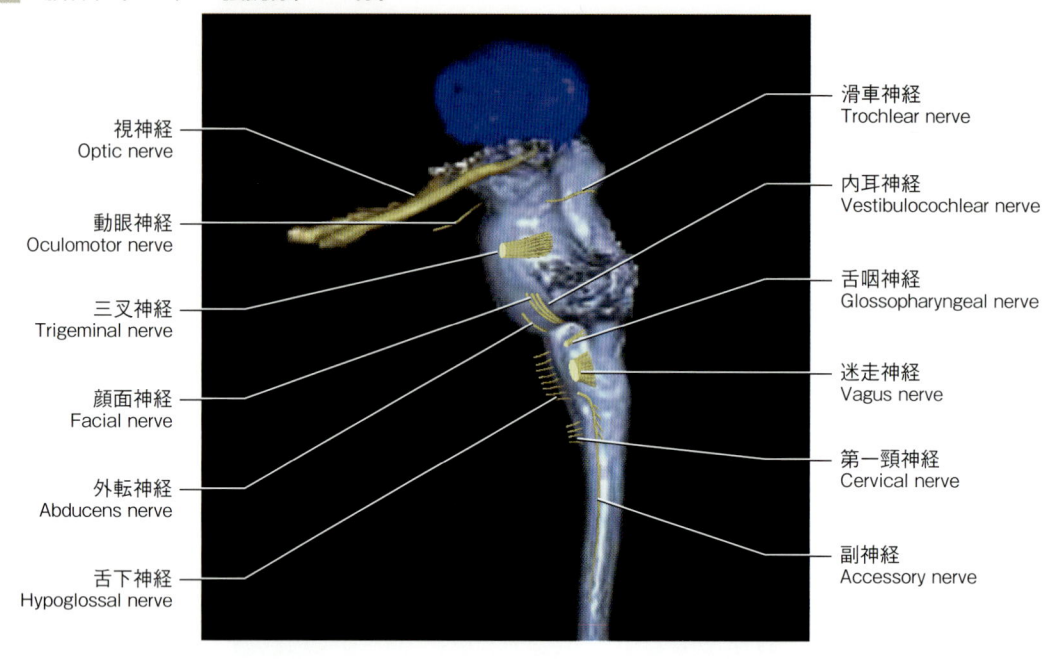

視神経 Optic nerve
動眼神経 Oculomotor nerve
三叉神経 Trigeminal nerve
顔面神経 Facial nerve
外転神経 Abducens nerve
舌下神経 Hypoglossal nerve
滑車神経 Trochlear nerve
内耳神経 Vestibulocochlear nerve
舌咽神経 Glossopharyngeal nerve
迷走神経 Vagus nerve
第一頸神経 Cervical nerve
副神経 Accessory nerve

1-80 脳神経の分類

CN I	嗅神経（Olfactory nerve）	知覚線維	嗅覚
CN II	視神経（Optic nerve）	知覚線維	視覚
CN III	動眼神経（Oculomotor nerve）	運動線維	眼球運動
		自律神経線維	瞳孔縮小, 遠近調節
CN IV	滑車神経（Trochlear nerve）	運動線維	眼球運動
CN V	三叉神経（Trigeminal nerve）	知覚線維	顔面の知覚, 温痛覚, 深部覚
		運動線維	咀嚼
CN VI	外転神経（Abducens nerve）	運動線維	眼球運動
CN VII	顔面神経（Facial nerve）	運動線維	顔面表情筋の運動
		知覚線維	舌前方2/3の味覚
		自律神経線維	唾液, 涙液の分泌
CN VIII	内耳神経（Vestibulocochlear nerve）	知覚線維	平衡感覚, 加速度感覚, 聴覚
CN IX	舌咽神経（Glossopharyngeal nerve）	知覚線維	咽喉頭知覚
		運動線維	咽喉頭の運動
		自律神経線維	唾液の分泌
CN X	迷走神経（Vagus nerve）	自律神経線維	内臓支配
		運動線維	咽喉頭の運動
		知覚線維	耳の温痛覚
CN XI	副神経（Accessory nerve）	運動線維	首の運動
CN XII	舌下神経（Hypoglossal nerve）	運動線維	舌の運動

NOTE 脳神経の描出にはheavy T2強調像（特に3DでのMR cisternography）が有効である．比較的太い三叉神経や視神経の一部などはルーチンの撮像でも同定可能である．

脳神経の断層解剖 [横・矢状断像（MRI, 白黒反転 heavy T2 強調像）]

1-81 嗅神経（CN I）

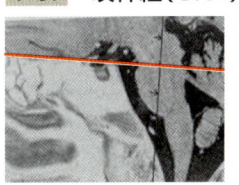

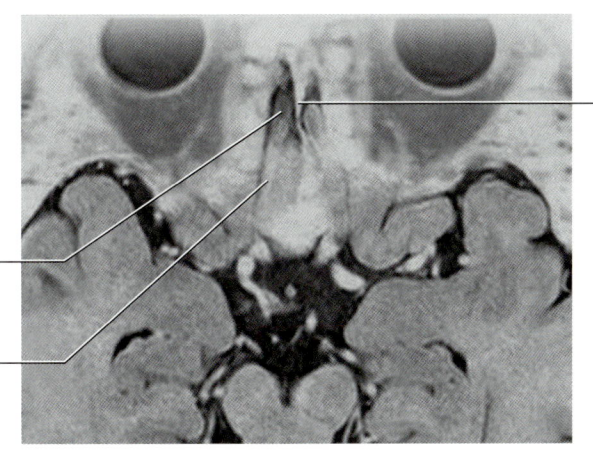

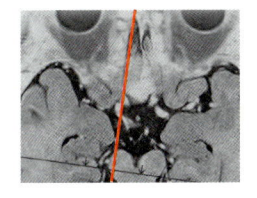

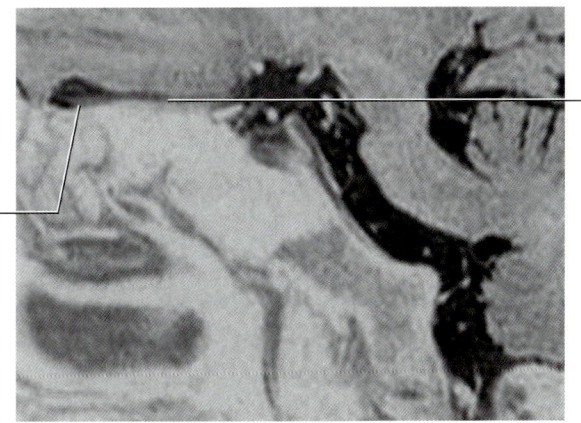

- 鶏冠 Crista galli
- 嗅球 Olfactory bulb
- 嗅神経（嗅索）Olfactory nerve
- 嗅神経（嗅索）Olfactory nerve
- 嗅球 Olfactory bulb

1-82 視神経（CN II）

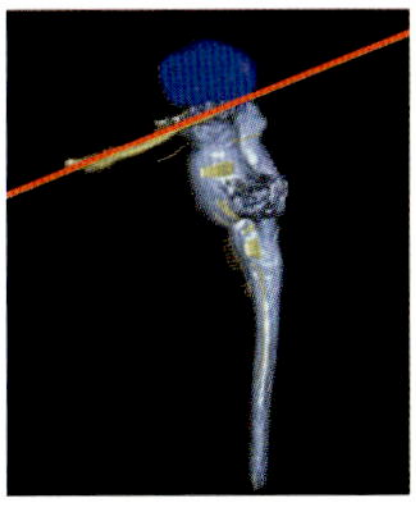

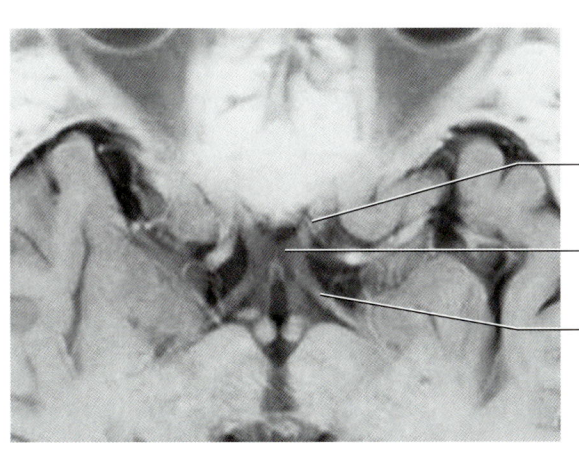

- 視神経 Optic nerve
- 視交叉 Optic chiasm
- 視索 Optic tract

> **NOTE** 鼻腔天蓋に存在する嗅細胞が束状になり，篩骨篩板を貫通したのちに前頭蓋底正中部の鶏冠両側に存在する嗅球へ至る．嗅球からは嗅索とよばれる嗅神経が背側方向に伸び嗅覚中枢に入る．嗅神経と視神経は末梢神経ではなく，終脳由来の中枢神経の一部である．

46　脳神経の断層解剖［横・矢状断像（MRI, 白黒反転 heavy T2 強調像）］

1-83　動眼神経（CN III）

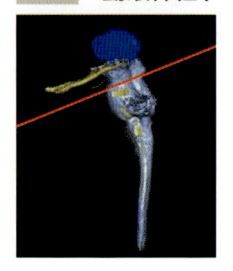

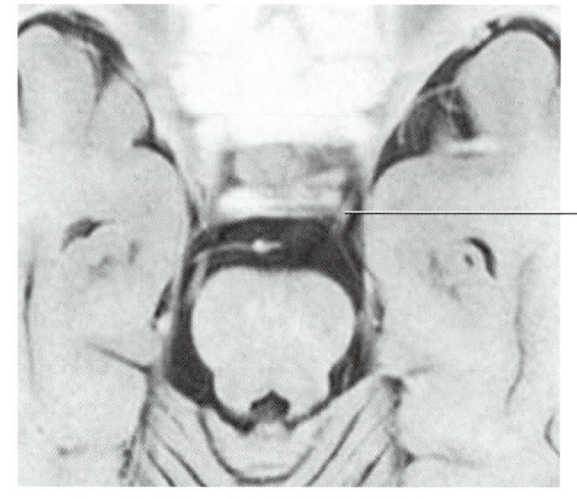

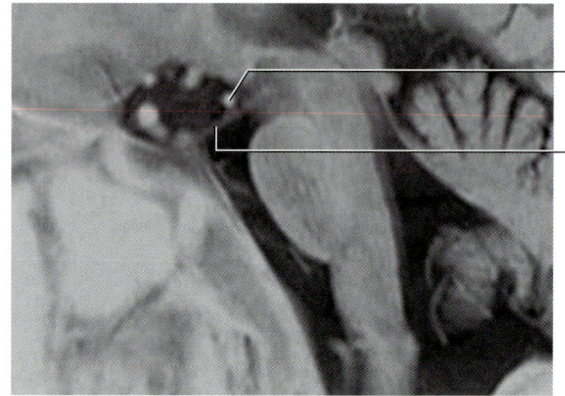

動眼神経
Oculomotor nerve

後大脳動脈
Posterior cerebral artery

動眼神経
Oculomotor nerve

1-84　滑車神経（CN IV）

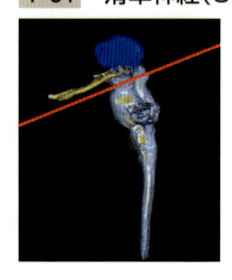

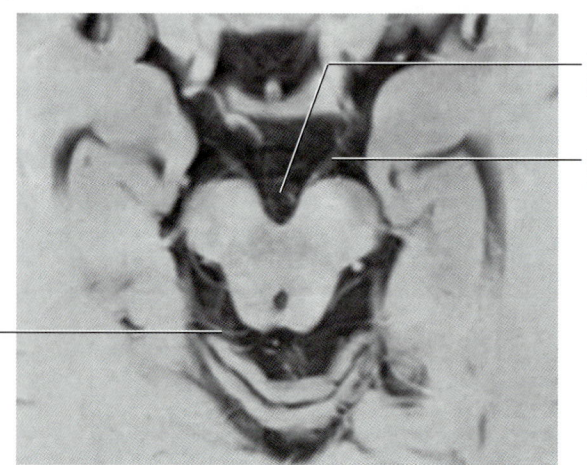

脚間窩
Interpeduncular fossa

動眼神経
Oculomotor nerve

滑車神経
Trochlear nerve

> **NOTE**　動眼神経は中脳脚間窩から起始し，前下方へ向かう．
> 　一方，滑車神経は下丘直下の中脳背側で交叉したのち背側面から起始し，中脳外側に沿って前方へ向かう．いずれも後大脳動脈と上小脳動脈の間を通り海綿静脈洞へ入り，上眼窩裂から眼窩内に至る．眼窩内で動眼神経は上直筋と上眼瞼挙筋に達する上枝と下直筋と内側直筋，下斜筋に達する下枝に分かれ，滑車神経は上斜筋に至る．

脳神経の断層解剖［横・矢状断像（MRI, 白黒反転 heavy T2 強調像）］

1-85 三叉神経（CN V）

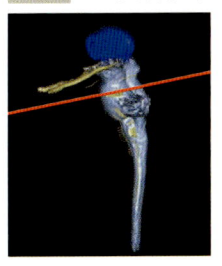

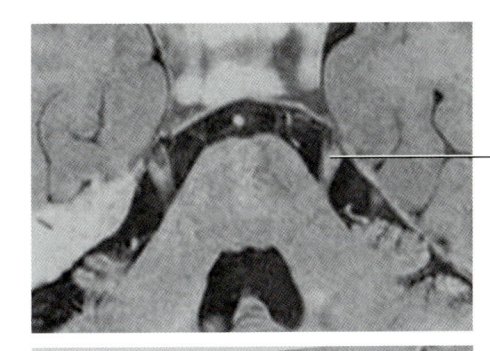

三叉神経
Trigeminal nerve

三叉神経
Trigeminal nerve

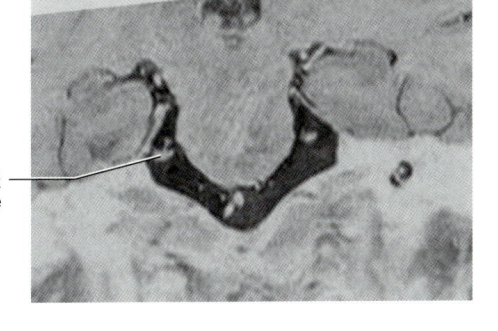

1-86 外転神経（CN VI）

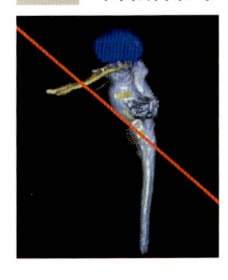

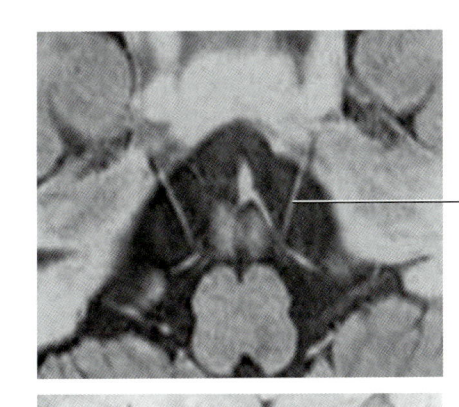

外転神経
Abducens nerve

外転神経
Abducens nerve

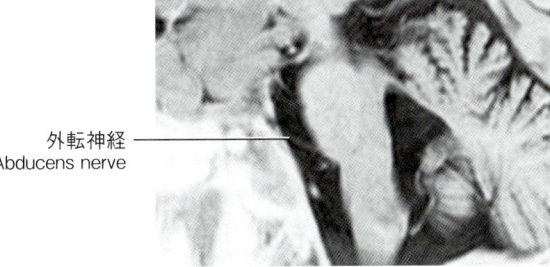

> **NOTE** 三叉神経は橋と中小脳脚移行部から起始し Meckel（メッケル）腔へ入り三叉神経節となったのち，眼神経・上顎神経・下顎神経に分かれる．
> 三叉神経への血管などによる圧迫は，三叉神経痛の原因としてしばしば MRI 検査の対象になる．3D-TOF MRA の元画像も有用である．

48　脳神経の断層解剖［横・矢状断像（MRI，白黒反転 heavy T2 強調像）］

1-87　顔面神経（CN VII），内耳神経（CN VIII）

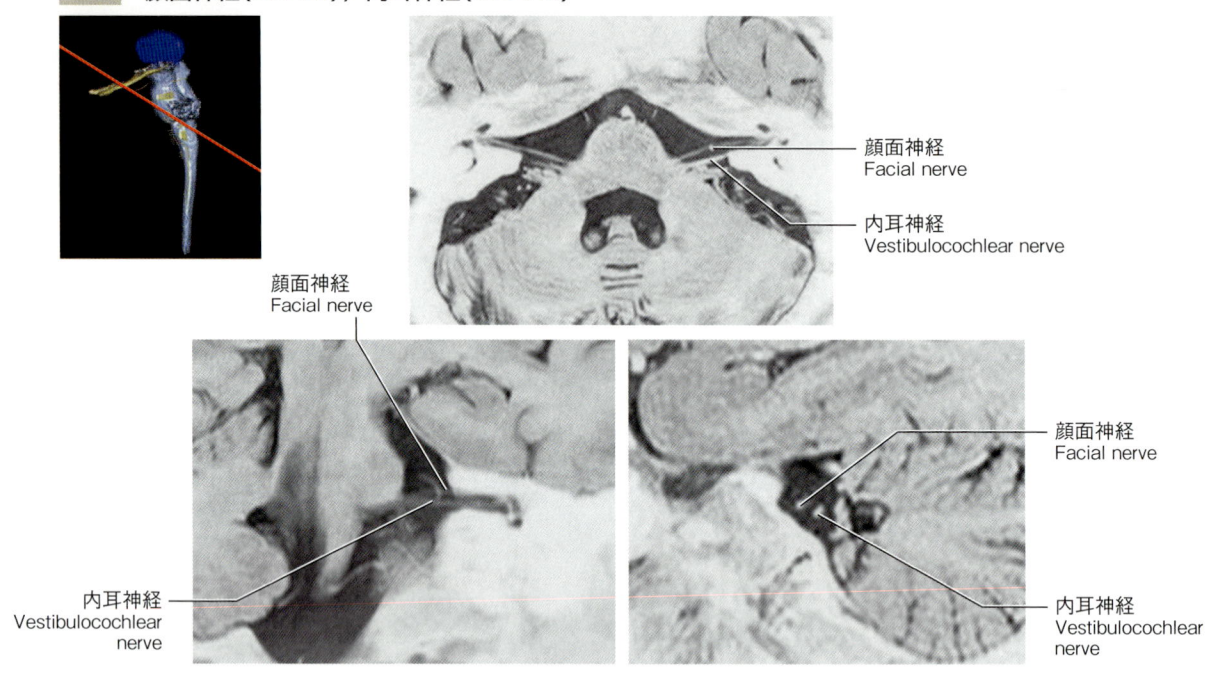

- 顔面神経 Facial nerve
- 内耳神経 Vestibulocochlear nerve

1-88　舌咽神経（CN IX），迷走神経（CN X）

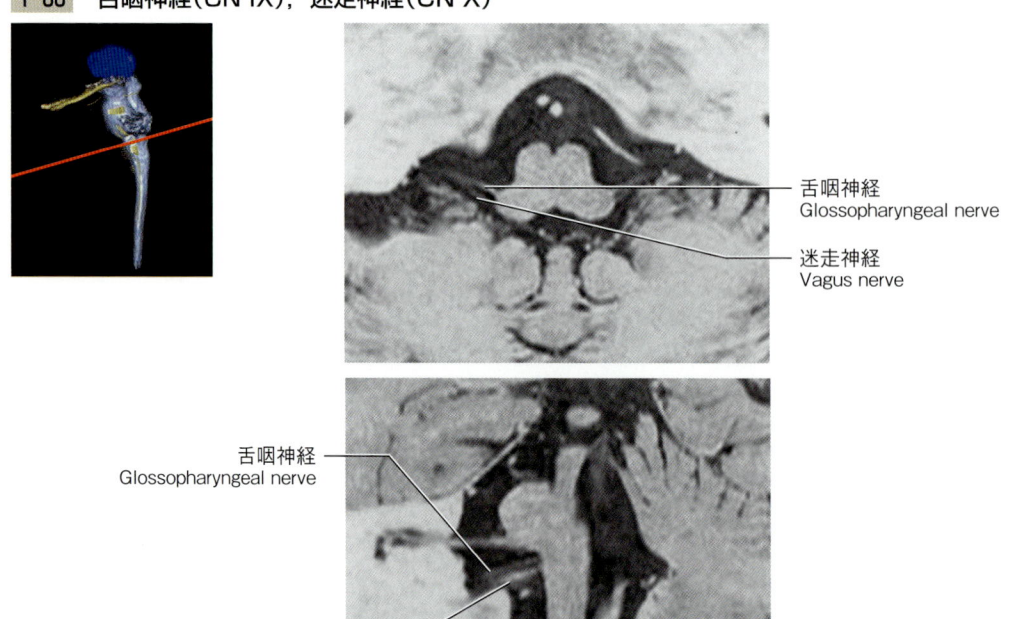

- 舌咽神経 Glossopharyngeal nerve
- 迷走神経 Vagus nerve

> **NOTE**　顔面神経への血管などによる圧迫は，片側顔面痙攣の原因としてしばしばMRI検査の対象になる．三叉神経痛の場合と同様に3D-TOF MRAの元画像も有用である．

脳神経の断層解剖［横・矢状断像（MRI, 白黒反転 heavy T2 強調像）］

1-89　副神経（CN XI）

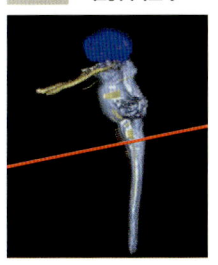

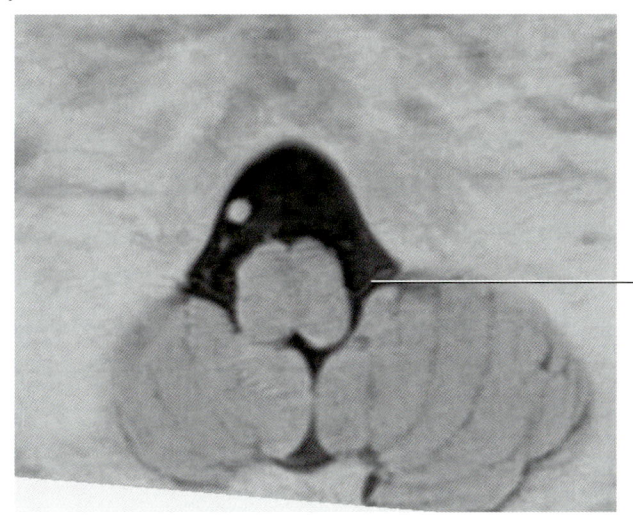

副神経
Accessory nerve

1-90　舌下神経（CN XII）

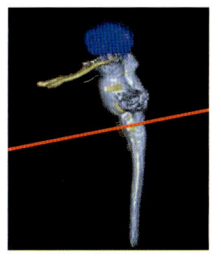

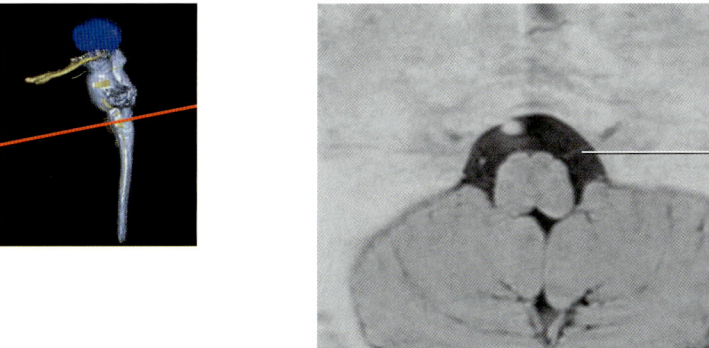

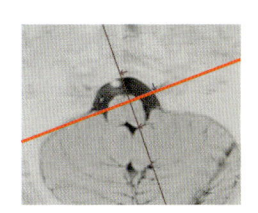

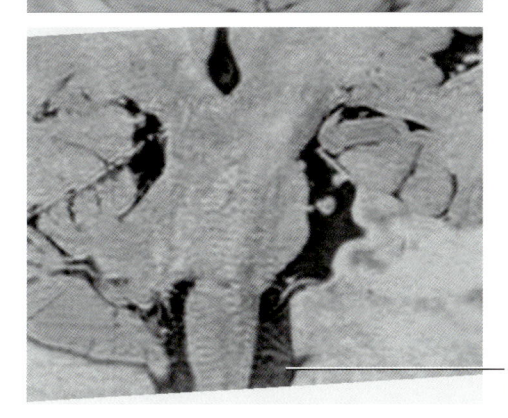

舌下神経
Hypoglossal nerve

舌下神経
Hypoglossal nerve

50 脳幹部の断層解剖 [横断像（MRI, 白黒反転 heavy T2 強調像）]

1-91

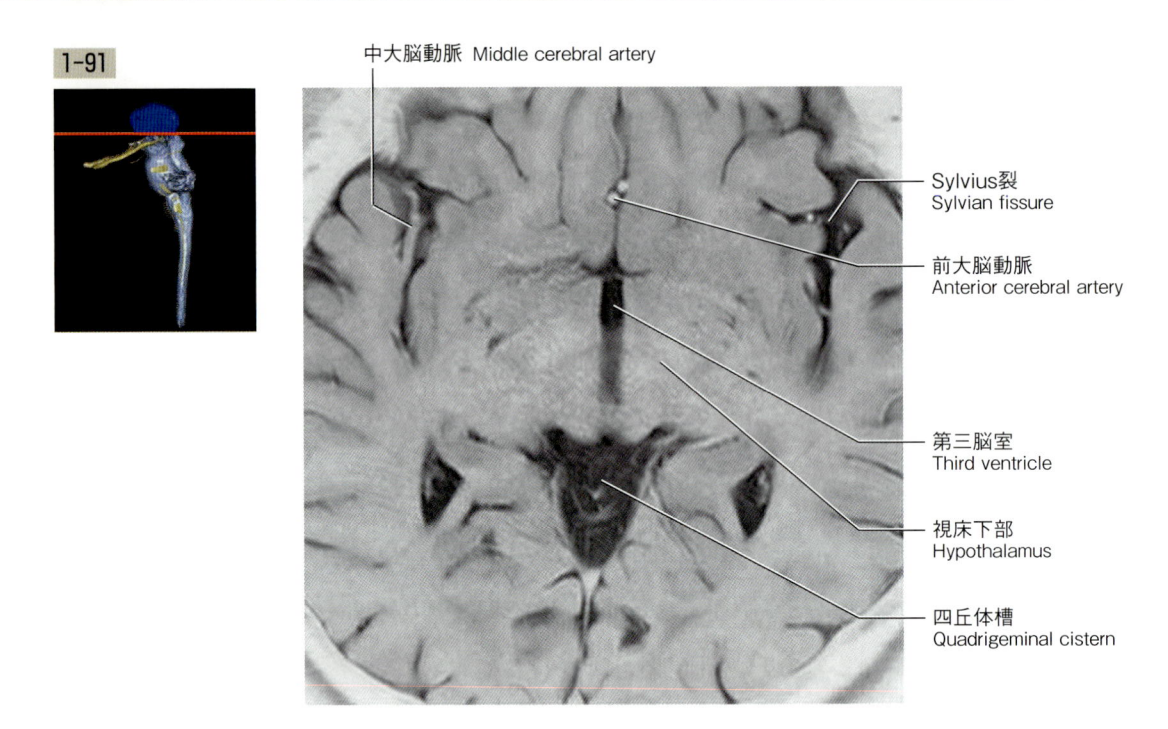

- 中大脳動脈 Middle cerebral artery
- Sylvius裂 Sylvian fissure
- 前大脳動脈 Anterior cerebral artery
- 第三脳室 Third ventricle
- 視床下部 Hypothalamus
- 四丘体槽 Quadrigeminal cistern

1-92

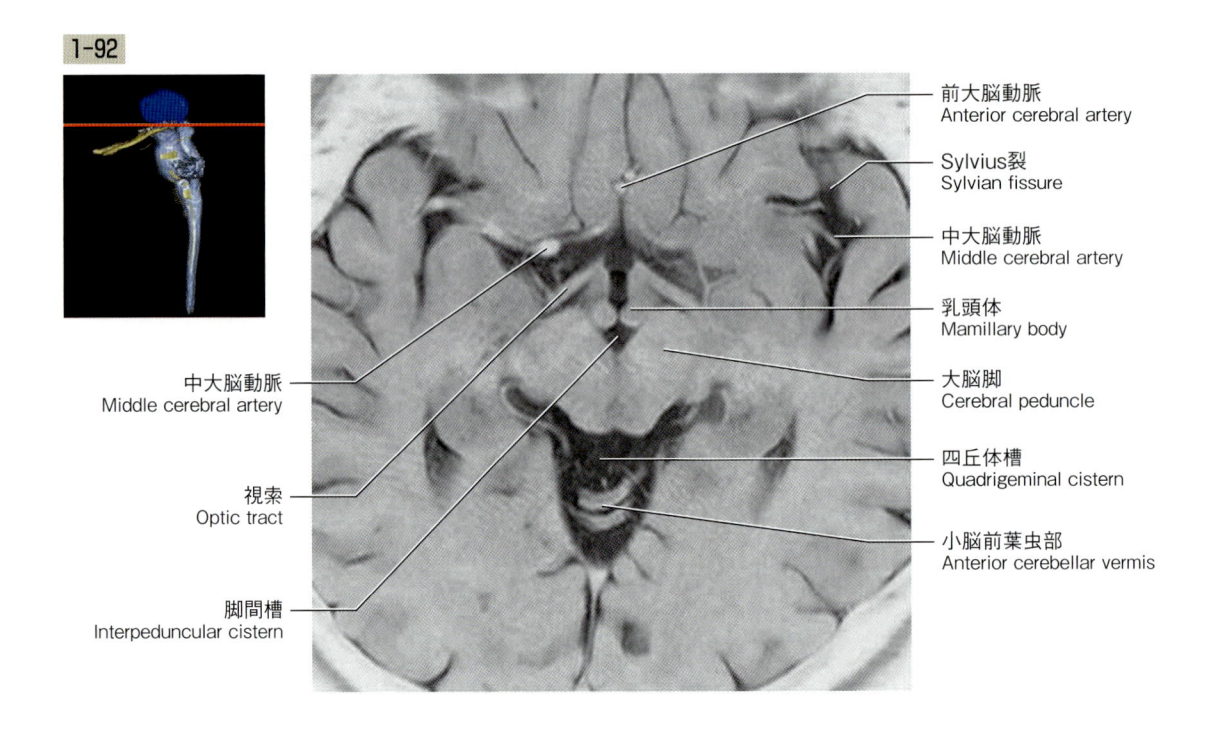

- 前大脳動脈 Anterior cerebral artery
- Sylvius裂 Sylvian fissure
- 中大脳動脈 Middle cerebral artery
- 乳頭体 Mamillary body
- 大脳脚 Cerebral peduncle
- 四丘体槽 Quadrigeminal cistern
- 小脳前葉虫部 Anterior cerebellar vermis
- 中大脳動脈 Middle cerebral artery
- 視索 Optic tract
- 脚間槽 Interpeduncular cistern

NOTE 中大脳動脈本幹部は Sylvius 裂の下方で数本に分かれ，島に沿って上行したのち，Sylvius 裂から外側へ向かい大脳表面へ達する．

脳幹部の断層解剖　[横断像（MRI, 白黒反転 heavy T2 強調像）]

1-93

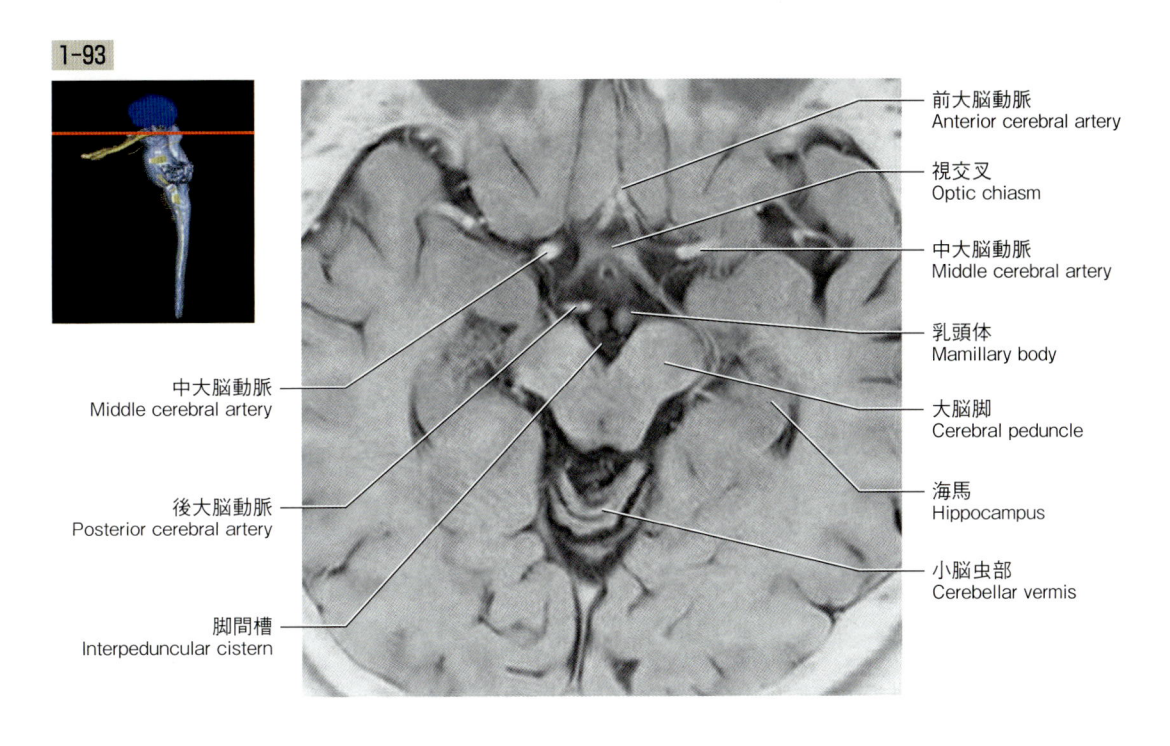

- 前大脳動脈　Anterior cerebral artery
- 視交叉　Optic chiasm
- 中大脳動脈　Middle cerebral artery
- 乳頭体　Mamillary body
- 大脳脚　Cerebral peduncle
- 海馬　Hippocampus
- 小脳虫部　Cerebellar vermis
- 中大脳動脈　Middle cerebral artery
- 後大脳動脈　Posterior cerebral artery
- 脚間槽　Interpeduncular cistern

1-94

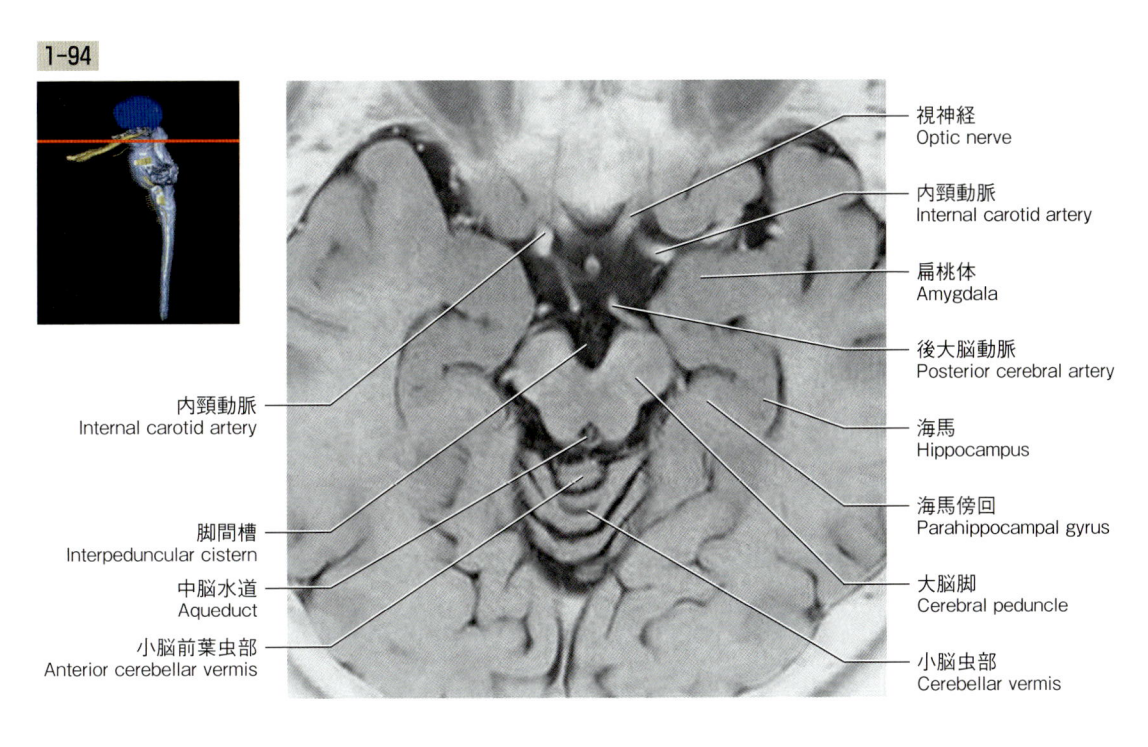

- 視神経　Optic nerve
- 内頸動脈　Internal carotid artery
- 扁桃体　Amygdala
- 後大脳動脈　Posterior cerebral artery
- 海馬　Hippocampus
- 海馬傍回　Parahippocampal gyrus
- 大脳脚　Cerebral peduncle
- 小脳虫部　Cerebellar vermis
- 内頸動脈　Internal carotid artery
- 脚間槽　Interpeduncular cistern
- 中脳水道　Aqueduct
- 小脳前葉虫部　Anterior cerebellar vermis

NOTE 脳幹上部の正確な評価は，トルコ鞍近傍病変の術前評価にしばしば重要である（特に病変と視交叉の関係）．

脳幹部の断層解剖 ［横断像（MRI，白黒反転 heavy T2 強調像）］

1-95

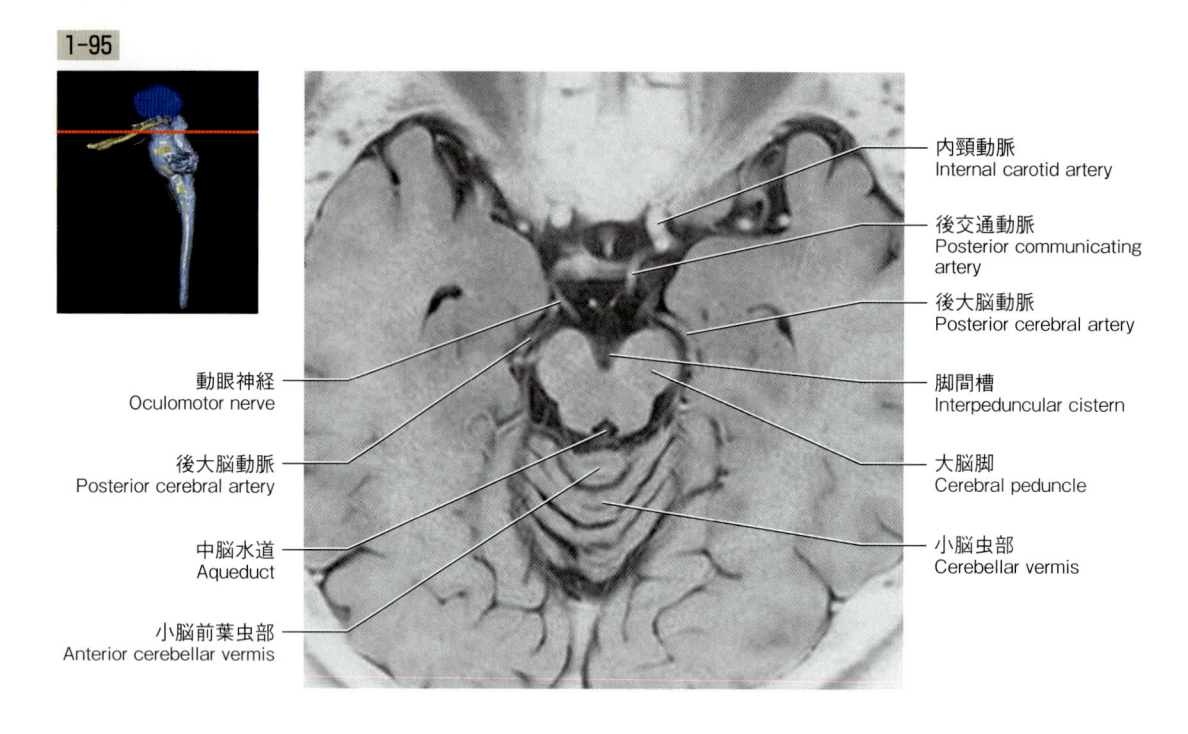

- 内頸動脈 Internal carotid artery
- 後交通動脈 Posterior communicating artery
- 後大脳動脈 Posterior cerebral artery
- 脚間槽 Interpeduncular cistern
- 大脳脚 Cerebral peduncle
- 小脳虫部 Cerebellar vermis
- 動眼神経 Oculomotor nerve
- 後大脳動脈 Posterior cerebral artery
- 中脳水道 Aqueduct
- 小脳前葉虫部 Anterior cerebellar vermis

1-96

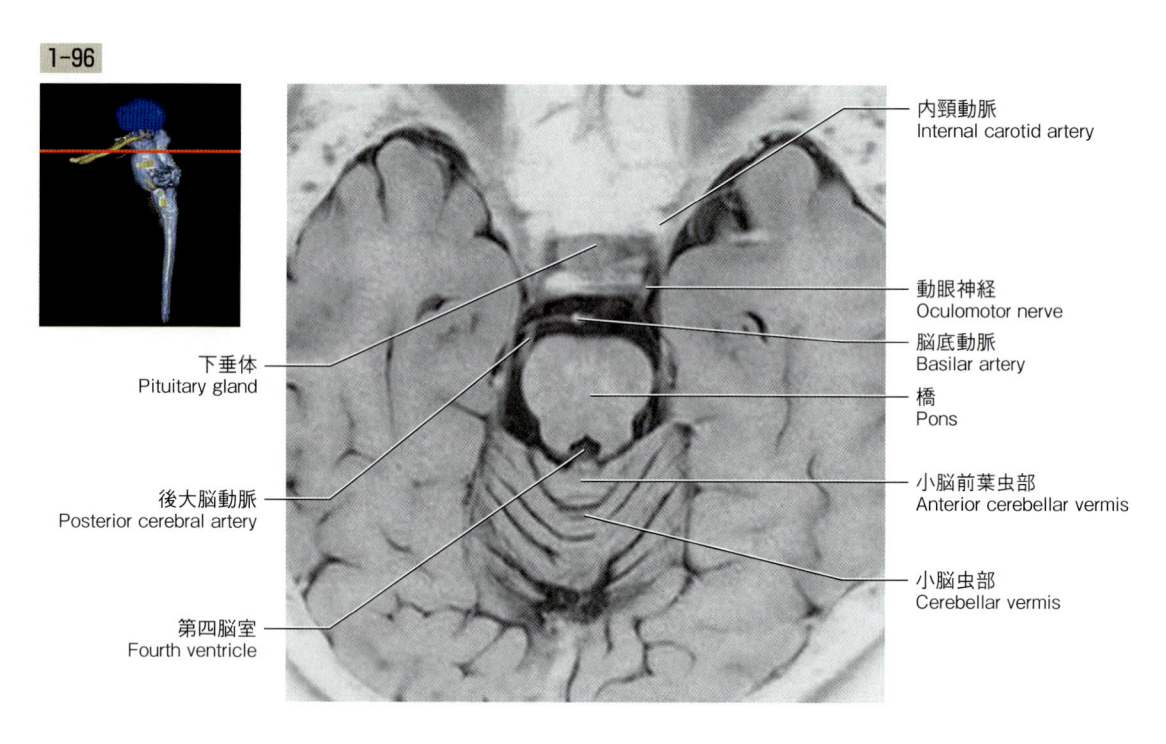

- 内頸動脈 Internal carotid artery
- 動眼神経 Oculomotor nerve
- 脳底動脈 Basilar artery
- 橋 Pons
- 小脳前葉虫部 Anterior cerebellar vermis
- 小脳虫部 Cerebellar vermis
- 下垂体 Pituitary gland
- 後大脳動脈 Posterior cerebral artery
- 第四脳室 Fourth ventricle

> **NOTE** 中脳水道 Aqueduct
> ductus（管）は，ducere（導く，引く）から由来した語である．induce（勧誘する），introduce（紹介する），educe（引き出す）など，現在の英語にも通ずる．「education（教育）とは"引き出す"ことから始まる」との箴言（しんげん）もある．

52

脳幹部の断層解剖 ［横断像（MRI, 白黒反転 heavy T2 強調像）］

1-97

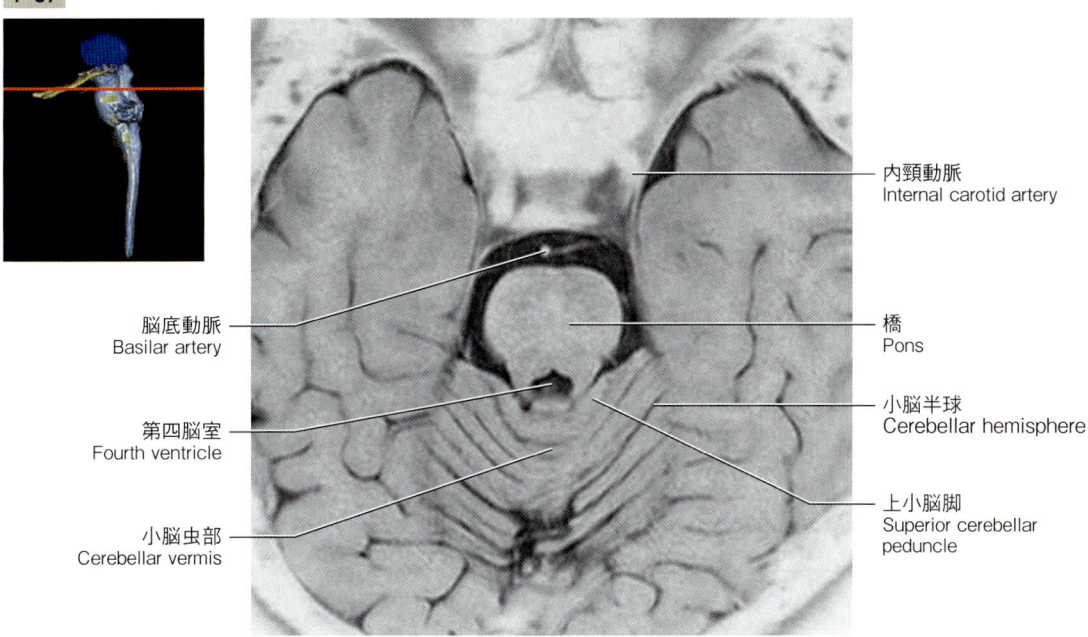

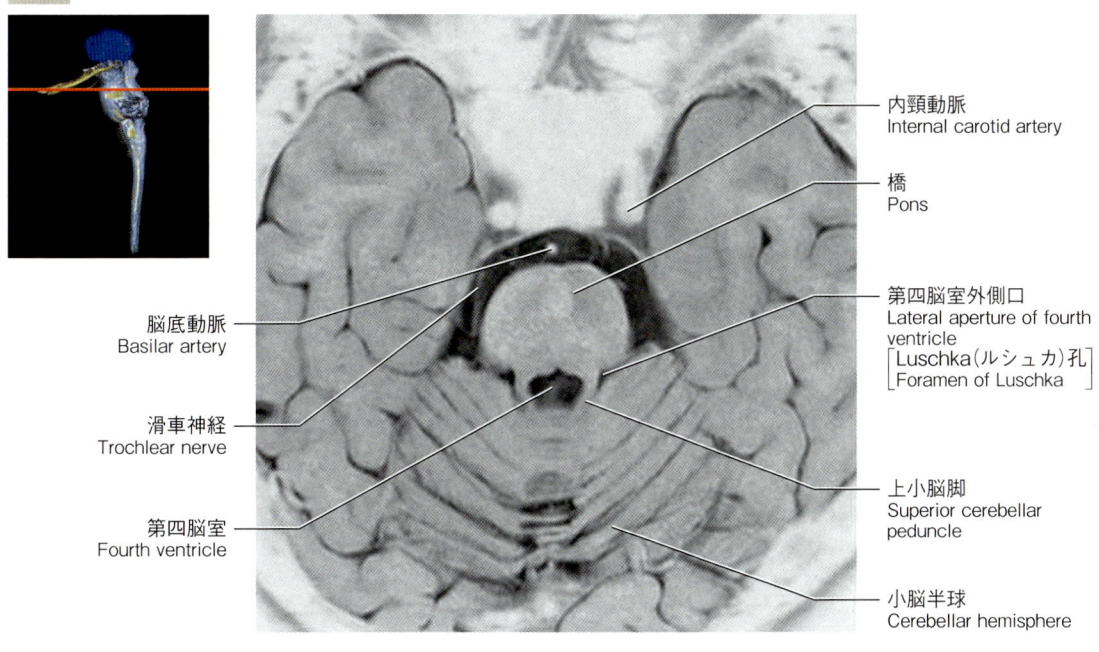

- 脳底動脈 Basilar artery
- 第四脳室 Fourth ventricle
- 小脳虫部 Cerebellar vermis
- 内頸動脈 Internal carotid artery
- 橋 Pons
- 小脳半球 Cerebellar hemisphere
- 上小脳脚 Superior cerebellar peduncle

1-98

- 脳底動脈 Basilar artery
- 滑車神経 Trochlear nerve
- 第四脳室 Fourth ventricle
- 内頸動脈 Internal carotid artery
- 橋 Pons
- 第四脳室外側口 Lateral aperture of fourth ventricle ［Luschka（ルシュカ）孔 Foramen of Luschka］
- 上小脳脚 Superior cerebellar peduncle
- 小脳半球 Cerebellar hemisphere

54 脳幹部の断層解剖 ［横断像（MRI，白黒反転 heavy T2 強調像）］

1-99

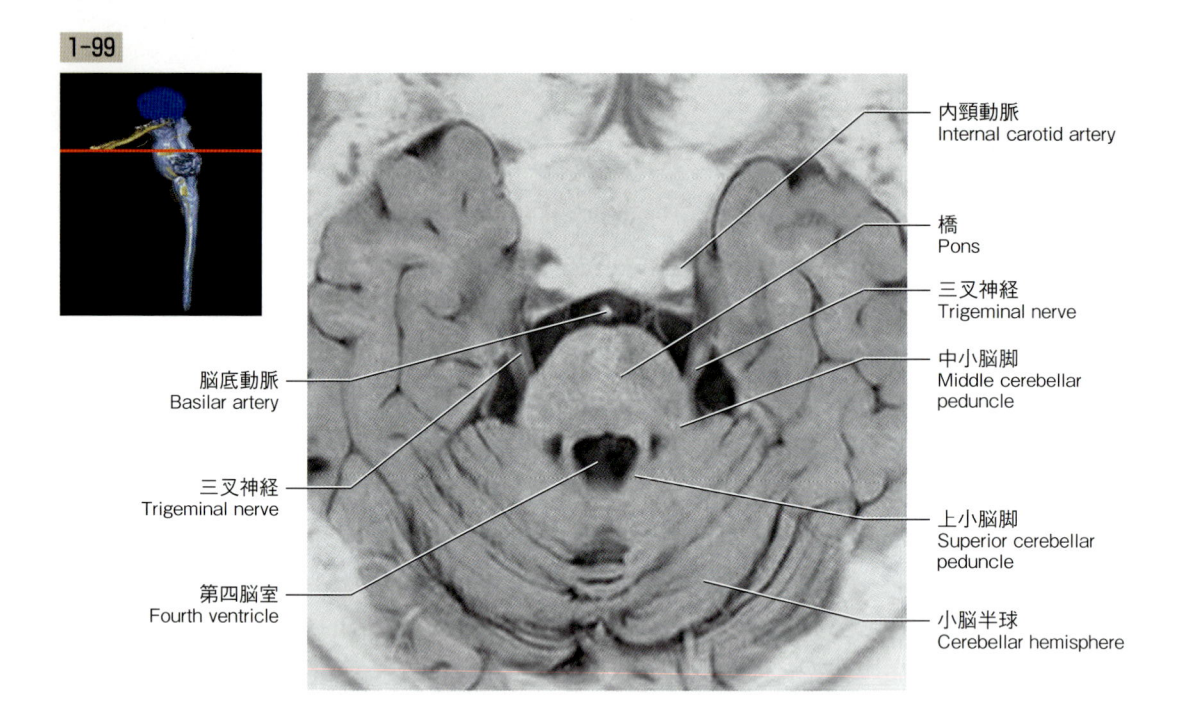

- 内頸動脈 Internal carotid artery
- 橋 Pons
- 三叉神経 Trigeminal nerve
- 中小脳脚 Middle cerebellar peduncle
- 上小脳脚 Superior cerebellar peduncle
- 小脳半球 Cerebellar hemisphere
- 脳底動脈 Basilar artery
- 三叉神経 Trigeminal nerve
- 第四脳室 Fourth ventricle

1-100

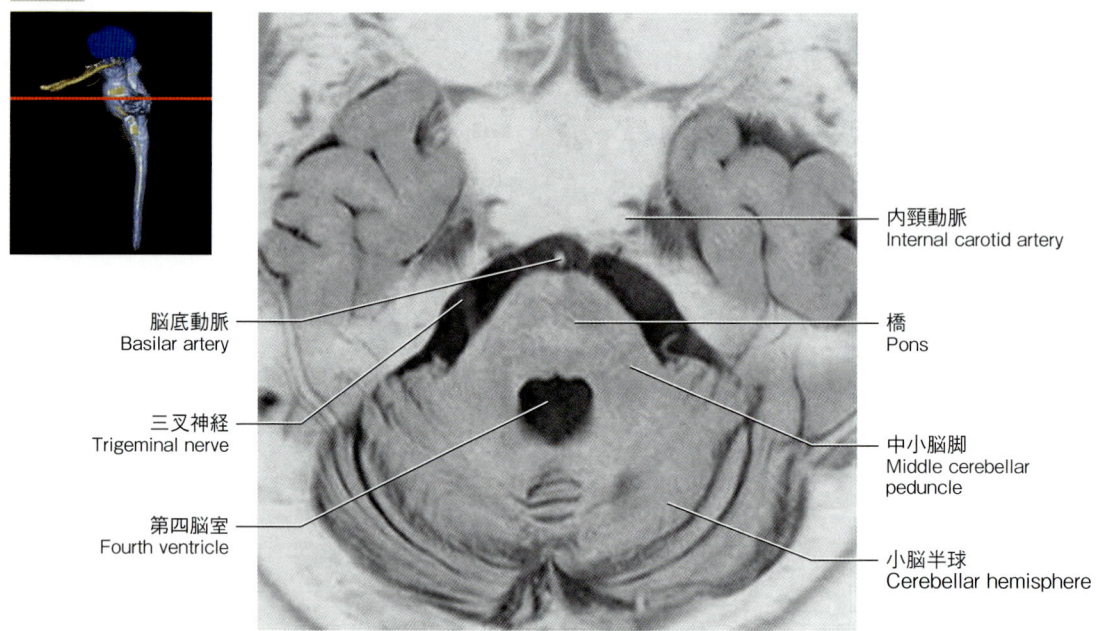

- 内頸動脈 Internal carotid artery
- 橋 Pons
- 中小脳脚 Middle cerebellar peduncle
- 小脳半球 Cerebellar hemisphere
- 脳底動脈 Basilar artery
- 三叉神経 Trigeminal nerve
- 第四脳室 Fourth ventricle

> **NOTE** 脳室 Ventricle
> Ventricle とは，小部屋の意味である．venter はもともと"腹"の意味で，ventral（腹側）となって残っているが，これから胃を ventriculus とよび，嚢の意味をもつようになり，脳室，喉頭室，心室などにも使われるようになった．-cle は小さいものを表す語尾である．ちなみに atrium とは，家の中心にある大広間の意味．心臓での役割を考えると興味はつきない．

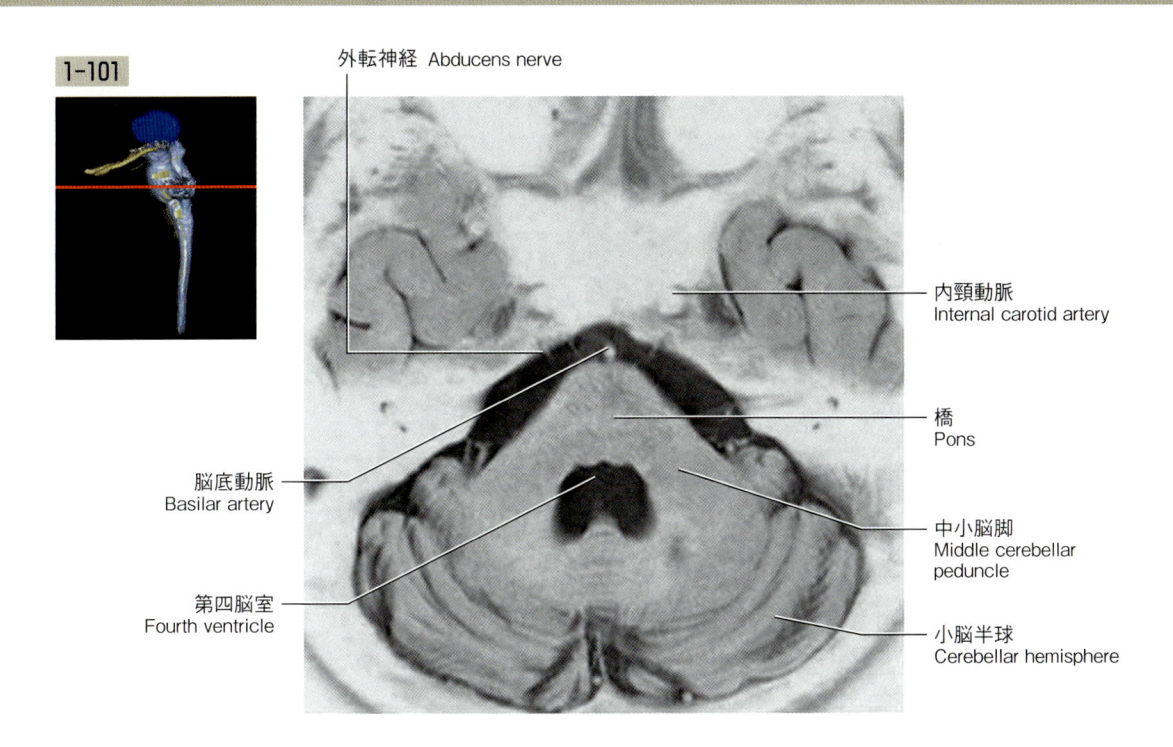

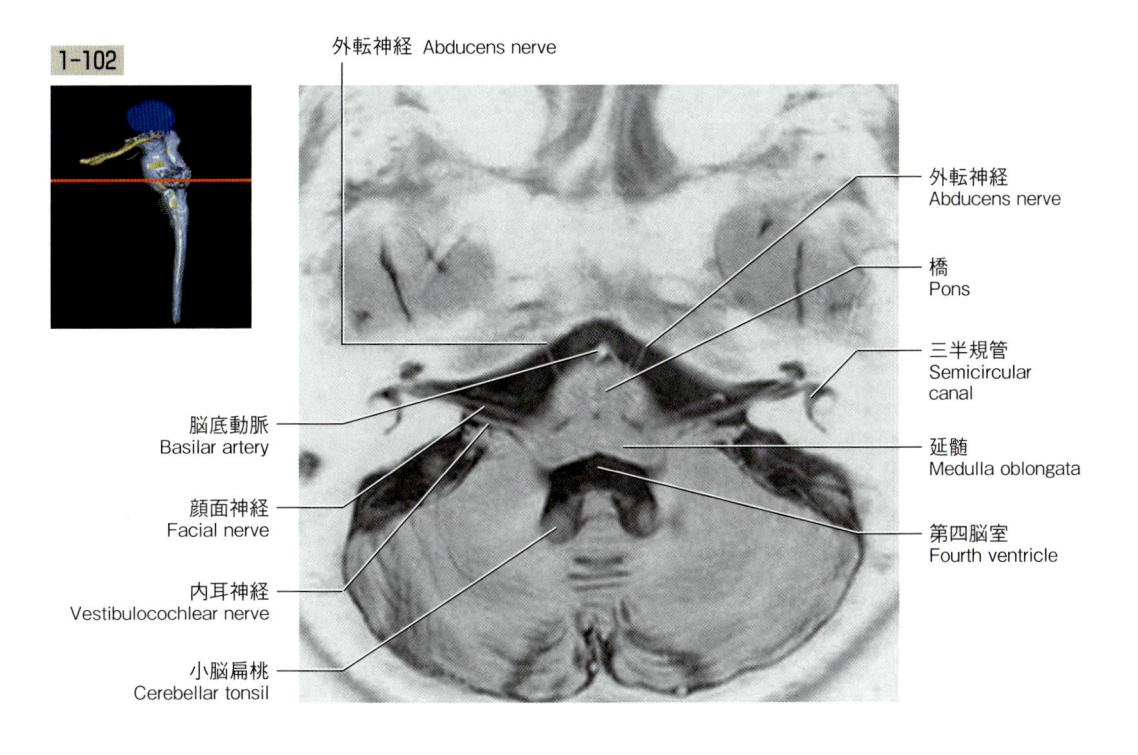

脳幹部の断層解剖　[横断像（MRI, 白黒反転 heavy T2 強調像）]

1-101

- 外転神経　Abducens nerve
- 内頸動脈　Internal carotid artery
- 橋　Pons
- 脳底動脈　Basilar artery
- 中小脳脚　Middle cerebellar peduncle
- 第四脳室　Fourth ventricle
- 小脳半球　Cerebellar hemisphere

1-102

- 外転神経　Abducens nerve
- 外転神経　Abducens nerve
- 橋　Pons
- 三半規管　Semicircular canal
- 脳底動脈　Basilar artery
- 延髄　Medulla oblongata
- 顔面神経　Facial nerve
- 第四脳室　Fourth ventricle
- 内耳神経　Vestibulocochlear nerve
- 小脳扁桃　Cerebellar tonsil

> **NOTE**　内耳神経をターゲットにした 1-102 のレベルの MR cisternography は，聴神経腫瘍の疑いの症例で頻繁に行われる．

脳幹部の断層解剖 ［横断像（MRI, 白黒反転 heavy T2 強調像）］

1-103

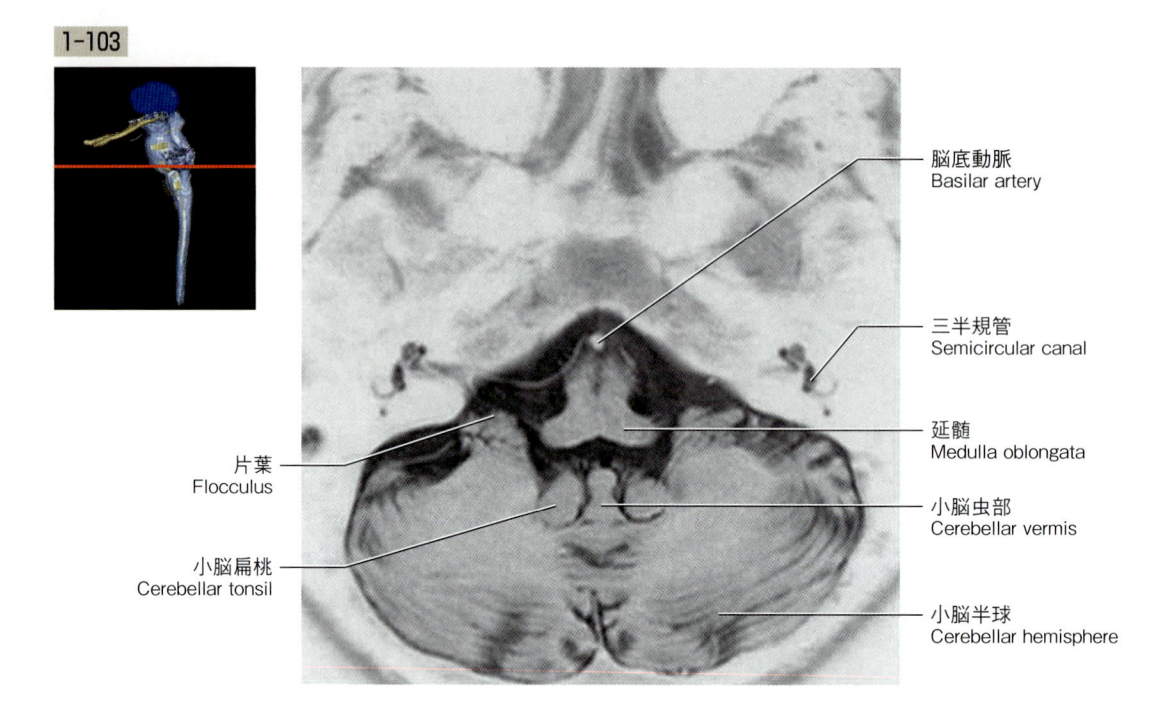

- 脳底動脈 Basilar artery
- 三半規管 Semicircular canal
- 延髄 Medulla oblongata
- 小脳虫部 Cerebellar vermis
- 小脳半球 Cerebellar hemisphere
- 片葉 Flocculus
- 小脳扁桃 Cerebellar tonsil

1-104

- 椎骨動脈 Vertebral artery
- 延髄錐体 Medullary pyramid
- 舌咽神経 Glossopharyngeal nerve
- 延髄 Medulla oblongata
- 小脳虫部 Cerebellar vermis
- 小脳半球 Cerebellar hemisphere
- 前正中裂 Ventral median fissure
- 舌咽神経 Glossopharyngeal nerve
- 小脳扁桃 Cerebellar tonsil

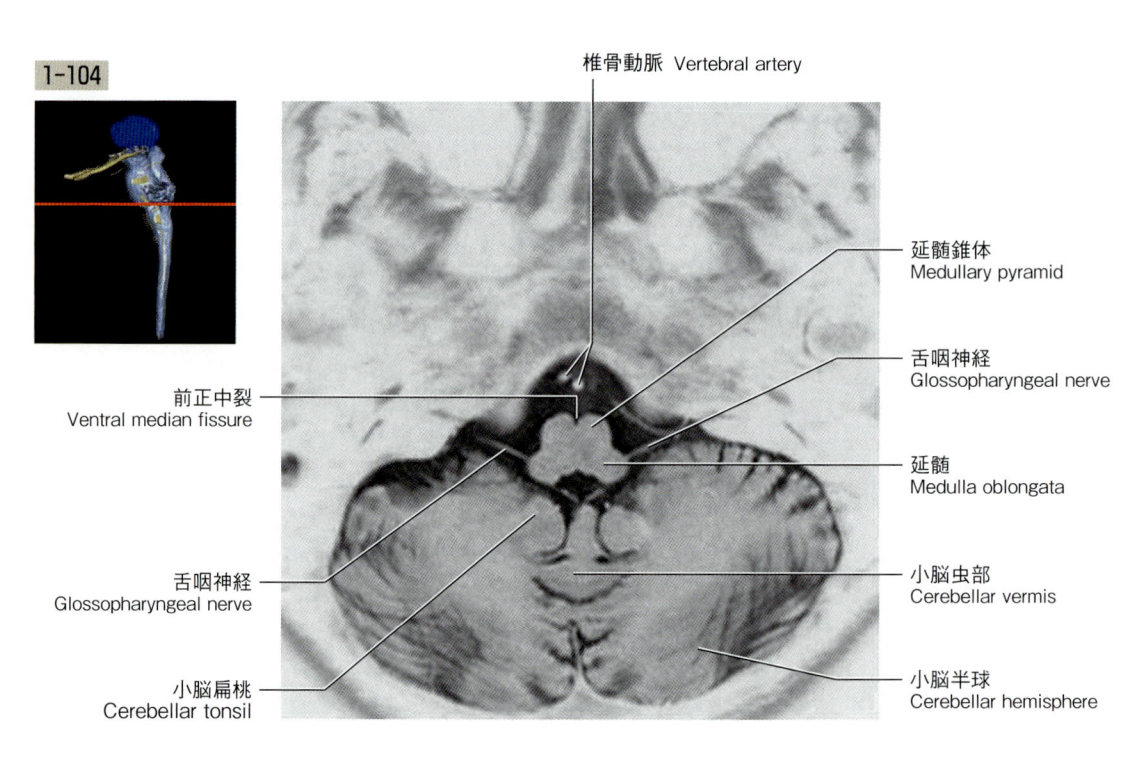

NOTE 延髄前面正中には脊髄から連続する前正中裂とよばれる溝があり，延髄上端部で盲孔となる．この前正中裂の左右には錐体とよばれる隆起があり，錐体路の通過経路となっている．錐体以外の延髄背側が延髄被蓋であり多数の脳神経核が存在する．

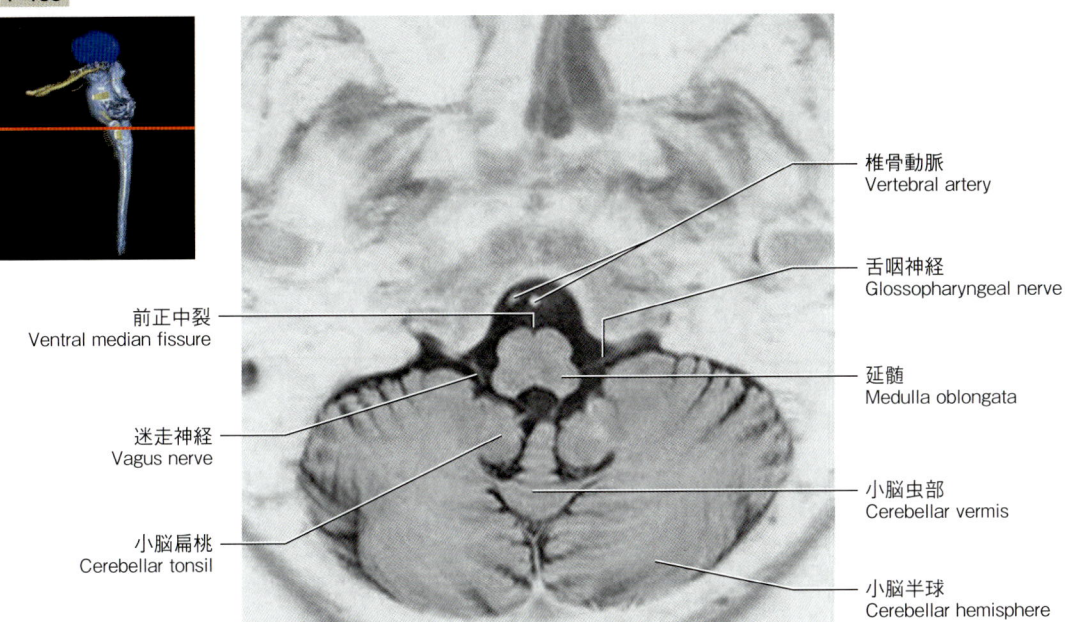

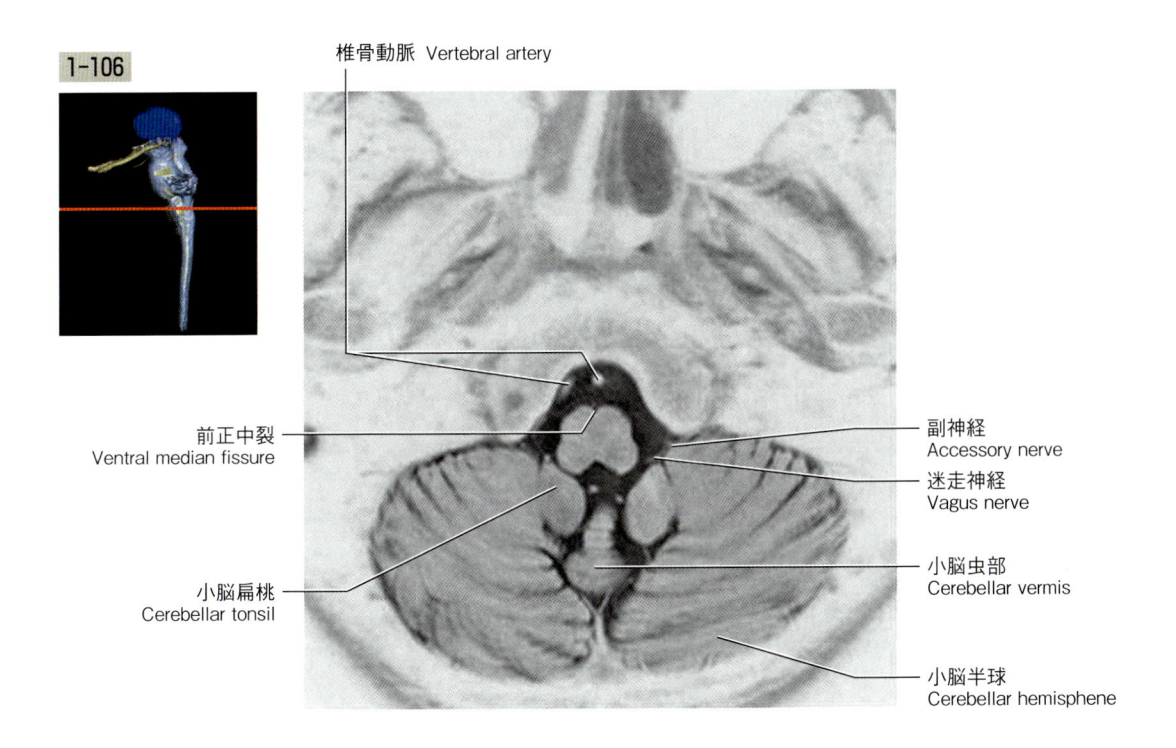

脳幹部の断層解剖 ［横断像（MRI, 白黒反転 heavy T2 強調像）］

1-105

- 前正中裂 Ventral median fissure
- 迷走神経 Vagus nerve
- 小脳扁桃 Cerebellar tonsil
- 椎骨動脈 Vertebral artery
- 舌咽神経 Glossopharyngeal nerve
- 延髄 Medulla oblongata
- 小脳虫部 Cerebellar vermis
- 小脳半球 Cerebellar hemisphere

1-106

- 椎骨動脈 Vertebral artery
- 前正中裂 Ventral median fissure
- 小脳扁桃 Cerebellar tonsil
- 副神経 Accessory nerve
- 迷走神経 Vagus nerve
- 小脳虫部 Cerebellar vermis
- 小脳半球 Cerebellar hemisphene

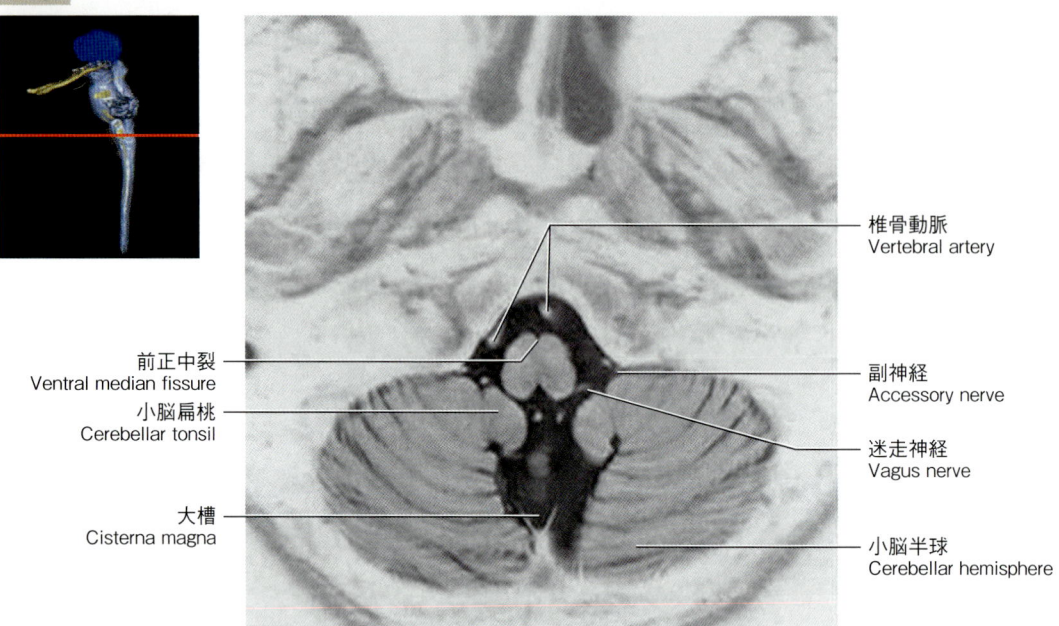

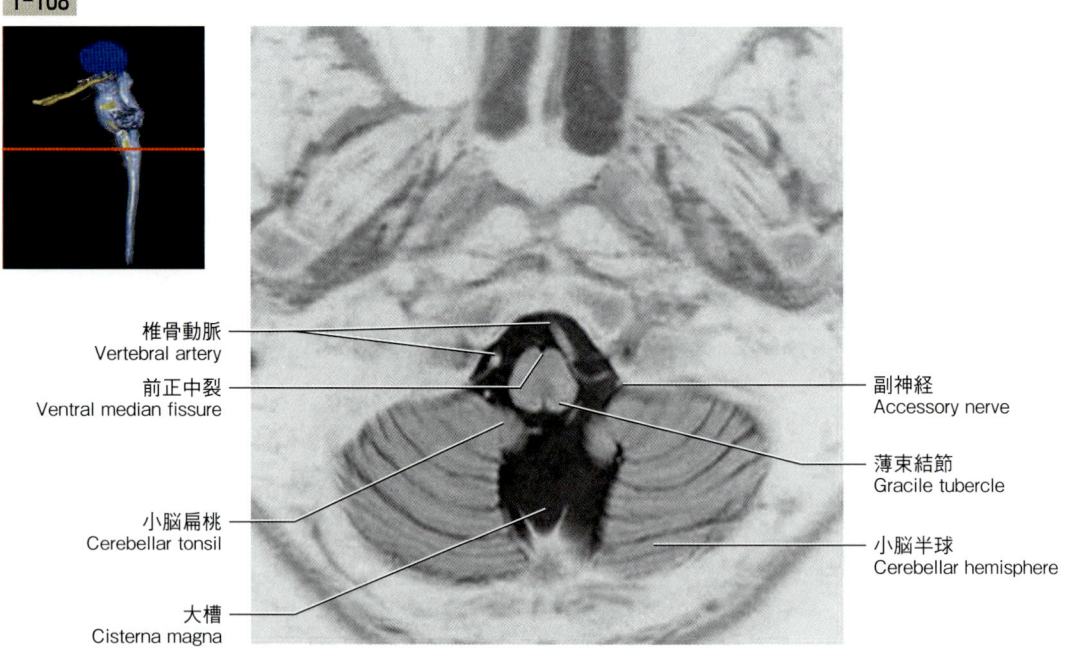

脳幹部の断層解剖　[横断像（MRI, 白黒反転 heavy T2 強調像）]

1-107

- 前正中裂 Ventral median fissure
- 小脳扁桃 Cerebellar tonsil
- 大槽 Cisterna magna
- 椎骨動脈 Vertebral artery
- 副神経 Accessory nerve
- 迷走神経 Vagus nerve
- 小脳半球 Cerebellar hemisphere

1-108

- 椎骨動脈 Vertebral artery
- 前正中裂 Ventral median fissure
- 小脳扁桃 Cerebellar tonsil
- 大槽 Cisterna magna
- 副神経 Accessory nerve
- 薄束結節 Gracile tubercle
- 小脳半球 Cerebellar hemisphere

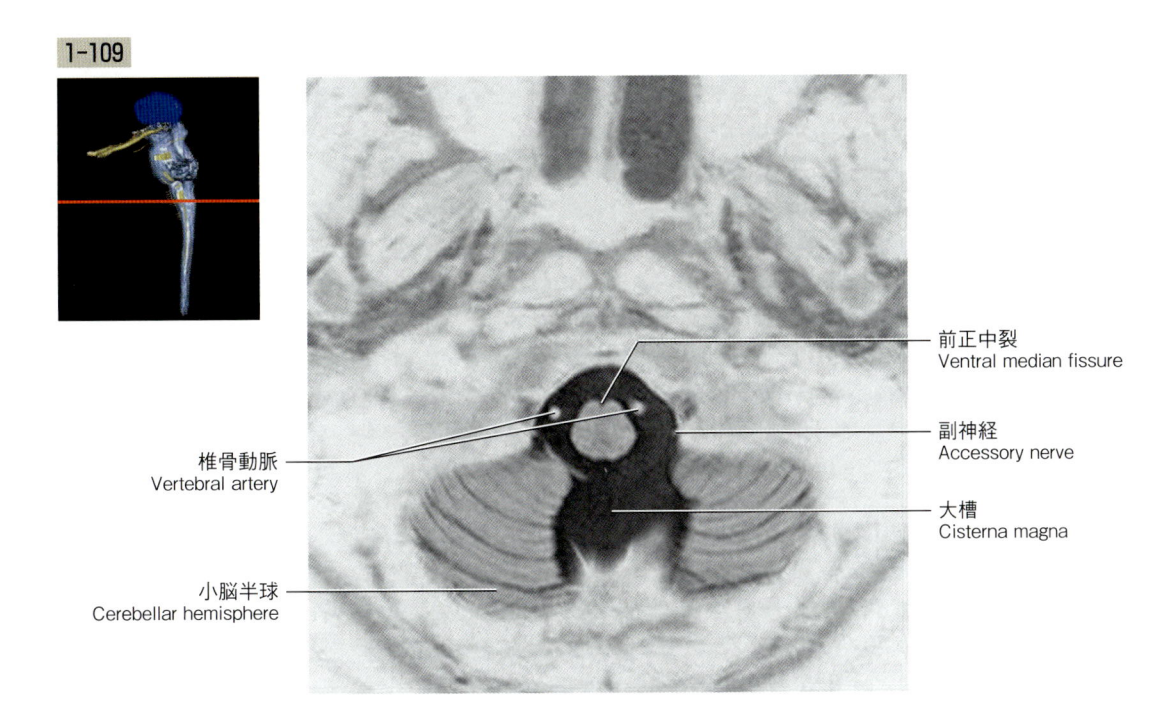

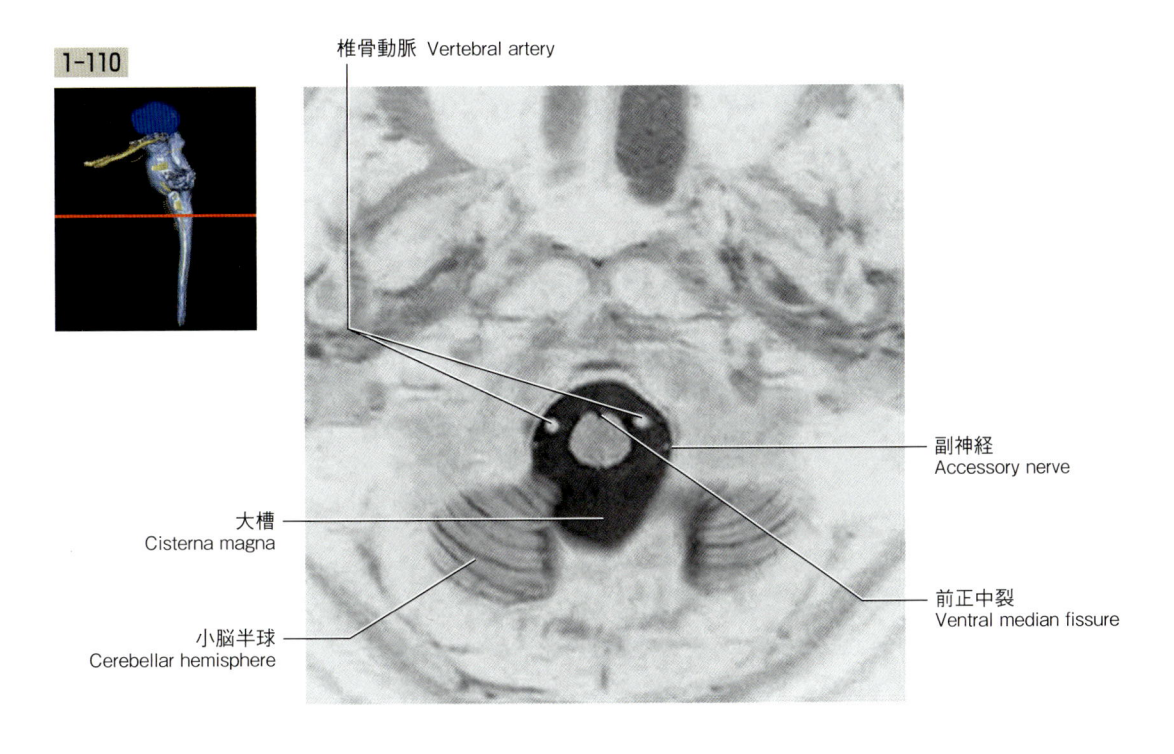

脳幹部の断層解剖 ［横断像（MRI, 白黒反転 heavy T2 強調像）］

1-109

- 前正中裂 Ventral median fissure
- 副神経 Accessory nerve
- 大槽 Cisterna magna
- 椎骨動脈 Vertebral artery
- 小脳半球 Cerebellar hemisphere

1-110

- 椎骨動脈 Vertebral artery
- 副神経 Accessory nerve
- 前正中裂 Ventral median fissure
- 大槽 Cisterna magna
- 小脳半球 Cerebellar hemisphere

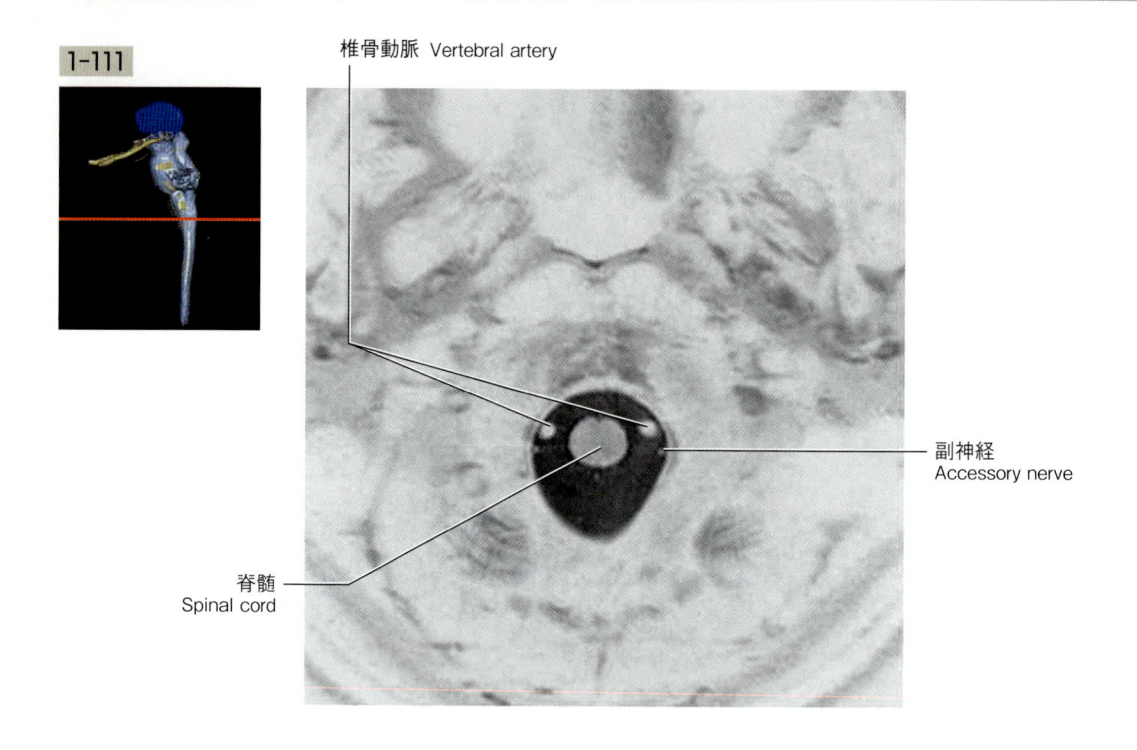

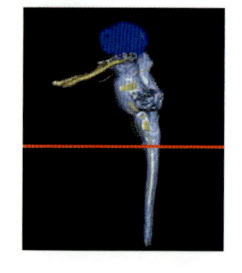

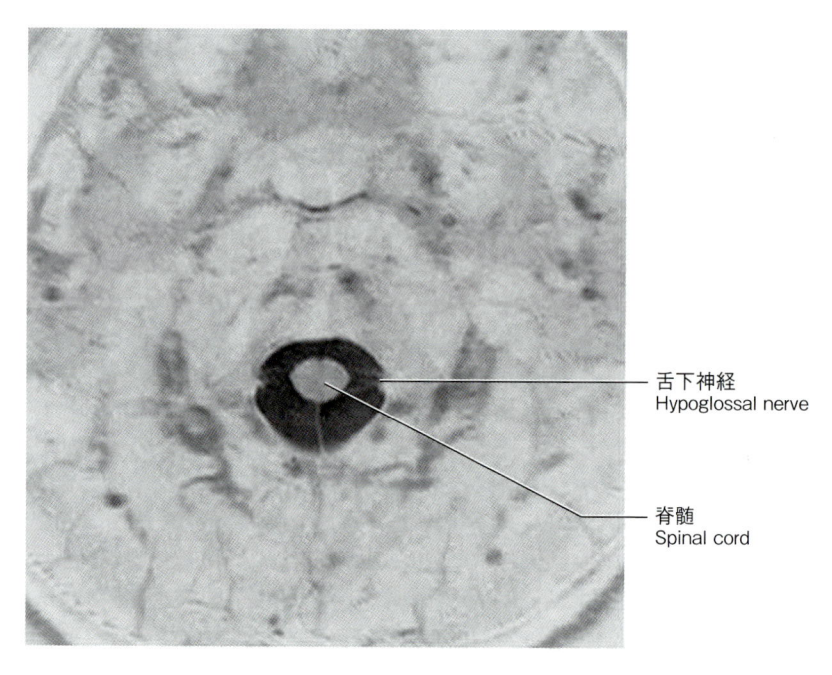

脳幹部の断層解剖　[横断像(MRI, 白黒反転 heavy T2 強調像)]

1-111

椎骨動脈 Vertebral artery
副神経 Accessory nerve
脊髄 Spinal cord

1-112

舌下神経 Hypoglossal nerve
脊髄 Spinal cord

脳幹部の断層解剖 [矢状断像（MRI, 白黒反転 heavy T2 強調像）]

1-113

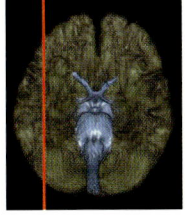

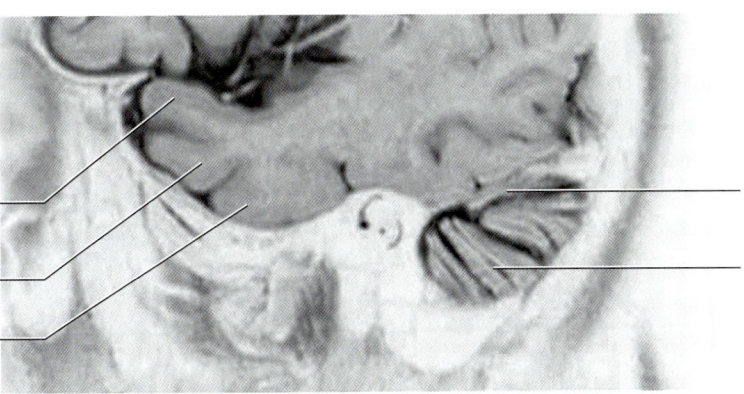

- 上側頭回 Superior temporal gyrus
- 中側頭回 Middle temporal gyrus
- 下側頭回 Inferior temporal gyrus
- 小脳テント Tentorium cerebelli
- 小脳半球 Cerebellar hemisphere

1-114

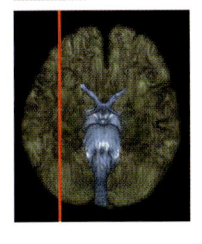

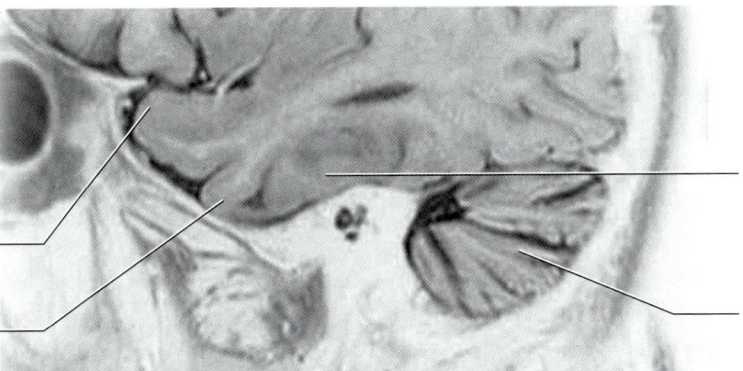

- 中側頭回 Middle temporal gyrus
- 下側頭回 Inferior temporal gyrus
- 外側後頭側頭回 Lateral occipitotemporal gyrus
- 小脳半球 Cerebellar hemisphere

1-115

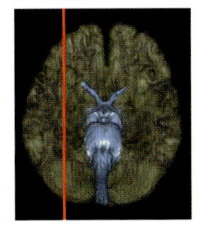

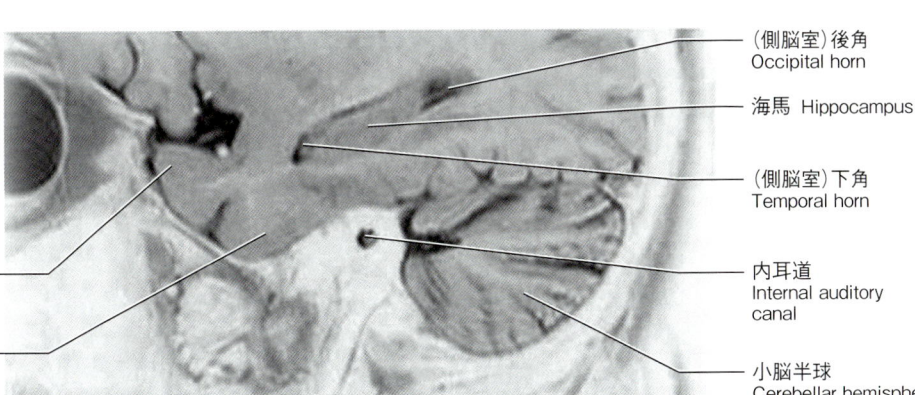

- 中側頭回 Middle temporal gyrus
- 下側頭回 Inferior temporal gyrus
- （側脳室）後角 Occipital horn
- 海馬 Hippocampus
- （側脳室）下角 Temporal horn
- 内耳道 Internal auditory canal
- 小脳半球 Cerebellar hemisphere

> **NOTE** 白質 White matter と灰白質 Grey matter
> 脳の白質，灰白質は英語／ラテン語でそれぞれ White matter/Substantia alba, Grey matter/Substantia grisea という．albus は"白い"の意であり，album（アルバム），albino（アルビノ：白子症）などはこれからの派生語である．

脳幹部の断層解剖　[矢状断像（MRI, 白黒反転 heavy T2 強調像）]

1-116

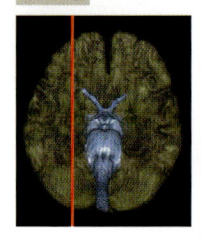

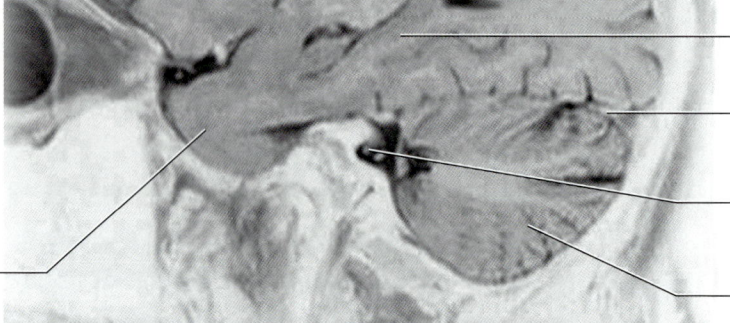

- 脈絡叢　Choroid plexus
- 海馬　Hippocampus
- 小脳テント　Tentorium cerebelli
- 内耳神経，顔面神経　Vestibulocochlear nerve, facial nerve
- 小脳半球　Cerebellar hemisphere
- 海馬傍回　Parahippocampal gyrus

1-117

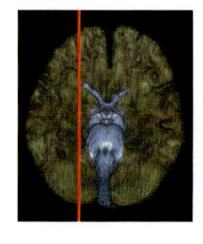

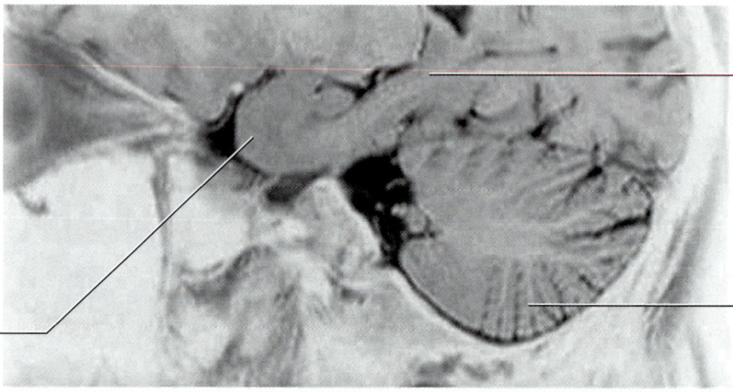

- 海馬体尾部　Hippocampus tail
- 小脳半球　Cerebellar hemisphere
- 海馬傍回　Parahippocampal gyrus

1-118

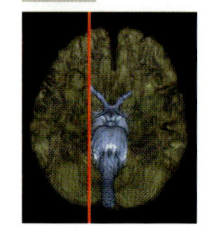

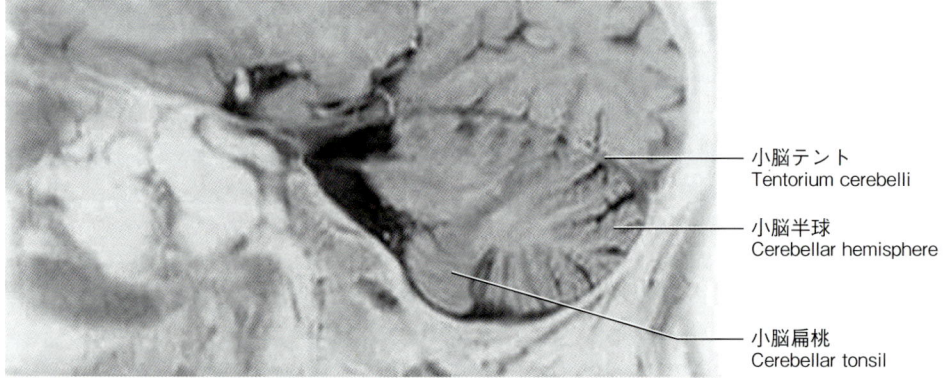

- 小脳テント　Tentorium cerebelli
- 小脳半球　Cerebellar hemisphere
- 小脳扁桃　Cerebellar tonsil

脳幹部の断層解剖 ［矢状断像（MRI，白黒反転 heavy T2 強調像）］

1-119

- 大脳脚 Cerebral peduncle
- 橋 Pons
- 斜台 Clivus
- 中小脳脚 Middle cerebellar peduncle
- 小脳テント Tentorium cerebelli
- 小脳半球 Cerebellar hemisphere
- 小脳扁桃 Cerebellar tonsil

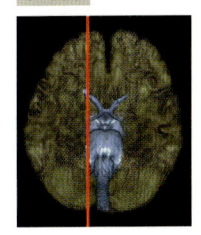

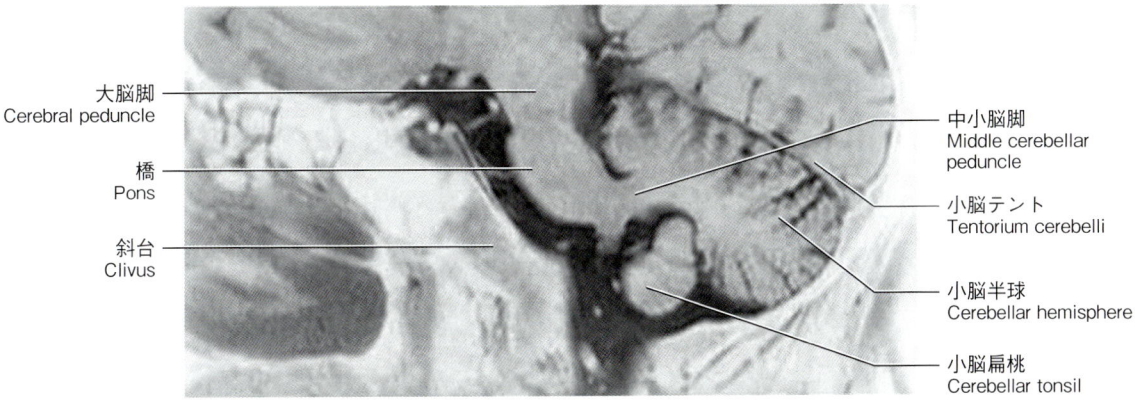

1-120

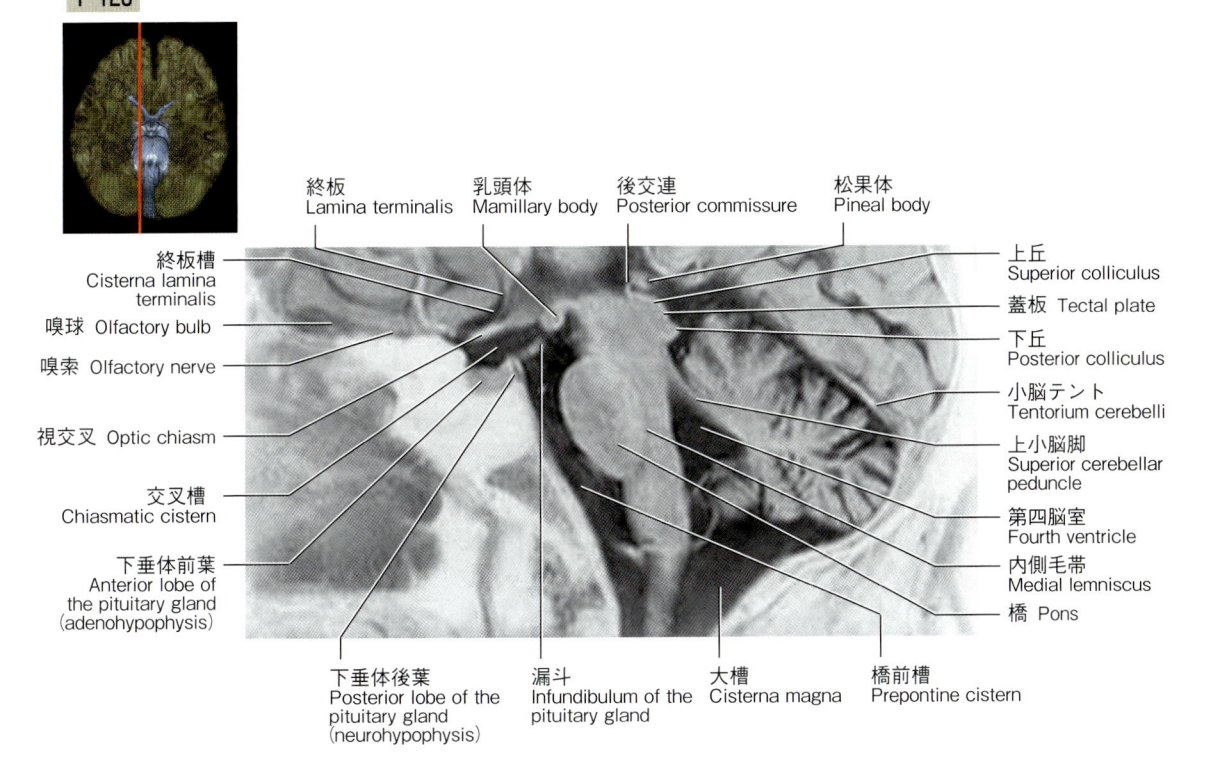

- 終板 Lamina terminalis
- 乳頭体 Mamillary body
- 後交連 Posterior commissure
- 松果体 Pineal body
- 終板槽 Cisterna lamina terminalis
- 嗅球 Olfactory bulb
- 嗅索 Olfactory nerve
- 視交叉 Optic chiasm
- 交叉槽 Chiasmatic cistern
- 下垂体前葉 Anterior lobe of the pituitary gland (adenohypophysis)
- 上丘 Superior colliculus
- 蓋板 Tectal plate
- 下丘 Posterior colliculus
- 小脳テント Tentorium cerebelli
- 上小脳脚 Superior cerebellar peduncle
- 第四脳室 Fourth ventricle
- 内側毛帯 Medial lemniscus
- 橋 Pons
- 下垂体後葉 Posterior lobe of the pituitary gland (neurohypophysis)
- 漏斗 Infundibulum of the pituitary gland
- 大槽 Cisterna magna
- 橋前槽 Prepontine cistern

NOTE 橋は内側毛帯により，前側の橋底部と背側の橋被蓋に分けられる．橋底部は縦走線維である橋縦束と，横走線維である横橋線維および横走線維の中に存在する神経細胞群の橋核から構成される．橋縦束は橋底部の中央にあり，錐体路の通過経路となっている．また，橋底部は大量の横走線維の存在により前側へ大きく膨隆する形状となっている．

脳幹部の断層解剖　［矢状断像（MRI, 白黒反転 heavy T2 強調像）］

1-121

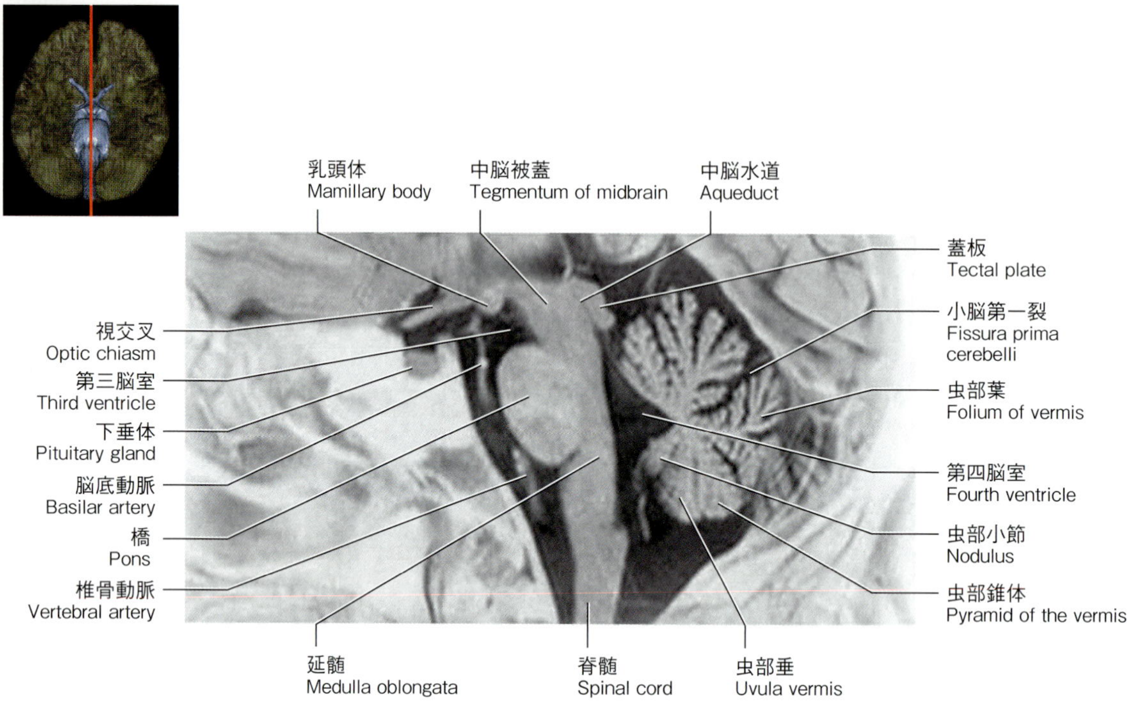

- 乳頭体 Mamillary body
- 中脳被蓋 Tegmentum of midbrain
- 中脳水道 Aqueduct
- 蓋板 Tectal plate
- 小脳第一裂 Fissura prima cerebelli
- 視交叉 Optic chiasm
- 第三脳室 Third ventricle
- 下垂体 Pituitary gland
- 虫部葉 Folium of vermis
- 脳底動脈 Basilar artery
- 第四脳室 Fourth ventricle
- 橋 Pons
- 虫部小節 Nodulus
- 椎骨動脈 Vertebral artery
- 虫部錐体 Pyramid of the vermis
- 延髄 Medulla oblongata
- 脊髄 Spinal cord
- 虫部垂 Uvula vermis

1-122

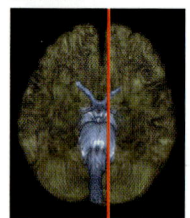

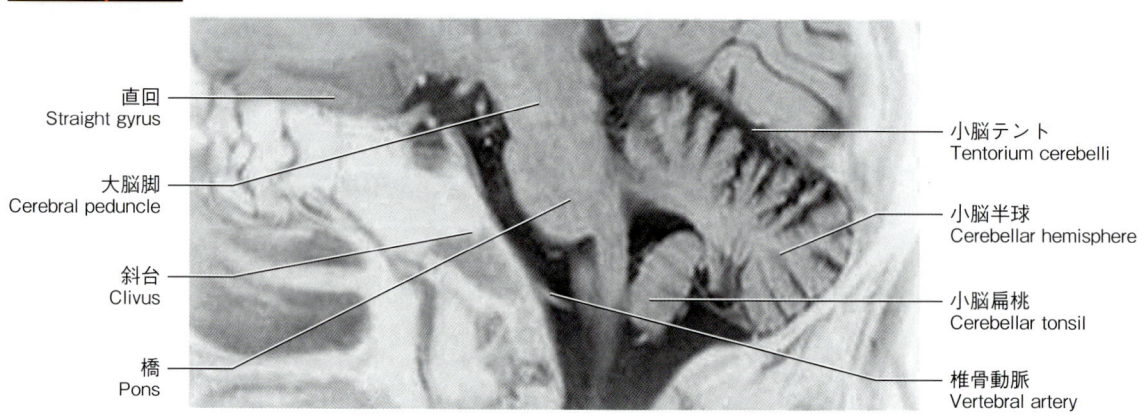

- 直回 Straight gyrus
- 小脳テント Tentorium cerebelli
- 大脳脚 Cerebral peduncle
- 小脳半球 Cerebellar hemisphere
- 斜台 Clivus
- 小脳扁桃 Cerebellar tonsil
- 橋 Pons
- 椎骨動脈 Vertebral artery

NOTE 中脳後部中央には中脳水道があり，第三脳室と第四脳室とを結んでいる．中脳水道よりも前側が広義の大脳脚，背側が中脳蓋に相当する．中脳蓋後面には上丘，下丘による上下一対の合計4つの隆起があり，四丘体あるいは蓋板とよばれる．上丘は視覚刺激を追跡する頭と眼の反射運動である視覚反射に，下丘は聴覚反射にかかわる．

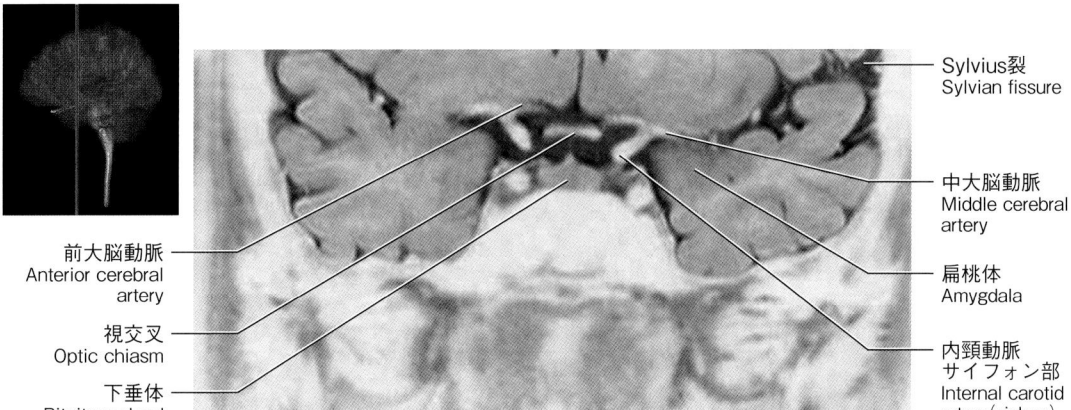

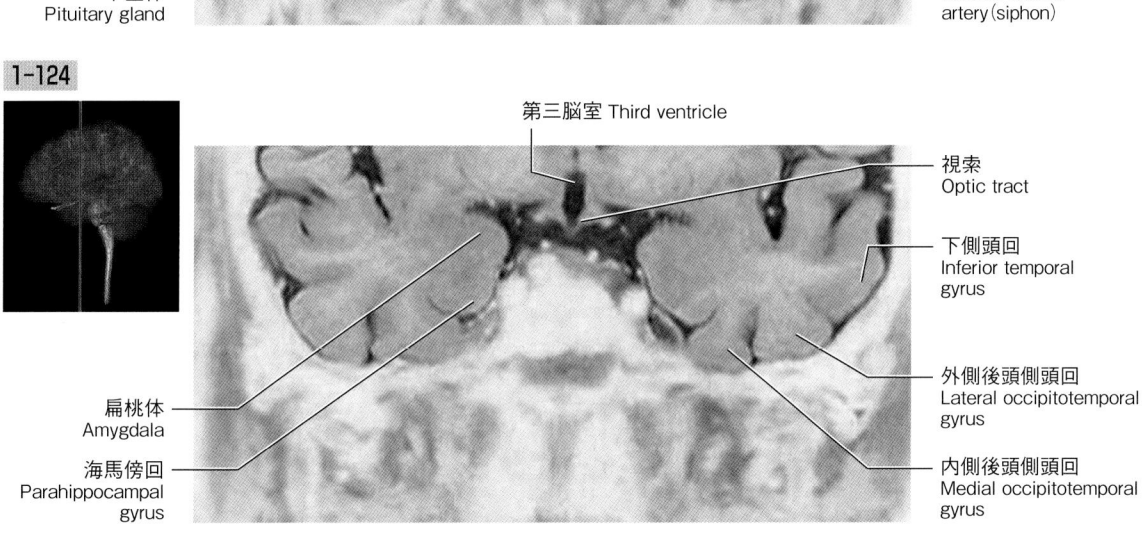

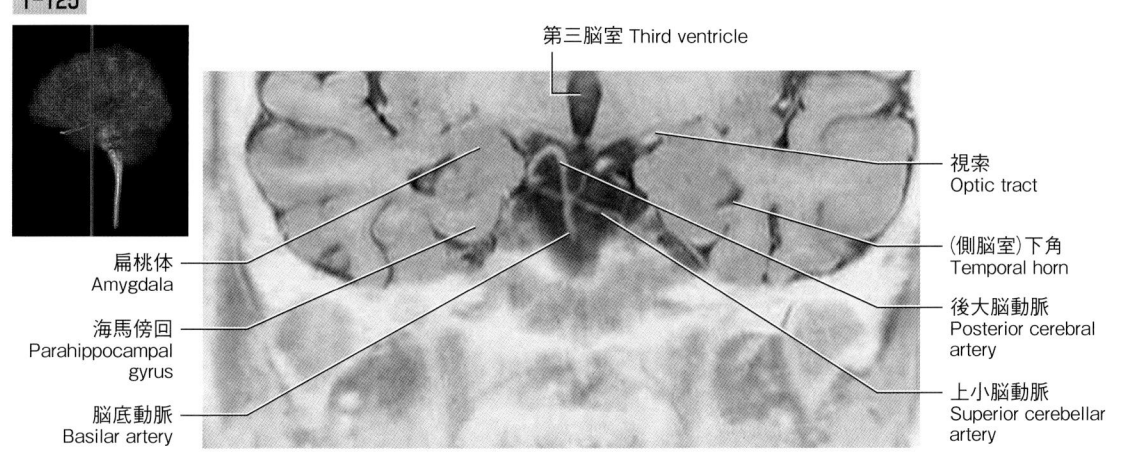

脳幹部の断層解剖［冠状断像（MRI, 白黒反転 heavy T2 強調像）］

1-123

- Sylvius裂 Sylvian fissure
- 中大脳動脈 Middle cerebral artery
- 扁桃体 Amygdala
- 内頸動脈サイフォン部 Internal carotid artery (siphon)
- 前大脳動脈 Anterior cerebral artery
- 視交叉 Optic chiasm
- 下垂体 Pituitary gland

1-124

- 第三脳室 Third ventricle
- 視索 Optic tract
- 下側頭回 Inferior temporal gyrus
- 外側後頭側頭回 Lateral occipitotemporal gyrus
- 内側後頭側頭回 Medial occipitotemporal gyrus
- 扁桃体 Amygdala
- 海馬傍回 Parahippocampal gyrus

1-125

- 第三脳室 Third ventricle
- 視索 Optic tract
- （側脳室）下角 Temporal horn
- 後大脳動脈 Posterior cerebral artery
- 上小脳動脈 Superior cerebellar artery
- 扁桃体 Amygdala
- 海馬傍回 Parahippocampal gyrus
- 脳底動脈 Basilar artery

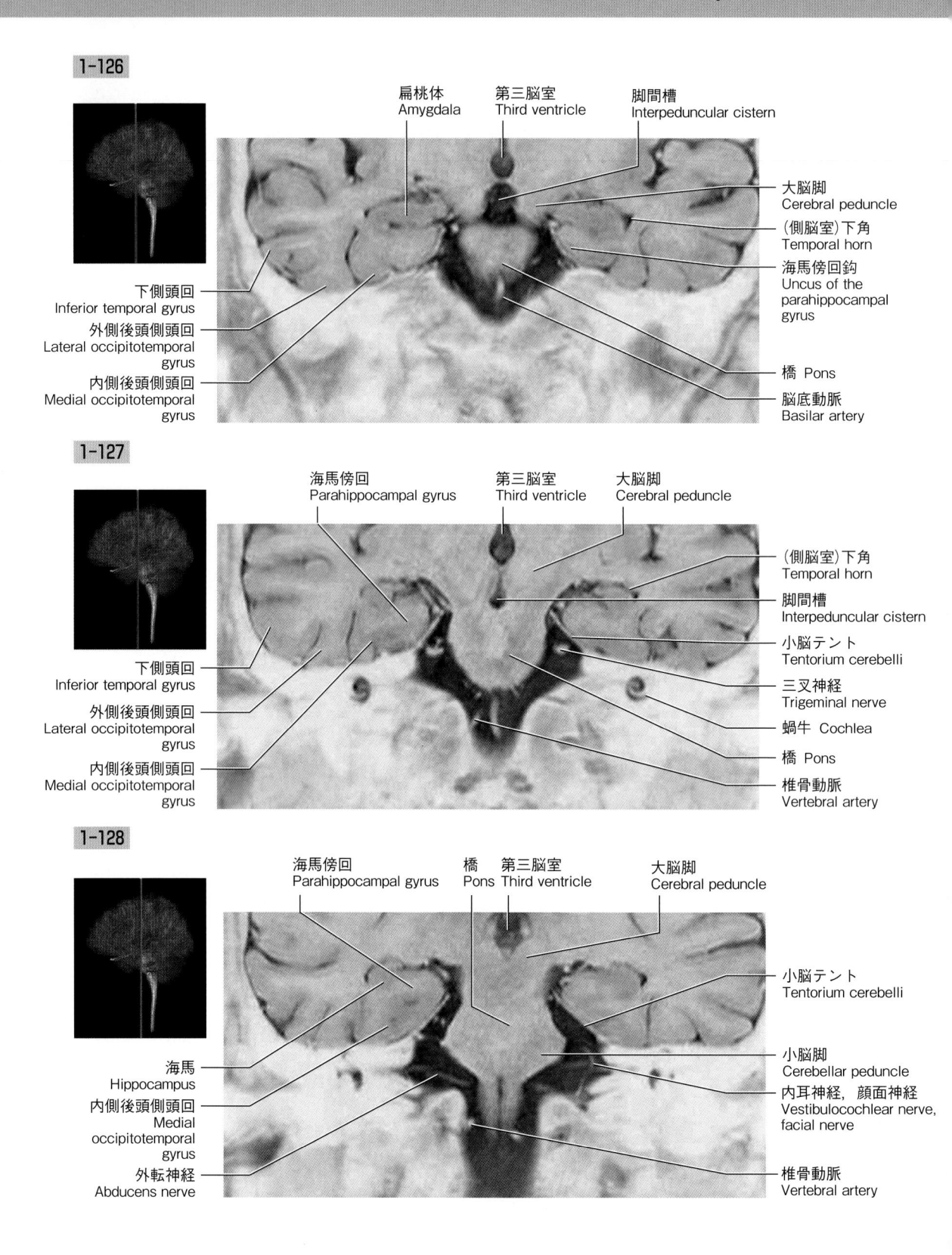

脳幹部の断層解剖 ［冠状断像（MRI，白黒反転 heavy T2 強調像）］

1-126

- 扁桃体 Amygdala
- 第三脳室 Third ventricle
- 脚間槽 Interpeduncular cistern
- 大脳脚 Cerebral peduncle
- （側脳室）下角 Temporal horn
- 海馬傍回鈎 Uncus of the parahippocampal gyrus
- 下側頭回 Inferior temporal gyrus
- 外側後頭側頭回 Lateral occipitotemporal gyrus
- 内側後頭側頭回 Medial occipitotemporal gyrus
- 橋 Pons
- 脳底動脈 Basilar artery

1-127

- 海馬傍回 Parahippocampal gyrus
- 第三脳室 Third ventricle
- 大脳脚 Cerebral peduncle
- （側脳室）下角 Temporal horn
- 脚間槽 Interpeduncular cistern
- 小脳テント Tentorium cerebelli
- 三叉神経 Trigeminal nerve
- 蝸牛 Cochlea
- 下側頭回 Inferior temporal gyrus
- 外側後頭側頭回 Lateral occipitotemporal gyrus
- 内側後頭側頭回 Medial occipitotemporal gyrus
- 橋 Pons
- 椎骨動脈 Vertebral artery

1-128

- 海馬傍回 Parahippocampal gyrus
- 橋 Pons
- 第三脳室 Third ventricle
- 大脳脚 Cerebral peduncle
- 小脳テント Tentorium cerebelli
- 小脳脚 Cerebellar peduncle
- 内耳神経，顔面神経 Vestibulocochlear nerve, facial nerve
- 海馬 Hippocampus
- 内側後頭側頭回 Medial occipitotemporal gyrus
- 外転神経 Abducens nerve
- 椎骨動脈 Vertebral artery

脳幹部の断層解剖 ［冠状断像（MRI, 白黒反転 heavy T2 強調像）］

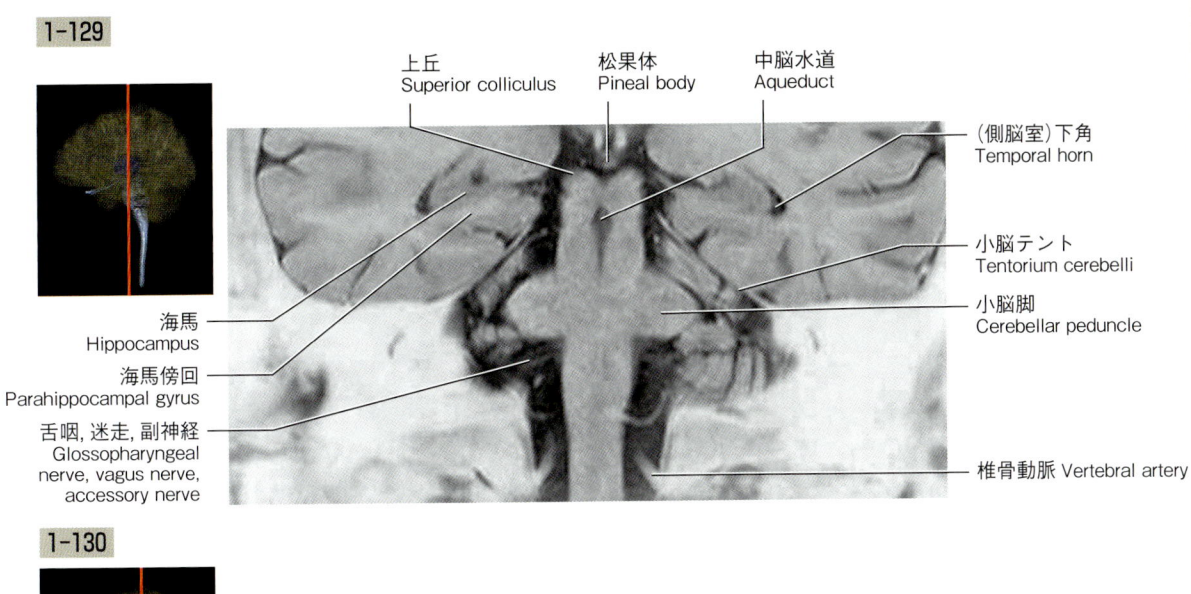

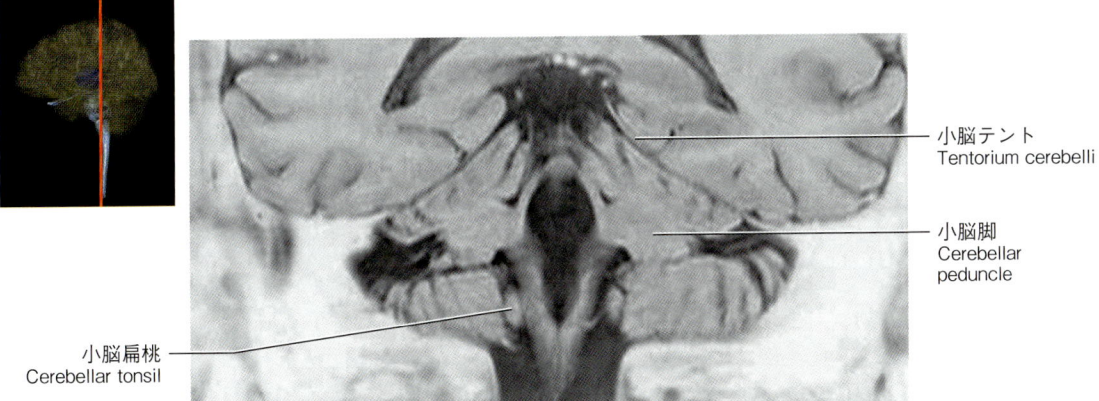

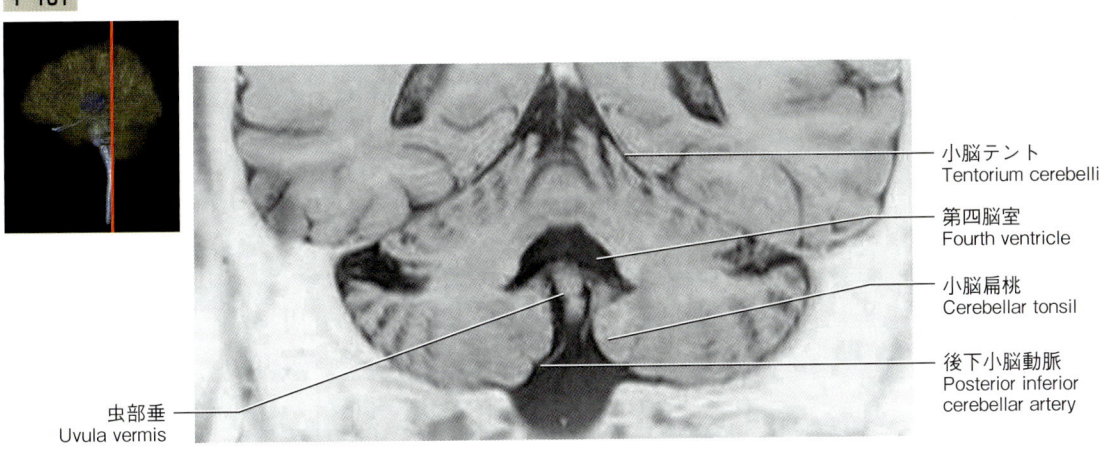

1-129

- 上丘 Superior colliculus
- 松果体 Pineal body
- 中脳水道 Aqueduct
- （側脳室）下角 Temporal horn
- 小脳テント Tentorium cerebelli
- 小脳脚 Cerebellar peduncle
- 海馬 Hippocampus
- 海馬傍回 Parahippocampal gyrus
- 舌咽, 迷走, 副神経 Glossopharyngeal nerve, vagus nerve, accessory nerve
- 椎骨動脈 Vertebral artery

1-130

- 小脳テント Tentorium cerebelli
- 小脳脚 Cerebellar peduncle
- 小脳扁桃 Cerebellar tonsil

1-131

- 小脳テント Tentorium cerebelli
- 第四脳室 Fourth ventricle
- 小脳扁桃 Cerebellar tonsil
- 後下小脳動脈 Posterior inferior cerebellar artery
- 虫部垂 Uvula vermis

脳幹部の断層解剖 ［冠状断像（MRI, 白黒反転 heavy T2 強調像）］

1-132

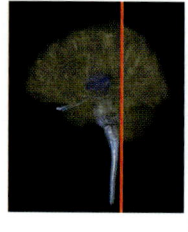

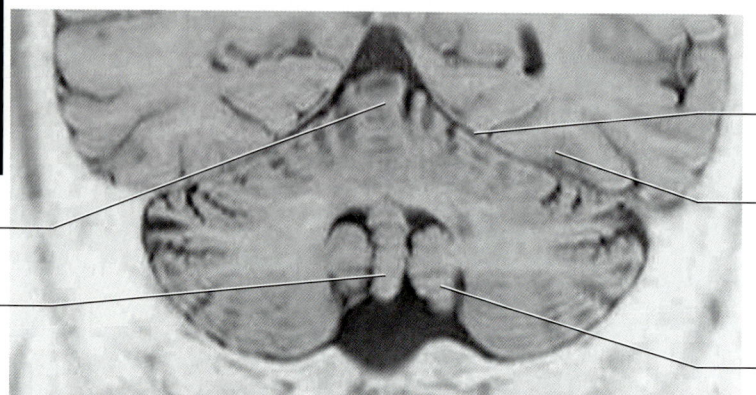

- 小脳虫部 Cerebellar vermis
- 虫部垂 Uvula vermis
- 小脳テント Tentorium cerebelli
- 外側後頭側頭回 Lateral occipitotemporal gyrus
- 小脳扁桃 Cerebellar tonsil

1-133

- 小脳虫部 Cerebellar vermis
- 虫部垂 Uvula vermis
- 内側後頭側頭回 Medial occipitotemporal gyrus
- 下側頭回 Inferior temporal gyrus
- 外側後頭側頭回 Lateral occipitotemporal gyrus
- 小脳テント Tentorium cerebelli

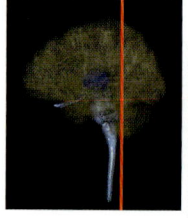

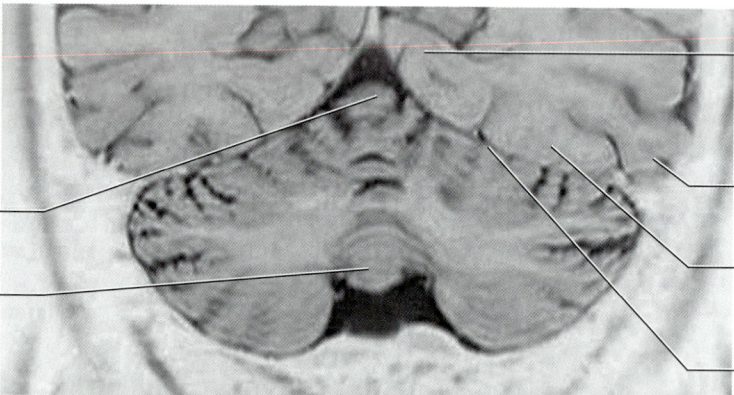

> **NOTE** 小脳虫部 Cerebellar vermis
> vermis はラテン語の"虫"の意味である．また虫垂はラテン語名"vermiform appendix"からの和訳である．appendix は"突起"の意味で古代ローマの司祭帽の先端に付いていた羊毛の房の apex からの派生であり，尖端や頂点を意味するようになった．

II

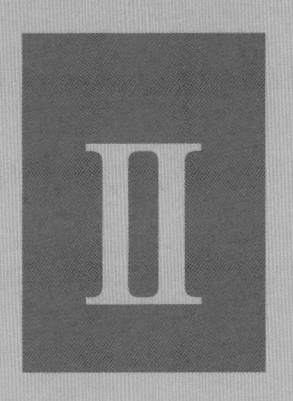

頭頸部
Head and Neck

頭頸部 (MDCT, VR 像)

2-1 副鼻腔・唾液腺・甲状腺（正面）

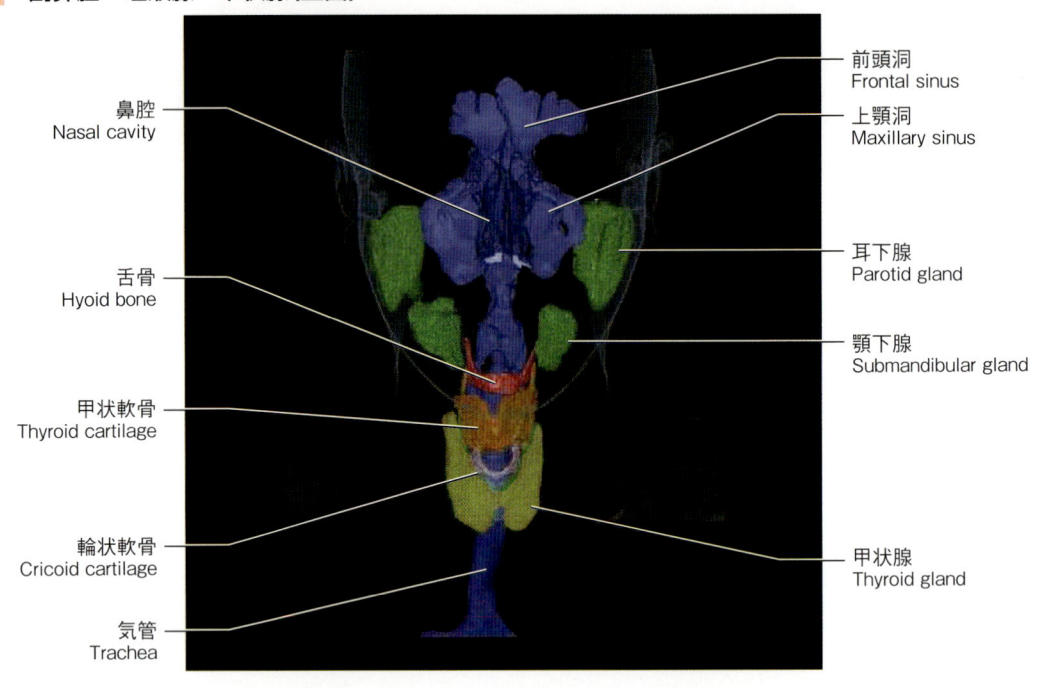

- 鼻腔 Nasal cavity
- 舌骨 Hyoid bone
- 甲状軟骨 Thyroid cartilage
- 輪状軟骨 Cricoid cartilage
- 気管 Trachea
- 前頭洞 Frontal sinus
- 上顎洞 Maxillary sinus
- 耳下腺 Parotid gland
- 顎下腺 Submandibular gland
- 甲状腺 Thyroid gland

2-2 副鼻腔・唾液腺・甲状腺（側面）

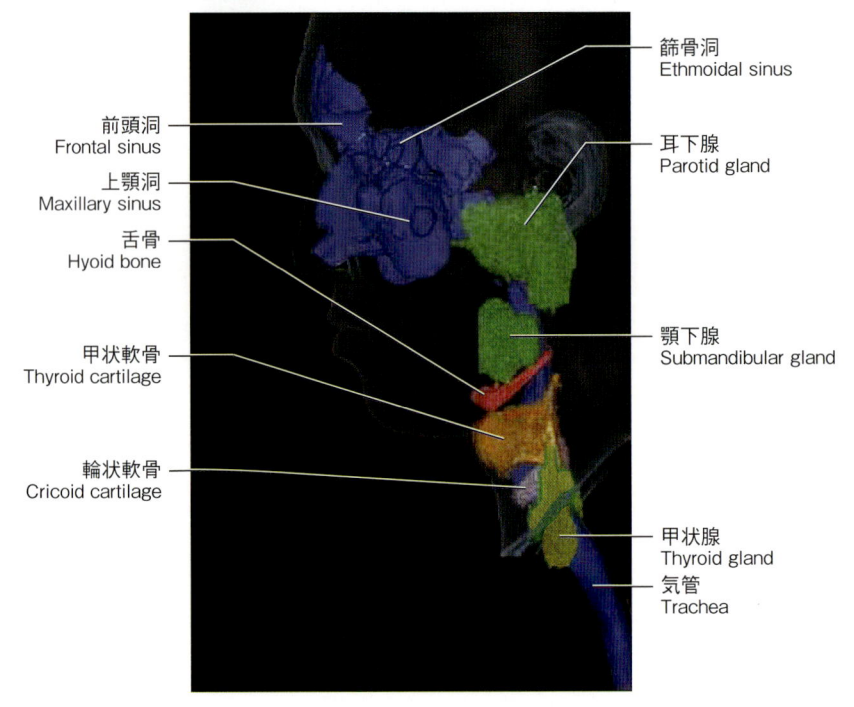

- 前頭洞 Frontal sinus
- 上顎洞 Maxillary sinus
- 舌骨 Hyoid bone
- 甲状軟骨 Thyroid cartilage
- 輪状軟骨 Cricoid cartilage
- 篩骨洞 Ethmoidal sinus
- 耳下腺 Parotid gland
- 顎下腺 Submandibular gland
- 甲状腺 Thyroid gland
- 気管 Trachea

頭頸部 (MDCT, VR 像)

2-3 副鼻腔・咽喉頭

正面

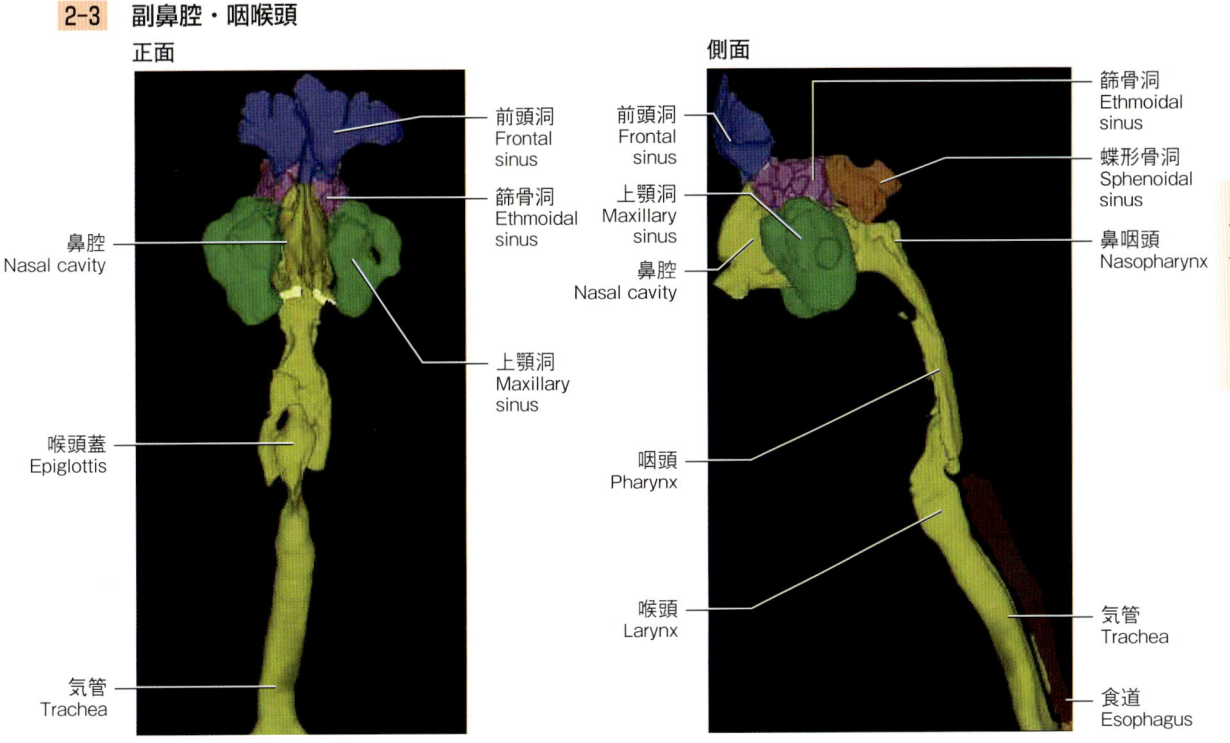

- 前頭洞 Frontal sinus
- 篩骨洞 Ethmoidal sinus
- 鼻腔 Nasal cavity
- 上顎洞 Maxillary sinus
- 喉頭蓋 Epiglottis
- 気管 Trachea

側面

- 前頭洞 Frontal sinus
- 篩骨洞 Ethmoidal sinus
- 蝶形骨洞 Sphenoidal sinus
- 上顎洞 Maxillary sinus
- 鼻腔 Nasal cavity
- 鼻咽頭 Nasopharynx
- 咽頭 Pharynx
- 喉頭 Larynx
- 気管 Trachea
- 食道 Esophagus

2-4 舌骨・甲状軟骨・輪状軟骨

正面

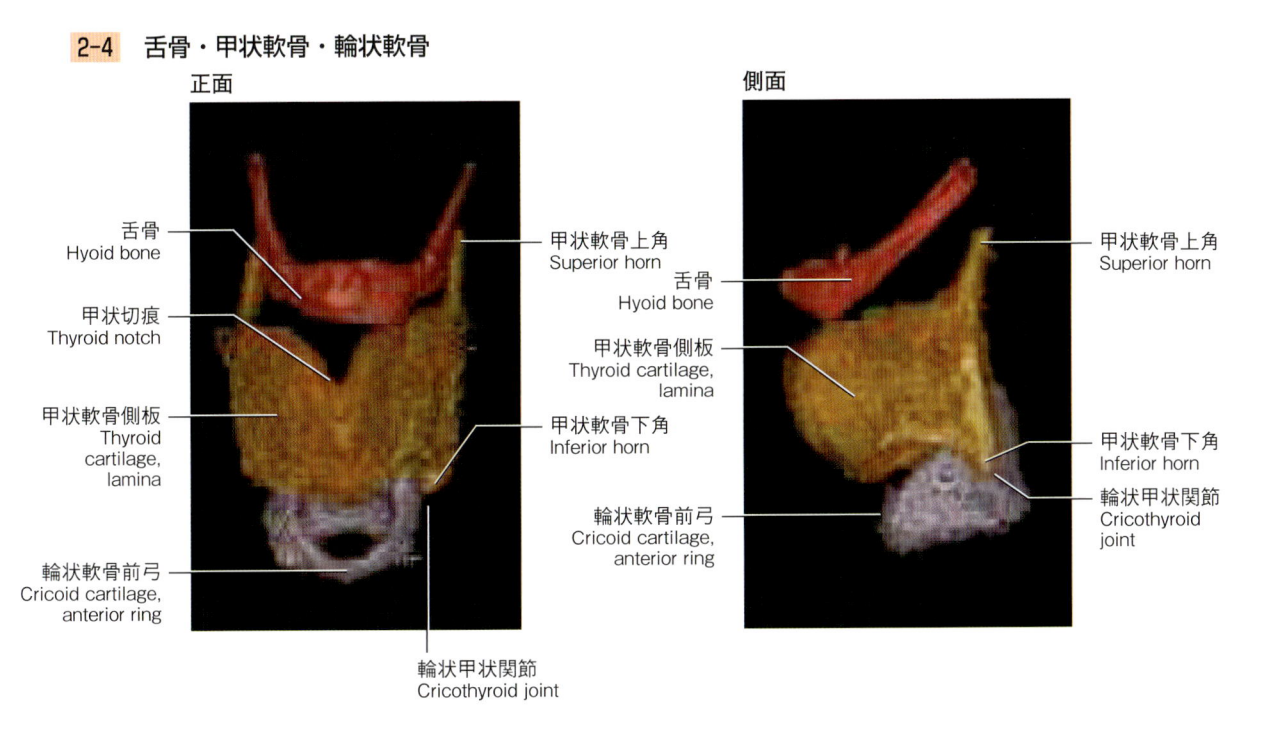

- 舌骨 Hyoid bone
- 甲状切痕 Thyroid notch
- 甲状軟骨上角 Superior horn
- 甲状軟骨側板 Thyroid cartilage, lamina
- 甲状軟骨下角 Inferior horn
- 輪状軟骨前弓 Cricoid cartilage, anterior ring
- 輪状甲状関節 Cricothyroid joint

側面

- 甲状軟骨上角 Superior horn
- 舌骨 Hyoid bone
- 甲状軟骨側板 Thyroid cartilage, lamina
- 甲状軟骨下角 Inferior horn
- 輪状甲状関節 Cricothyroid joint

頭頸部の断層解剖 ［横断像（造影CT）］

2-5 眼窩上方レベル

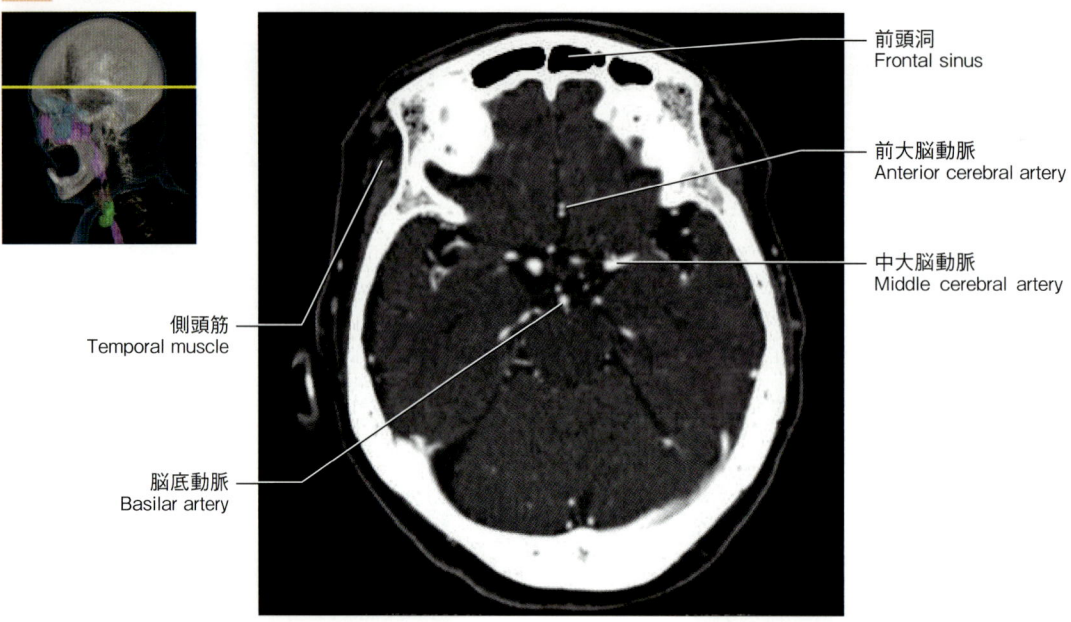

- 前頭洞 Frontal sinus
- 前大脳動脈 Anterior cerebral artery
- 中大脳動脈 Middle cerebral artery
- 側頭筋 Temporal muscle
- 脳底動脈 Basilar artery

2-6 眼窩レベル

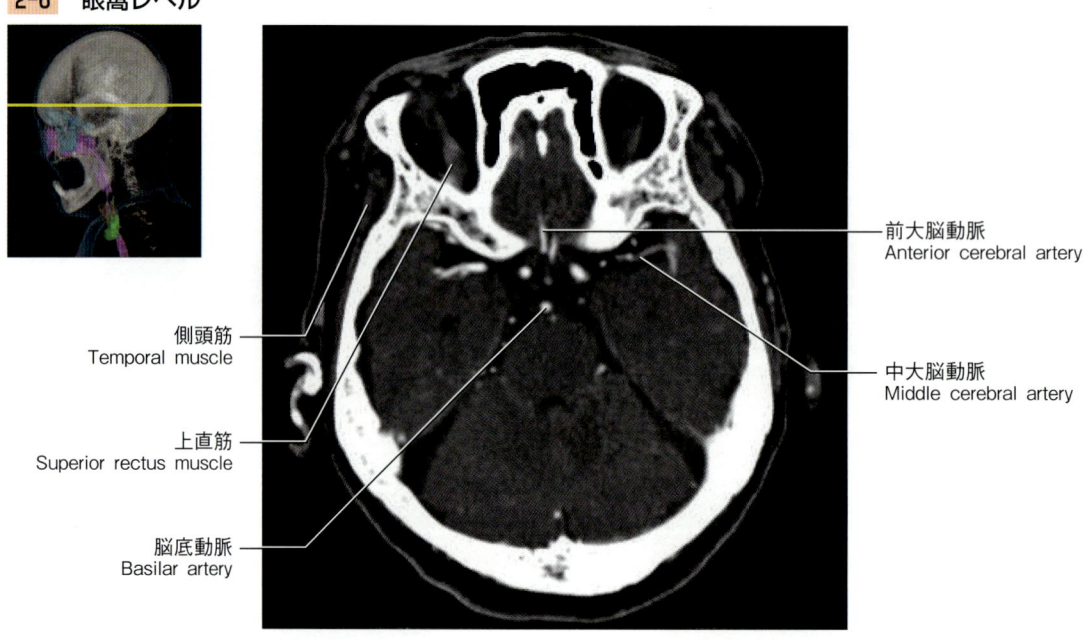

- 前大脳動脈 Anterior cerebral artery
- 中大脳動脈 Middle cerebral artery
- 側頭筋 Temporal muscle
- 上直筋 Superior rectus muscle
- 脳底動脈 Basilar artery

頭頸部の断層解剖 ［横断像（造影 CT）］

2-7 眼窩レベル

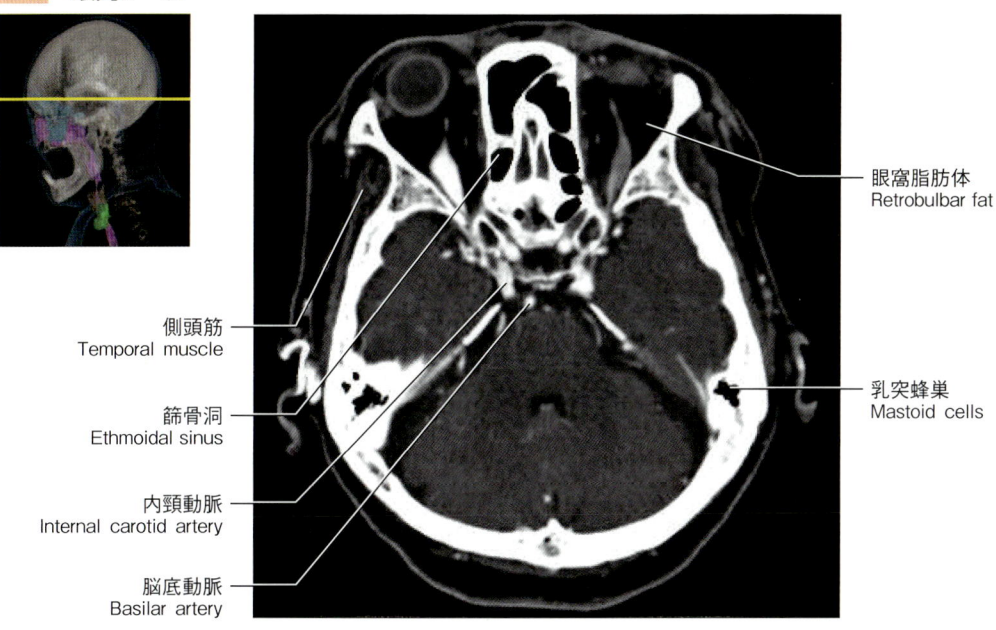

- 眼窩脂肪体 Retrobulbar fat
- 側頭筋 Temporal muscle
- 篩骨洞 Ethmoidal sinus
- 乳突蜂巣 Mastoid cells
- 内頸動脈 Internal carotid artery
- 脳底動脈 Basilar artery

2-8 眼窩レベル

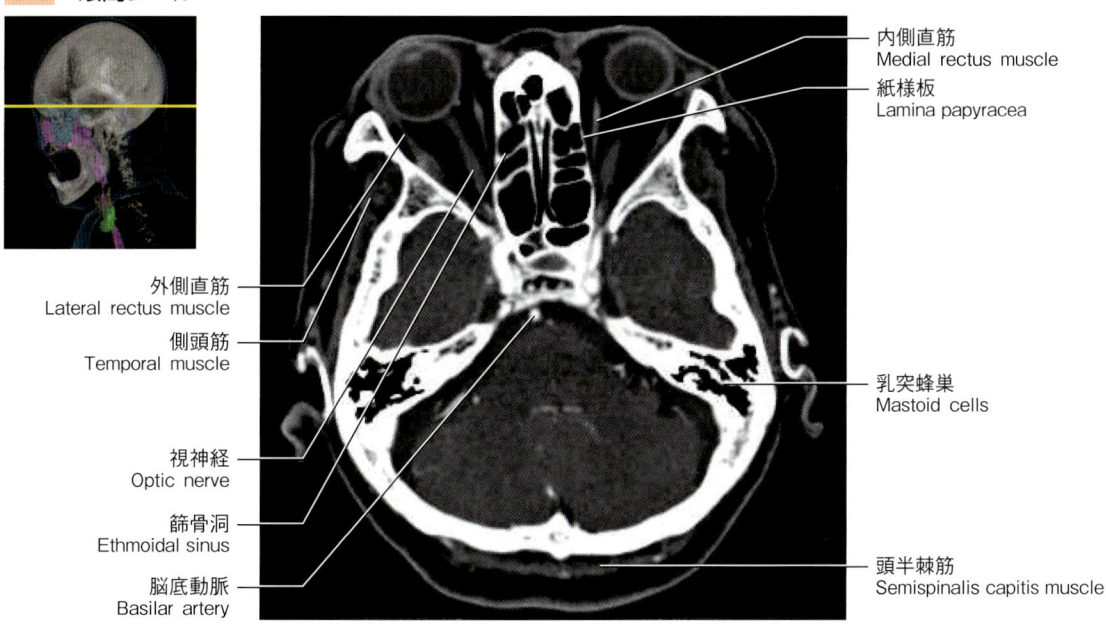

- 内側直筋 Medial rectus muscle
- 紙様板 Lamina papyracea
- 外側直筋 Lateral rectus muscle
- 側頭筋 Temporal muscle
- 乳突蜂巣 Mastoid cells
- 視神経 Optic nerve
- 篩骨洞 Ethmoidal sinus
- 頭半棘筋 Semispinalis capitis muscle
- 脳底動脈 Basilar artery

NOTE 眼窩内側壁は紙様板（Lamina papyracea）ともいわれ，大変薄い構造である．眼窩吹き抜け骨折の好発部位であり，鼻内内視鏡手術の操作の際に注意を要する箇所である．

頭頸部の断層解剖 ［横断像（造影CT）］

2-9 眼窩レベル

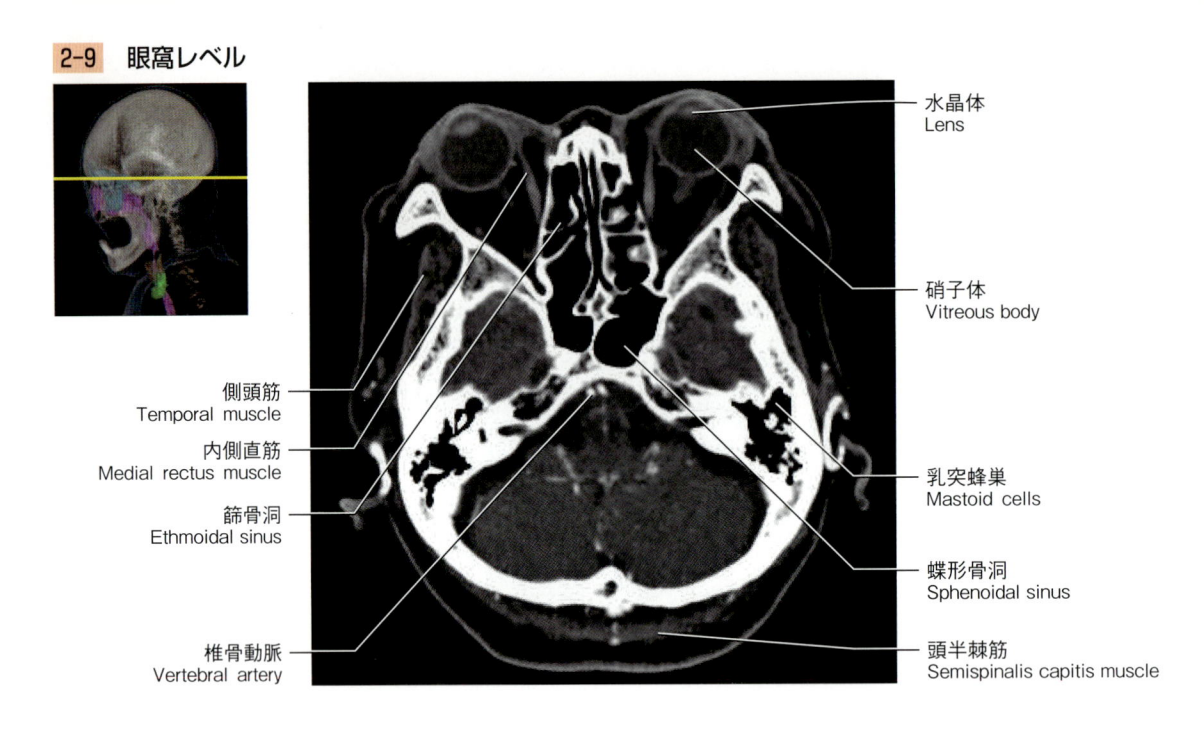

- 水晶体 Lens
- 硝子体 Vitreous body
- 側頭筋 Temporal muscle
- 内側直筋 Medial rectus muscle
- 篩骨洞 Ethmoidal sinus
- 乳突蜂巣 Mastoid cells
- 蝶形骨洞 Sphenoidal sinus
- 椎骨動脈 Vertebral artery
- 頭半棘筋 Semispinalis capitis muscle

2-10 眼窩レベル

- 篩骨洞 Ethmoidal sinus
- 蝶篩陥凹 Sphenoethmoidal recess
- 蝶形骨洞 Sphenoidal sinus

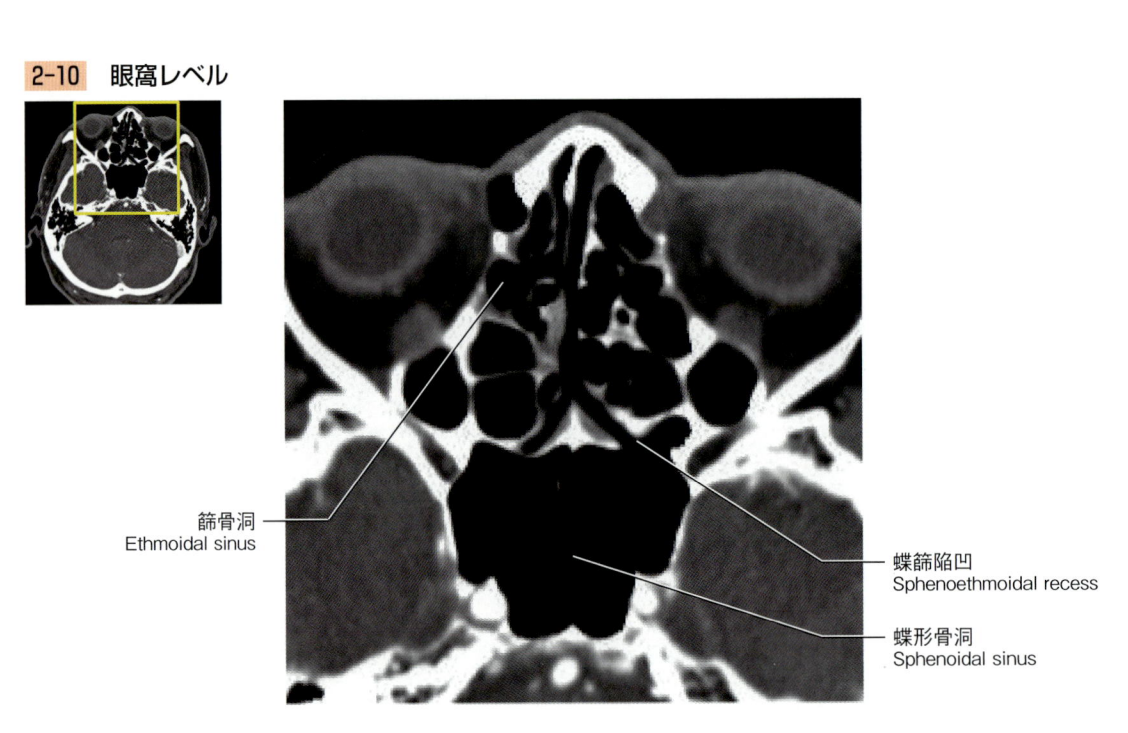

NOTE 蝶篩陥凹は鼻腔後方に位置し，後篩骨洞と蝶形骨洞からの排泄口となる．

頭頸部の断層解剖 ［横断像（造影CT）］

2-11 眼窩レベル

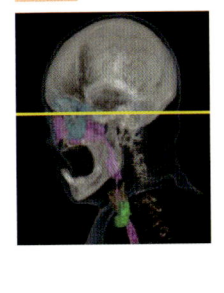

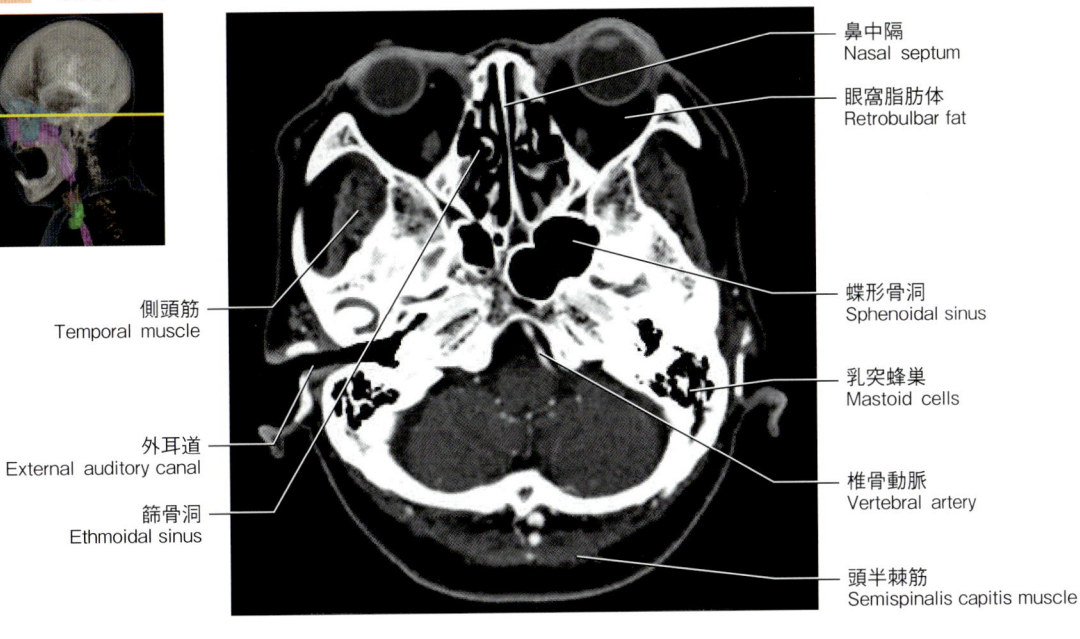

- 鼻中隔 Nasal septum
- 眼窩脂肪体 Retrobulbar fat
- 蝶形骨洞 Sphenoidal sinus
- 乳突蜂巣 Mastoid cells
- 椎骨動脈 Vertebral artery
- 頭半棘筋 Semispinalis capitis muscle
- 側頭筋 Temporal muscle
- 外耳道 External auditory canal
- 篩骨洞 Ethmoidal sinus

2-12 眼窩レベル

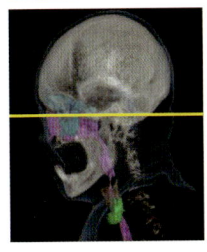

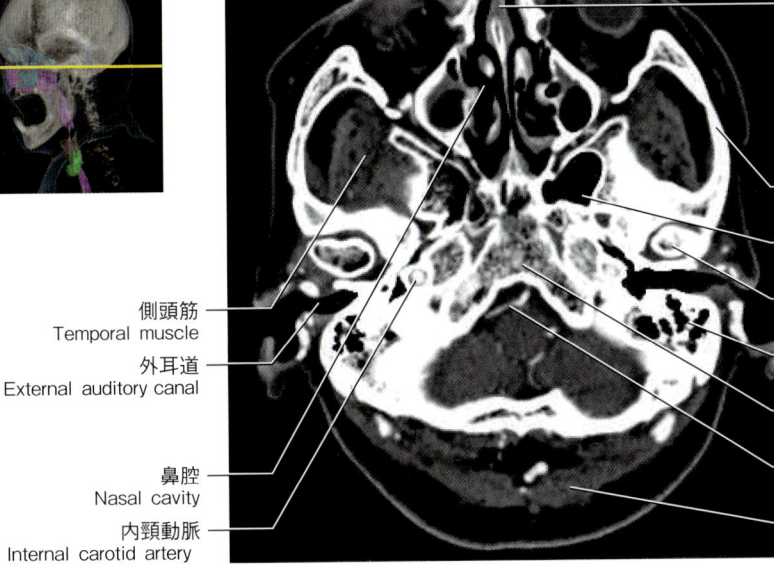

- 鼻骨 Nasal bone
- 鼻中隔 Nasal septum
- 頬骨弓 Zygomatic arch
- 蝶形骨洞 Sphenoidal sinus
- 下顎頭 Head of mandible
- 乳突蜂巣 Mastoid cells
- 斜台 Clivus
- 椎骨動脈 Vertebral artery
- 頭半棘筋 Semispinalis capitis muscle
- 側頭筋 Temporal muscle
- 外耳道 External auditory canal
- 鼻腔 Nasal cavity
- 内頸動脈 Internal carotid artery

NOTE 頬骨弓は頬骨の単独骨折の好発部位である．

頭頸部の断層解剖 ［横断像（造影CT）］

2-13 眼窩下縁・上顎洞レベル

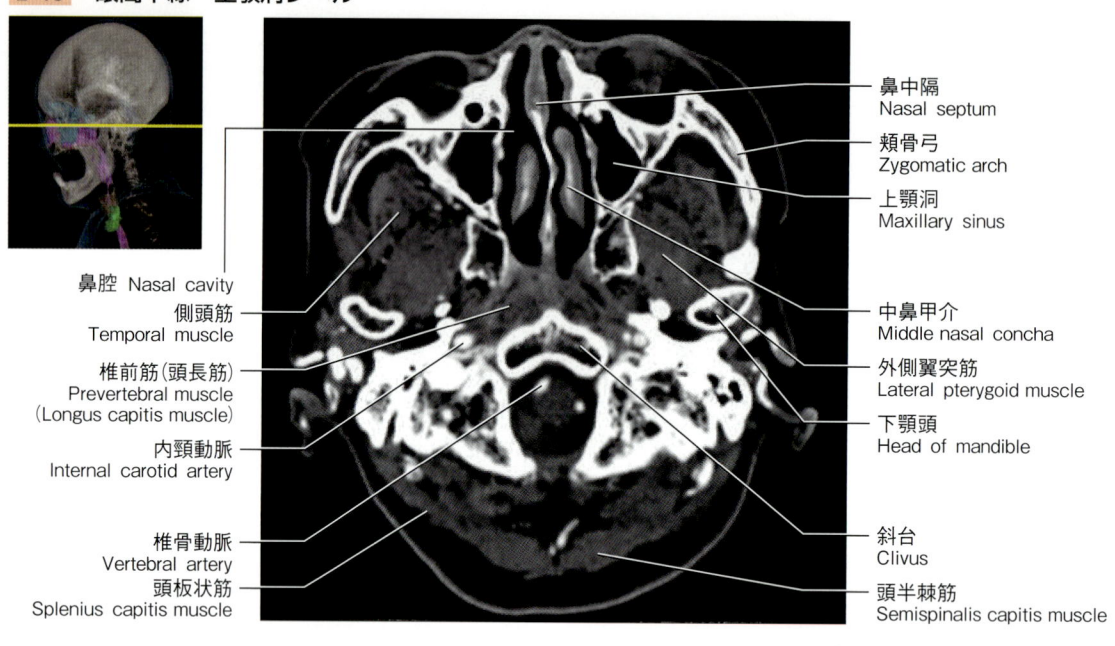

- 鼻中隔 Nasal septum
- 頬骨弓 Zygomatic arch
- 上顎洞 Maxillary sinus
- 鼻腔 Nasal cavity
- 側頭筋 Temporal muscle
- 中鼻甲介 Middle nasal concha
- 椎前筋（頭長筋）Prevertebral muscle (Longus capitis muscle)
- 外側翼突筋 Lateral pterygoid muscle
- 内頸動脈 Internal carotid artery
- 下顎頭 Head of mandible
- 椎骨動脈 Vertebral artery
- 斜台 Clivus
- 頭板状筋 Splenius capitis muscle
- 頭半棘筋 Semispinalis capitis muscle

2-14 上顎洞レベル

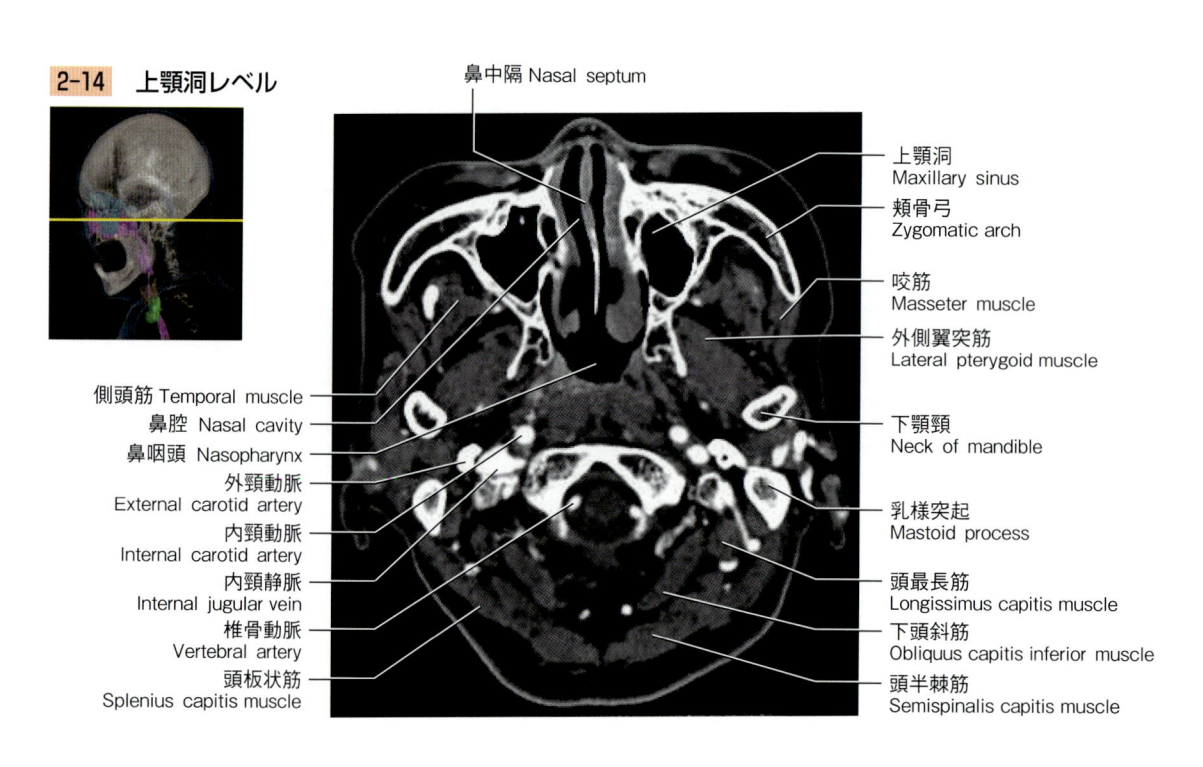

- 鼻中隔 Nasal septum
- 上顎洞 Maxillary sinus
- 頬骨弓 Zygomatic arch
- 咬筋 Masseter muscle
- 外側翼突筋 Lateral pterygoid muscle
- 側頭筋 Temporal muscle
- 鼻腔 Nasal cavity
- 鼻咽頭 Nasopharynx
- 下顎頸 Neck of mandible
- 外頸動脈 External carotid artery
- 内頸動脈 Internal carotid artery
- 乳様突起 Mastoid process
- 内頸静脈 Internal jugular vein
- 頭最長筋 Longissimus capitis muscle
- 椎骨動脈 Vertebral artery
- 下頭斜筋 Obliquus capitis inferior muscle
- 頭板状筋 Splenius capitis muscle
- 頭半棘筋 Semispinalis capitis muscle

> **NOTE** 頬骨 Zygoma
> Zygomaは，ギリシャ語のzygonくびき（一対のウシなどを首のところでつなぐ農具）からの派生語で，左右一対を表す意味．左右対称の骨はほかにも多数あるが，最も目立つものだから代表したのであろう．ちなみに左右不対である静脈をazygosとよび，和訳は奇数(不対)の意を込めて奇静脈となったとされる(191頁のNOTEを参照).

頭頸部の断層解剖 ［横断像（造影CT）］

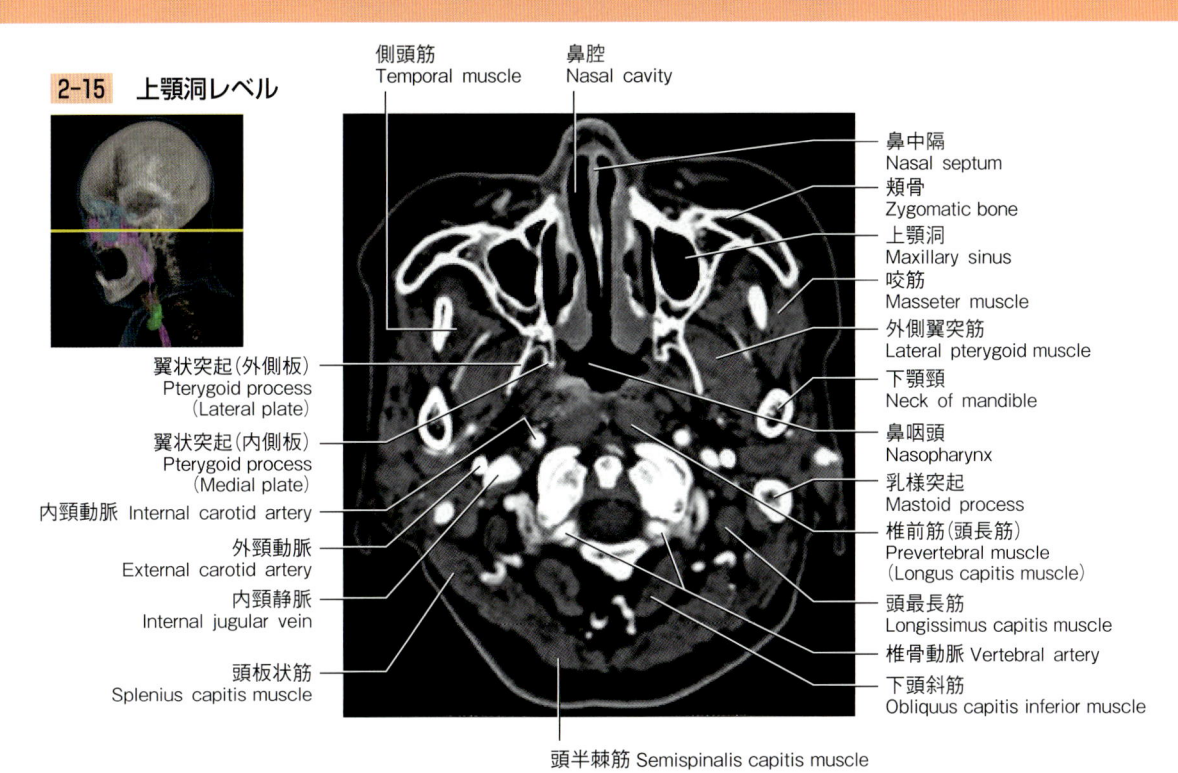

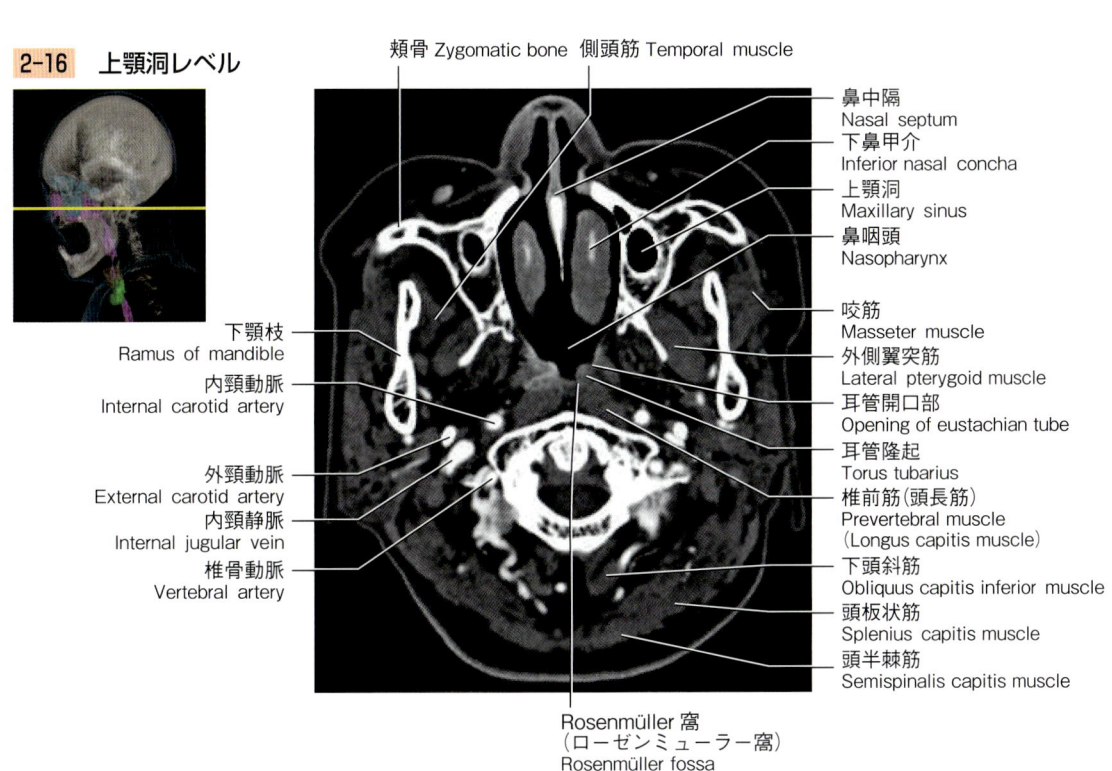

2-15 上顎洞レベル

- 側頭筋 Temporal muscle
- 鼻腔 Nasal cavity
- 鼻中隔 Nasal septum
- 頬骨 Zygomatic bone
- 上顎洞 Maxillary sinus
- 咬筋 Masseter muscle
- 外側翼突筋 Lateral pterygoid muscle
- 下顎頸 Neck of mandible
- 鼻咽頭 Nasopharynx
- 乳様突起 Mastoid process
- 椎前筋（頭長筋）Prevertebral muscle（Longus capitis muscle）
- 頭最長筋 Longissimus capitis muscle
- 椎骨動脈 Vertebral artery
- 下頭斜筋 Obliquus capitis inferior muscle
- 翼状突起（外側板）Pterygoid process（Lateral plate）
- 翼状突起（内側板）Pterygoid process（Medial plate）
- 内頸動脈 Internal carotid artery
- 外頸動脈 External carotid artery
- 内頸静脈 Internal jugular vein
- 頭板状筋 Splenius capitis muscle
- 頭半棘筋 Semispinalis capitis muscle

2-16 上顎洞レベル

- 頬骨 Zygomatic bone
- 側頭筋 Temporal muscle
- 鼻中隔 Nasal septum
- 下鼻甲介 Inferior nasal concha
- 上顎洞 Maxillary sinus
- 鼻咽頭 Nasopharynx
- 咬筋 Masseter muscle
- 外側翼突筋 Lateral pterygoid muscle
- 耳管開口部 Opening of eustachian tube
- 耳管隆起 Torus tubarius
- 椎前筋（頭長筋）Prevertebral muscle（Longus capitis muscle）
- 下頭斜筋 Obliquus capitis inferior muscle
- 頭板状筋 Splenius capitis muscle
- 頭半棘筋 Semispinalis capitis muscle
- 下顎枝 Ramus of mandible
- 内頸動脈 Internal carotid artery
- 外頸動脈 External carotid artery
- 内頸静脈 Internal jugular vein
- 椎骨動脈 Vertebral artery
- Rosenmüller窩（ローゼンミューラー窩）Rosenmüller fossa

NOTE Rosenmüller（ローゼンミューラー）窩は上咽頭癌の好発部位である．ここに腫瘍が発生すると，前方の耳管開口部が閉塞し中耳炎を発症する．

頭頸部の断層解剖 ［横断像（造影CT）］

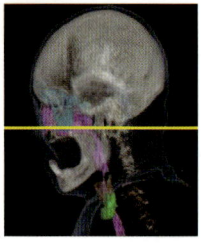

2-17 上顎洞下縁レベル

- 鼻咽頭 Nasopharynx
- 咬筋 Masseter muscle
- 内側翼突筋 Medial pterygoid muscle
- 椎前筋（頭長筋） Prevertebral muscle (Longus capitis muscle)
- 下顎枝 Ramus of mandible
- 耳下腺 Parotid gland
- 外頸動脈 External carotid artery
- 下頭斜筋 Obliquus capitis inferior muscle
- 内頸動脈 Internal carotid artery
- 頭半棘筋 Semispinalis capitis muscle
- 椎骨動脈 Vertebral artery
- 頭板状筋 Splenius capitis muscle

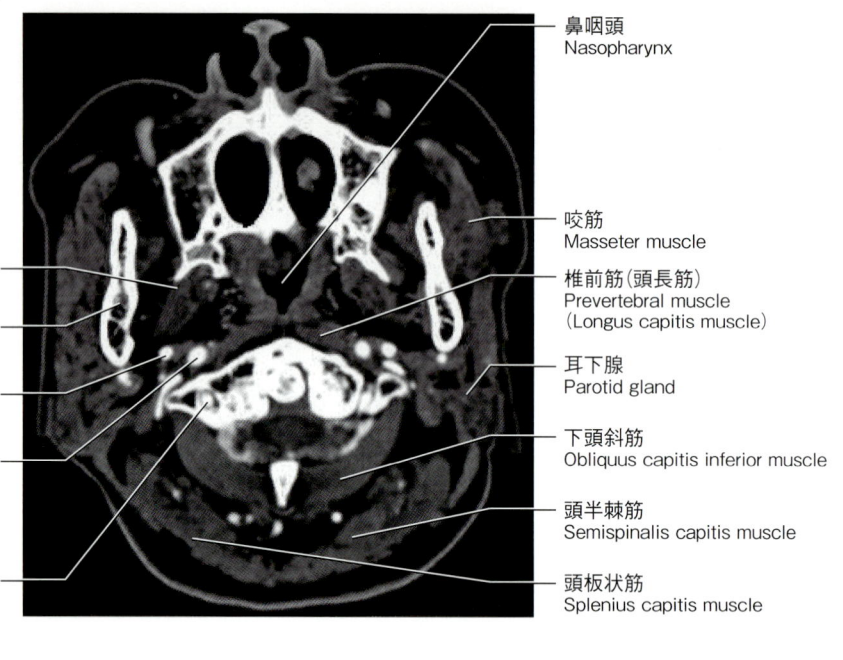

2-18 歯槽突起レベル

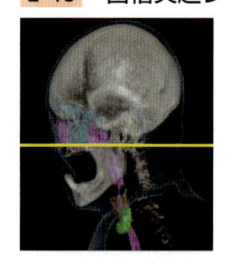

- 歯槽突起 Alveolar process
- 上咽頭, 中咽頭 Epipharynx, mesopharynx
- 口蓋扁桃 Palatine tonsil
- 頬筋 Buccinator muscle
- 咬筋 Masseter muscle
- 下顎枝 Ramus of mandible
- 下顎後静脈 Retromandibular vein
- 内頸動脈 Internal carotid artery
- 耳下腺 Parotid gland
- 内頸静脈 Internal jugular vein
- 胸鎖乳突筋 Sternocleidomastoid muscle
- 椎骨動脈 Vertebral artery
- 頭板状筋 Splenius capitis muscle
- 下頭斜筋 Obliquus capitis inferior muscle
- 頭半棘筋 Semispinalis capitis muscle

> **NOTE** 頭頸部における原発不明癌の"原発"は鼻咽頭・扁桃・舌根部・梨状窩であることが多い．

頭頸部の断層解剖 ［横断像（造影CT）］

2-19 歯槽突起下縁レベル

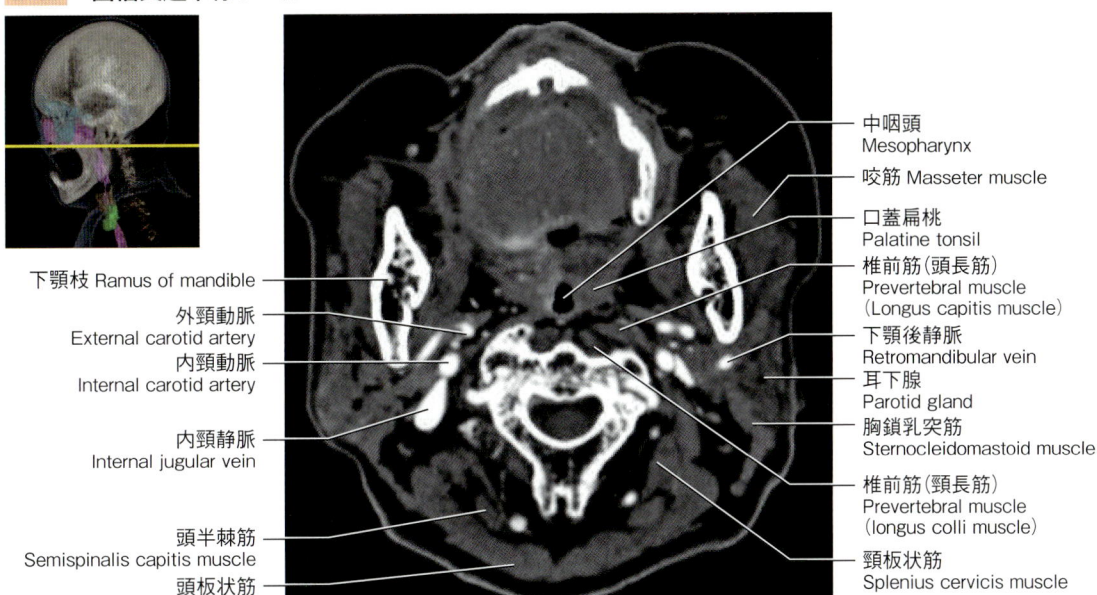

- 下顎枝 Ramus of mandible
- 外頸動脈 External carotid artery
- 内頸動脈 Internal carotid artery
- 内頸静脈 Internal jugular vein
- 頭半棘筋 Semispinalis capitis muscle
- 頭板状筋 Splenius capitis muscle
- 中咽頭 Mesopharynx
- 咬筋 Masseter muscle
- 口蓋扁桃 Palatine tonsil
- 椎前筋（頭長筋）Prevertebral muscle (Longus capitis muscle)
- 下顎後静脈 Retromandibular vein
- 耳下腺 Parotid gland
- 胸鎖乳突筋 Sternocleidomastoid muscle
- 椎前筋（頸長筋）Prevertebral muscle (longus colli muscle)
- 頸板状筋 Splenius cervicis muscle

2-20 口腔レベル

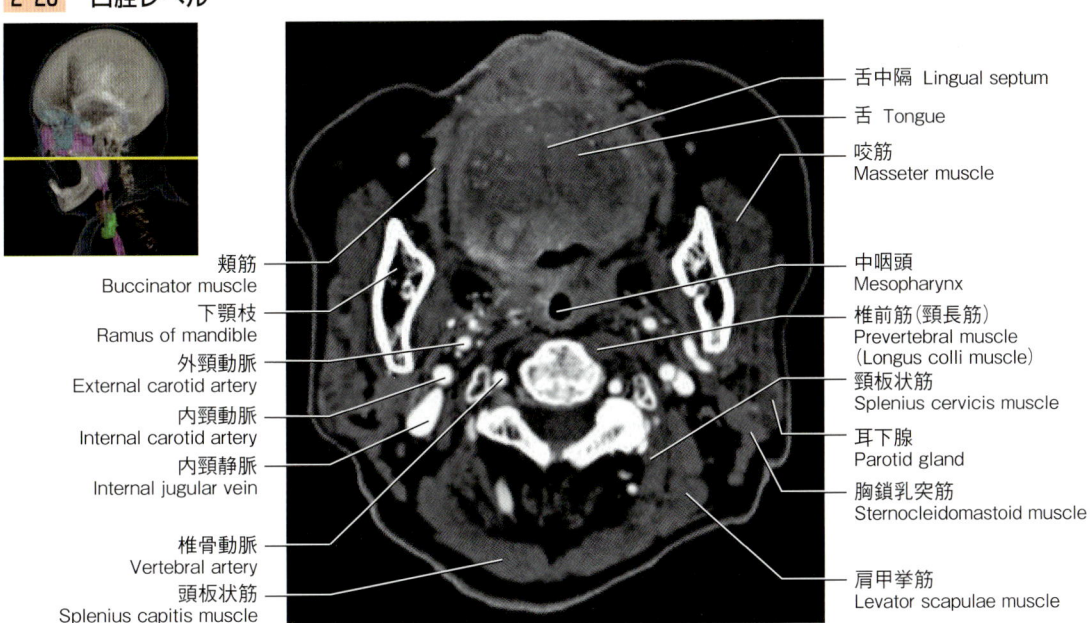

- 頬筋 Buccinator muscle
- 下顎枝 Ramus of mandible
- 外頸動脈 External carotid artery
- 内頸動脈 Internal carotid artery
- 内頸静脈 Internal jugular vein
- 椎骨動脈 Vertebral artery
- 頭板状筋 Splenius capitis muscle
- 舌中隔 Lingual septum
- 舌 Tongue
- 咬筋 Masseter muscle
- 中咽頭 Mesopharynx
- 椎前筋（頸長筋）Prevertebral muscle (Longus colli muscle)
- 頸板状筋 Splenius cervicis muscle
- 耳下腺 Parotid gland
- 胸鎖乳突筋 Sternocleidomastoid muscle
- 肩甲挙筋 Levator scapulae muscle

> **NOTE** 傍神経節腫のうち頸動脈小体由来のものは，内頸・外頸動脈を離開させるのが特徴的である．

頭頸部の断層解剖 ［横断像（造影 CT）］

2-21 口腔レベル

- 舌中隔 Lingual septum
- 舌 Tongue
- 咬筋 Masseter muscle
- 中咽頭 Mesopharynx
- 耳下腺 Parotid gland
- 胸鎖乳突筋 Sternocleidomastoid muscle
- 肩甲挙筋 Levator scapulae muscle
- 頸板状筋 Splenius cervicis muscle
- 頸半棘筋 Semispinalis capitis muscle
- 頬筋 Buccinator muscle
- 下顎枝 Ramus of mandible
- 外頸動脈 External carotid artery
- 内頸動脈 Internal carotid artery
- 内頸静脈 Internal jugular vein
- 椎骨動脈 Vertebral artery
- 頭板状筋 Splenius capitis muscle

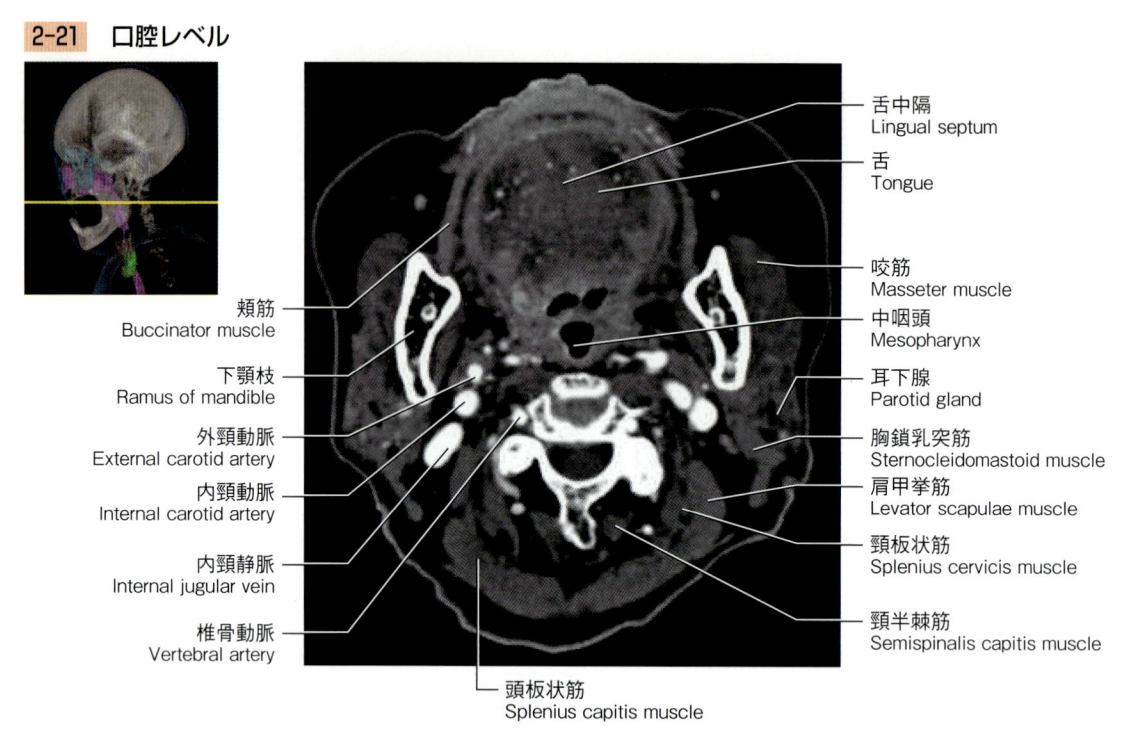

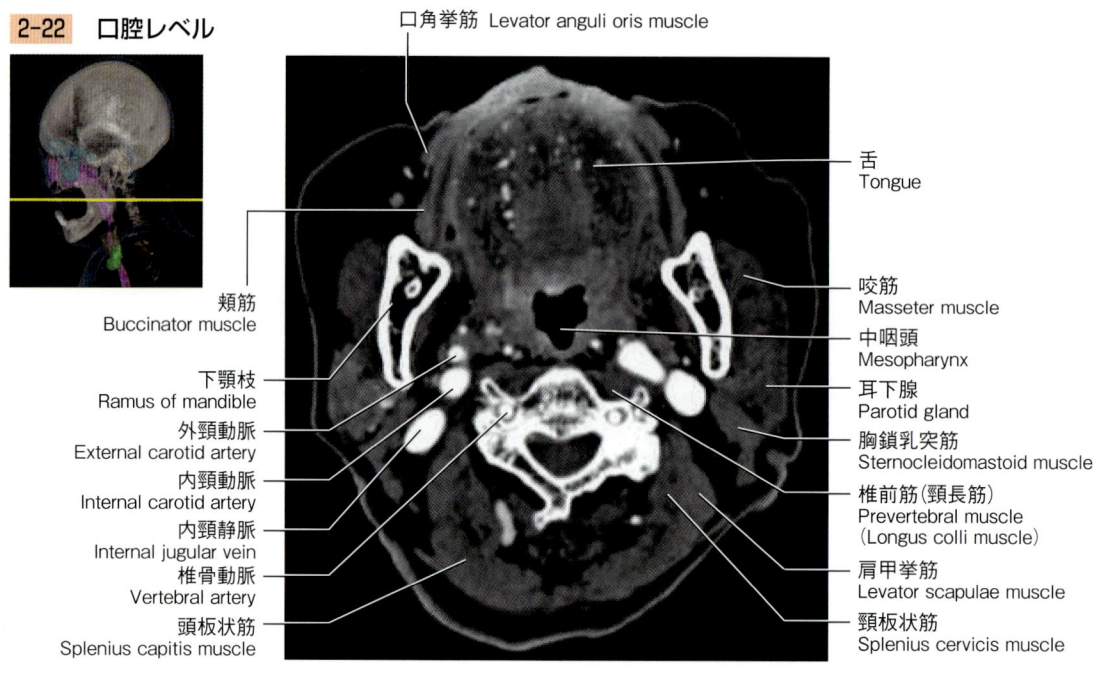

2-22 口腔レベル

- 口角挙筋 Levator anguli oris muscle
- 舌 Tongue
- 咬筋 Masseter muscle
- 中咽頭 Mesopharynx
- 耳下腺 Parotid gland
- 胸鎖乳突筋 Sternocleidomastoid muscle
- 椎前筋（頸長筋）Prevertebral muscle（Longus colli muscle）
- 肩甲挙筋 Levator scapulae muscle
- 頸板状筋 Splenius cervicis muscle
- 頬筋 Buccinator muscle
- 下顎枝 Ramus of mandible
- 外頸動脈 External carotid artery
- 内頸動脈 Internal carotid artery
- 内頸静脈 Internal jugular vein
- 椎骨動脈 Vertebral artery
- 頭板状筋 Splenius capitis muscle

頭頸部の断層解剖 ［横断像（造影 CT）］

2-23 口腔・口腔底レベル

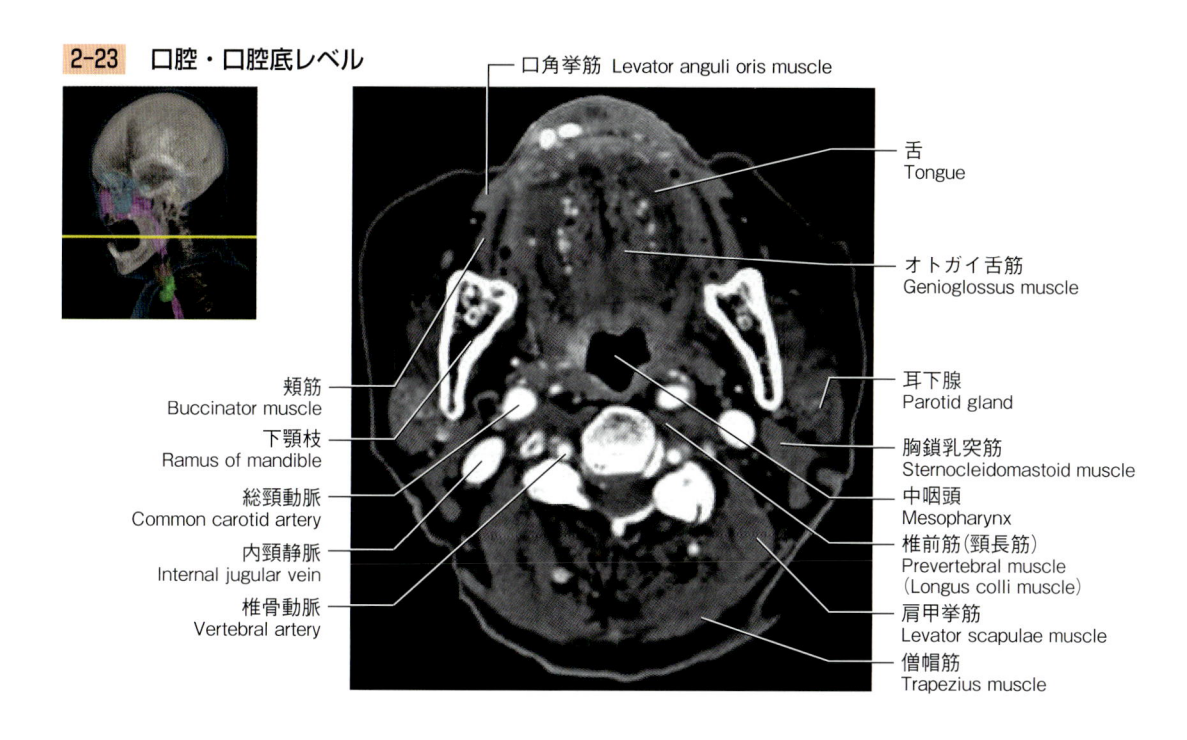

- 口角挙筋 Levator anguli oris muscle
- 舌 Tongue
- オトガイ舌筋 Genioglossus muscle
- 頬筋 Buccinator muscle
- 下顎枝 Ramus of mandible
- 総頸動脈 Common carotid artery
- 内頸静脈 Internal jugular vein
- 椎骨動脈 Vertebral artery
- 耳下腺 Parotid gland
- 胸鎖乳突筋 Sternocleidomastoid muscle
- 中咽頭 Mesopharynx
- 椎前筋（頸長筋）Prevertebral muscle（Longus colli muscle）
- 肩甲挙筋 Levator scapulae muscle
- 僧帽筋 Trapezius muscle

2-24 口腔・口腔底レベル

- 口角挙筋 Levator anguli oris muscle
- オトガイ舌筋 Genioglossus muscle
- 中咽頭 Mesopharynx
- 下顎管 Mandibular canal
- 下顎枝 Ramus of mandible
- 総頸動脈 Common carotid artery
- 内頸静脈 Internal jugular vein
- 椎骨動脈 Vertebral artery
- 耳下腺 Parotid gland
- 胸鎖乳突筋 Sternocleidomastoid muscle
- 椎前筋（頸長筋）Prevertebral muscle（Longus colli muscle）
- 肩甲挙筋 Levator scapulae muscle
- 僧帽筋 Trapezius muscle

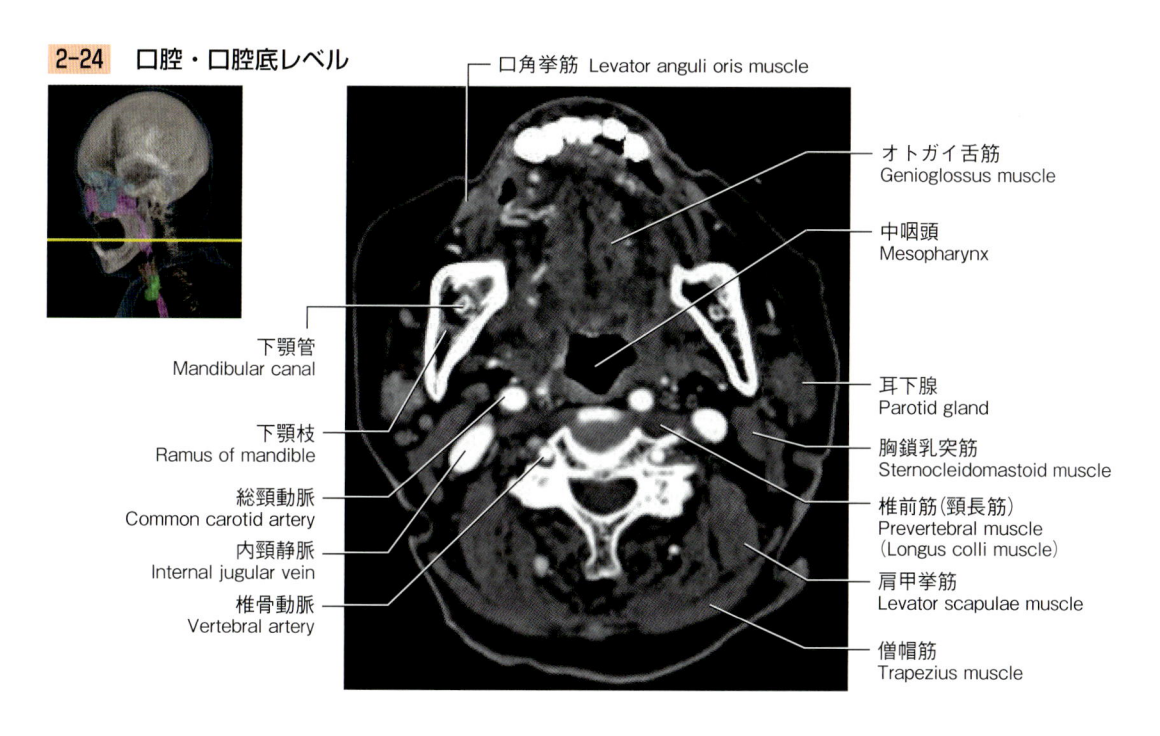

NOTE オトガイ舌筋は舌の筋肉のうち外舌筋（舌以外に起始部をもつ）の1つである．このほか，外舌筋には舌骨舌筋・茎突舌筋・口蓋舌筋がある．

頭頸部の断層解剖 ［横断像（造影CT）］

2-25 口腔・口腔底レベル

- 口角挙筋 Levator anguli oris muscle
- オトガイ舌筋 Genioglossus muscle
- 喉頭蓋 Epiglottis
- 中咽頭 Mesopharynx
- 総頸動脈 Common carotid artery
- 胸鎖乳突筋 Sternocleidomastoid muscle
- 椎前筋（頸長筋） Prevertebral muscle（Longus colli muscle）
- 内頸静脈 Internal jugular vein
- 肩甲挙筋 Levator scapulae muscle
- 椎骨動脈 Vertebral artery
- 僧帽筋 Trapezius muscle

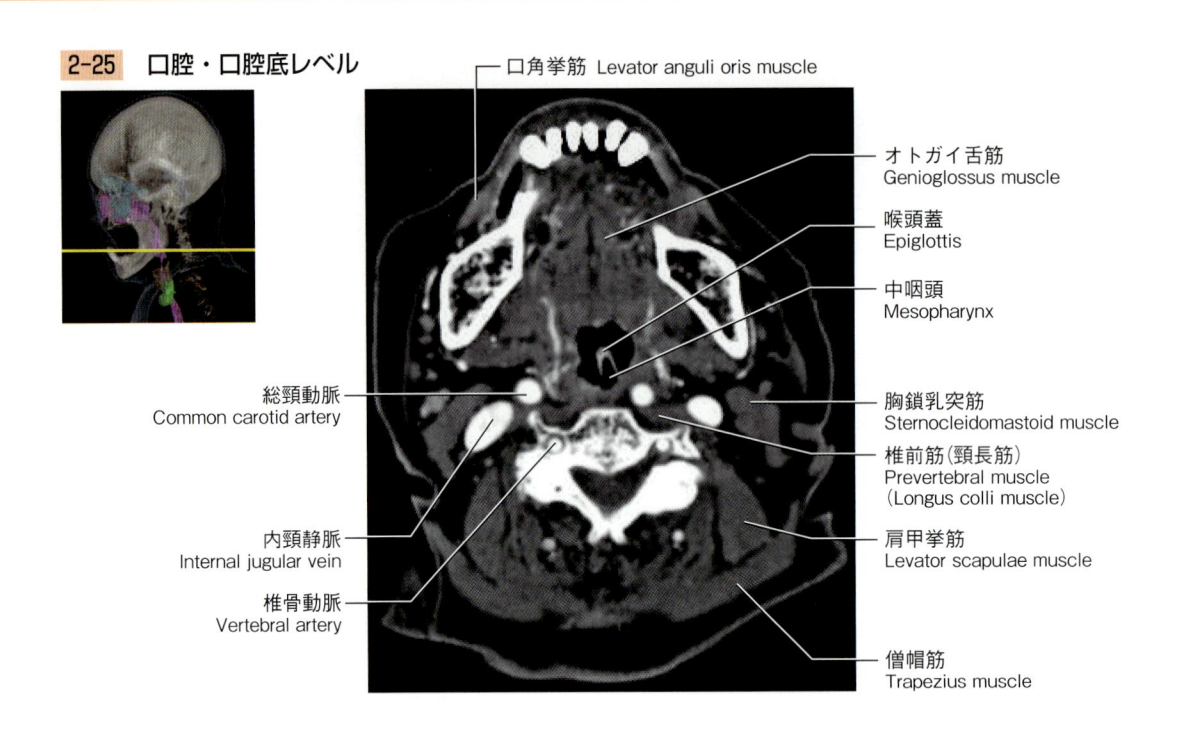

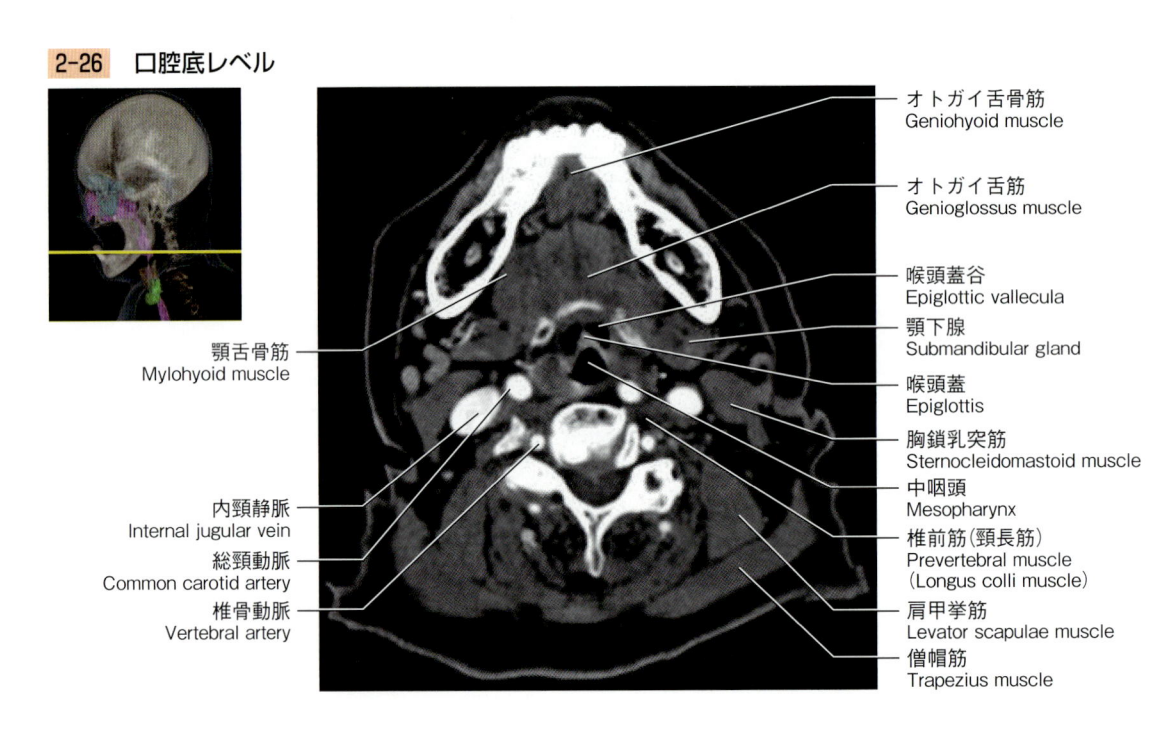

2-26 口腔底レベル

- オトガイ舌骨筋 Geniohyoid muscle
- オトガイ舌筋 Genioglossus muscle
- 喉頭蓋谷 Epiglottic vallecula
- 顎下腺 Submandibular gland
- 顎舌骨筋 Mylohyoid muscle
- 喉頭蓋 Epiglottis
- 胸鎖乳突筋 Sternocleidomastoid muscle
- 中咽頭 Mesopharynx
- 内頸静脈 Internal jugular vein
- 椎前筋（頸長筋） Prevertebral muscle（Longus colli muscle）
- 総頸動脈 Common carotid artery
- 肩甲挙筋 Levator scapulae muscle
- 椎骨動脈 Vertebral artery
- 僧帽筋 Trapezius muscle

NOTE 動脈硬化などにより一側あるいは両側の総頸動脈（もしくは内頸動脈）が咽頭後間隙を走行することがあり，"Ectatic carotid artery"とよばれる．両側にみられる場合は"Kissing carotids"とよばれる．

頭頸部の断層解剖 ［横断像（造影 CT）］

2-27 口腔底レベル

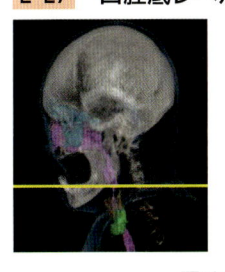

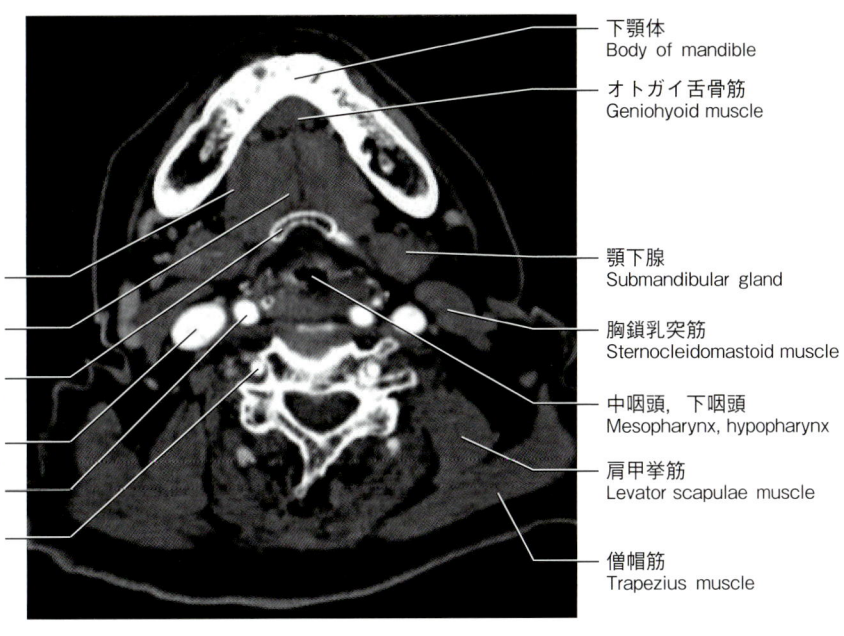

- 下顎体 Body of mandible
- オトガイ舌骨筋 Geniohyoid muscle
- 顎舌骨筋 Mylohyoid muscle
- オトガイ舌筋 Genioglossus muscle
- 舌骨 Hyoid bone
- 内頸静脈 Internal jugular vein
- 総頸動脈 Common carotid artery
- 椎骨動脈 Vertebral artery
- 顎下腺 Submandibular gland
- 胸鎖乳突筋 Sternocleidomastoid muscle
- 中咽頭，下咽頭 Mesopharynx, hypopharynx
- 肩甲挙筋 Levator scapulae muscle
- 僧帽筋 Trapezius muscle

2-28 口腔底レベル

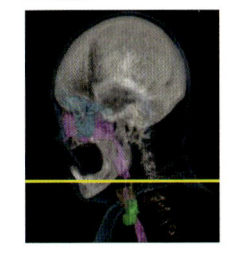

- 下顎体 Body of mandible
- 顎舌骨筋 Mylohyoid muscle
- オトガイ舌筋 Genioglossus muscle
- 舌骨下筋群 Infrahyoid muscles
- 内頸静脈 Internal jugular vein
- 総頸動脈 Common carotid artery
- 椎骨動脈 Vertebral artery
- 胸鎖乳突筋 Sternocleidomastoid muscle
- 下咽頭 Hypopharynx
- 肩甲挙筋 Levator scapulae muscle
- 僧帽筋 Trapezius muscle

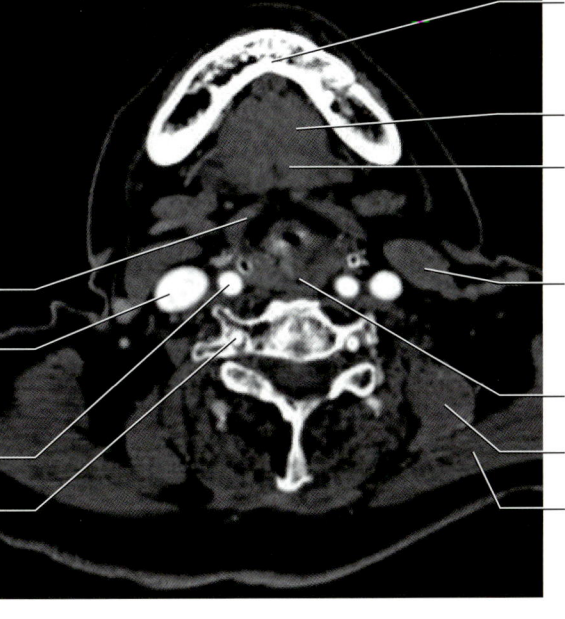

NOTE 頸動脈 Carotid artery

ラテン語の caros は「眠る」，「昏睡」の意味で，この動脈を圧迫すると意識がなくなることから，両者に強い関連を感じて Carotid artery と名付けたとされる（84, 88 頁の NOTE を参照）．

頭頸部の断層解剖 ［横断像（造影 CT）］

2-29 口腔底レベル

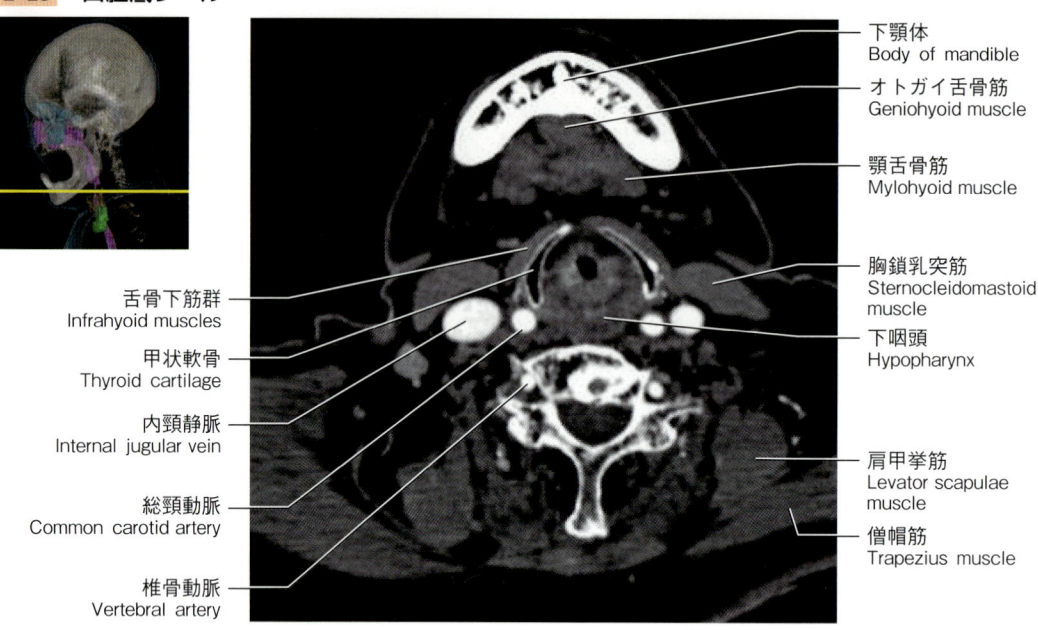

- 下顎体 Body of mandible
- オトガイ舌骨筋 Geniohyoid muscle
- 顎舌骨筋 Mylohyoid muscle
- 胸鎖乳突筋 Sternocleidomastoid muscle
- 下咽頭 Hypopharynx
- 肩甲挙筋 Levator scapulae muscle
- 僧帽筋 Trapezius muscle
- 舌骨下筋群 Infrahyoid muscles
- 甲状軟骨 Thyroid cartilage
- 内頸静脈 Internal jugular vein
- 総頸動脈 Common carotid artery
- 椎骨動脈 Vertebral artery

2-30 下顎骨下縁レベル

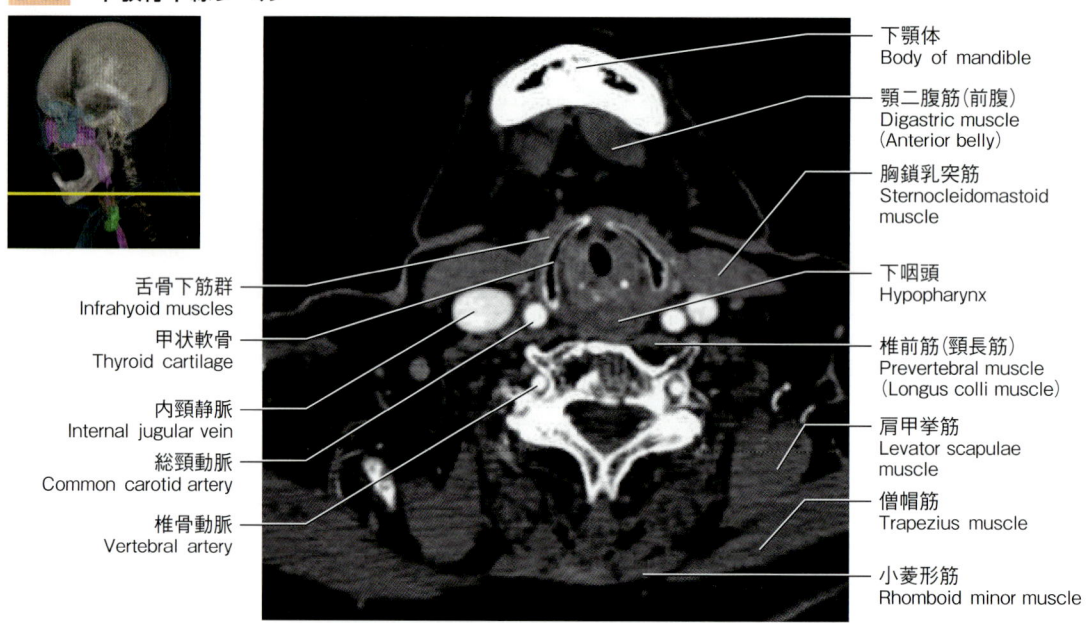

- 下顎体 Body of mandible
- 顎二腹筋（前腹） Digastric muscle (Anterior belly)
- 胸鎖乳突筋 Sternocleidomastoid muscle
- 下咽頭 Hypopharynx
- 椎前筋（頸長筋） Prevertebral muscle (Longus colli muscle)
- 肩甲挙筋 Levator scapulae muscle
- 僧帽筋 Trapezius muscle
- 小菱形筋 Rhomboid minor muscle
- 舌骨下筋群 Infrahyoid muscles
- 甲状軟骨 Thyroid cartilage
- 内頸静脈 Internal jugular vein
- 総頸動脈 Common carotid artery
- 椎骨動脈 Vertebral artery

NOTE 頸静脈 Jugular vein

ラテン語の jugularis，iugulum は「首」，「咽」の意．carotid が動作・行為を表す語であるのに対し，jugular は部位を表す語（83，88 頁の NOTE を参照）．

頭頸部の断層解剖 ［横断像（造影CT）］

2-31 声門レベル

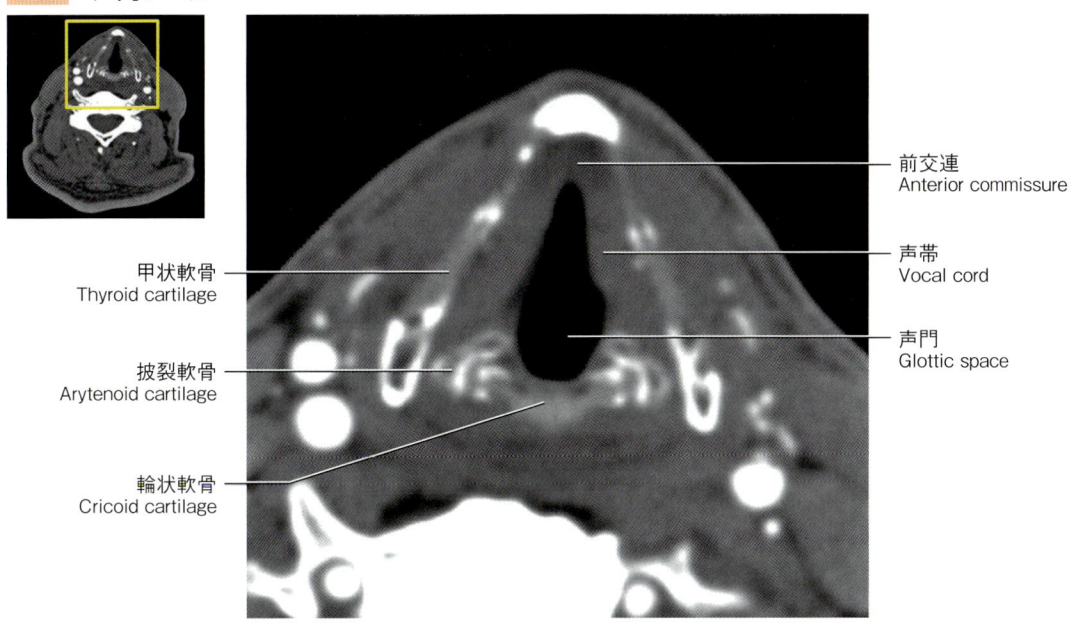

- 甲状軟骨 Thyroid cartilage
- 披裂軟骨 Arytenoid cartilage
- 輪状軟骨 Cricoid cartilage
- 前交連 Anterior commissure
- 声帯 Vocal cord
- 声門 Glottic space

2-32 下顎骨下縁レベル

- 胸鎖乳突筋 Sternocleidomastoid muscle
- 鎖骨 Clavicle
- 内頸静脈 Internal jugular vein
- 甲状軟骨 Thyroid cartilage
- 総頸動脈 Common carotid artery
- 椎骨動脈 Vertebral artery
- 輪状軟骨 Cricoid cartilage
- 下咽頭 Hypopharynx
- 椎前筋（頸長筋） Prevertebral muscle（Longus colli muscle）
- 肩甲挙筋 Levator scapulae muscle
- 僧帽筋 Trapezius muscle
- 小菱形筋 Rhomboid minor muscle

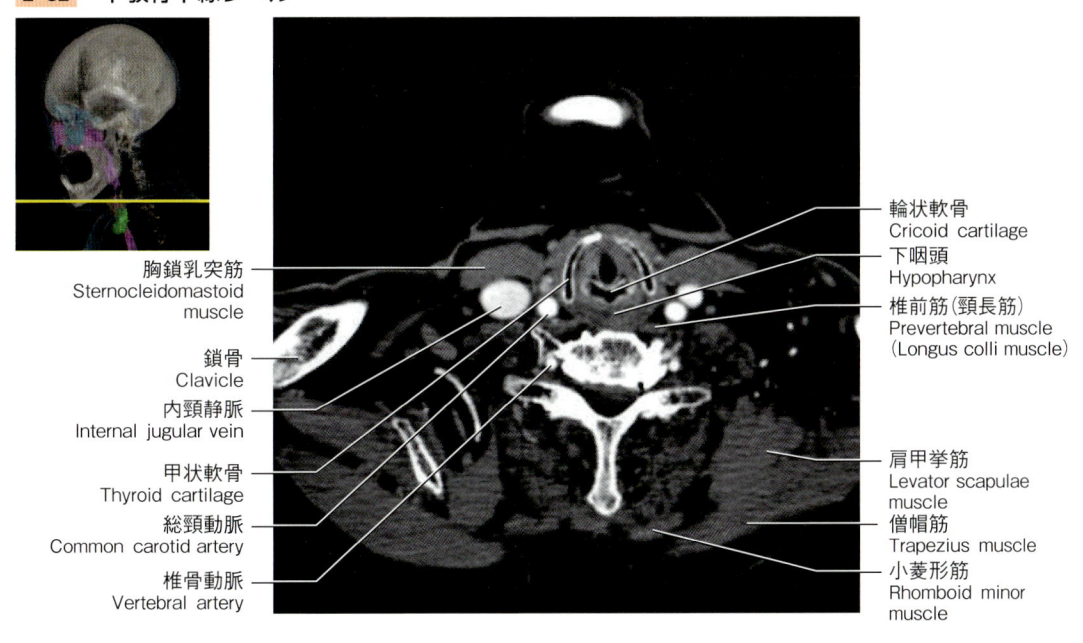

NOTE 喉頭軟骨には甲状軟骨・輪状軟骨・披裂軟骨・角状軟骨・楔状軟骨・喉頭蓋軟骨がある．披裂軟骨は声門の開閉に関与しており，発声に最も重要な軟骨である．

頭頸部の断層解剖［横断像（造影 CT）］

2-33 鎖骨上窩レベル

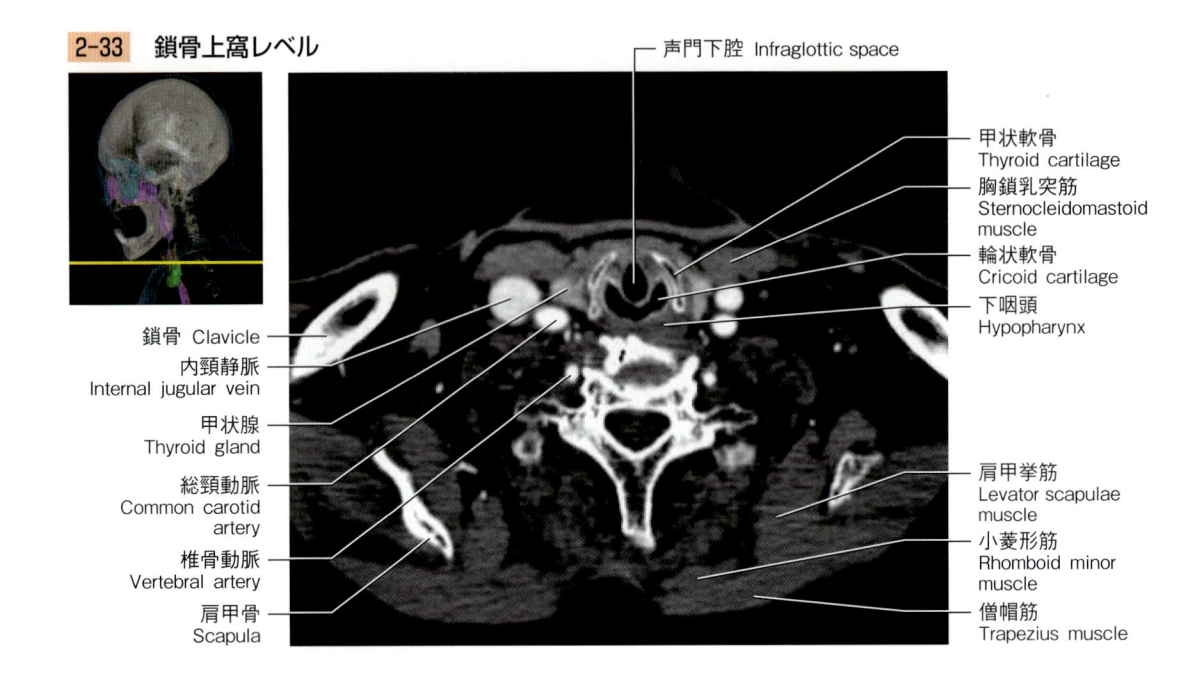

ラベル:
- 声門下腔 Infraglottic space
- 甲状軟骨 Thyroid cartilage
- 胸鎖乳突筋 Sternocleidomastoid muscle
- 輪状軟骨 Cricoid cartilage
- 下咽頭 Hypopharynx
- 肩甲挙筋 Levator scapulae muscle
- 小菱形筋 Rhomboid minor muscle
- 僧帽筋 Trapezius muscle
- 鎖骨 Clavicle
- 内頸静脈 Internal jugular vein
- 甲状腺 Thyroid gland
- 総頸動脈 Common carotid artery
- 椎骨動脈 Vertebral artery
- 肩甲骨 Scapula

2-34 鎖骨上窩レベル

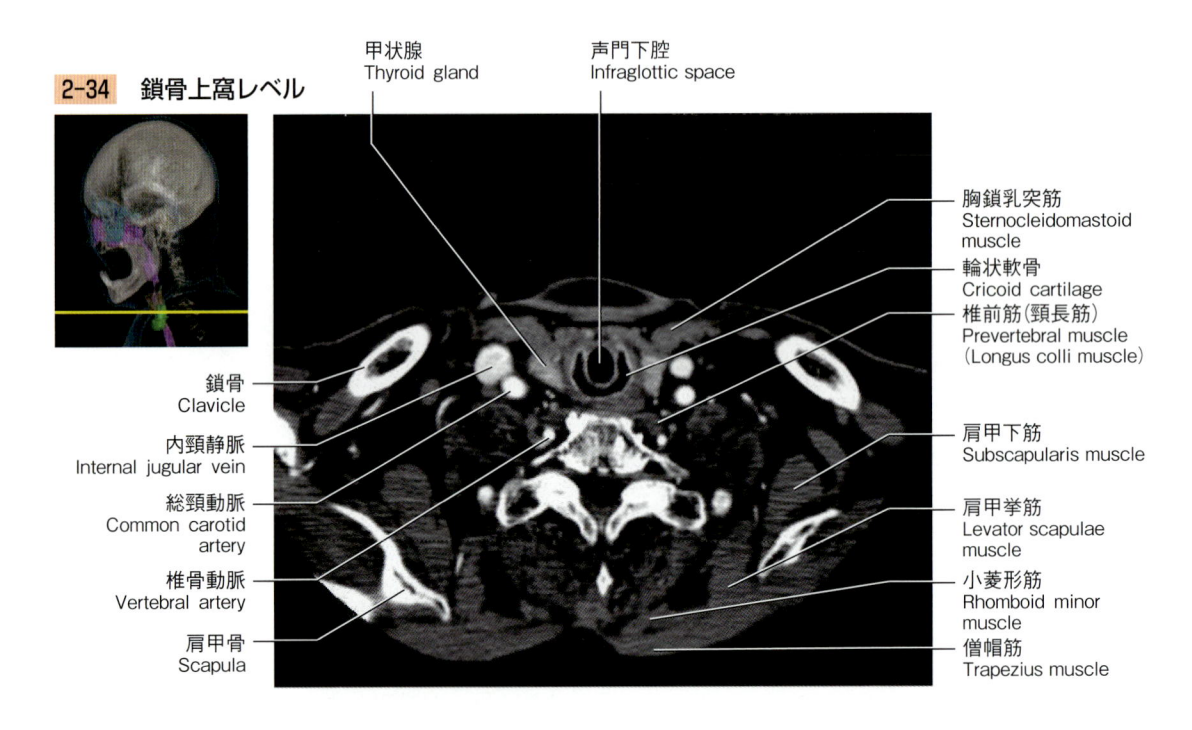

ラベル:
- 甲状腺 Thyroid gland
- 声門下腔 Infraglottic space
- 胸鎖乳突筋 Sternocleidomastoid muscle
- 輪状軟骨 Cricoid cartilage
- 椎前筋（頸長筋）Prevertebral muscle (Longus colli muscle)
- 肩甲下筋 Subscapularis muscle
- 肩甲挙筋 Levator scapulae muscle
- 小菱形筋 Rhomboid minor muscle
- 僧帽筋 Trapezius muscle
- 鎖骨 Clavicle
- 内頸静脈 Internal jugular vein
- 総頸動脈 Common carotid artery
- 椎骨動脈 Vertebral artery
- 肩甲骨 Scapula

> **NOTE 僧帽筋 Trapezius（muscle）**
> Trapezius（muscle）は，いずれの辺も平行でない四辺形を表す trapezium（ギリシャ語）からきた語．背部にあるこの筋は左右2つを合わせると不平行四辺形を呈する．日本名はドイツ語の Kapuzenmuskel の訳であり，Kapuze は頭巾，フード付きマントを表す．カトリック フランチェスコ派の貧しい僧衣についた帽子で，心臓の僧帽弁（Mitral valve）とはまったく異なる僧帽（223 頁の NOTE も参照）．

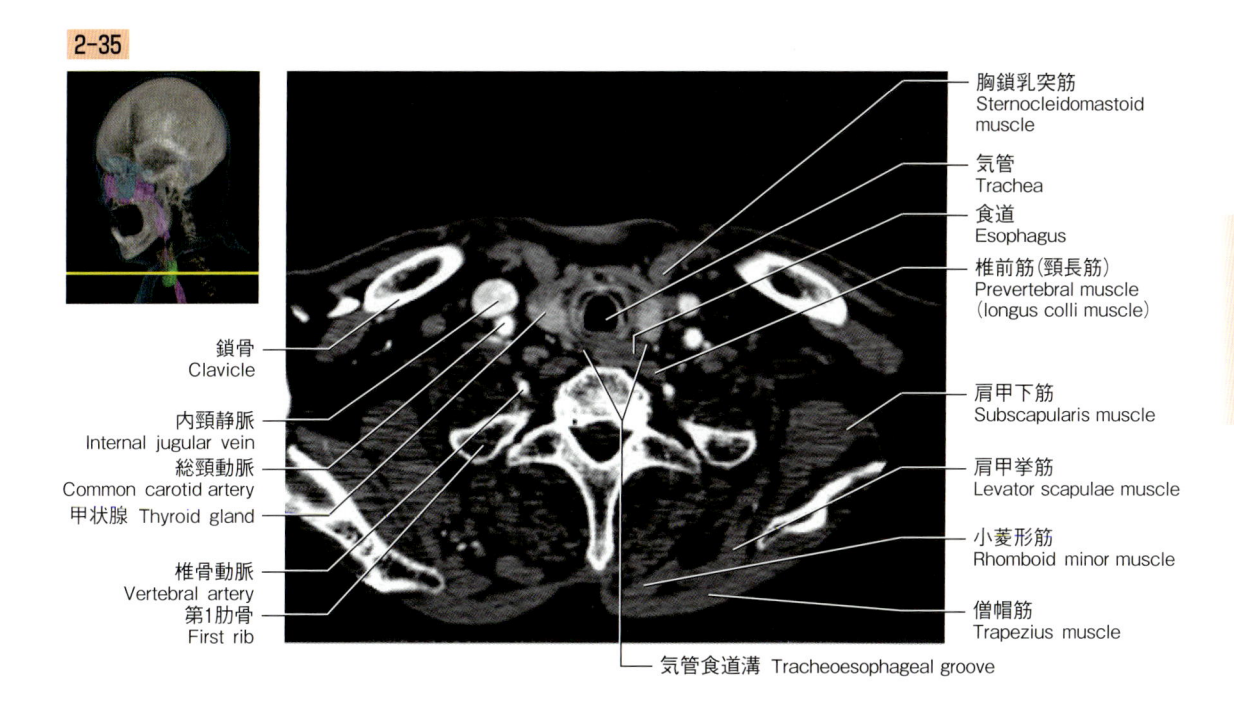

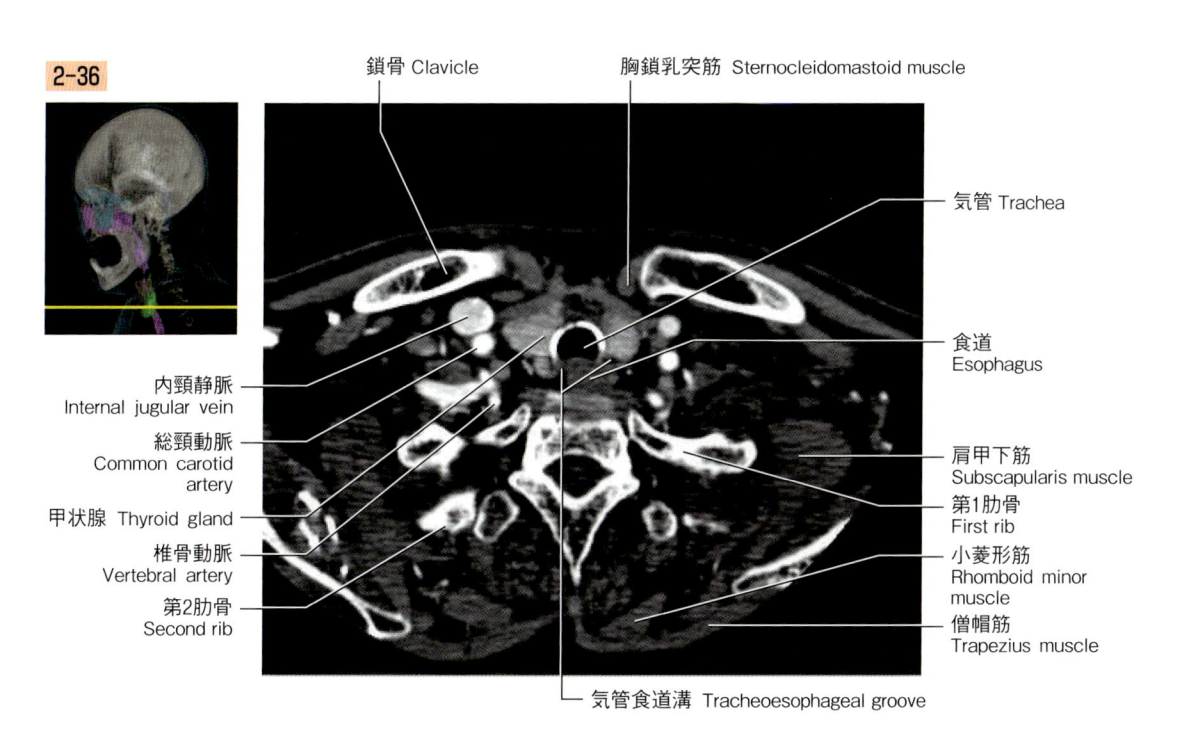

頭頸部の断層解剖 ［横断像（造影CT）］

2-35

- 胸鎖乳突筋 Sternocleidomastoid muscle
- 気管 Trachea
- 食道 Esophagus
- 椎前筋（頸長筋）Prevertebral muscle (longus colli muscle)
- 肩甲下筋 Subscapularis muscle
- 肩甲挙筋 Levator scapulae muscle
- 小菱形筋 Rhomboid minor muscle
- 僧帽筋 Trapezius muscle
- 鎖骨 Clavicle
- 内頸静脈 Internal jugular vein
- 総頸動脈 Common carotid artery
- 甲状腺 Thyroid gland
- 椎骨動脈 Vertebral artery
- 第1肋骨 First rib
- 気管食道溝 Tracheoesophageal groove

2-36

- 鎖骨 Clavicle
- 胸鎖乳突筋 Sternocleidomastoid muscle
- 気管 Trachea
- 食道 Esophagus
- 肩甲下筋 Subscapularis muscle
- 第1肋骨 First rib
- 小菱形筋 Rhomboid minor muscle
- 僧帽筋 Trapezius muscle
- 内頸静脈 Internal jugular vein
- 総頸動脈 Common carotid artery
- 甲状腺 Thyroid gland
- 椎骨動脈 Vertebral artery
- 第2肋骨 Second rib
- 気管食道溝 Tracheoesophageal groove

NOTE 反回神経は，右は鎖骨下動脈，左は大動脈弓部下面を反回したのち，同側の気管食道溝に沿って上行する．

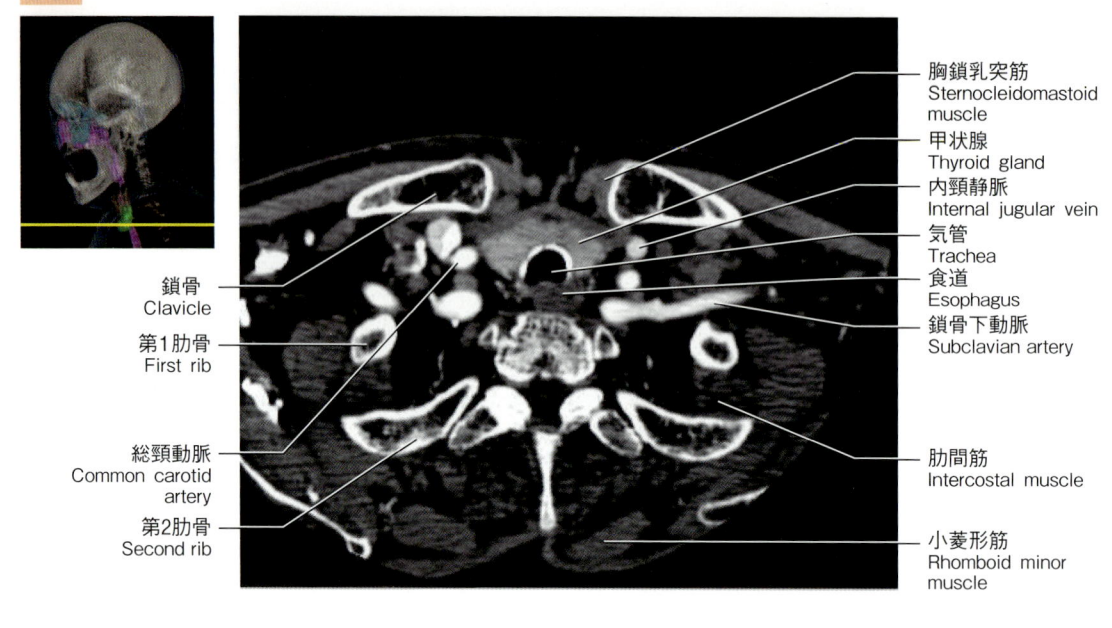

頭頸部の断層解剖　[横断像（造影CT）]

2-37

- 胸鎖乳突筋 Sternocleidomastoid muscle
- 甲状腺 Thyroid gland
- 内頸静脈 Internal jugular vein
- 気管 Trachea
- 食道 Esophagus
- 鎖骨下動脈 Subclavian artery
- 肋間筋 Intercostal muscle
- 小菱形筋 Rhomboid minor muscle
- 鎖骨 Clavicle
- 第1肋骨 First rib
- 総頸動脈 Common carotid artery
- 第2肋骨 Second rib

> **NOTE** 伴行静脈　Accompanying vein, Companion vein
> 　体循環の静脈は浅静脈と深静脈に分かれ，深静脈は一般に同名動脈に伴行し，通常，同名動脈より太く，逆転すると病的状態である（252頁のNOTEを参照）．頸部の動静脈は，"Carotid artery"と"Jugular vein"と別の名をもつ．古くからすでに広く一般に使われている用語を後世の解剖学者が統一化することは至難であったのか．頸部血管は神への生贄（いけにえ）処理の際に重要な臓器であっただろうと想像は尽きない（83, 84頁のNOTEを参照）．

頭頸部の断層解剖 ［矢状断像（造影CT）］

2-38 大頬骨弓やや内側

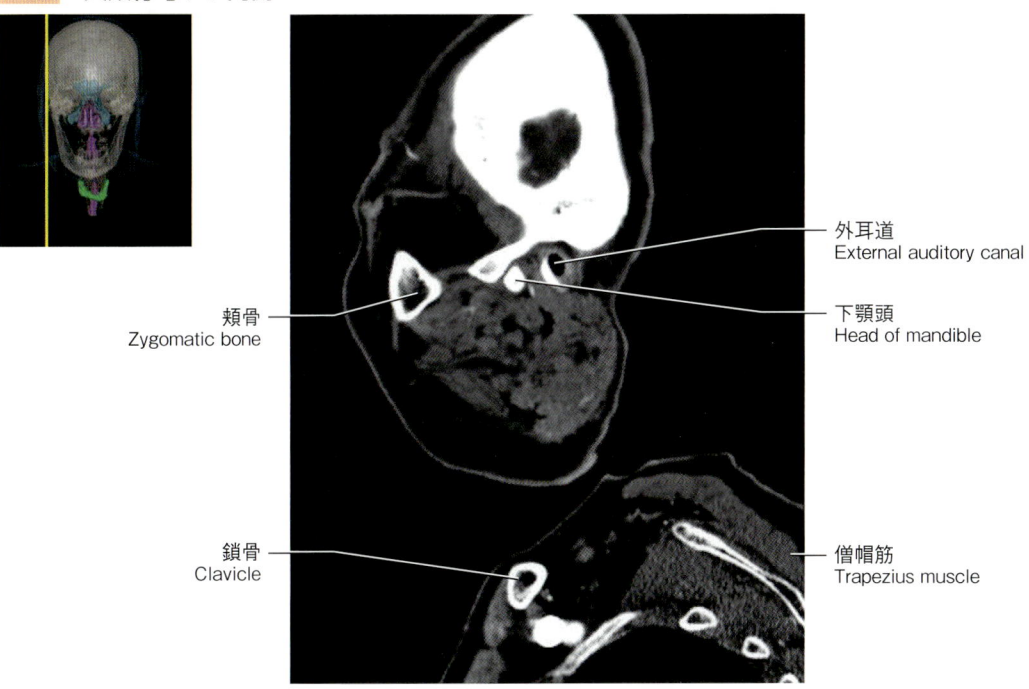

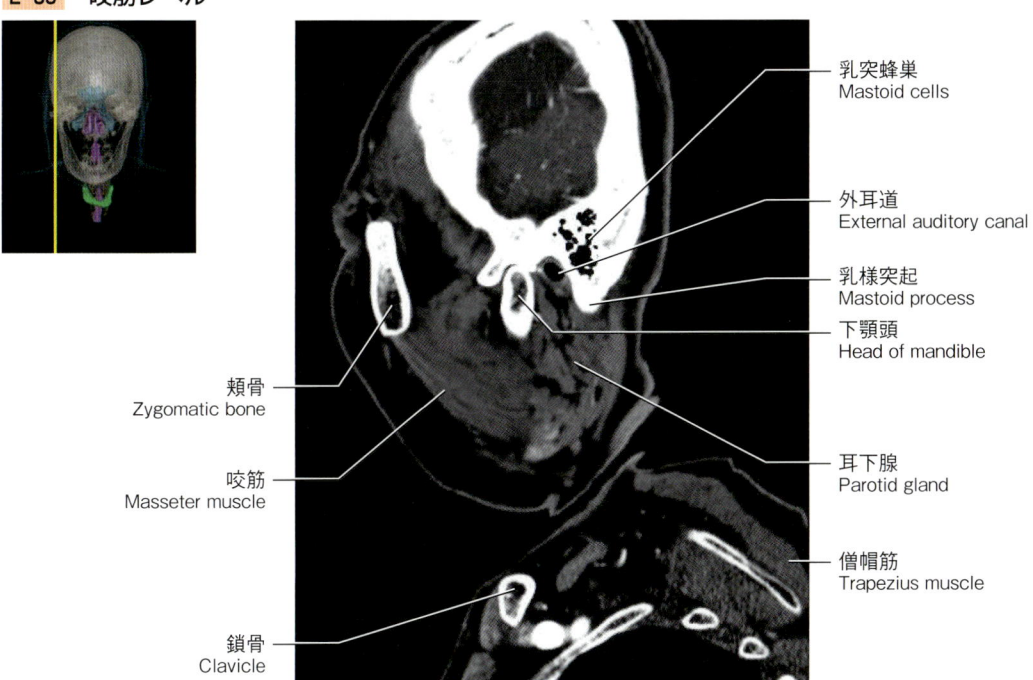

- 頬骨 / Zygomatic bone
- 外耳道 / External auditory canal
- 下顎頭 / Head of mandible
- 鎖骨 / Clavicle
- 僧帽筋 / Trapezius muscle

2-39 咬筋レベル

- 乳突蜂巣 / Mastoid cells
- 外耳道 / External auditory canal
- 乳様突起 / Mastoid process
- 下顎頭 / Head of mandible
- 頬骨 / Zygomatic bone
- 咬筋 / Masseter muscle
- 耳下腺 / Parotid gland
- 僧帽筋 / Trapezius muscle
- 鎖骨 / Clavicle

NOTE 咬筋の起始は頬骨弓，停止は下顎枝・下顎角・下顎体後部の外側縁であり，下顎骨の挙上を担う．

頭頸部の断層解剖 ［矢状断像（造影 CT）］

2-40 顎関節レベル

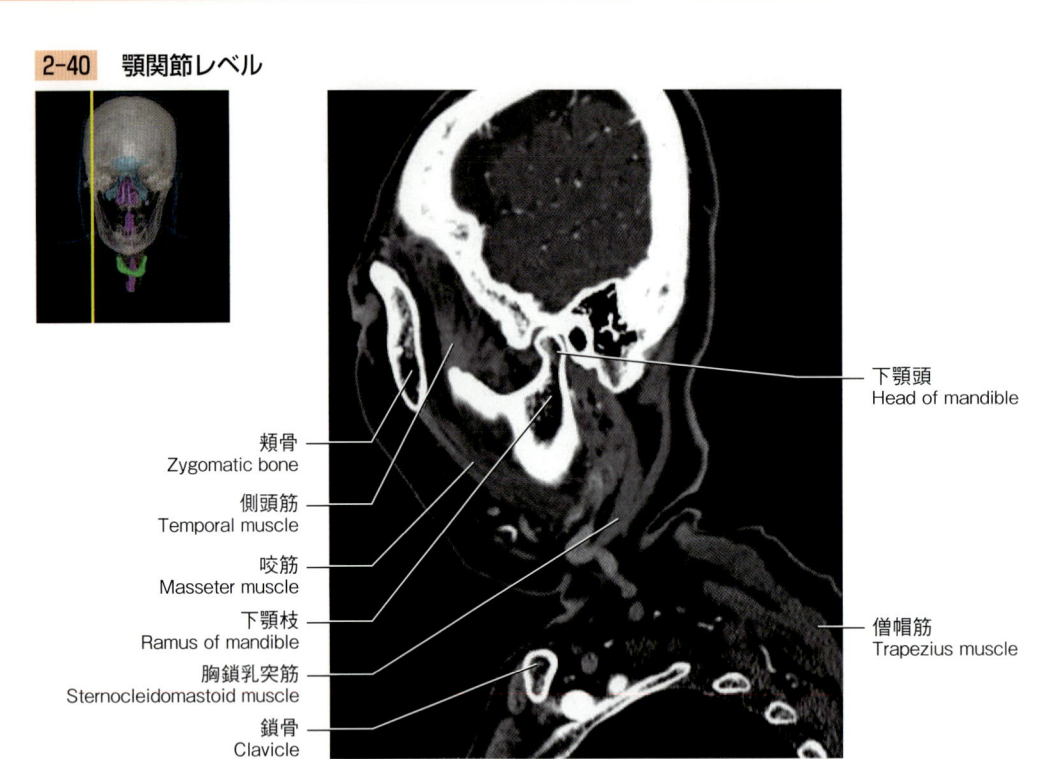

- 頬骨 / Zygomatic bone
- 側頭筋 / Temporal muscle
- 咬筋 / Masseter muscle
- 下顎枝 / Ramus of mandible
- 胸鎖乳突筋 / Sternocleidomastoid muscle
- 鎖骨 / Clavicle
- 下顎頭 / Head of mandible
- 僧帽筋 / Trapezius muscle

2-41 顎関節レベル

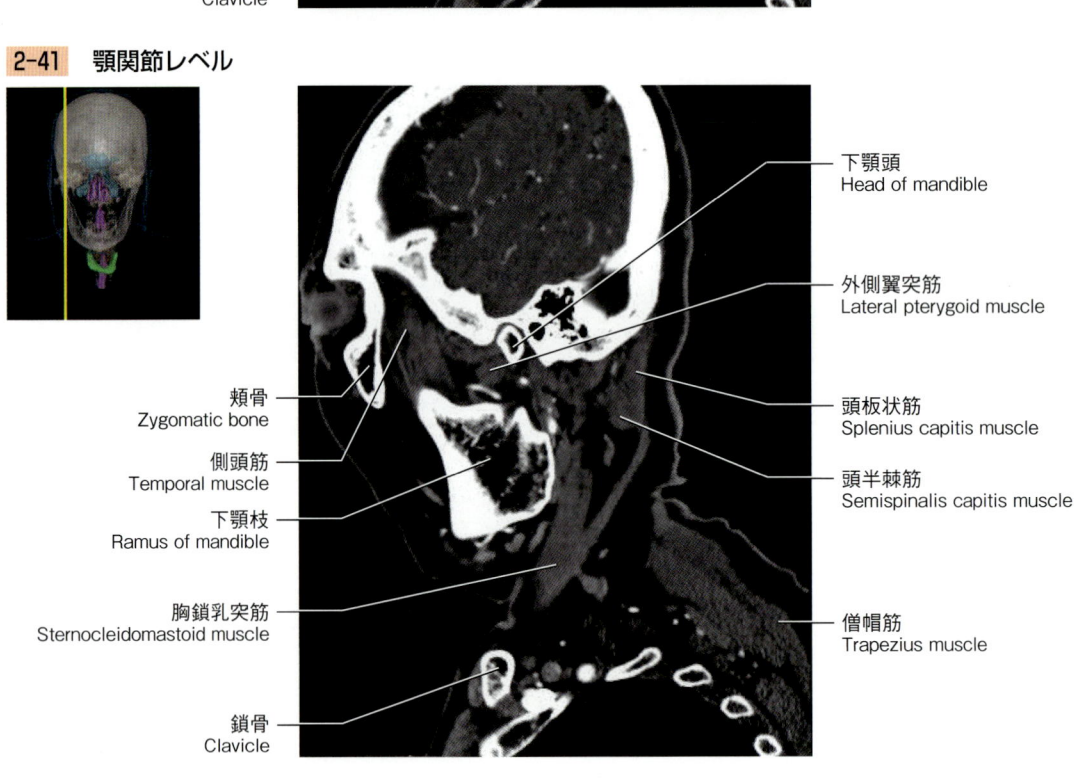

- 頬骨 / Zygomatic bone
- 側頭筋 / Temporal muscle
- 下顎枝 / Ramus of mandible
- 胸鎖乳突筋 / Sternocleidomastoid muscle
- 鎖骨 / Clavicle
- 下顎頭 / Head of mandible
- 外側翼突筋 / Lateral pterygoid muscle
- 頭板状筋 / Splenius capitis muscle
- 頭半棘筋 / Semispinalis capitis muscle
- 僧帽筋 / Trapezius muscle

NOTE 側頭筋の起始は側頭窩，停止は下顎角筋突起，下顎枝前縁である．下顎を挙上し後方へ引く作用を有する．

頭頸部の断層解剖 ［矢状断像（造影CT）］

2-42 下顎角レベル

- 硝子体 Vitreous body
- 側頭筋 Temporal muscle
- 外側翼突筋 Lateral pterygoid muscle
- 顎二腹筋（後腹） Digastric muscle (Posterior belly)
- 頭板状筋 Splenius capitis muscle
- 頭半棘筋 Semispinalis capitis muscle
- 内側翼突筋 Medial pterygoid muscle
- 僧帽筋 Trapezius muscle
- 内頸静脈 Internal jugular vein
- 水晶体 Lens
- 眼球 Eyeball
- 頬骨 Zygomatic bone
- 下顎枝 Ramus of mandible
- 下顎管 Mandibular canal
- 下顎角 Angle of mandible
- 胸鎖乳突筋 Sternocleidomastoid muscle
- 鎖骨 Clavicle

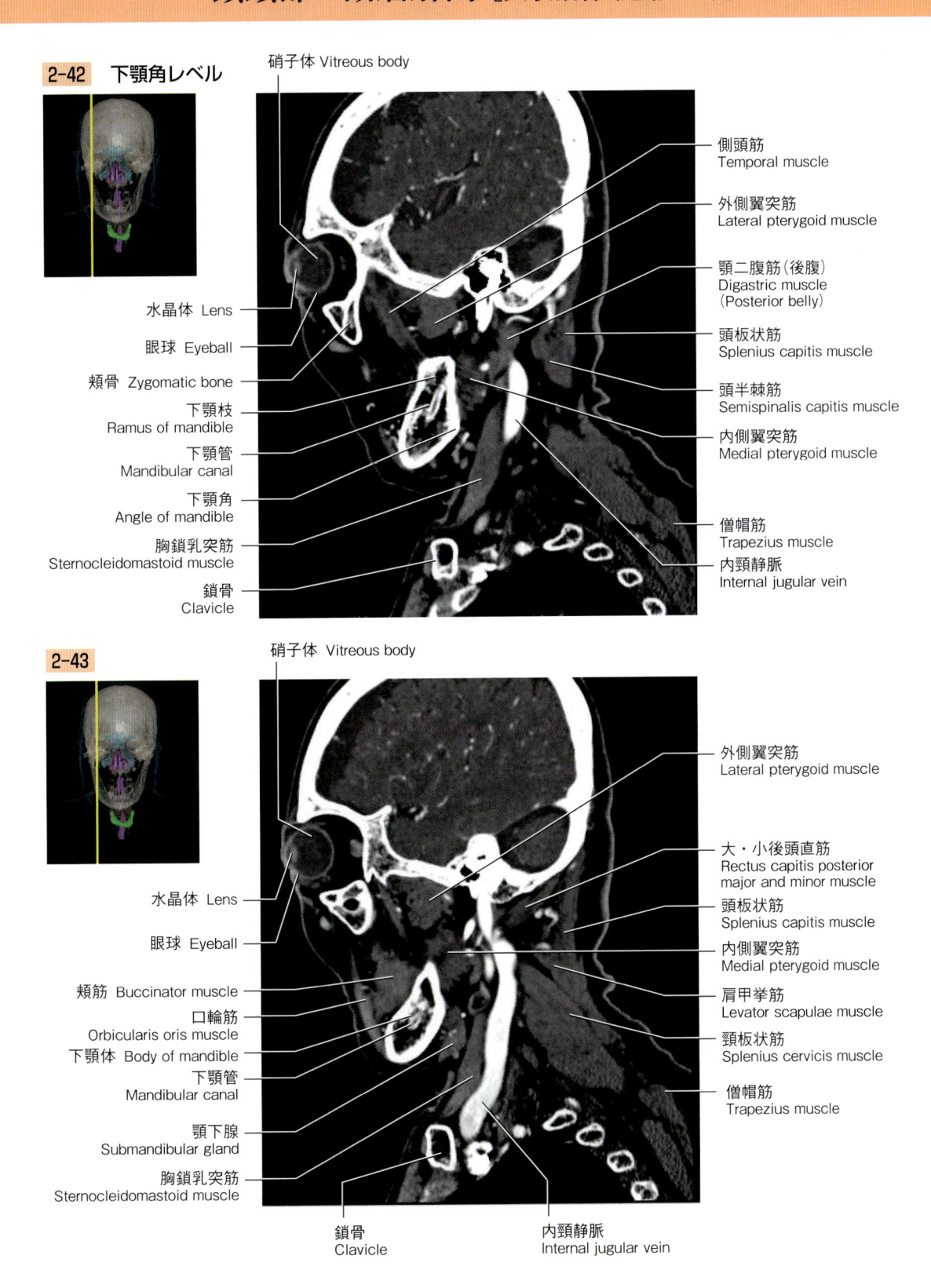

2-43

- 硝子体 Vitreous body
- 外側翼突筋 Lateral pterygoid muscle
- 大・小後頭直筋 Rectus capitis posterior major and minor muscle
- 頭板状筋 Splenius capitis muscle
- 内側翼突筋 Medial pterygoid muscle
- 肩甲挙筋 Levator scapulae muscle
- 頸板状筋 Splenius cervicis muscle
- 僧帽筋 Trapezius muscle
- 水晶体 Lens
- 眼球 Eyeball
- 頬筋 Buccinator muscle
- 口輪筋 Orbicularis oris muscle
- 下顎体 Body of mandible
- 下顎管 Mandibular canal
- 顎下腺 Submandibular gland
- 胸鎖乳突筋 Sternocleidomastoid muscle
- 鎖骨 Clavicle
- 内頸静脈 Internal jugular vein

NOTE 下顎管内には下歯槽神経・下歯槽動脈・下歯槽静脈が走行している．下顎智歯や下顎第二大臼歯根尖部は下顎管近傍に位置しており，これらの歯科治療の際には注意が必要である．

頭頸部の断層解剖 ［矢状断像（造影 CT）］

2-44 下顎体・上顎洞レベル

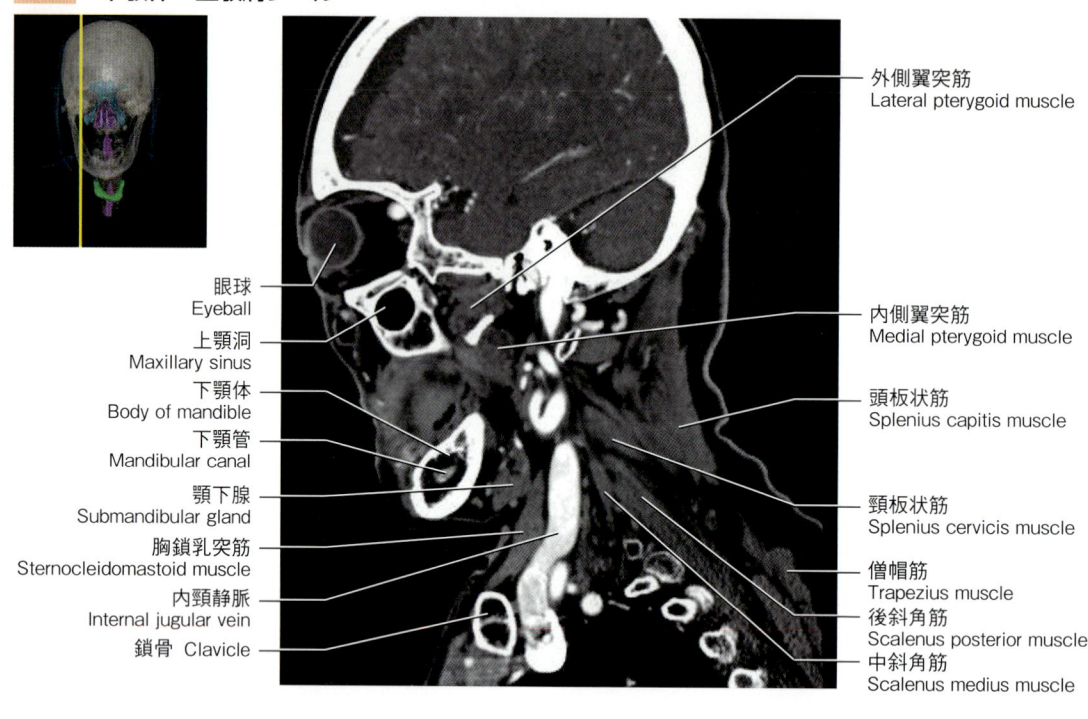

- 眼球 Eyeball
- 上顎洞 Maxillary sinus
- 下顎体 Body of mandible
- 下顎管 Mandibular canal
- 顎下腺 Submandibular gland
- 胸鎖乳突筋 Sternocleidomastoid muscle
- 内頸静脈 Internal jugular vein
- 鎖骨 Clavicle
- 外側翼突筋 Lateral pterygoid muscle
- 内側翼突筋 Medial pterygoid muscle
- 頭板状筋 Splenius capitis muscle
- 頸板状筋 Splenius cervicis muscle
- 僧帽筋 Trapezius muscle
- 後斜角筋 Scalenus posterior muscle
- 中斜角筋 Scalenus medius muscle

2-45 下顎体・上顎洞レベル

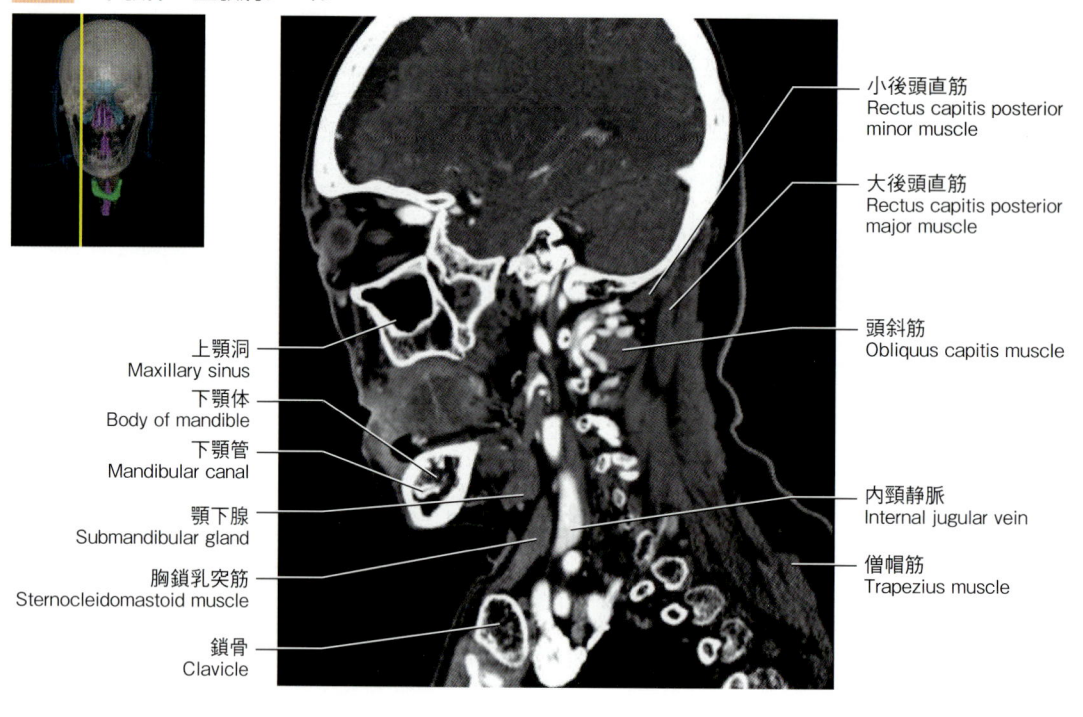

- 上顎洞 Maxillary sinus
- 下顎体 Body of mandible
- 下顎管 Mandibular canal
- 顎下腺 Submandibular gland
- 胸鎖乳突筋 Sternocleidomastoid muscle
- 鎖骨 Clavicle
- 小後頭直筋 Rectus capitis posterior minor muscle
- 大後頭直筋 Rectus capitis posterior major muscle
- 頭斜筋 Obliquus capitis muscle
- 内頸静脈 Internal jugular vein
- 僧帽筋 Trapezius muscle

頭頸部の断層解剖 ［矢状断像（造影CT）］

2-46　下顎体・上顎洞レベル

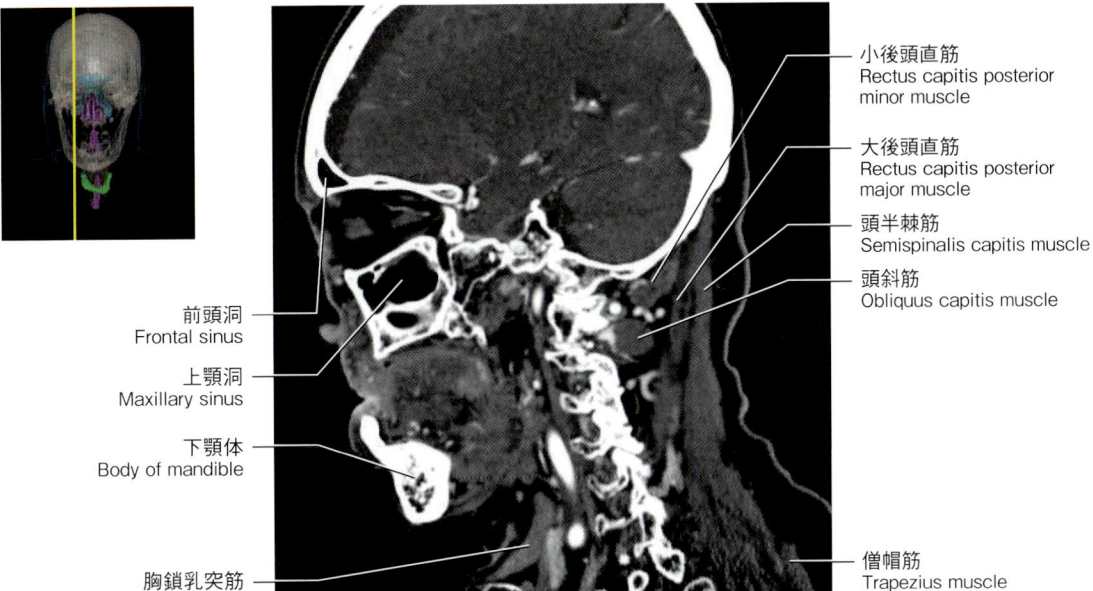

- 前頭洞　Frontal sinus
- 上顎洞　Maxillary sinus
- 下顎体　Body of mandible
- 胸鎖乳突筋　Sternocleidomastoid muscle
- 鎖骨　Clavicle
- 小後頭直筋　Rectus capitis posterior minor muscle
- 大後頭直筋　Rectus capitis posterior major muscle
- 頭半棘筋　Semispinalis capitis muscle
- 頭斜筋　Obliquus capitis muscle
- 僧帽筋　Trapezius muscle

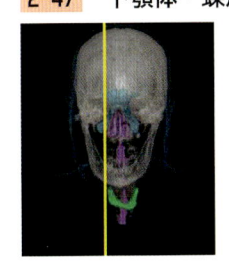

2-47　下顎体・蝶形骨洞レベル

- 前頭洞　Frontal sinus
- 顎舌骨筋　Mylohyoid muscle
- 下顎体　Body of mandible
- 顎二腹筋（前腹）　Digastric muscle (Anterior belly)
- 蝶形骨洞　Sphenoidal sinus
- 頭半棘筋　Semispinalis capitis muscle
- 頭斜筋　Obliquus capitis muscle
- 甲状腺　Thyroid gland

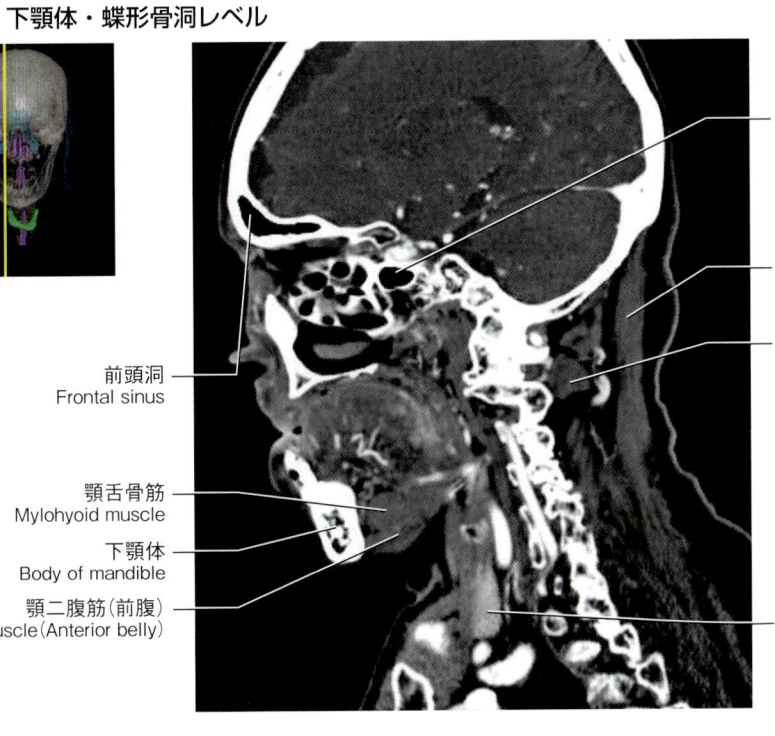

頭頸部の断層解剖 [矢状断像（造影CT）]

2-48 下顎体・篩骨洞レベル

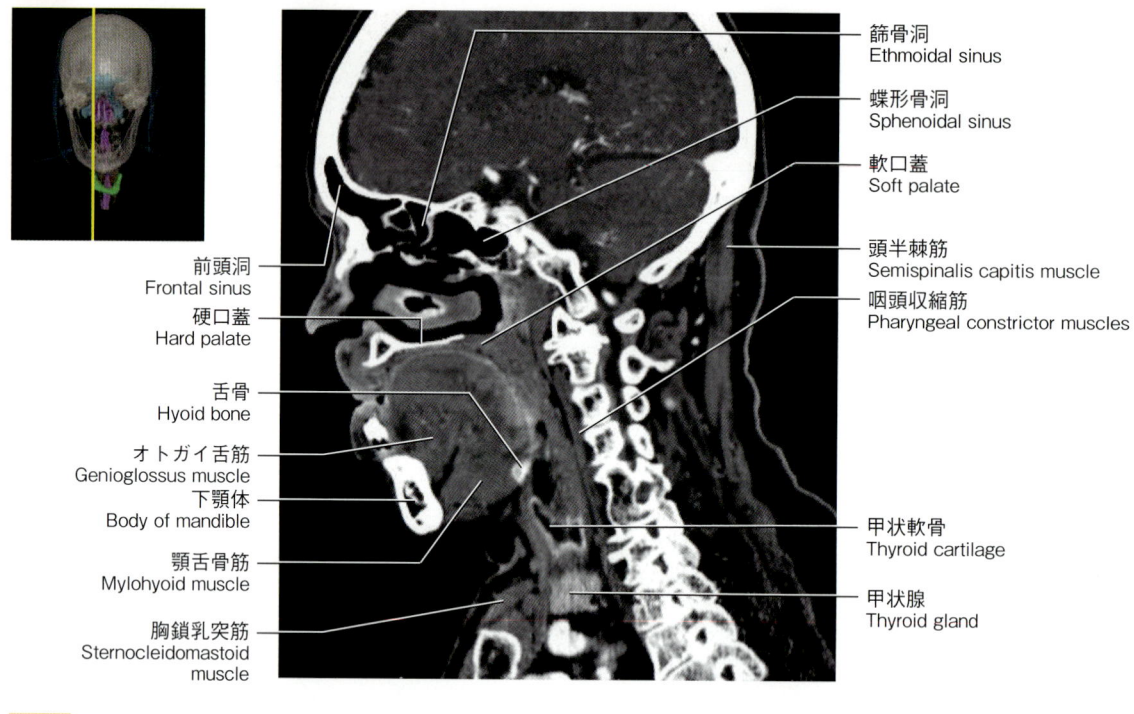

- 篩骨洞 / Ethmoidal sinus
- 蝶形骨洞 / Sphenoidal sinus
- 軟口蓋 / Soft palate
- 頭半棘筋 / Semispinalis capitis muscle
- 咽頭収縮筋 / Pharyngeal constrictor muscles
- 前頭洞 / Frontal sinus
- 硬口蓋 / Hard palate
- 舌骨 / Hyoid bone
- オトガイ舌筋 / Genioglossus muscle
- 下顎体 / Body of mandible
- 顎舌骨筋 / Mylohyoid muscle
- 胸鎖乳突筋 / Sternocleidomastoid muscle
- 甲状軟骨 / Thyroid cartilage
- 甲状腺 / Thyroid gland

2-49 下顎体・篩骨洞レベル

- 篩骨洞 / Ethmoidal sinus
- 蝶形骨洞 / Sphenoidal sinus
- 頭半棘筋 / Semispinalis capitis muscle
- 軟口蓋 / Soft palate
- 前頭洞 / Frontal sinus
- 硬口蓋 / Hard palate
- オトガイ舌筋 / Genioglossus muscle
- 舌骨 / Hyoid bone
- 下顎体 / Body of mandible
- 顎舌骨筋 / Mylohyoid muscle
- 甲状軟骨 / Thyroid cartilage
- 輪状軟骨 / Cricoid cartilage
- 気管 / Trachea

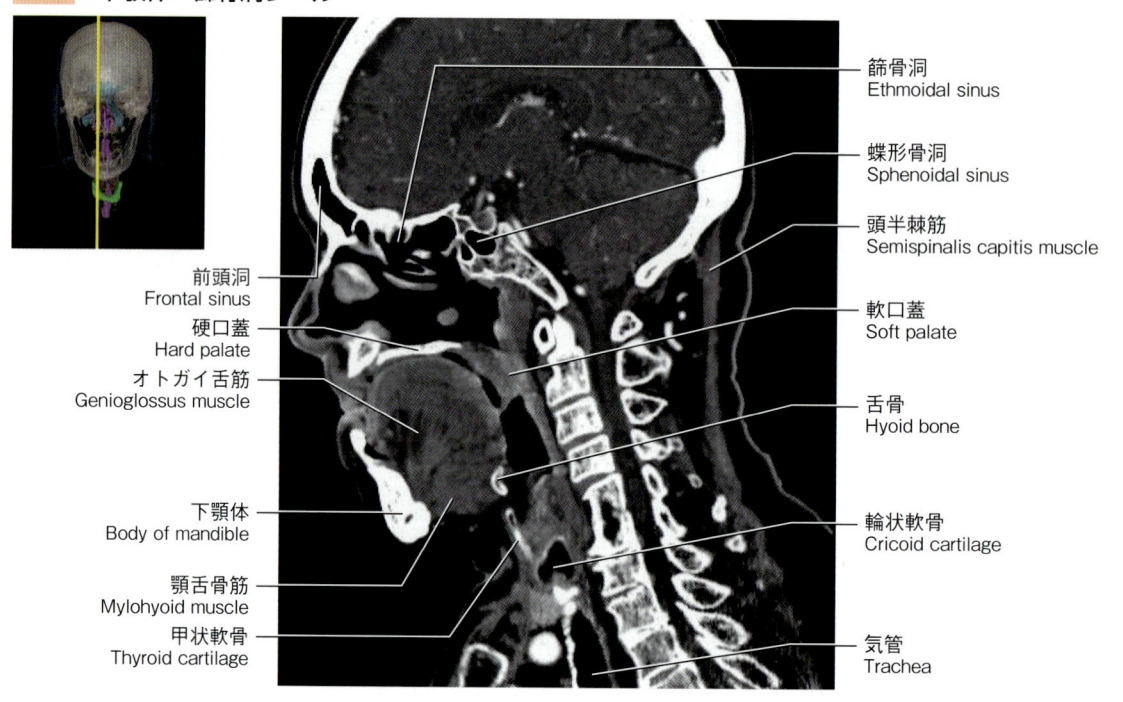

NOTE 舌骨・甲状軟骨間には甲状舌骨間膜が，甲状軟骨・輪状軟骨間には輪状甲状間膜があり，喉頭癌の喉頭外軟部組織浸潤の進展経路となる．

頭頸部の断層解剖　[矢状断像（造影CT）]

2-50　下顎体・蝶形骨洞レベル

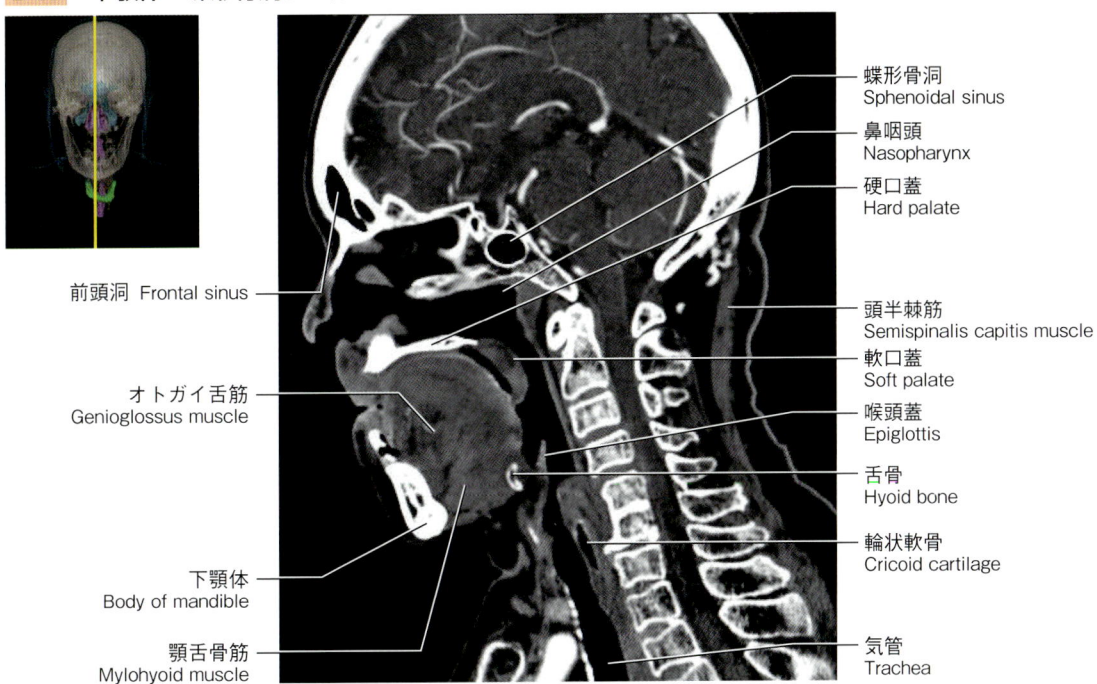

- 蝶形骨洞　Sphenoidal sinus
- 鼻咽頭　Nasopharynx
- 硬口蓋　Hard palate
- 前頭洞　Frontal sinus
- 頭半棘筋　Semispinalis capitis muscle
- 軟口蓋　Soft palate
- オトガイ舌筋　Genioglossus muscle
- 喉頭蓋　Epiglottis
- 舌骨　Hyoid bone
- 輪状軟骨　Cricoid cartilage
- 下顎体　Body of mandible
- 顎舌骨筋　Mylohyoid muscle
- 気管　Trachea

2-51　下顎体・蝶形骨洞・篩骨洞レベル

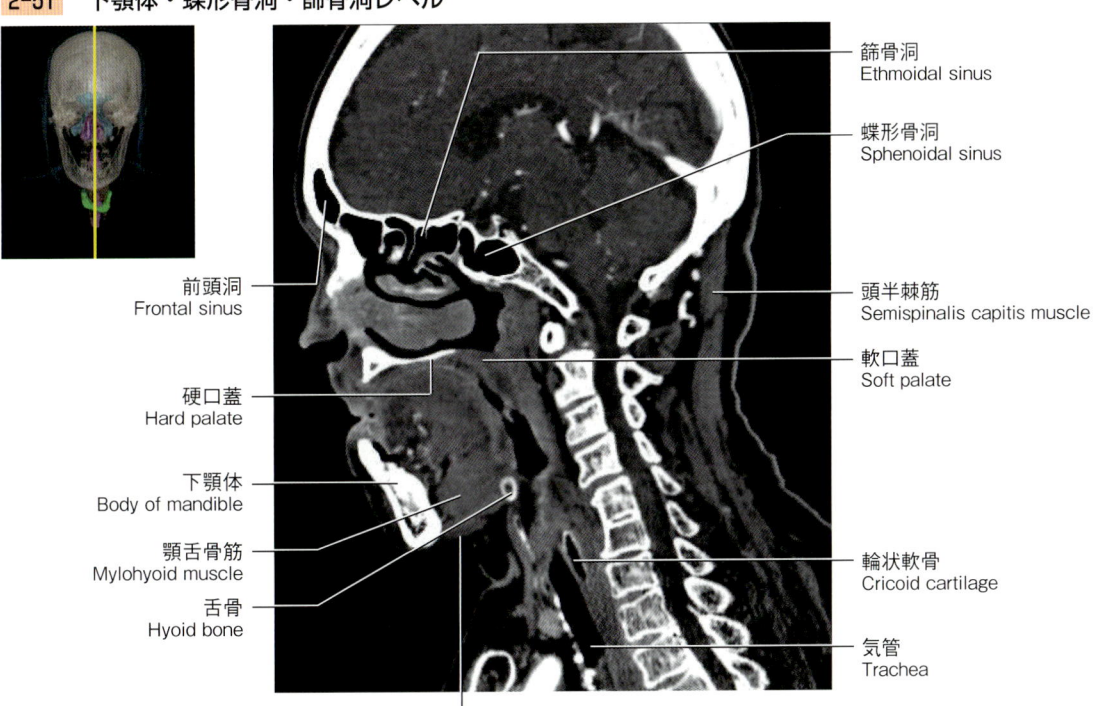

- 篩骨洞　Ethmoidal sinus
- 蝶形骨洞　Sphenoidal sinus
- 前頭洞　Frontal sinus
- 頭半棘筋　Semispinalis capitis muscle
- 軟口蓋　Soft palate
- 硬口蓋　Hard palate
- 下顎体　Body of mandible
- 顎舌骨筋　Mylohyoid muscle
- 輪状軟骨　Cricoid cartilage
- 舌骨　Hyoid bone
- 気管　Trachea
- 顎二腹筋（前腹）　Digastric muscle（Anterior belly）

NOTE 篩骨蜂巣のうち，蜂巣を前方・後方に区分する隔壁がいくつかあり，これらを基板とよぶ．第3基板は最も大きく，中鼻甲介をつり下げる．

頭頸部の断層解剖 ［冠状断像（造影 CT）］

2-52 眼窩口レベル

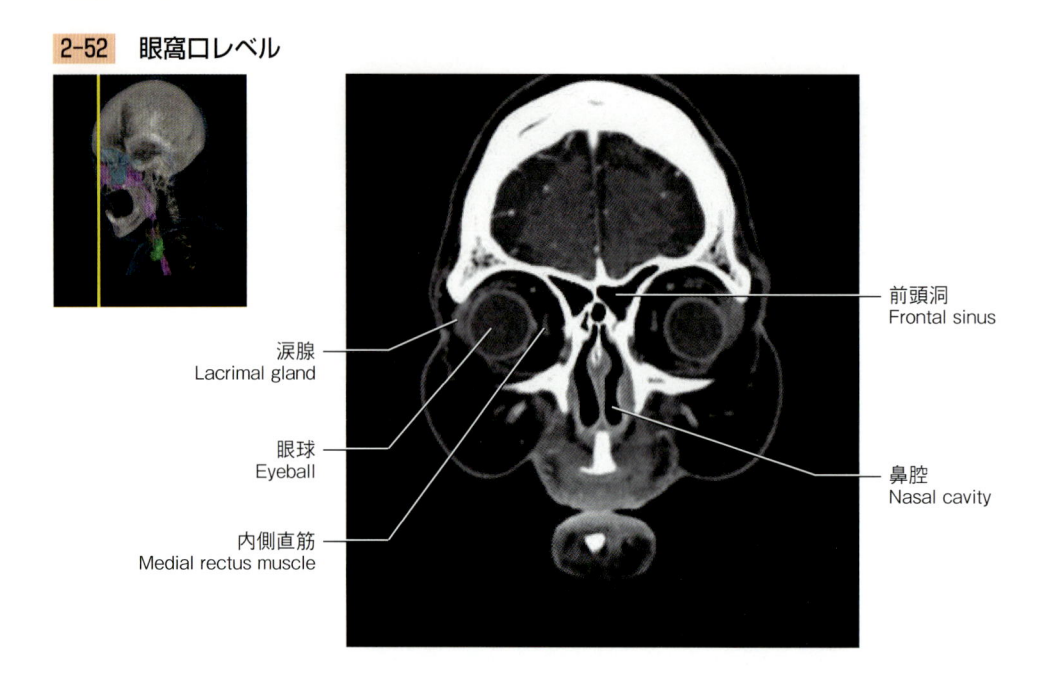

- 前頭洞 Frontal sinus
- 涙腺 Lacrimal gland
- 眼球 Eyeball
- 鼻腔 Nasal cavity
- 内側直筋 Medial rectus muscle

2-53

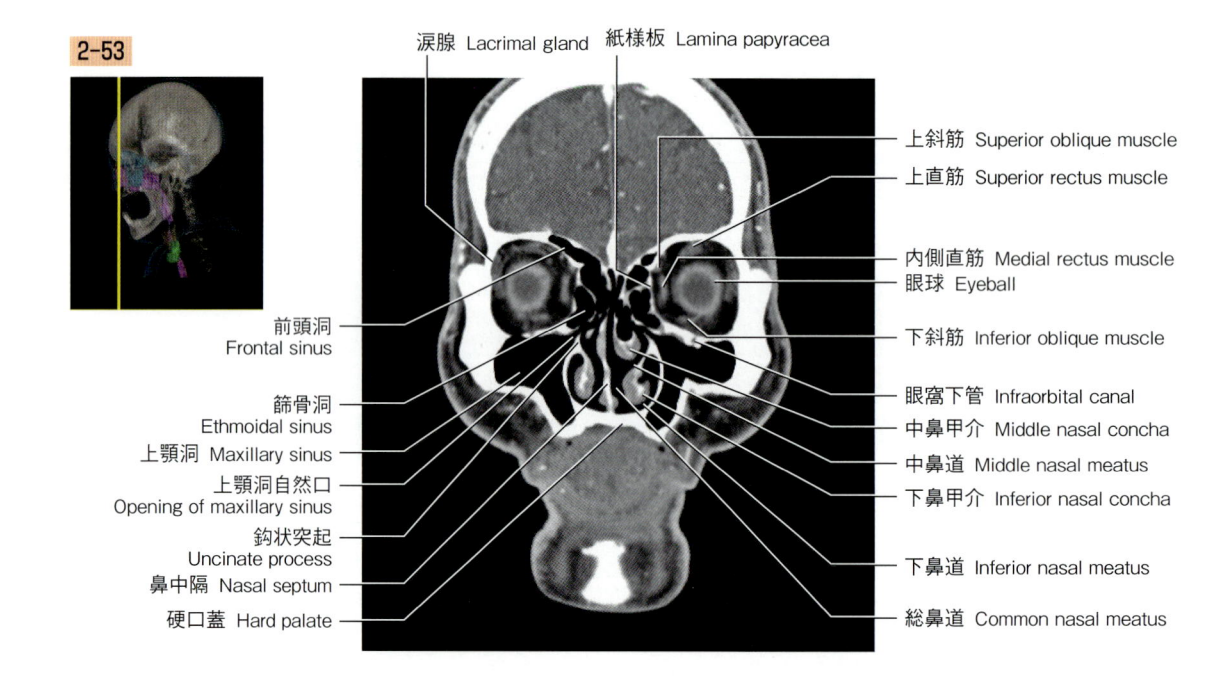

- 涙腺 Lacrimal gland
- 紙様板 Lamina papyracea
- 上斜筋 Superior oblique muscle
- 上直筋 Superior rectus muscle
- 内側直筋 Medial rectus muscle
- 眼球 Eyeball
- 下斜筋 Inferior oblique muscle
- 眼窩下管 Infraorbital canal
- 中鼻甲介 Middle nasal concha
- 中鼻道 Middle nasal meatus
- 下鼻甲介 Inferior nasal concha
- 下鼻道 Inferior nasal meatus
- 総鼻道 Common nasal meatus
- 前頭洞 Frontal sinus
- 篩骨洞 Ethmoidal sinus
- 上顎洞 Maxillary sinus
- 上顎洞自然口 Opening of maxillary sinus
- 鈎状突起 Uncinate process
- 鼻中隔 Nasal septum
- 硬口蓋 Hard palate

NOTE 眼窩骨折の好発部位は，下壁・側壁である．眼窩脂肪織脱出や外眼筋の牽引のほか，下壁では眼窩下管損傷にも留意する（眼窩下管内を眼窩下神経，眼窩下動脈が走行する）．

頭頸部の断層解剖［冠状断像（造影 CT）］

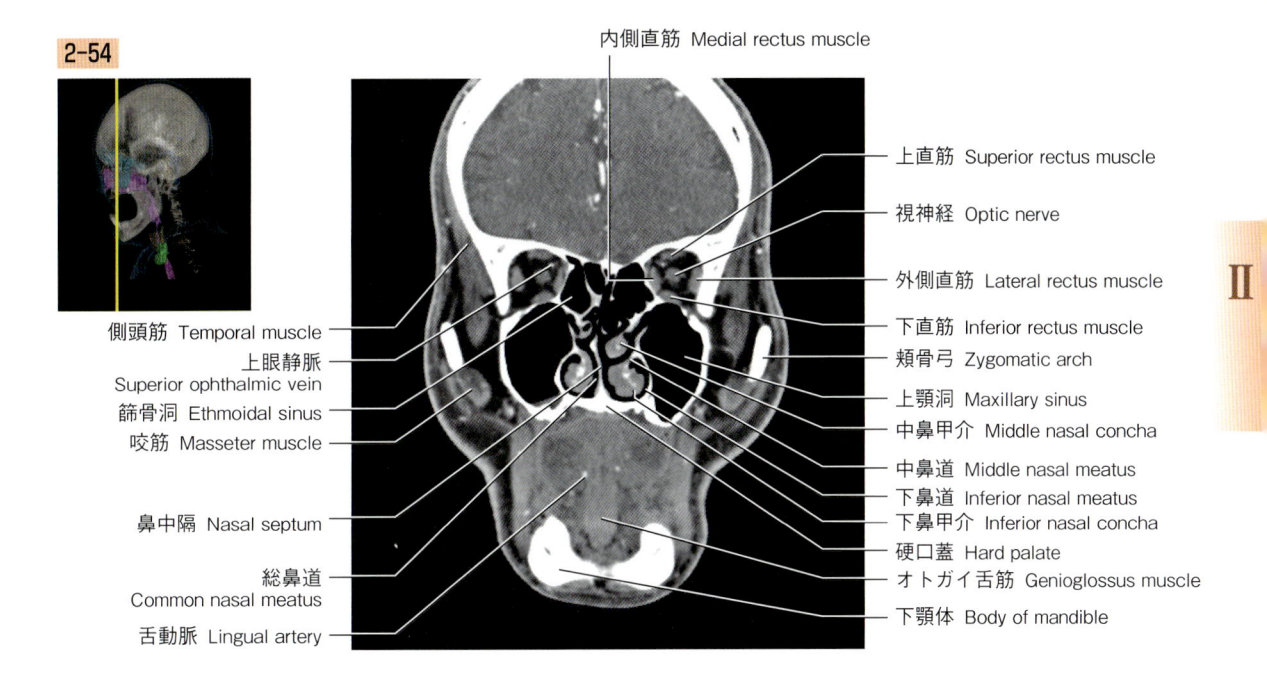

2-54

- 内側直筋 Medial rectus muscle
- 上直筋 Superior rectus muscle
- 視神経 Optic nerve
- 外側直筋 Lateral rectus muscle
- 下直筋 Inferior rectus muscle
- 頬骨弓 Zygomatic arch
- 上顎洞 Maxillary sinus
- 中鼻甲介 Middle nasal concha
- 中鼻道 Middle nasal meatus
- 下鼻道 Inferior nasal meatus
- 下鼻甲介 Inferior nasal concha
- 硬口蓋 Hard palate
- オトガイ舌筋 Genioglossus muscle
- 下顎体 Body of mandible
- 側頭筋 Temporal muscle
- 上眼静脈 Superior ophthalmic vein
- 篩骨洞 Ethmoidal sinus
- 咬筋 Masseter muscle
- 鼻中隔 Nasal septum
- 総鼻道 Common nasal meatus
- 舌動脈 Lingual artery

2-55 眼球後方・上顎洞レベル

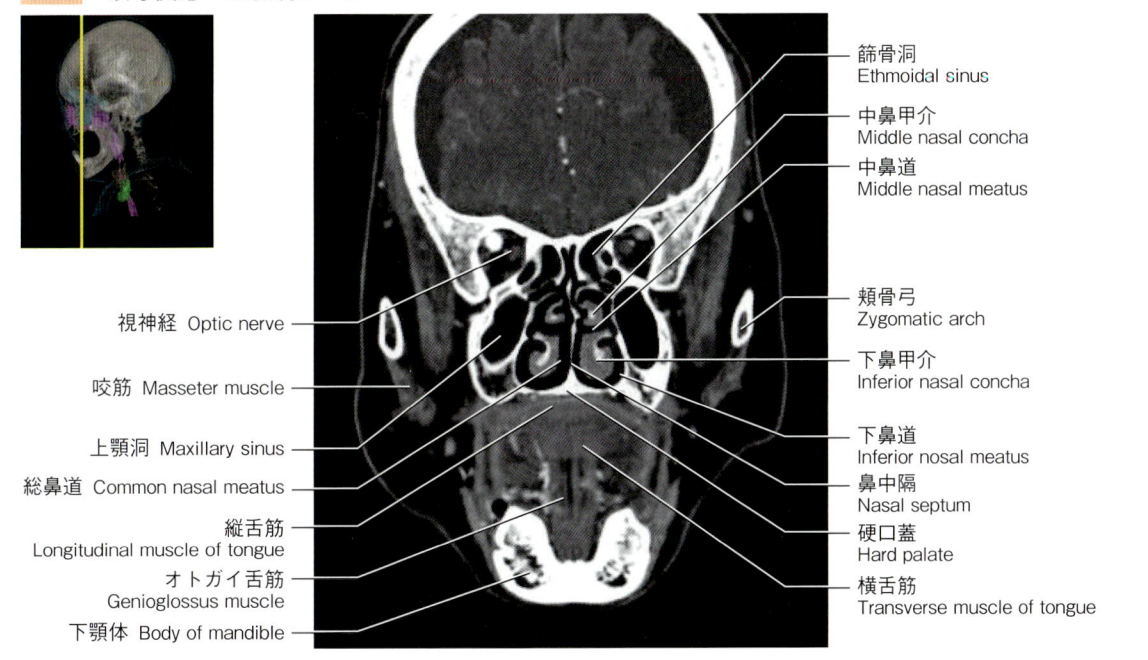

- 篩骨洞 Ethmoidal sinus
- 中鼻甲介 Middle nasal concha
- 中鼻道 Middle nasal meatus
- 頬骨弓 Zygomatic arch
- 下鼻甲介 Inferior nasal concha
- 下鼻道 Inferior nosal meatus
- 鼻中隔 Nasal septum
- 硬口蓋 Hard palate
- 横舌筋 Transverse muscle of tongue
- 視神経 Optic nerve
- 咬筋 Masseter muscle
- 上顎洞 Maxillary sinus
- 総鼻道 Common nasal meatus
- 縦舌筋 Longitudinal muscle of tongue
- オトガイ舌筋 Genioglossus muscle
- 下顎体 Body of mandible

NOTE
- 内頸動脈・海綿静脈洞瘻では上眼静脈の拡張がみられる．
- 中鼻甲介内部に篩骨蜂巣が進展して含気を伴うものを"Concha bullosa"という．大きなものでは中鼻道の狭小化をきたし，二次性副鼻腔炎の原因となりうる．

頭頸部の断層解剖 ［冠状断像（造影CT）］

2-56 眼窩先端レベル

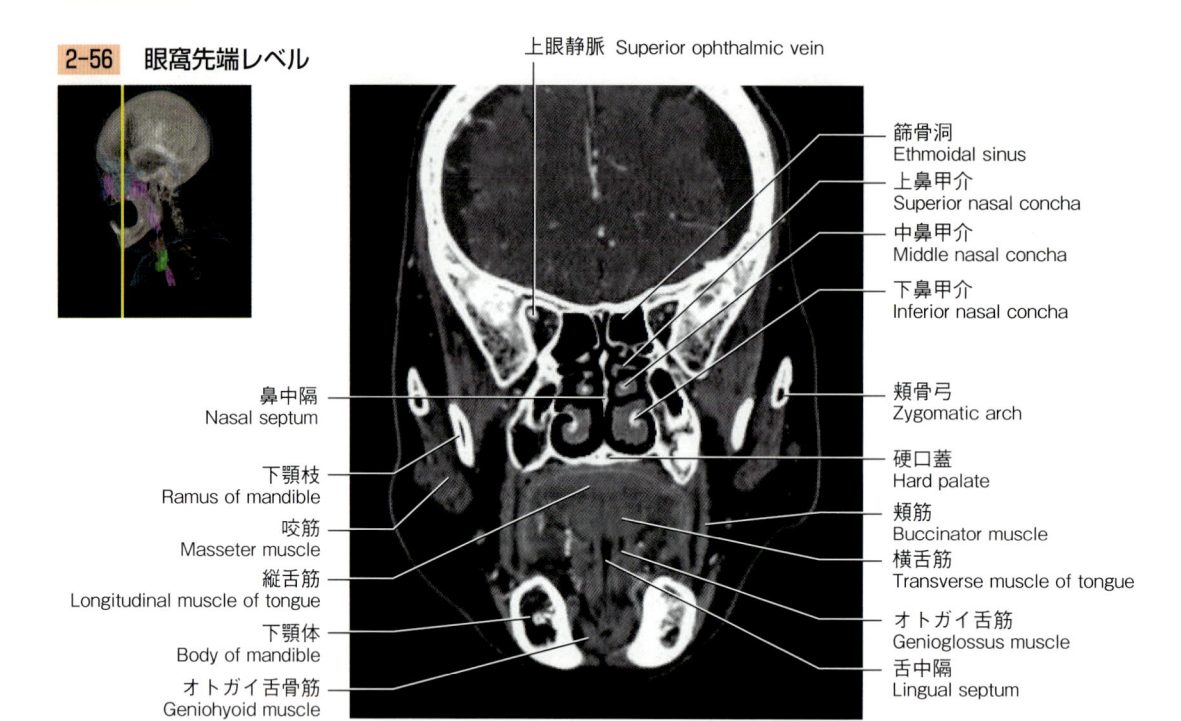

上眼静脈 Superior ophthalmic vein
篩骨洞 Ethmoidal sinus
上鼻甲介 Superior nasal concha
中鼻甲介 Middle nasal concha
下鼻甲介 Inferior nasal concha
鼻中隔 Nasal septum
頬骨弓 Zygomatic arch
下顎枝 Ramus of mandible
硬口蓋 Hard palate
咬筋 Masseter muscle
頬筋 Buccinator muscle
横舌筋 Transverse muscle of tongue
縦舌筋 Longitudinal muscle of tongue
オトガイ舌筋 Genioglossus muscle
下顎体 Body of mandible
舌中隔 Lingual septum
オトガイ舌骨筋 Geniohyoid muscle

2-57 眼窩先端レベル

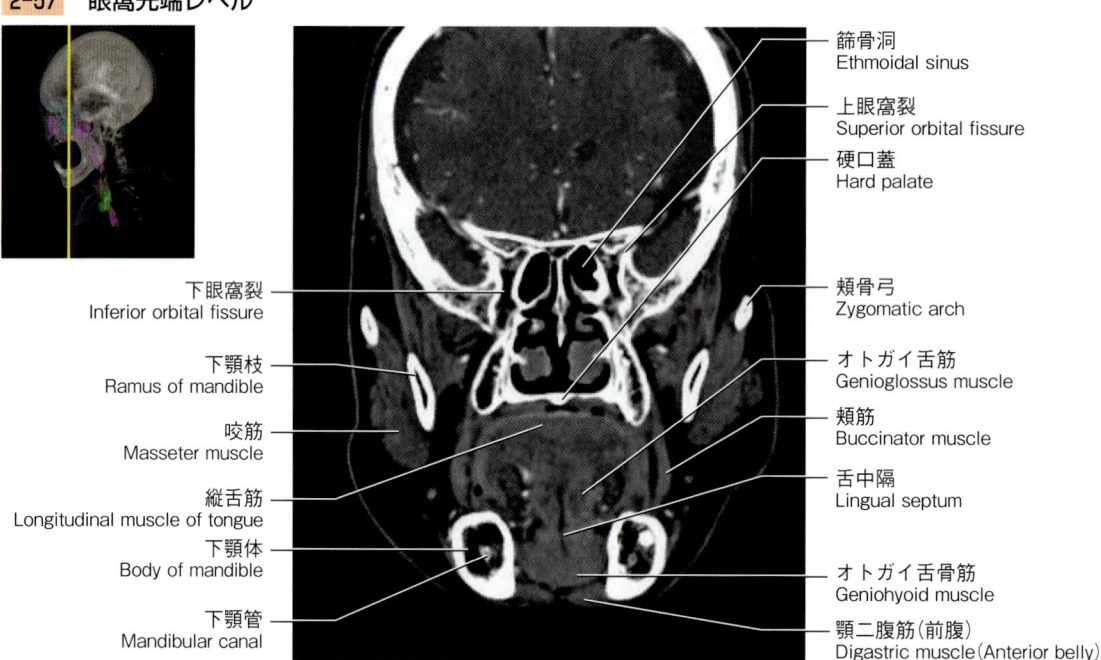

篩骨洞 Ethmoidal sinus
上眼窩裂 Superior orbital fissure
硬口蓋 Hard palate
下眼窩裂 Inferior orbital fissure
頬骨弓 Zygomatic arch
下顎枝 Ramus of mandible
オトガイ舌筋 Genioglossus muscle
咬筋 Masseter muscle
頬筋 Buccinator muscle
縦舌筋 Longitudinal muscle of tongue
舌中隔 Lingual septum
下顎体 Body of mandible
オトガイ舌骨筋 Geniohyoid muscle
下顎管 Mandibular canal
顎二腹筋（前腹）Digastric muscle (Anterior belly)

NOTE 硬口蓋は骨腫の好発部位であり，同部の骨腫は口蓋隆起ともよばれる．

頭頸部の断層解剖 ［冠状断像（造影CT）］

2-58　眼窩先端部後方レベル

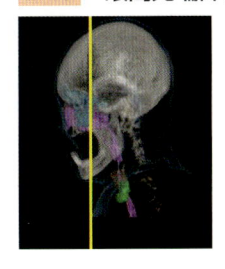

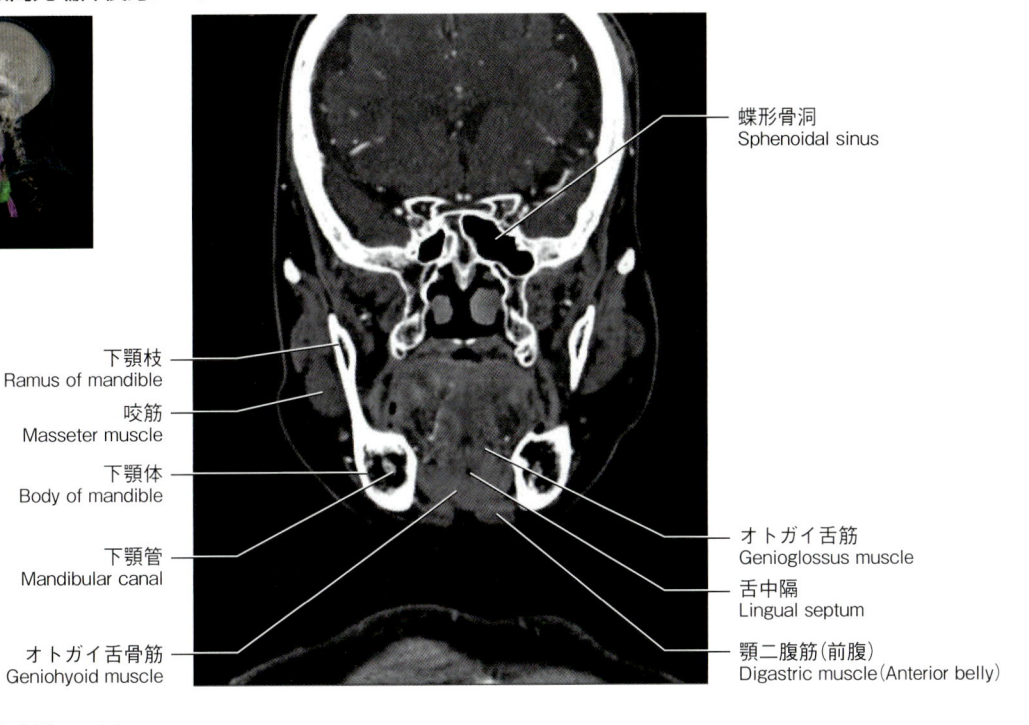

- 蝶形骨洞 Sphenoidal sinus
- 下顎枝 Ramus of mandible
- 咬筋 Masseter muscle
- 下顎体 Body of mandible
- 下顎管 Mandibular canal
- オトガイ舌骨筋 Geniohyoid muscle
- オトガイ舌筋 Genioglossus muscle
- 舌中隔 Lingual septum
- 顎二腹筋（前腹） Digastric muscle（Anterior belly）

2-59　後鼻孔レベル

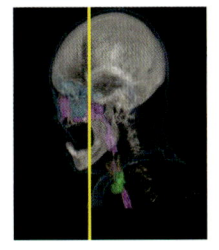

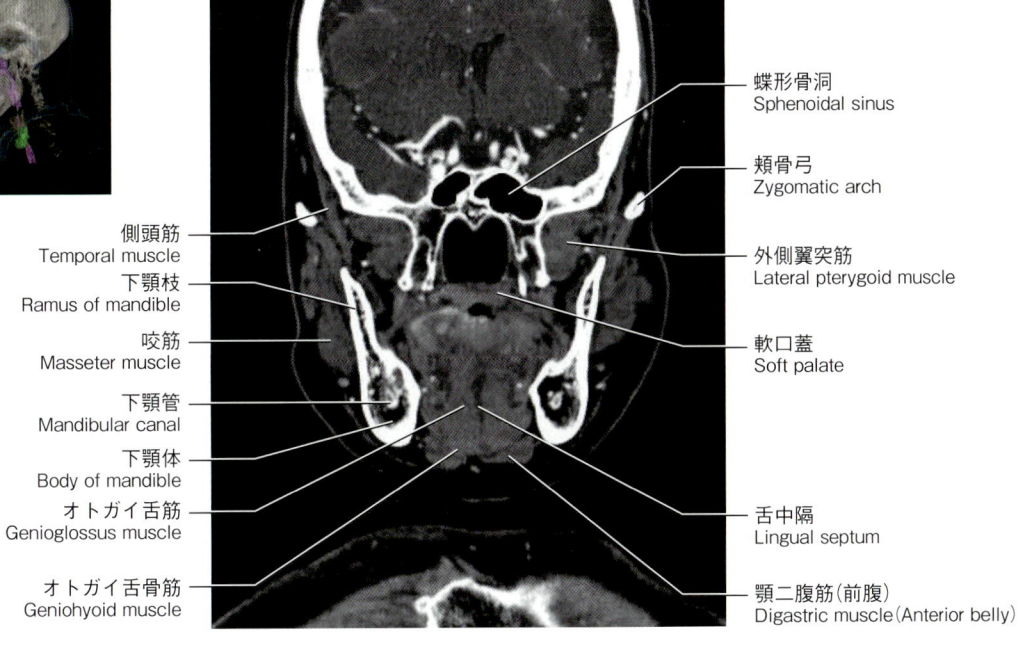

- 蝶形骨洞 Sphenoidal sinus
- 頬骨弓 Zygomatic arch
- 側頭筋 Temporal muscle
- 下顎枝 Ramus of mandible
- 咬筋 Masseter muscle
- 下顎管 Mandibular canal
- 下顎体 Body of mandible
- オトガイ舌筋 Genioglossus muscle
- オトガイ舌骨筋 Geniohyoid muscle
- 外側翼突筋 Lateral pterygoid muscle
- 軟口蓋 Soft palate
- 舌中隔 Lingual septum
- 顎二腹筋（前腹） Digastric muscle（Anterior belly）

頭頸部の断層解剖 [冠状断像（造影CT）]

2-60 後鼻孔・下顎枝レベル

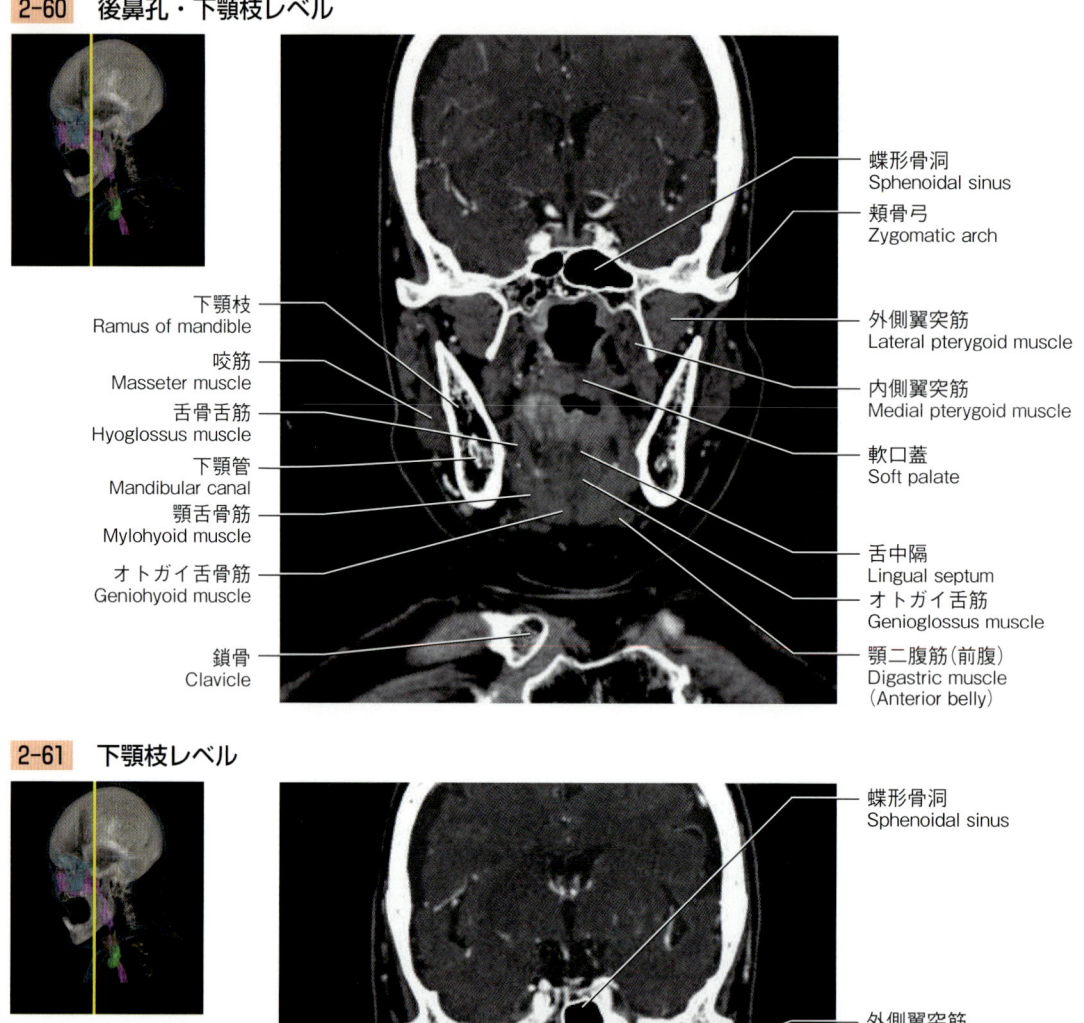

- 蝶形骨洞 Sphenoidal sinus
- 頬骨弓 Zygomatic arch
- 下顎枝 Ramus of mandible
- 咬筋 Masseter muscle
- 舌骨舌筋 Hyoglossus muscle
- 下顎管 Mandibular canal
- 顎舌骨筋 Mylohyoid muscle
- オトガイ舌骨筋 Geniohyoid muscle
- 鎖骨 Clavicle
- 外側翼突筋 Lateral pterygoid muscle
- 内側翼突筋 Medial pterygoid muscle
- 軟口蓋 Soft palate
- 舌中隔 Lingual septum
- オトガイ舌筋 Genioglossus muscle
- 顎二腹筋（前腹）Digastric muscle（Anterior belly）

2-61 下顎枝レベル

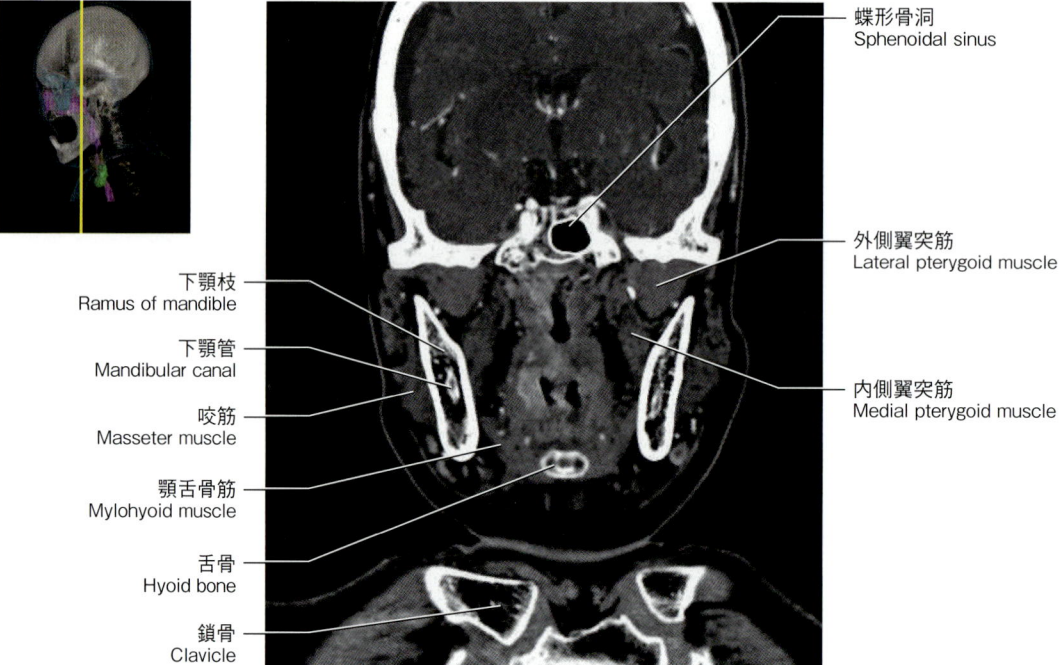

- 蝶形骨洞 Sphenoidal sinus
- 下顎枝 Ramus of mandible
- 下顎管 Mandibular canal
- 咬筋 Masseter muscle
- 顎舌骨筋 Mylohyoid muscle
- 舌骨 Hyoid bone
- 鎖骨 Clavicle
- 外側翼突筋 Lateral pterygoid muscle
- 内側翼突筋 Medial pterygoid muscle

NOTE 内側翼突筋の起始は翼状突起内・外側板の間，停止は下顎角内側面である．下顎骨の挙上を担う．外側翼突筋の起始は側頭下稜と翼状突起外側板で，停止は下顎骨翼突筋窩である．下顎の前方運動を担う．

頭頸部の断層解剖　[冠状断像（造影CT）]

2-62　顎関節レベル

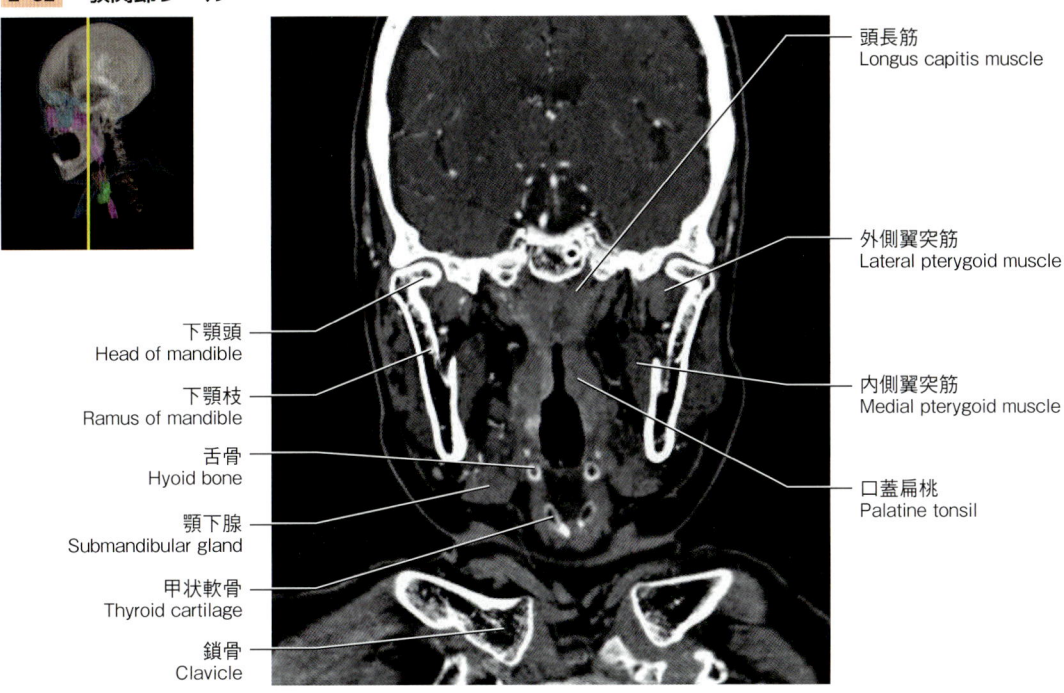

図中ラベル：
- 頭長筋　Longus capitis muscle
- 外側翼突筋　Lateral pterygoid muscle
- 内側翼突筋　Medial pterygoid muscle
- 口蓋扁桃　Palatine tonsil
- 下顎頭　Head of mandible
- 下顎枝　Ramus of mandible
- 舌骨　Hyoid bone
- 顎下腺　Submandibular gland
- 甲状軟骨　Thyroid cartilage
- 鎖骨　Clavicle

2-63　顎関節レベル

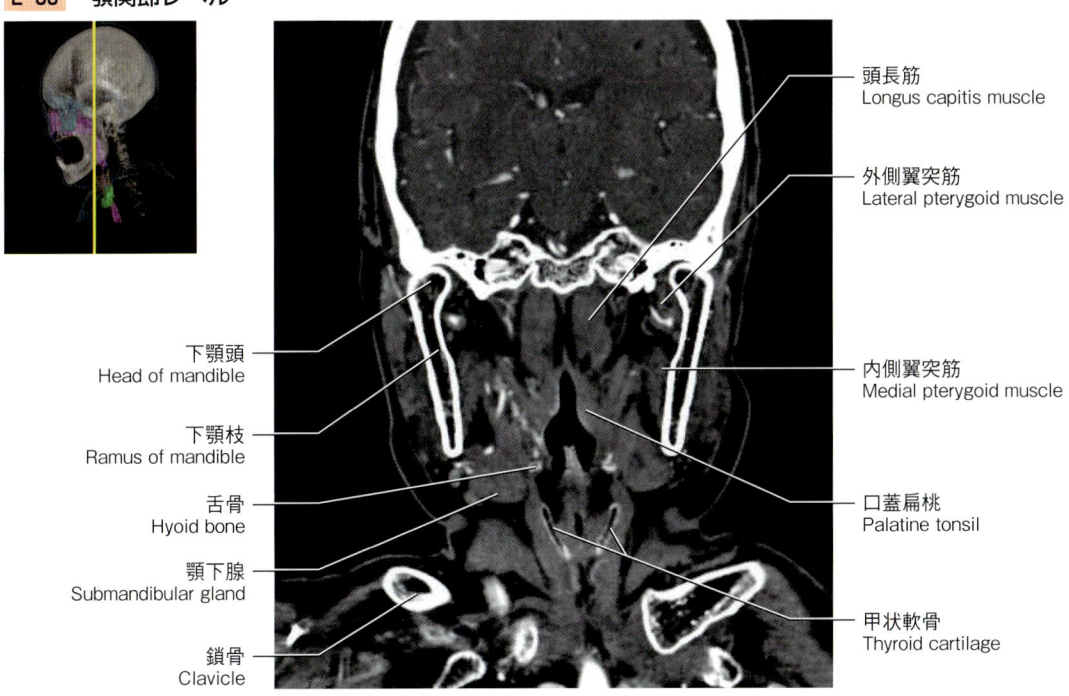

図中ラベル：
- 頭長筋　Longus capitis muscle
- 外側翼突筋　Lateral pterygoid muscle
- 内側翼突筋　Medial pterygoid muscle
- 口蓋扁桃　Palatine tonsil
- 甲状軟骨　Thyroid cartilage
- 下顎頭　Head of mandible
- 下顎枝　Ramus of mandible
- 舌骨　Hyoid bone
- 顎下腺　Submandibular gland
- 鎖骨　Clavicle

> **NOTE**　顎関節強直症は感染や外傷により生じ，下顎頭・側頭骨の変形，関節裂隙狭小化などがみられる．著明な開口障害をきたす．

頭頸部の断層解剖 ［冠状断像（造影CT）］

2-64 顎関節後方レベル

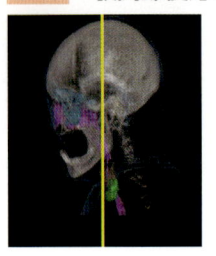

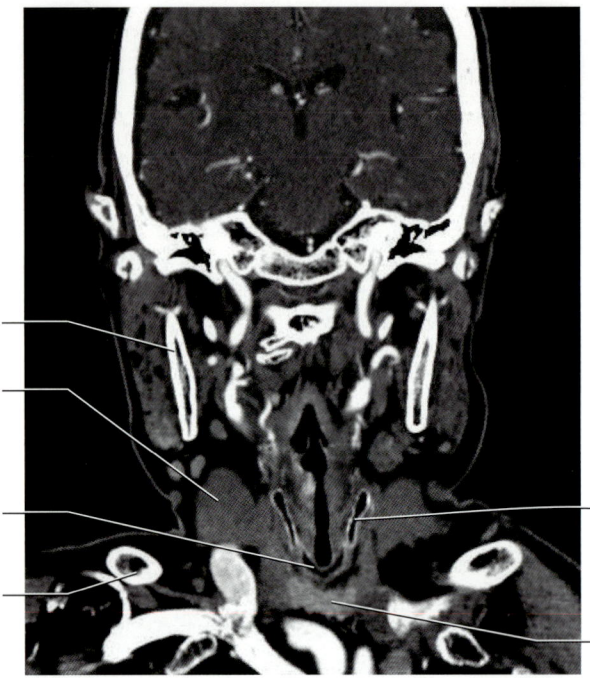

- 下顎枝 Ramus of mandible
- 胸鎖乳突筋 Sternocleidomastoid muscle
- 輪状軟骨 Cricoid cartilage
- 鎖骨 Clavicle
- 甲状軟骨 Thyroid cartilage
- 甲状腺 Thyroid gland

2-65 外耳道レベル

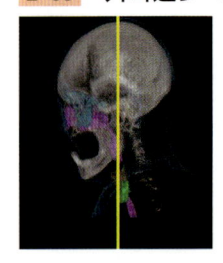

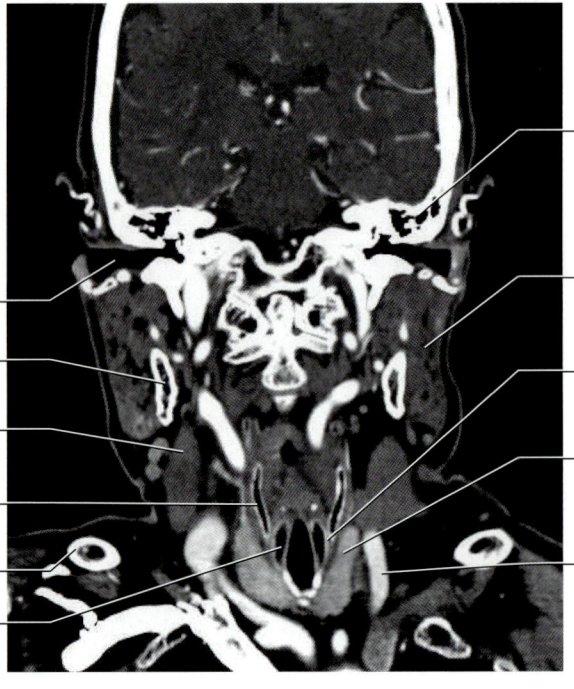

- 外耳道 External auditory canal
- 下顎枝 Ramus of mandible
- 胸鎖乳突筋 Sternocleidomastoid muscle
- 甲状軟骨 Thyroid cartilage
- 鎖骨 Clavicle
- 輪状軟骨 Cricoid cartilage
- 乳突蜂巣 Mastoid cells
- 耳下腺 Parotid gland
- 輪状甲状関節 Cricothyroid joint
- 甲状腺 Thyroid gland
- 内頸静脈 Internal jugular vein

NOTE 甲状軟骨は喉頭軟骨で最大の軟骨であり，喉頭の前壁から外側壁を形成する．

頭頸部の断層解剖 ［冠状断像（造影CT）］

2-66 外耳道後方レベル

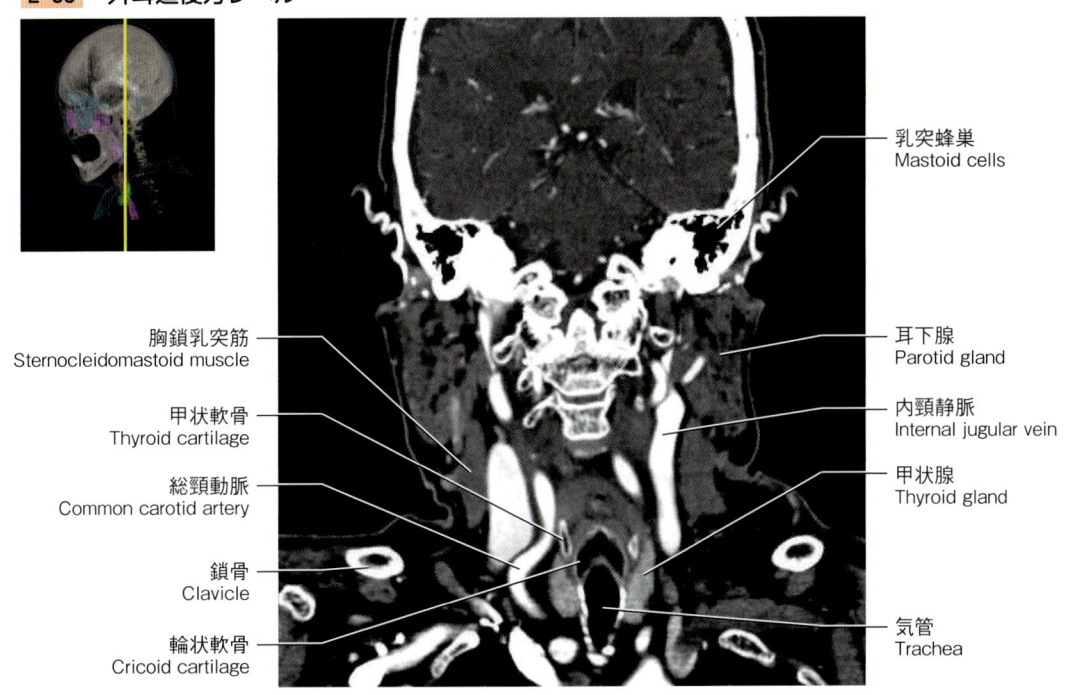

- 乳突蜂巣 Mastoid cells
- 耳下腺 Parotid gland
- 内頸静脈 Internal jugular vein
- 甲状腺 Thyroid gland
- 気管 Trachea
- 胸鎖乳突筋 Sternocleidomastoid muscle
- 甲状軟骨 Thyroid cartilage
- 総頸動脈 Common carotid artery
- 鎖骨 Clavicle
- 輪状軟骨 Cricoid cartilage

2-67 外耳道後方・乳突蜂巣レベル

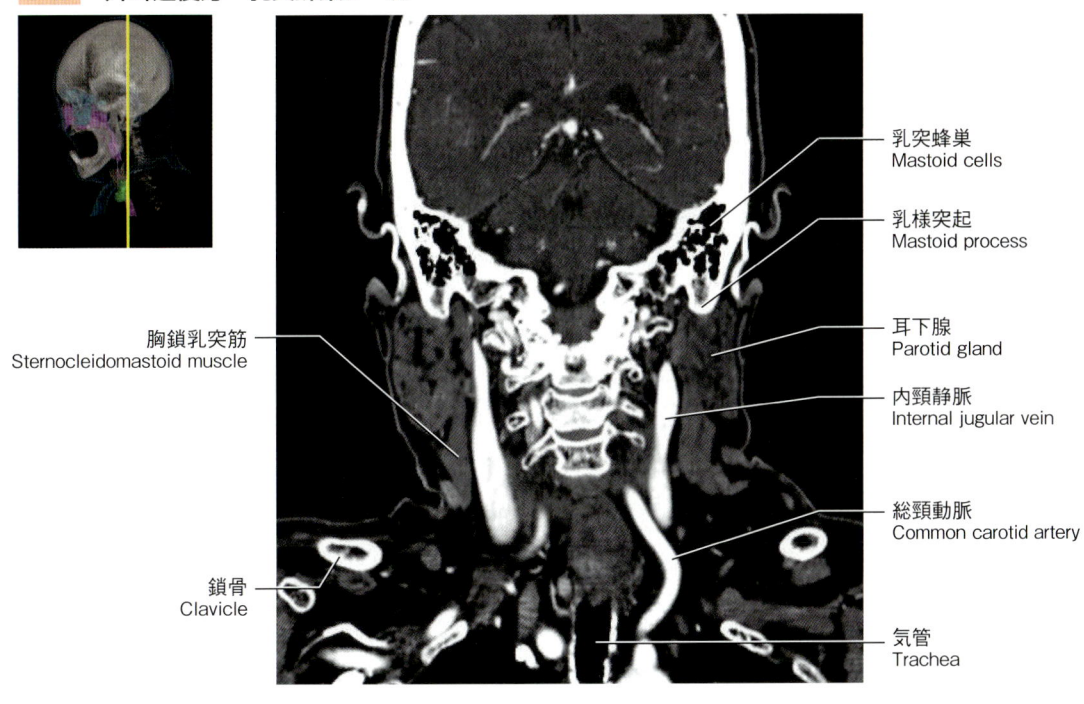

- 乳突蜂巣 Mastoid cells
- 乳様突起 Mastoid process
- 耳下腺 Parotid gland
- 内頸静脈 Internal jugular vein
- 総頸動脈 Common carotid artery
- 気管 Trachea
- 胸鎖乳突筋 Sternocleidomastoid muscle
- 鎖骨 Clavicle

> **NOTE** 内頸静脈には，中心静脈カテーテルの留置や頸部感染性リンパ筋炎，悪性腫瘍などで血栓性静脈炎が起こりうるが，頭尾側方向に長く伸びる場合もあり，造影CT冠状断や矢状断など多方向での評価が肝要である．

頭頸部の断層解剖 ［冠状断像（造影CT）］

2-68 乳突蜂巣後方・乳様突起レベル

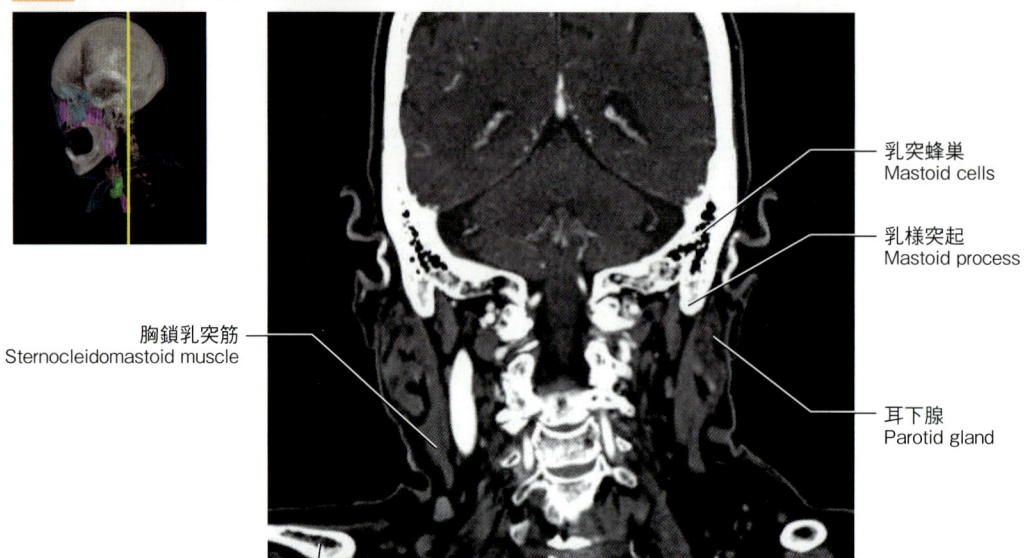

- 乳突蜂巣 Mastoid cells
- 乳様突起 Mastoid process
- 胸鎖乳突筋 Sternocleidomastoid muscle
- 耳下腺 Parotid gland
- 鎖骨 Clavicle
- 気管 Trachea

2-69 乳様突起レベル

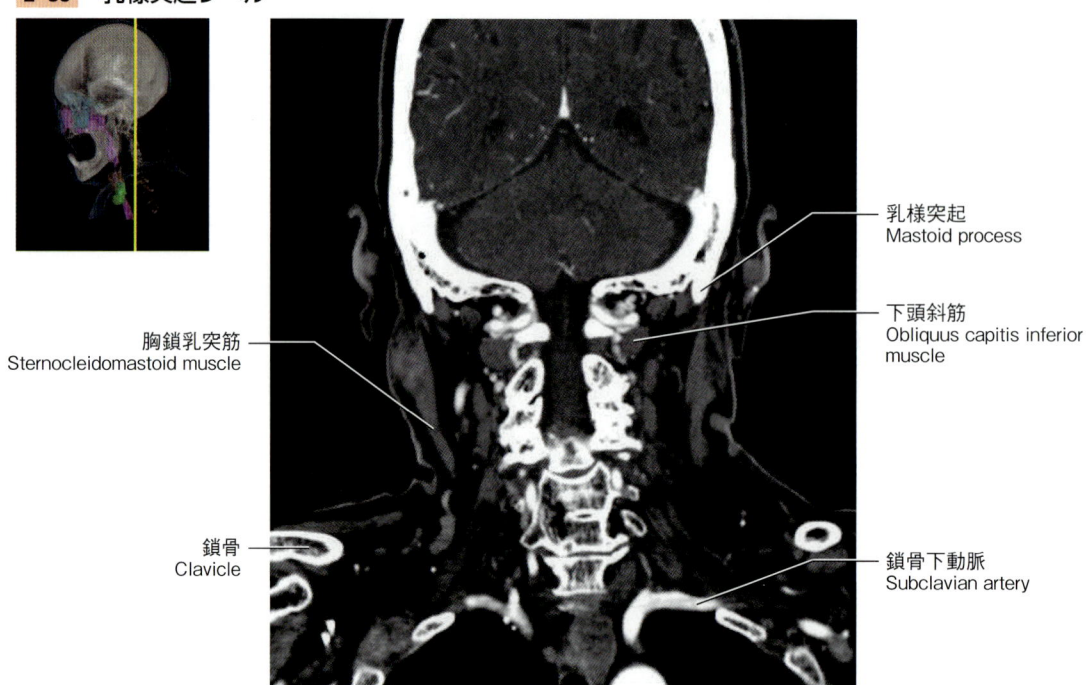

- 乳様突起 Mastoid process
- 胸鎖乳突筋 Sternocleidomastoid muscle
- 下頭斜筋 Obliquus capitis inferior muscle
- 鎖骨 Clavicle
- 鎖骨下動脈 Subclavian artery

> **NOTE** 急性中耳炎の合併症で乳突蜂巣炎から骨破壊をきたすことがあるが，骨破壊が乳様突起に及び，乳様突起周囲から胸鎖乳突筋に沿って膿瘍が形成されることがある．これをBezold（ベツォルド）膿瘍という．

頭頸部の断層解剖 ［冠状断像（造影 CT）］

2-70

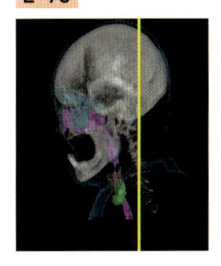

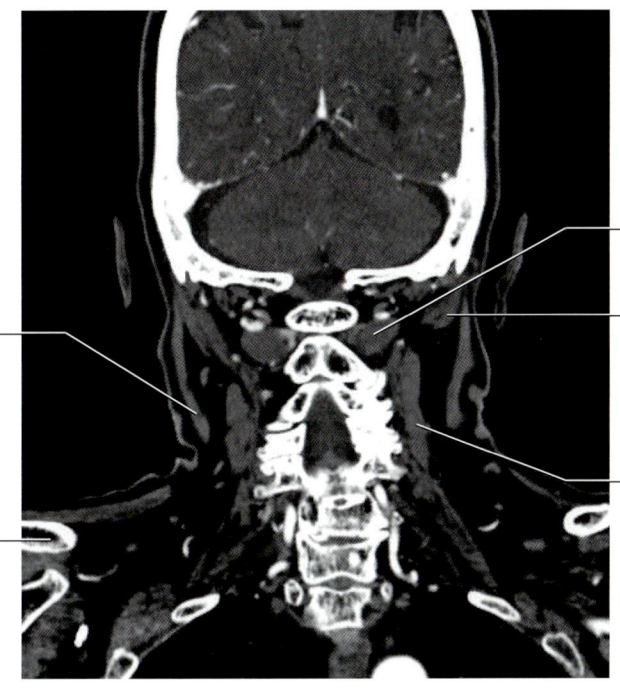

胸鎖乳突筋
Sternocleidomastoid muscle

鎖骨
Clavicle

下頭斜筋
Obliquus capitis inferior muscle

頭板状筋
Splenius capitis muscle

肩甲挙筋
Levator scapulae muscle

2-71

胸鎖乳突筋
Sternocleidomastoid muscle

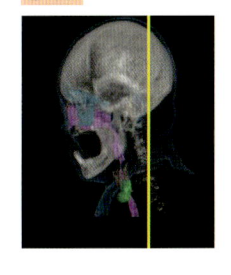

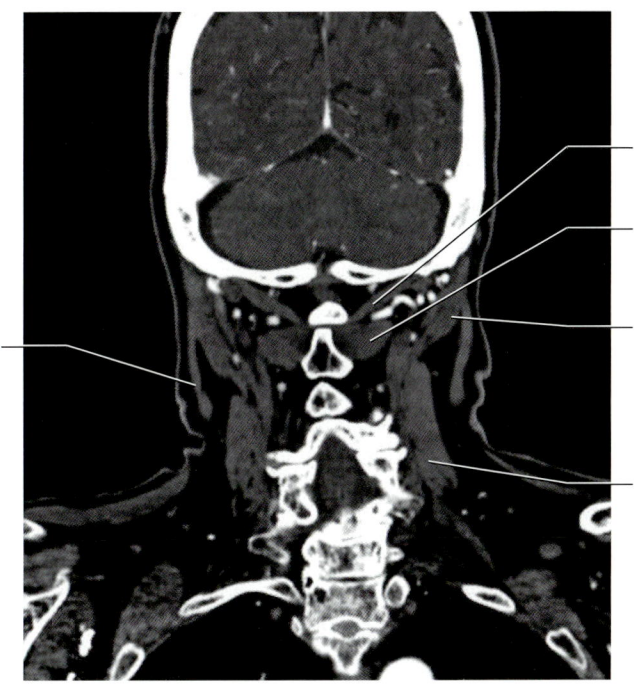

大後頭直筋
Rectus capitis posterior major muscle

下頭斜筋
Obliquus capitis inferior muscle

頭板状筋
Splenius capitis muscle

肩甲挙筋
Levator scapulae muscle

頭頸部の断層解剖 ［冠状断像（造影 CT）］

2-72

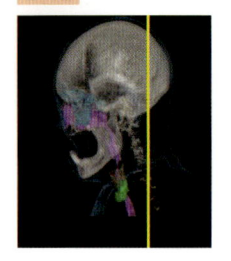

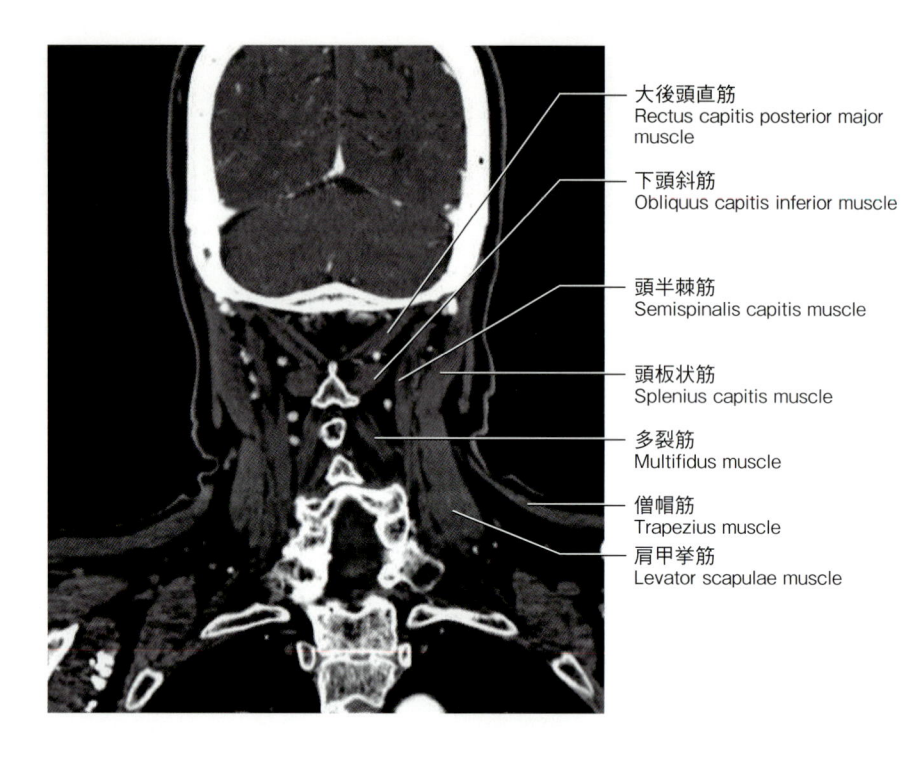

大後頭直筋
Rectus capitis posterior major muscle

下頭斜筋
Obliquus capitis inferior muscle

頭半棘筋
Semispinalis capitis muscle

頭板状筋
Splenius capitis muscle

多裂筋
Multifidus muscle

僧帽筋
Trapezius muscle

肩甲挙筋
Levator scapulae muscle

2-73

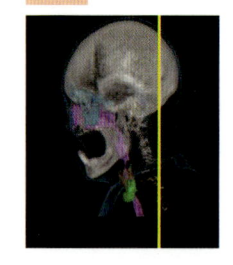

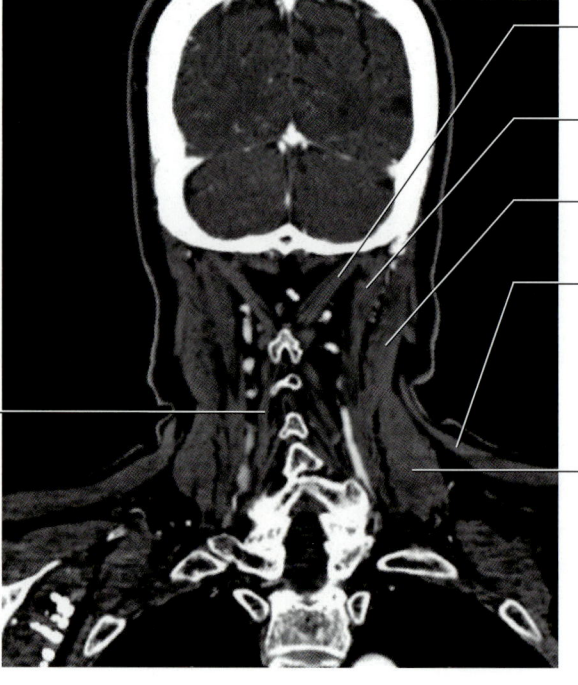

大後頭直筋
Rectus capitis posterior major muscle

頭半棘筋
Semispinalis capitis muscle

頭板状筋
Splenius capitis muscle

僧帽筋
Trapezius muscle

多裂筋
Multifidus muscle

肩甲挙筋
Levator scapulae muscle

頸部リンパ節のレベルシステム

2-74

レベル IA	オトガイ下リンパ節
レベル IB	顎下リンパ節
レベル IIA	上内深頸リンパ節
レベル IIB	最上部レベルの副神経リンパ節
レベル III	中内深頸リンパ節
レベル IV	下内深頸リンパ節
レベル VA	上部レベルの副神経リンパ節
レベル VB	下部レベルの副神経リンパ節
レベル VI	喉頭前リンパ節，気管前リンパ節，気管傍リンパ節などの臓側リンパ節
レベル VII	上縦隔リンパ節

2-75

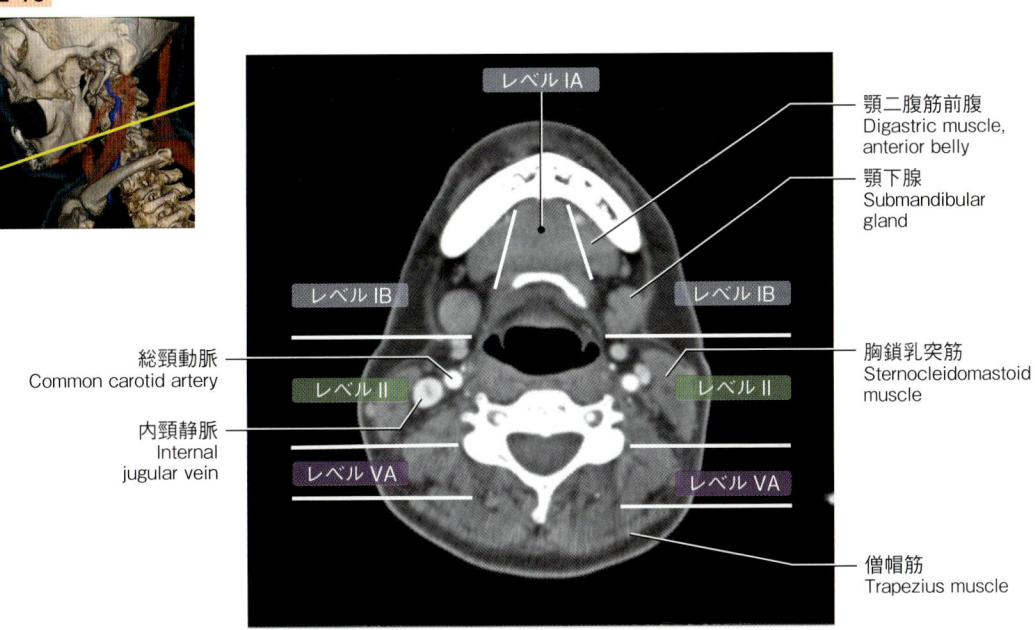

レベル IA
顎二腹筋前腹 Digastric muscle, anterior belly
顎下腺 Submandibular gland
レベル IB
レベル IB
総頸動脈 Common carotid artery
胸鎖乳突筋 Sternocleidomastoid muscle
レベル II
レベル II
内頸静脈 Internal jugular vein
レベル VA
レベル VA
僧帽筋 Trapezius muscle

NOTE 頭頸部領域のリンパ節の評価には，Som らによって紹介されたレベルシステムが広く用いられている．各リンパ節との対応は 2-74 の表に示した通りである．なお，レベル IIA は顎二腹筋後腹と舌骨間の高さ，レベル III は舌骨と輪状軟骨の間の高さ，レベル IV は輪状軟骨より下方で鎖骨上窩より上方の高さ，レベル VA は頭蓋底から輪状軟骨下縁の高さ，レベル VB は輪状軟骨下縁から鎖骨上縁の高さが目安となる．

頸部リンパ節のレベルシステム

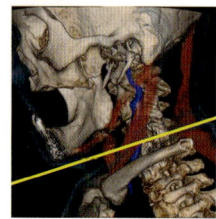

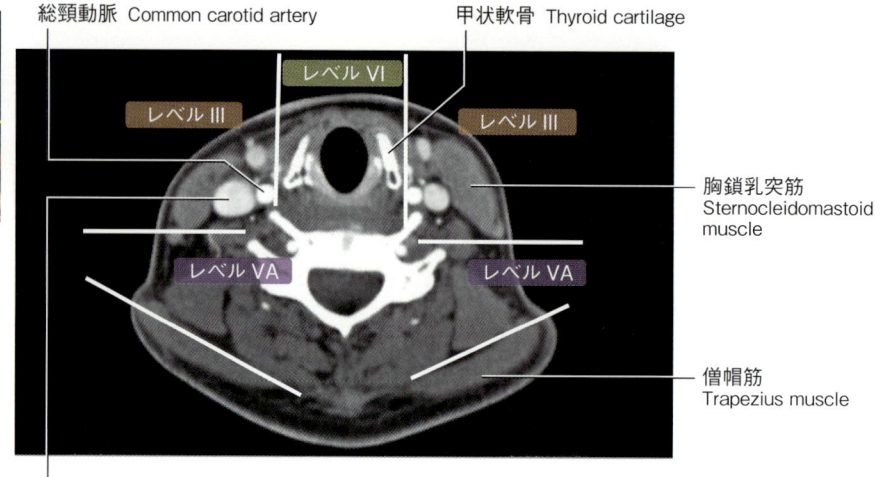

2-76

- 総頸動脈 Common carotid artery
- 甲状軟骨 Thyroid cartilage
- レベルVI
- レベルIII
- レベルIII
- 胸鎖乳突筋 Sternocleidomastoid muscle
- レベルVA
- レベルVA
- 僧帽筋 Trapezius muscle
- 内頸静脈 Internal jugular vein

2-77

- 内頸静脈 Internal jugular vein
- 胸鎖乳突筋 Sternocleidomastoid muscle
- レベルVI
- レベルIV
- レベルIV
- 前斜角筋 Scalenus anterior muscle
- レベルVB
- レベルVB
- 僧帽筋 Trapezius muscle
- 総頸動脈 Common carotid artery

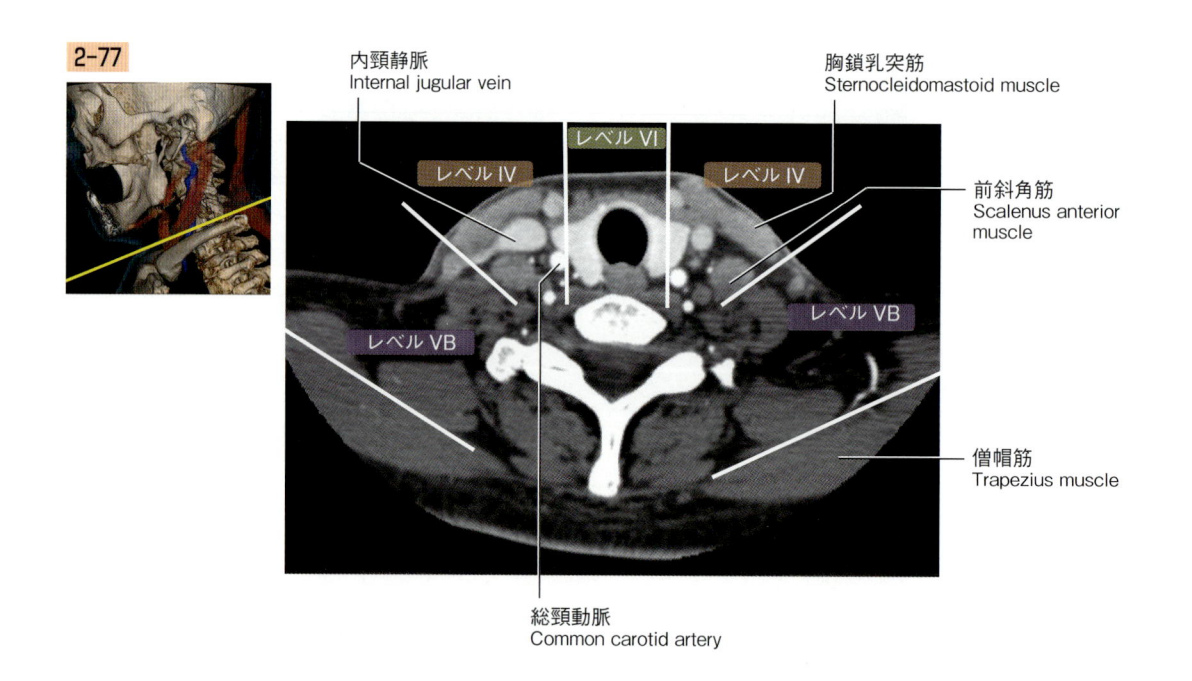

NOTE 中咽頭レベル，顎二腹筋後腹直下には，深頸リンパ節最高位のリンパ節あり，内頸静脈二腹筋リンパ節［Küttner（キュットナー）リンパ節］とよばれる．顔面・頭頸部のリンパ系が集まるところであり，リンパ節転移の好発部位として知られている．

耳小骨・三半規管

2-78 下方から

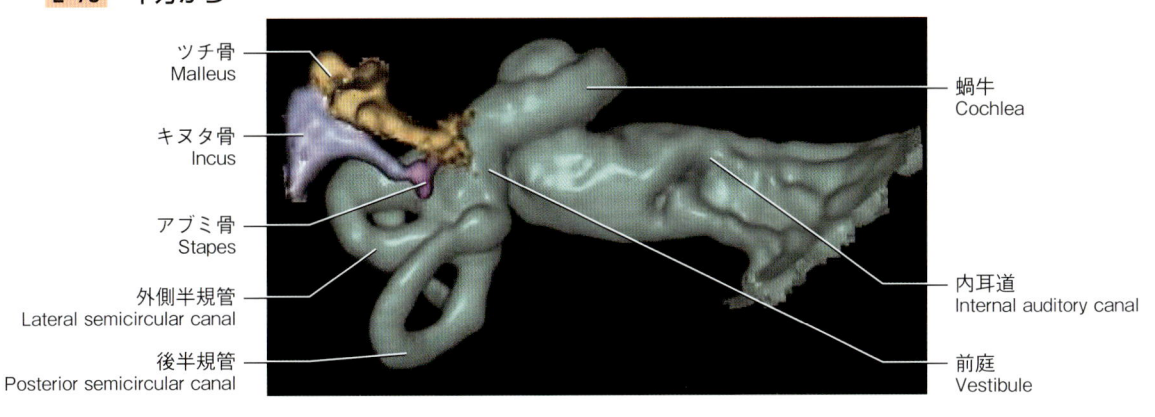

- ツチ骨 Malleus
- キヌタ骨 Incus
- アブミ骨 Stapes
- 外側半規管 Lateral semicircular canal
- 後半規管 Posterior semicircular canal
- 蝸牛 Cochlea
- 内耳道 Internal auditory canal
- 前庭 Vestibule

2-79 前方から

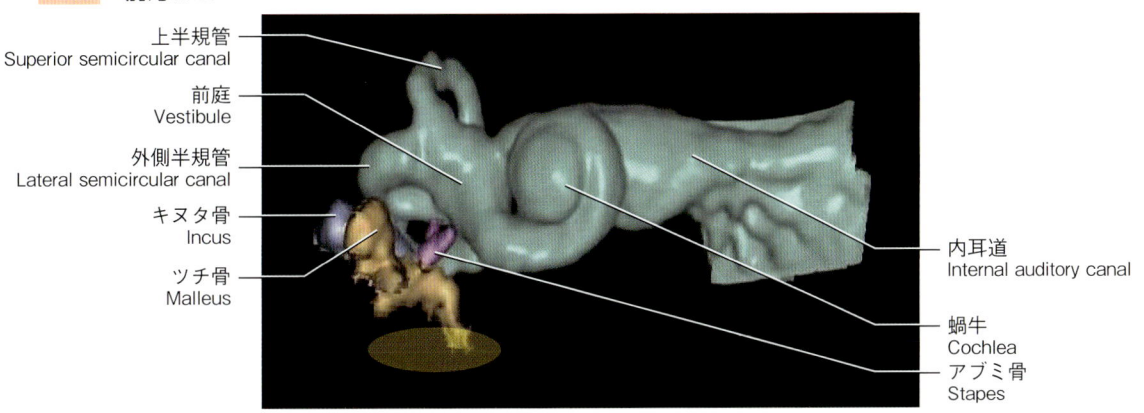

- 上半規管 Superior semicircular canal
- 前庭 Vestibule
- 外側半規管 Lateral semicircular canal
- キヌタ骨 Incus
- ツチ骨 Malleus
- 内耳道 Internal auditory canal
- 蝸牛 Cochlea
- アブミ骨 Stapes

2-80 外側から

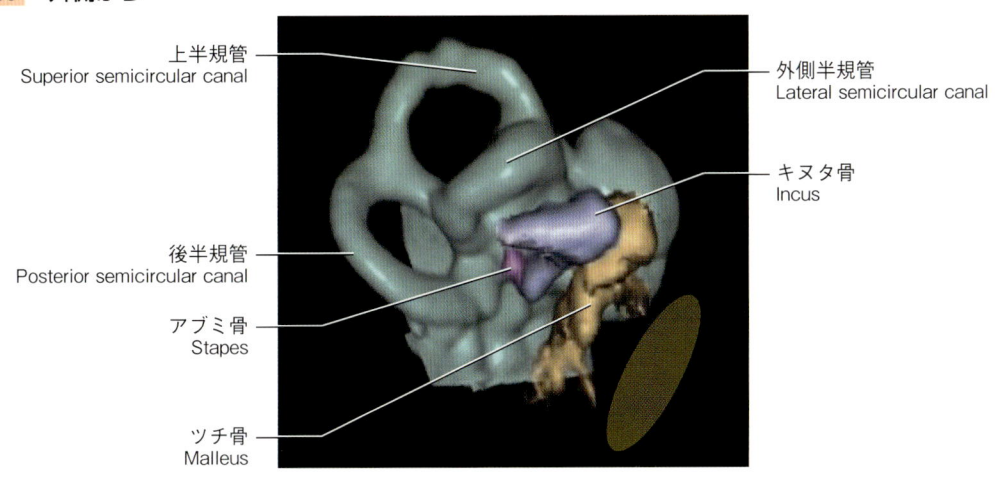

- 上半規管 Superior semicircular canal
- 後半規管 Posterior semicircular canal
- アブミ骨 Stapes
- ツチ骨 Malleus
- 外側半規管 Lateral semicircular canal
- キヌタ骨 Incus

NOTE 2-78〜80は，MDCTより作成した耳小骨のVR像とMR cisternographyより作成した三半規管のVR像のfusion画像である．2-79, 80の ● は，鼓膜に相当する部分を示している．

側頭骨の断層解剖 [横断像，頭頂から頭蓋底に向かって(CT)]

2-81 内耳道上方レベル

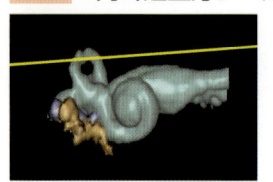

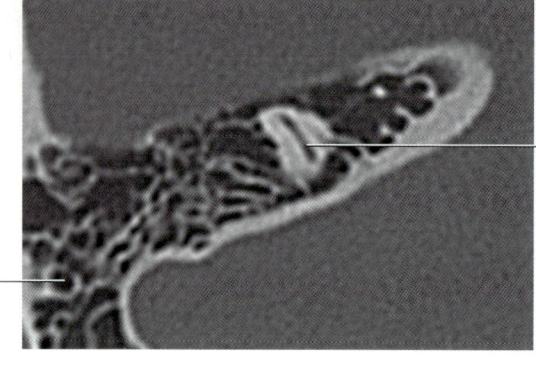

上半規管
Superior semicircular canal

乳突蜂巣
Mastoid cells

2-82 内耳道上方レベル

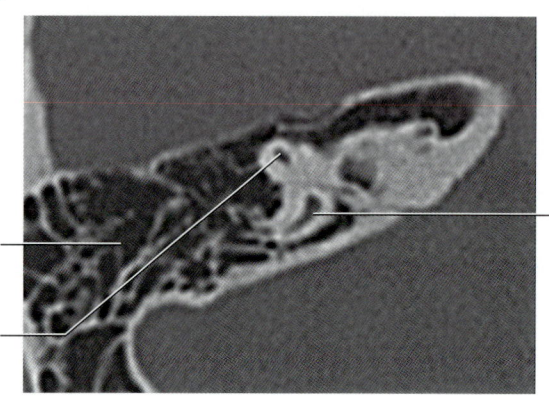

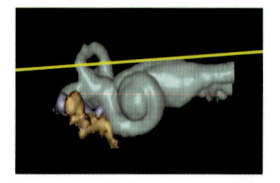

乳突蜂巣
Mastoid cells

上半規管
Superior semicircular canal

後半規管
Posterior semicircular canal

2-83 内耳道上方レベル

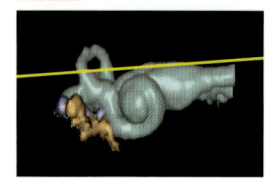

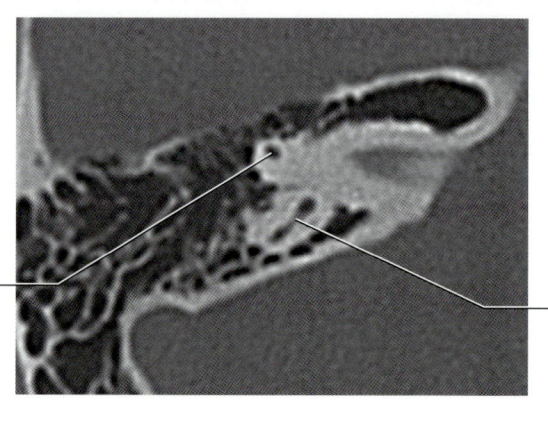

上半規管
Superior semicircular canal

後半規管
Posterior semicircular canal

側頭骨の断層解剖 [横断像，頭頂から頭蓋底に向かって(CT)]

2-84 内耳道レベル

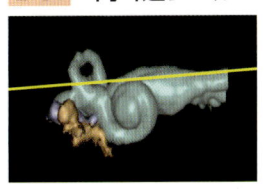

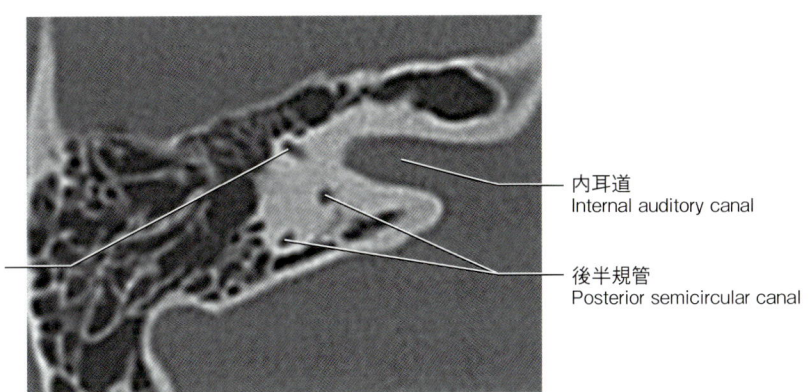

- 上半規管 Superior semicircular canal
- 内耳道 Internal auditory canal
- 後半規管 Posterior semicircular canal

2-85 内耳道レベル

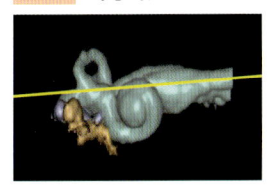

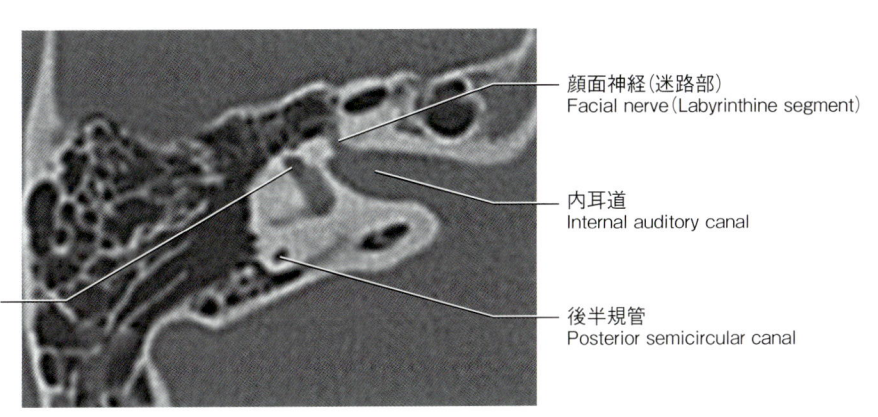

- 上半規管 Superior semicircular canal
- 顔面神経（迷路部）Facial nerve (Labyrinthine segment)
- 内耳道 Internal auditory canal
- 後半規管 Posterior semicircular canal

2-86 内耳道レベル

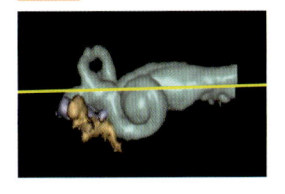

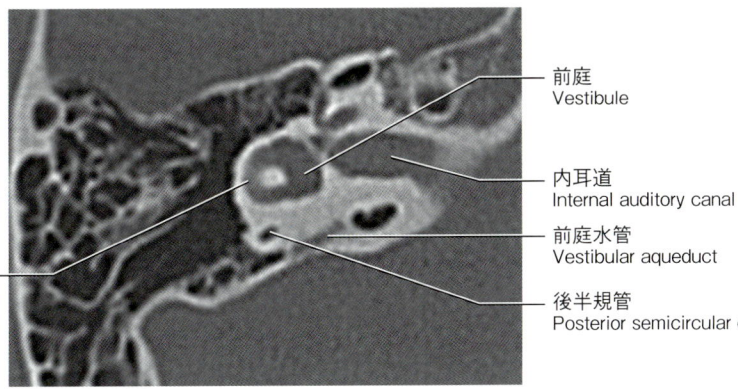

- 外側半規管 Lateral semicircular canal
- 前庭 Vestibule
- 内耳道 Internal auditory canal
- 前庭水管 Vestibular aqueduct
- 後半規管 Posterior semicircular canal

> **NOTE** 半規管の奇形で最も多いのは Vestibule-lateral semicircular canal dysplasia であり，外側半規管と前庭が1つの腔を形成している病態である．この場合，外側半規管の Central bone island は認められない．

側頭骨の断層解剖 ［横断像，頭頂から頭蓋底に向かって（CT）］

2-87 内耳道・蝸牛レベル

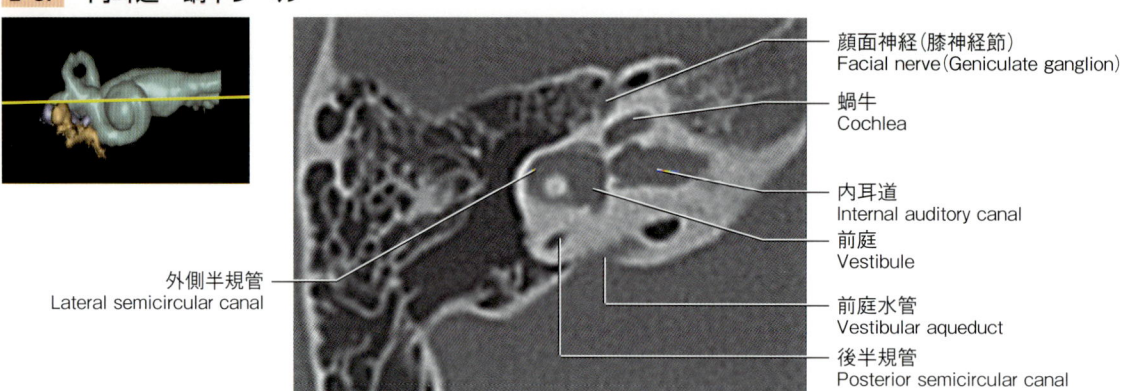

- 顔面神経（膝神経節） Facial nerve (Geniculate ganglion)
- 蝸牛 Cochlea
- 内耳道 Internal auditory canal
- 前庭 Vestibule
- 前庭水管 Vestibular aqueduct
- 後半規管 Posterior semicircular canal
- 外側半規管 Lateral semicircular canal

2-88 蝸牛レベル

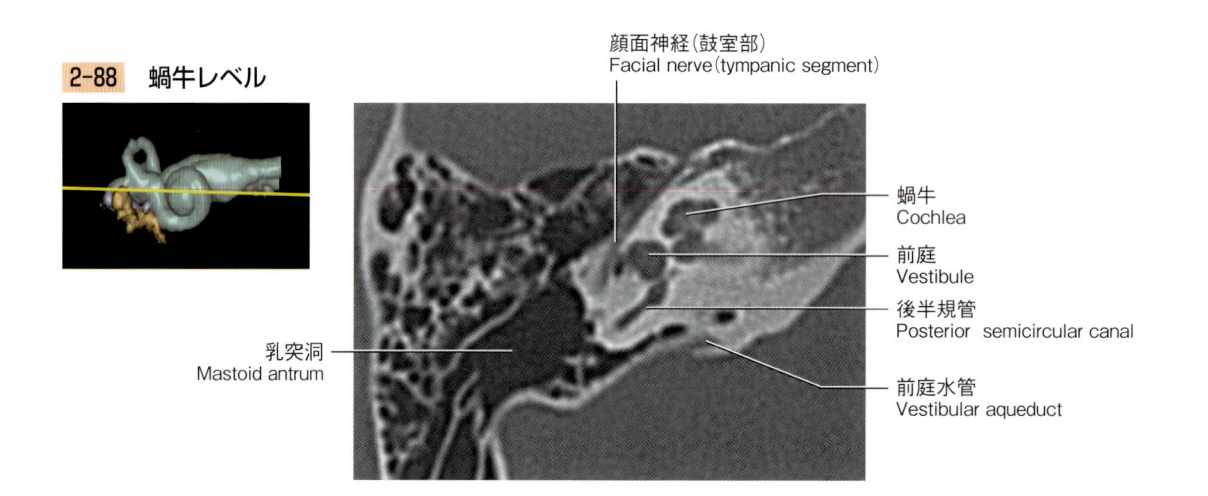

- 顔面神経（鼓室部） Facial nerve (tympanic segment)
- 蝸牛 Cochlea
- 前庭 Vestibule
- 後半規管 Posterior semicircular canal
- 前庭水管 Vestibular aqueduct
- 乳突洞 Mastoid antrum

2-89 ツチ・キヌタ関節レベル

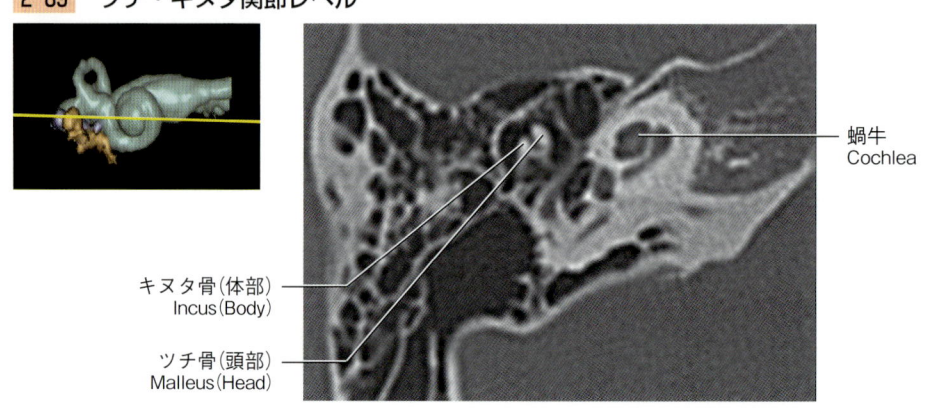

- 蝸牛 Cochlea
- キヌタ骨（体部） Incus (Body)
- ツチ骨（頭部） Malleus (Head)

NOTE 前庭水管は内リンパ腔である膜迷路（内リンパ管嚢）を入れる骨管であり，前後径が 1.5 mm を超えると拡張と見なすが，これ以下でも管外の内リンパ嚢が拡張していることがあり，内リンパ管，嚢拡張症の診断には原則 MRI が必要である．

側頭骨の断層解剖 ［横断像，頭頂から頭蓋底に向かって（CT）］

2-90 キヌタ・アブミ関節レベル

- 前鼓室陥凹 Epitympanic recess
- ツチ骨（頭部） Malleus (Head)
- キヌタ骨（体部） Incus (Body)
- キヌタ骨（短脚） Incus (Short crus)
- 蝸牛 Cochlea
- アブミ骨 Stapes

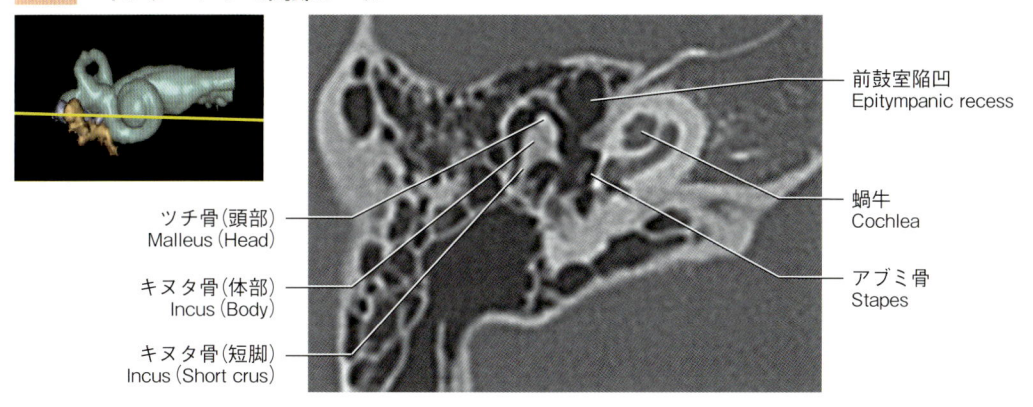

2-91 キヌタ・アブミ関節レベル

- ツチ骨（頭部） Malleus (Head)
- キヌタ骨（長脚） Incus (Long crus)
- 蝸牛 Cochlea
- アブミ骨 Stapes

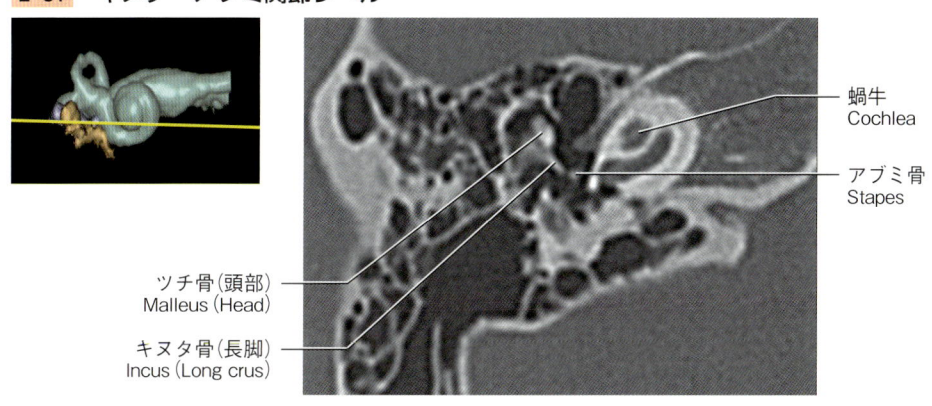

2-92 ツチ骨柄・キヌタ骨長脚レベル

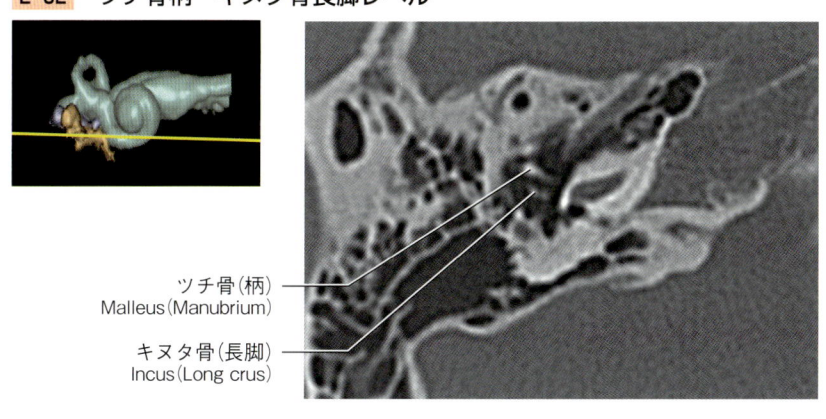

- ツチ骨（柄） Malleus (Manubrium)
- キヌタ骨（長脚） Incus (Long crus)

NOTE
- キヌタ骨はツチ骨，アブミ骨に比べ重く，靱帯でのみ固定されていることより脱臼しやすい．ツチ・キヌタ骨関節離断が多く，次いでキヌタ・アブミ骨関節離断が多い．
- 軸位断像ではツチ骨柄とキヌタ骨長脚はほぼ平行に走行する（Parallel line）．

側頭骨の断層解剖 ［横断像，頭頂から頭蓋底に向かって（CT）］

2-93 ツチ骨柄レベル

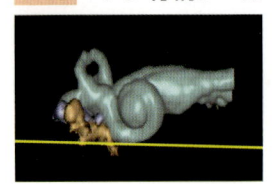

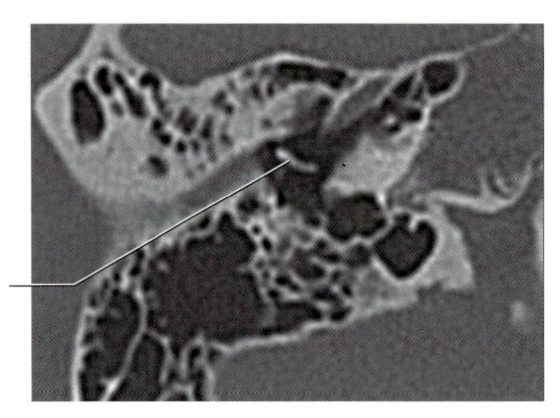

ツチ骨（柄）
Malleus (Manubrium)

2-94 外耳道レベル

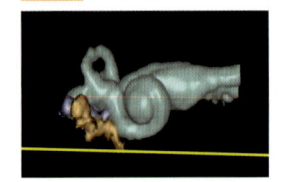

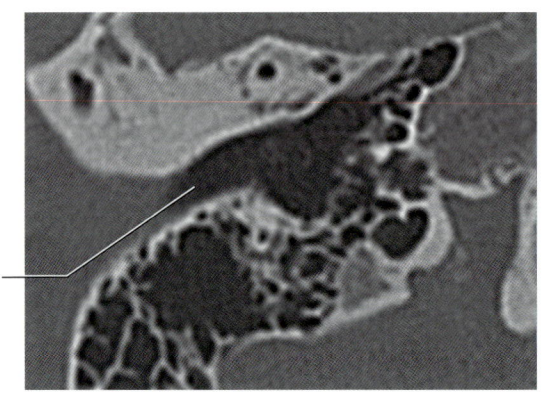

外耳道
External auditory canal

> **NOTE** 外耳に好発する代表的な病変として外耳道深部から発生する骨性増殖，外骨腫がある．サーフィンなどで長時間冷水に曝された際の温度刺激に伴う反応性の変化であり，"Surfer's ear"ともよばれる．

側頭骨の断層解剖 ［冠状断像，前方から後方へ（CT）］

2-95 蝸牛レベル

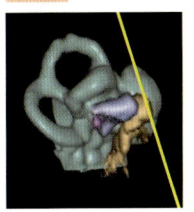

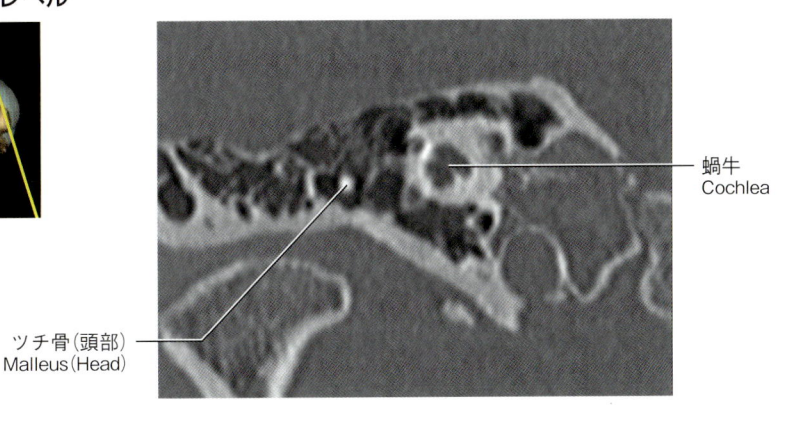

蝸牛 Cochlea
ツチ骨（頭部） Malleus（Head）

2-96 蝸牛レベル

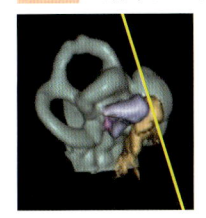

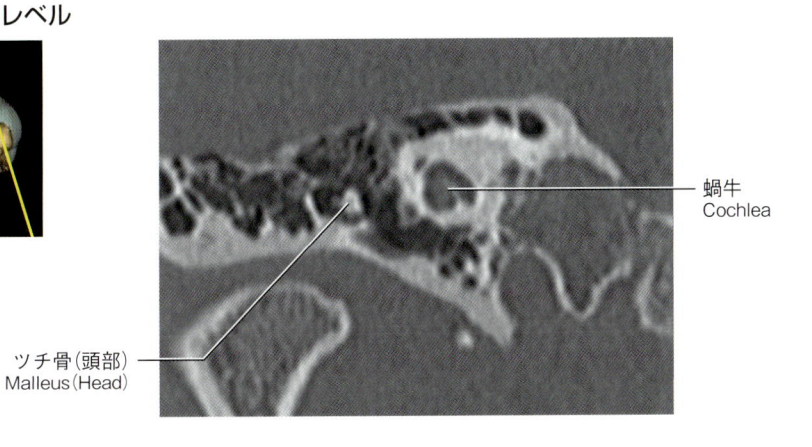

蝸牛 Cochlea
ツチ骨（頭部） Malleus（Head）

2-97 ツチ・キヌタ関節レベル

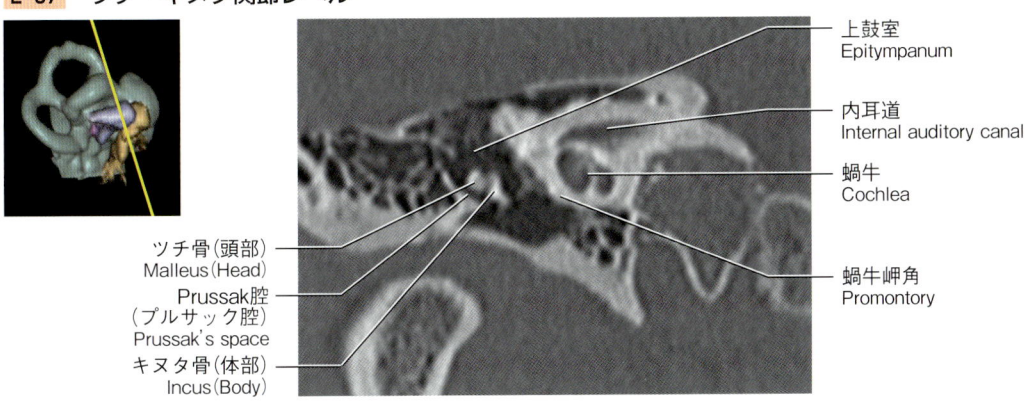

上鼓室 Epitympanum
内耳道 Internal auditory canal
蝸牛 Cochlea
蝸牛岬角 Promontory
ツチ骨（頭部） Malleus（Head）
Prussak腔（プルサック腔） Prussak's space
キヌタ骨（体部） Incus（Body）

NOTE Prussak（プルサック）腔とは上鼓室外側の鼓膜弛緩部，ツチ骨外側突起，ツチ骨頸部，外側ツチ骨靱帯に囲まれた部位で，弛緩部（上鼓室）型真珠腫の好発部位である．

側頭骨の断層解剖［冠状断像，前方から後方へ（CT）］

2-98 内耳道レベル

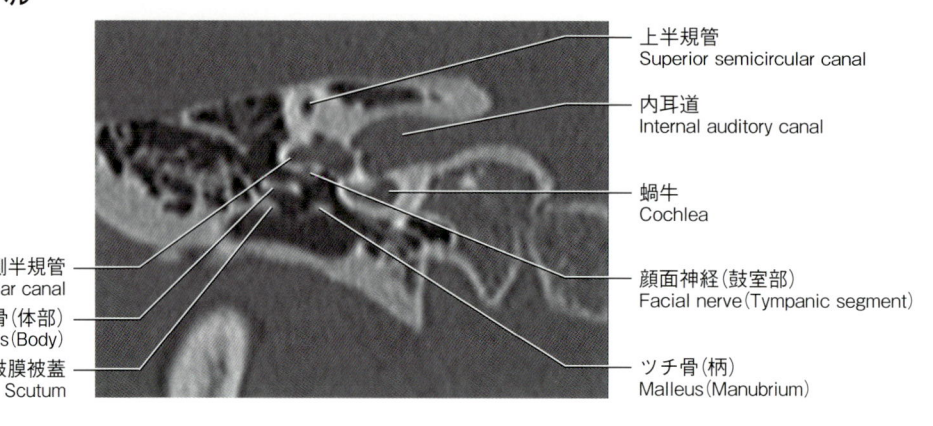

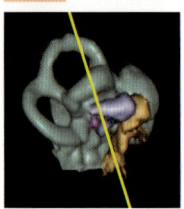

- 上半規管 Superior semicircular canal
- 内耳道 Internal auditory canal
- 蝸牛 Cochlea
- 顔面神経（鼓室部） Facial nerve（Tympanic segment）
- ツチ骨（柄） Malleus（Manubrium）
- 外側半規管 Lateral semicircular canal
- キヌタ骨（体部） Incus（Body）
- 鼓膜被蓋 Scutum

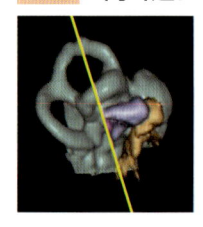

2-99 内耳道レベル

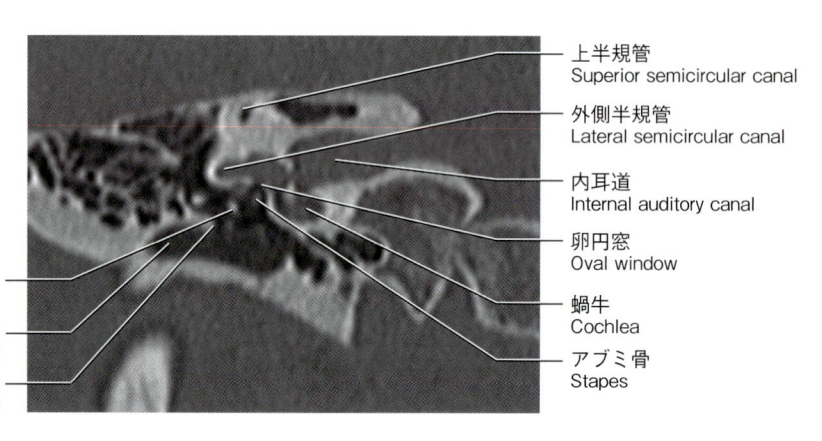

- 上半規管 Superior semicircular canal
- 外側半規管 Lateral semicircular canal
- 内耳道 Internal auditory canal
- 卵円窓 Oval window
- 蝸牛 Cochlea
- アブミ骨 Stapes
- キヌタ骨（長脚） Incus（Long crus）
- 外耳道 External auditory canal
- 鼓膜被蓋 Scutum

2-100 内耳道レベル

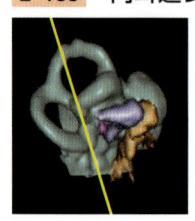

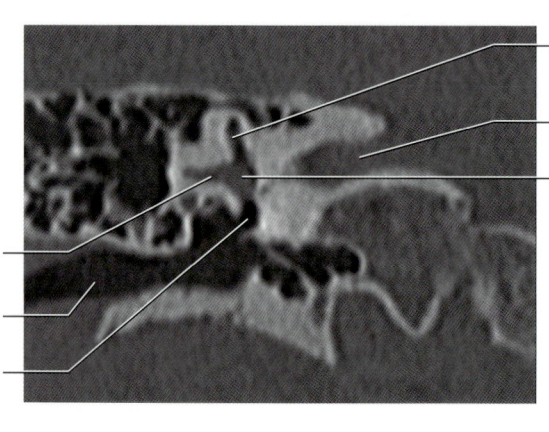

- 上半規管 Superior semicircular canal
- 内耳道 Internal auditory canal
- 前庭 Vestibule
- 外側半規管 Lateral semicircular canal
- 外耳道 External auditory canal
- 正円窓 Round window

NOTE 弛緩部（上鼓室）型真珠腫では鼓膜被蓋の鈍化がみられる．

側頭骨の断層解剖 [冠状断像，前方から後方へ(CT)]

2-101 内耳道後方・後半規管レベル

後半規管
Posterior semicircular canal

外耳道
External auditory canal

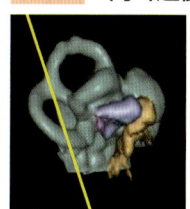

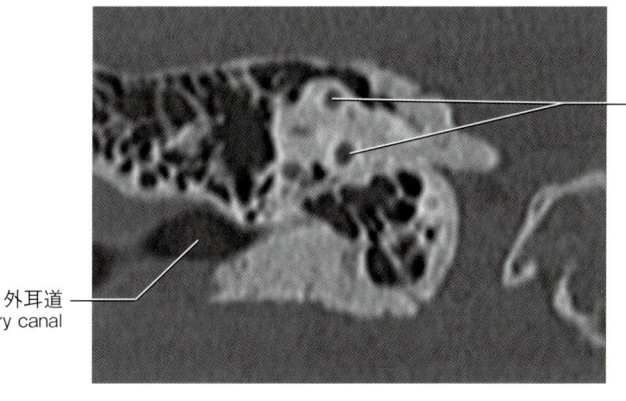

2-102 内耳道後方・後半規管レベル

後半規管
Posterior semicircular canal

外耳道
External auditory canal

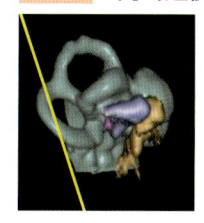

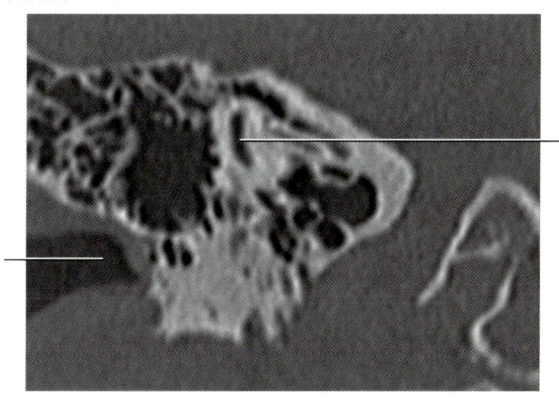

NOTE 耳管 Eustachian tube
　耳管は，中耳と咽頭をつなぐ管．発見した解剖学者B. Eustachiの名前をとり，Eustachian tube あるいは，Auditory tubeが英語名で，日本ではユースタキオ管とされる．なお，tubaとは"ラッパが原意の管"の意味に使う語．早くは旧約聖書にあらわれるが，現代オーケストラの最大の金管楽器の名と，耳管・卵管の解剖学用語に残る．

側頭骨の断層解剖 ［矢状断像，右外側から左外側（CT）］

2-103 ツチ・キヌタ関節レベル

- 外側半規管 Lateral semicircular canal
- ツチ骨（頭部） Malleus(Head)
- キヌタ骨（体部） Incus(Body)

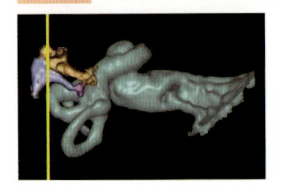

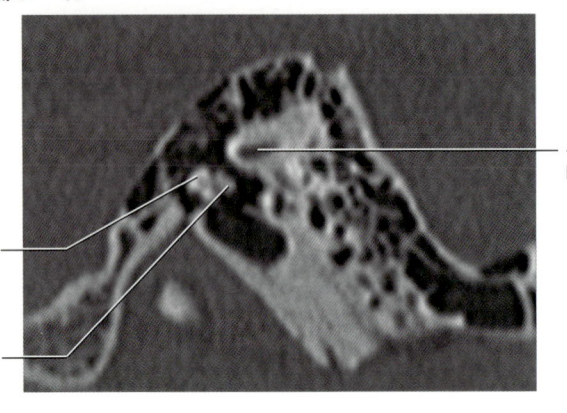

2-104 ツチ・キヌタ関節レベル

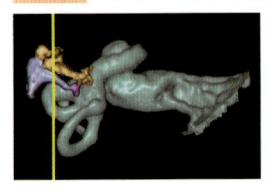

- 外側半規管 Lateral semicircular canal
- キヌタ骨（体部） Incus(Body)
- ツチ骨（頭部） Malleus(Head)
- ツチ骨（頸部） Malleus(Neck)
- ツチ骨（柄） Malleus(Manubrium)

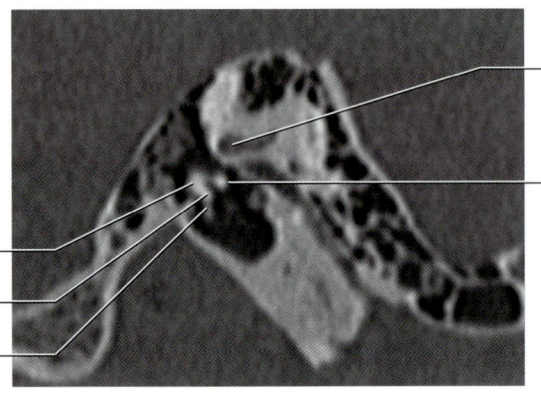

2-105 ツチ・キヌタ関節内側レベル

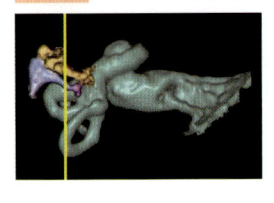

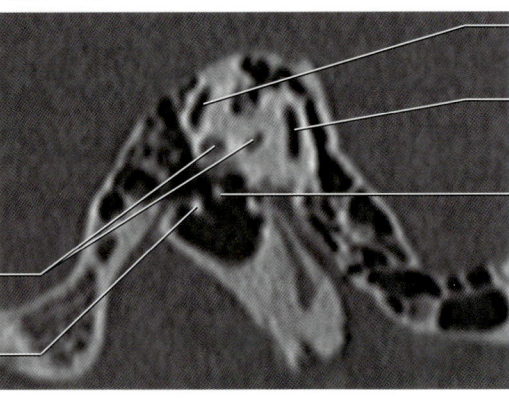

- 上半規管 Superior semicircular canal
- 後半規管 Posterior semicircular canal
- キヌタ骨（体部） Incus(Body)
- 外側半規管 Lateral semicircular canal
- ツチ骨（柄） Malleus(Manubrium)

側頭骨の断層解剖 ［矢状断像，右外側から左外側(CT)］

2-106 ツチ・キヌタ関節内側レベル

- 上半規管 Superior semicircular canal
- 後半規管 Posterior semicircular canal
- キヌタ骨（豆状突起） Incus (Lenticular process)
- 外側半規管 Lateral semicircular canal
- ツチ骨（柄） Malleus (Manubrium)

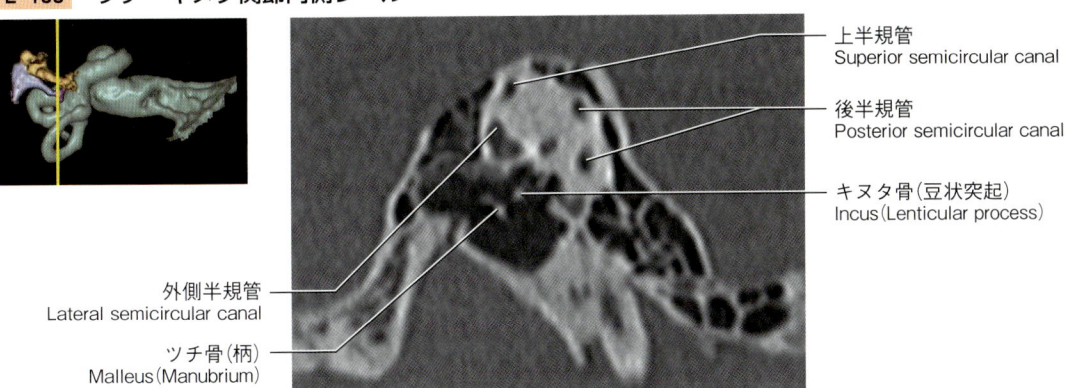

2-107 ツチ・キヌタ関節内側レベル

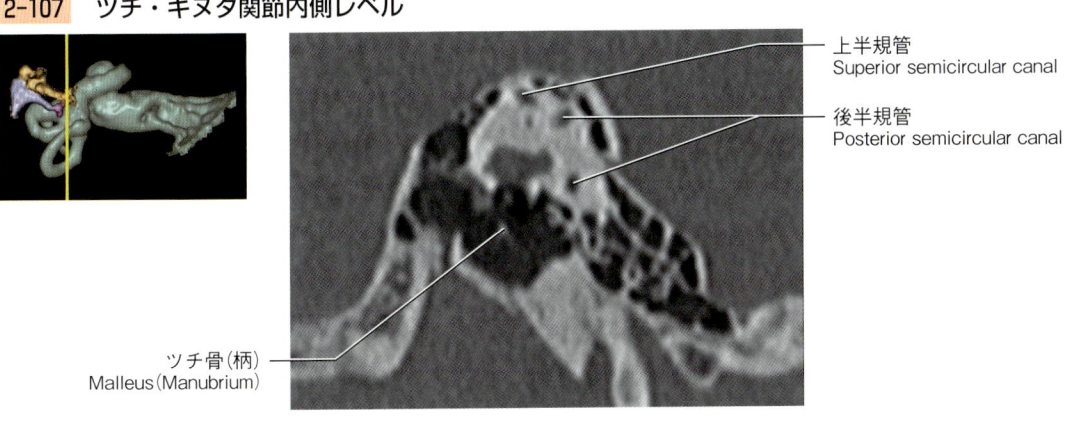

- 上半規管 Superior semicircular canal
- 後半規管 Posterior semicircular canal
- ツチ骨（柄） Malleus (Manubrium)

2-108 前庭レベル

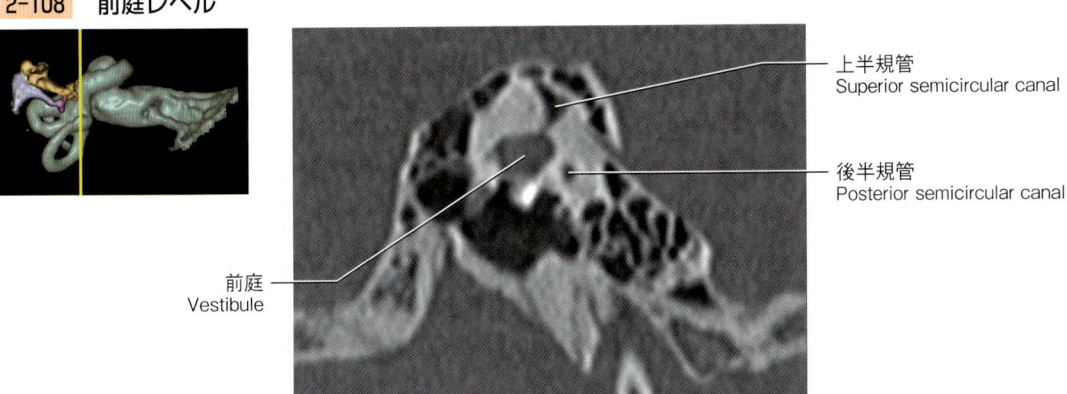

- 上半規管 Superior semicircular canal
- 後半規管 Posterior semicircular canal
- 前庭 Vestibule

NOTE 上半規管の骨壁が先天的に欠損し，迷路リンパ液の動きが頭蓋内に抜けてしまう病態を上半規管裂隙症候群という．症状として大きな音で引き起こされるめまいが特徴的である．

側頭骨の断層解剖　[矢状断像，右外側から左外側(CT)]

2-109　前庭レベル

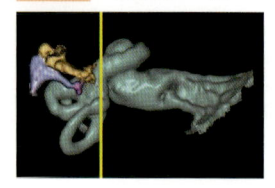

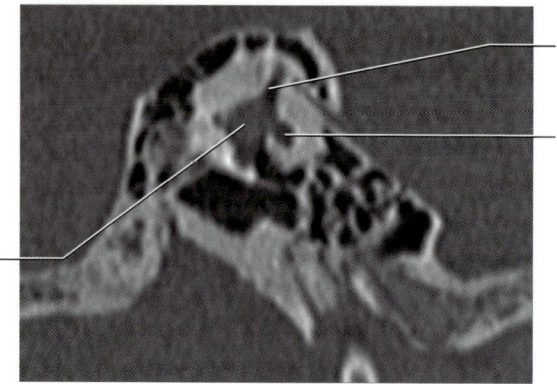

- 上半規管　Superior semicircular canal
- 後半規管　Posterior semicircular canal
- 前庭　Vestibule

2-110　蝸牛レベル

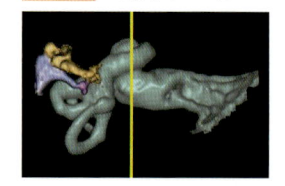

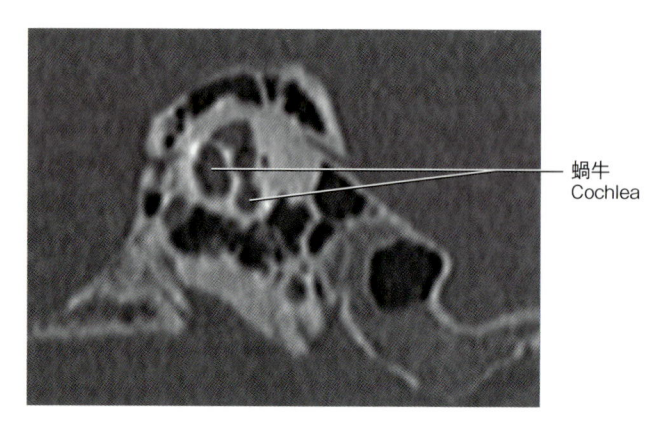

- 蝸牛　Cochlea

2-111　蝸牛・内耳道レベル

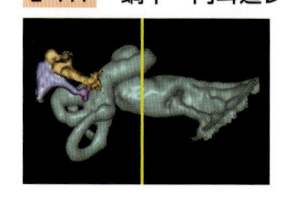

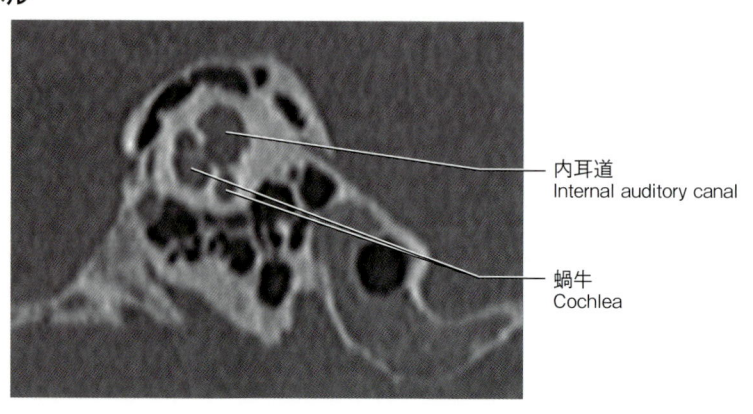

- 内耳道　Internal auditory canal
- 蝸牛　Cochlea

> **NOTE**　内耳道の前上方を顔面神経，前下方を蝸牛神経，後上方を上前庭神経，後下方を下前庭神経が走行する．これらはMR cisternographyで明瞭に描出される．

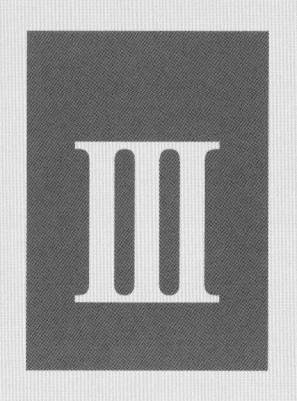

III

脊　椎
Spine

脊　柱

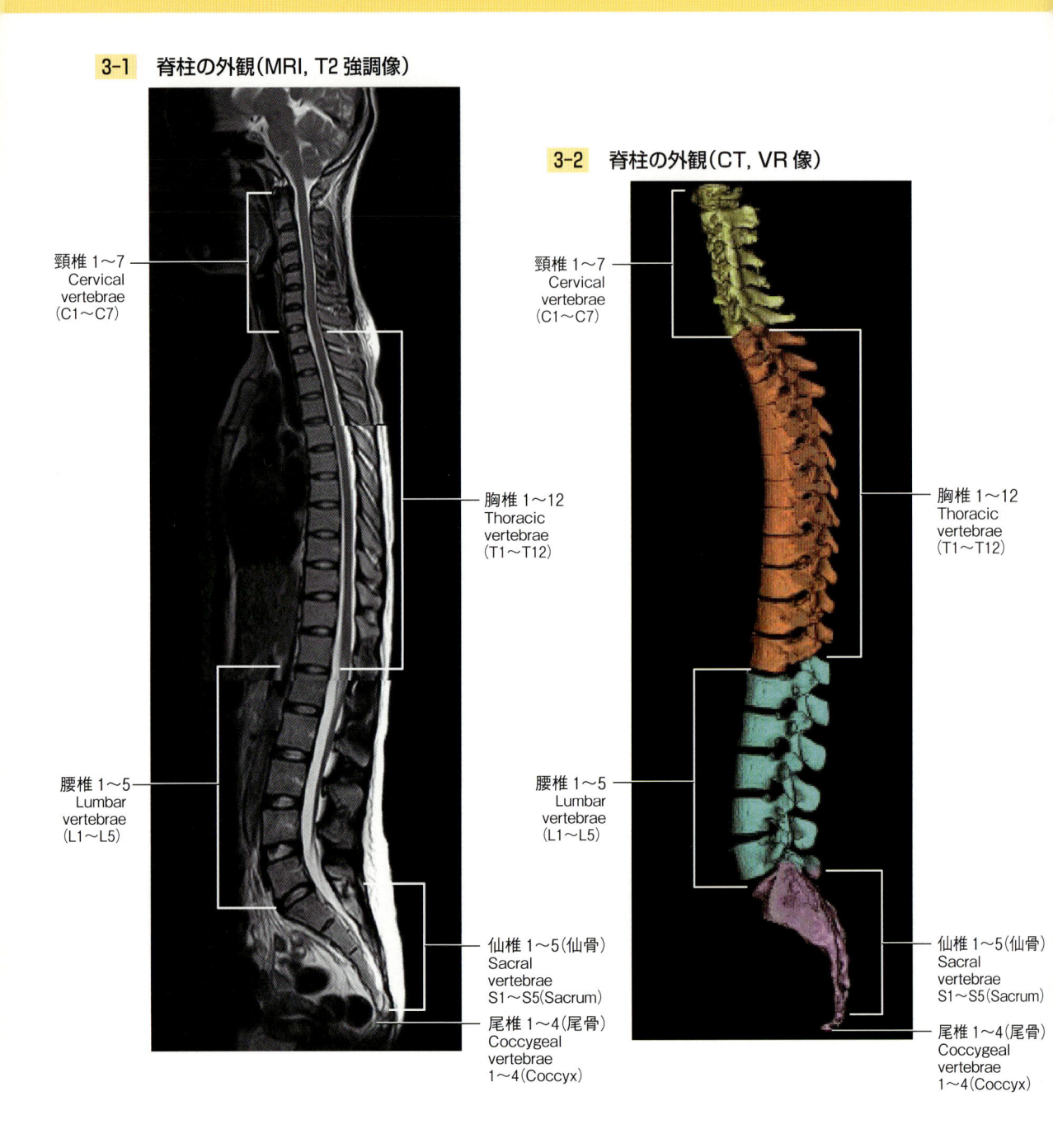

3-1　脊柱の外観（MRI, T2強調像）

- 頸椎 1～7 Cervical vertebrae（C1～C7）
- 胸椎 1～12 Thoracic vertebrae（T1～T12）
- 腰椎 1～5 Lumbar vertebrae（L1～L5）
- 仙椎 1～5（仙骨）Sacral vertebrae S1～S5（Sacrum）
- 尾椎 1～4（尾骨）Coccygeal vertebrae 1～4（Coccyx）

3-2　脊柱の外観（CT, VR像）

- 頸椎 1～7 Cervical vertebrae（C1～C7）
- 胸椎 1～12 Thoracic vertebrae（T1～T12）
- 腰椎 1～5 Lumbar vertebrae（L1～L5）
- 仙椎 1～5（仙骨）Sacral vertebrae S1～S5（Sacrum）
- 尾椎 1～4（尾骨）Coccygeal vertebrae 1～4（Coccyx）

> **NOTE** 成人の脊柱は一般に33個の椎骨からなり，頸椎，胸椎，腰椎，仙椎，尾椎の5つの部分に分けられる．頸椎は7個，胸椎は12個，腰椎は5個，仙椎は5個，尾椎は4個の椎骨で形成され，仙椎と尾椎の各椎骨は癒合してそれぞれ仙骨と尾骨になる．仙骨に至るまで脊椎骨は下方へ向かうにつれ大きくなるが，これは人間が二足歩行のため，下方へ向かうほど支えなければならない体重が増加するためである．

頸椎 (CT, VR像)

3-3 頸椎（正面）

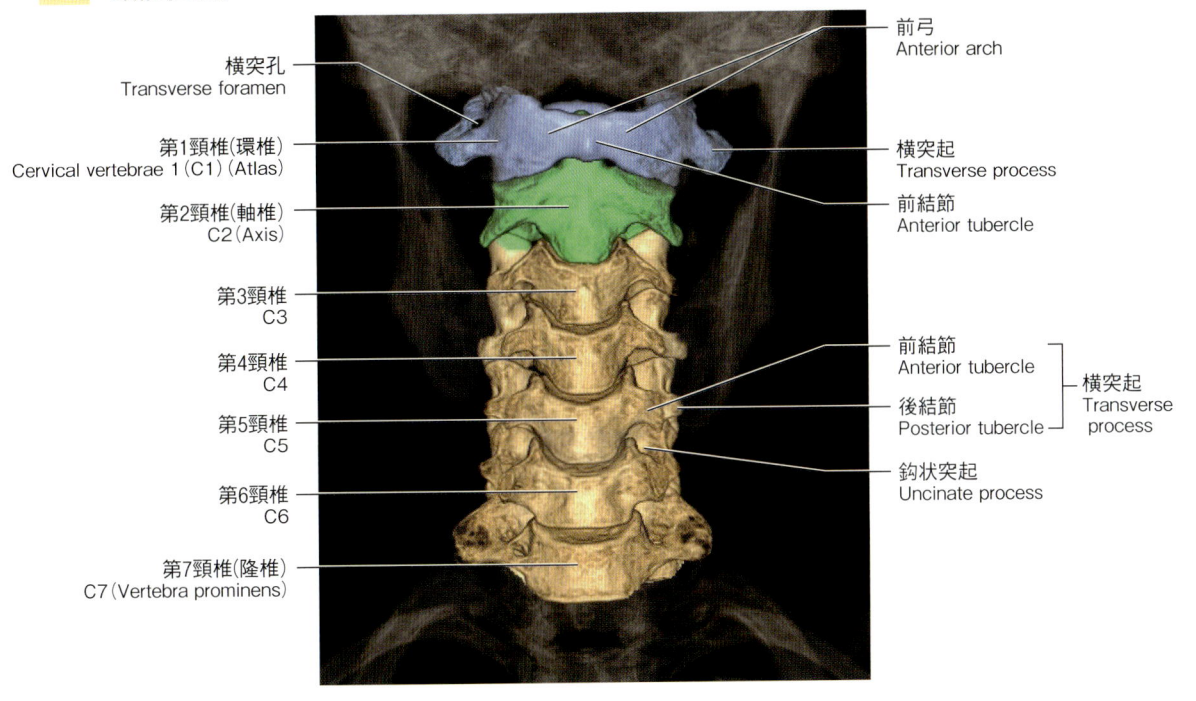

- 横突孔 Transverse foramen
- 第1頸椎（環椎）Cervical vertebrae 1 (C1) (Atlas)
- 第2頸椎（軸椎）C2 (Axis)
- 第3頸椎 C3
- 第4頸椎 C4
- 第5頸椎 C5
- 第6頸椎 C6
- 第7頸椎（隆椎）C7 (Vertebra prominens)
- 前弓 Anterior arch
- 横突起 Transverse process
- 前結節 Anterior tubercle
- 前結節 Anterior tubercle
- 後結節 Posterior tubercle
- 横突起 Transverse process
- 鉤状突起 Uncinate process

3-4 頸椎（側面）

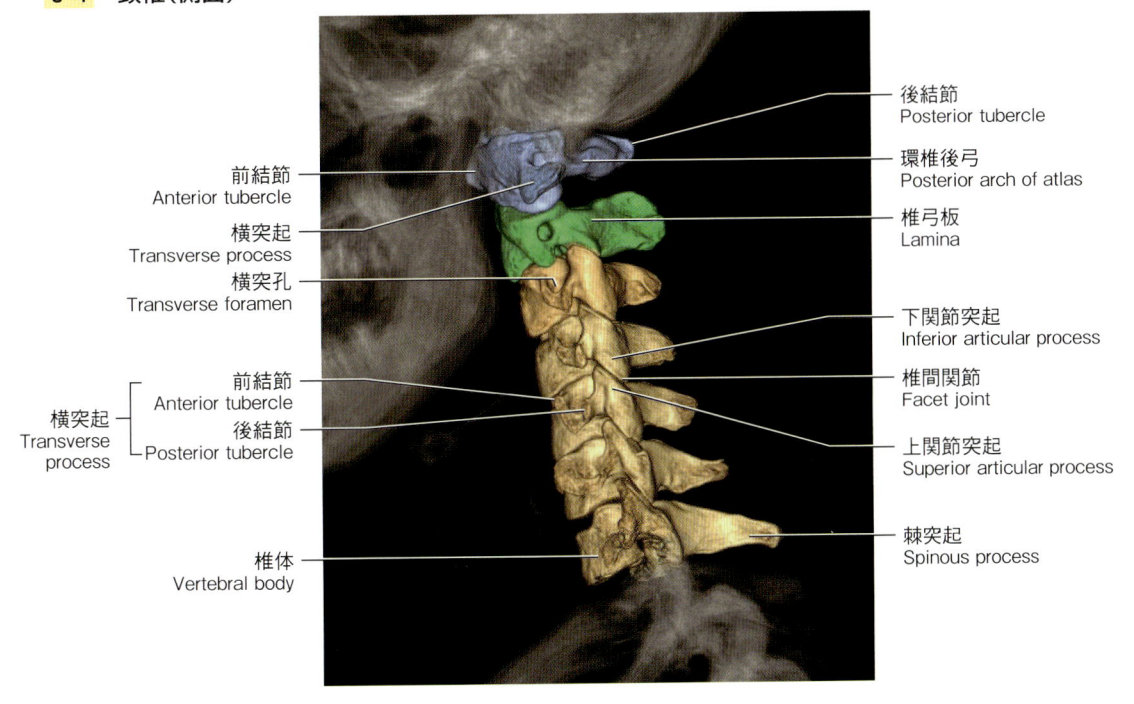

- 前結節 Anterior tubercle
- 横突起 Transverse process
- 横突孔 Transverse foramen
- 横突起 Transverse process
  - 前結節 Anterior tubercle
  - 後結節 Posterior tubercle
- 椎体 Vertebral body
- 後結節 Posterior tubercle
- 環椎後弓 Posterior arch of atlas
- 椎弓板 Lamina
- 下関節突起 Inferior articular process
- 椎間関節 Facet joint
- 上関節突起 Superior articular process
- 棘突起 Spinous process

NOTE 頸椎は第1頸椎～第7頸椎まで7個の椎骨で構成される．第1頸椎は環椎，第2頸椎は軸椎とよばれ，第3頸椎以下の椎骨と形状を異にしている．また，第7頸椎は後方に突出する棘突起が長く隆椎ともよばれる．指を頸部背側正中で後頭部との付け根に置き，そこから下方へ正中に沿って降ろした際，はじめに最もはっきりと触れることのできる突起が隆椎の棘突起である．

頸椎（CT，VR像）

3-5 頸椎（斜位）

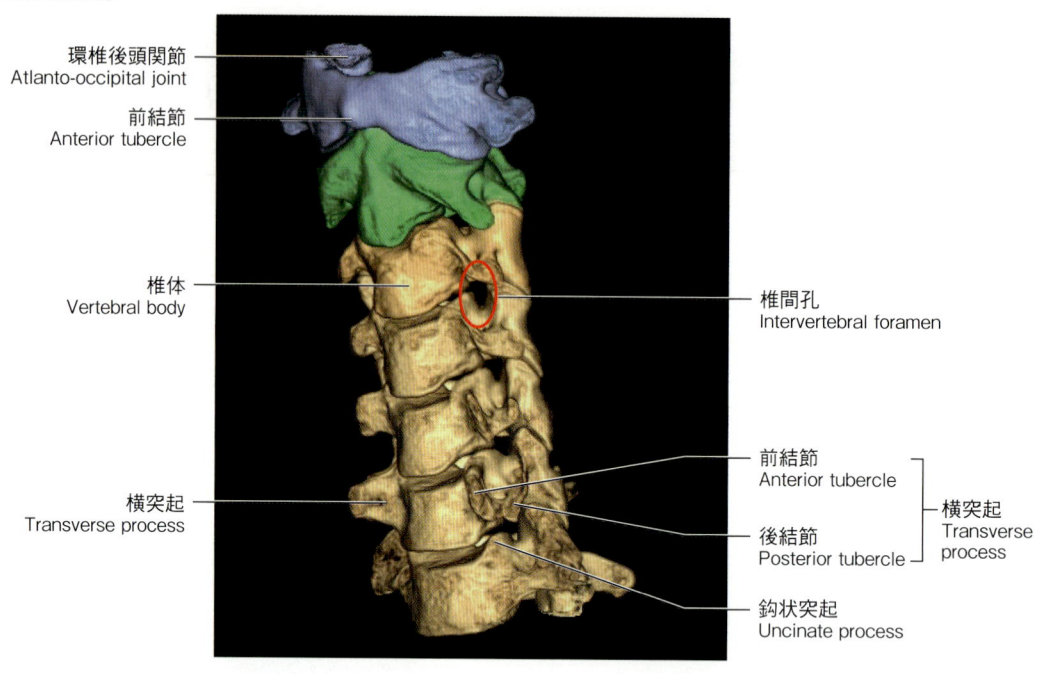

- 環椎後頭関節 Atlanto-occipital joint
- 前結節 Anterior tubercle
- 椎体 Vertebral body
- 椎間孔 Intervertebral foramen
- 横突起 Transverse process
- 前結節 Anterior tubercle ┐ 横突起 Transverse process
- 後結節 Posterior tubercle ┘
- 鉤状突起 Uncinate process

3-6 第1頸椎（環椎），第2頸椎（軸椎）（矢状断）

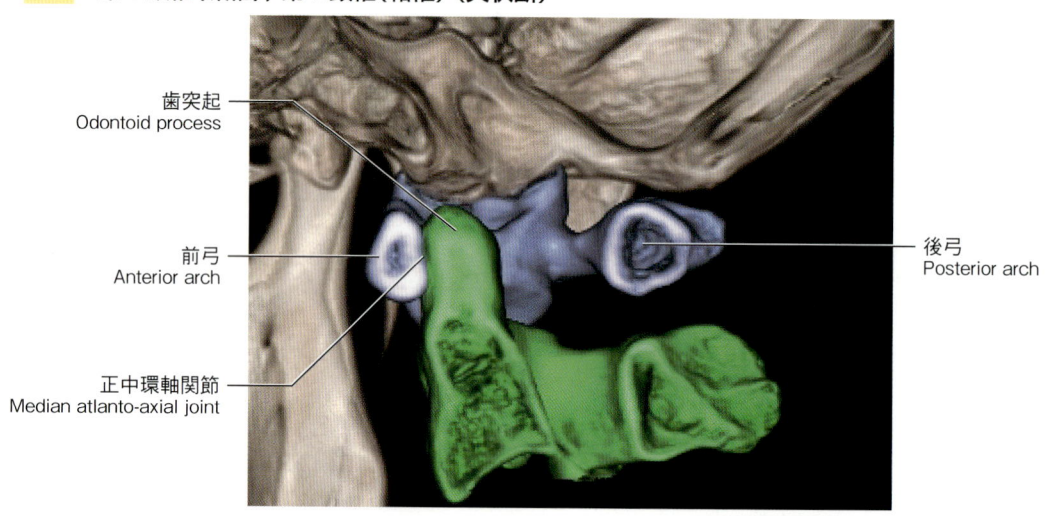

- 歯突起 Odontoid process
- 前弓 Anterior arch
- 正中環軸関節 Median atlanto-axial joint
- 後弓 Posterior arch

NOTE 環椎 Atlas

　Atlas（アトラス）は，アフリカ北西部の山脈名，メルカトール以来の地図帳の意味として古く，また解剖図譜の意味，NASAのロケット名などにも広く使われる語だが，もちろんすべてギリシャ神話の神の名からである．ゼウスに敗れ，地球・天体を支え続ける罰を受けた巨神で，その様子から頭蓋骨を支える環椎（C1）の名前となった．

頸椎（CT, VR像） 125

3-7 第1頸椎（環椎），第2頸椎（軸椎）（冠状断）

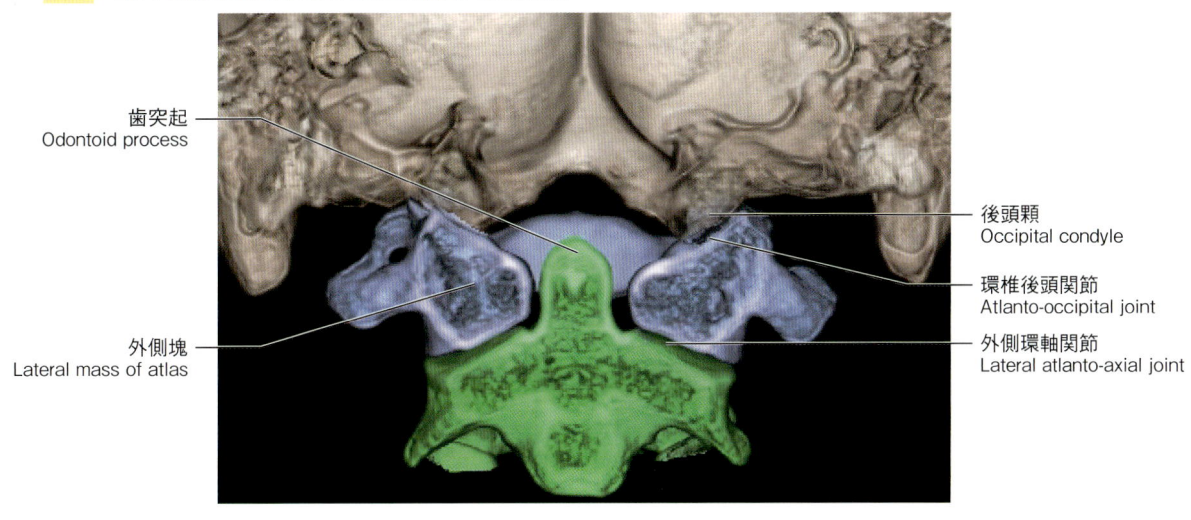

- 歯突起 Odontoid process
- 外側塊 Lateral mass of atlas
- 後頭顆 Occipital condyle
- 環椎後頭関節 Atlanto-occipital joint
- 外側環軸関節 Lateral atlanto-axial joint

3-8 第1頸椎（環椎），第2頸椎（軸椎）（上方）

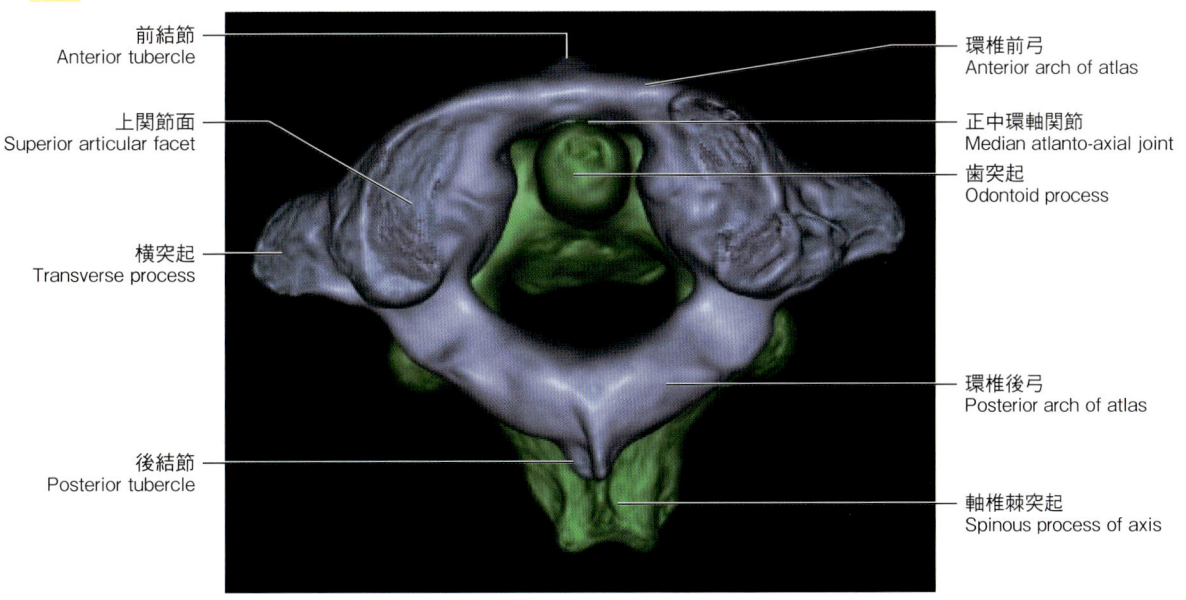

- 前結節 Anterior tubercle
- 上関節面 Superior articular facet
- 横突起 Transverse process
- 後結節 Posterior tubercle
- 環椎前弓 Anterior arch of atlas
- 正中環軸関節 Median atlanto-axial joint
- 歯突起 Odontoid process
- 環椎後弓 Posterior arch of atlas
- 軸椎棘突起 Spinous process of axis

> **NOTE** 環椎の外側塊は，上面にある上関節面で頭蓋骨の大後頭孔の両側にある後頭顆とよばれる隆起と環椎後頭関節を，下面にある下関節面で軸椎の上関節面と外側環軸関節をそれぞれ形成し，前・後屈や回旋に際し広い可動域を可能としている．

頸　椎（CT, VR 像）

3-9　第1頸椎（環椎）

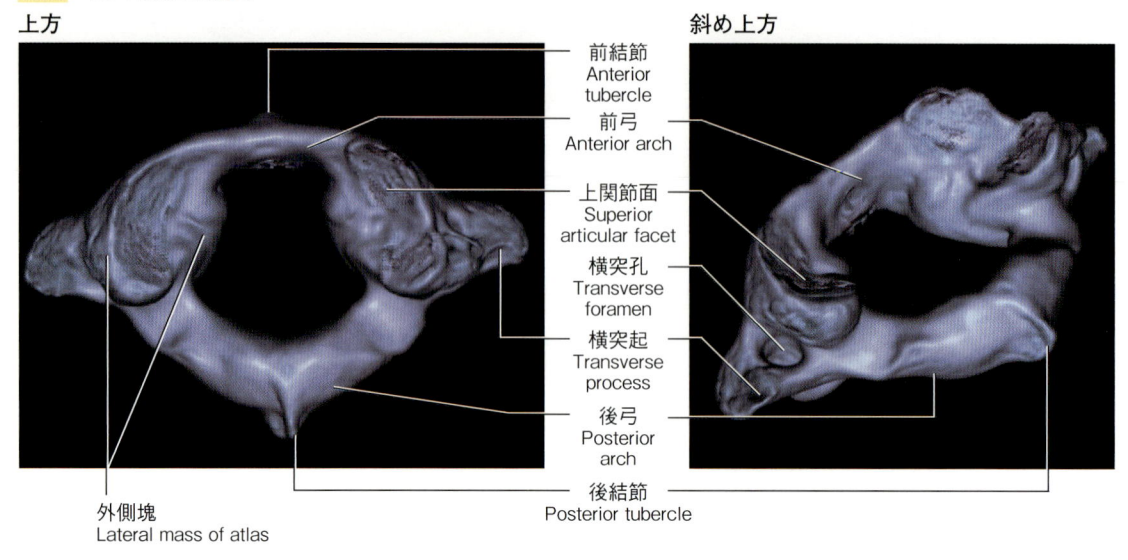

上方／斜め上方

- 前結節 Anterior tubercle
- 前弓 Anterior arch
- 上関節面 Superior articular facet
- 横突孔 Transverse foramen
- 横突起 Transverse process
- 後弓 Posterior arch
- 後結節 Posterior tubercle
- 外側塊 Lateral mass of atlas

3-10　第2頸椎（軸椎）

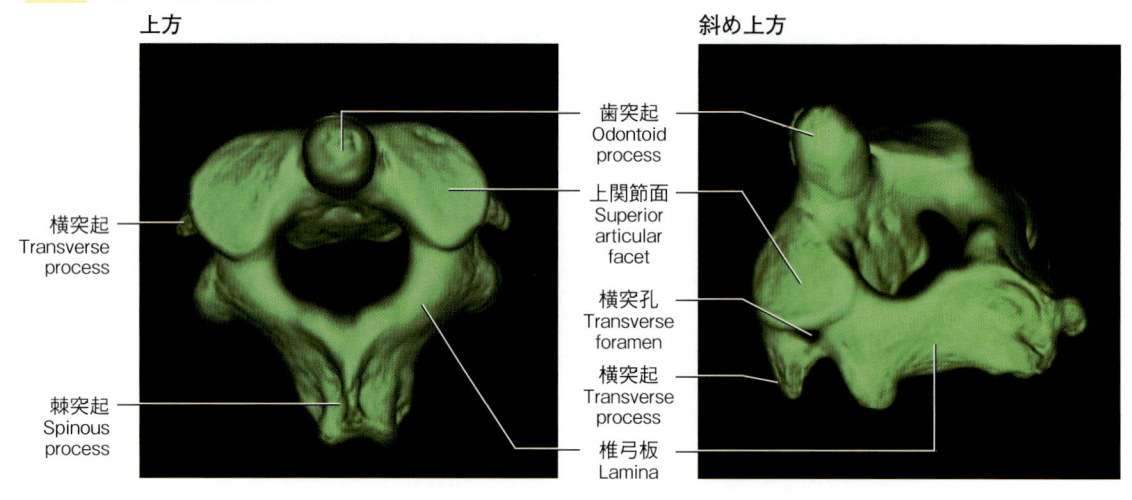

上方／斜め上方

- 歯突起 Odontoid process
- 上関節面 Superior articular facet
- 横突孔 Transverse foramen
- 横突起 Transverse process
- 椎弓板 Lamina
- 横突起 Transverse process
- 棘突起 Spinous process

> **NOTE**　環椎は椎体と棘突起をもたず，前弓・後弓・外側塊から構成される輪状の形状を呈している．環椎の外側塊は大きく，転落した際などに後頭窩と軸椎の間で圧排されバラバラになる Jefferson 骨折あるいは破裂骨折を生じる（3-9）．軸椎には歯突起とよばれる突起が椎体から上方へ向かい垂直に伸びている．"No" の意思表示をする際，軸椎の上関節面の上を環椎が回旋するための軸となる（3-10）．

頸椎の断層解剖 ［横断像(CT)］

3-11　第1頸椎(環椎)レベル

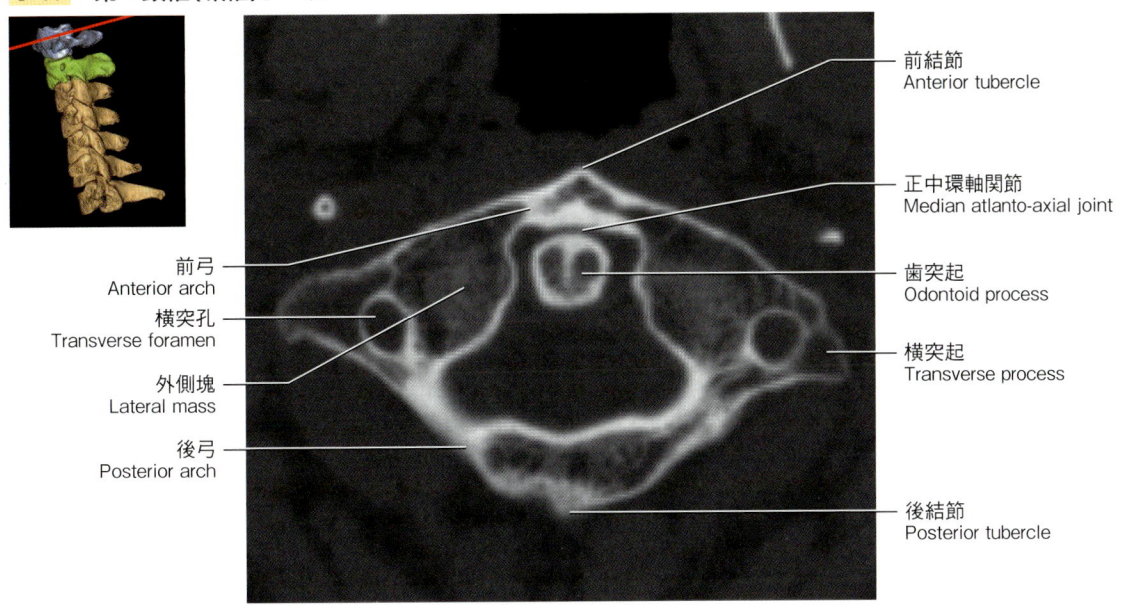

- 前結節 Anterior tubercle
- 正中環軸関節 Median atlanto-axial joint
- 歯突起 Odontoid process
- 横突起 Transverse process
- 後結節 Posterior tubercle
- 前弓 Anterior arch
- 横突孔 Transverse foramen
- 外側塊 Lateral mass
- 後弓 Posterior arch

3-12　第2頸椎(軸椎)レベル

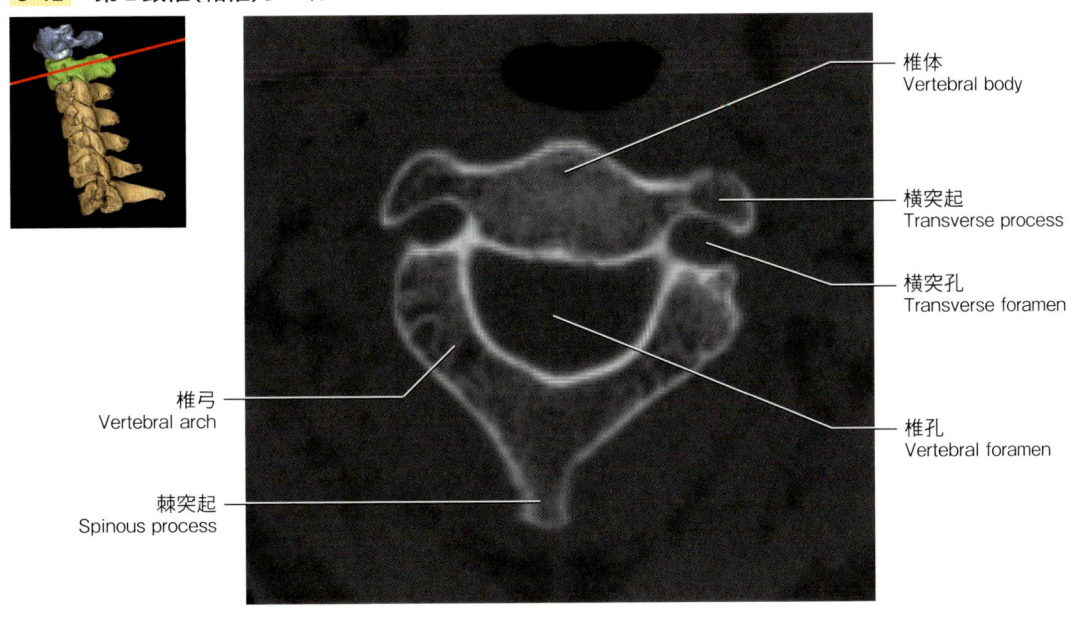

- 椎体 Vertebral body
- 横突起 Transverse process
- 横突孔 Transverse foramen
- 椎孔 Vertebral foramen
- 椎弓 Vertebral arch
- 棘突起 Spinous process

> **NOTE** 椎体と椎弓によって形成される孔を椎孔とよび，各椎骨が関節で連続し脊柱を形成することで椎孔も連続し脊柱管が形成される．脊髄はこの脊柱管の中にあり，周りを強固な骨で囲まれ守られている．

頸椎の断層解剖 [横断像(CT)]

3-13 第2-第3頸椎椎間レベル

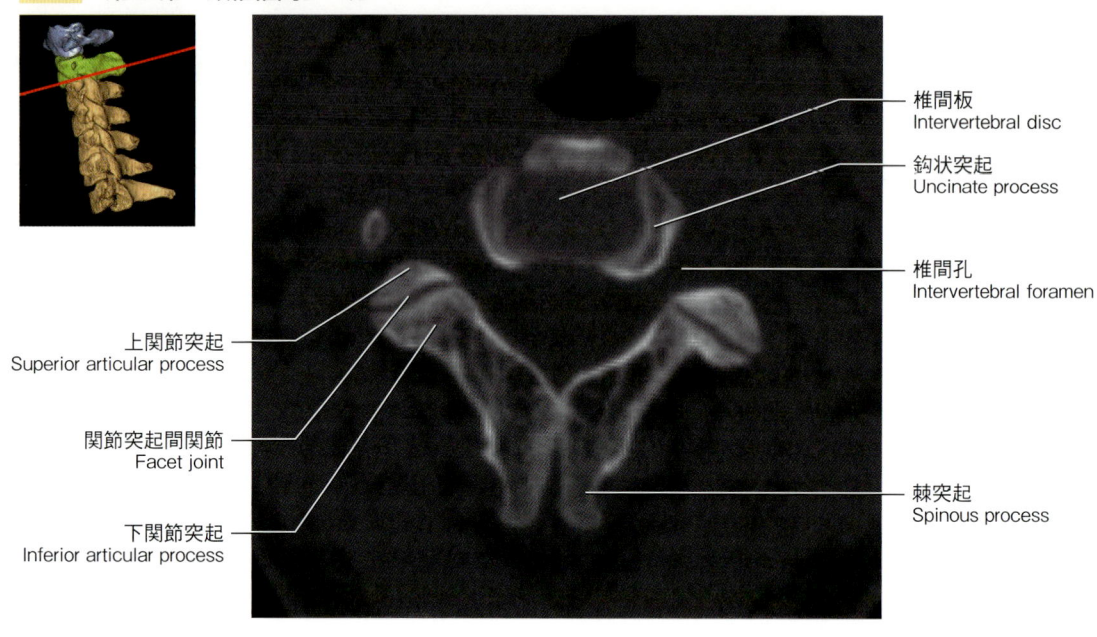

- 椎間板 Intervertebral disc
- 鉤状突起 Uncinate process
- 椎間孔 Intervertebral foramen
- 上関節突起 Superior articular process
- 関節突起間関節 Facet joint
- 下関節突起 Inferior articular process
- 棘突起 Spinous process

3-14 第3頸椎レベル

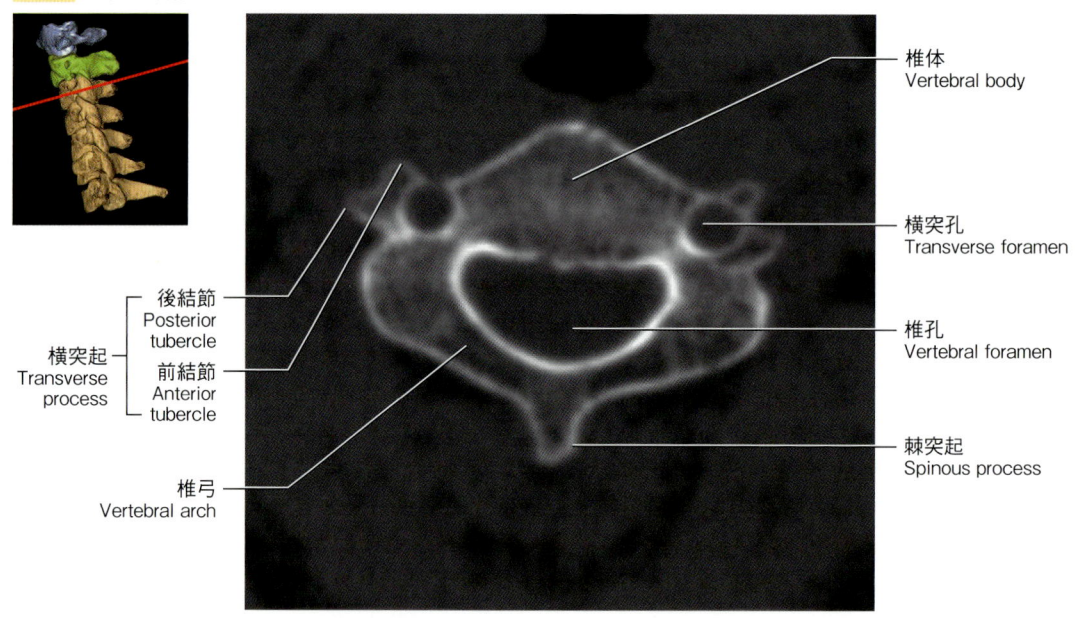

- 椎体 Vertebral body
- 横突孔 Transverse foramen
- 椎孔 Vertebral foramen
- 横突起 Transverse process
  - 後結節 Posterior tubercle
  - 前結節 Anterior tubercle
- 椎弓 Vertebral arch
- 棘突起 Spinous process

NOTE 脊椎 Spine

Spine の元となった spina は本来，棘(トゲ)の意味をもつラテン語．古代ローマの長円状の大競技場"チルクス"の中央にある塀の上には尖塔や彫像が飾られ，たくさんのトゲを並べたようにみえたことから，脊柱のことを Spine とよぶようになったとの有力な説がある．

頸椎の断層解剖 ［冠状断像（CT, MPR像）］

3-15　椎体中央部レベル

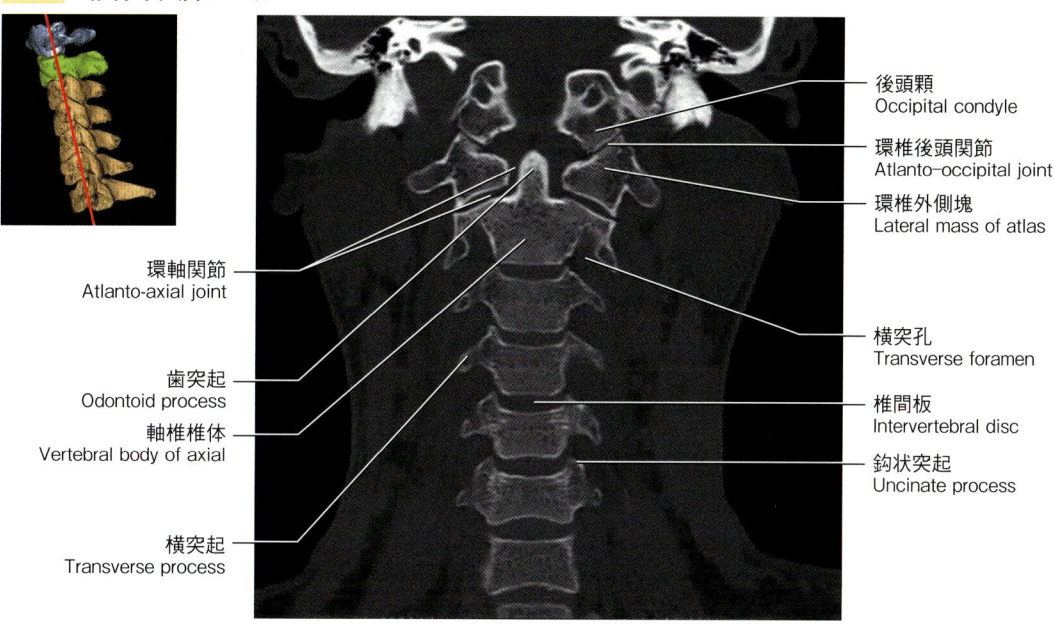

- 後頭顆　Occipital condyle
- 環椎後頭関節　Atlanto-occipital joint
- 環椎外側塊　Lateral mass of atlas
- 環軸関節　Atlanto-axial joint
- 歯突起　Odontoid process
- 軸椎椎体　Vertebral body of axial
- 横突孔　Transverse foramen
- 椎間板　Intervertebral disc
- 鉤状突起　Uncinate process
- 横突起　Transverse process

3-16　椎体後部レベル

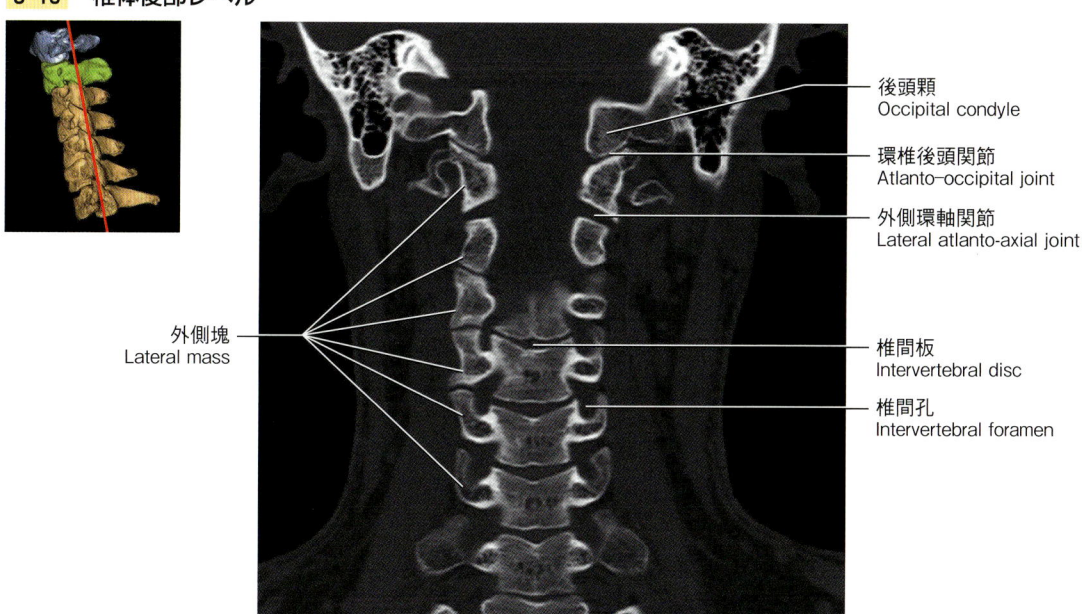

- 後頭顆　Occipital condyle
- 環椎後頭関節　Atlanto-occipital joint
- 外側環軸関節　Lateral atlanto-axial joint
- 外側塊　Lateral mass
- 椎間板　Intervertebral disc
- 椎間孔　Intervertebral foramen

> **NOTE**　環椎の外側塊は大きく，ここから横突起が伸びているため，これより下の脊椎の横突起よりも外側に位置している（3-15）．また，胎生期に下位頸椎から出ていた肋骨が遺残したものを"頸肋"とよぶ．

頸椎の断層解剖 ［矢状断像（CT, MPR 像）］

3-17 関節突起間関節レベル

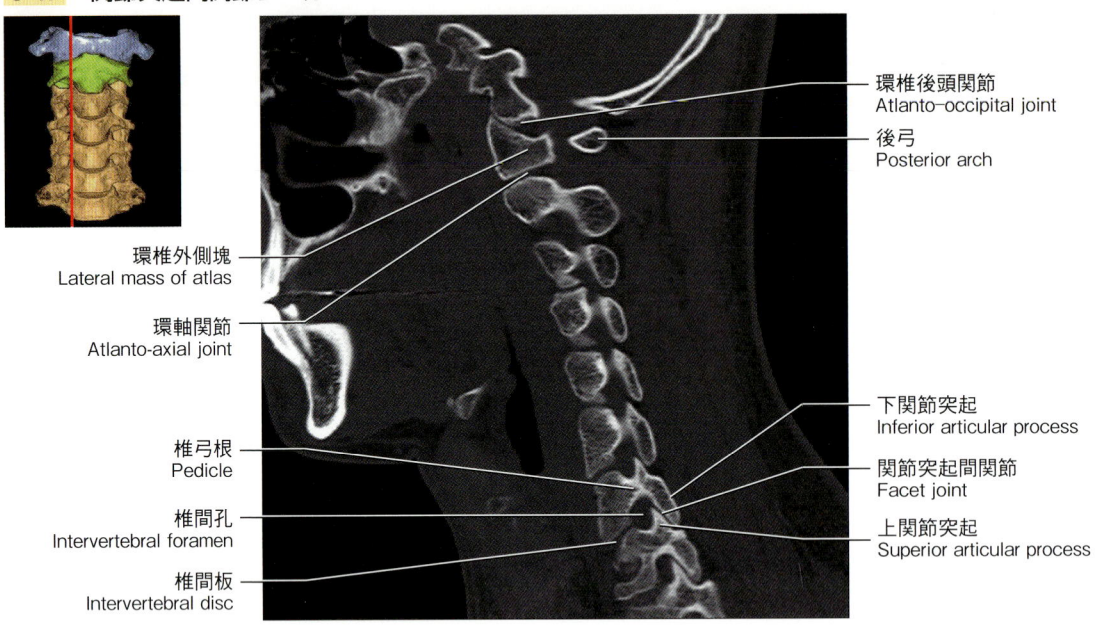

- 環椎後頭関節 Atlanto-occipital joint
- 後弓 Posterior arch
- 環椎外側塊 Lateral mass of atlas
- 環軸関節 Atlanto-axial joint
- 下関節突起 Inferior articular process
- 椎弓根 Pedicle
- 関節突起間関節 Facet joint
- 椎間孔 Intervertebral foramen
- 上関節突起 Superior articular process
- 椎間板 Intervertebral disc

3-18 脊柱管レベル

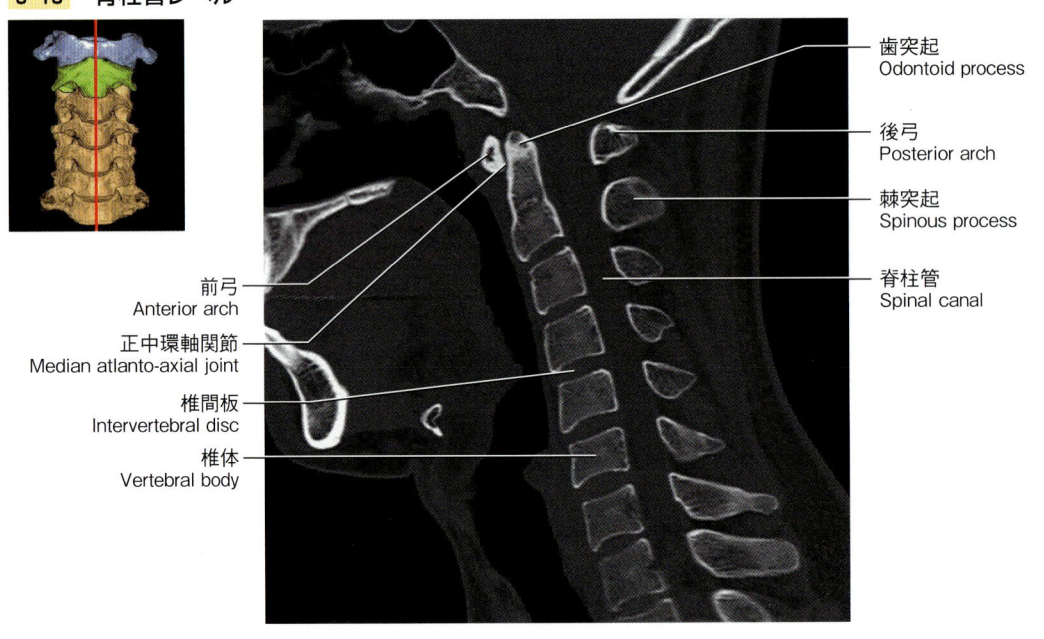

- 歯突起 Odontoid process
- 後弓 Posterior arch
- 棘突起 Spinous process
- 前弓 Anterior arch
- 脊柱管 Spinal canal
- 正中環軸関節 Median atlanto-axial joint
- 椎間板 Intervertebral disc
- 椎体 Vertebral body

> **NOTE** 椎間孔は上下縁を椎弓根，後縁を椎間関節，前縁上部を椎体，前縁下部を椎間板によって構成された孔であり，この中を脊髄神経が脊柱から出ていく（3-17）．第2頸椎である軸椎には上方へ突出する歯突起があることが特徴であり，これは矢状断像で高位を決定するうえでの指標となる（3-18）．

頸椎の断層解剖 ［横断像（MRI，T1強調像）］

3-19 第1頸椎（環椎）下縁レベル

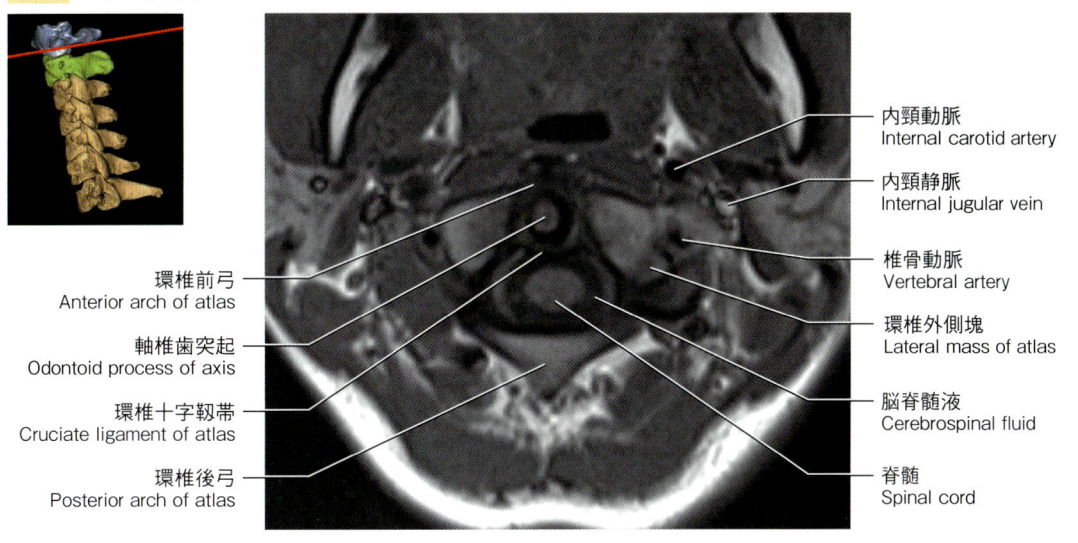

- 環椎前弓 Anterior arch of atlas
- 軸椎歯突起 Odontoid process of axis
- 環椎十字靱帯 Cruciate ligament of atlas
- 環椎後弓 Posterior arch of atlas
- 内頸動脈 Internal carotid artery
- 内頸静脈 Internal jugular vein
- 椎骨動脈 Vertebral artery
- 環椎外側塊 Lateral mass of atlas
- 脳脊髄液 Cerebrospinal fluid
- 脊髄 Spinal cord

3-20 第1頸椎（環椎）下縁レベル

- 下頭斜筋 Obliquus capitis inferior muscle
- 後頭直筋 Rectus capitis posterior muscle
- 椎前筋 Prevertebral muscle
- 頸最長筋 Longissimus cervicis muscle
- 胸鎖乳突筋 Sternocleidomastoid muscle
- 頭板状筋 Splenius capitis muscle
- 頭半棘筋 Semispinalis capitis muscle
- 僧帽筋 Trapezius muscle

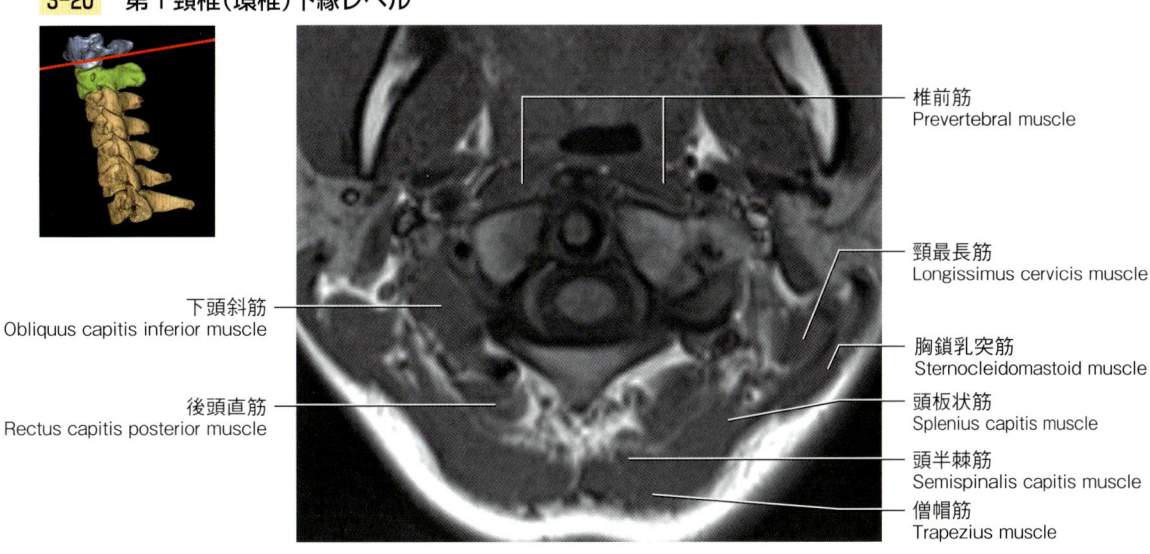

> **NOTE** 環椎十字靱帯は一側の外側塊から対側の外側塊をつなぎ，かつ歯突起を背側から覆う靱帯で，環椎前弓が前方へずれたり，歯突起が後方へずれることを防いでいる（3-19）．

頸椎の断層解剖 ［横断像（MRI, T1強調像）］

3-21　第2-第3頸椎椎間レベル

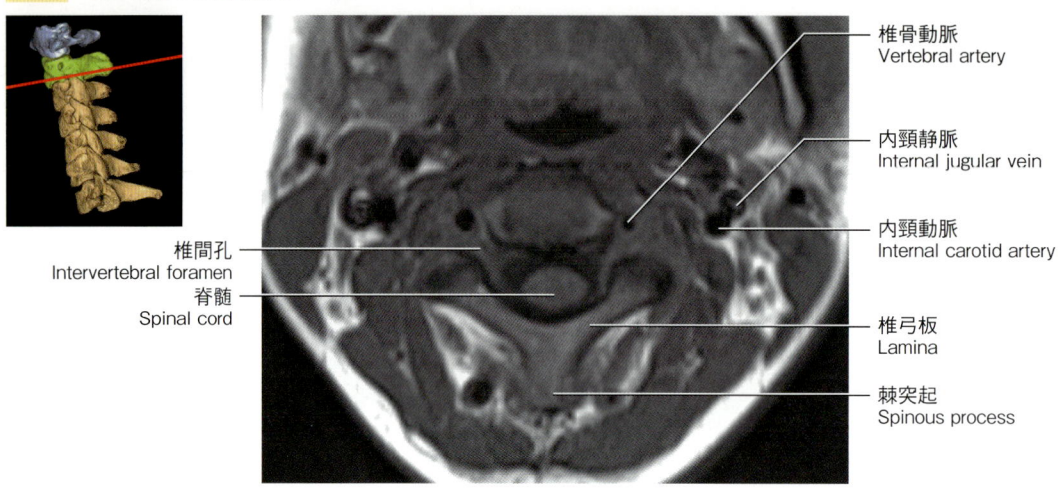

椎骨動脈　Vertebral artery
内頸静脈　Internal jugular vein
内頸動脈　Internal carotid artery
椎弓板　Lamina
棘突起　Spinous process

椎間孔　Intervertebral foramen
脊髄　Spinal cord

3-22　第2-第3頸椎椎間レベル

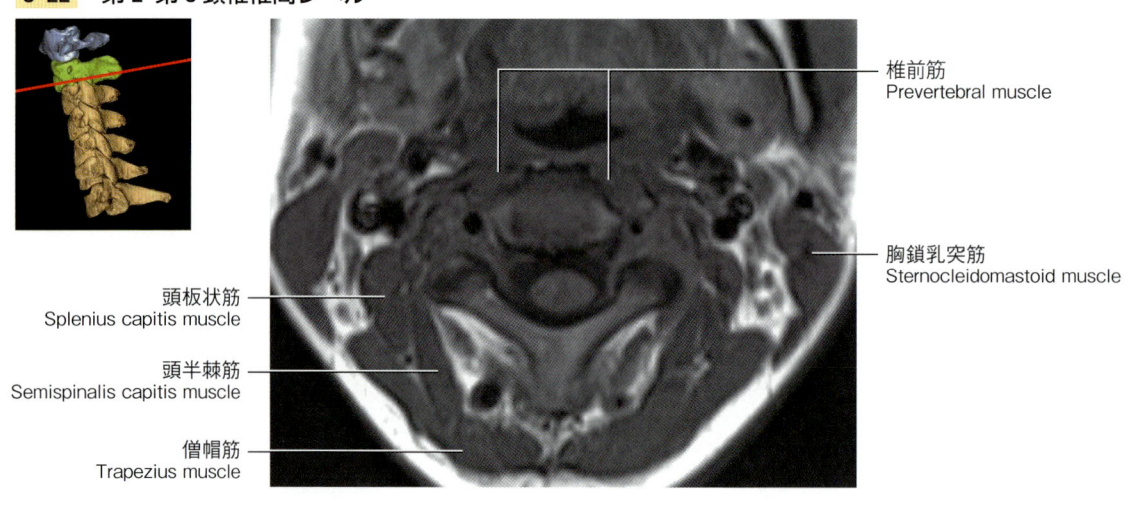

椎前筋　Prevertebral muscle
胸鎖乳突筋　Sternocleidomastoid muscle

頭板状筋　Splenius capitis muscle
頭半棘筋　Semispinalis capitis muscle
僧帽筋　Trapezius muscle

頸椎の断層解剖 ［横断像（MRI，T1・T2強調像）］

3-23　第3頸椎上縁レベル（T1強調像）

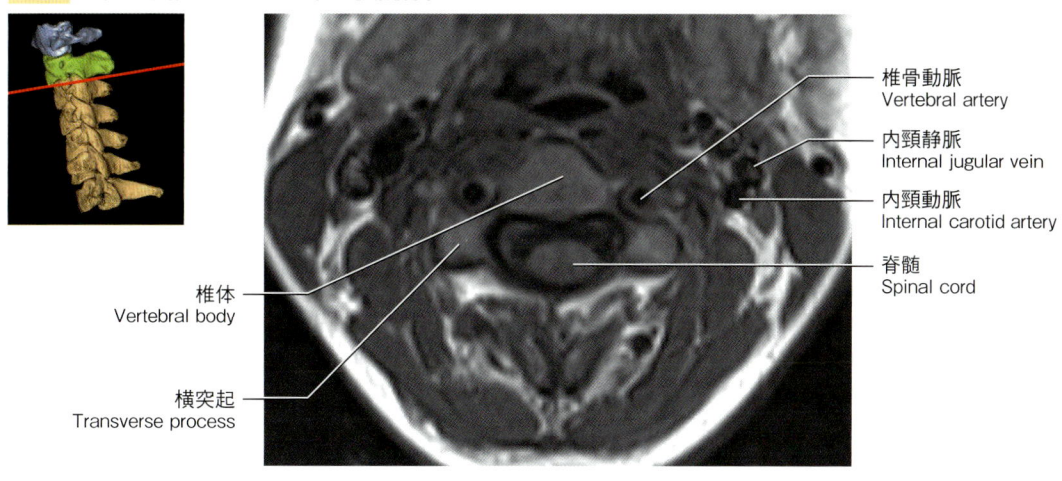

- 椎骨動脈 Vertebral artery
- 内頸静脈 Internal jugular vein
- 内頸動脈 Internal carotid artery
- 脊髄 Spinal cord
- 椎体 Vertebral body
- 横突起 Transverse process

3-24　第3頸椎上縁レベル（T2強調像）

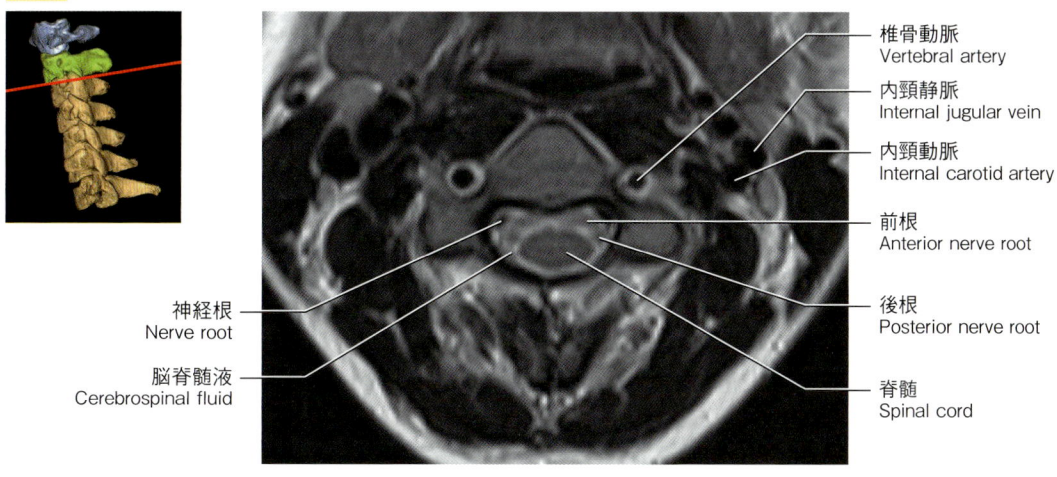

- 椎骨動脈 Vertebral artery
- 内頸静脈 Internal jugular vein
- 内頸動脈 Internal carotid artery
- 前根 Anterior nerve root
- 後根 Posterior nerve root
- 脊髄 Spinal cord
- 神経根 Nerve root
- 脳脊髄液 Cerebrospinal fluid

> **NOTE**　神経根は前根と後根が遠位で同一の神経上膜内に合したもので，頸神経8対，胸神経12対，腰神経5対，仙骨神経5対，尾骨神経1対の左右計31対存在する．後頭骨と第1頸椎との間から数えるため，頸椎レベルでは同じ番号の脊椎直上の椎間孔から，胸椎レベル以下では同じ番号の脊椎直下の椎間孔から出ることになる（3-24）．

頸椎の断層解剖 ［冠状断像（MRI, T1強調像）］

3-25 椎体前部レベル

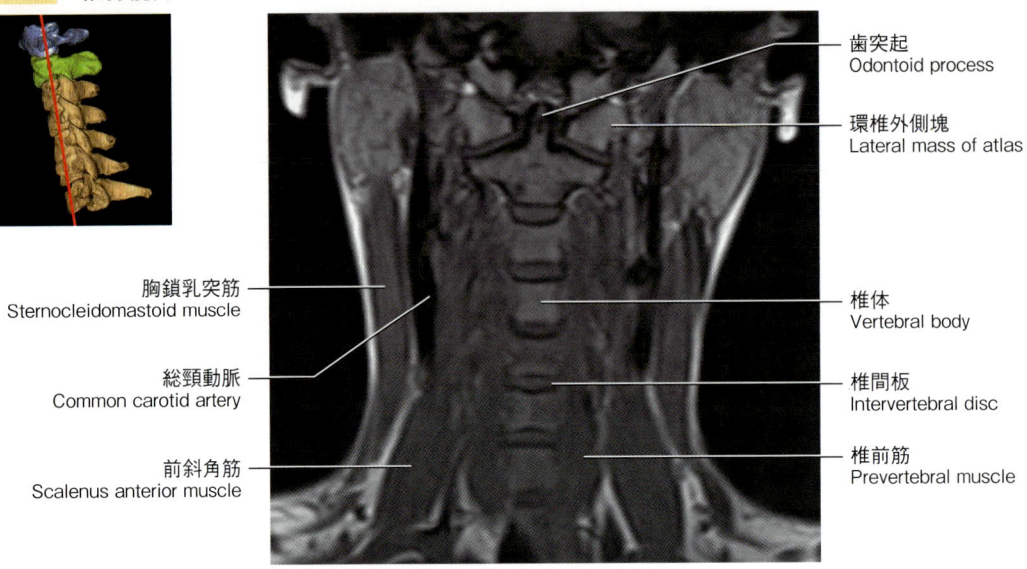

- 歯突起 Odontoid process
- 環椎外側塊 Lateral mass of atlas
- 胸鎖乳突筋 Sternocleidomastoid muscle
- 総頸動脈 Common carotid artery
- 前斜角筋 Scalenus anterior muscle
- 椎体 Vertebral body
- 椎間板 Intervertebral disc
- 椎前筋 Prevertebral muscle

3-26 椎体後部レベル

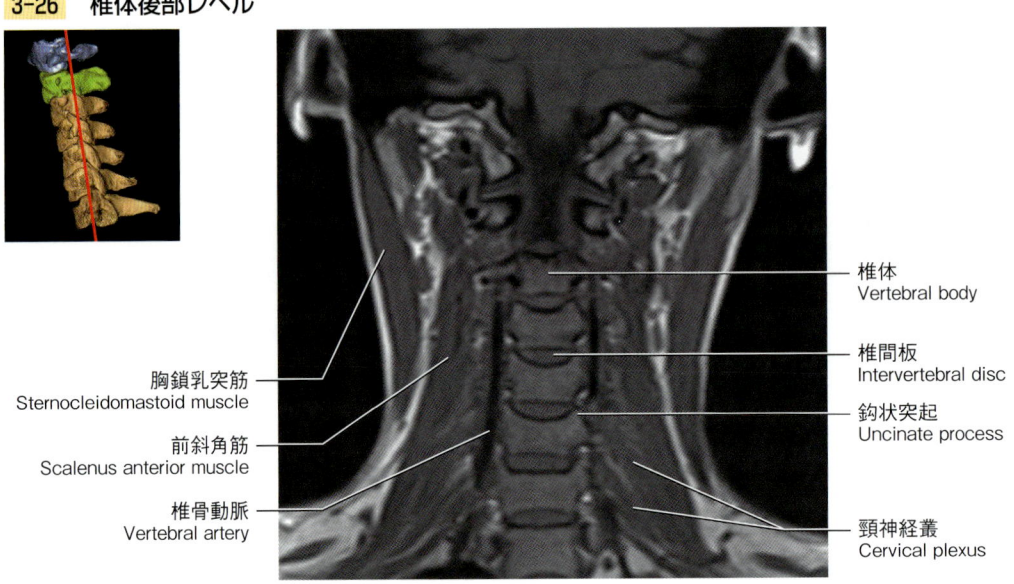

- 胸鎖乳突筋 Sternocleidomastoid muscle
- 前斜角筋 Scalenus anterior muscle
- 椎骨動脈 Vertebral artery
- 椎体 Vertebral body
- 椎間板 Intervertebral disc
- 鉤状突起 Uncinate process
- 頸神経叢 Cervical plexus

> **NOTE** 神経根は椎間孔から出たのち，前枝と後枝に分かれ，一部の前枝は神経叢をつくり末梢へ向かう．頸神経叢は第1～第4頸神経の前枝からなり，このほか第5頸神経～第1胸神経の前枝からは腕神経叢，第12胸神経～第4腰神経の前枝から腰神経叢，第4腰神経～第5腰神経の前枝から仙骨神経叢が形成される．

頸椎の断層解剖　[冠状断像（MRI，T1 強調像）]

3-27　脊柱管レベル

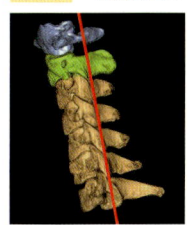

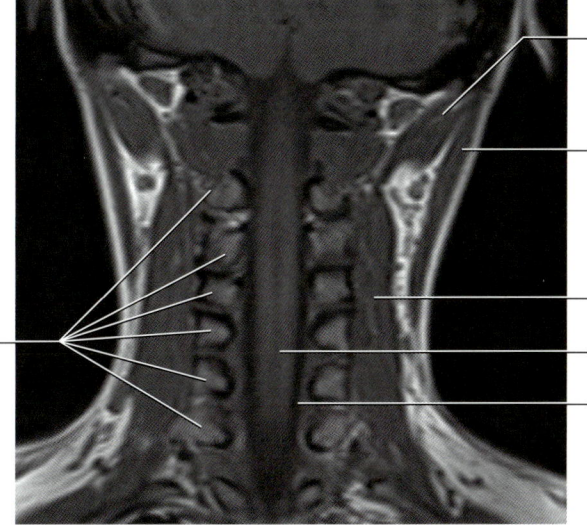

- 下頭斜筋　Obliquus capitis inferior muscle
- 胸鎖乳突筋　Sternocleidomastoid muscle
- 前斜角筋　Scalenus anterior muscle
- 脊髄　Spinal cord
- 脳脊髄液　Cerebrospinal fluid
- 外側塊　Lateral mass

NOTE　椎骨 Vertebra

vert，vers は「回す」の意味のラテン語で，Vertebra は回転する骨の意味．convert は「転換させる」の英語で，vertigo は「めまい」．

頸椎の断層解剖 ［矢状断像（MRI，T1強調像）］

3-28 椎間関節レベル

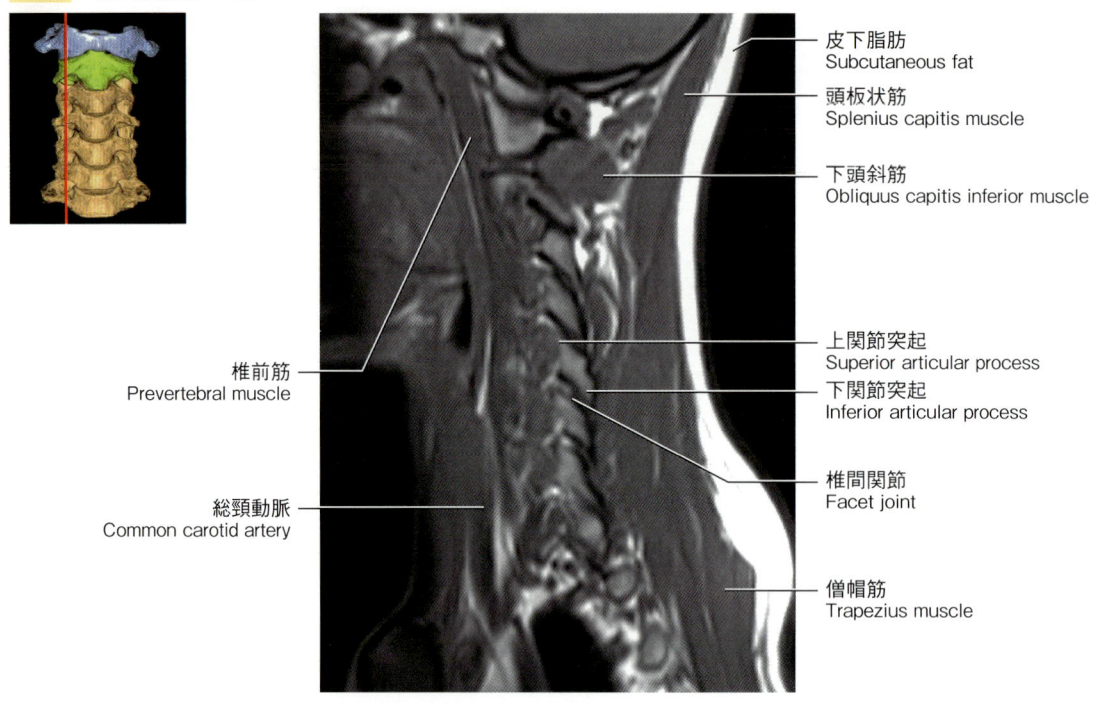

- 皮下脂肪 Subcutaneous fat
- 頭板状筋 Splenius capitis muscle
- 下頭斜筋 Obliquus capitis inferior muscle
- 上関節突起 Superior articular process
- 下関節突起 Inferior articular process
- 椎間関節 Facet joint
- 僧帽筋 Trapezius muscle
- 椎前筋 Prevertebral muscle
- 総頸動脈 Common carotid artery

3-29 脊柱管レベル

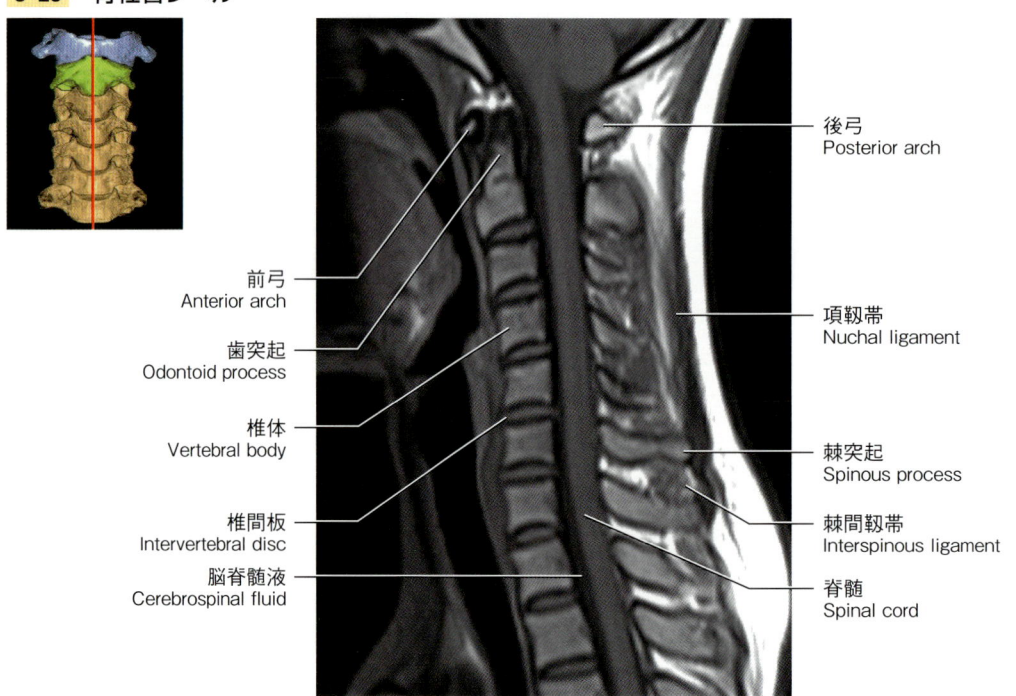

- 後弓 Posterior arch
- 項靱帯 Nuchal ligament
- 棘突起 Spinous process
- 棘間靱帯 Interspinous ligament
- 脊髄 Spinal cord
- 前弓 Anterior arch
- 歯突起 Odontoid process
- 椎体 Vertebral body
- 椎間板 Intervertebral disc
- 脳脊髄液 Cerebrospinal fluid

NOTE 項靱帯は肥厚した線維弾性組織であり，外後頭隆起および大後頭孔後縁から頸椎棘突起まで伸びている．第3頸椎〜第5頸椎までの棘突起は短いため，項靱帯が棘突起の代わりに筋肉の付着部位となっている．棘間靱帯は棘突起間を連結する膜状の構造物である．

頸椎の断層解剖 ［矢状断像（MRI，T2強調像）］

3-30　脊柱管レベル

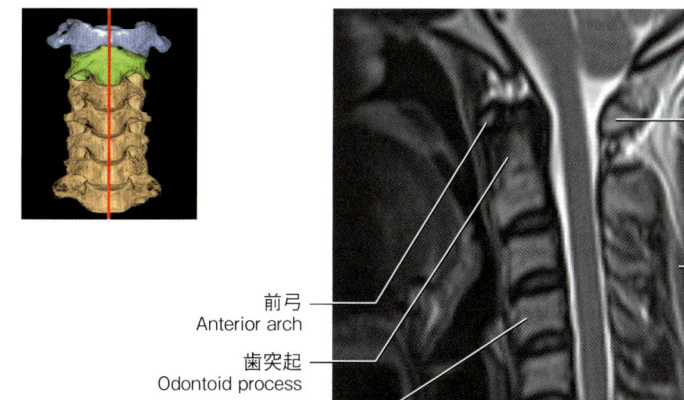

- 皮下脂肪 Subcutaneous fat
- 後弓 Posterior arch
- 項靱帯 Nuchal ligament
- 棘突起 Spinous process
- 棘間靱帯 Interspinous ligament
- 前弓 Anterior arch
- 歯突起 Odontoid process
- 椎体 Vertebral body
- 椎間板 Intervertebral disc
- 脳脊髄液 Cerebrospinal fluid
- 脊髄 Spinal cord

NOTE　正面衝突など，頸部に強制的に過屈曲が生じると椎間板が後方へ脱出することがある．頸部では椎間板は椎間孔前縁の正中に位置しているため，突出した椎間板により椎間孔を走行する脊髄神経が圧迫される．脊髄神経は同じ番号の椎体の上から出るため，突出した椎間板と圧迫される神経の高位は同一となる．たとえば，第5-第6頸椎椎間板の突出は6番の神経根を圧迫することになる．

胸椎（CT, VR像）

3-31 胸椎（側面）

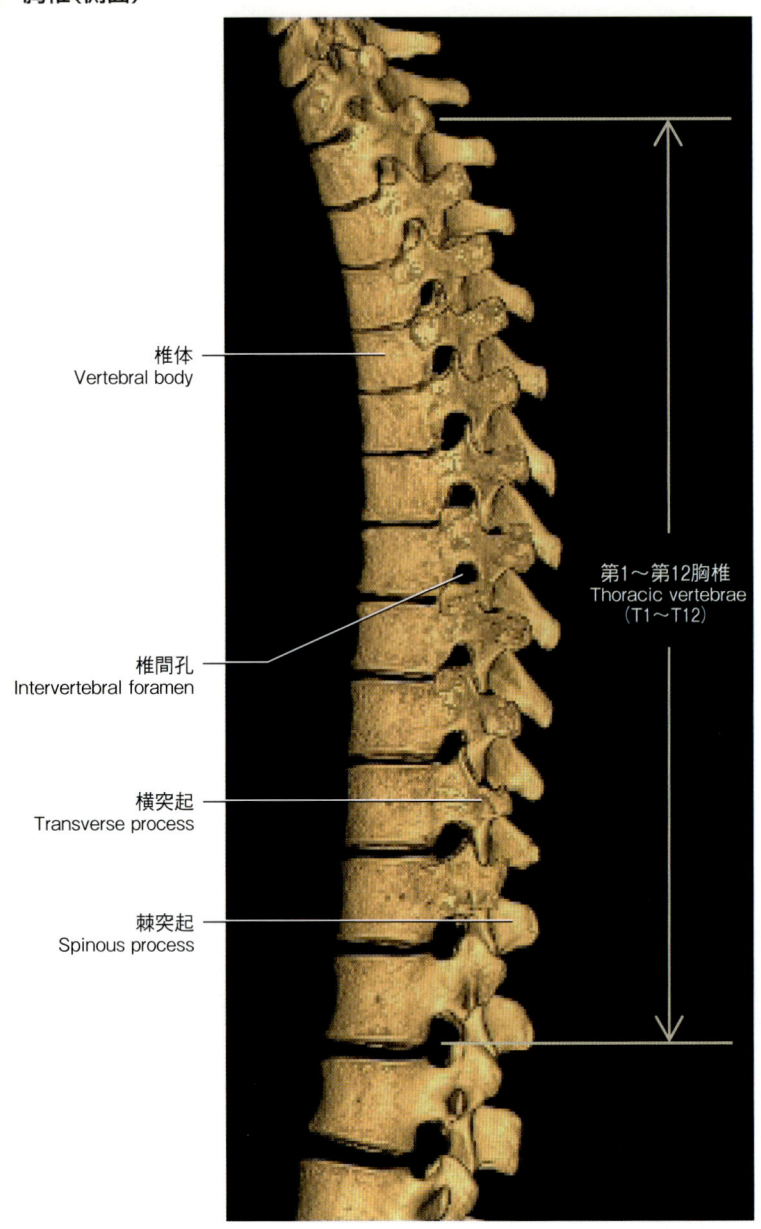

椎体
Vertebral body

第1～第12胸椎
Thoracic vertebrae
(T1～T12)

椎間孔
Intervertebral foramen

横突起
Transverse process

棘突起
Spinous process

> **NOTE** 胸椎の主な特徴は胸郭を形成する肋骨が付着する肋骨窩が存在することである．胸椎の関節突起は縦に伸びており，棘突起は長く，後下方に傾斜し先端部は下の椎体の高さに達する．これらが胸椎の側屈や屈曲，伸展に制限を加えている．

胸椎（CT, VR像）

3-32 胸椎椎骨（側面）

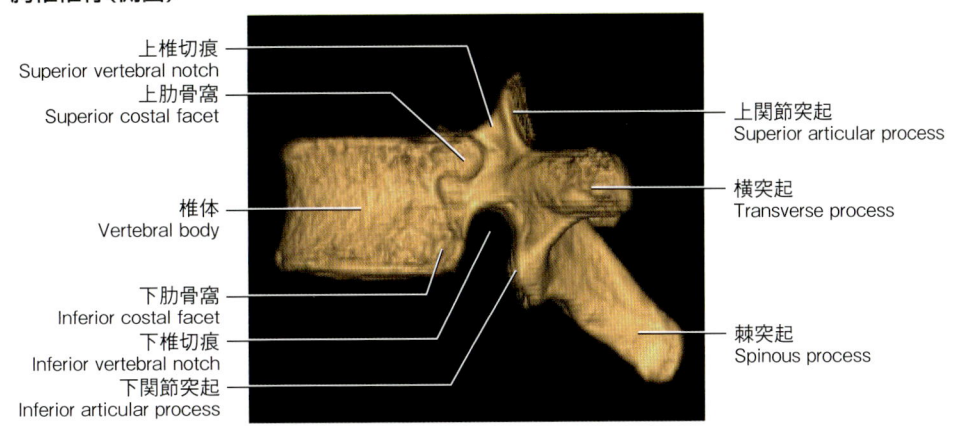

- 上椎切痕 Superior vertebral notch
- 上肋骨窩 Superior costal facet
- 椎体 Vertebral body
- 下肋骨窩 Inferior costal facet
- 下椎切痕 Inferior vertebral notch
- 下関節突起 Inferior articular process
- 上関節突起 Superior articular process
- 横突起 Transverse process
- 棘突起 Spinous process

3-33 胸椎椎骨（前面）

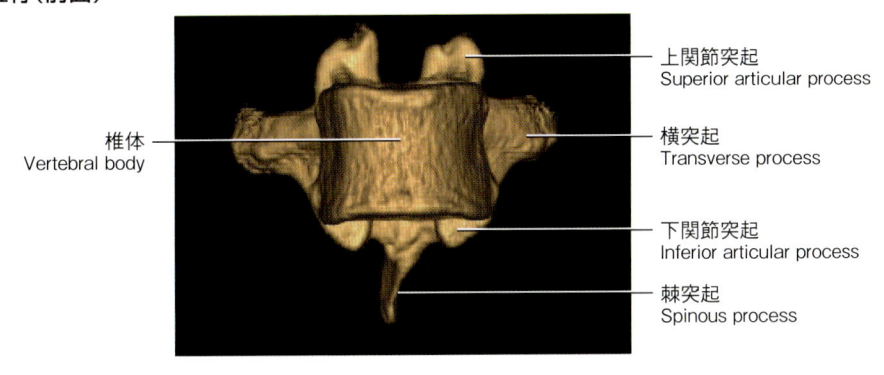

- 椎体 Vertebral body
- 上関節突起 Superior articular process
- 横突起 Transverse process
- 下関節突起 Inferior articular process
- 棘突起 Spinous process

3-34 胸椎椎骨（下面）

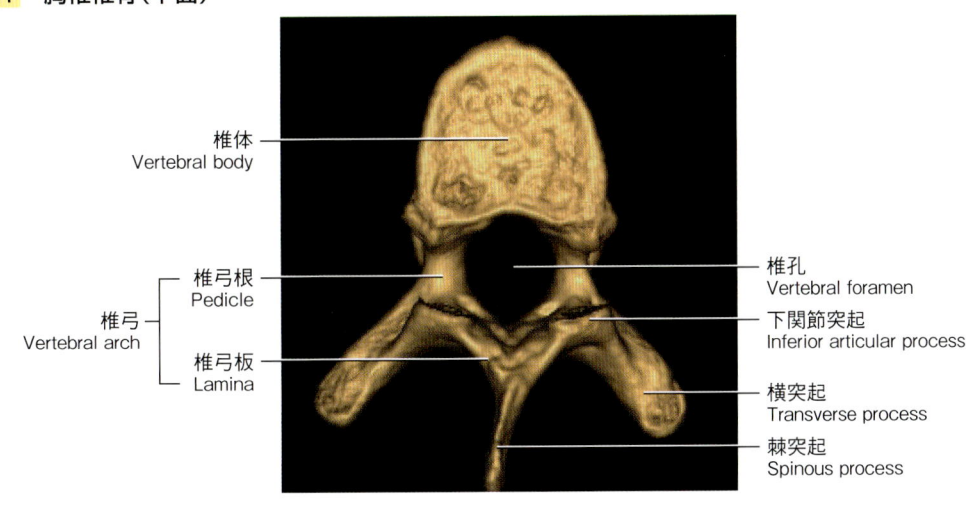

- 椎体 Vertebral body
- 椎弓 Vertebral arch
  - 椎弓根 Pedicle
  - 椎弓板 Lamina
- 椎孔 Vertebral foramen
- 下関節突起 Inferior articular process
- 横突起 Transverse process
- 棘突起 Spinous process

NOTE 椎体は椎骨の前の部分を構成する円柱状の構造で，主に体重を支える部分になる．このため下方へ向かうほど椎体は大きく，第4胸椎以下で顕著となり，第5腰椎で最大となる．椎弓は椎体後部の左右にある椎弓根と椎弓板からなり，左右の椎弓板結合部から後方へ突出するのが棘突起である．

胸椎の断層解剖 ［横断像（CT）］

3-35 第8胸椎レベル

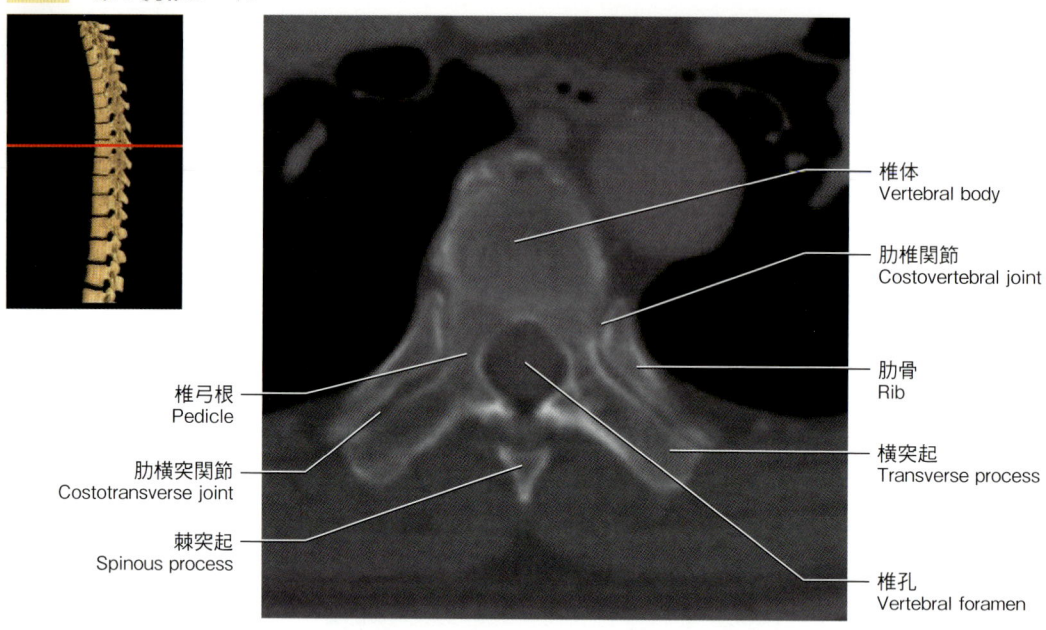

- 椎体 Vertebral body
- 肋椎関節 Costovertebral joint
- 肋骨 Rib
- 横突起 Transverse process
- 椎孔 Vertebral foramen
- 椎弓根 Pedicle
- 肋横突関節 Costotransverse joint
- 棘突起 Spinous process

3-36 第8胸椎下部レベル

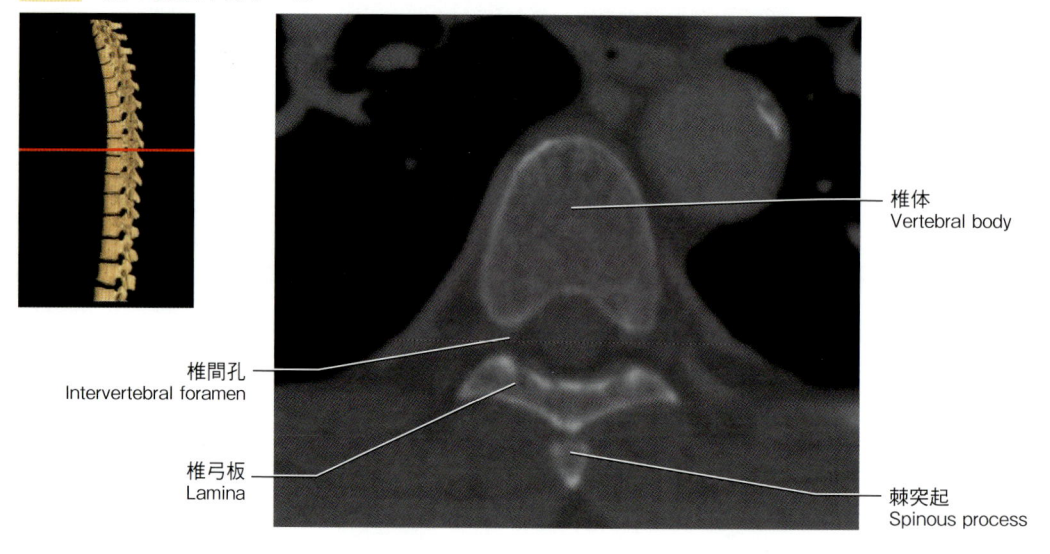

- 椎体 Vertebral body
- 椎間孔 Intervertebral foramen
- 椎弓板 Lamina
- 棘突起 Spinous process

> **NOTE** 胸椎の椎体と横突起はそれぞれ肋骨と肋椎関節，肋横突関節を形成している．胸椎横突起は長く後外側に伸び，下方の椎骨ほど短くなる．

胸椎の断層解剖 ［横断像（CT）］

3-37　第8-第9胸椎椎間レベル

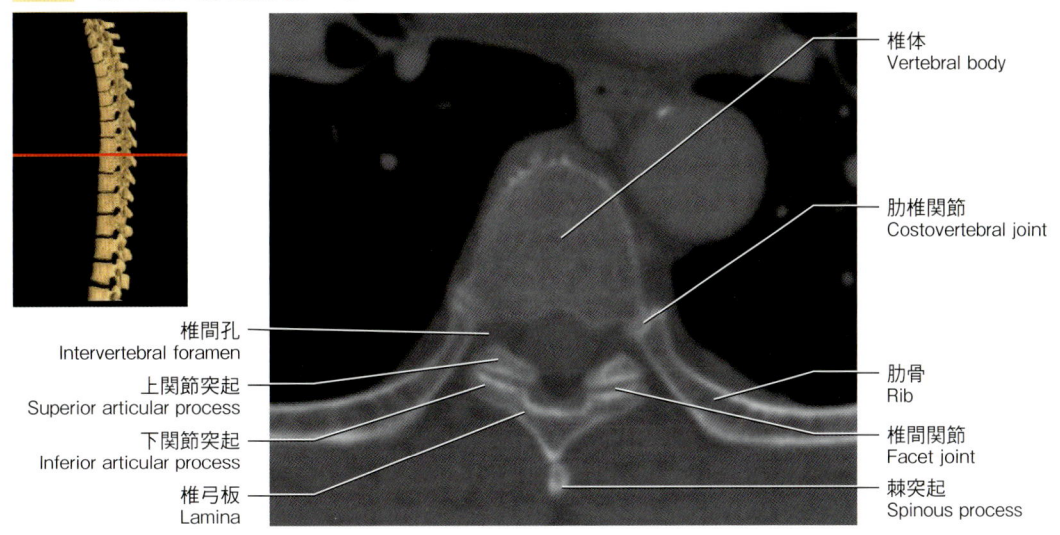

- 椎体 / Vertebral body
- 肋椎関節 / Costovertebral joint
- 椎間孔 / Intervertebral foramen
- 上関節突起 / Superior articular process
- 下関節突起 / Inferior articular process
- 椎弓板 / Lamina
- 肋骨 / Rib
- 椎間関節 / Facet joint
- 棘突起 / Spinous process

胸椎の断層解剖 ［冠状断像（CT, MPR像）］

3-38 椎体レベル

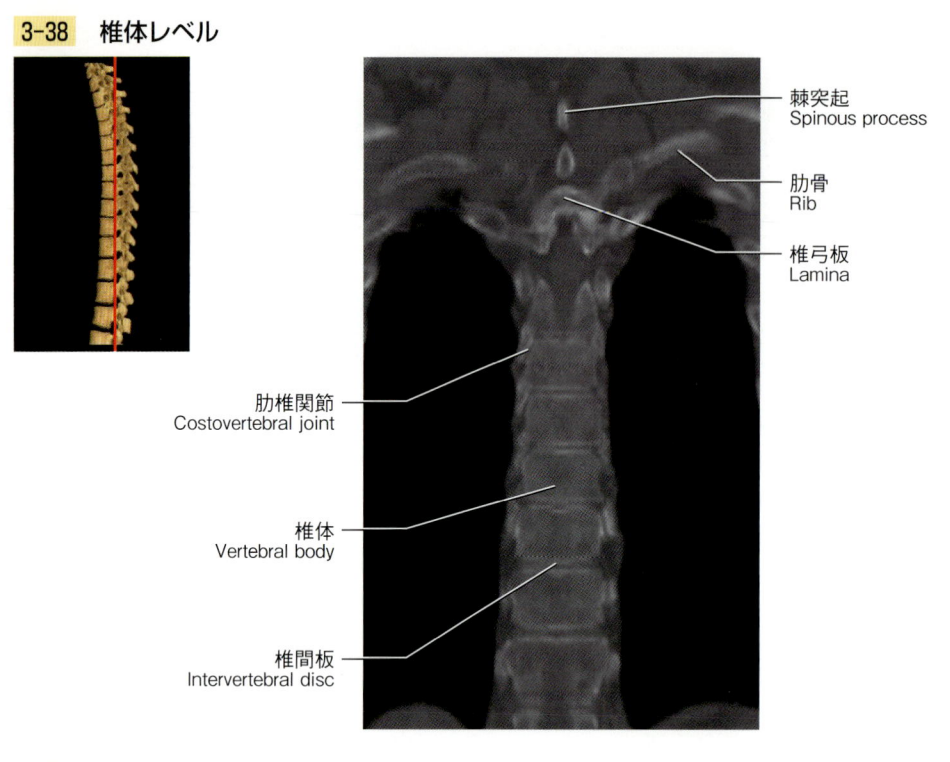

- 棘突起 Spinous process
- 肋骨 Rib
- 椎弓板 Lamina
- 肋椎関節 Costovertebral joint
- 椎体 Vertebral body
- 椎間板 Intervertebral disc

3-39 椎間孔レベル

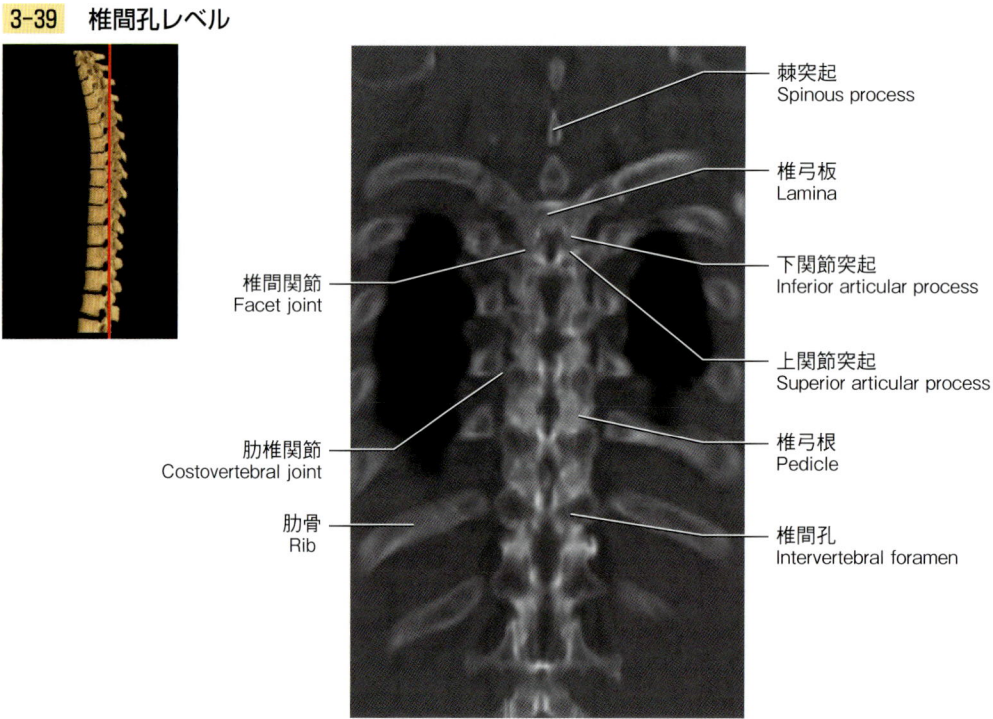

- 棘突起 Spinous process
- 椎弓板 Lamina
- 下関節突起 Inferior articular process
- 上関節突起 Superior articular process
- 椎間関節 Facet joint
- 椎弓根 Pedicle
- 肋椎関節 Costovertebral joint
- 肋骨 Rib
- 椎間孔 Intervertebral foramen

胸椎の断層解剖 ［冠状断像（CT, MPR 像）］

3-40　棘突起レベル

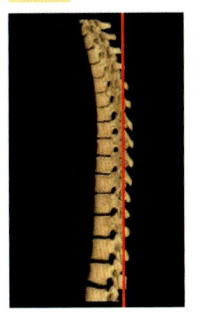

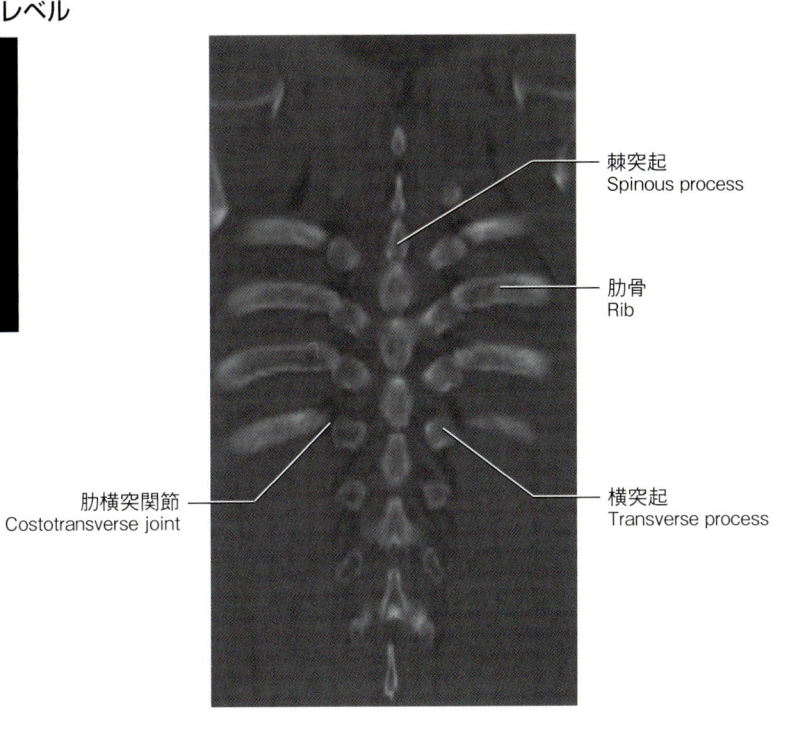

- 棘突起　Spinous process
- 肋骨　Rib
- 肋横突関節　Costotransverse joint
- 横突起　Transverse process

胸椎の断層解剖 ［矢状断像（CT, MPR 像）］

3-41 肋横突関節レベル

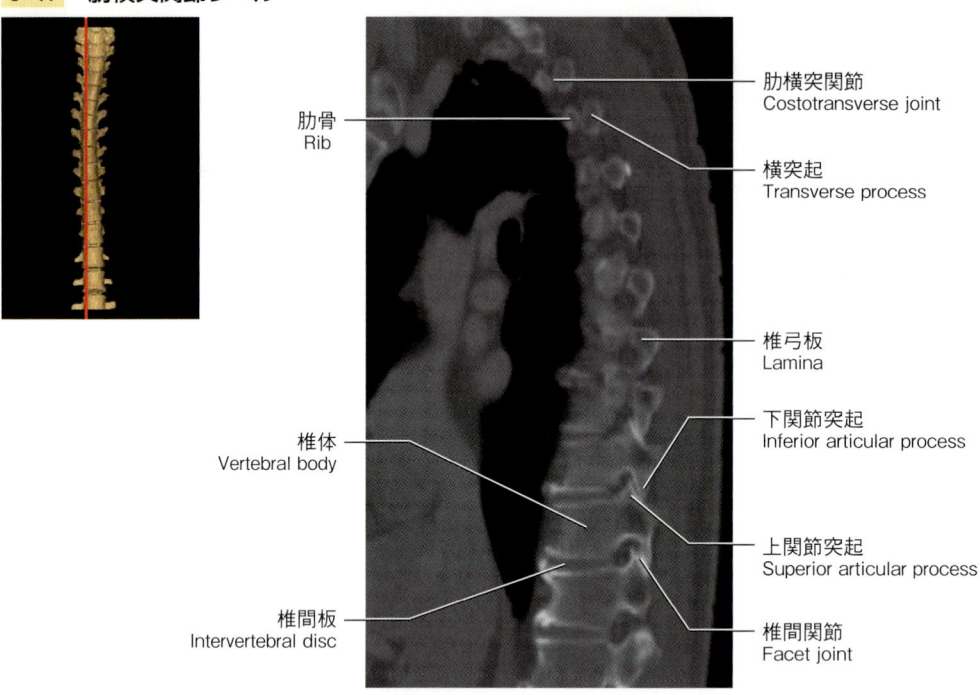

- 肋骨 Rib
- 肋横突関節 Costotransverse joint
- 横突起 Transverse process
- 椎弓板 Lamina
- 下関節突起 Inferior articular process
- 椎体 Vertebral body
- 上関節突起 Superior articular process
- 椎間板 Intervertebral disc
- 椎間関節 Facet joint

3-42 脊柱管レベル

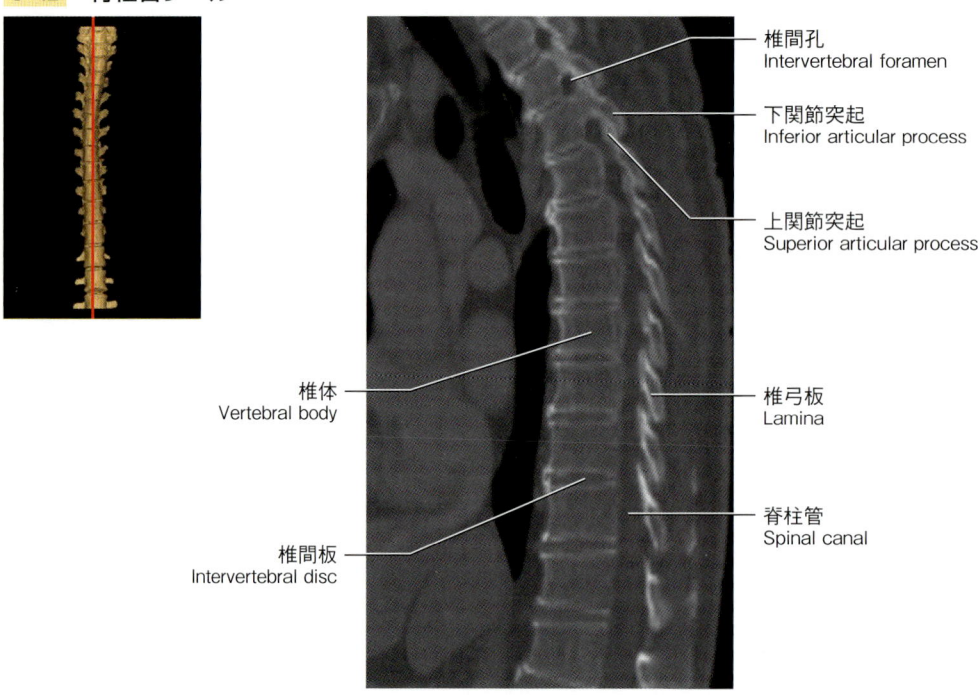

- 椎間孔 Intervertebral foramen
- 下関節突起 Inferior articular process
- 上関節突起 Superior articular process
- 椎体 Vertebral body
- 椎弓板 Lamina
- 椎間板 Intervertebral disc
- 脊柱管 Spinal canal

> **NOTE 矢状 Sagittal**
> Sagittal はもともと頭蓋骨縫合の Suture sagittalis（矢状縫合）からできた語とされる．つまり冠状縫合と左右頭頂骨間の縫合を合わせてみると，弓と矢の形となることからできた．この使用範囲が広がって，矢状縫合に平行な方向，つまり矢が体を前後に貫く方向を示す語として使われるようになったとの説がある．

胸椎の断層解剖 ［矢状断像（CT, MPR 像）］

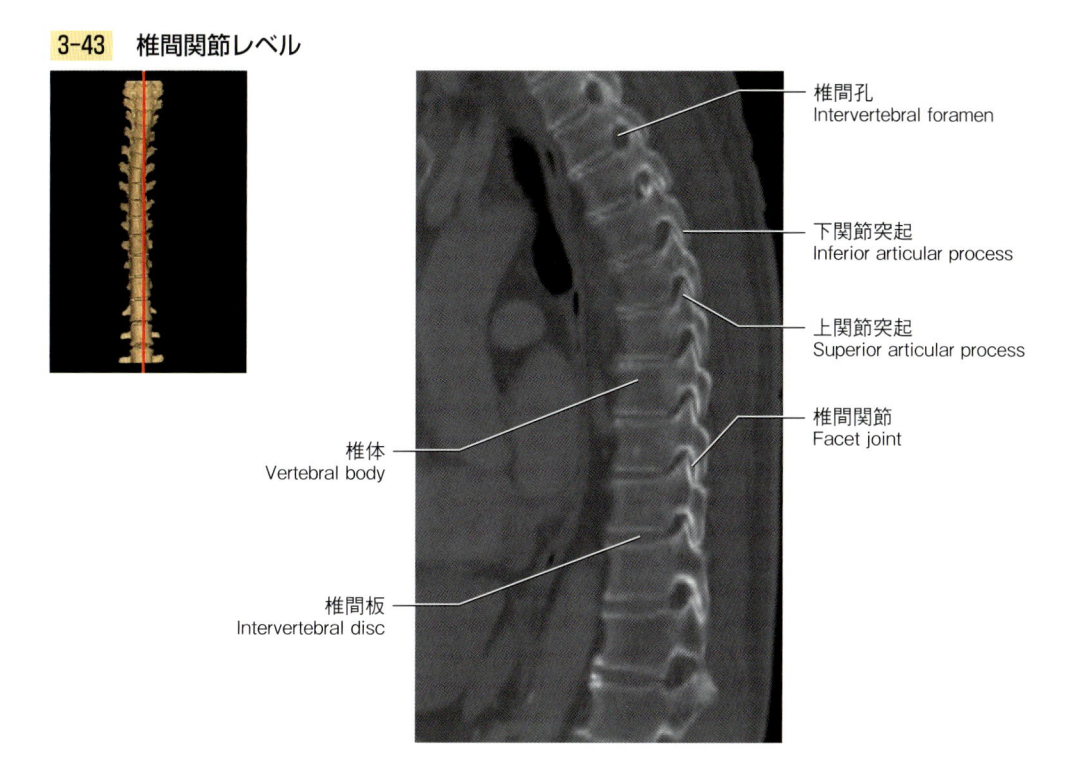

3-43　椎間関節レベル

- 椎間孔　Intervertebral foramen
- 下関節突起　Inferior articular process
- 上関節突起　Superior articular process
- 椎間関節　Facet joint
- 椎体　Vertebral body
- 椎間板　Intervertebral disc

NOTE　椎間孔の後縁は椎間関節が構成しているため，加齢性変化により椎間関節に骨棘が生じると椎間孔を走行する脊髄神経が圧迫され，関連する皮膚分節の分布に沿って疼痛が生じることになる．

胸椎の断層解剖 ［横断像（MRI, T2強調像）］

3-44 第6胸椎下部レベル

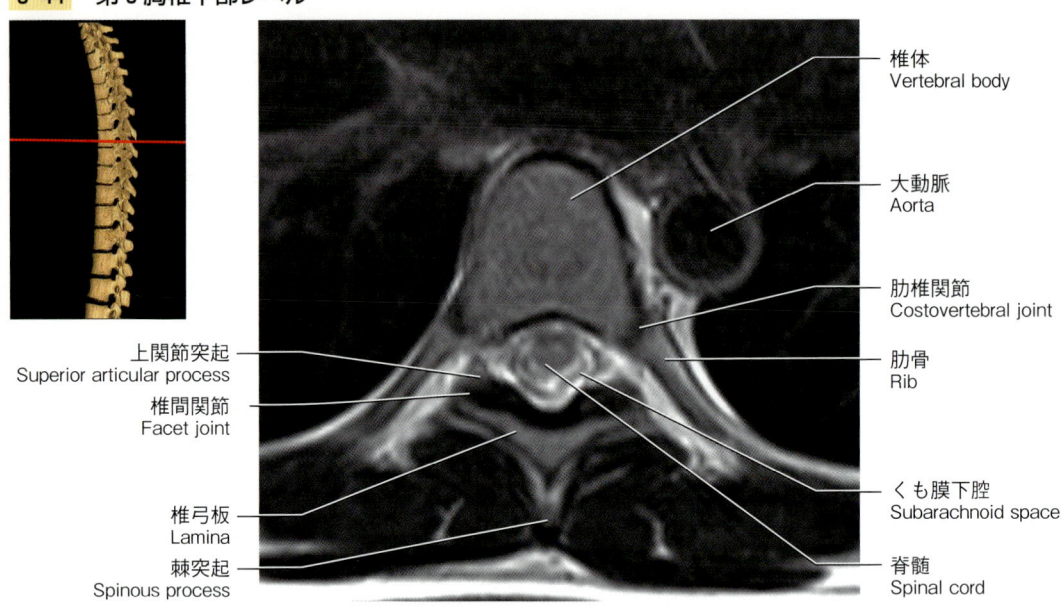

- 椎体 Vertebral body
- 大動脈 Aorta
- 肋椎関節 Costovertebral joint
- 肋骨 Rib
- くも膜下腔 Subarachnoid space
- 脊髄 Spinal cord
- 上関節突起 Superior articular process
- 椎間関節 Facet joint
- 椎弓板 Lamina
- 棘突起 Spinous process

3-45 第6-第7胸椎椎間レベル

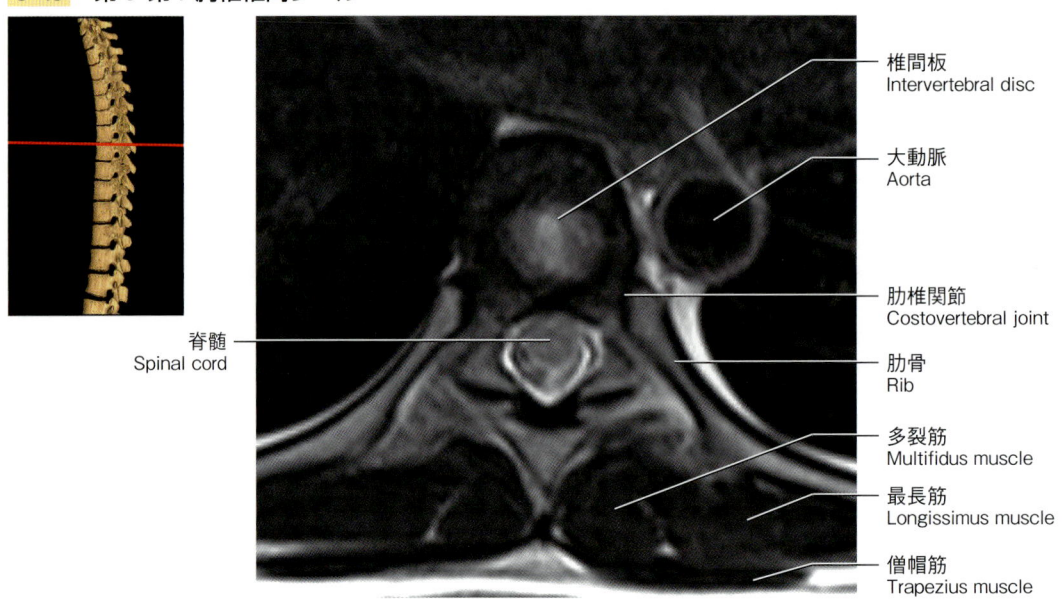

- 椎間板 Intervertebral disc
- 大動脈 Aorta
- 肋椎関節 Costovertebral joint
- 肋骨 Rib
- 多裂筋 Multifidus muscle
- 最長筋 Longissimus muscle
- 僧帽筋 Trapezius muscle
- 脊髄 Spinal cord

胸椎の断層解剖 ［横断像（MRI, T2・T1 強調像）］

3-46　第7胸椎上部レベル（T2強調像）

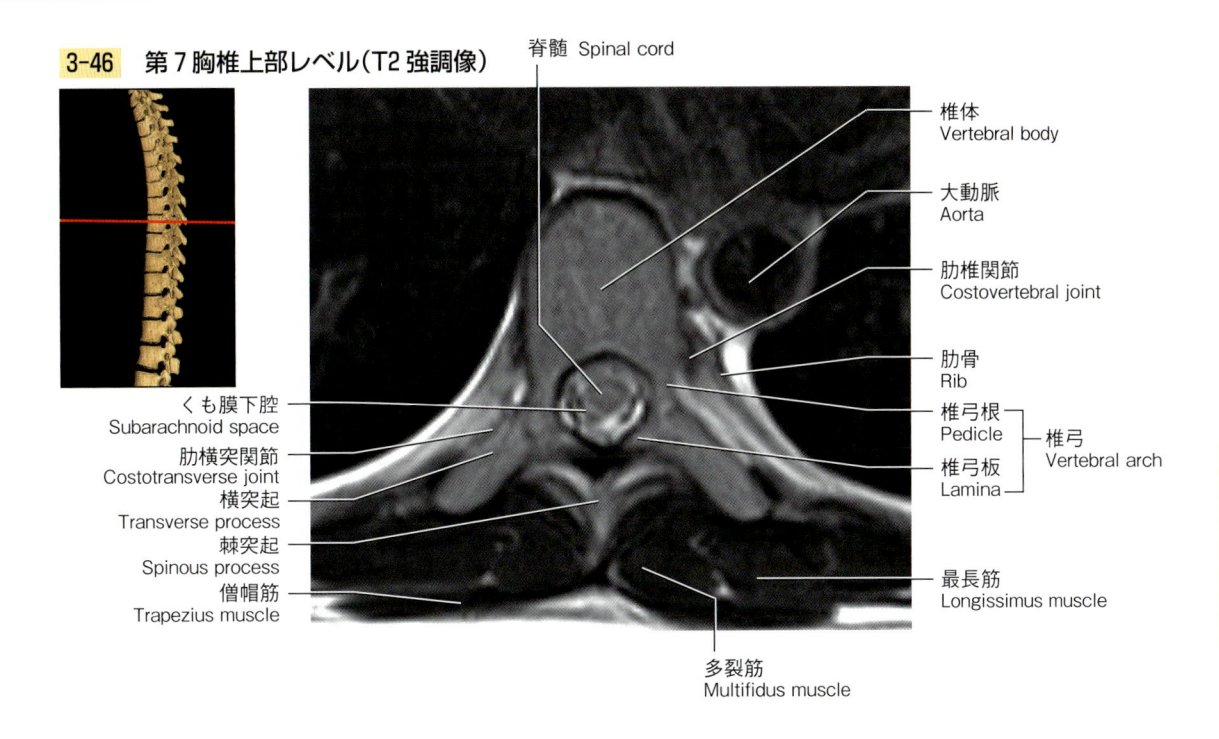

- 脊髄　Spinal cord
- 椎体　Vertebral body
- 大動脈　Aorta
- 肋椎関節　Costovertebral joint
- 肋骨　Rib
- 椎弓根　Pedicle ┐ 椎弓 Vertebral arch
- 椎弓板　Lamina ┘
- くも膜下腔　Subarachnoid space
- 肋横突関節　Costotransverse joint
- 横突起　Transverse process
- 棘突起　Spinous process
- 僧帽筋　Trapezius muscle
- 最長筋　Longissimus muscle
- 多裂筋　Multifidus muscle

3-47　第7胸椎上部レベル（T1強調像）

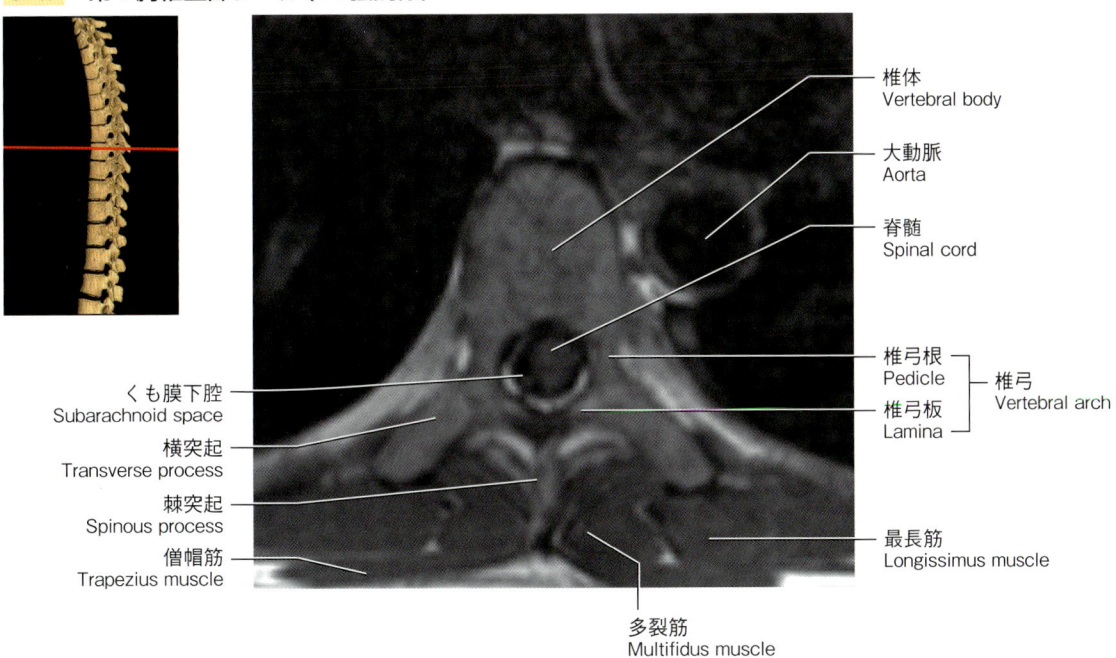

- 椎体　Vertebral body
- 大動脈　Aorta
- 脊髄　Spinal cord
- 椎弓根　Pedicle ┐ 椎弓 Vertebral arch
- 椎弓板　Lamina ┘
- くも膜下腔　Subarachnoid space
- 横突起　Transverse process
- 棘突起　Spinous process
- 僧帽筋　Trapezius muscle
- 最長筋　Longissimus muscle
- 多裂筋　Multifidus muscle

> **NOTE**　棘突起と椎弓板を外科的に切除することを椎弓切除術とよぶ．これにより椎骨の後方部分が開放されるため，腫瘍や椎間板ヘルニアなどで脊柱管が狭窄している場合や，脊髄神経根が圧迫されている場合に，これらの程度を軽減することができる．

胸椎の断層解剖 ［冠状断像（MRI, T1強調像）］

3-48 椎体レベル

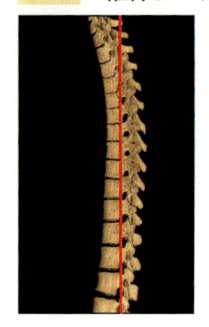

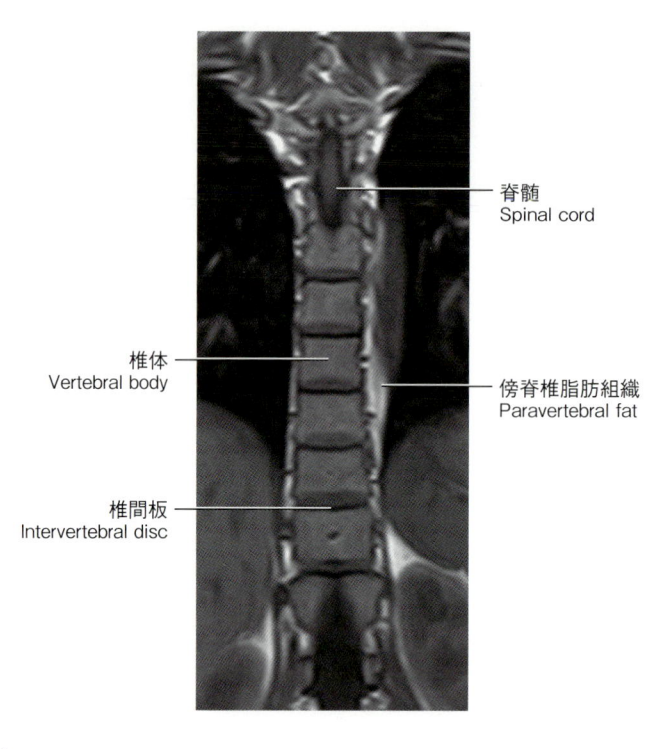

- 脊髄 Spinal cord
- 椎体 Vertebral body
- 傍脊椎脂肪組織 Paravertebral fat
- 椎間板 Intervertebral disc

3-49 脊柱管レベル

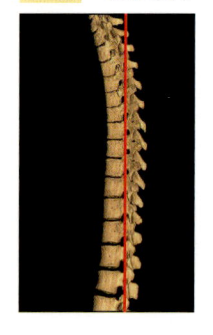

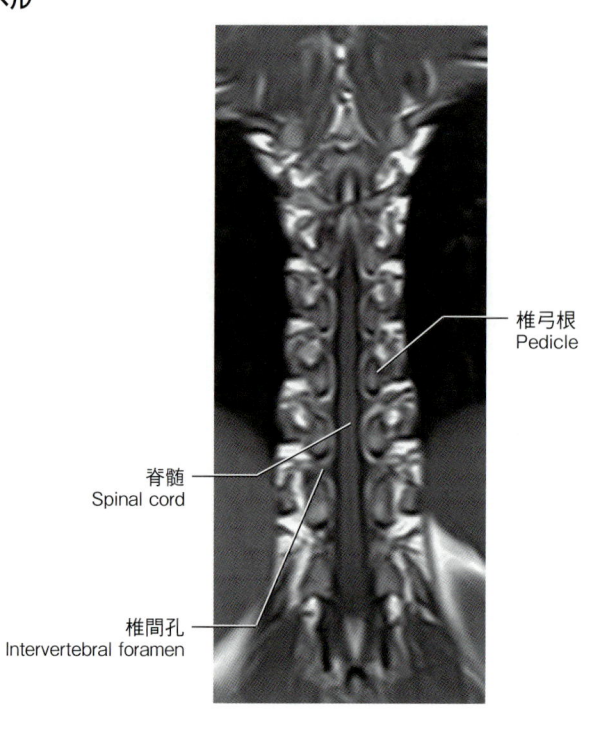

- 椎弓根 Pedicle
- 脊髄 Spinal cord
- 椎間孔 Intervertebral foramen

胸椎の断層解剖 ［矢状断像（MRI, T1強調像）］

3-50 椎弓根レベル

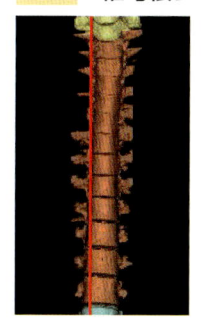

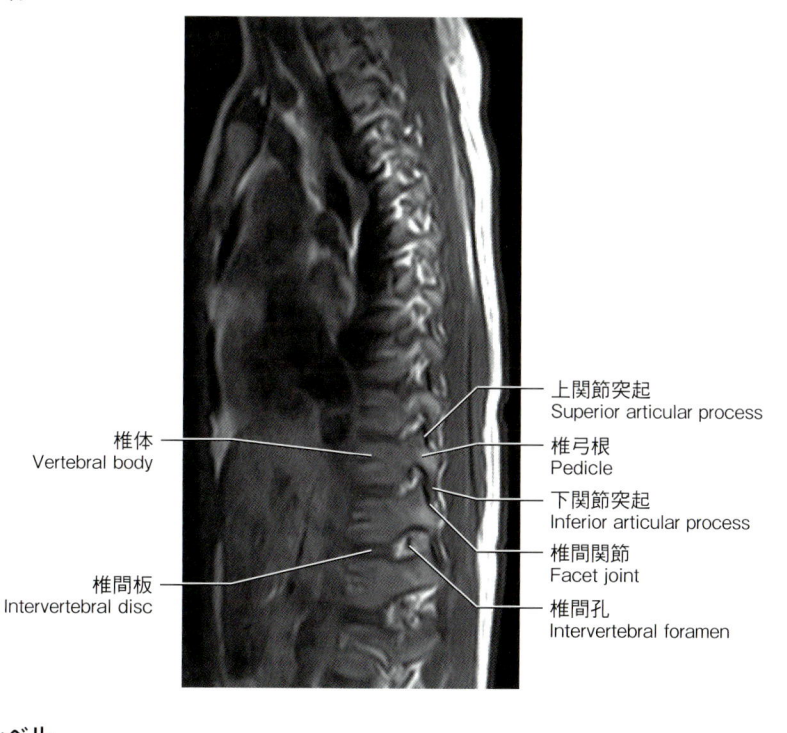

- 椎体 Vertebral body
- 上関節突起 Superior articular process
- 椎弓根 Pedicle
- 下関節突起 Inferior articular process
- 椎間板 Intervertebral disc
- 椎間関節 Facet joint
- 椎間孔 Intervertebral foramen

3-51 椎間関節レベル

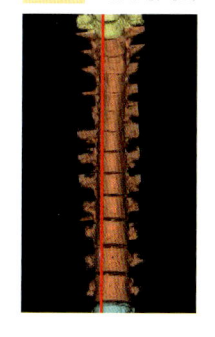

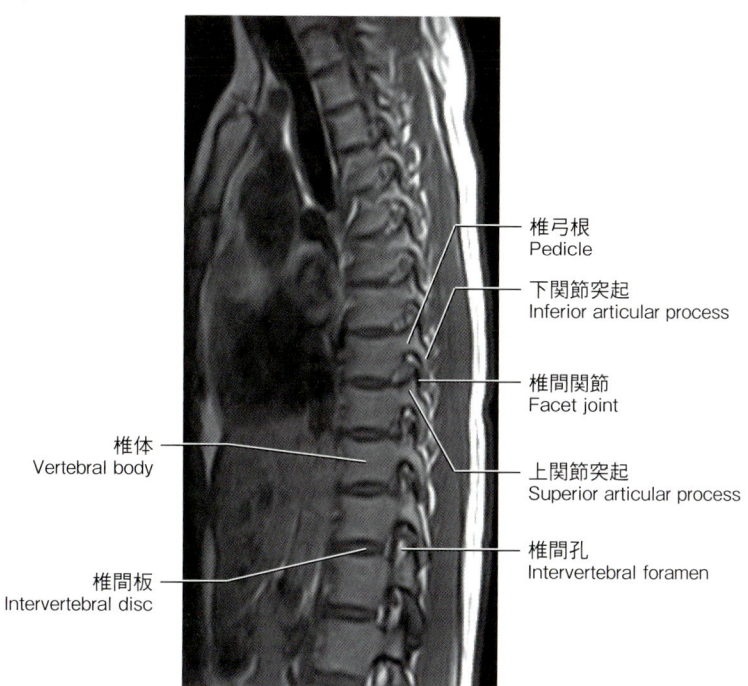

- 椎弓根 Pedicle
- 下関節突起 Inferior articular process
- 椎間関節 Facet joint
- 椎体 Vertebral body
- 上関節突起 Superior articular process
- 椎間板 Intervertebral disc
- 椎間孔 Intervertebral foramen

> **NOTE** 椎間孔内部を神経根や神経節，動静脈が走行する．脂肪組織が高信号を示すため，これらの構造は低信号として描出される．

胸椎の断層解剖　[矢状断像（MRI, T1・T2 強調像）]

3-52　脊柱管レベル（T1 強調像）

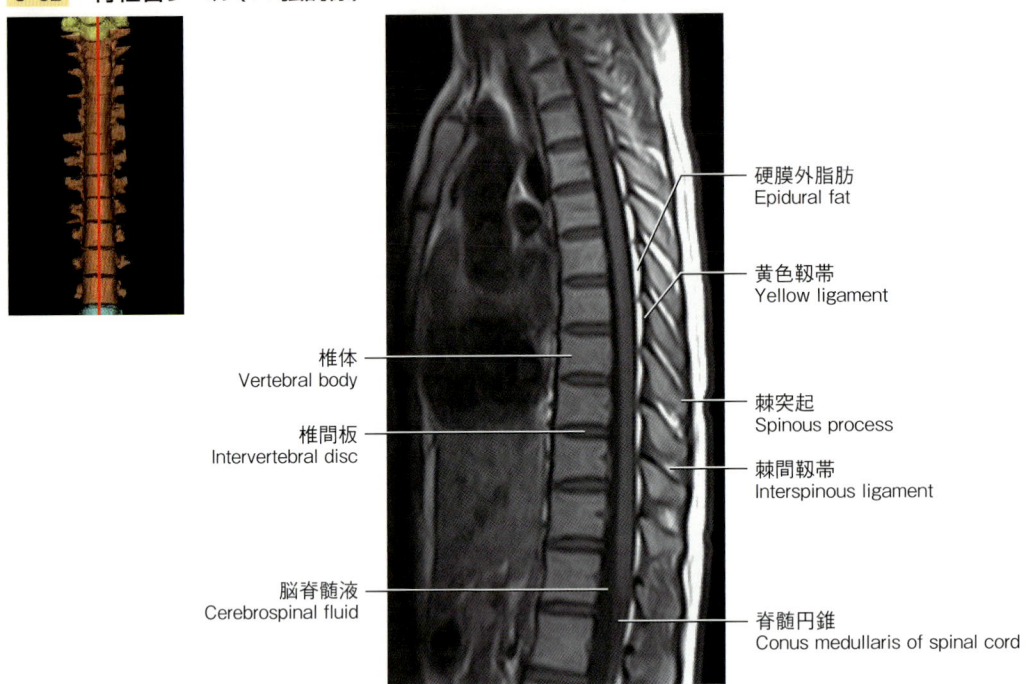

- 椎体　Vertebral body
- 椎間板　Intervertebral disc
- 脳脊髄液　Cerebrospinal fluid
- 硬膜外脂肪　Epidural fat
- 黄色靱帯　Yellow ligament
- 棘突起　Spinous process
- 棘間靱帯　Interspinous ligament
- 脊髄円錐　Conus medullaris of spinal cord

3-53　脊柱管レベル（T2 強調像）

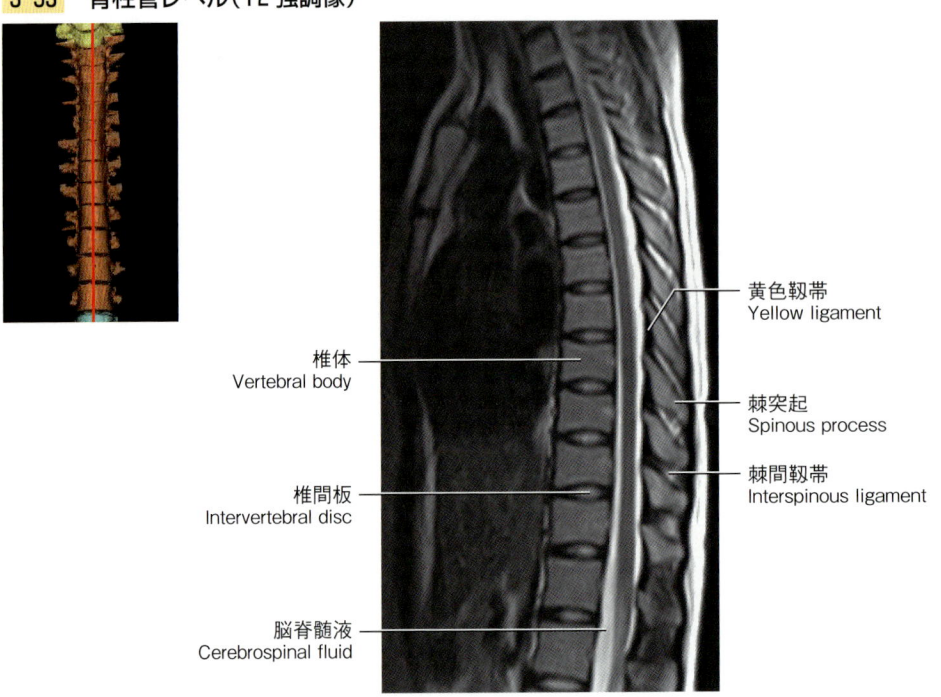

- 椎体　Vertebral body
- 椎間板　Intervertebral disc
- 脳脊髄液　Cerebrospinal fluid
- 黄色靱帯　Yellow ligament
- 棘突起　Spinous process
- 棘間靱帯　Interspinous ligament

> **NOTE**　脊髄はいくつかの膜によって包まれている．最外層が硬膜であり，脊柱管を形成する．骨と硬膜との間が硬膜外腔で硬膜外脂肪が存在する．硬膜の内側にはくも膜がある．くも膜は血管を欠く膜であり，脳脊髄液で満たされたくも膜下腔を覆っている．くも膜は脳脊髄液の圧により硬膜へ押しつけられている．くも膜の内側が脊髄表面を覆う軟膜である．

腰　椎（CT, VR 像）

3-54 腰椎（正面）

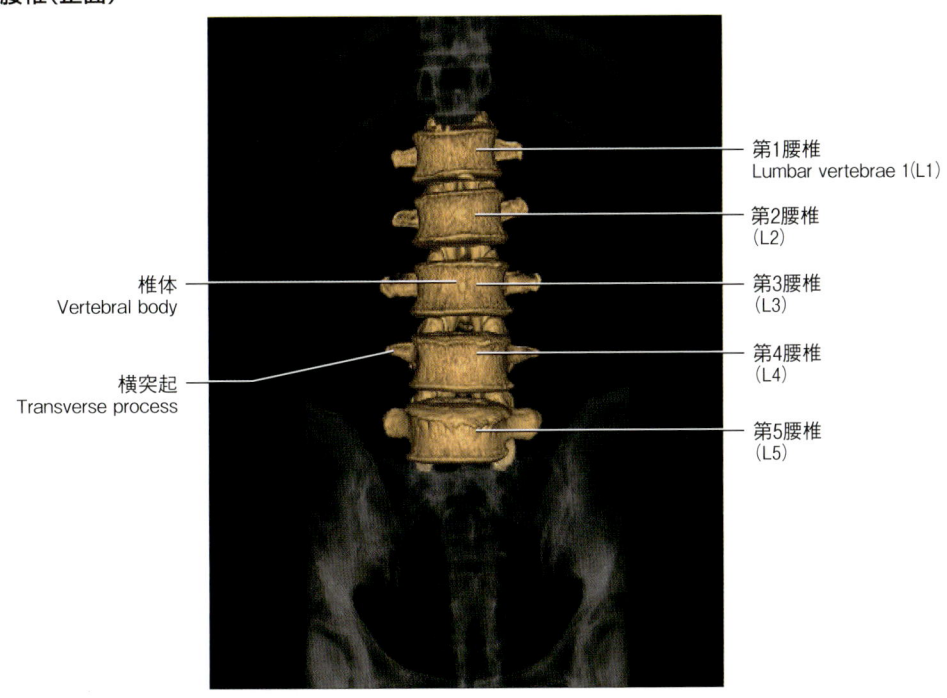

- 椎体 Vertebral body
- 横突起 Transverse process
- 第1腰椎 Lumbar vertebrae 1（L1）
- 第2腰椎（L2）
- 第3腰椎（L3）
- 第4腰椎（L4）
- 第5腰椎（L5）

3-55 腰椎（側面）

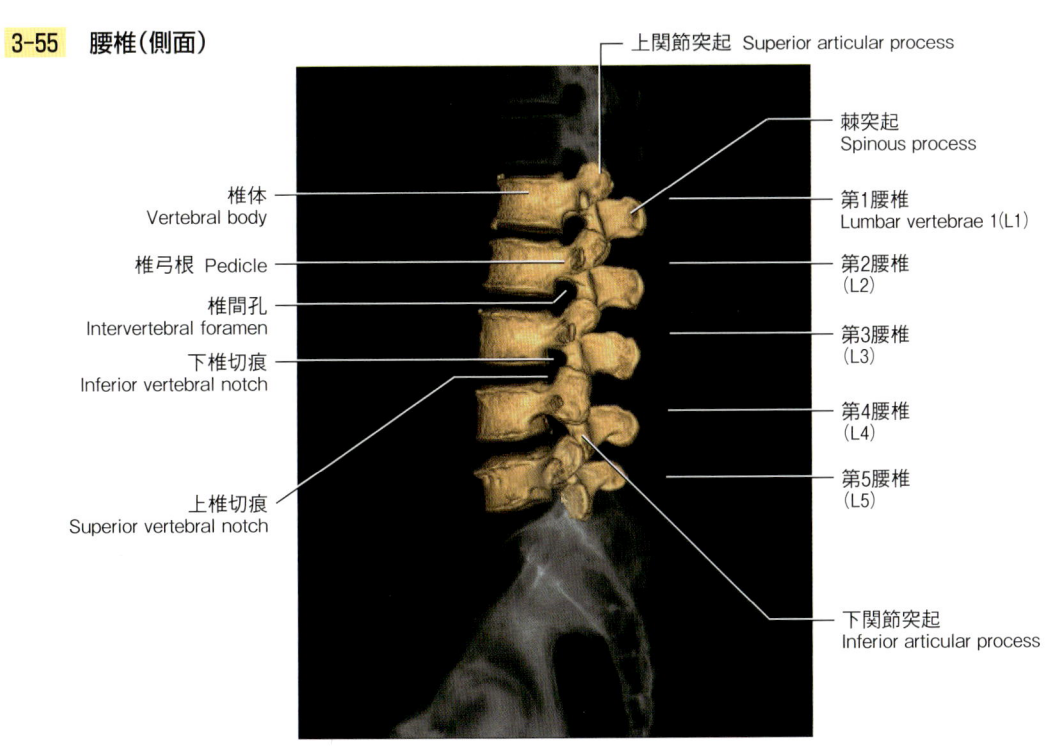

- 椎体 Vertebral body
- 椎弓根 Pedicle
- 椎間孔 Intervertebral foramen
- 下椎切痕 Inferior vertebral notch
- 上椎切痕 Superior vertebral notch
- 上関節突起 Superior articular process
- 棘突起 Spinous process
- 第1腰椎 Lumbar vertebrae 1（L1）
- 第2腰椎（L2）
- 第3腰椎（L3）
- 第4腰椎（L4）
- 第5腰椎（L5）
- 下関節突起 Inferior articular process

NOTE 腰椎は，頸椎や胸椎と比し体重を支えるために必要な，幅広く厚い椎体が特徴である．関節突起は縦方向に伸び，関節面は矢状方向を向いているため回旋が制限される．腰椎の中でも第5腰椎と第1仙椎の関節面は冠状方向を向いている．

腰 椎（CT, VR 像）

3-56 第3腰椎（側面）

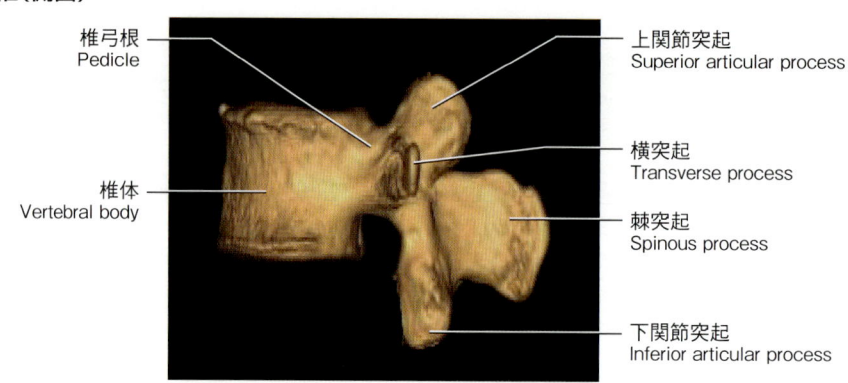

- 椎弓根 Pedicle
- 椎体 Vertebral body
- 上関節突起 Superior articular process
- 横突起 Transverse process
- 棘突起 Spinous process
- 下関節突起 Inferior articular process

3-57 第3腰椎（後面）

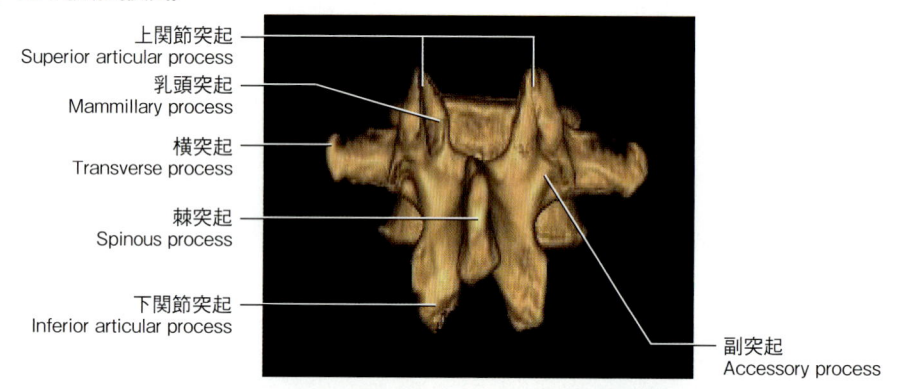

- 上関節突起 Superior articular process
- 乳頭突起 Mammillary process
- 横突起 Transverse process
- 棘突起 Spinous process
- 下関節突起 Inferior articular process
- 副突起 Accessory process

3-58 第3腰椎（上面）

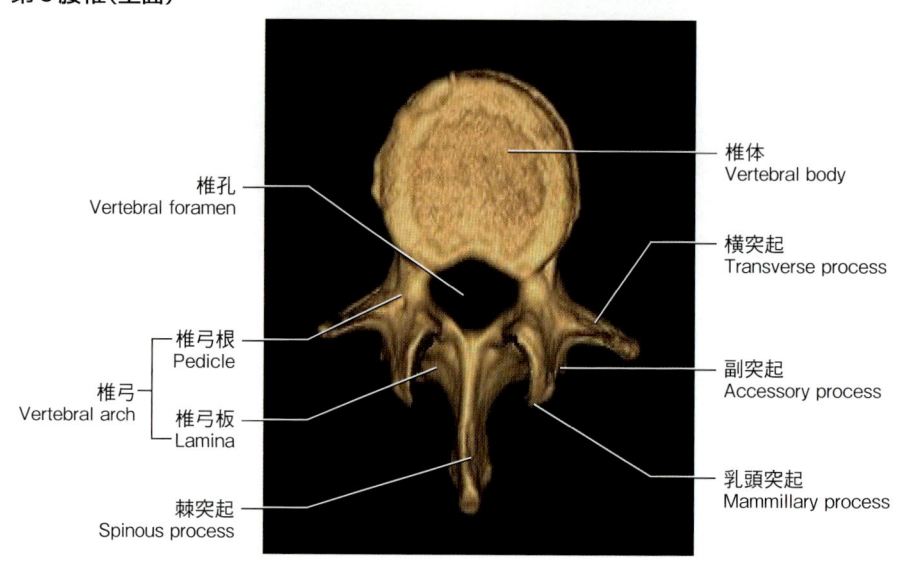

- 椎孔 Vertebral foramen
- 椎弓根 Pedicle
- 椎弓 Vertebral arch
- 椎弓板 Lamina
- 棘突起 Spinous process
- 椎体 Vertebral body
- 横突起 Transverse process
- 副突起 Accessory process
- 乳頭突起 Mammillary process

> **NOTE** 腰椎の横突起は外側やや後上方へ向かって伸びている．横突起の基部後面には小さな突起があり副突起とよばれ腰内側横突間筋（背筋）が付着する．また，上関節突起の後面にも乳頭突起とよばれる突起があり，多裂筋や背筋が付着している．

腰椎の断層解剖 ［横断像（CT）］

3-59　第1腰椎レベル

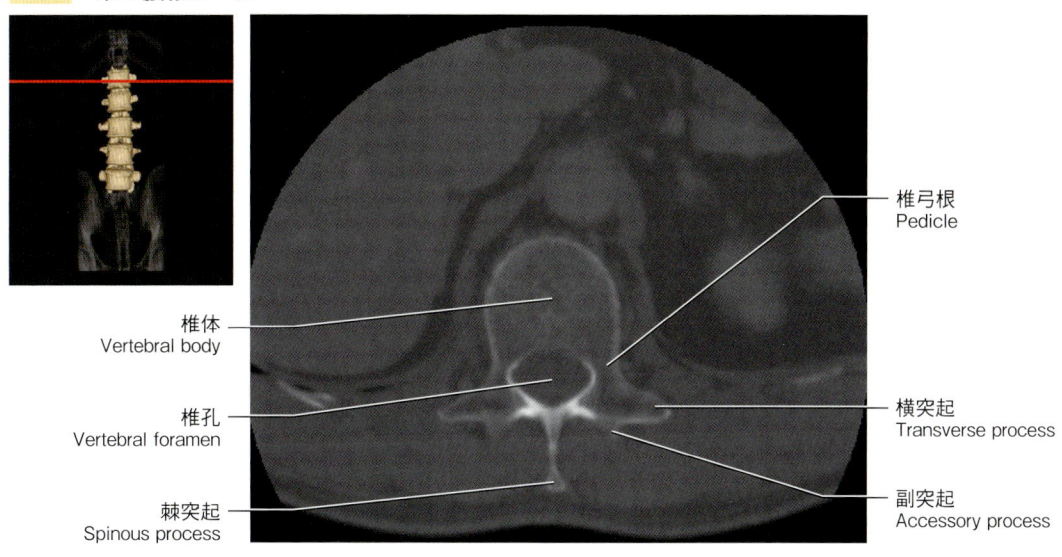

- 椎体 Vertebral body
- 椎孔 Vertebral foramen
- 棘突起 Spinous process
- 椎弓根 Pedicle
- 横突起 Transverse process
- 副突起 Accessory process

3-60　第1-第2腰椎椎間レベル

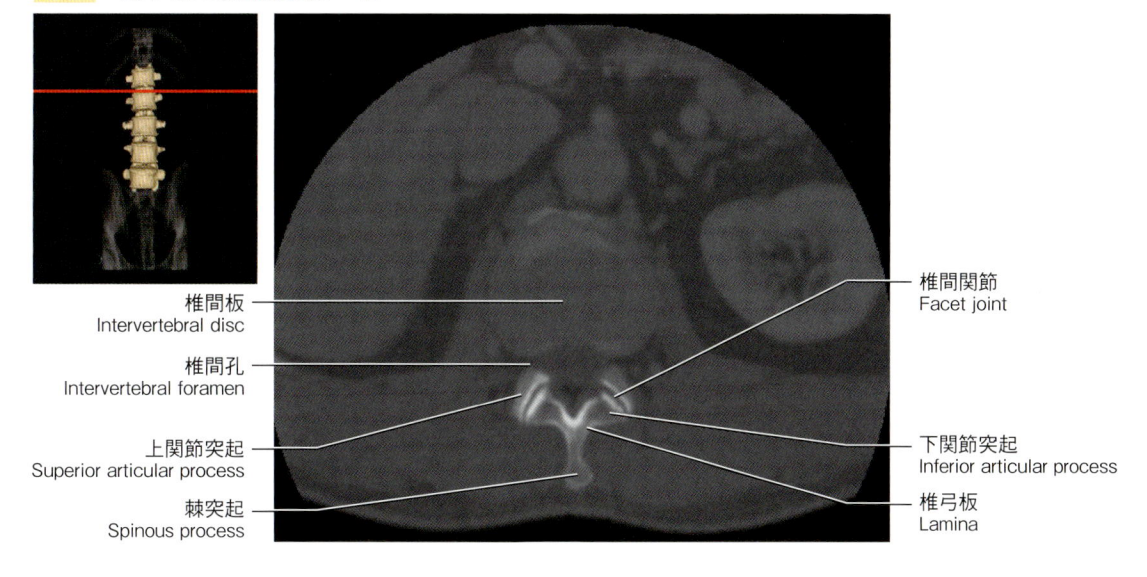

- 椎間板 Intervertebral disc
- 椎間孔 Intervertebral foramen
- 上関節突起 Superior articular process
- 棘突起 Spinous process
- 椎間関節 Facet joint
- 下関節突起 Inferior articular process
- 椎弓板 Lamina

腰椎の断層解剖 ［冠状断像（CT, MPR像）］

3-61 椎体中央レベル

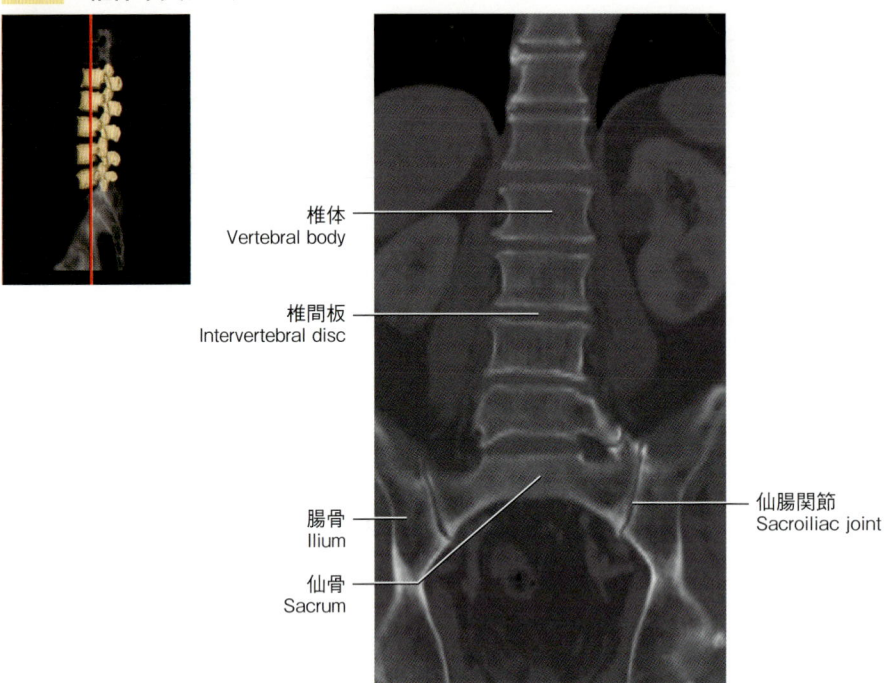

- 椎体 Vertebral body
- 椎間板 Intervertebral disc
- 腸骨 Ilium
- 仙骨 Sacrum
- 仙腸関節 Sacroiliac joint

3-62 脊柱管レベル

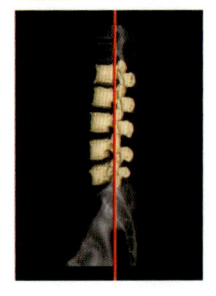

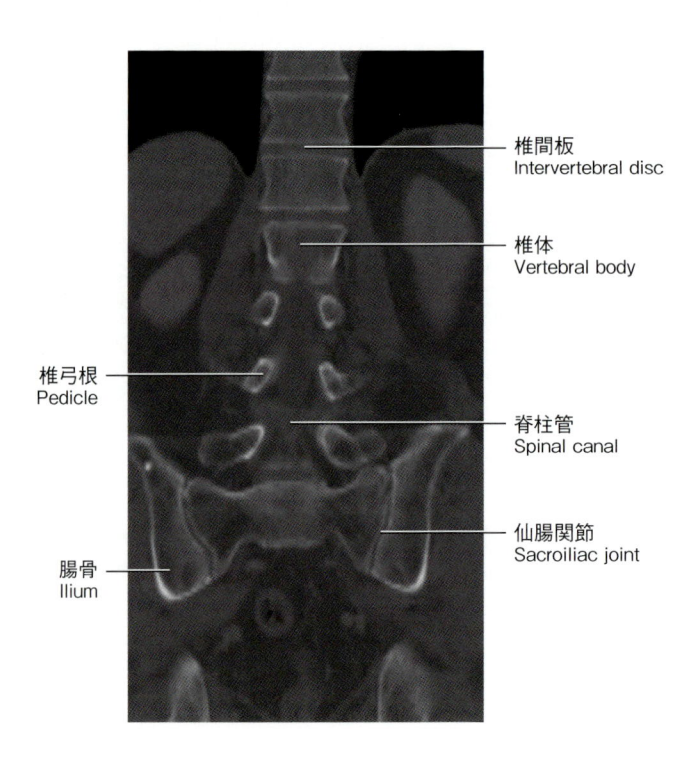

- 椎間板 Intervertebral disc
- 椎体 Vertebral body
- 椎弓根 Pedicle
- 脊柱管 Spinal canal
- 仙腸関節 Sacroiliac joint
- 腸骨 Ilium

腰椎の断層解剖 ［冠状断像（CT，MPR像）］

3-63 椎間関節レベル

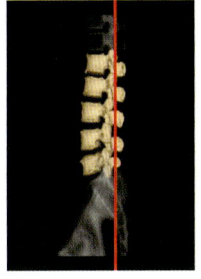

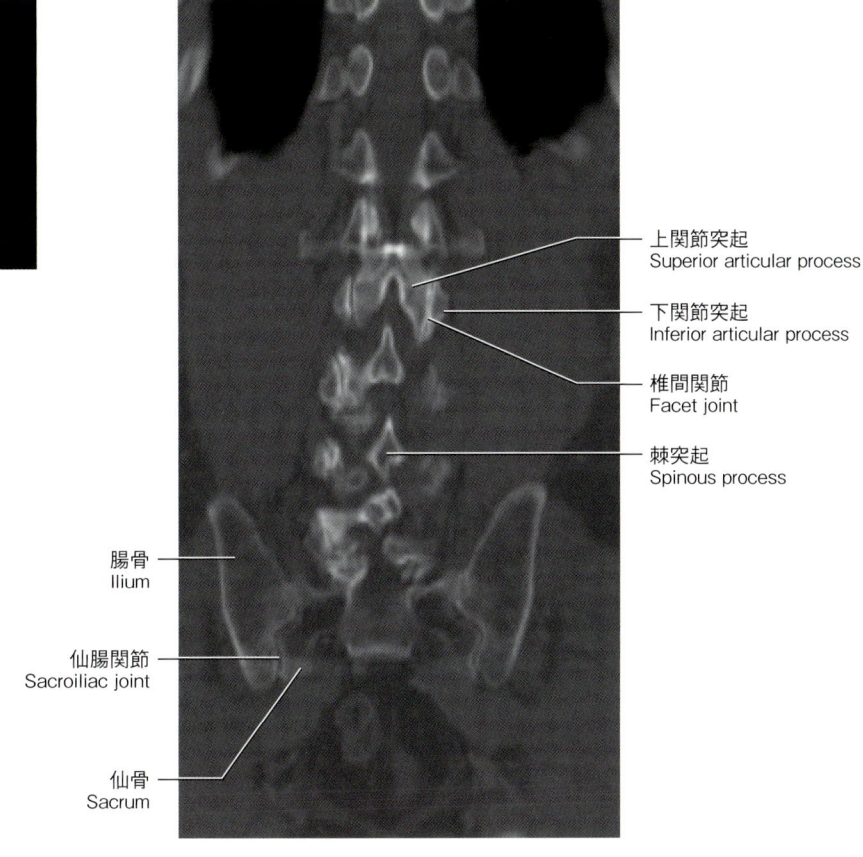

- 上関節突起 Superior articular process
- 下関節突起 Inferior articular process
- 椎間関節 Facet joint
- 棘突起 Spinous process
- 腸骨 Ilium
- 仙腸関節 Sacroiliac joint
- 仙骨 Sacrum

NOTE 隣接する上下の関節突起によって構成される平面滑膜関節が椎間関節であり，関節突起間のすべり運動を可能としている．各関節は関節包によって包まれている．

腰椎の断層解剖 ［矢状断像（CT, MPR像）］

3-64 椎間関節レベル

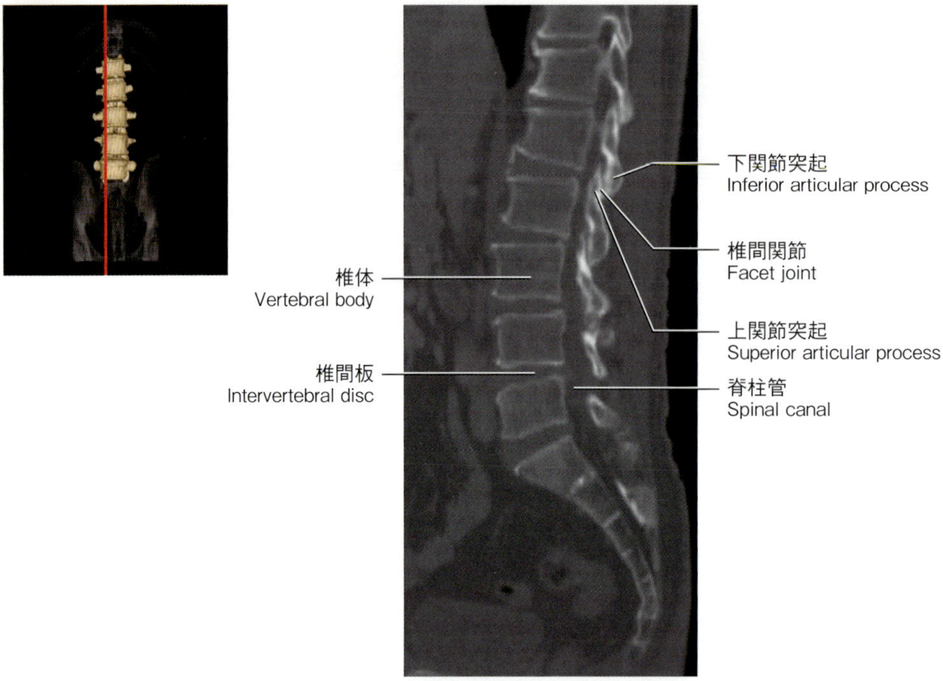

- 椎体 Vertebral body
- 椎間板 Intervertebral disc
- 下関節突起 Inferior articular process
- 椎間関節 Facet joint
- 上関節突起 Superior articular process
- 脊柱管 Spinal canal

3-65 脊柱管レベル

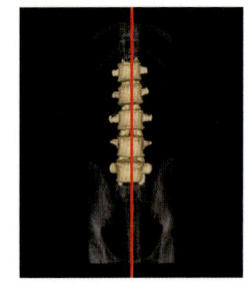

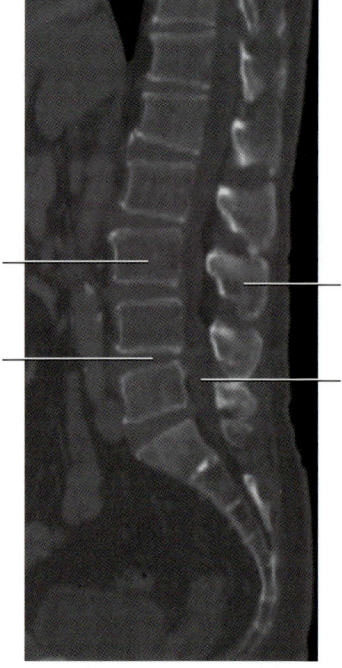

- 椎体 Vertebral body
- 椎間板 Intervertebral disc
- 棘突起 Spinous process
- 脊柱管 Spinal canal

腰椎の断層解剖 ［矢状断像（CT, MPR 像）］

3-66 椎弓根レベル

- 椎体 Vertebral body
- 椎間板 Intervertebral disc
- 椎弓根 Pedicle
- 下椎切痕 Inferior vertebral notch
- 上椎切痕 Superior vertebral notch
- 椎間孔 Intervertebral foramen

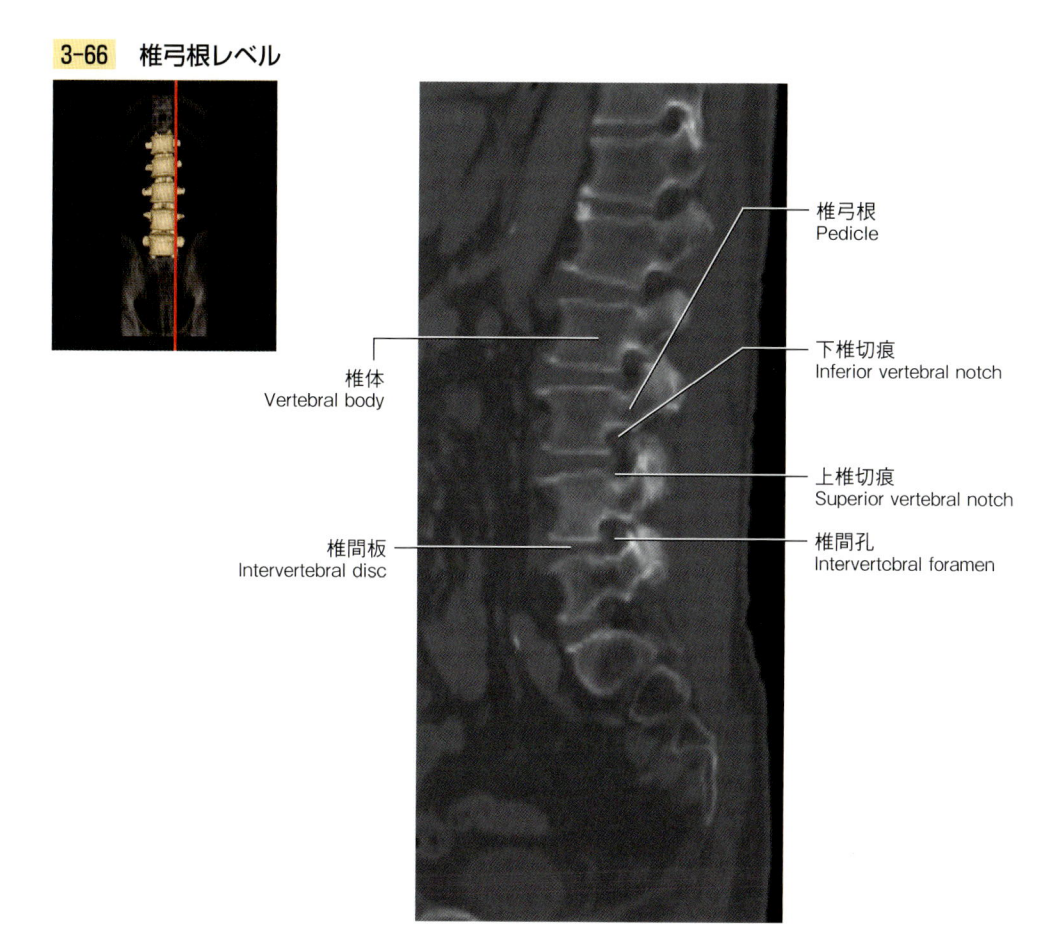

NOTE 上・下椎切痕 Superior/Inferior vertebral notch

　superior, inferior, anteior, posterior は, super, infra, ante, post の位置を示す前置詞から導かれたラテン語形容詞の比較級．「上の」に限定すると，superus, superior, superimus が，その原級，比較級，最上級．最上級は解剖名では最上肋間動脈の英名 Supreme intercostal artery（Highest intercostal artery）にあらわれる．

腰椎の断層解剖 ［横断像（MRI, T2強調像）］

3-67 第1腰椎下部レベル

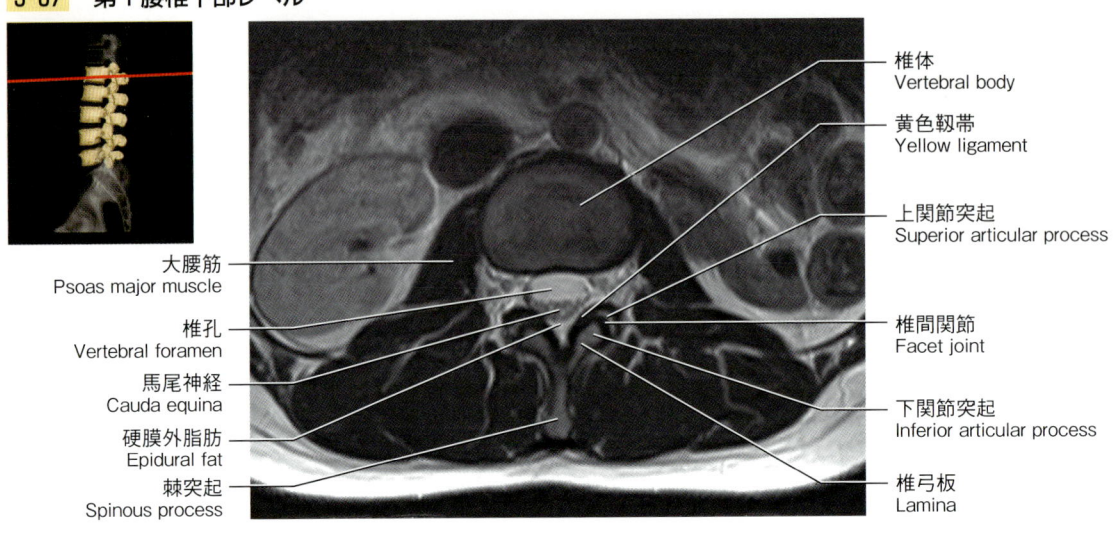

- 椎体 Vertebral body
- 黄色靱帯 Yellow ligament
- 上関節突起 Superior articular process
- 椎間関節 Facet joint
- 下関節突起 Inferior articular process
- 椎弓板 Lamina
- 大腰筋 Psoas major muscle
- 椎孔 Vertebral foramen
- 馬尾神経 Cauda equina
- 硬膜外脂肪 Epidural fat
- 棘突起 Spinous process

3-68 第1-第2腰椎椎間レベル

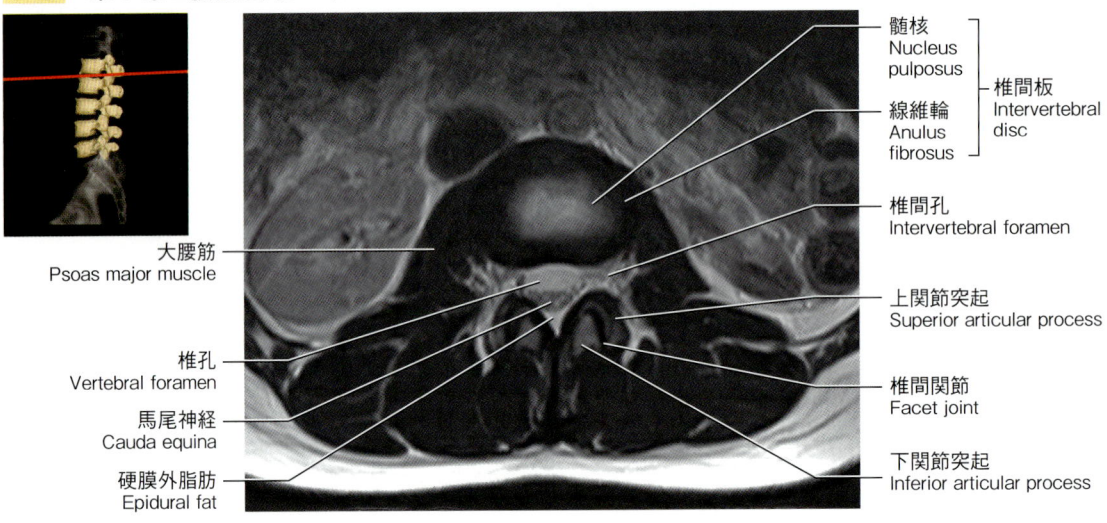

- 髄核 Nucleus pulposus
- 線維輪 Anulus fibrosus
- 椎間板 Intervertebral disc
- 椎間孔 Intervertebral foramen
- 上関節突起 Superior articular process
- 椎間関節 Facet joint
- 下関節突起 Inferior articular process
- 大腰筋 Psoas major muscle
- 椎孔 Vertebral foramen
- 馬尾神経 Cauda equina
- 硬膜外脂肪 Epidural fat

NOTE 椎間板は外側を線維性の部分からなる線維輪，中心部を水分量の多いゼラチン様部分からなる髄核で構成される．椎間板は隣接する椎体同士を結びつける接着装置としての役割のほか，中心部の髄核が柔らかく弾力性があるためさまざまな動きに対する椎骨間の衝撃吸収装置の役割を果たす．椎間板は圧迫されると広がり，伸展では引き延ばされ薄くなる．これにより脊椎の多彩な動きを可能にしている．

腰椎の断層解剖　[横断像（MRI, T2・T1 強調像）]

3-69　第 2 腰椎上部レベル（T2 強調像）

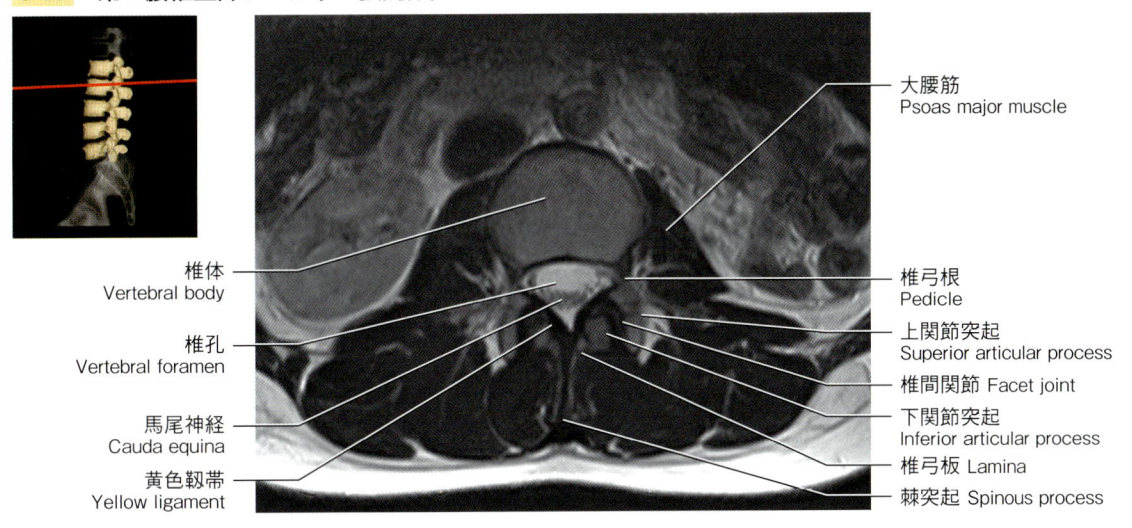

- 椎体 Vertebral body
- 椎孔 Vertebral foramen
- 馬尾神経 Cauda equina
- 黄色靱帯 Yellow ligament
- 大腰筋 Psoas major muscle
- 椎弓根 Pedicle
- 上関節突起 Superior articular process
- 椎間関節 Facet joint
- 下関節突起 Inferior articular process
- 椎弓板 Lamina
- 棘突起 Spinous process

3-70　第 2 腰椎上部レベル（T1 強調像）

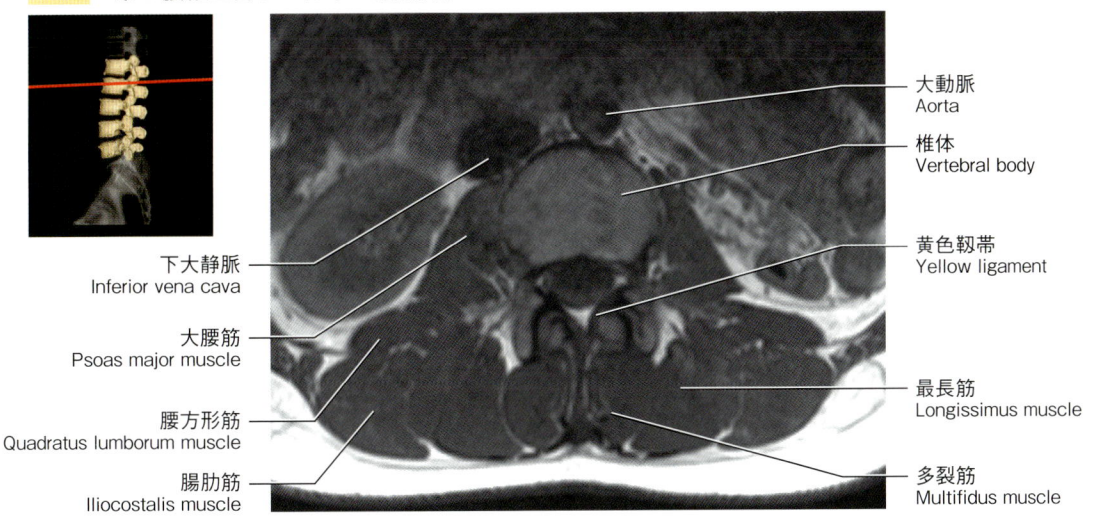

- 下大静脈 Inferior vena cava
- 大腰筋 Psoas major muscle
- 腰方形筋 Quadratus lumborum muscle
- 腸肋筋 Iliocostalis muscle
- 大動脈 Aorta
- 椎体 Vertebral body
- 黄色靱帯 Yellow ligament
- 最長筋 Longissimus muscle
- 多裂筋 Multifidus muscle

NOTE 隣り合う椎弓板を連結する幅の広い黄色の靱帯を黄色靱帯とよぶ．左右に 1 対ずつあり，正中で混ざり垂直に伸びており，隣接する脊椎の椎弓板を連結している．黄色靱帯は頸部で幅広く，腰部で最も厚くなる．

NOTE 黄色靱帯　Yellow ligament
　黄色靱帯は英語名では Yellow ligament だが，ラテン語の Ligament flavum のほうが一般的である．flavum は"黄色の，金色の"の意味．flamma（炎，火）に連なる語で，英語の flame（炎，白熱）に至る．

腰椎の断層解剖 ［冠状断像（MRI, T1強調像）］

3-71 椎体レベル

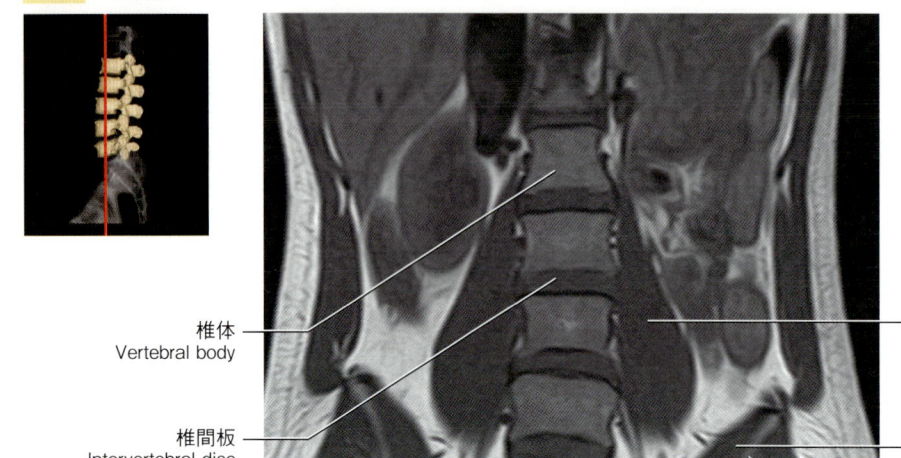

- 椎体 Vertebral body
- 椎間板 Intervertebral disc
- 大殿筋 Gluteus maximus muscle
- 大腰筋 Psoas major muscle
- 腸骨筋 Iliacus muscle
- 腸骨 Ilium

3-72 脊柱管レベル

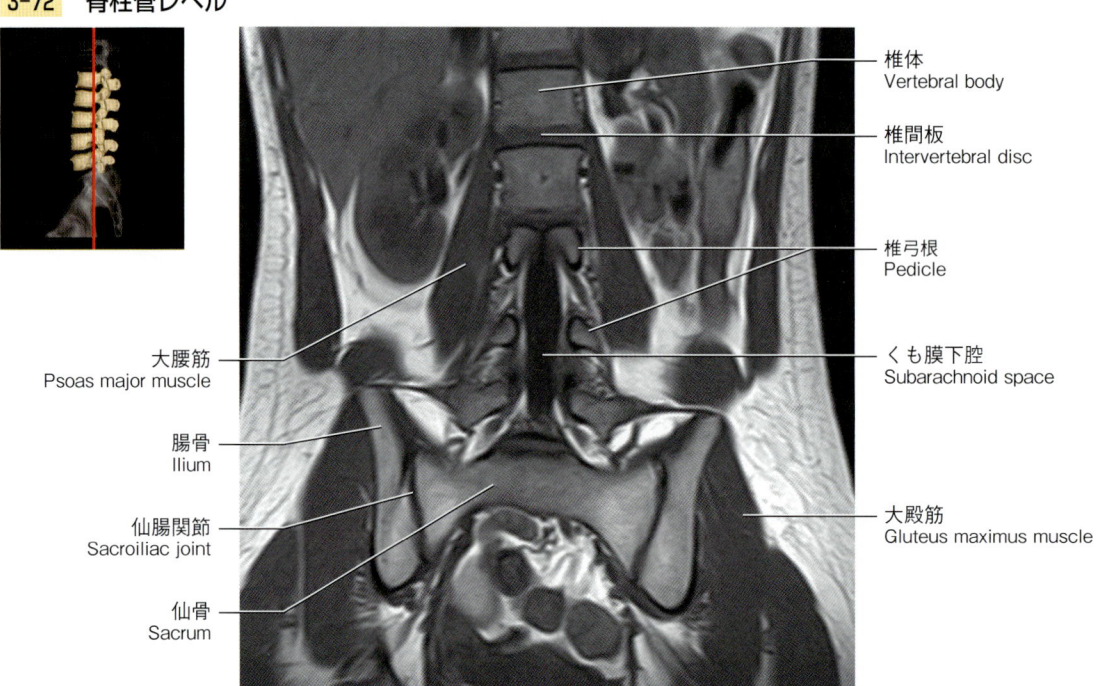

- 椎体 Vertebral body
- 椎間板 Intervertebral disc
- 椎弓根 Pedicle
- くも膜下腔 Subarachnoid space
- 大腰筋 Psoas major muscle
- 腸骨 Ilium
- 仙腸関節 Sacroiliac joint
- 仙骨 Sacrum
- 大殿筋 Gluteus maximus muscle

腰椎の断層解剖 ［冠状断像（MRI，T2強調像）］

3-73 脊柱管レベル

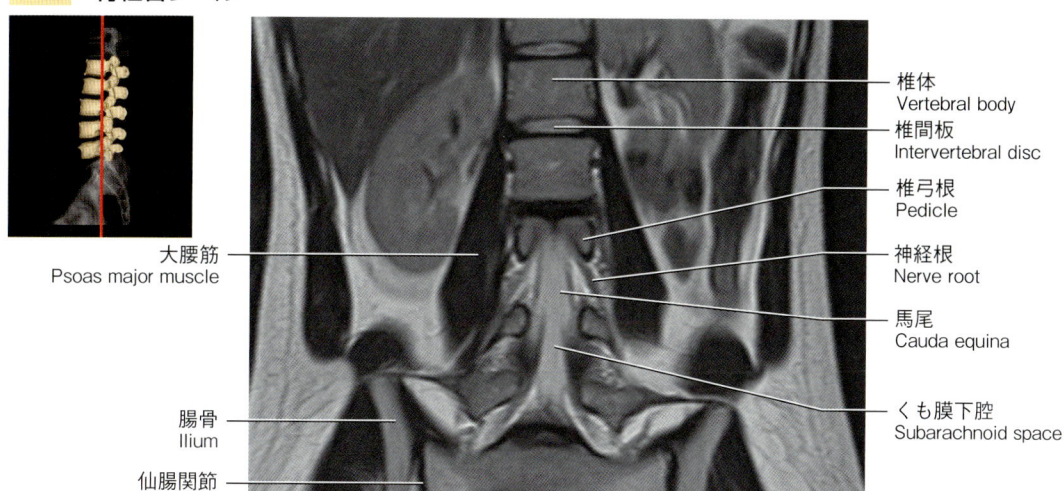

- 大腰筋 Psoas major muscle
- 腸骨 Ilium
- 仙腸関節 Sacroiliac joint
- 仙骨 Sacrum
- 椎体 Vertebral body
- 椎間板 Intervertebral disc
- 椎弓根 Pedicle
- 神経根 Nerve root
- 馬尾 Cauda equina
- くも膜下腔 Subarachnoid space
- 大殿筋 Gluteus maximus muscle

NOTE 脊髄は延髄から連続し第1腰椎あるいは第2腰椎付近で先細りし，脊髄円錐とよばれる終末部となる．この脊髄円錐から尾側方向に脊髄神経根の束が伸びており，馬の尻尾のようにみえることから馬尾と名付けられた．脊髄円錐から起こり，馬尾の脊髄神経の中を尾側方向へ走行し，尾骨背側に付着するのが終糸であり，脊髄下端を固定する役割を果たす．

腰椎の断層解剖 [矢状断像（MRI，T1強調像）]

3-74 椎間関節レベル

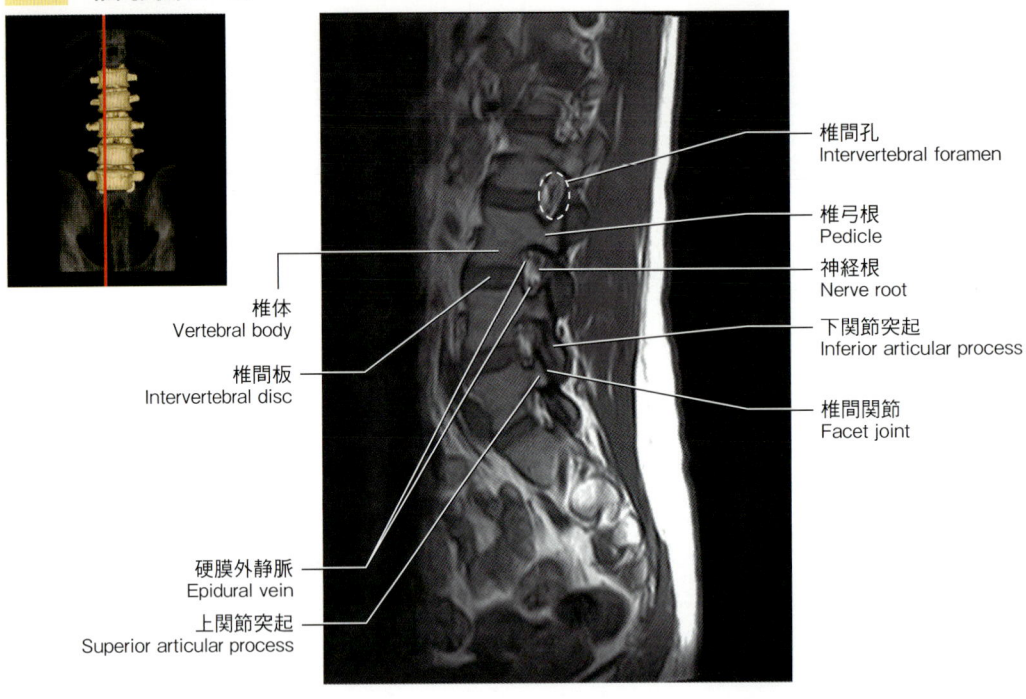

- 椎間孔 Intervertebral foramen
- 椎弓根 Pedicle
- 神経根 Nerve root
- 下関節突起 Inferior articular process
- 椎間関節 Facet joint
- 椎体 Vertebral body
- 椎間板 Intervertebral disc
- 硬膜外静脈 Epidural vein
- 上関節突起 Superior articular process

3-75 脊柱管レベル

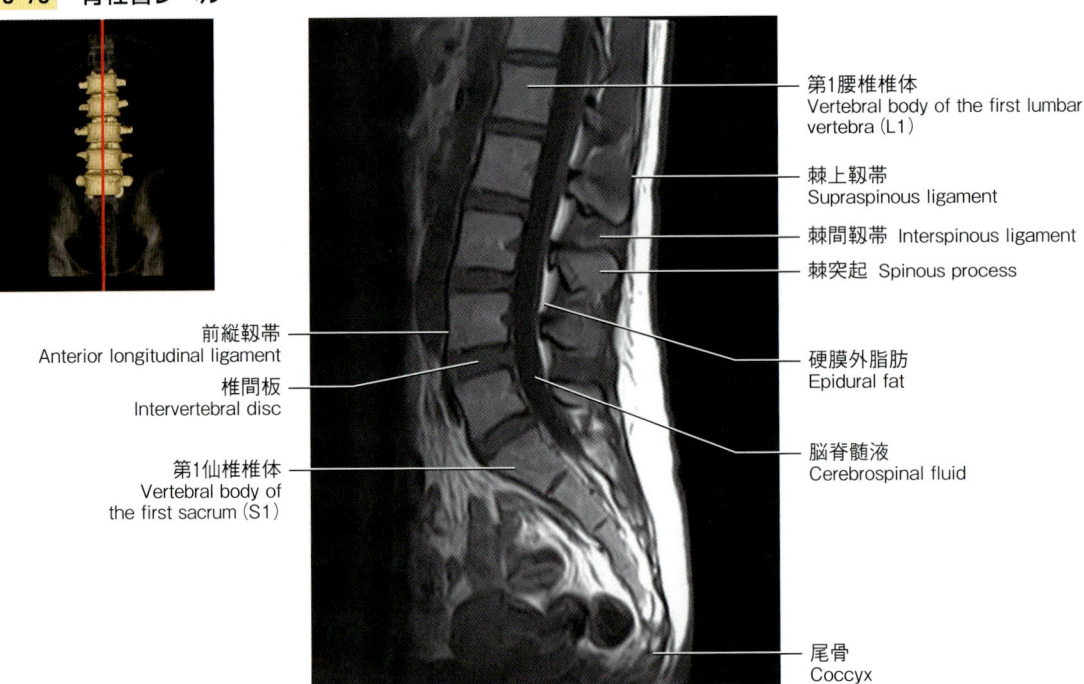

- 第1腰椎椎体 Vertebral body of the first lumbar vertebra（L1）
- 棘上靱帯 Supraspinous ligament
- 棘間靱帯 Interspinous ligament
- 棘突起 Spinous process
- 前縦靱帯 Anterior longitudinal ligament
- 椎間板 Intervertebral disc
- 第1仙椎椎体 Vertebral body of the first sacrum（S1）
- 硬膜外脂肪 Epidural fat
- 脳脊髄液 Cerebrospinal fluid
- 尾骨 Coccyx

腰椎の断層解剖　[矢状断像（MRI, T2 強調像）]

3-76　脊柱管レベル

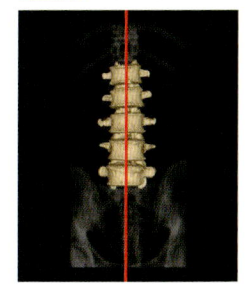

- 第1腰椎椎体　Vertebral body of L1
- 脊髄円錐　Conus medullaris of spiral cord
- 棘上靱帯　Supraspinous ligament
- 棘突起　Spinous process
- 棘間靱帯　Interspinous ligament
- 黄色靱帯　Yellow ligament
- 硬膜外脂肪　Epidural fat
- 馬尾神経　Cauda equina
- くも膜下腔　Subarachnoid space
- 尾骨　Coccyx
- 前縦靱帯　Anterior longitudinal ligament
- 後縦靱帯　Posterior longitudinal ligament
- 椎間板　Intervertebral disc
- 髄核　Nucleus pulposus
- 線維輪　Anulus fibrosus
- 髄核内裂　Intranuclear cleft
- 第1仙椎椎体　Vertebral body of S1

NOTE　脊椎の過屈曲により椎間板の前方は圧迫，後方は伸展される．この伸展により引き伸ばされた後側の線維輪に亀裂が生じることで中心部の髄核が脱出することを椎間板ヘルニアとよぶ．椎間板は椎間孔前壁の構成成分のひとつであるため，後方へ突出することで神経根を圧排し，限局した背部痛を訴える．

仙椎 (CT, VR像)

3-77 仙椎（正面）

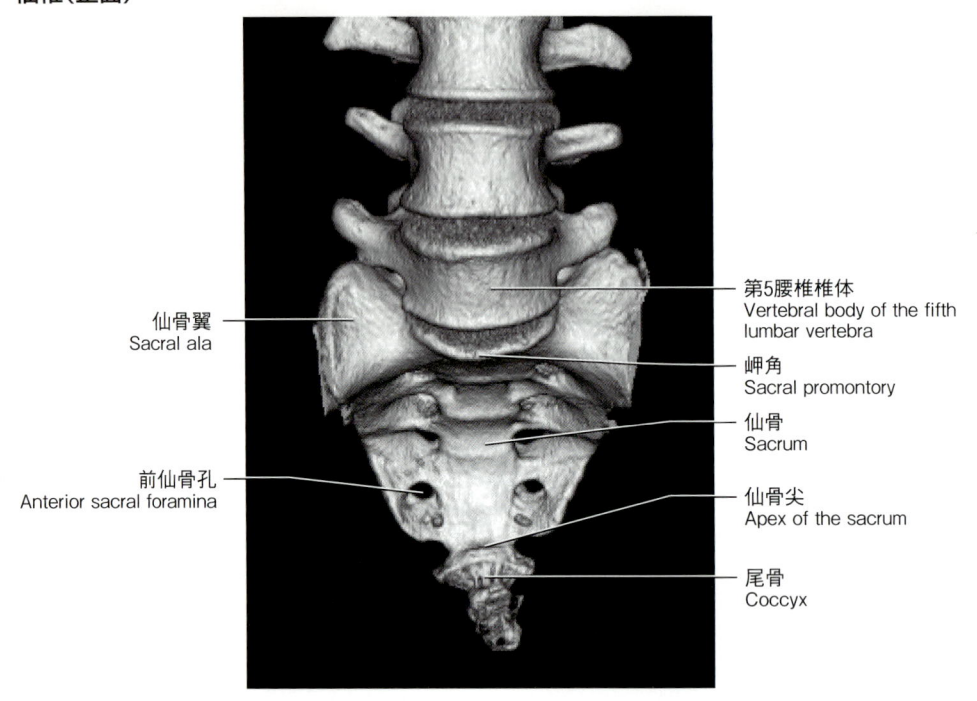

- 仙骨翼 Sacral ala
- 前仙骨孔 Anterior sacral foramina
- 第5腰椎椎体 Vertebral body of the fifth lumbar vertebra
- 岬角 Sacral promontory
- 仙骨 Sacrum
- 仙骨尖 Apex of the sacrum
- 尾骨 Coccyx

3-78 仙椎（後面）

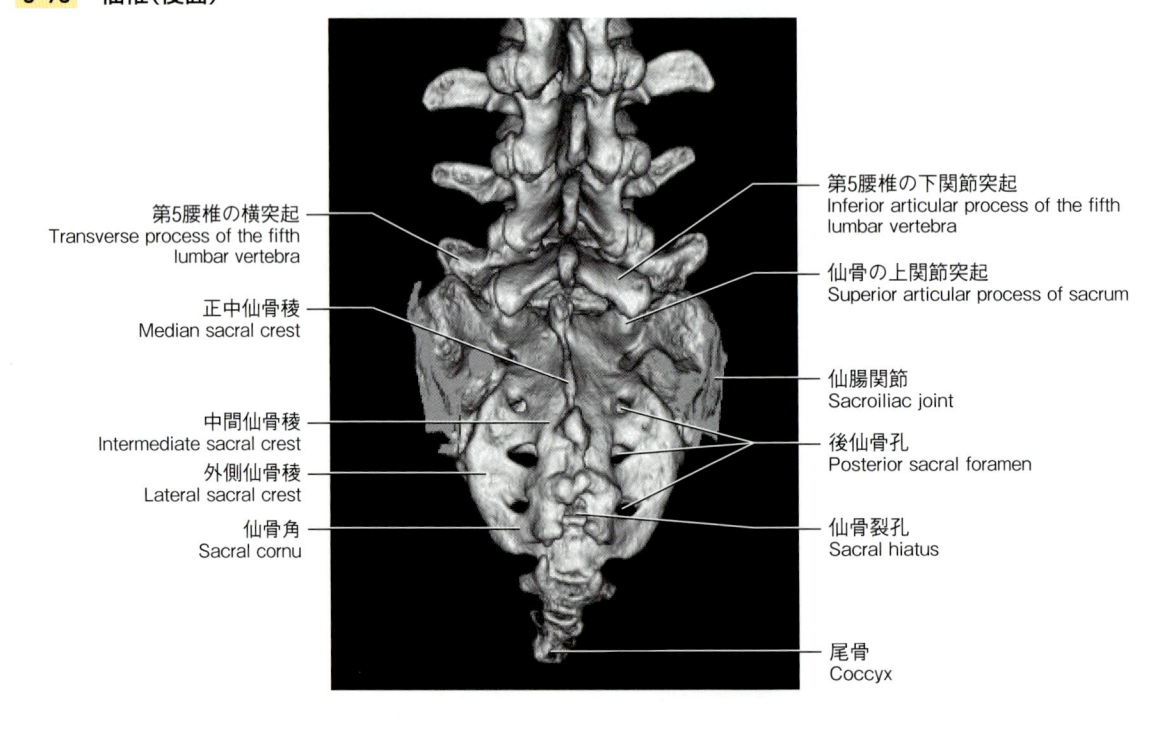

- 第5腰椎の横突起 Transverse process of the fifth lumbar vertebra
- 正中仙骨稜 Median sacral crest
- 中間仙骨稜 Intermediate sacral crest
- 外側仙骨稜 Lateral sacral crest
- 仙骨角 Sacral cornu
- 第5腰椎の下関節突起 Inferior articular process of the fifth lumbar vertebra
- 仙骨の上関節突起 Superior articular process of sacrum
- 仙腸関節 Sacroiliac joint
- 後仙骨孔 Posterior sacral foramen
- 仙骨裂孔 Sacral hiatus
- 尾骨 Coccyx

> **NOTE** 小児期には各仙椎は椎間板で隔てられているが，20歳ごろから仙椎の癒合が始まり，中年期以降に椎間板が骨化する．成人では5つの仙椎は癒合し，全体として三角形の仙骨を形成する．仙骨は背側に凸の緩やかなカーブを描き骨盤の後壁を形成している．

仙椎の断層解剖 ［横断像（CT），斜冠状断像（CT, MPR像）］

3-79　第1仙椎レベル（横断像）

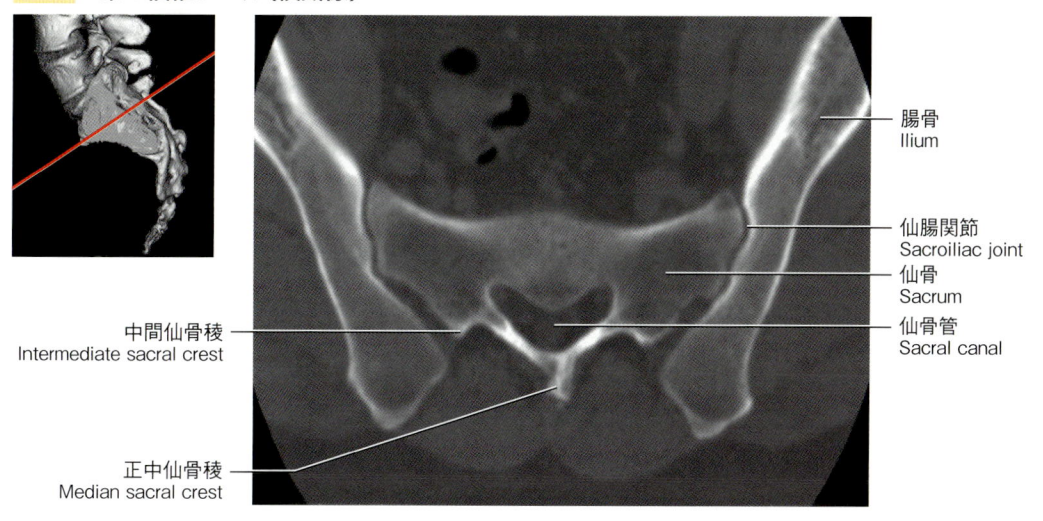

- 腸骨 Ilium
- 仙腸関節 Sacroiliac joint
- 仙骨 Sacrum
- 仙骨管 Sacral canal
- 中間仙骨稜 Intermediate sacral crest
- 正中仙骨稜 Median sacral crest

3-80　仙骨レベル（斜冠状断像）

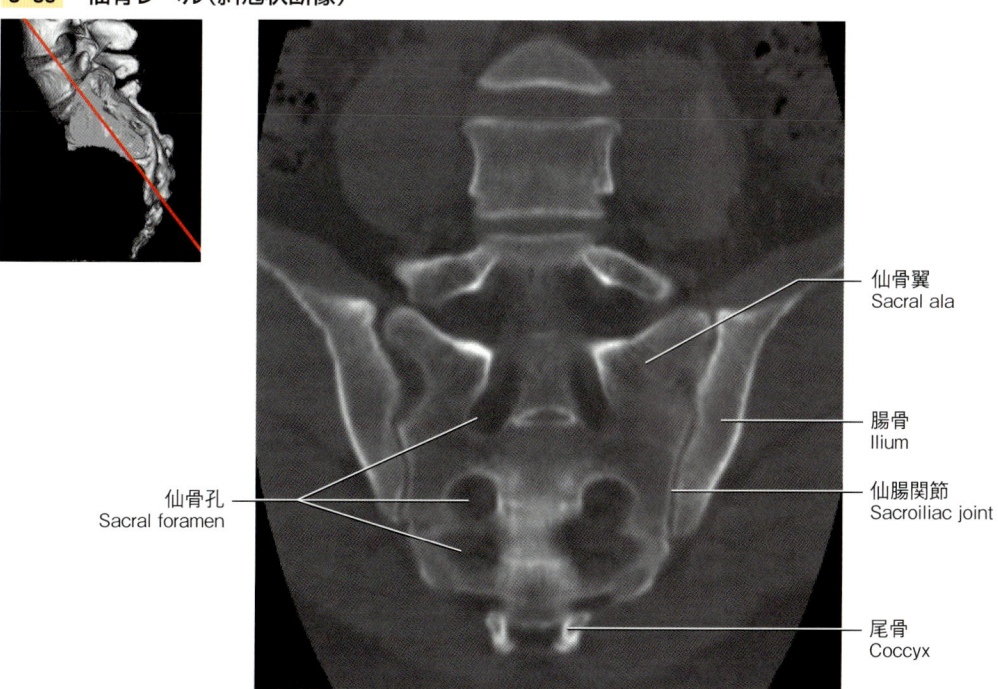

- 仙骨翼 Sacral ala
- 腸骨 Ilium
- 仙腸関節 Sacroiliac joint
- 尾骨 Coccyx
- 仙骨孔 Sacral foramen

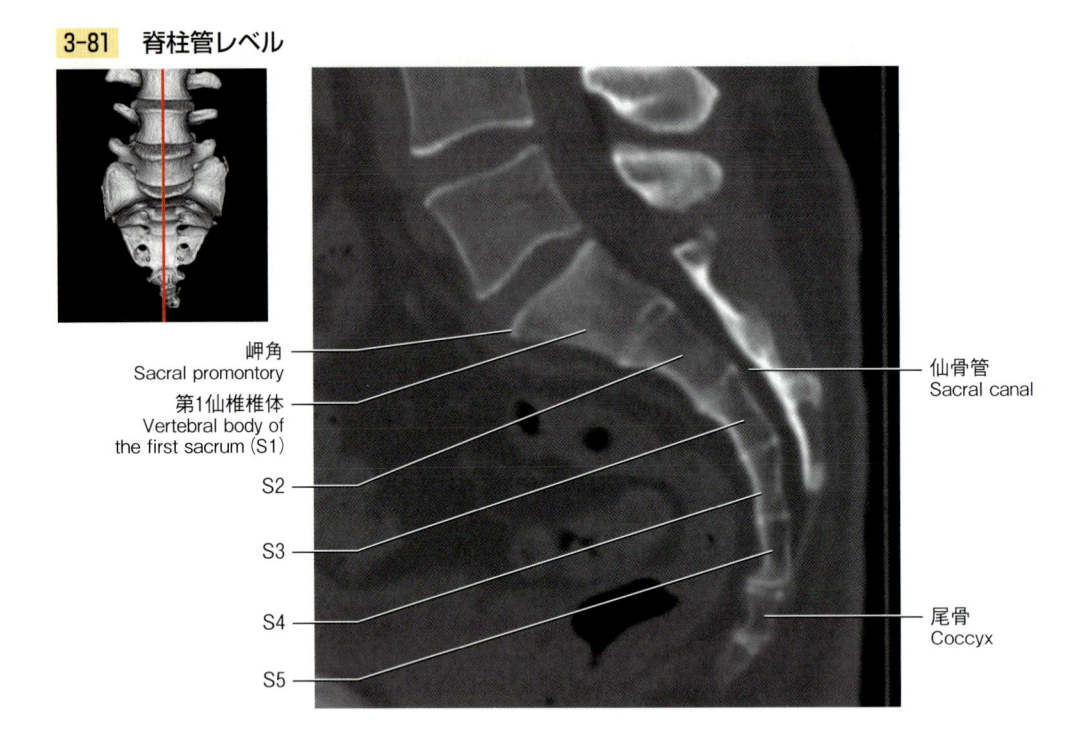

仙椎の断層解剖 ［矢状断像（CT, MPR像）］

3-81 脊柱管レベル

- 岬角 Sacral promontory
- 第1仙椎椎体 Vertebral body of the first sacrum（S1）
- S2
- S3
- S4
- S5
- 仙骨管 Sacral canal
- 尾骨 Coccyx

NOTE 仙骨管は脊柱管が仙椎にまで連続したものであり，馬尾が走行している．

仙椎の断層解剖　[横断像（MRI, T1 強調像）]

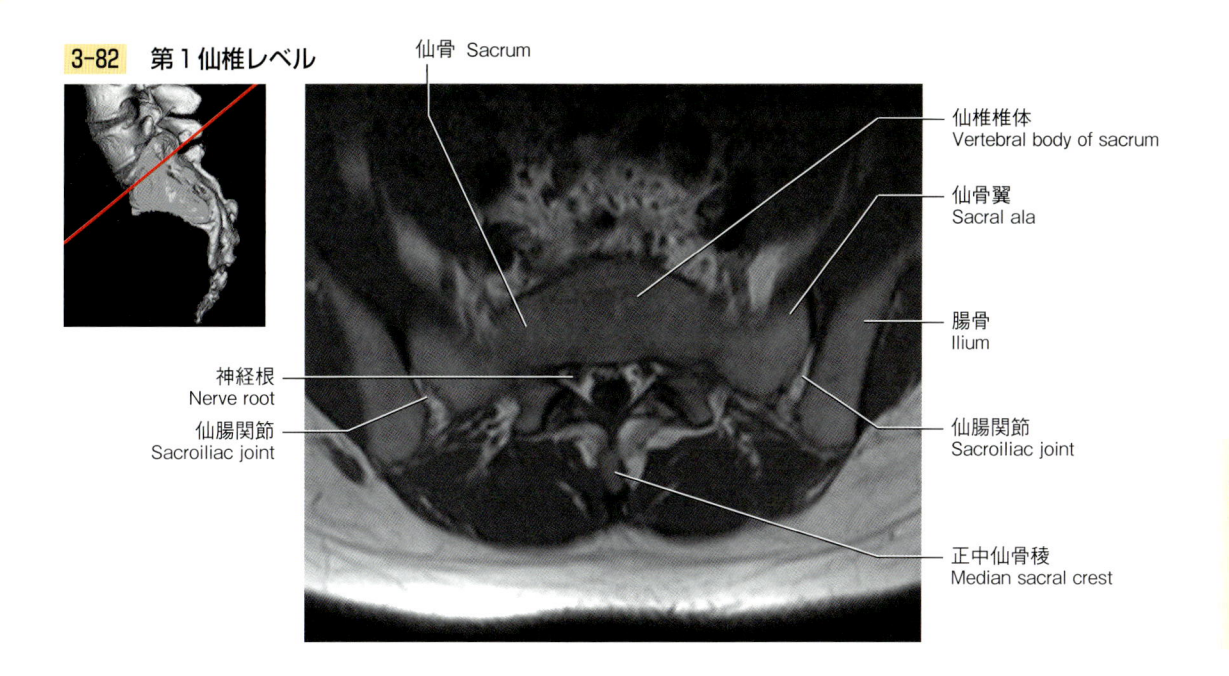

3-82　第1仙椎レベル

- 仙骨　Sacrum
- 仙椎椎体　Vertebral body of sacrum
- 仙骨翼　Sacral ala
- 腸骨　Ilium
- 神経根　Nerve root
- 仙腸関節　Sacroiliac joint
- 仙腸関節　Sacroiliac joint
- 正中仙骨稜　Median sacral crest

3-83　第2仙椎レベル

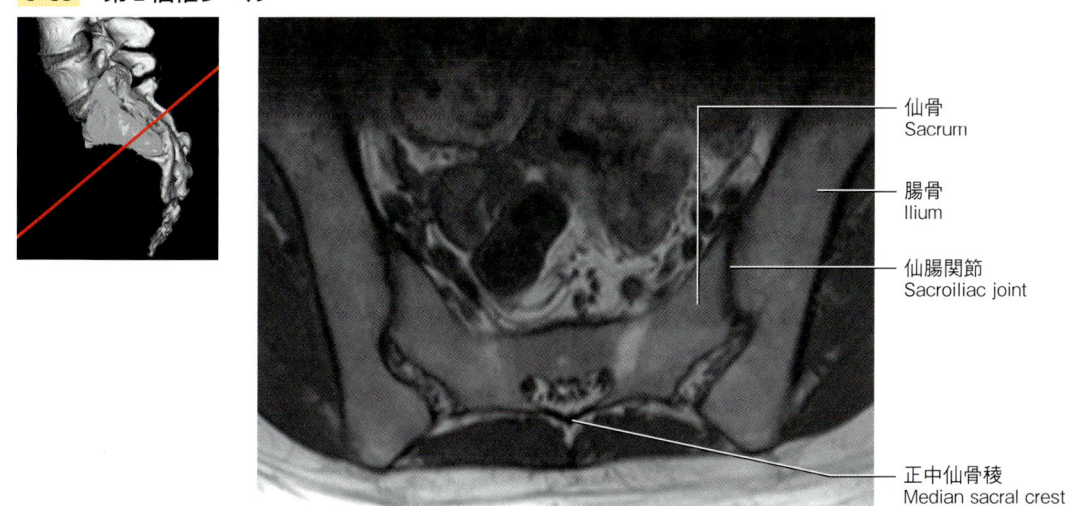

- 仙骨　Sacrum
- 腸骨　Ilium
- 仙腸関節　Sacroiliac joint
- 正中仙骨稜　Median sacral crest

仙椎の断層解剖 ［冠状断像（MRI, T1強調像）］

3-84 仙骨レベル

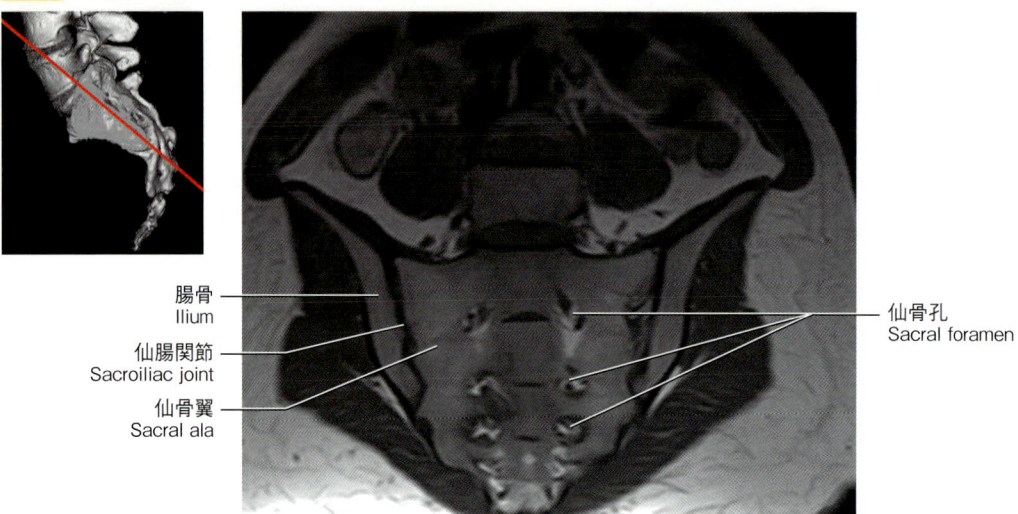

- 腸骨 Ilium
- 仙腸関節 Sacroiliac joint
- 仙骨翼 Sacral ala
- 仙骨孔 Sacral foramen

3-85 仙骨管レベル

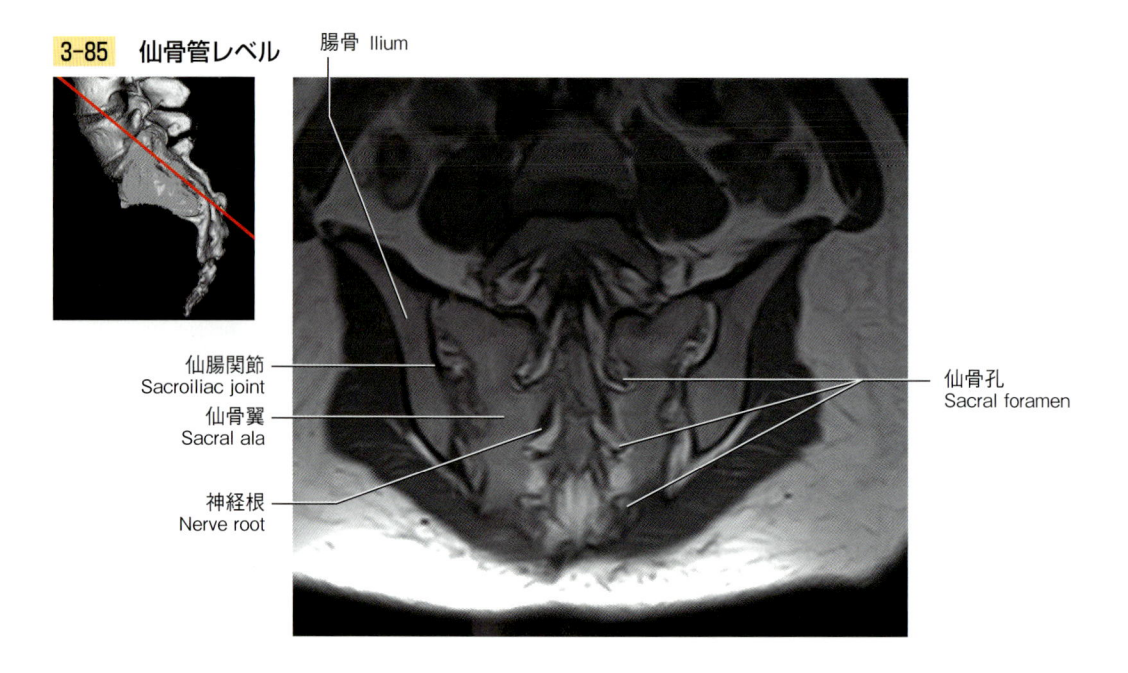

- 腸骨 Ilium
- 仙腸関節 Sacroiliac joint
- 仙骨翼 Sacral ala
- 神経根 Nerve root
- 仙骨孔 Sacral foramen

NOTE 仙骨の前面と後面にそれぞれ仙骨孔があり，それぞれ脊髄神経の前枝と後枝が出る．

IV

胸部
Chest

胸　郭 (CT, VR像)

4-1 胸郭の構成（前面）

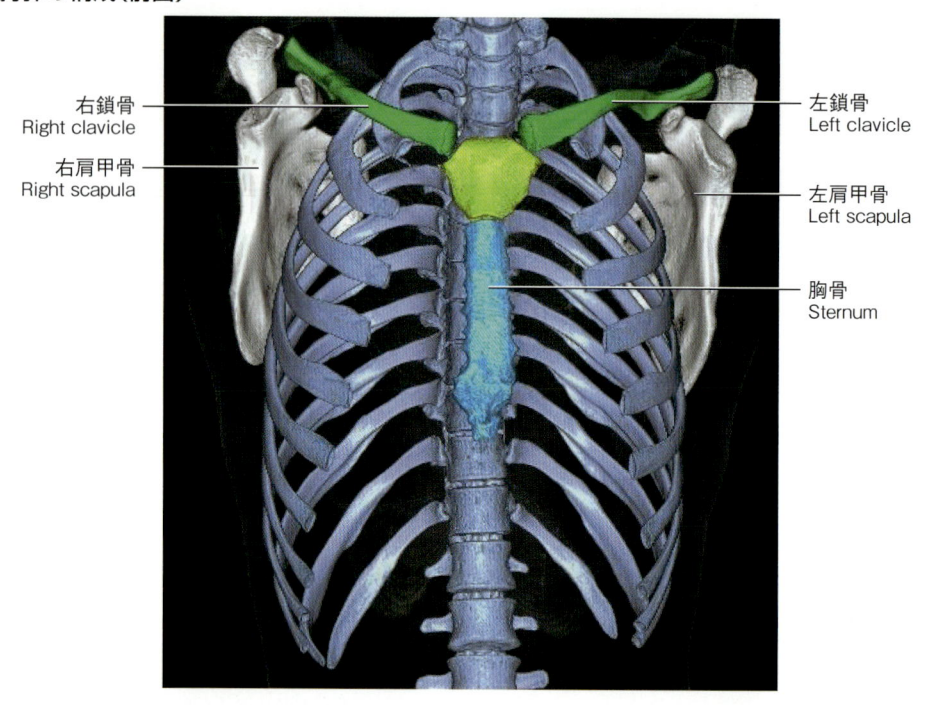

- 右鎖骨 Right clavicle
- 右肩甲骨 Right scapula
- 左鎖骨 Left clavicle
- 左肩甲骨 Left scapula
- 胸骨 Sternum

4-2 胸郭の構成（後面）

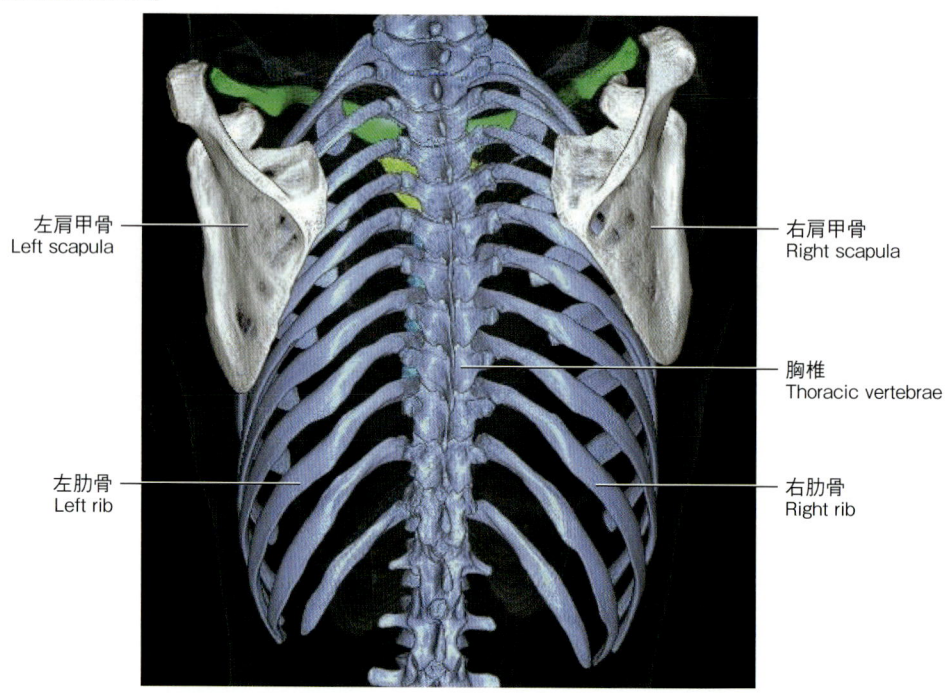

- 左肩甲骨 Left scapula
- 右肩甲骨 Right scapula
- 胸椎 Thoracic vertebrae
- 左肋骨 Left rib
- 右肋骨 Right rib

NOTE 胸部は，胸腔およびその内容物と，これらを囲む胸壁からなる．このうち骨軟骨性の胸郭は12個の胸椎，12対の肋骨，および1個の胸骨で構成される．これらは心臓，肺，食道などを保護し，胸筋による働きで呼吸運動を助けている．胸郭は上方が狭く，前後に圧平された樽状を呈し，前後径より左右径が大きいが，加齢により胸郭の横径に上下で差がなくなり，前後径が増す．さらに胸椎の後弯も加わり，全体として丸みを帯びた状態になる．

胸　郭（CT, VR 像）

4-3　胸郭の構成（左側面）

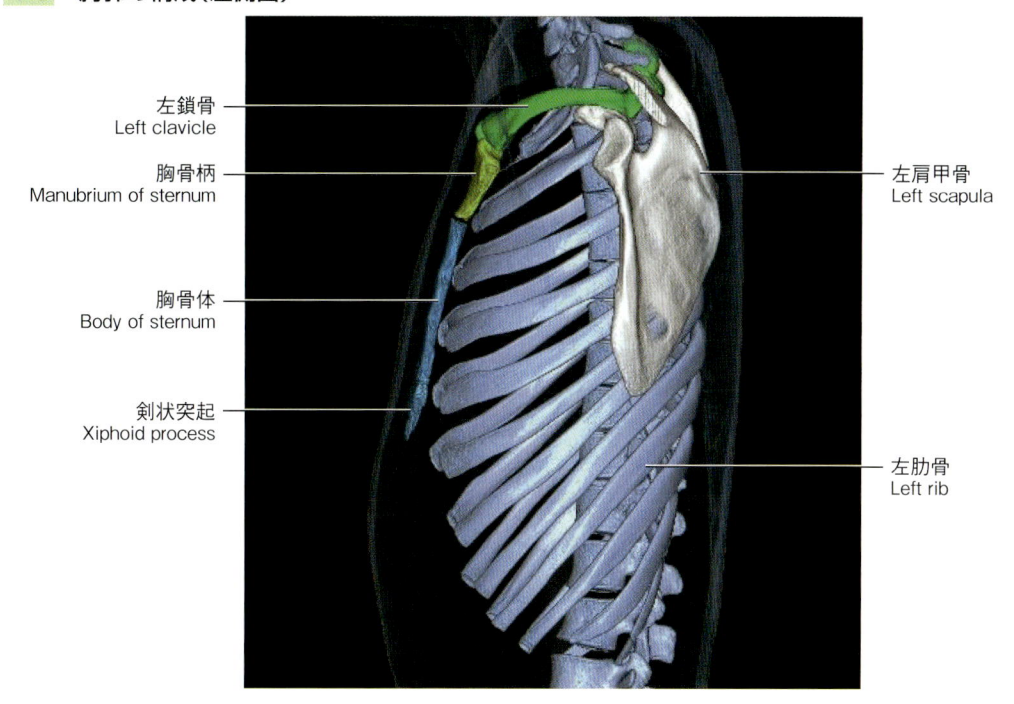

- 左鎖骨 Left clavicle
- 胸骨柄 Manubrium of sternum
- 胸骨体 Body of sternum
- 剣状突起 Xiphoid process
- 左肩甲骨 Left scapula
- 左肋骨 Left rib

4-4　胸郭・肋骨（後面）

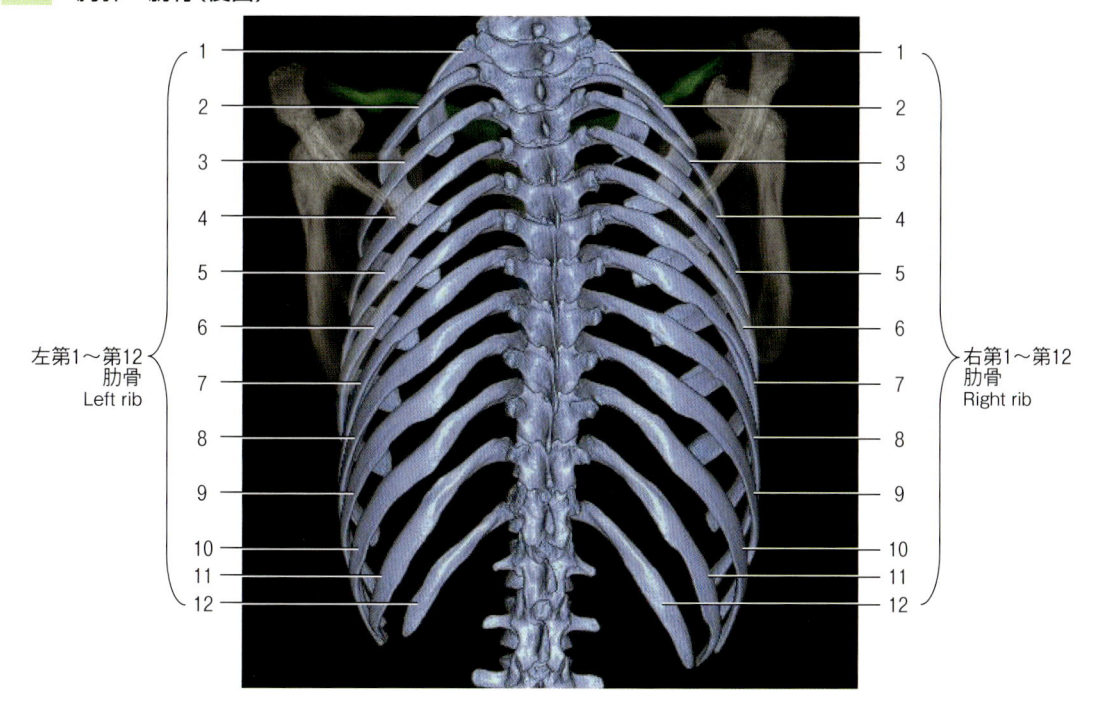

- 左第1～第12肋骨 Left rib
- 右第1～第12肋骨 Right rib

> **NOTE**　肋骨は扁平長骨で，左右12対あり，後方で胸椎と連結して胸郭を構成する．椎体の両側に肋骨窩があり，上肋骨窩と下肋骨窩が肋骨頭と関節を形成する．第1～第7肋骨は直接肋軟骨を介して胸骨につく（真肋）．第8～第10肋骨は，肋軟骨が上位の肋軟骨と結合して肋骨弓を形成する（仮肋）．第11，第12肋骨は自由端で終わる（浮肋）．

胸　郭（CT, VR 像）

4-5　鎖骨・胸骨・肩甲骨（前面）

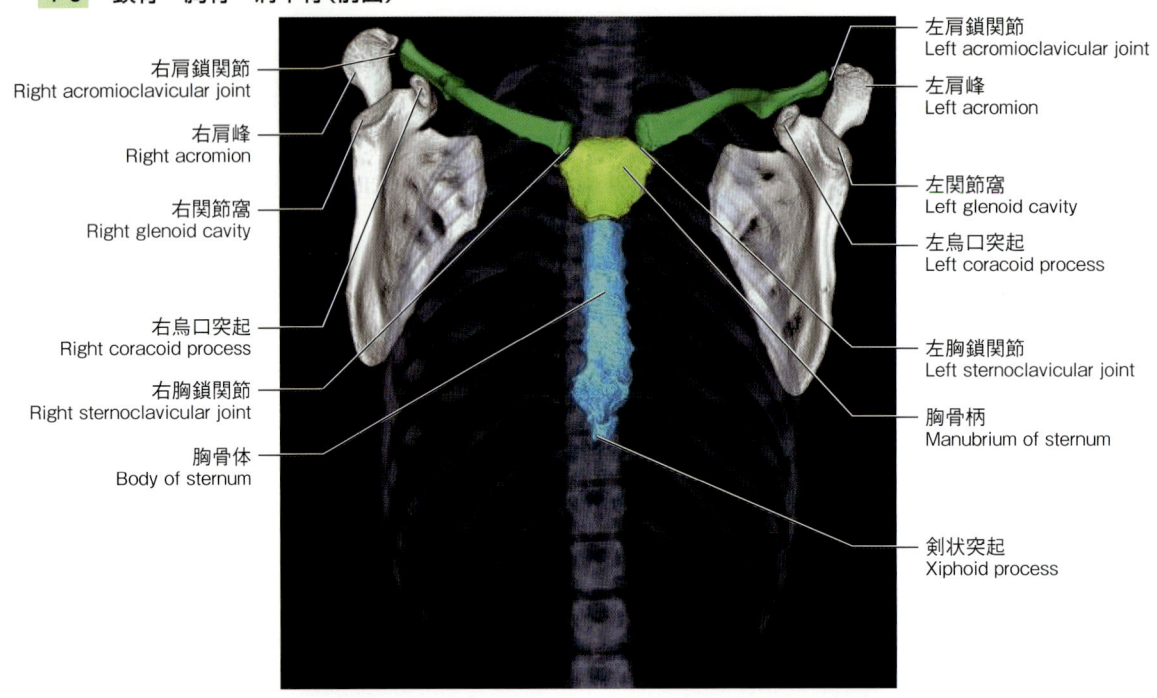

- 右肩鎖関節　Right acromioclavicular joint
- 右肩峰　Right acromion
- 右関節窩　Right glenoid cavity
- 右烏口突起　Right coracoid process
- 右胸鎖関節　Right sternoclavicular joint
- 胸骨体　Body of sternum
- 左肩鎖関節　Left acromioclavicular joint
- 左肩峰　Left acromion
- 左関節窩　Left glenoid cavity
- 左烏口突起　Left coracoid process
- 左胸鎖関節　Left sternoclavicular joint
- 胸骨柄　Manubrium of sternum
- 剣状突起　Xiphoid process

4-6　鎖骨・胸骨・肩甲骨（後面）

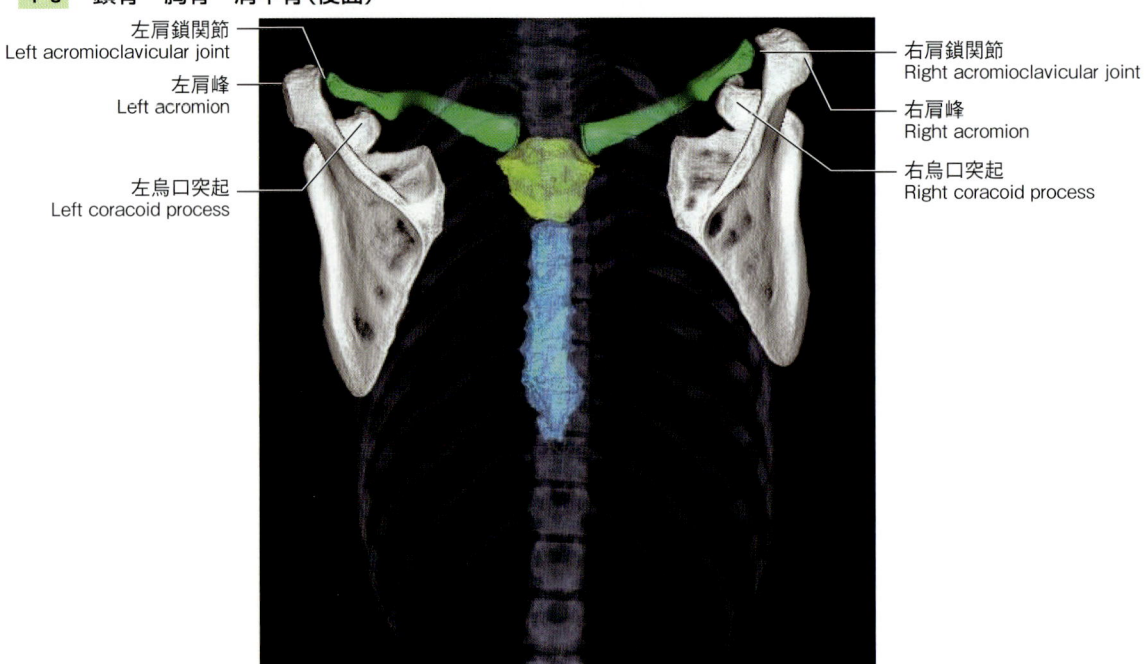

- 左肩鎖関節　Left acromioclavicular joint
- 左肩峰　Left acromion
- 左烏口突起　Left coracoid process
- 右肩鎖関節　Right acromioclavicular joint
- 右肩峰　Right acromion
- 右烏口突起　Right coracoid process

NOTE　胸鎖関節は，胸骨の鎖骨切痕と鎖骨の胸骨端との間の関節で，線維軟骨性の関節円板が介在している．一方，肩鎖関節は肩峰関節面と鎖骨肩峰端との間の関節で，しばしば関節円板があるが，不完全なことが多い．胸鎖関節と共同して働き，肩甲骨が肩関節の運動に伴って動くことを可能にしている．

胸　郭（CT, VR 像）

4-7　鎖骨・胸骨・肩甲骨（右側面）

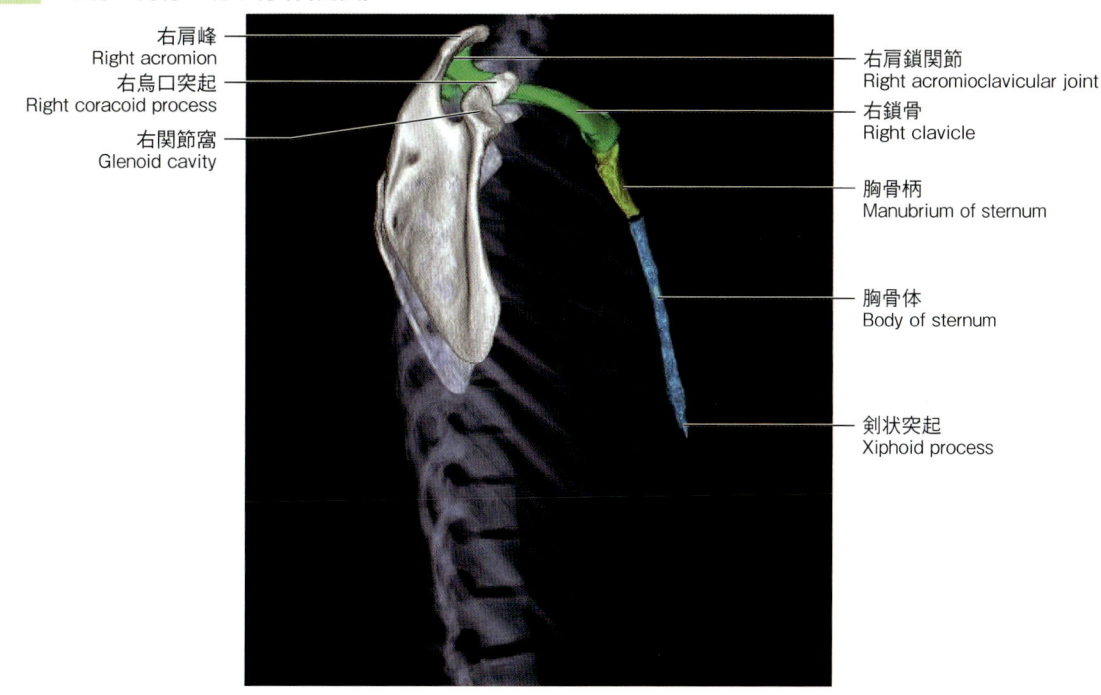

- 右肩峰　Right acromion
- 右烏口突起　Right coracoid process
- 右関節窩　Glenoid cavity
- 右肩鎖関節　Right acromioclavicular joint
- 右鎖骨　Right clavicle
- 胸骨柄　Manubrium of sternum
- 胸骨体　Body of sternum
- 剣状突起　Xiphoid process

4-8　鎖骨・胸骨・肩甲骨（左側面）

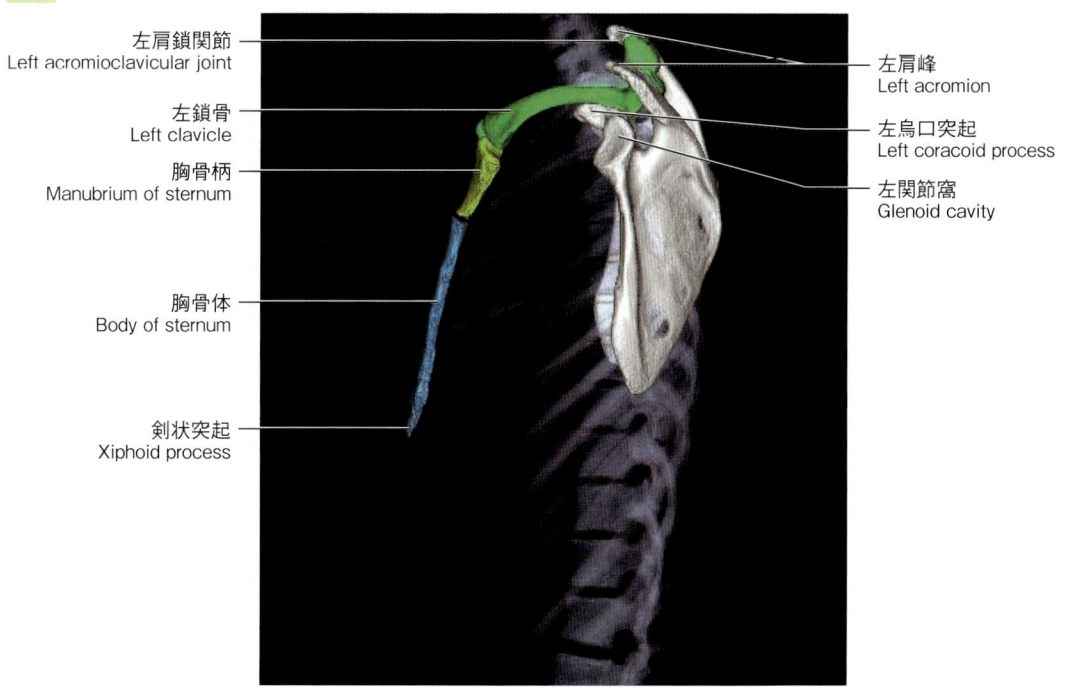

- 左肩鎖関節　Left acromioclavicular joint
- 左鎖骨　Left clavicle
- 胸骨柄　Manubrium of sternum
- 胸骨体　Body of sternum
- 剣状突起　Xiphoid process
- 左肩峰　Left acromion
- 左烏口突起　Left coracoid process
- 左関節窩　Glenoid cavity

NOTE　胸骨は，胸骨柄，胸骨体，および剣状突起からなる．胸骨柄と胸骨体の軟骨結合部（胸骨柄結合部）は，前方にやや突出し胸骨角をなす．

胸　郭（CT，VR像）

4-9　右肩甲骨（前面）

- 肩峰 Acromion
- 烏口突起 Coracoid process
- 関節窩 Glenoid cavity
- 外側縁 Lateral border
- 内側縁 Medial border

4-10　右肩甲骨（側面）

- 烏口突起 Coracoid process
- 肩峰 Acromion
- 関節窩 Glenoid cavity
- 外側縁 Lateral border

4-11　右肩甲骨（後面）

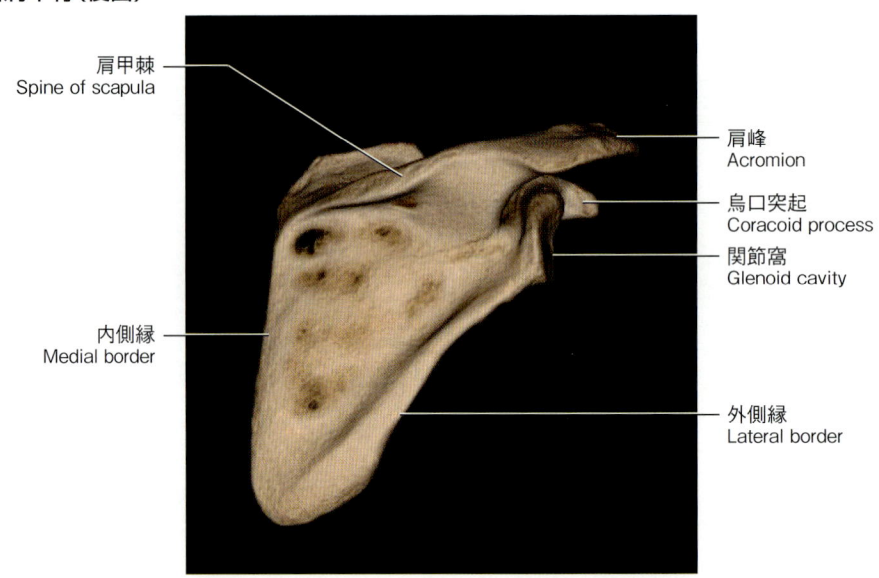

- 肩甲棘 Spine of scapula
- 肩峰 Acromion
- 烏口突起 Coracoid process
- 関節窩 Glenoid cavity
- 内側縁 Medial border
- 外側縁 Lateral border

> **NOTE** 肩甲骨は，胸郭の後方上外側に存在する扁平骨である．外側角の部分は上縁と外側縁の合するところで肥厚しており，その外側端に楕円形の関節窩がある．肋骨面は全体に浅く凹んでおり肩甲下窩という．後面の上部には肩甲棘というほぼ水平に走る隆起があり，その尖端は大きく扁平な突起となって関節窩の外方へ突き出していて肩峰となる．また鉤状の烏口突起が前方に突き出している．

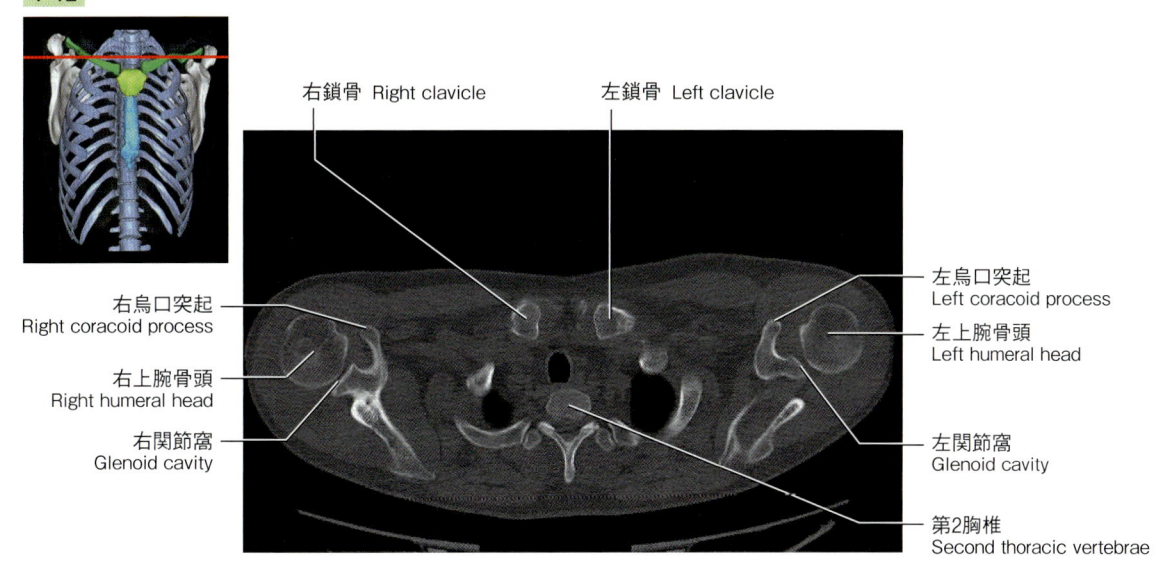

胸郭の断層解剖 ［横断像(CT)］

4-12

- 右鎖骨 Right clavicle
- 左鎖骨 Left clavicle
- 右烏口突起 Right coracoid process
- 右上腕骨頭 Right humeral head
- 右関節窩 Glenoid cavity
- 左烏口突起 Left coracoid process
- 左上腕骨頭 Left humeral head
- 左関節窩 Glenoid cavity
- 第2胸椎 Second thoracic vertebrae

4-13

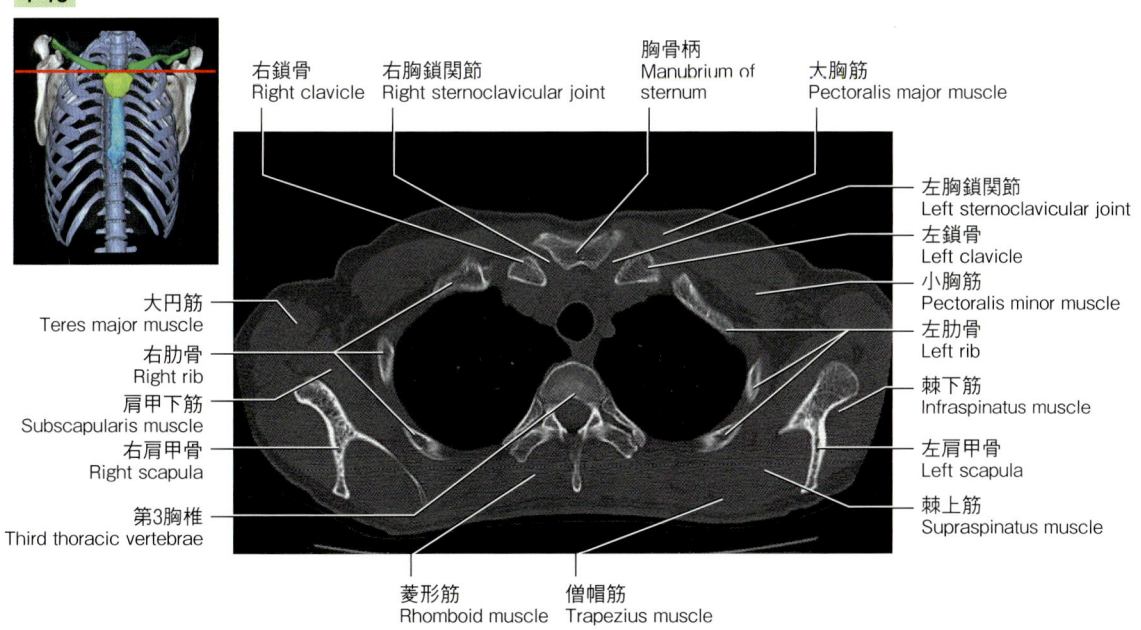

- 右鎖骨 Right clavicle
- 右胸鎖関節 Right sternoclavicular joint
- 胸骨柄 Manubrium of sternum
- 大胸筋 Pectoralis major muscle
- 左胸鎖関節 Left sternoclavicular joint
- 左鎖骨 Left clavicle
- 小胸筋 Pectoralis minor muscle
- 大円筋 Teres major muscle
- 右肋骨 Right rib
- 肩甲下筋 Subscapularis muscle
- 右肩甲骨 Right scapula
- 第3胸椎 Third thoracic vertebrae
- 左肋骨 Left rib
- 棘下筋 Infraspinatus muscle
- 左肩甲骨 Left scapula
- 棘上筋 Supraspinatus muscle
- 菱形筋 Rhomboid muscle
- 僧帽筋 Trapezius muscle

> **NOTE** 胸郭上口は，胸腔と頸部および上肢の間の出入り口であり，第1胸椎椎体，左右の第1肋骨とその肋軟骨，胸骨柄上縁により囲まれている．一方，胸郭下口は第12胸椎，第12肋骨，および軟骨性肋骨弓により囲まれている．

胸郭の断層解剖 ［横断像（CT）］

4-14

- 右肋骨 Right rib
- 胸骨体 Body of sternum
- 右肋骨 Right rib
- 左肋骨 Left rib
- 右肩甲骨 Right scapula
- 左肩甲骨 SLeft scapula
- 右肋骨 Right rib
- 第7胸椎 Seventh thoracic vertebrae

4-15

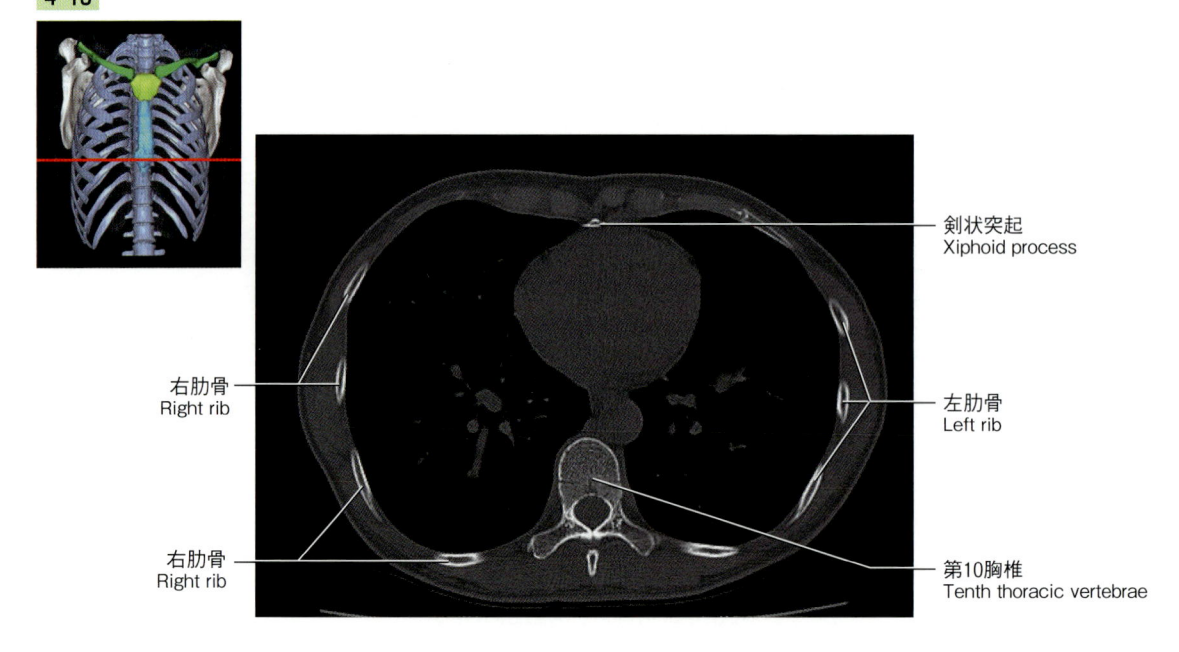

- 剣状突起 Xiphoid process
- 右肋骨 Right rib
- 左肋骨 Left rib
- 右肋骨 Right rib
- 第10胸椎 Tenth thoracic vertebrae

> **NOTE** 胸郭変形のうち最も頻度が高いものが漏斗胸であり，胸骨とそれに接合する肋軟骨の陥凹偏位を呈する．一方，鳩胸は胸骨の突出偏位である．両者ともに肋軟骨の過剰成長が一般的な原因と考えられている．

胸郭の断層解剖 ［冠状断像（CT）］

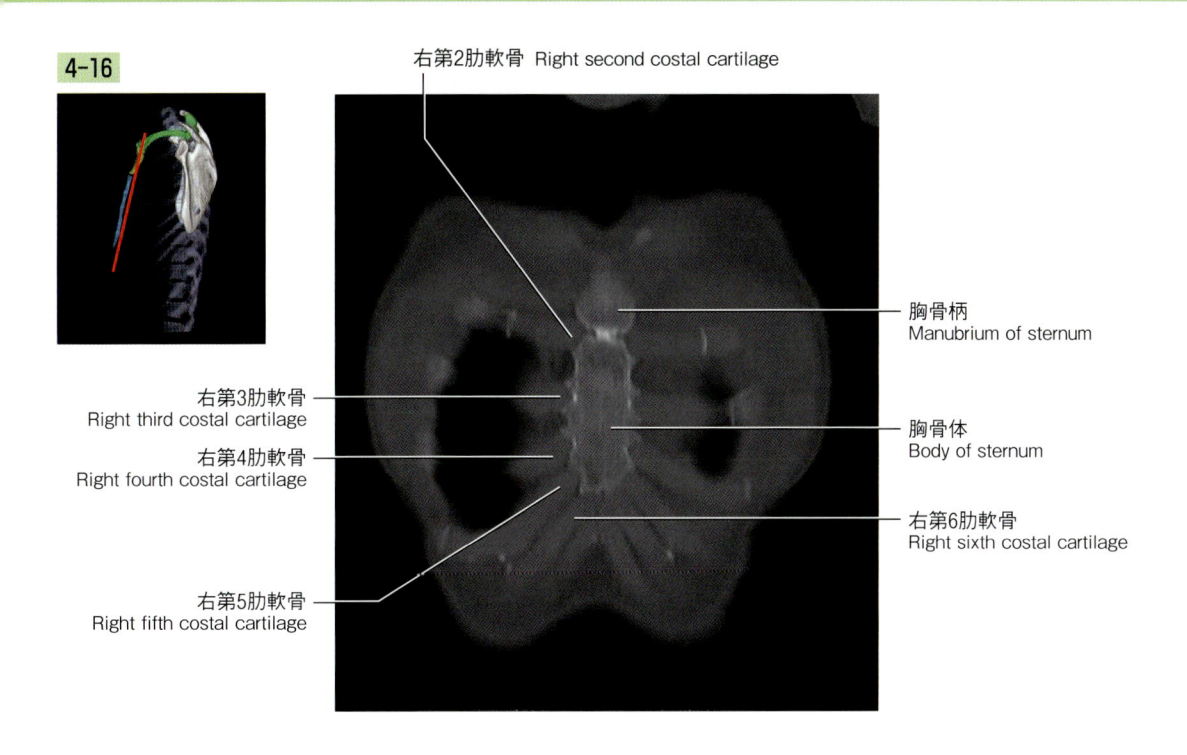

4-16

右第2肋軟骨 Right second costal cartilage

胸骨柄
Manubrium of sternum

右第3肋軟骨
Right third costal cartilage

右第4肋軟骨
Right fourth costal cartilage

胸骨体
Body of sternum

右第6肋軟骨
Right sixth costal cartilage

右第5肋軟骨
Right fifth costal cartilage

NOTE 胸骨柄と胸骨体（胸骨柄結合）および胸骨体と剣状突起（胸骨剣結合）の軟骨結合部は，加齢とともに骨化する．胸骨柄結合には第2肋軟骨がつき，肋骨を体表から数えるときの重要な指標となる．胸骨体には第3〜第6肋軟骨が結合する．

胸郭の断層解剖 ［冠状断像（CT）］

4-17

- 左鎖骨 Left clavicle
- 左胸鎖関節 Left sternoclavicular joint
- 右鎖骨 Right clavicle
- 右胸鎖関節 Right sternoclavicular joint

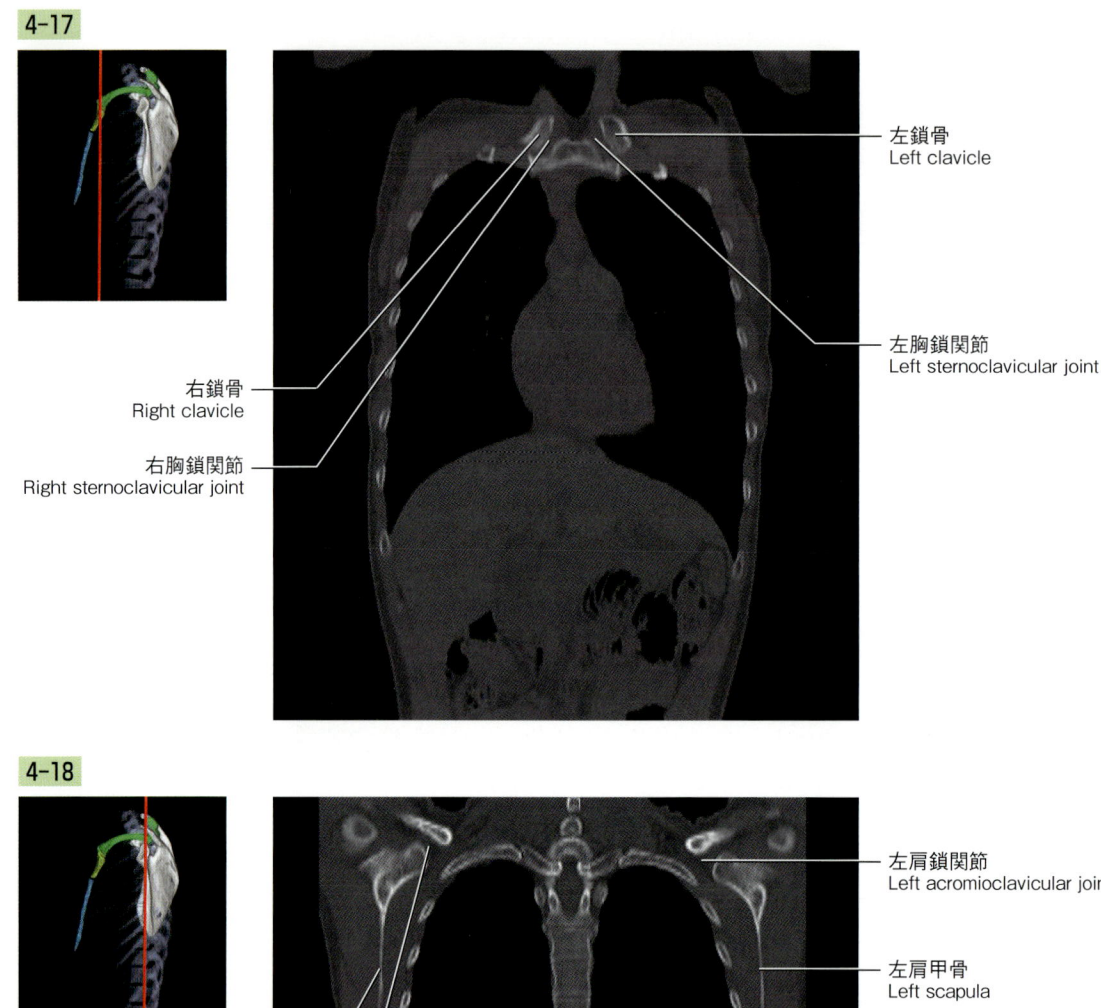

4-18

- 左肩鎖関節 Left acromioclavicular joint
- 左肩甲骨 Left scapula
- 胸椎椎体 Vertebral body
- 右肩甲骨 Right scapula
- 右肩鎖関節 Right acromioclavicular joint

> **NOTE** 胸椎の椎体は下位にいくほど大きい．高齢者では，椎体辺縁に変形性脊椎症による骨棘を認めることが多いが，この変化は下位胸椎右側にみられる傾向にある．胸部下行大動脈の拍動により，椎体左側の骨棘形成が抑制されるためと考えられている．

胸郭の断層解剖 ［矢状断像(CT)］

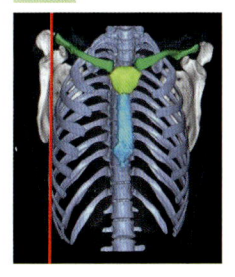

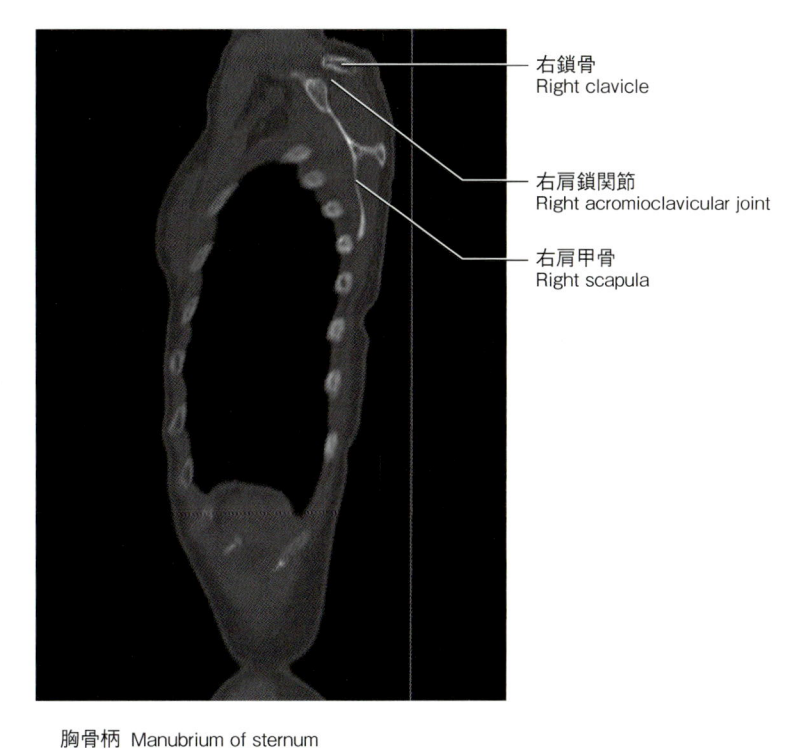

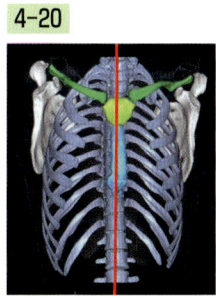

4-19

- 右鎖骨 Right clavicle
- 右肩鎖関節 Right acromioclavicular joint
- 右肩甲骨 Right scapula

4-20

- 胸骨柄 Manubrium of sternum
- 胸骨体 Body of sternum
- 剣状突起 Xiphoid process
- 胸椎椎体 Vertebral body
- 胸椎棘突起 Spinous process

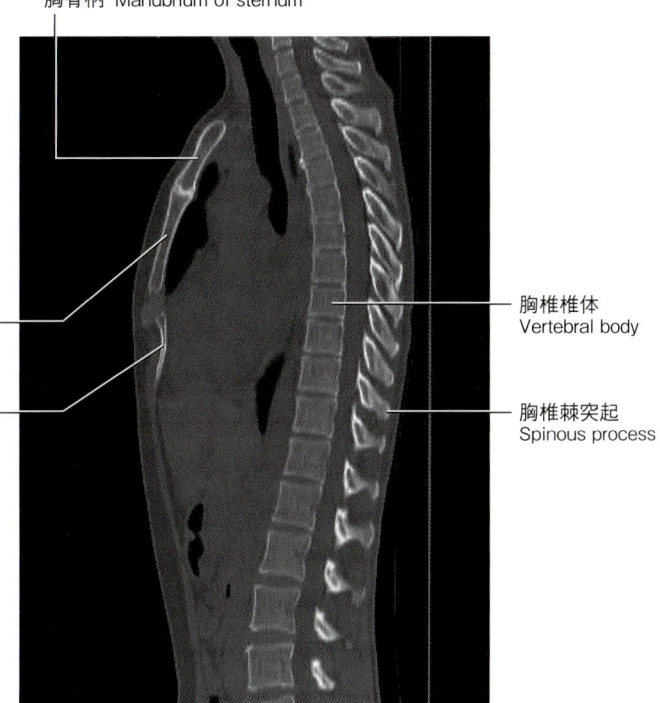

> **NOTE** 胸椎は生理的弯曲として後弯を呈しており，加齢によりこの後弯が強くなる傾向にある．棘突起は下方に傾斜しており，第8胸椎までは傾斜が強くなるが，その後は次第に傾斜が弱まり，第12胸椎ではほとんど水平となる．

肺（CT, VR像）

4-21 肺区域（前面）

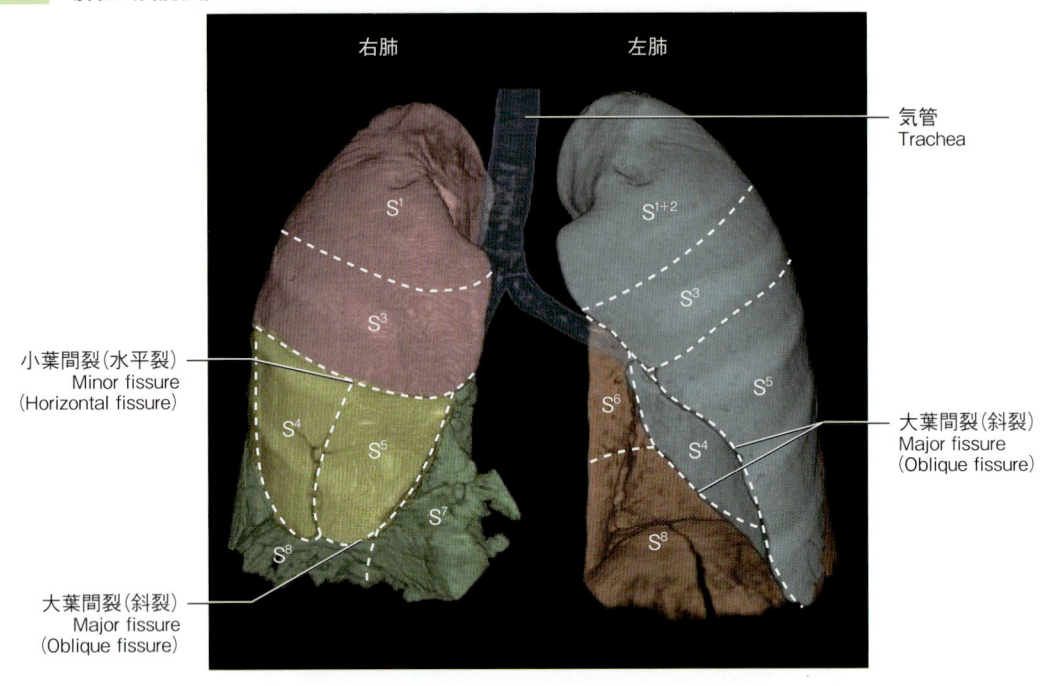

4-22 肺区域（後面）

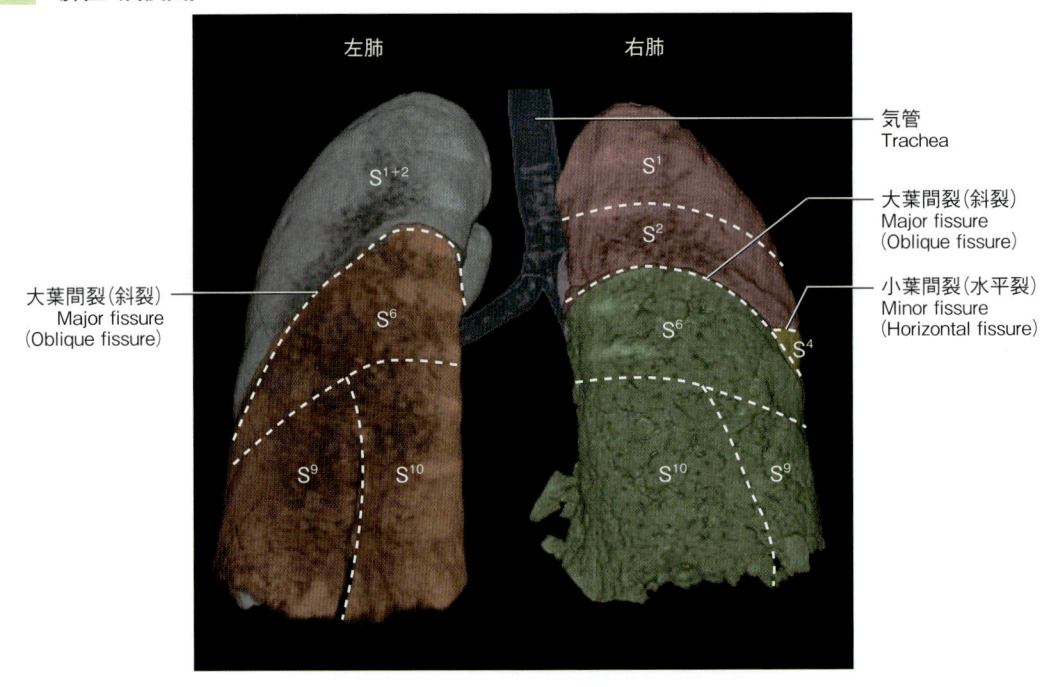

NOTE 右肺は上葉，中葉，下葉の3葉からなり，おのおのは小葉間裂（水平裂），大葉間裂（斜裂）によって区切られる．また左肺は上葉，下葉の2葉からなり，大葉間裂（斜裂）によって区切られる．左肺は右肺よりも小さい．左右肺の前縁では，心臓の縁に沿って削られるようになっており，特に左肺前縁では顕著で心切痕とよばれる．

肺（CT, VR像）

4-23　肺区域（内側面）

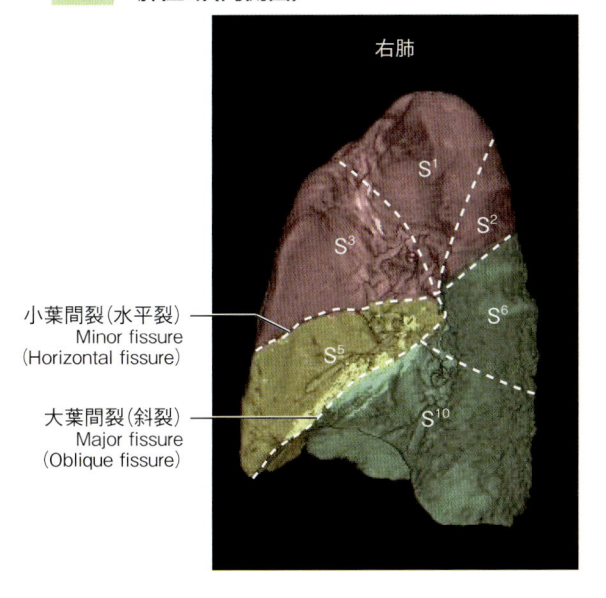

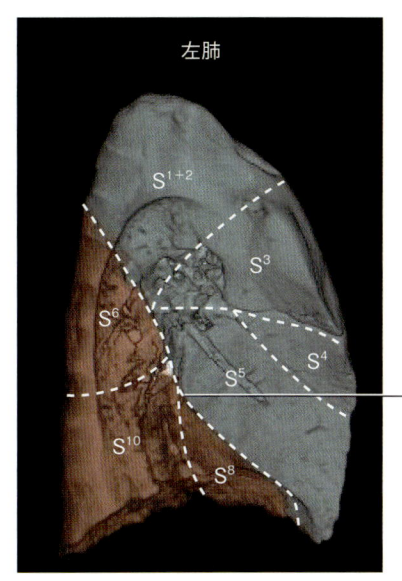

右肺 / 左肺

小葉間裂（水平裂）
Minor fissure
(Horizontal fissure)

大葉間裂（斜裂）
Major fissure
(Oblique fissure)

大葉間裂（斜裂）
Major fissure
(Oblique fissure)

4-24　肺区域（外側面）

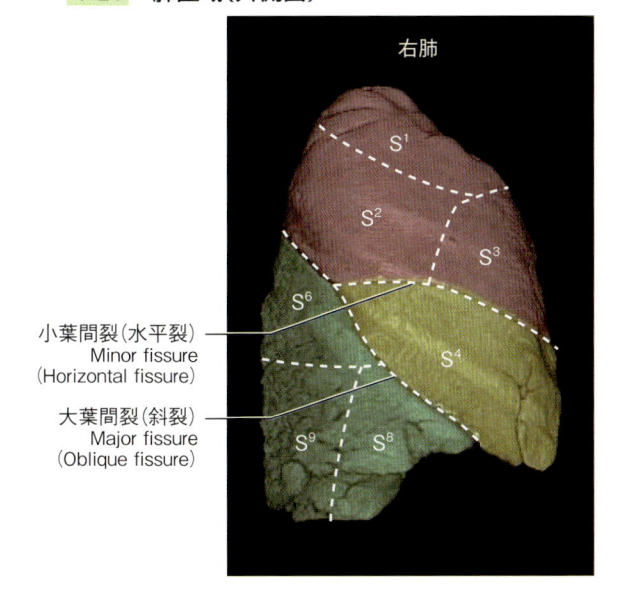

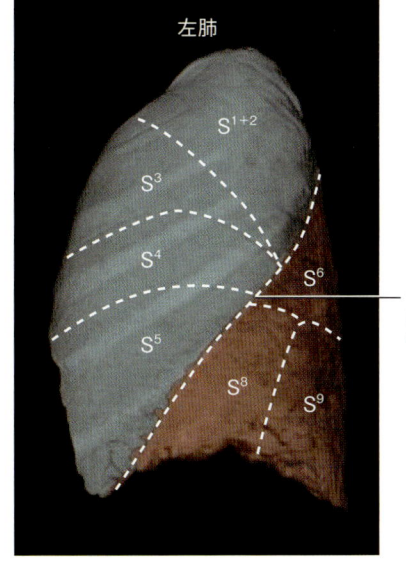

右肺 / 左肺

小葉間裂（水平裂）
Minor fissure
(Horizontal fissure)

大葉間裂（斜裂）
Major fissure
(Oblique fissure)

大葉間裂（斜裂）
Major fissure
(Oblique fissure)

> **NOTE**　肺の表面は主に3つに分けられる．縦隔面（内側面）は，心膜と心臓を含む縦隔の中部と接しているため陥凹している．縦隔面には肺門があり，気管支，血管（肺動脈，肺静脈，気管支動脈，気管支静脈）が出入りする．外側面は弧を描くように突出し，肋骨と接するため，肋骨面ともよばれる．横隔面は凹面を呈しており，横隔膜の天井部に乗るように肺の底部をなす．

気管・血管（CT, VR 像）

4-25　胸部の血管（前面）

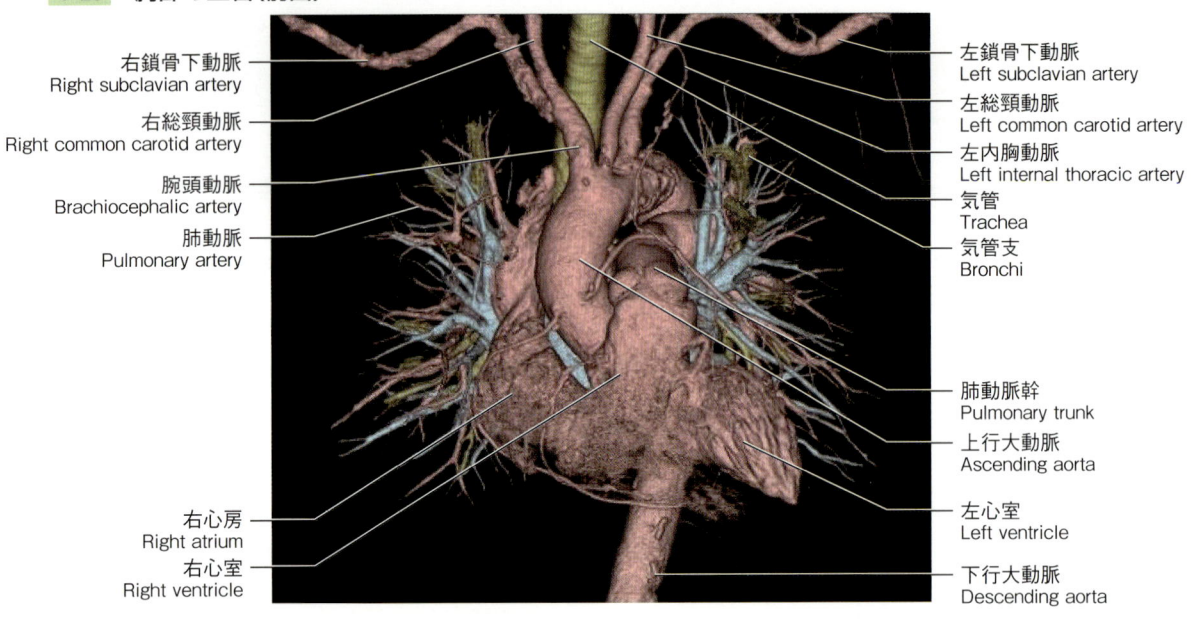

- 右鎖骨下動脈　Right subclavian artery
- 右総頸動脈　Right common carotid artery
- 腕頭動脈　Brachiocephalic artery
- 肺動脈　Pulmonary artery
- 左鎖骨下動脈　Left subclavian artery
- 左総頸動脈　Left common carotid artery
- 左内胸動脈　Left internal thoracic artery
- 気管　Trachea
- 気管支　Bronchi
- 肺動脈幹　Pulmonary trunk
- 上行大動脈　Ascending aorta
- 右心房　Right atrium
- 右心室　Right ventricle
- 左心室　Left ventricle
- 下行大動脈　Descending aorta

4-26　胸部の血管（後面）

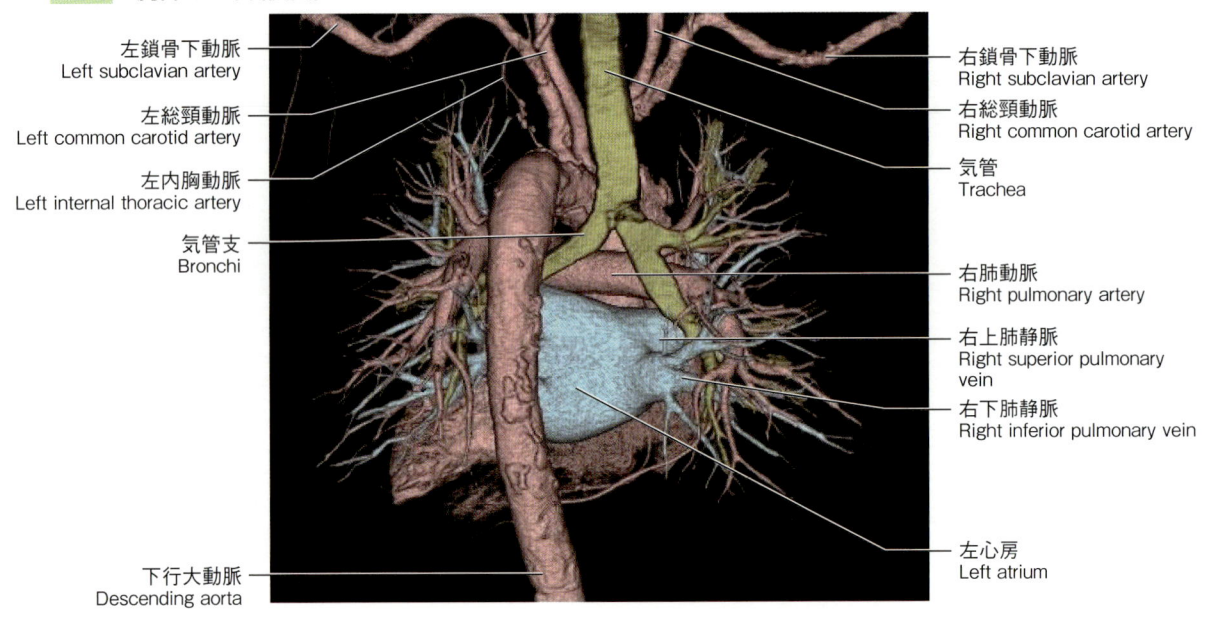

- 左鎖骨下動脈　Left subclavian artery
- 左総頸動脈　Left common carotid artery
- 左内胸動脈　Left internal thoracic artery
- 気管支　Bronchi
- 右鎖骨下動脈　Right subclavian artery
- 右総頸動脈　Right common carotid artery
- 気管　Trachea
- 右肺動脈　Right pulmonary artery
- 右上肺静脈　Right superior pulmonary vein
- 右下肺静脈　Right inferior pulmonary vein
- 左心房　Left atrium
- 下行大動脈　Descending aorta

> **NOTE**　肺動脈は右心室から起始し，比較的太く短い肺動脈幹を経たのち，左右の肺動脈に分かれ，それぞれ左右の肺に静脈血を運ぶ．肺内では肺動脈は気管支と伴走する．一方，肺静脈は一般的に肺動脈より太く，肺動脈との間を直線状に走行する．肺静脈は通常は最終的に左右2本ずつとなり，心臓の後面寄りにある左心房に流入する．

気管・血管（CT, VR 像）

4-27 区域気管支

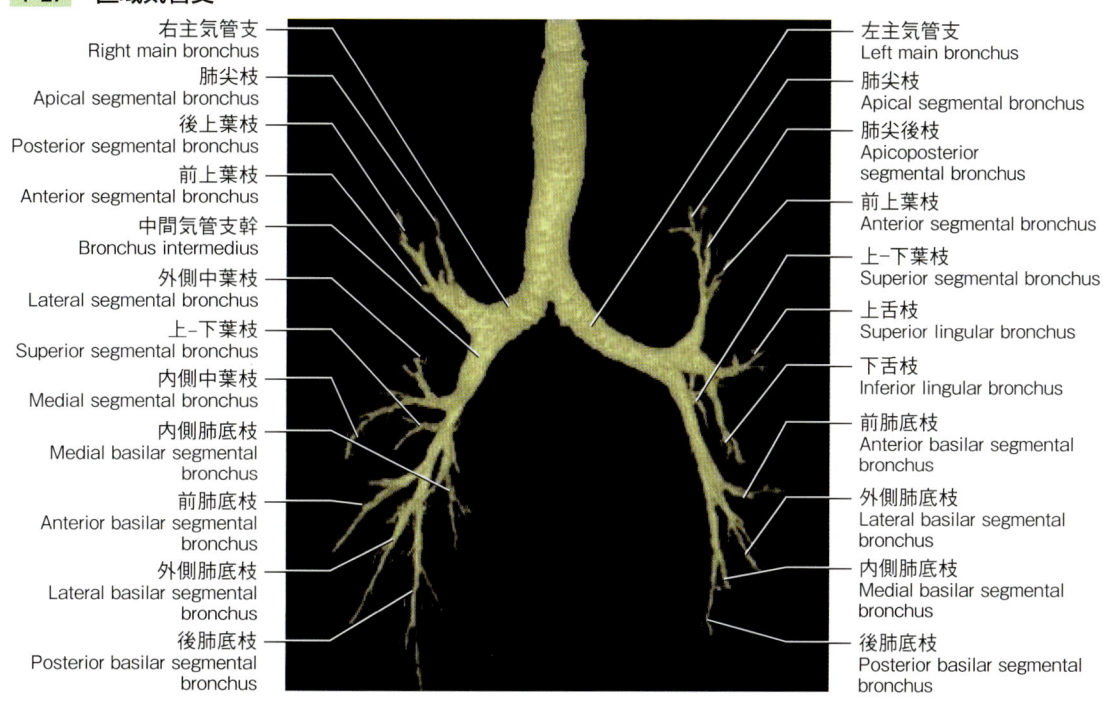

- 右主気管支 Right main bronchus
- 肺尖枝 Apical segmental bronchus
- 後上葉枝 Posterior segmental bronchus
- 前上葉枝 Anterior segmental bronchus
- 中間気管支幹 Bronchus intermedius
- 外側中葉枝 Lateral segmental bronchus
- 上-下葉枝 Superior segmental bronchus
- 内側中葉枝 Medial segmental bronchus
- 内側肺底枝 Medial basilar segmental bronchus
- 前肺底枝 Anterior basilar segmental bronchus
- 外側肺底枝 Lateral basilar segmental bronchus
- 後肺底枝 Posterior basilar segmental bronchus

- 左主気管支 Left main bronchus
- 肺尖枝 Apical segmental bronchus
- 肺尖後枝 Apicoposterior segmental bronchus
- 前上葉枝 Anterior segmental bronchus
- 上-下葉枝 Superior segmental bronchus
- 上舌枝 Superior lingular bronchus
- 下舌枝 Inferior lingular bronchus
- 前肺底枝 Anterior basilar segmental bronchus
- 外側肺底枝 Lateral basilar segmental bronchus
- 内側肺底枝 Medial basilar segmental bronchus
- 後肺底枝 Posterior basilar segmental bronchus

4-28 気管支と肺動静脈の関係

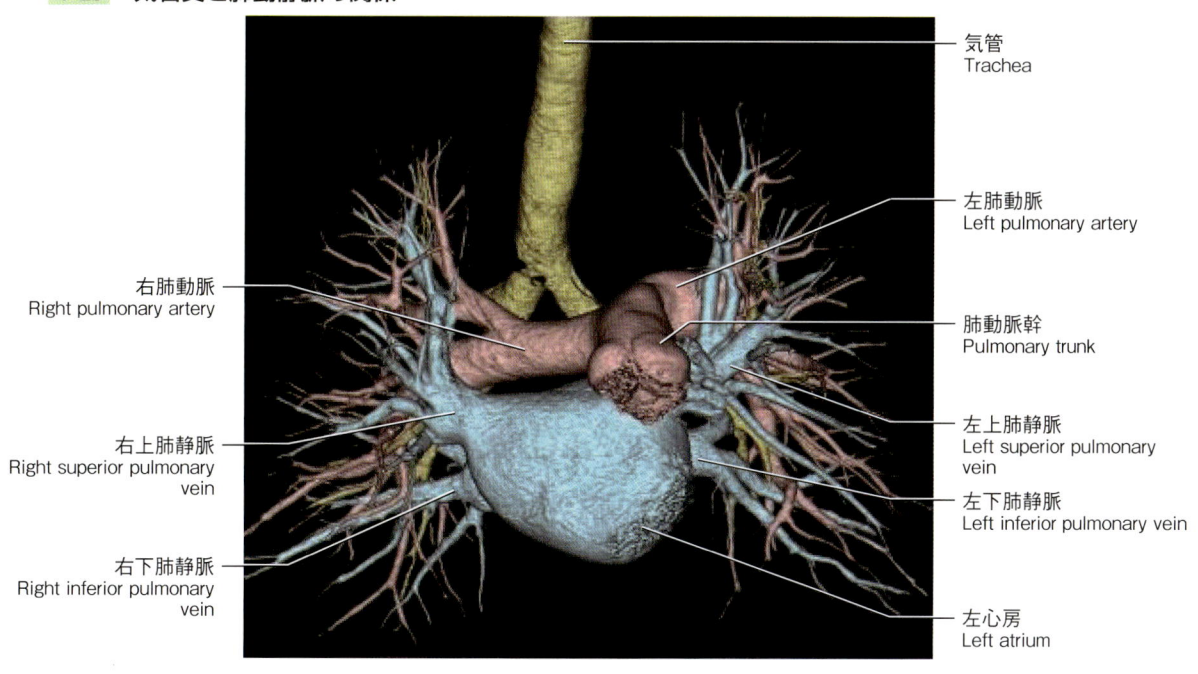

- 気管 Trachea
- 右肺動脈 Right pulmonary artery
- 右上肺静脈 Right superior pulmonary vein
- 右下肺静脈 Right inferior pulmonary vein
- 左肺動脈 Left pulmonary artery
- 肺動脈幹 Pulmonary trunk
- 左上肺静脈 Left superior pulmonary vein
- 左下肺静脈 Left inferior pulmonary vein
- 左心房 Left atrium

> **NOTE** 気管は胸骨角の高さで二分し主気管支となり，肺門部から左右の肺に入る．右主気管支のほうが左主気管支と比べ，幅広く短い．また垂直方向に走行するため，気管支異物は左側より右側に生じる頻度が高いとされる．それぞれの主気管支は右で3つ，左で2つの葉気管支に分かれ，肺葉に対応して分布する．さらに，それぞれの葉気管支はいくつかの区域気管支に分かれ，肺区域に対応して分布する．

気管・血管（CT, VR像）

4-29　気管支と肺動静脈の関係

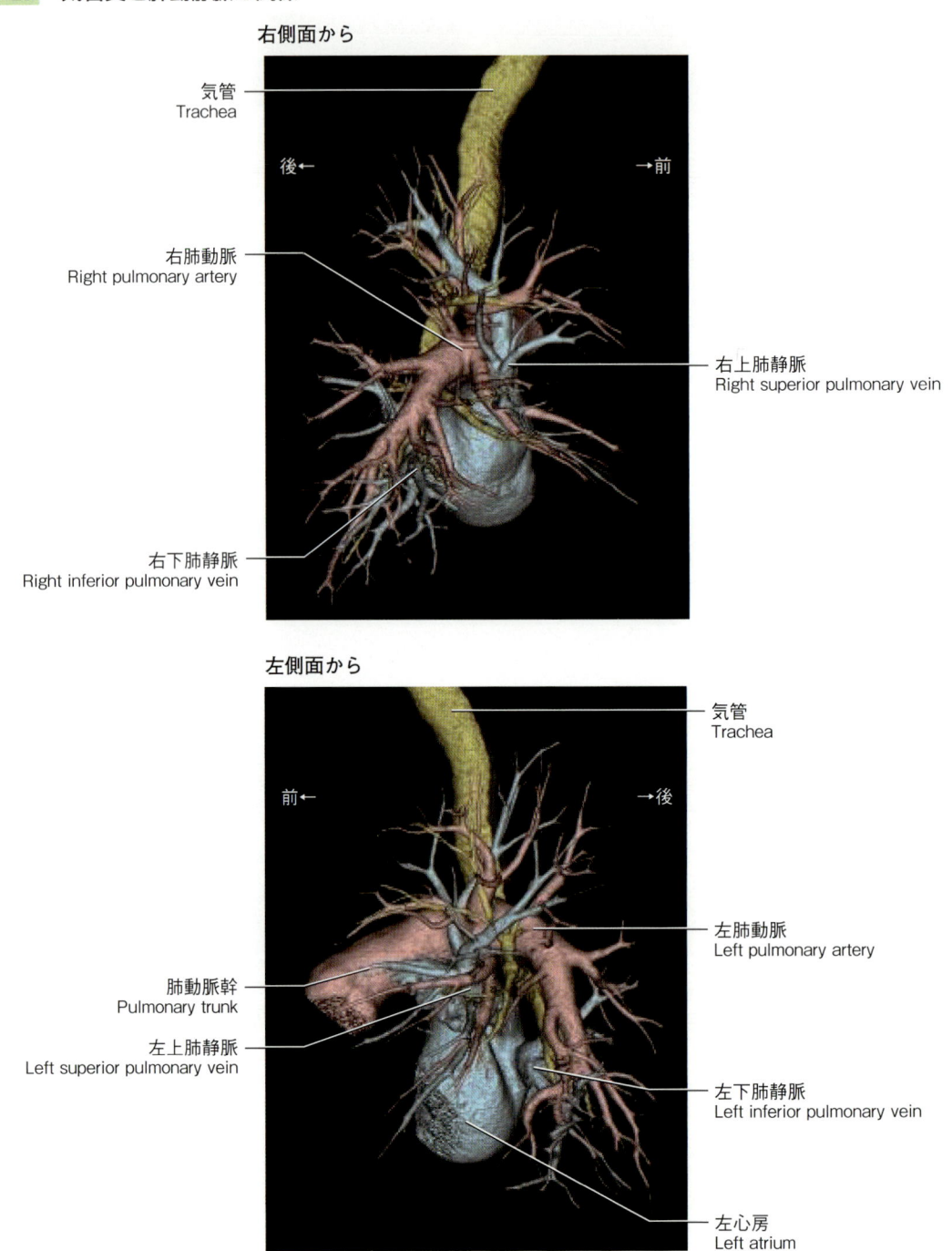

右側面から

- 気管 Trachea
- 後← →前
- 右肺動脈 Right pulmonary artery
- 右上肺静脈 Right superior pulmonary vein
- 右下肺静脈 Right inferior pulmonary vein

左側面から

- 気管 Trachea
- 前← →後
- 肺動脈幹 Pulmonary trunk
- 左上肺静脈 Left superior pulmonary vein
- 左肺動脈 Left pulmonary artery
- 左下肺静脈 Left inferior pulmonary vein
- 左心房 Left atrium

> **NOTE**　右肺動脈は気管分岐部の前下方から上幹動脈を出し，中間気管支幹の前方から外側へと回りながらこれに沿って下降し（中間肺動脈幹），中葉および下葉の各区域支の動脈に分かれる．一方，左肺動脈は後上方へ走行し，左主気管支を乗り越え下葉気管支の外側を下降する．胸部単純X線写真で，一般的に左肺門影が右側より高くみられるのは，この肺動脈の走行による．

縦隔の断層解剖 ［横断像（造影CT，縦隔条件）］

4-30

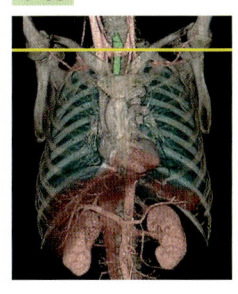

- 気管 Trachea
- 甲状腺 Thyroid gland
- 左内頸静脈 Left internal jugular vein
- 食道 Esophagus
- 右総頸動脈 Right common carotid artery

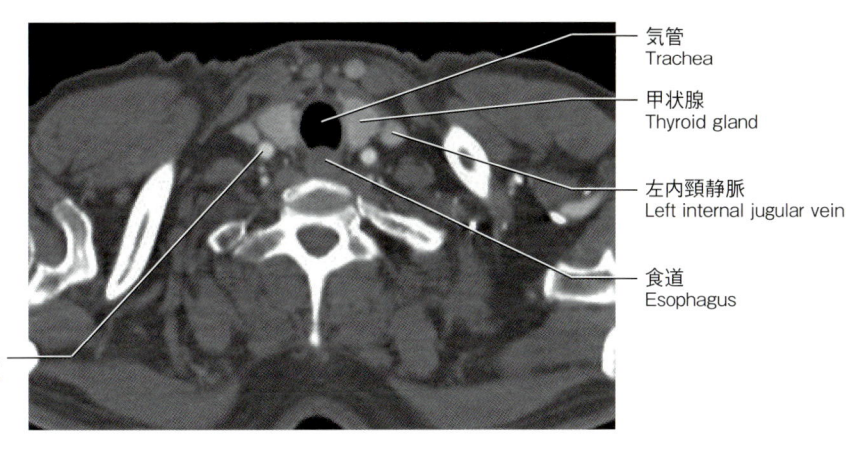

4-31

- 右腕頭静脈 Right brachiocephalic vein
- 気管 Trachea
- 左腕頭静脈 Left brachiocephalic vein
- 左総頸動脈 Left common carotid artery
- 左鎖骨下動脈 Left subclavian artery
- 食道 Esophagus
- 右総頸動脈 Right common carotid artery
- 右鎖骨下動脈 Right subclavian artery

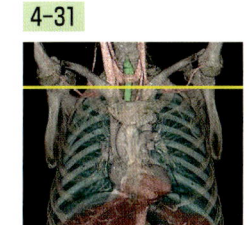

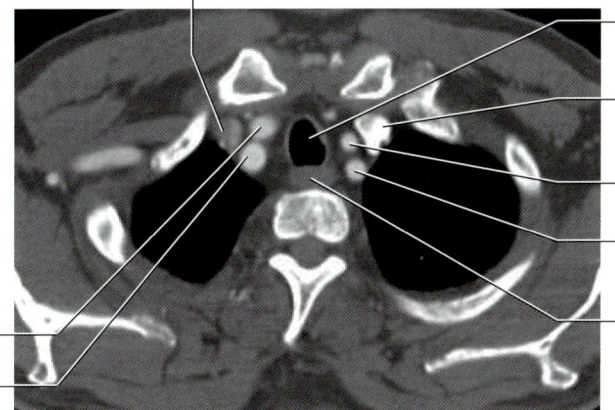

4-32

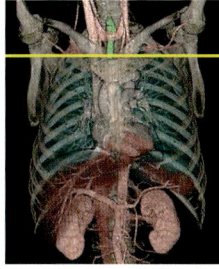

- 左腕頭静脈 Left brachiocephalic vein
- 左総頸動脈 Left common carotid artery
- 左鎖骨下動脈 Left subclavian artery
- 食道 Esophagus
- 右腕頭静脈 Right brachiocephalic vein
- 腕頭動脈 Brachiocephalic artery
- 気管 Trachea

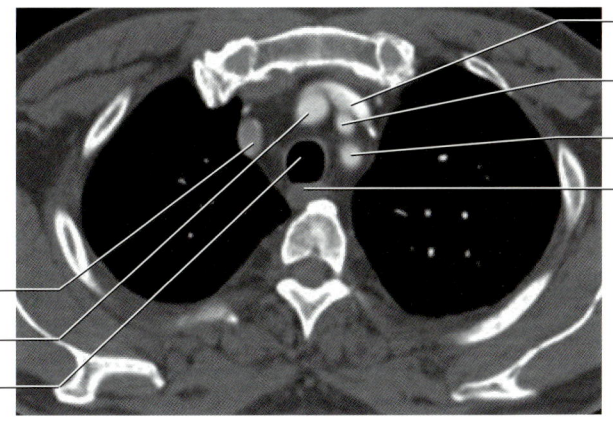

> **NOTE** 大動脈弓から分枝した腕頭動脈，左総頸動脈，および左鎖骨下動脈が，気管の前方から左側方を取り囲むように認められる（4-32）．腕頭動脈はさらに右総頸動脈と右鎖骨下動脈に分かれる（4-31）．前方には左右の腕頭静脈が存在する．左腕頭静脈は右よりも長く，左総頸動脈と腕頭動脈の前を横切り（4-32），その後に右腕頭静脈と合流し上大静脈となる（4-33）．

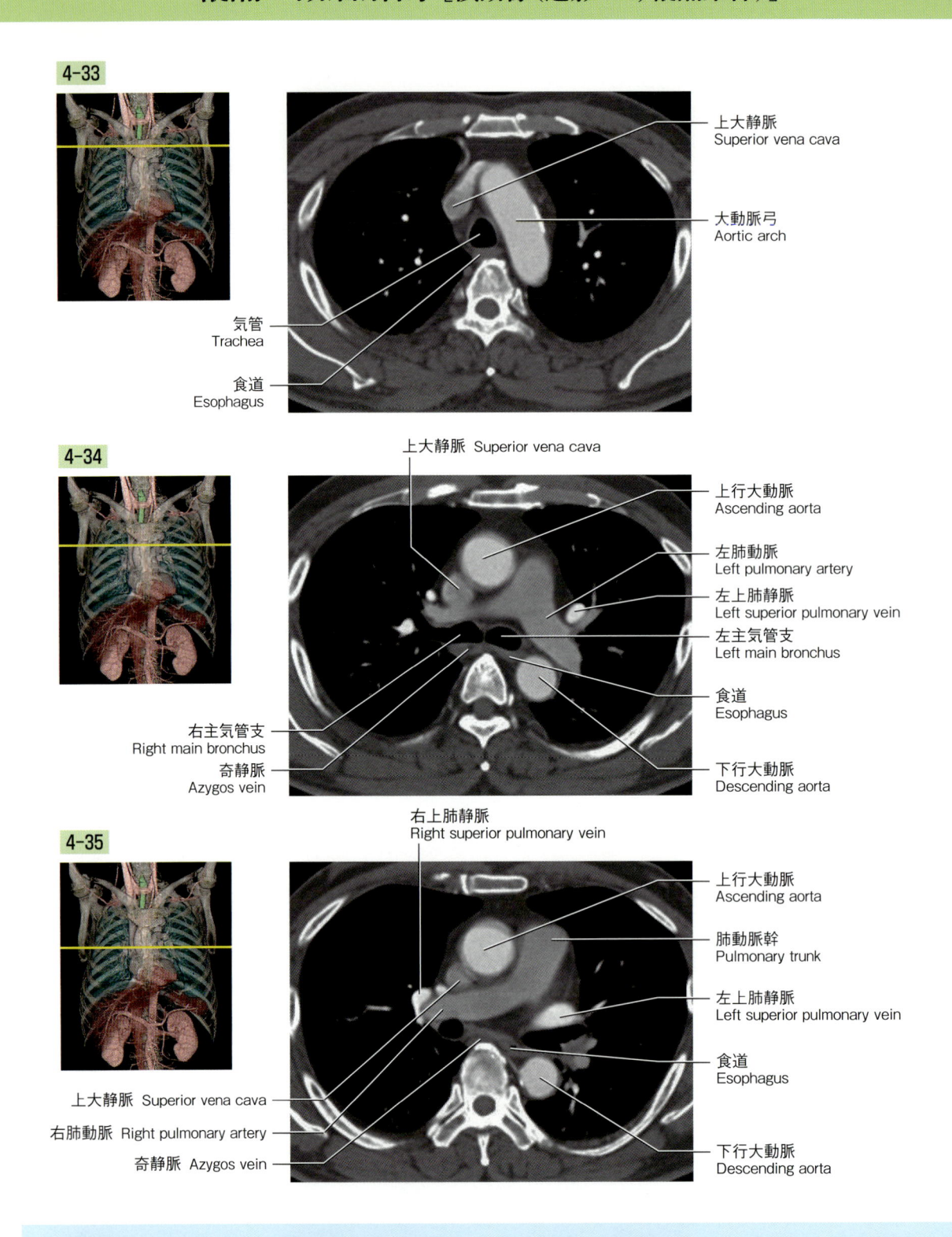

縦隔の断層解剖 ［横断像（造影CT，縦隔条件）］

4-33

- 上大静脈 Superior vena cava
- 大動脈弓 Aortic arch
- 気管 Trachea
- 食道 Esophagus

4-34

- 上大静脈 Superior vena cava
- 上行大動脈 Ascending aorta
- 左肺動脈 Left pulmonary artery
- 左上肺静脈 Left superior pulmonary vein
- 左主気管支 Left main bronchus
- 食道 Esophagus
- 下行大動脈 Descending aorta
- 右主気管支 Right main bronchus
- 奇静脈 Azygos vein

4-35

- 右上肺静脈 Right superior pulmonary vein
- 上行大動脈 Ascending aorta
- 肺動脈幹 Pulmonary trunk
- 左上肺静脈 Left superior pulmonary vein
- 食道 Esophagus
- 下行大動脈 Descending aorta
- 上大静脈 Superior vena cava
- 右肺動脈 Right pulmonary artery
- 奇静脈 Azygos vein

NOTE 肺動脈幹が右心室の動脈円錐から起始し，左上方へ向かい左右の肺動脈に分かれる(4-34, 35)．右肺動脈は大動脈弓部の下方を走行し，上大静脈の後方に認められる(4-35)．また右肺門部で右上肺静脈の後方に位置する(4-35)．左肺動脈は下行大動脈の前方に存在する(4-34)．奇静脈は，胸椎椎体の前面を上行し(4-34, 35)，奇静脈弓として右気管支の上方を越えて上大静脈に流入する．奇静脈や半奇静脈などの奇静脈系は縦隔や胸腹壁の血流を還流するが，下大静脈に閉塞が生じた場合に，その側副路として機能する．

縦隔の断層解剖　[横断像（造影 CT, 縦隔条件）]

4-36

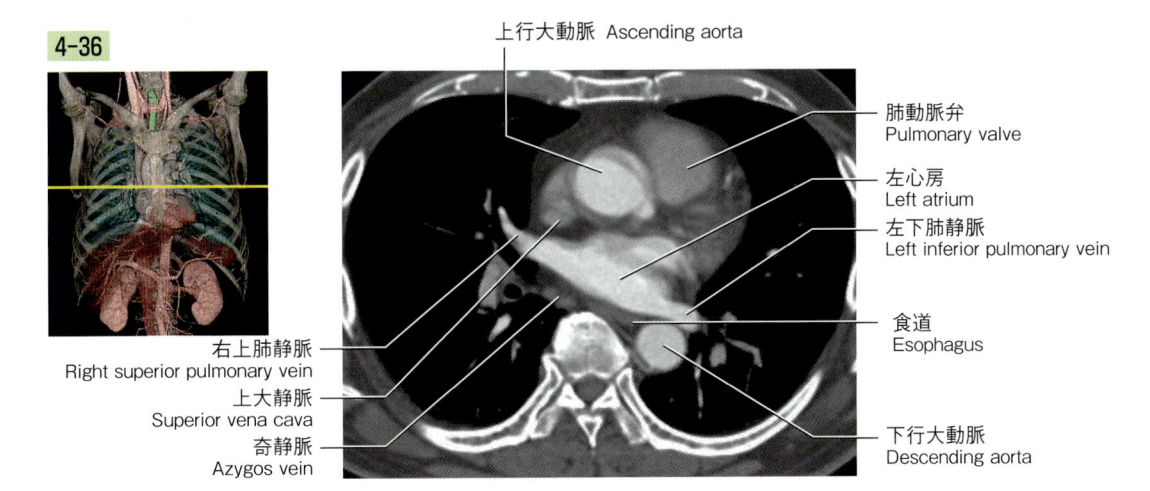

- 上行大動脈　Ascending aorta
- 肺動脈弁　Pulmonary valve
- 左心房　Left atrium
- 左下肺静脈　Left inferior pulmonary vein
- 食道　Esophagus
- 下行大動脈　Descending aorta
- 右上肺静脈　Right superior pulmonary vein
- 上大静脈　Superior vena cava
- 奇静脈　Azygos vein

4-37

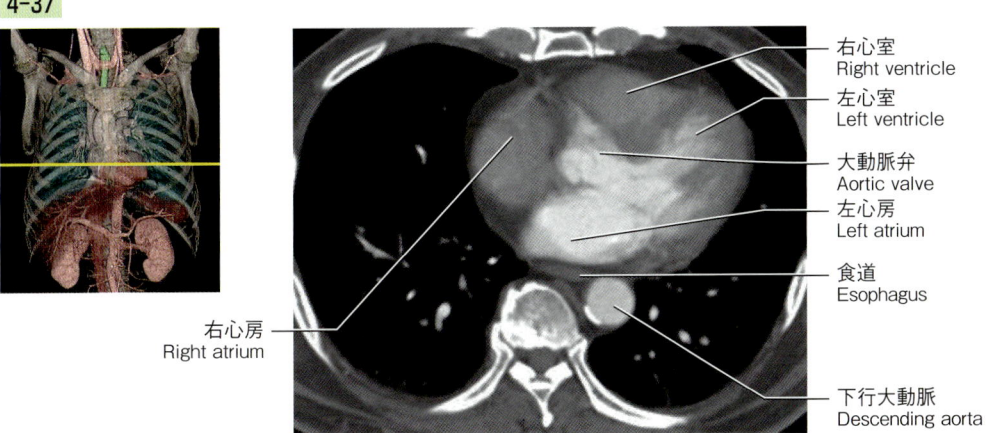

- 右心室　Right ventricle
- 左心室　Left ventricle
- 大動脈弁　Aortic valve
- 左心房　Left atrium
- 食道　Esophagus
- 下行大動脈　Descending aorta
- 右心房　Right atrium

4-38

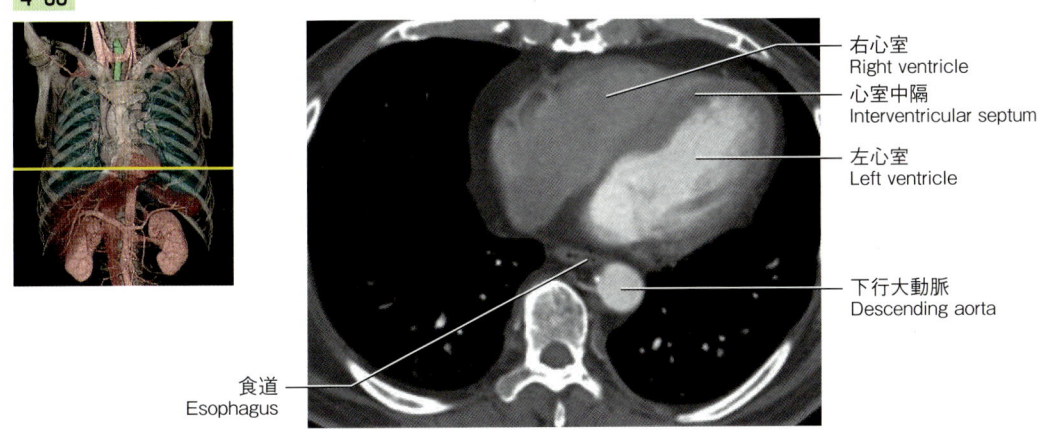

- 右心室　Right ventricle
- 心室中隔　Interventricular septum
- 左心室　Left ventricle
- 下行大動脈　Descending aorta
- 食道　Esophagus

> **NOTE**　上大静脈や下大静脈の血流は右心房に流入し（4-37），三尖弁を介し右心室へ入る．右心室は心臓の前面に位置し，上方で先細りし動脈円錐となって肺動脈幹につながる（4-36, 37）．左心室は心臓の最も左側にあり，心尖部を形成する（4-38）．壁は厚く，右心室との間に心室中隔を認める（4-38）．左心房は心臓の後面に位置し，肺静脈からの血流を受ける（4-36, 37）．

縦隔の断層解剖 ［冠状断像（造影CT，縦隔条件）］

4-39

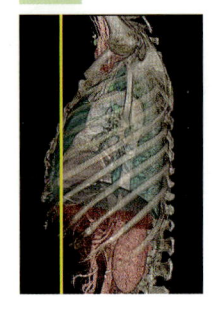

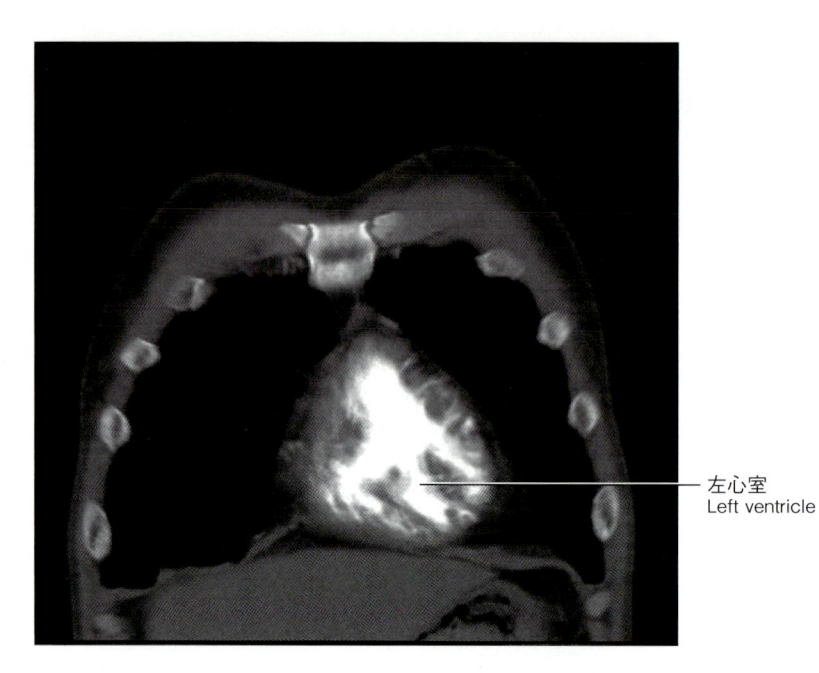

左心室
Left ventricle

4-40

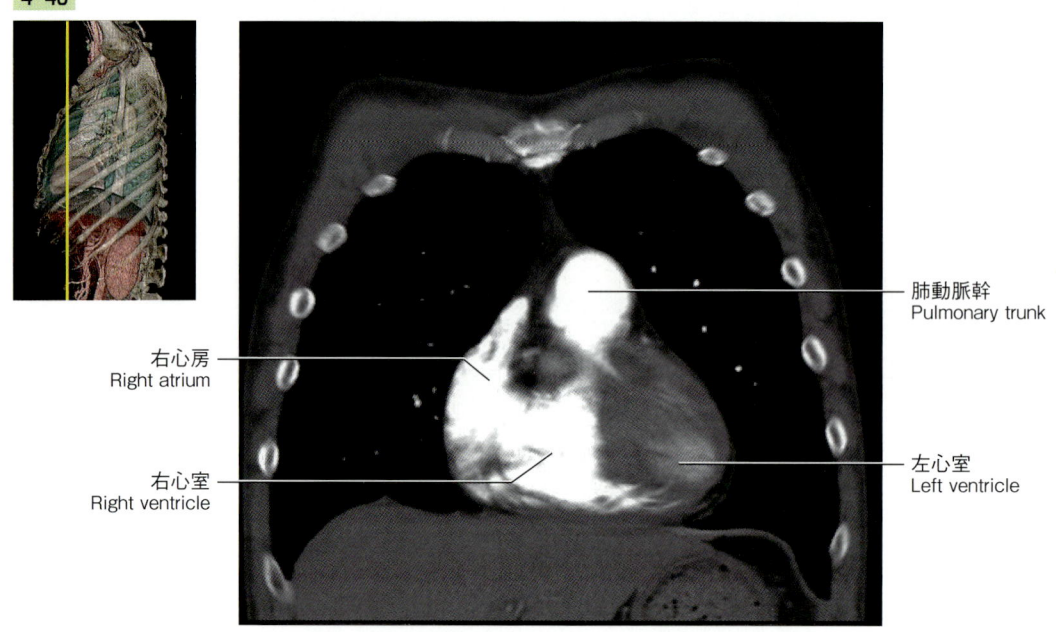

肺動脈幹
Pulmonary trunk

右心房
Right atrium

右心室
Right ventricle

左心室
Left ventricle

NOTE 冠状断像では，心臓の構造で左心室が最も前方に位置している．左心室は厚い筋層からなり，収縮時に高い内圧を作り出して血液循環のポンプ機能として働く．また右心室よりも繊細で数の多いメッシュ状の肉柱とよばれる構造が多数みられる．前および後乳頭筋も観察される．一方，右心室は左心室に比べて内圧が低いために，その壁は薄い．

縦隔の断層解剖 ［冠状断像（造影 CT, 縦隔条件）］

4-41

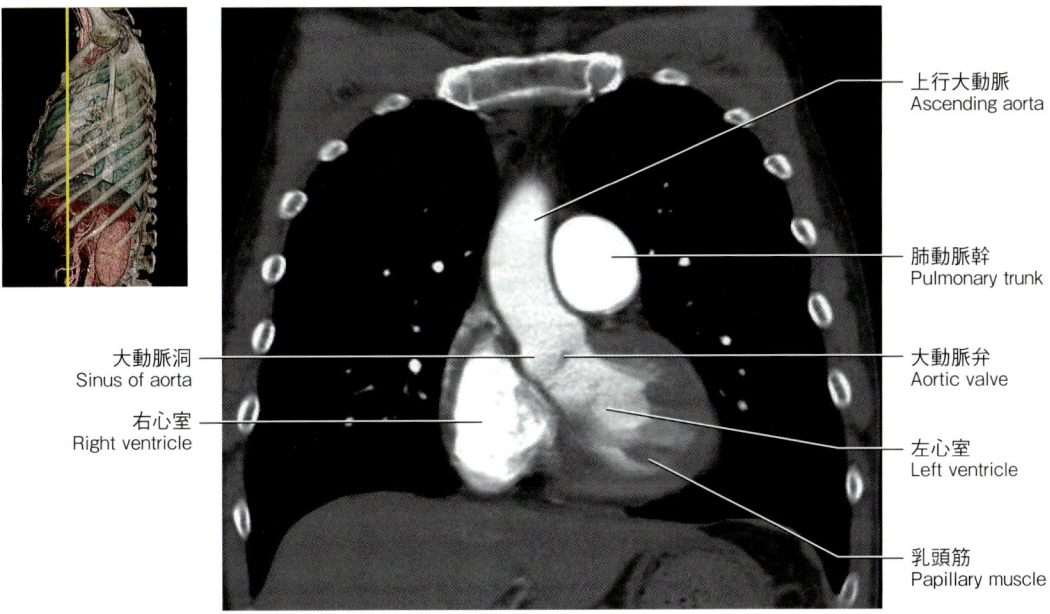

- 上行大動脈 Ascending aorta
- 肺動脈幹 Pulmonary trunk
- 大動脈洞 Sinus of aorta
- 大動脈弁 Aortic valve
- 右心室 Right ventricle
- 左心室 Left ventricle
- 乳頭筋 Papillary muscle

4-42

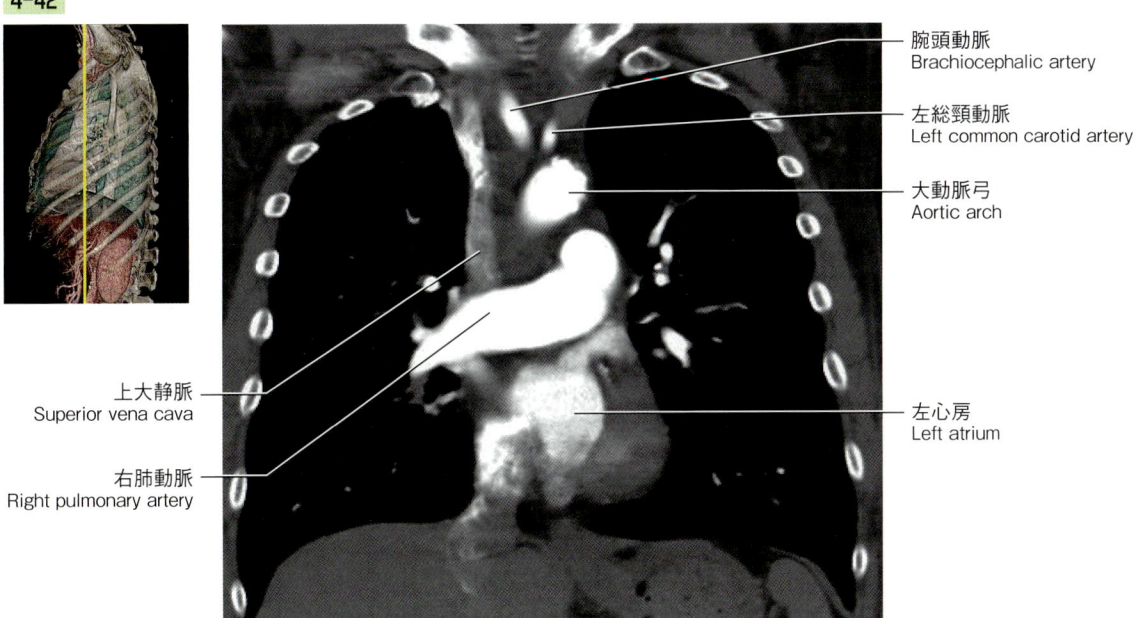

- 腕頭動脈 Brachiocephalic artery
- 左総頸動脈 Left common carotid artery
- 大動脈弓 Aortic arch
- 上大静脈 Superior vena cava
- 左心房 Left atrium
- 右肺動脈 Right pulmonary artery

NOTE 冠状断像では，左心室と上行大動脈の間に，大動脈弁が観察される．上行大動脈の起始部は球状に拡張しており，大動脈洞あるいは Valsalva（バルサルバ）洞とよばれ，ここから左右の冠動脈が起始している．

縦隔の断層解剖 ［冠状断像（造影 CT, 縦隔条件）］

4-43

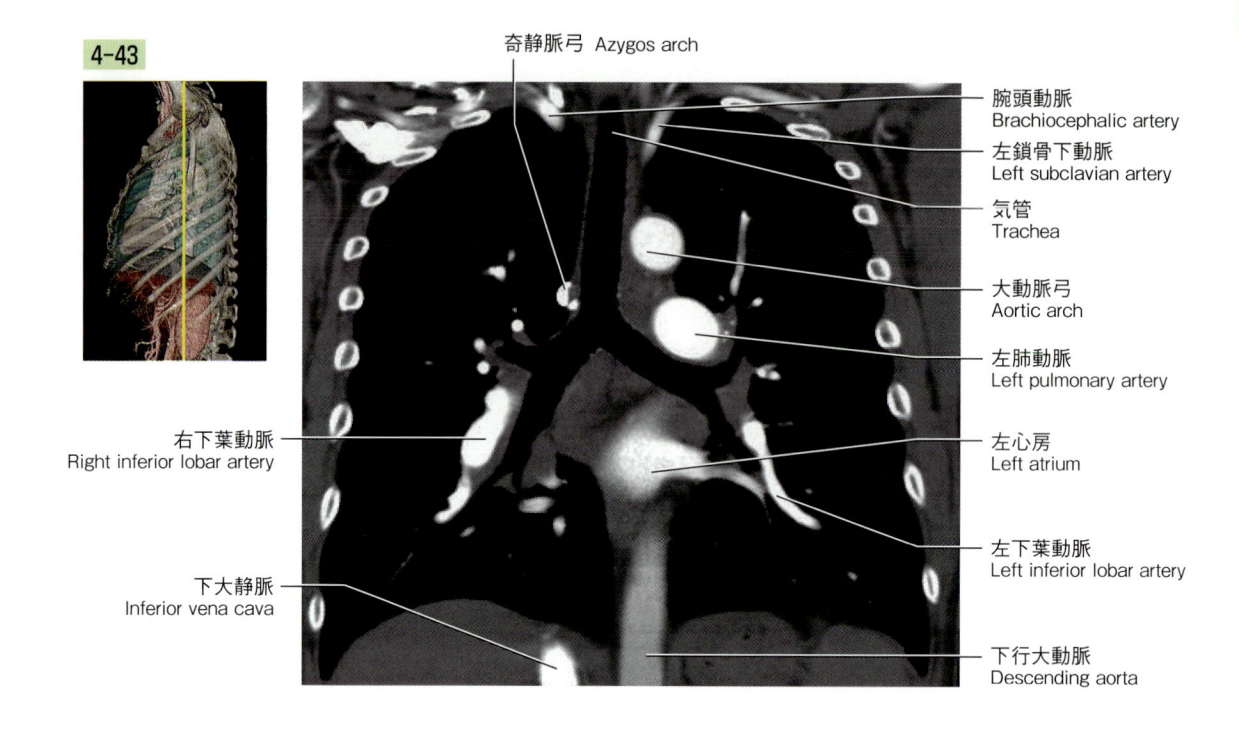

- 奇静脈弓 Azygos arch
- 腕頭動脈 Brachiocephalic artery
- 左鎖骨下動脈 Left subclavian artery
- 気管 Trachea
- 大動脈弓 Aortic arch
- 左肺動脈 Left pulmonary artery
- 右下葉動脈 Right inferior lobar artery
- 左心房 Left atrium
- 左下葉動脈 Left inferior lobar artery
- 下大静脈 Inferior vena cava
- 下行大動脈 Descending aorta

4-44

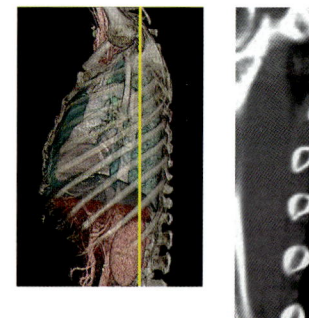

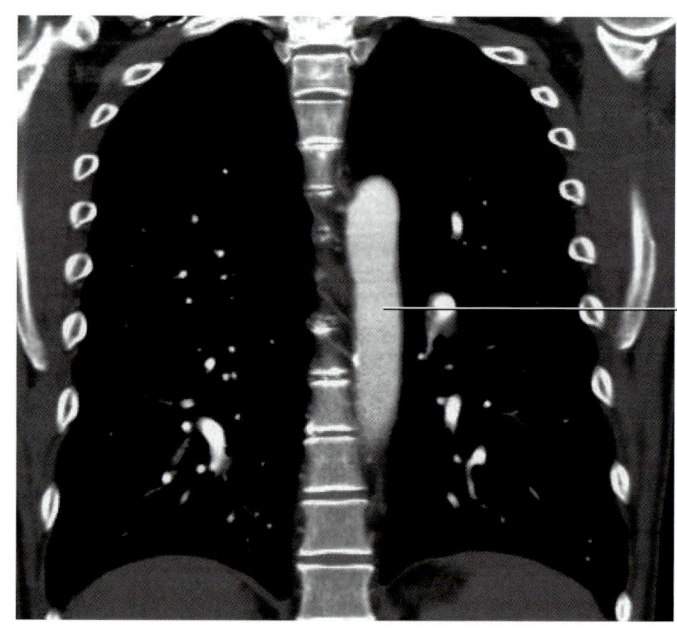

- 下行大動脈 Descending aorta

> **NOTE** 下行大動脈は，第 12 胸椎の高さで横隔膜を貫き，横隔膜の大動脈裂孔を通り腹腔内に入る．

縦隔の断層解剖 ［矢状断像（造影 CT，縦隔条件）］

4-45

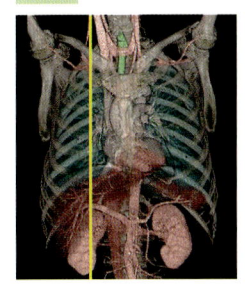

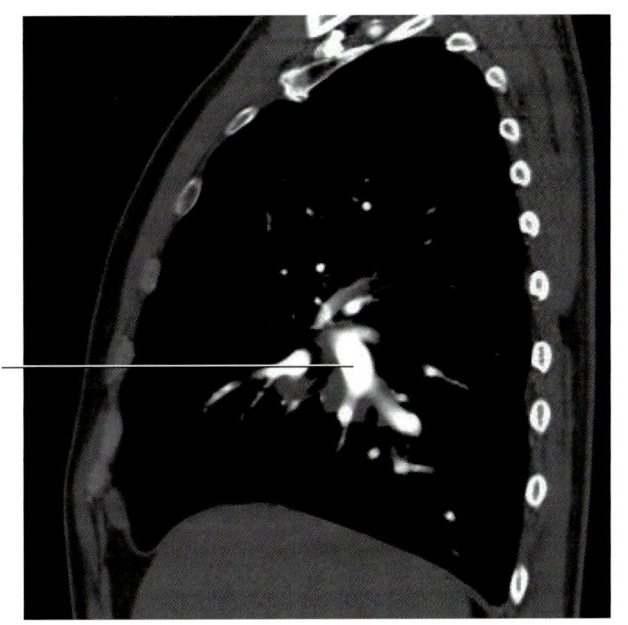

右肺動脈
Right pulmonary artery

4-46

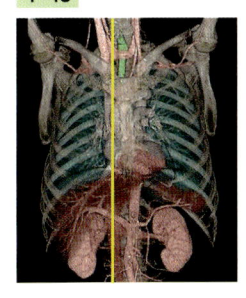

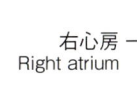

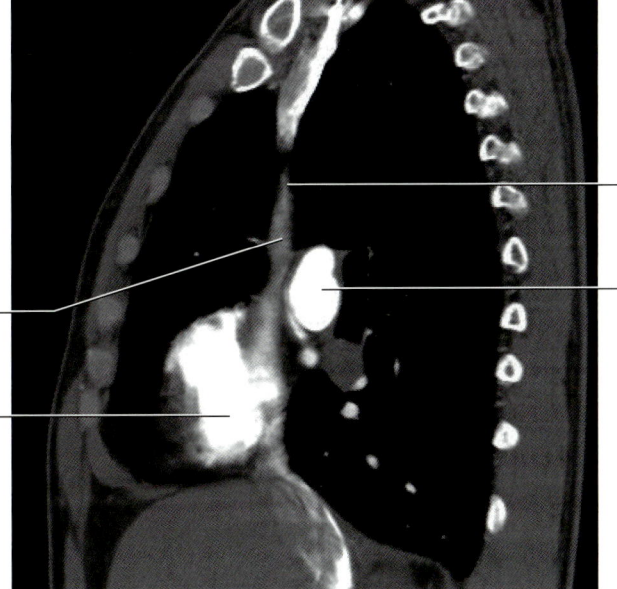

上大静脈
Superior vena cava

右肺動脈
Right pulmonary artery

奇静脈合流部
Orifice of azygos vein

右心房
Right atrium

NOTE　奇静脈 Azygos vein
　zygo-はギリシャ語の zygon（くびき）から発した左右一対の意味をもち，「～でない」のa-がつき，not being one of pair（不対）の意味の Azygos となった．和名は対の意味をもつ偶（数）の反対語，奇（数）をとって奇静脈となったもので，奇妙な静脈ではない．（副）半奇静脈は枝と考える（76, 186 頁の NOTE を参照）．

縦隔の断層解剖［矢状断像（造影CT，縦隔条件）］

4-47

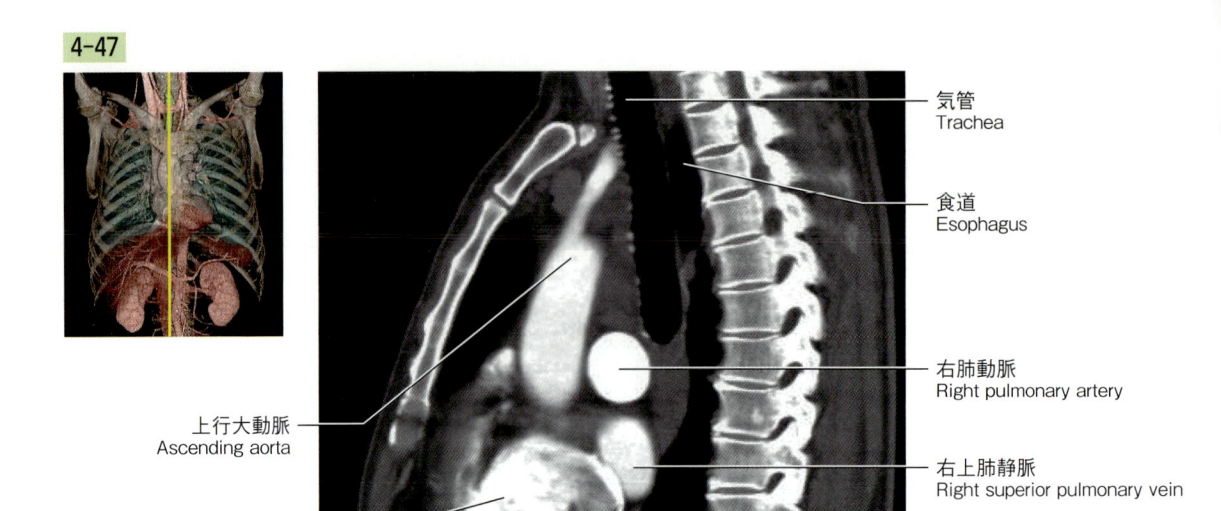

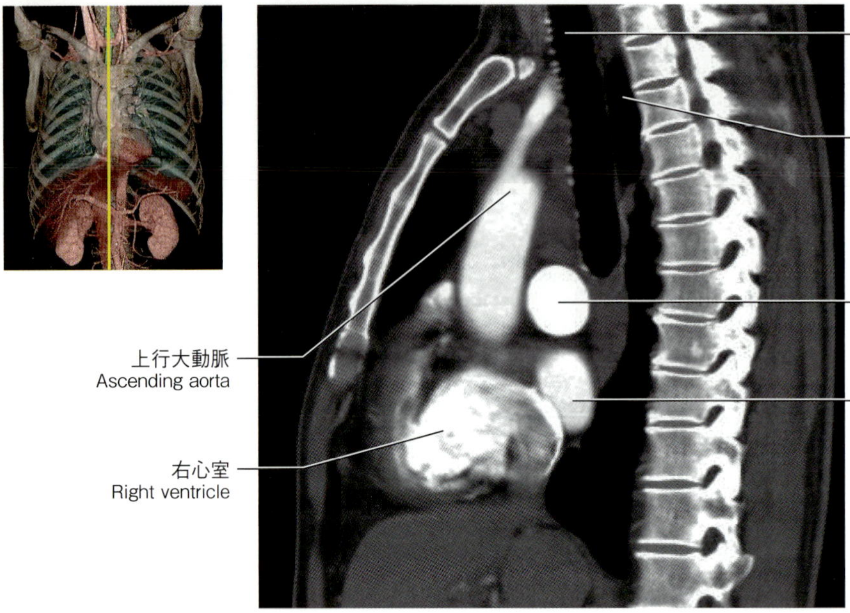

- 気管 Trachea
- 食道 Esophagus
- 右肺動脈 Right pulmonary artery
- 右上肺静脈 Right superior pulmonary vein
- 上行大動脈 Ascending aorta
- 右心室 Right ventricle

4-48

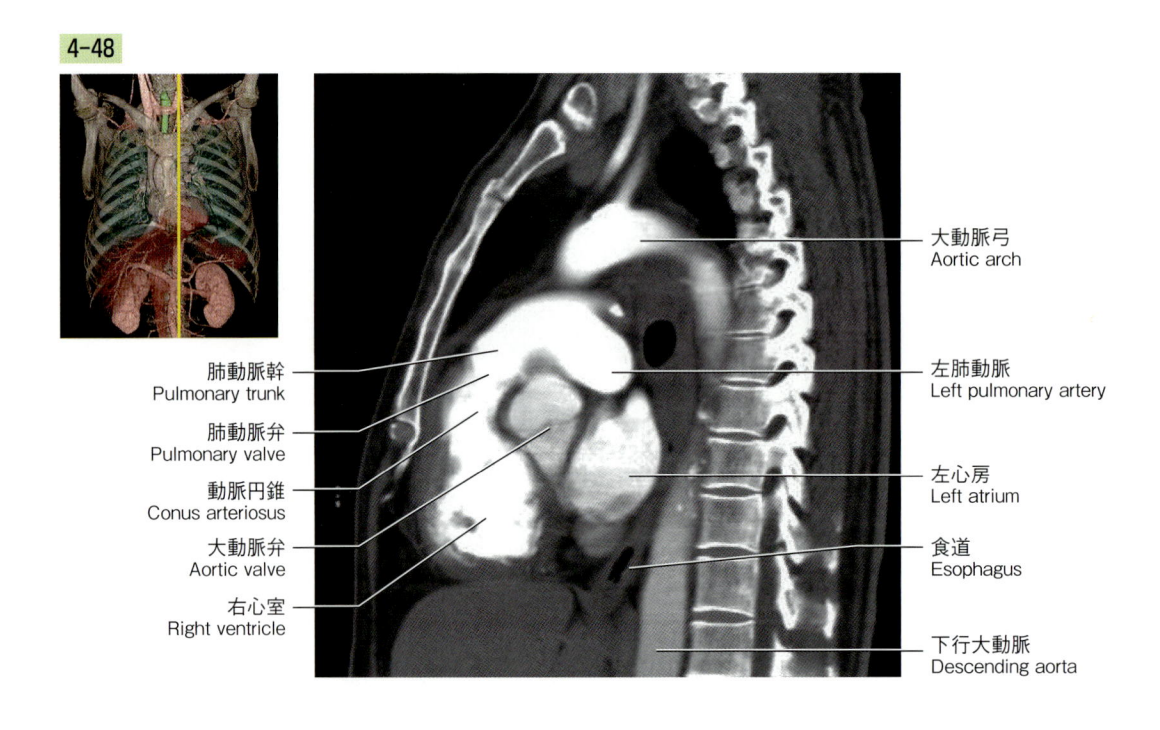

- 大動脈弓 Aortic arch
- 左肺動脈 Left pulmonary artery
- 左心房 Left atrium
- 食道 Esophagus
- 下行大動脈 Descending aorta
- 肺動脈幹 Pulmonary trunk
- 肺動脈弁 Pulmonary valve
- 動脈円錐 Conus arteriosus
- 大動脈弁 Aortic valve
- 右心室 Right ventricle

> **NOTE** 食道は気管の後方を走行し，食道裂孔を介して横隔膜を貫き，腹腔内に至る（4-47, 48）．右心室の流出路は，上方へ向かい円錐状を呈し，動脈円錐とよばれる（4-48, 49）．肺動脈弁は大動脈弁の前方かつ高位に位置していることがわかる（4-48）．

縦隔の断層解剖 ［矢状断像（造影 CT，縦隔条件）］

4-49

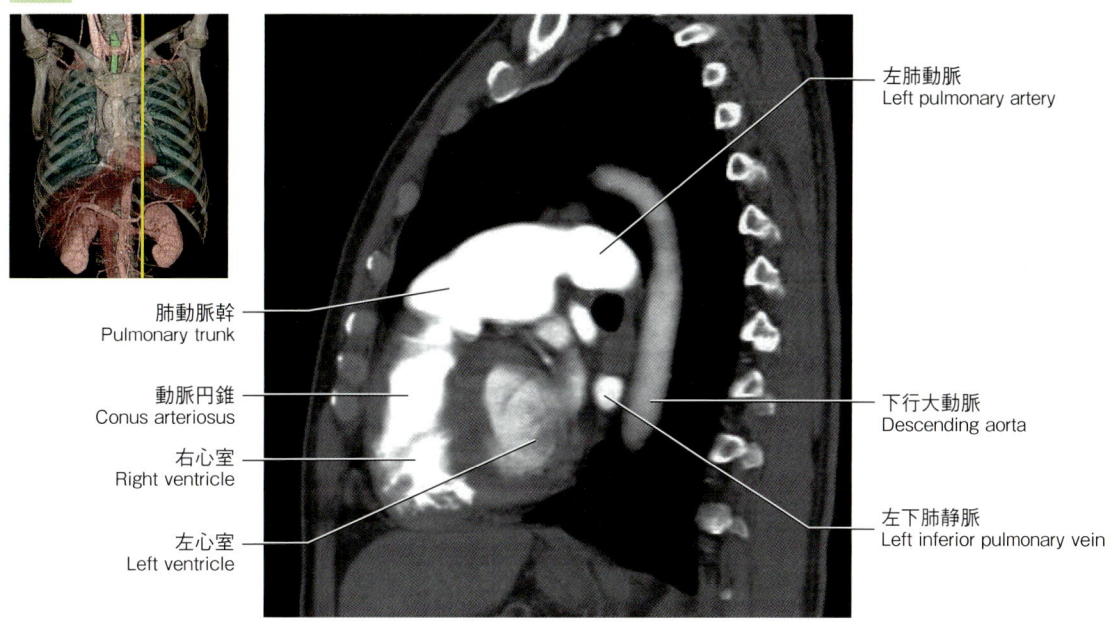

- 肺動脈幹 / Pulmonary trunk
- 動脈円錐 / Conus arteriosus
- 右心室 / Right ventricle
- 左心室 / Left ventricle
- 左肺動脈 / Left pulmonary artery
- 下行大動脈 / Descending aorta
- 左下肺静脈 / Left inferior pulmonary vein

4-50

- 右心室 / Right ventricle
- 左肺動脈 / Left pulmonary artery
- 左心室 / Left ventricle

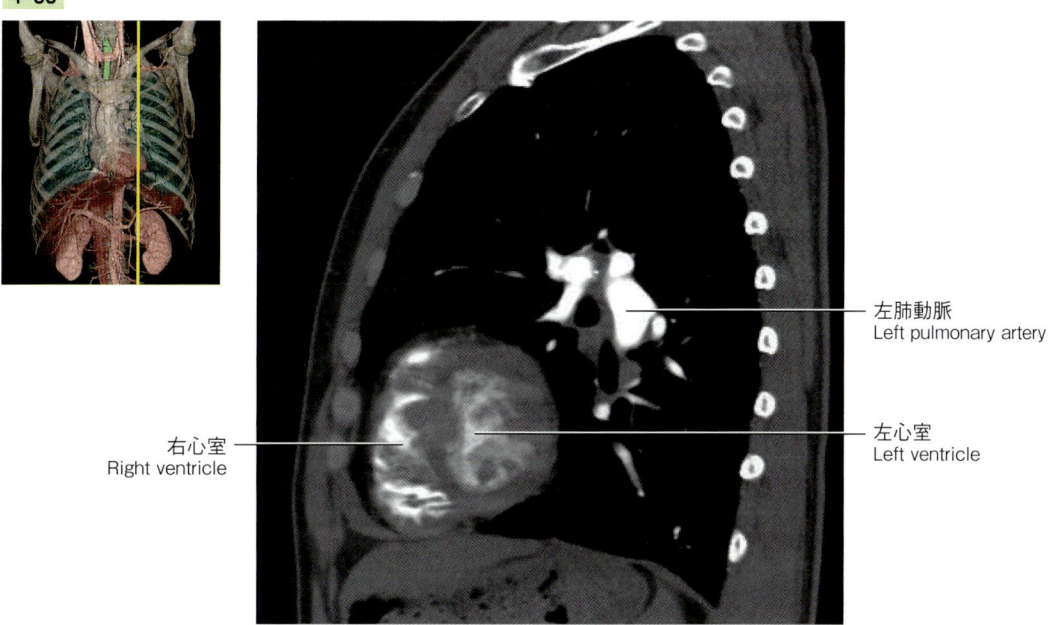

NOTE 肺動脈幹は，直径3cm，長さ約5cmの比較的太く短い構造を呈している．右心室の動脈円錐から続き，上後方へ走行したのち，左右の肺動脈に分かれる（4-48, 49）．

縦隔の断層解剖 ［矢状断像（造影CT, 縦隔条件）］

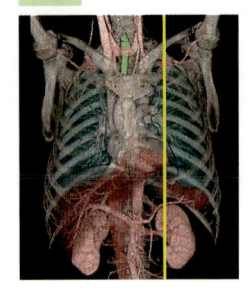

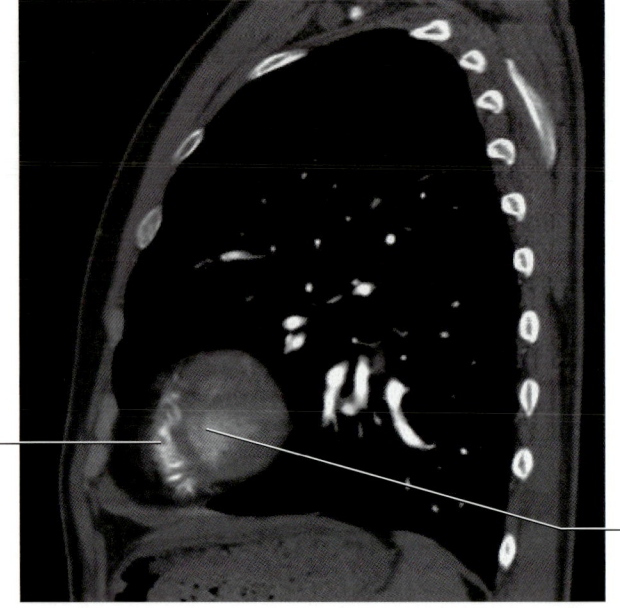

4-51

右心室
Right ventricle

左心室
Left ventricle

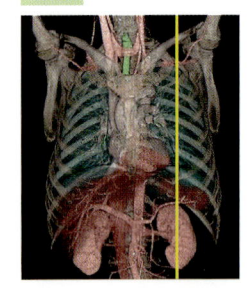

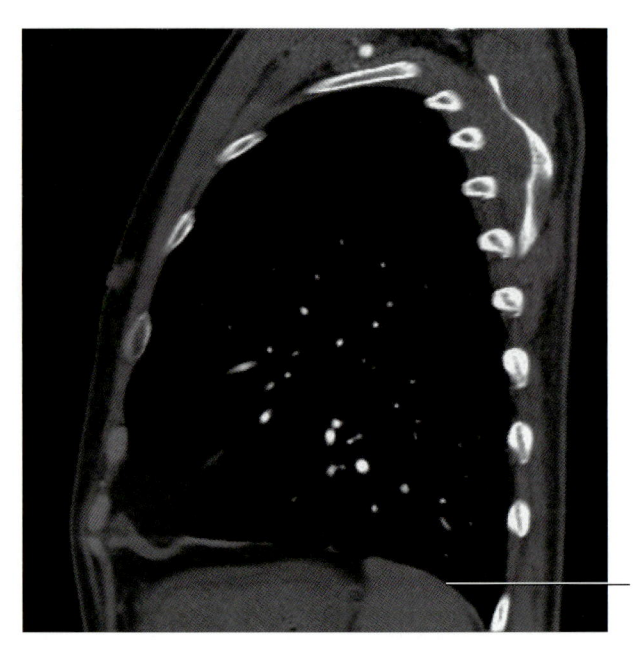

4-52

横隔膜
Diaphragm

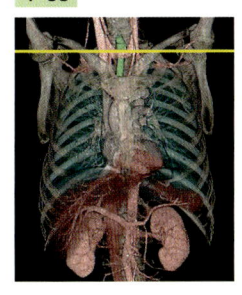

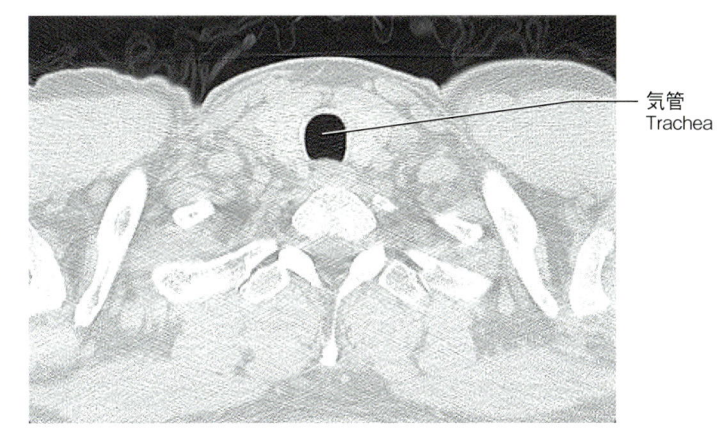

肺の断層解剖 ［横断像（造影 CT, 肺野条件）］

4-53

気管
Trachea

4-54

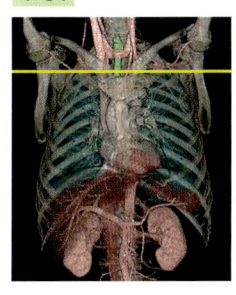

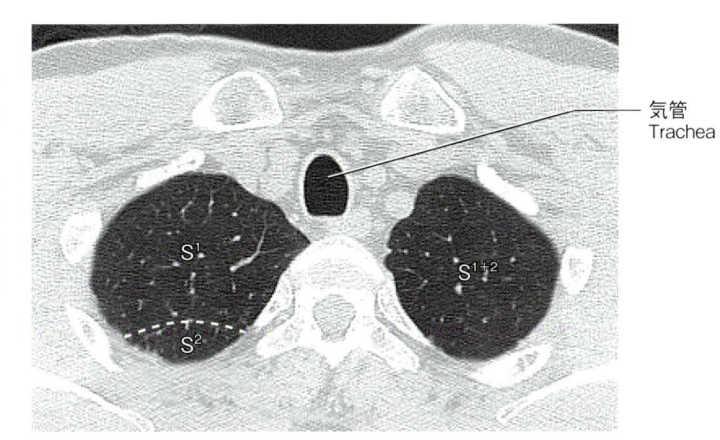

気管
Trachea

S¹ S¹⁺² S²

4-55

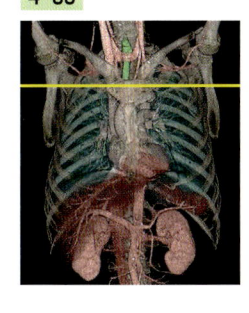

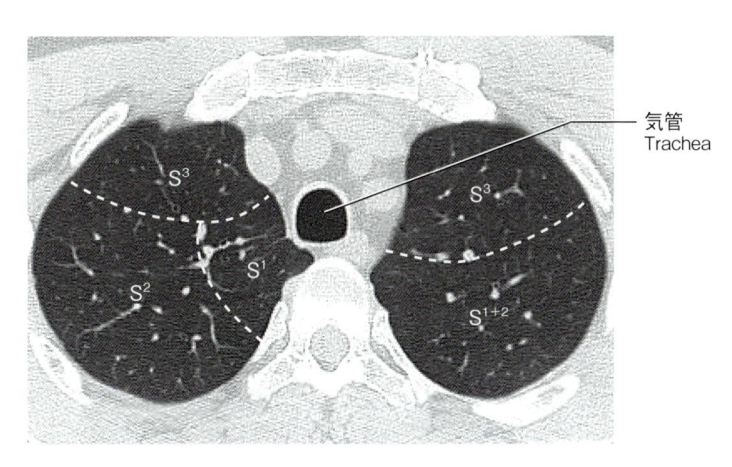

気管
Trachea

S³ S³
S¹
S² S¹⁺²

> **NOTE** CT で左右肺の各肺葉を同定する際には，その境界となる葉間裂（葉間胸膜）に注目するとよい．右では大葉間裂（斜裂）と小葉間裂（水平裂）(197 頁の 4-59) が，左では大葉間裂が存在し，各肺葉を分けている(4-57, 58)．ただし葉間裂にはさまざまな変異が存在し，副葉間裂に遭遇する機会も多い．比較的多く認められる副葉間裂として，右側では奇静脈裂・上副葉裂・下副葉裂，左側では上中葉間裂・上副葉裂・下副葉裂がある．

肺の断層解剖 ［横断像（造影 CT，肺野条件）］

4-56

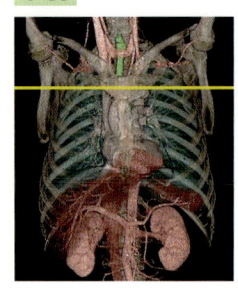

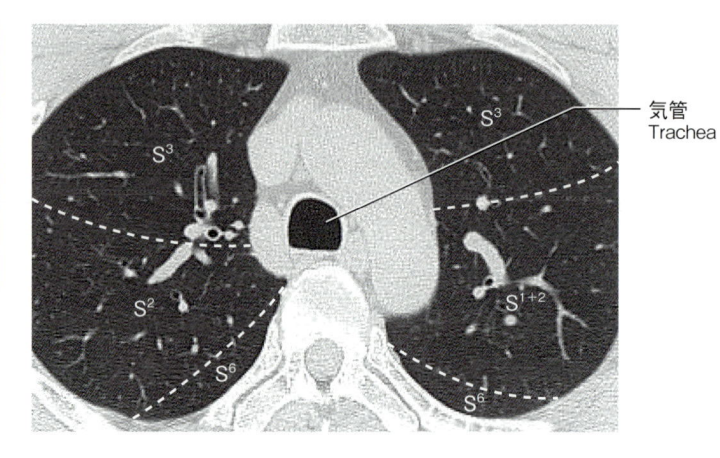

気管
Trachea

4-57

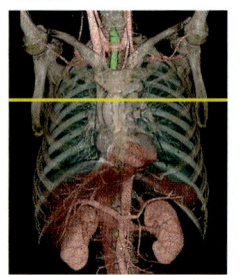

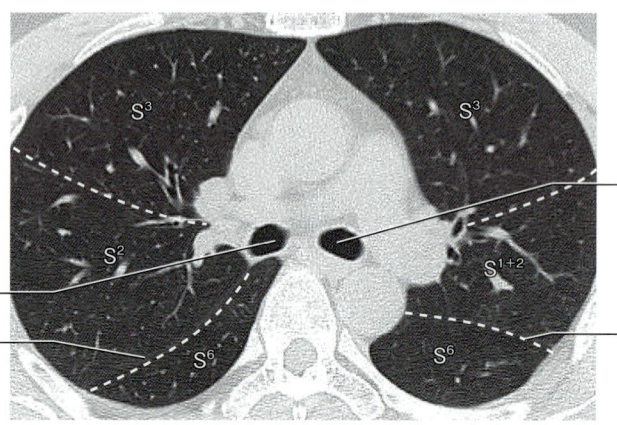

左主気管支
Left main bronchus

右主気管支
Right main bronchus

右大葉間裂
Right major fissure

左大葉間裂
Left major fissure

4-58

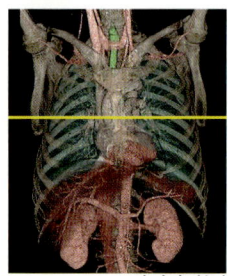

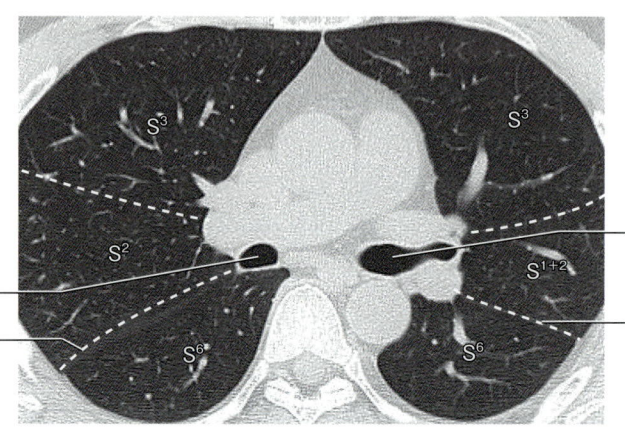

左主気管支
Left main bronchus

右主気管支
Right main bronchus

右大葉間裂
Right major fissure

左大葉間裂
Left major fissure

> **NOTE** 10 mm 程度の比較的厚いスライス厚の CT では，葉間裂は線状の構造として認識されず，いわゆる無血管帯といわれる索状の低吸収域として描出されることが多い．1〜2 mm スライス厚の高分解能 CT（high-resolution CT：HRCT）を用いると，葉間裂は線状の構造として明瞭に認識され，同定が容易となる．ただし，葉間裂全体が認識できる例は必ずしも多くなく，分葉が不全であることも多い．

肺の断層解剖 ［横断像（造影CT，肺野条件）］

4-59

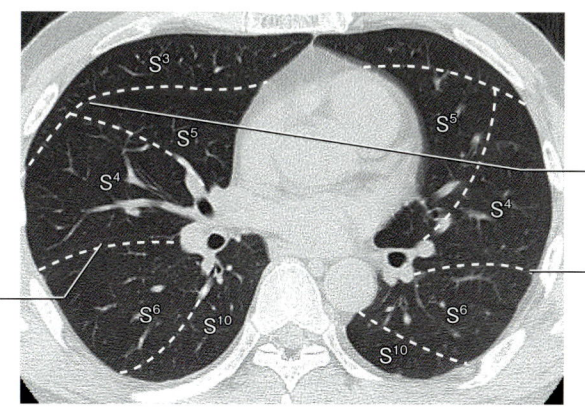

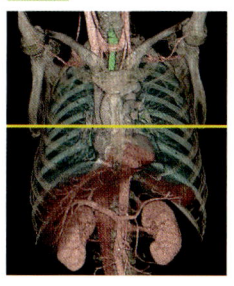

小葉間裂
Minor fissure

左大葉間裂
Left major fissure

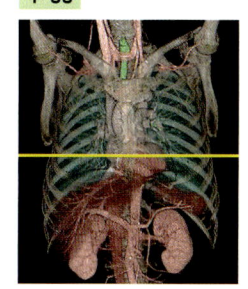

右大葉間裂
Right major fissure

4-60

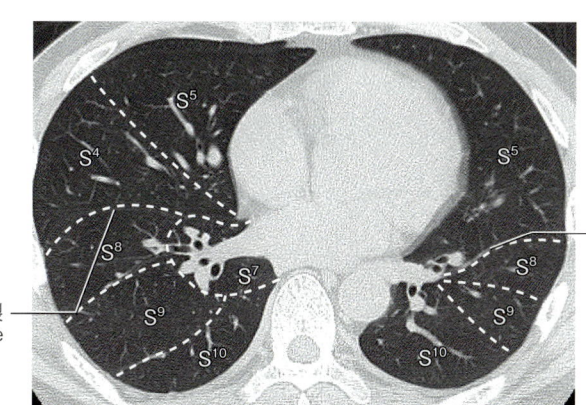

左大葉間裂
Left major fissure

右大葉間裂
Right major fissure

4-61

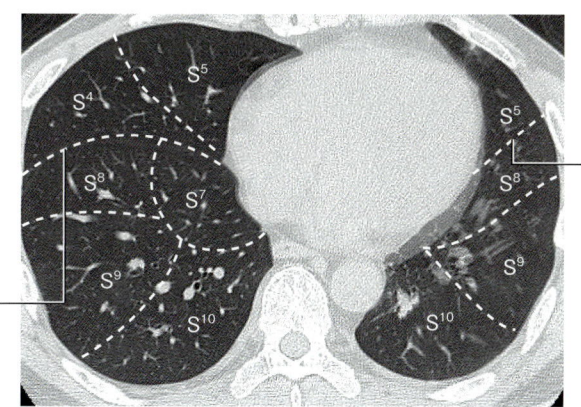

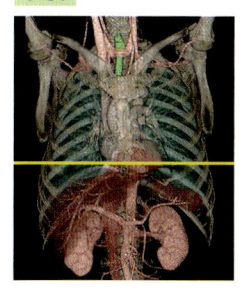

左大葉間裂
Left major fissure

右大葉間裂
Right major fissure

> **NOTE** 肺の区域や亜区域を同定するには，肺動静脈や気管支の走行に注目する．肺動脈はその分岐に多くの変異があるが，区域・亜区域レベルより末梢では気管支と伴走し，区域動脈，亜区域動脈となり，区域・亜区域の構造の中心を走行する．一方，肺静脈は肺動脈や気管支の走行とは独立しており，末梢で小葉間隔壁内を走行したのち，おのおのの亜区域や区域の境界を走行する．肺静脈の分岐にも多くの変異があるが，最終的に左右の上下肺静脈となり左心房に流入する．

肺の断層解剖　[冠状断像（造影 CT, 肺野条件）]

4-62

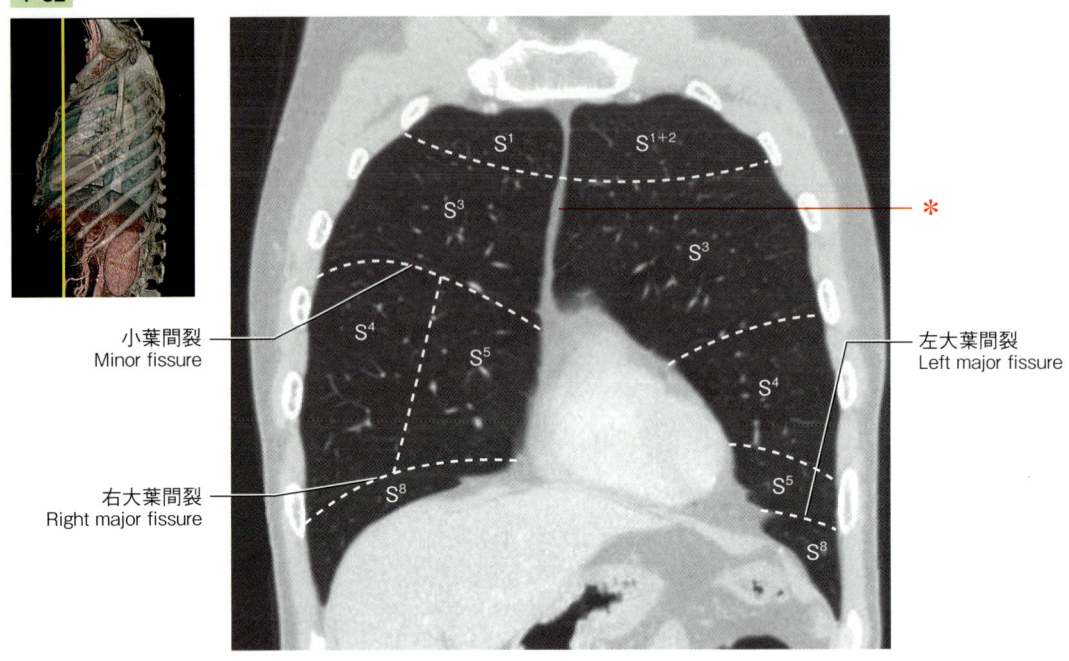

- 小葉間裂 Minor fissure
- 右大葉間裂 Right major fissure
- 左大葉間裂 Left major fissure
- ＊

4-63

- 小葉間裂 Minor fissure
- 右大葉間裂 Right major fissure
- 左大葉間裂 Left major fissure

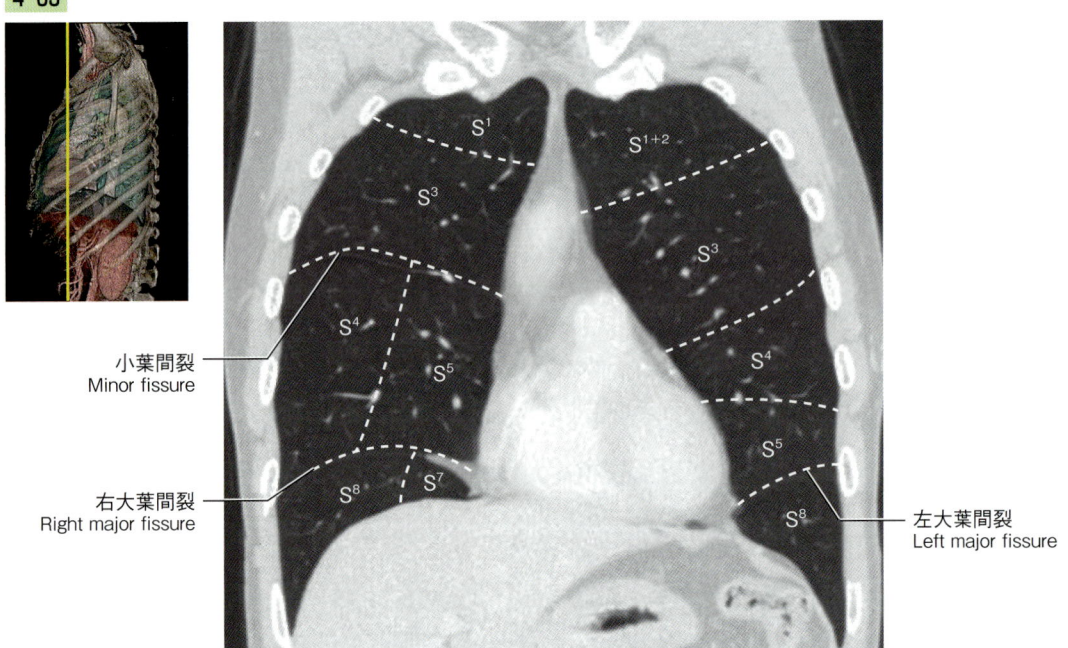

NOTE 両肺の前部は，胸骨の後方で接している．その境界部分は臓側胸膜と壁側胸膜が前内側で合わさることによる線状の構造として描出され（4-62の＊），胸部単純X線写真正面像では前接合線として知られている．この構造には，通常ごく少量の脂肪を含むことが多いが，脂肪が多い場合や若年者で胸腺組織が発達している場合には，さまざまな厚さの索状構造として認められる．

肺の断層解剖［冠状断像（造影 CT, 肺野条件）］

4-64

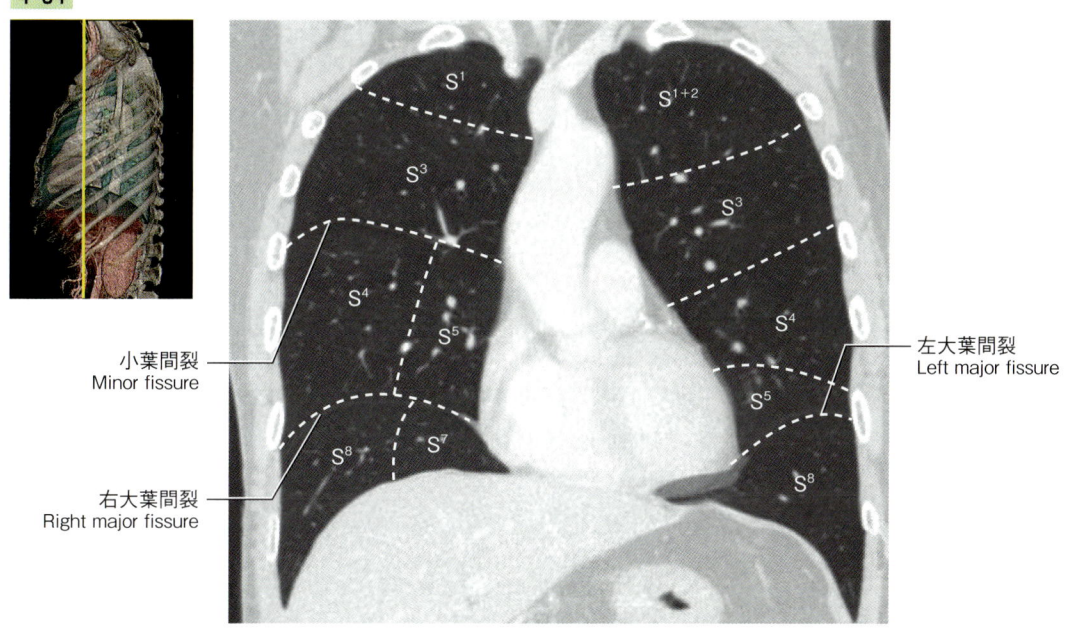

小葉間裂 Minor fissure
右大葉間裂 Right major fissure
左大葉間裂 Left major fissure

4-65

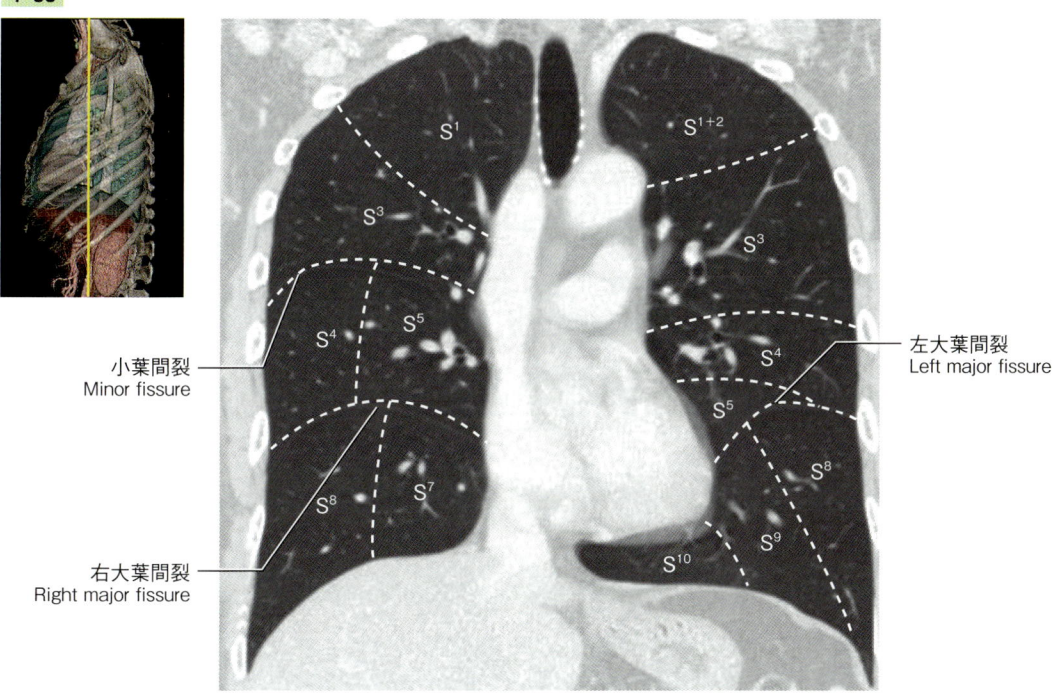

小葉間裂 Minor fissure
右大葉間裂 Right major fissure
左大葉間裂 Left major fissure

> **NOTE** 胸郭入口部から奇静脈弓や大動脈弓部上方のレベルで，両肺の後部は胸椎の直前で接している（4-66 の＊）．この境界部分は胸部単純 X 線写真正面像で後接合線として描出されることがあり，前接合線と同様に左右の臓側および壁側胸膜と脂肪組織から構成される．

肺の断層解剖 ［冠状断像（造影 CT, 肺野条件）］

4-66

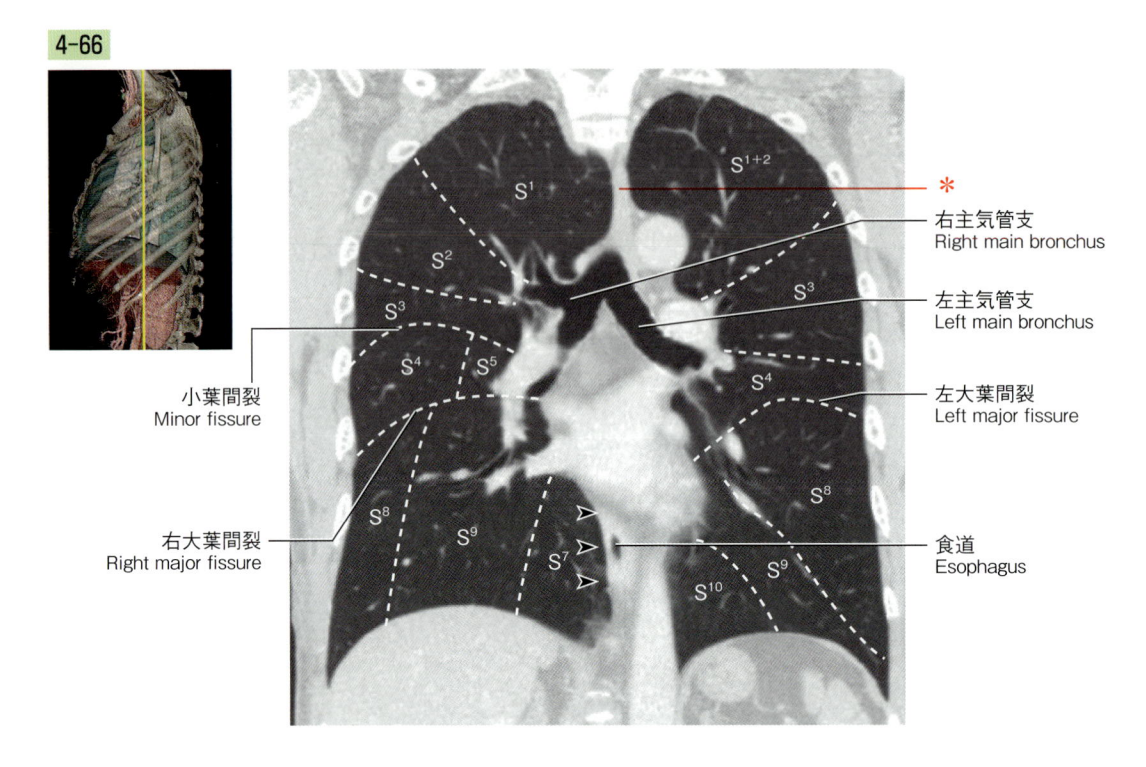

- 小葉間裂 Minor fissure
- 右大葉間裂 Right major fissure
- ＊
- 右主気管支 Right main bronchus
- 左主気管支 Left main bronchus
- 左大葉間裂 Left major fissure
- 食道 Esophagus

4-67

- 小葉間裂 Minor fissure
- 右大葉間裂 Right major fissure
- 左大葉間裂 Left major fissure

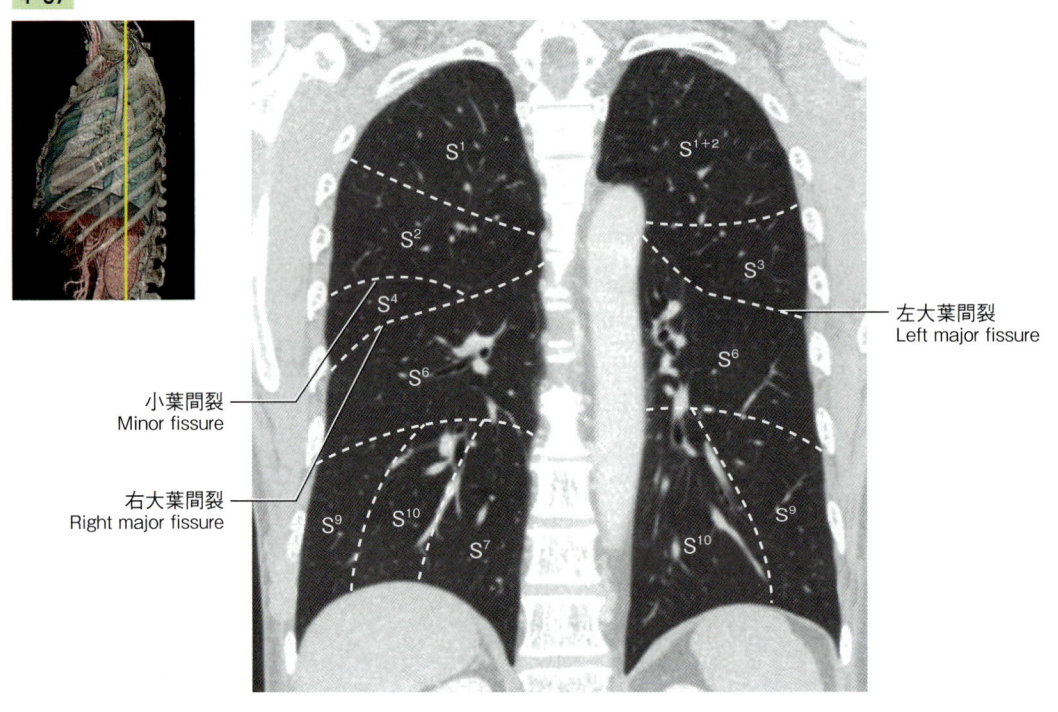

> **NOTE** 右肺下葉の後部は，心臓と胸椎の間で縦隔側に入り込むように存在する．この部位は食道や奇静脈の右側と境界されるため，食道奇静脈陥凹とよばれ（4-66 の ▶），胸部単純 X 線写真正面像においてもしばしばこの境界が認められる．

肺の断層解剖 ［矢状断像（造影 CT, 肺野条件）］

4-68

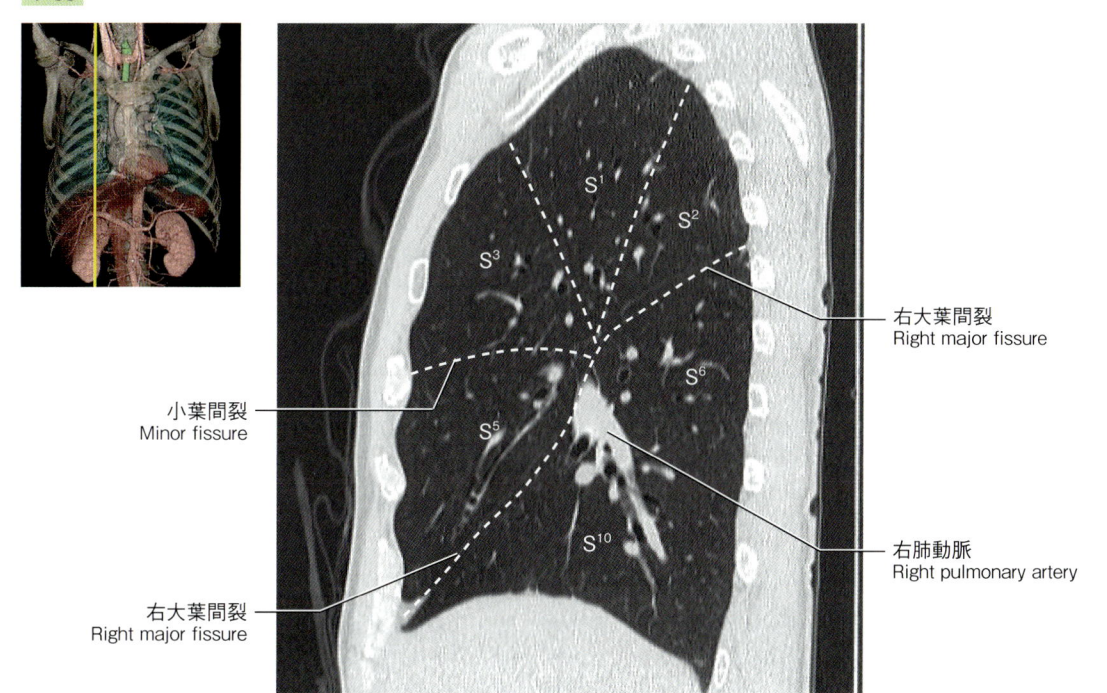

- 小葉間裂 Minor fissure
- 右大葉間裂 Right major fissure
- 右大葉間裂 Right major fissure
- 右肺動脈 Right pulmonary artery

4-69

- 小葉間裂 Minor fissure
- 右大葉間裂 Right major fissure
- 右主気管支 Right main bronchus

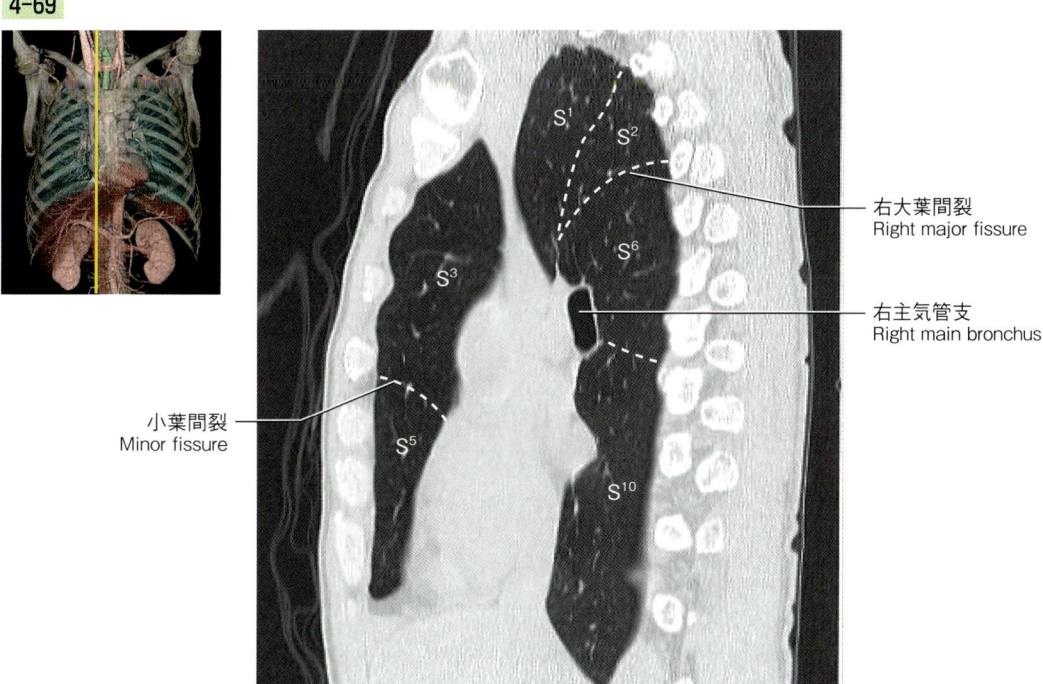

> **NOTE** 葉間裂は2枚の臓側胸膜が重なって形成されている．臓側胸膜の間質は胸膜下の小葉間隔壁と連続している．葉間胸膜は非常に薄い膜のため，スライス面に対する角度とスライス厚により描出が異なる．上葉と中葉間にある小葉間裂は，一般に水平方向に走行するため，横断像ではHRCTでも認識しづらいが，矢状断像や冠状断像ではその認識が容易となる．

肺の断層解剖　[矢状断像（造影 CT，肺野条件）]

4-70

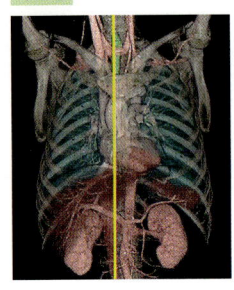

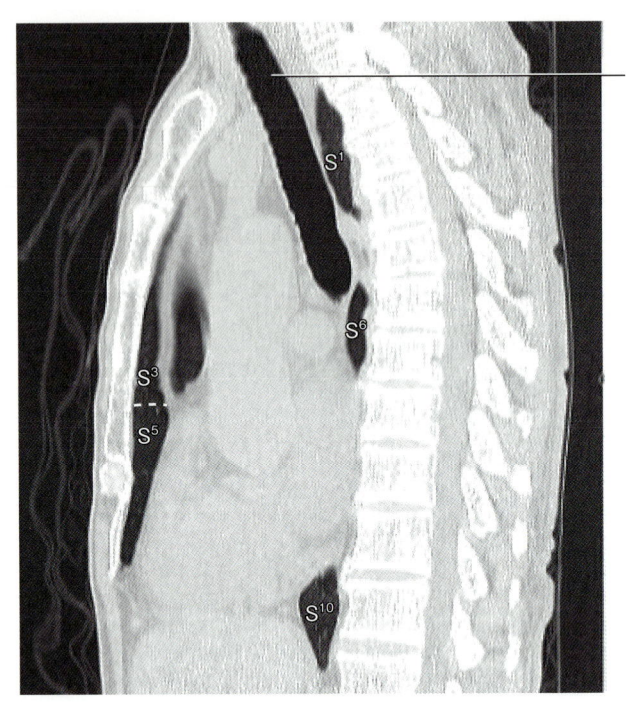

気管
Trachea

S¹
S⁶
S³
S⁵
S¹⁰

4-71

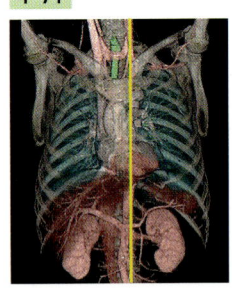

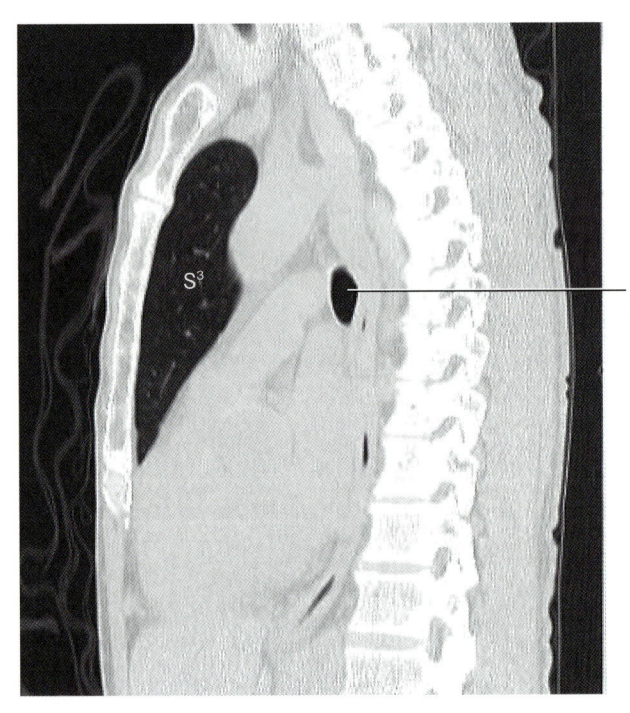

S³

左主気管支
Left main bronchus

> **NOTE** 気管は輪状軟骨下縁（第6頸椎レベル）から気管分岐部（第5胸椎レベル）までの構造で，長さは10〜12 cmである．気管横径の正常値は，成人男性で13〜25 mm，女性で10〜21 mm．前後径の正常値は，男性で13〜27 mm，女性で10〜23 mmである．一般的に吸気で撮影してものと比べ，呼気では横径で約15%，前後径で約30%減少する．

肺の断層解剖 ［矢状断像（造影CT, 肺野条件）］

4-72

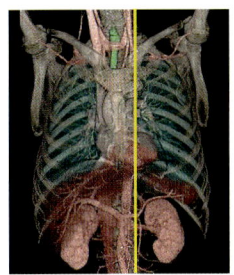

- 左肺動脈 Left pulmonary artery
- 下行大動脈 Descending aorta
- 左主気管支 Left main bronchus

4-73

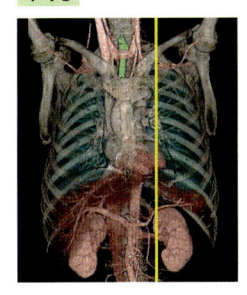

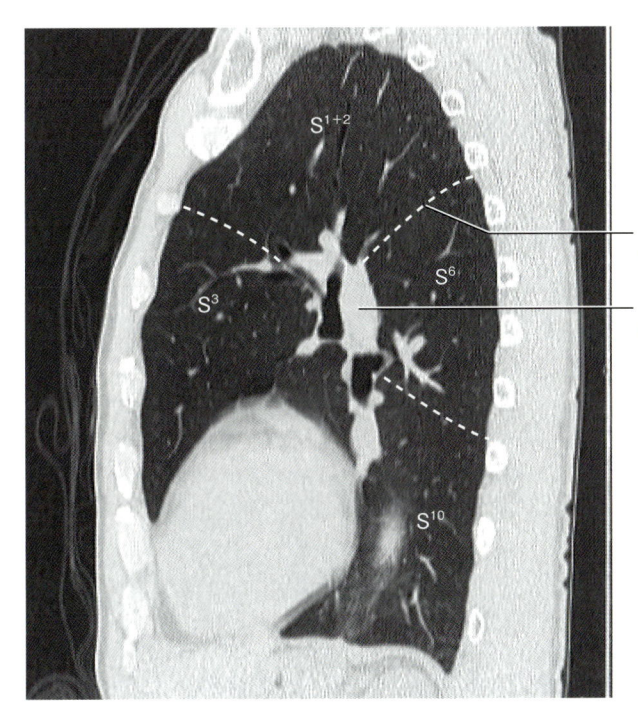

- 左大葉間裂 Left major fissue
- 左肺動脈 Left pulmonary artery

> **NOTE** 肺のリンパ管は，気管支周囲，肺血管周囲，小葉間隔壁，あるいは胸膜の間質に分布している．原則として肺の末梢から肺門のリンパ節に向かってリンパ流が存在する．リンパ管自体はCTで同定できないが，リンパ路の拡張が生じると（癌性リンパ管症や心不全による間質性肺水腫など），気管支壁の肥厚や血管影の拡大，小葉間隔壁の肥厚が生じ，容易に認識されるようになる．

肺の断層解剖　[矢状断像（造影 CT, 肺野条件）]

4-74

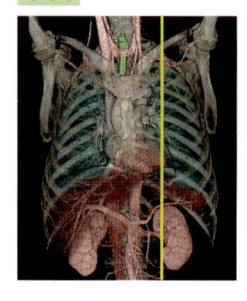

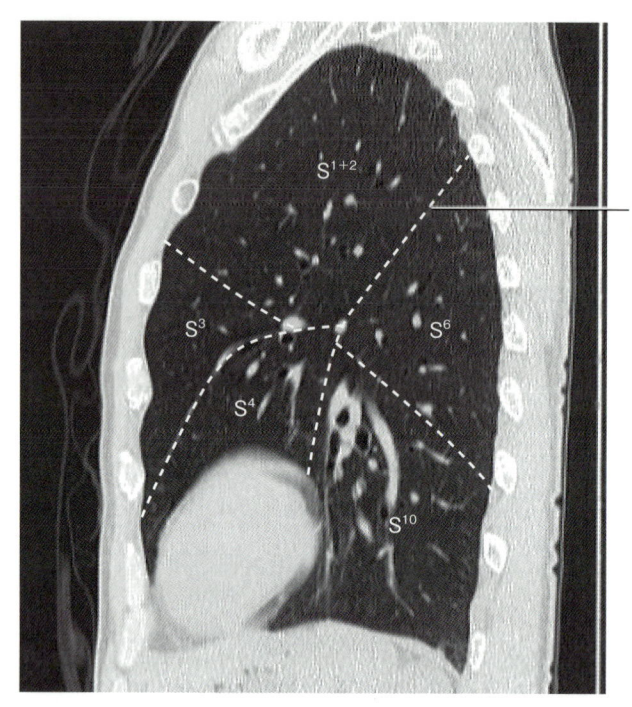

左大葉間裂
Left major fissure

S1+2, S3, S4, S6, S10

4-75

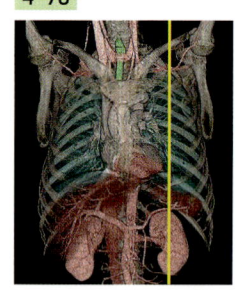

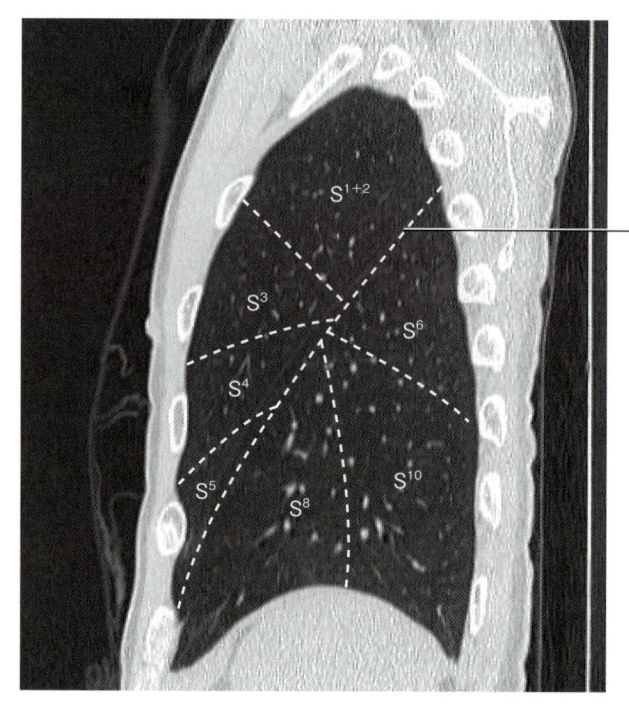

左大葉間裂
Left major fissure

S1+2, S3, S4, S5, S6, S8, S10

> **NOTE** 一般的に HRCT で認識できる構造は，二次小葉の中心を走行する肺動脈や，二次小葉の境界を走行する肺静脈のレベルまでで，さらに末梢の構造の認識は困難である．気管支の場合は，HRCT で確実に描出可能なのは亜区域枝レベルまでであり，次の分枝（第 4 分枝）は約半数程度でしか描出されないとされる．

心　臓（CT, VR像）

4-76　心臓の外観（前面）

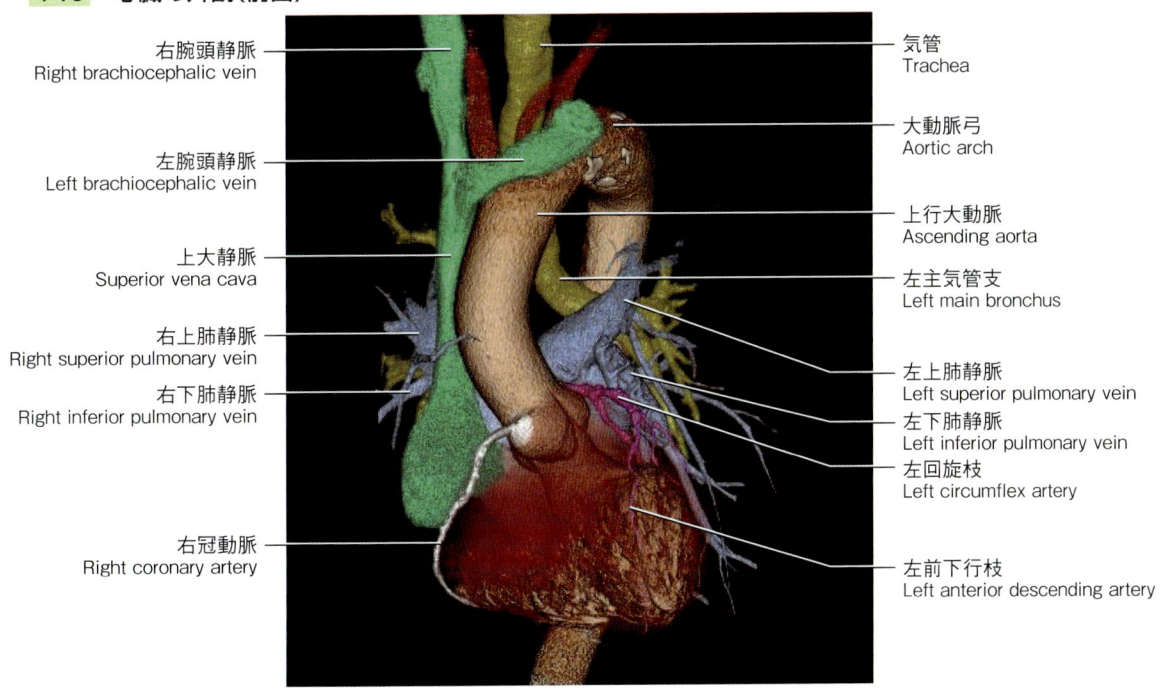

- 右腕頭静脈　Right brachiocephalic vein
- 左腕頭静脈　Left brachiocephalic vein
- 上大静脈　Superior vena cava
- 右上肺静脈　Right superior pulmonary vein
- 右下肺静脈　Right inferior pulmonary vein
- 右冠動脈　Right coronary artery
- 気管　Trachea
- 大動脈弓　Aortic arch
- 上行大動脈　Ascending aorta
- 左主気管支　Left main bronchus
- 左上肺静脈　Left superior pulmonary vein
- 左下肺静脈　Left inferior pulmonary vein
- 左回旋枝　Left circumflex artery
- 左前下行枝　Left anterior descending artery

4-77　心臓の外観（後面）

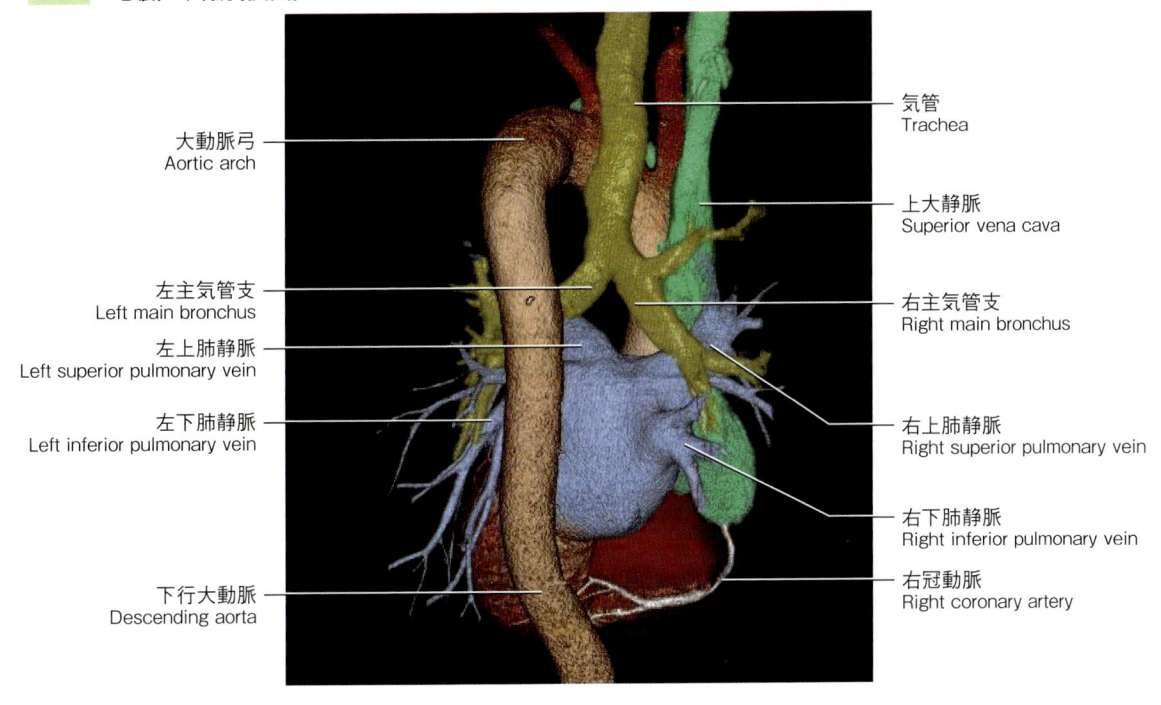

- 大動脈弓　Aortic arch
- 左主気管支　Left main bronchus
- 左上肺静脈　Left superior pulmonary vein
- 左下肺静脈　Left inferior pulmonary vein
- 下行大動脈　Descending aorta
- 気管　Trachea
- 上大静脈　Superior vena cava
- 右主気管支　Right main bronchus
- 右上肺静脈　Right superior pulmonary vein
- 右下肺静脈　Right inferior pulmonary vein
- 右冠動脈　Right coronary artery

> **NOTE**　最近のMDCT（multidetector-row CT）の進歩により，検出器の多列化やガントリー回転速度の高速化が急速に進み，胸部全体の詳細な解剖学的情報が非侵襲的に得られるようになった．1回の撮像で，心臓や冠動脈の形態のみでなく，大動脈や肺動静脈の情報も同時に得られることが可能で，臨床の場面でさまざまな応用がなされている．

心　臓（CT, VR像）

4-78　左心室短軸像

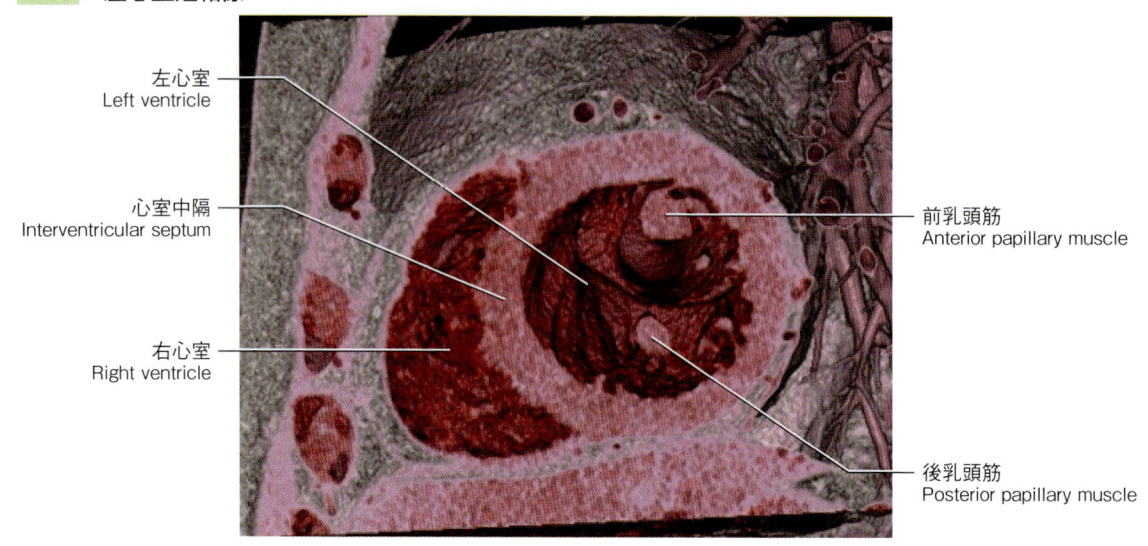

- 左心室 Left ventricle
- 心室中隔 Interventricular septum
- 右心室 Right ventricle
- 前乳頭筋 Anterior papillary muscle
- 後乳頭筋 Posterior papillary muscle

4-79　左心室長軸像

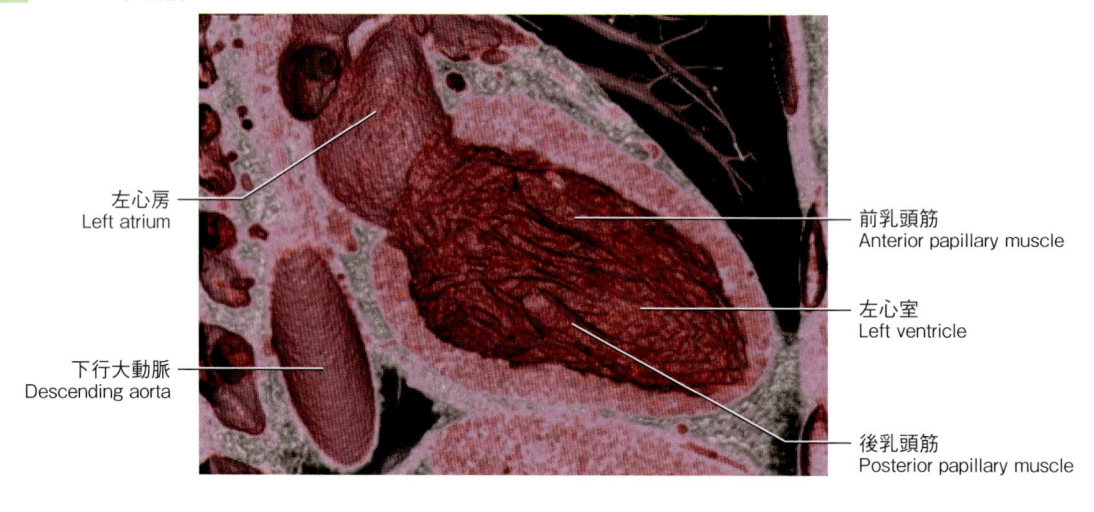

- 左心房 Left atrium
- 下行大動脈 Descending aorta
- 前乳頭筋 Anterior papillary muscle
- 左心室 Left ventricle
- 後乳頭筋 Posterior papillary muscle

> **NOTE**　心臓は4つの腔より構成され，線維性の心房中隔が左右の心房を分け，また筋性の心室中隔が左右の心室を分ける．これらの構造は漿膜性の心膜で包まれ，臓側心膜と壁側心膜間に少量の心膜液を含んでいる．MDCTはこれらの構造を詳細に描出可能で，心電同期を併用することにより，心周期による壁運動や壁厚の変化の把握も可能となる．

心　臓（CT, VR像） 207

4-80 四腔断像

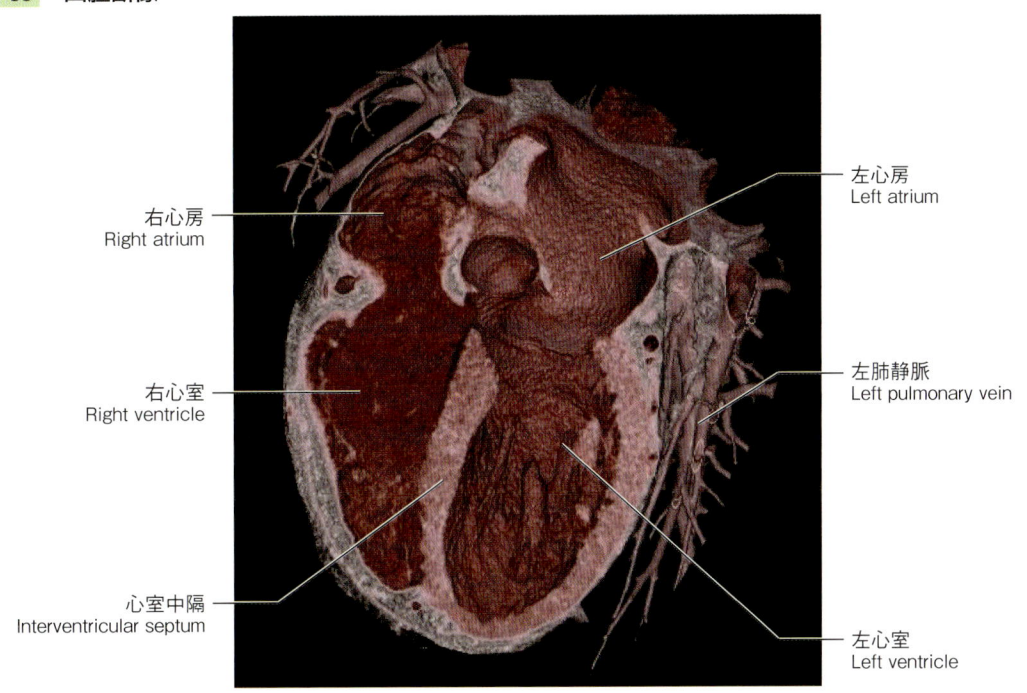

右心房 Right atrium
右心室 Right ventricle
心室中隔 Interventricular septum
左心房 Left atrium
左肺静脈 Left pulmonary vein
左心室 Left ventricle

4-81 三腔断像

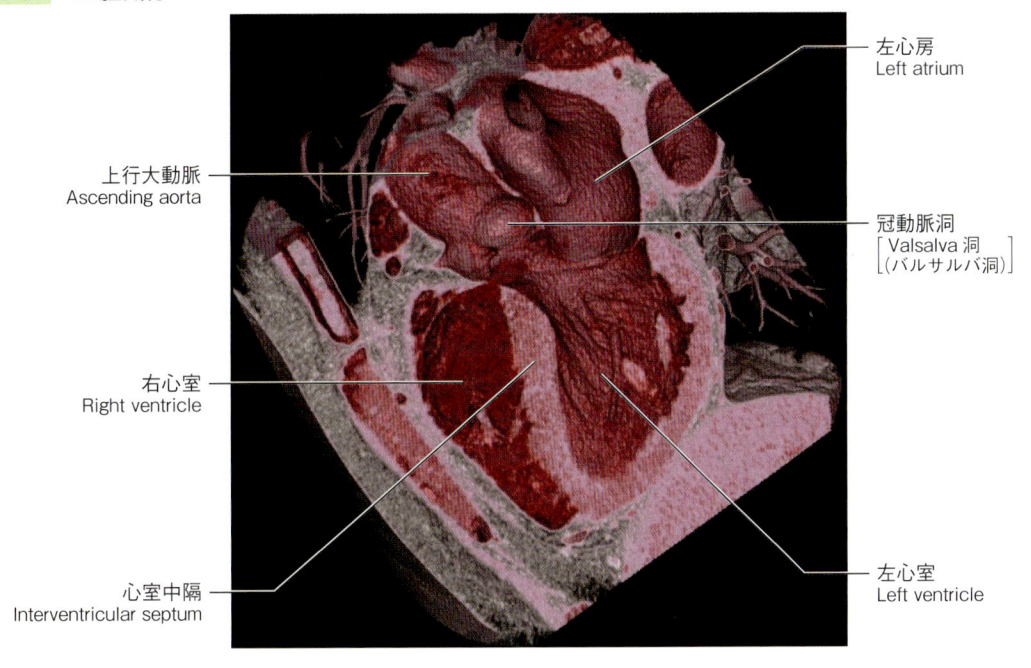

上行大動脈 Ascending aorta
右心室 Right ventricle
心室中隔 Interventricular septum
左心房 Left atrium
冠動脈洞 [Valsalva洞] [（バルサルバ洞）]
左心室 Left ventricle

冠動脈（CT，VR像）

4-82 心臓（前面から）

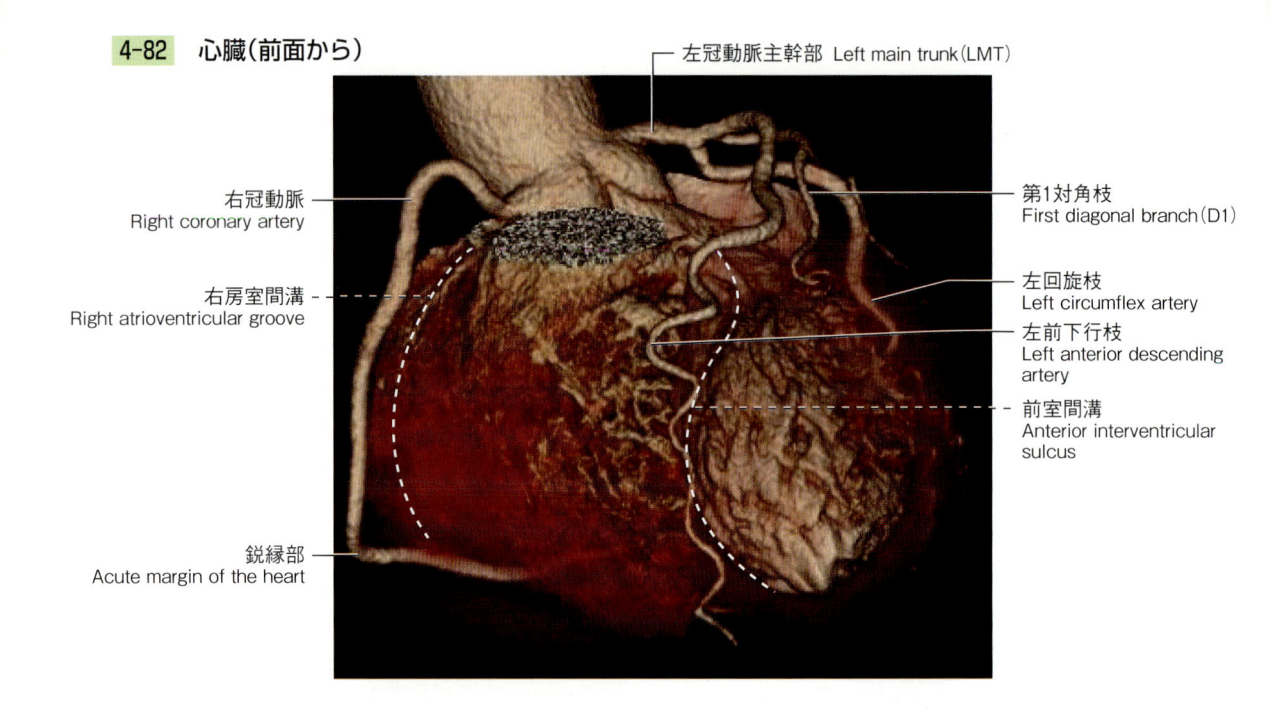

- 左冠動脈主幹部 Left main trunk (LMT)
- 右冠動脈 Right coronary artery
- 第1対角枝 First diagonal branch (D1)
- 右房室間溝 Right atrioventricular groove
- 左回旋枝 Left circumflex artery
- 左前下行枝 Left anterior descending artery
- 前室間溝 Anterior interventricular sulcus
- 鋭縁部 Acute margin of the heart

4-83 心臓（後面から）

- 左冠動脈主幹部 Left main trunk (LMT)
- 左前下行枝 Left anterior descending artery
- 第1対角枝 First diagonal branch (D1)
- 左回旋枝 Left circumflex artery
- 右冠動脈 Right coronary artery
- 左房室間溝 Left atrioventricular groove
- 後室間溝 Posterior interventricular sulcus
- 房室結節枝 Atrioventricular branch
- 後下行枝 Posterior descending branch

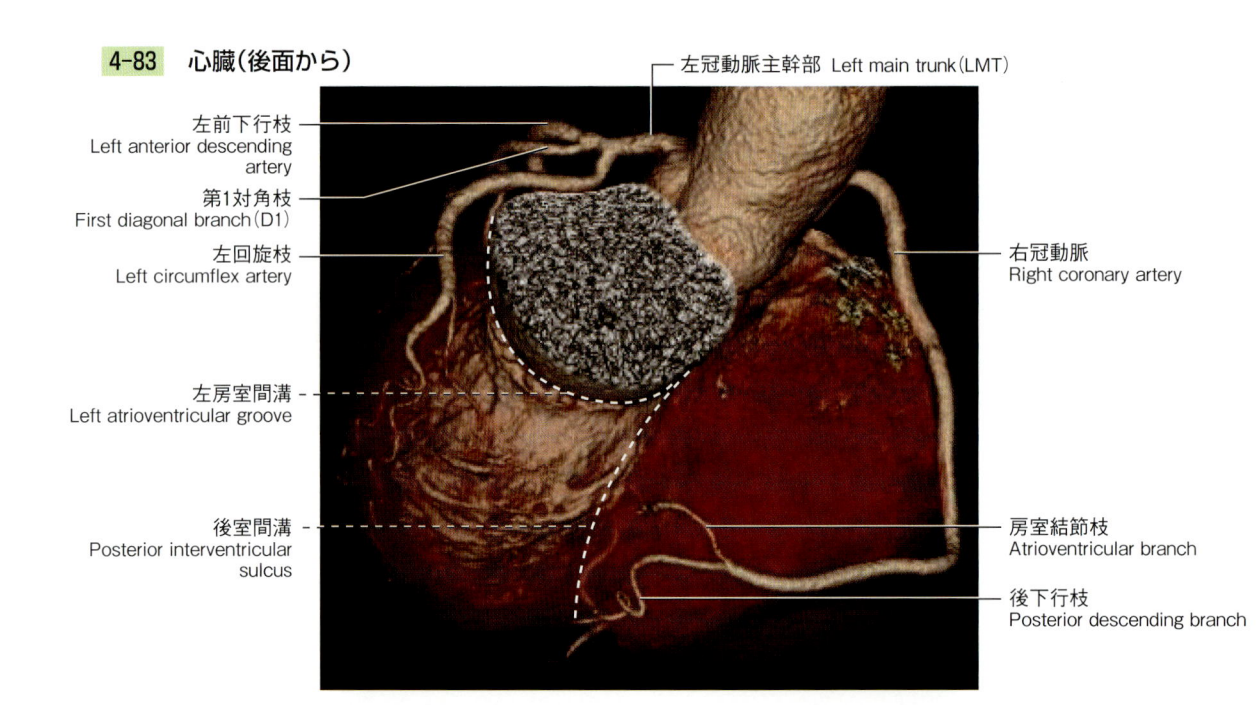

> **NOTE** 冠動脈は右冠動脈，左冠動脈の前下行枝および回旋枝という3つの主要な動脈により構成される．これらの走行を理解するには，心臓表面の構造を考えるとよい．心房と心室の関係に注目すると，その境目にある溝を房室間溝といい，右房と右室を分けるのが右房室間溝，左房と左室を分けるのが左房室間溝である．右房室間溝に右冠動脈が主に走行し，左房室間溝に左回旋枝が走行する．

冠動脈（CT, VR 像）

4-84　心臓（前面上方から）

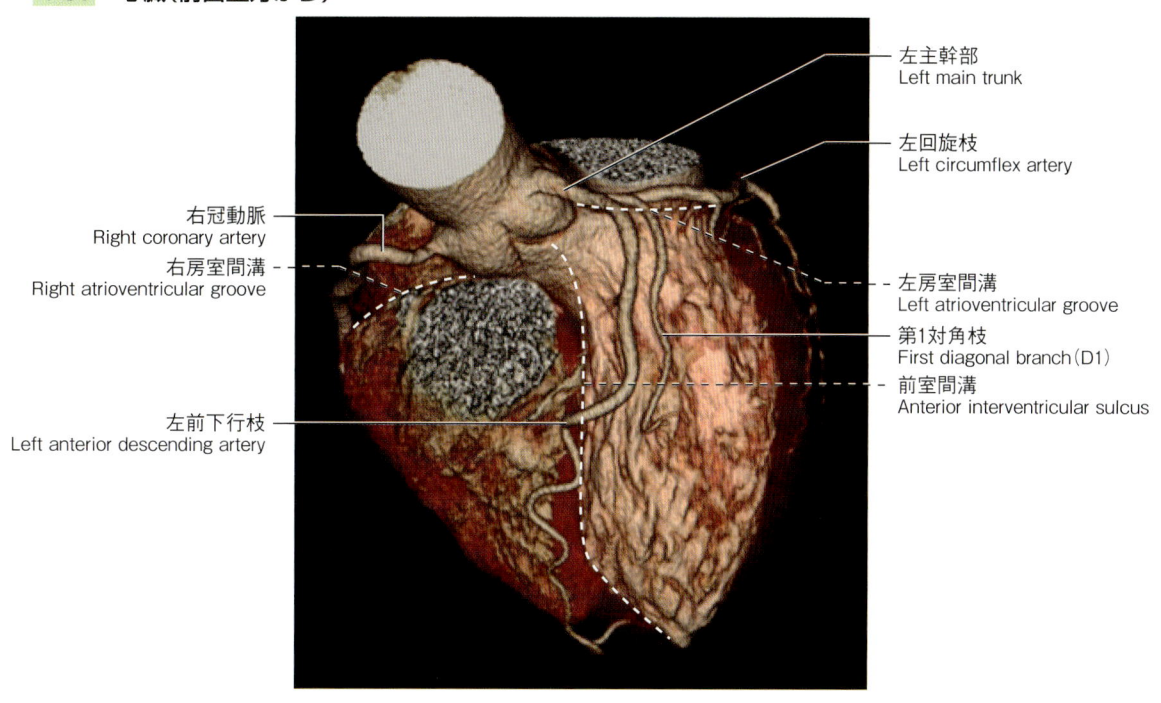

- 左主幹部　Left main trunk
- 左回旋枝　Left circumflex artery
- 右冠動脈　Right coronary artery
- 右房室間溝　Right atrioventricular groove
- 左房室間溝　Left atrioventricular groove
- 第1対角枝　First diagonal branch (D1)
- 前室間溝　Anterior interventricular sulcus
- 左前下行枝　Left anterior descending artery

4-85　心臓（後面下方から）

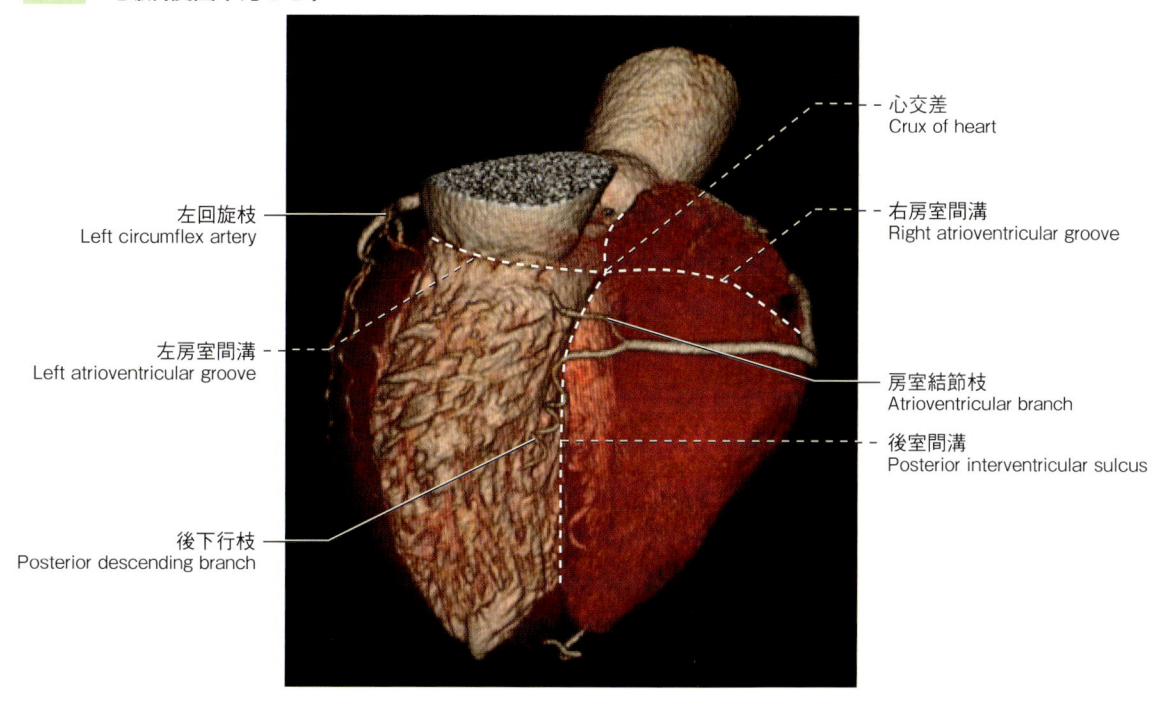

- 心交差　Crux of heart
- 左回旋枝　Left circumflex artery
- 右房室間溝　Right atrioventricular groove
- 左房室間溝　Left atrioventricular groove
- 房室結節枝　Atrioventricular branch
- 後室間溝　Posterior interventricular sulcus
- 後下行枝　Posterior descending branch

NOTE 右心室と左心室の関係に注目すると，心臓の前面で右心室と左心室を分けている溝が前室間溝で，心尖部より後面で右心室と左心室を分ける溝を後室間溝とよぶ．前室間溝に左前下行枝が主に走行する．ちなみに心房と心室を分ける左右の房室間溝と，後面で右心室と左心室を分ける後室間溝が交わる部分は心交差（心十字）とよばれる．

冠動脈（CT, VR像）

4-86　心臓（右前面から）

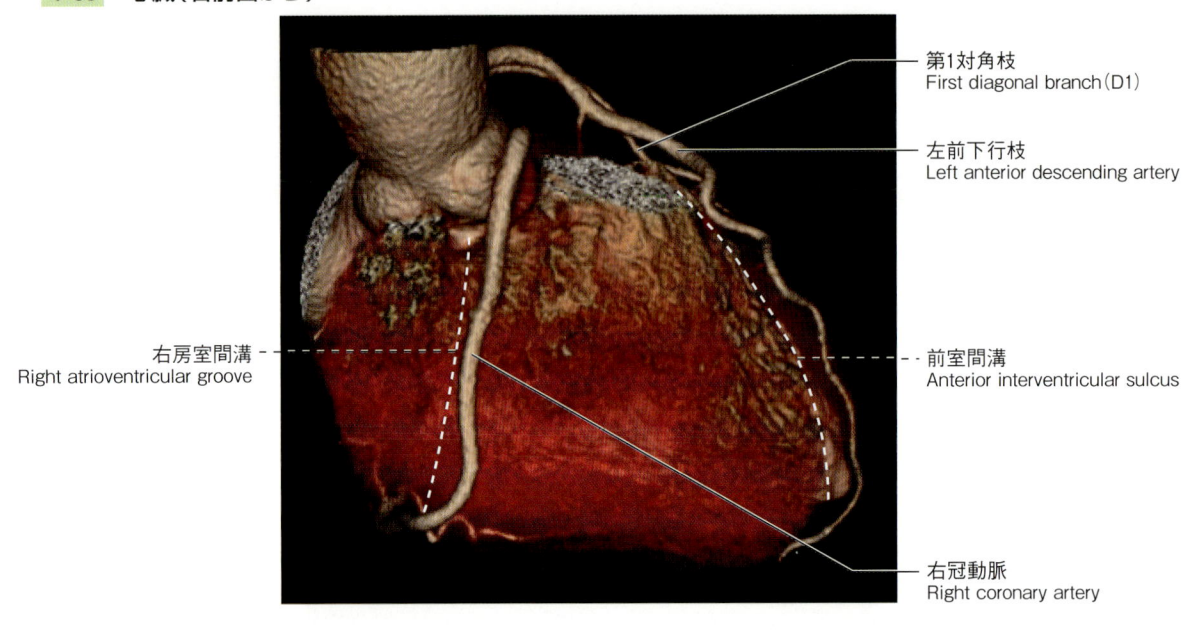

- 第1対角枝　First diagonal branch (D1)
- 左前下行枝　Left anterior descending artery
- 右房室間溝　Right atrioventricular groove
- 前室間溝　Anterior interventricular sulcus
- 右冠動脈　Right coronary artery

4-87　心臓（左前面から）

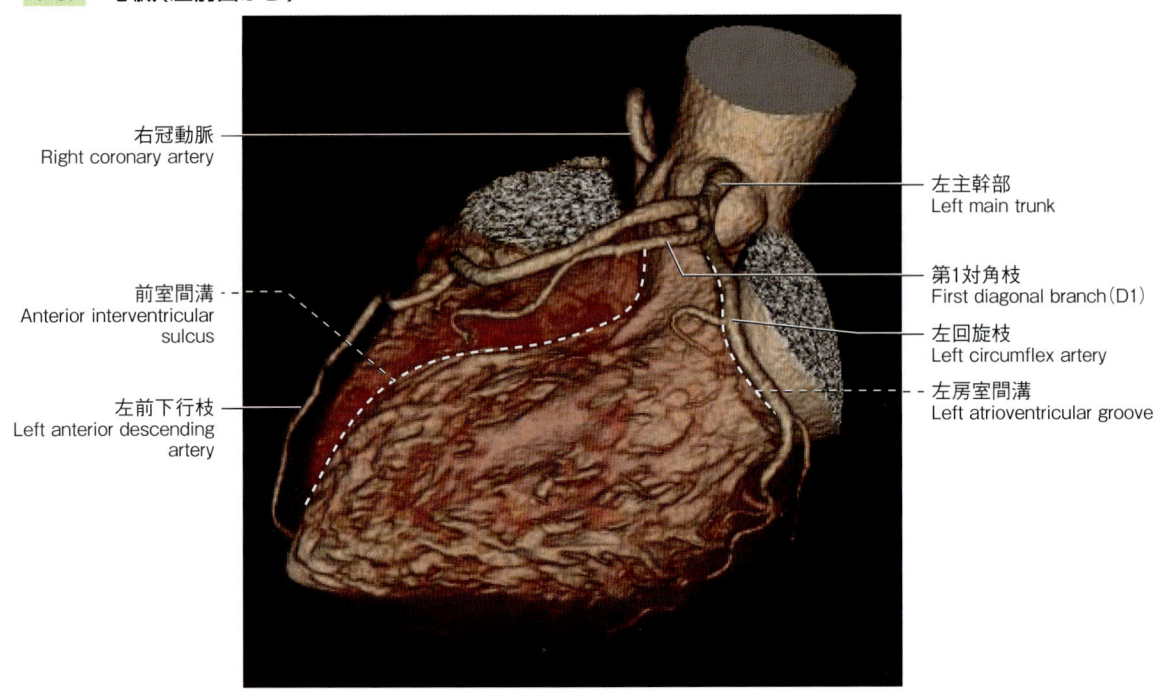

- 右冠動脈　Right coronary artery
- 左主幹部　Left main trunk
- 前室間溝　Anterior interventricular sulcus
- 第1対角枝　First diagonal branch (D1)
- 左回旋枝　Left circumflex artery
- 左前下行枝　Left anterior descending artery
- 左房室間溝　Left atrioventricular groove

> **NOTE**　心臓を前面から観察すると，右心室側は鋭い縁を形成し，鋭縁部とよばれる（4-82）．また左心室側は鈍い縁を形成し，鈍縁部とよばれる．右冠動脈は右冠動脈洞（Valsalva洞）から起始し，前述のように右房室間溝に沿って後面に向かうが，その後ろ側に回り込むところが鋭縁部となる．右冠動脈の分枝である鋭縁枝は鋭縁部付近を栄養する枝，左回旋枝の分枝である鈍縁枝は鈍縁部を栄養する枝となる．

冠動脈の AHA 分類 (CT, VR 像)

4-88 右冠動脈（RCA #1～4）

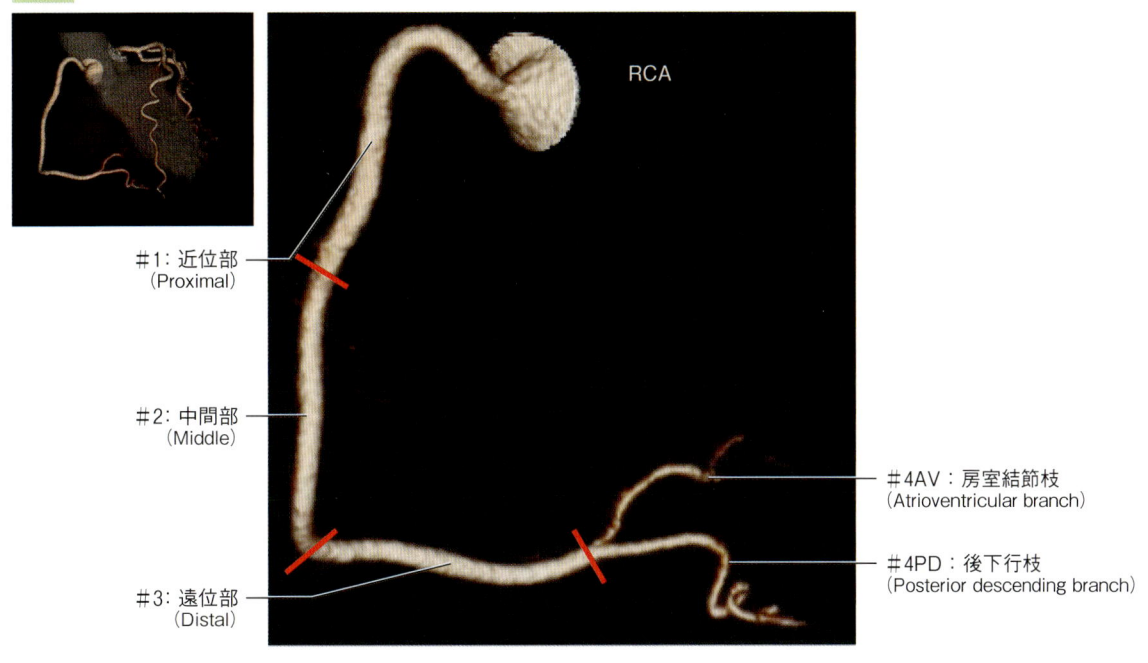

RCA

- #1：近位部（Proximal）
- #2：中間部（Middle）
- #3：遠位部（Distal）
- #4AV：房室結節枝（Atrioventricular branch）
- #4PD：後下行枝（Posterior descending branch）

4-89 左冠動脈（前面から）（LMT #5, LAD #6～10, LCX #11～15）

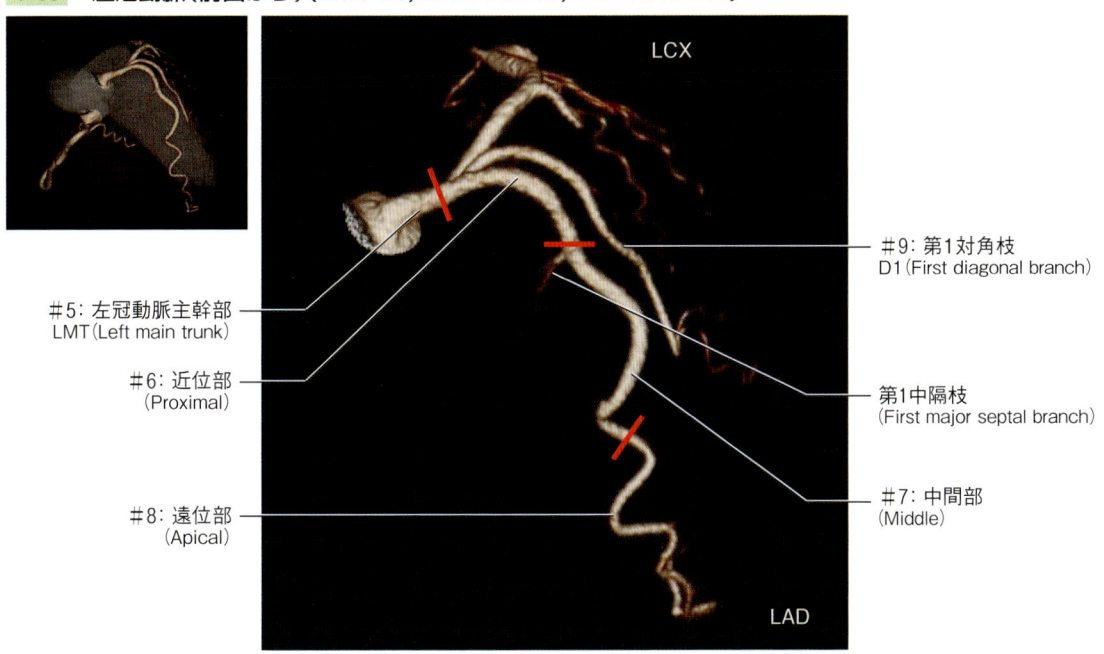

LCX

- #5：左冠動脈主幹部 LMT（Left main trunk）
- #6：近位部（Proximal）
- #8：遠位部（Apical）
- #9：第1対角枝 D1（First diagonal branch）
- 第1中隔枝（First major septal branch）
- #7：中間部（Middle）

LAD

> **NOTE** AHA（American Heart Association：米国心臓協会）分類では，冠動脈の主要な部分に，セグメント（segment）1（#1）から #15 までの番号を割り当てている．右冠動脈（RCA）は #1～4，左冠動脈主幹部（LMT）は #5，左冠動脈前下行枝（LAD）およびその分枝は #6～10，そして左冠動脈回旋枝（LCX）およびその分枝は #11～14 となっている．後室間溝を走行する後下行枝が，右冠動脈から支配される右優位型の場合は #4PD，左冠動脈から支配される場合は #15PD と表記される．

冠動脈の AHA 分類（CT, VR 像）

4-90 左冠動脈（後面から）(LMT #5, LAD #6〜10, LCX #11〜15)

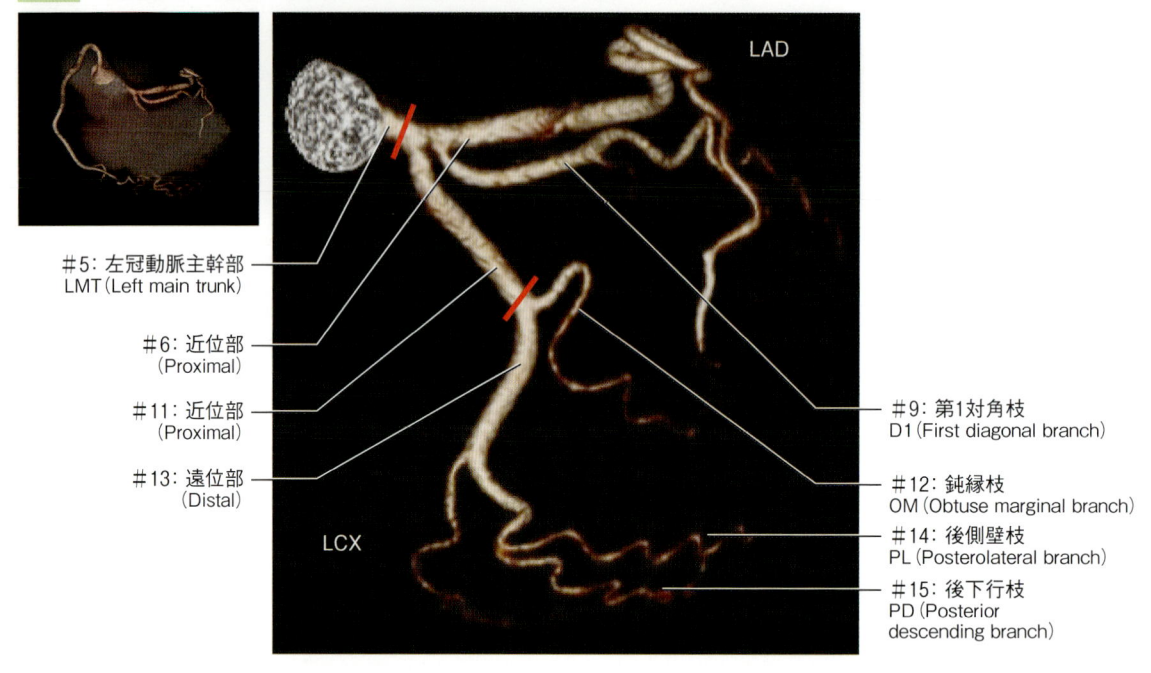

- #5: 左冠動脈主幹部 LMT (Left main trunk)
- #6: 近位部 (Proximal)
- #11: 近位部 (Proximal)
- #13: 遠位部 (Distal)
- #9: 第1対角枝 D1 (First diagonal branch)
- #12: 鈍縁枝 OM (Obtuse marginal branch)
- #14: 後側壁枝 PL (Posterolateral branch)
- #15: 後下行枝 PD (Posterior descending branch)

4-91 左冠動脈（側面から）(LMT #5, LAD #6〜10, LCX #11〜15)

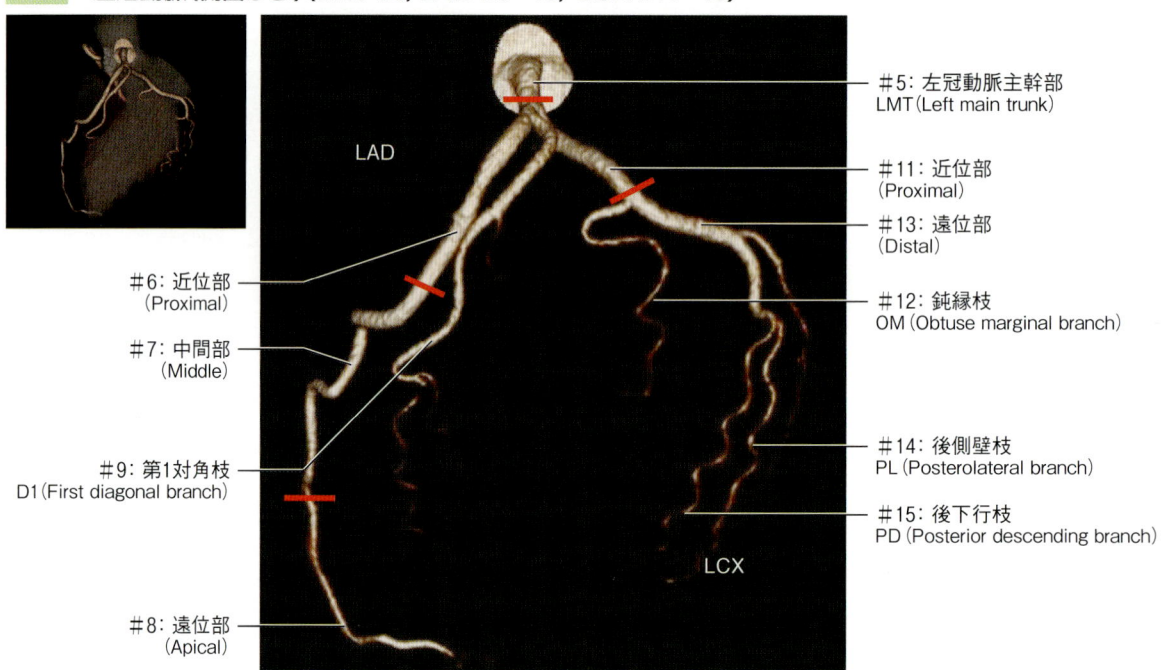

- #5: 左冠動脈主幹部 LMT (Left main trunk)
- #6: 近位部 (Proximal)
- #7: 中間部 (Middle)
- #9: 第1対角枝 D1 (First diagonal branch)
- #8: 遠位部 (Apical)
- #11: 近位部 (Proximal)
- #13: 遠位部 (Distal)
- #12: 鈍縁枝 OM (Obtuse marginal branch)
- #14: 後側壁枝 PL (Posterolateral branch)
- #15: 後下行枝 PD (Posterior descending branch)

> **NOTE** 右冠動脈(RCA)では，鋭縁部が #2(中間部)と #3(遠位部)の境界となり，起始部から鋭縁部を二等分すれば #1(近位部)と #2(中間部)となる(4-88)．左冠動脈前下行枝(LAD)では，最初に分枝した中隔枝(第1中隔枝)までが #6(近位部)，第1中隔枝の分枝から心尖部までを二等分したものが，#7(中間部)と #8(遠位部)になる(4-89)．#9(第1対角枝)と #10(第2対角枝)は前下行枝の分枝で，左室表面を走行する．左冠動脈回旋枝(LCX)は #11(近位部)と #13(遠位部)で，この境界が #12(鈍縁枝)，また #14(後側壁枝)が遠位部より分枝する(4-90, 91)．

心臓の断層解剖 ［横断像（造影CT）］

4-92

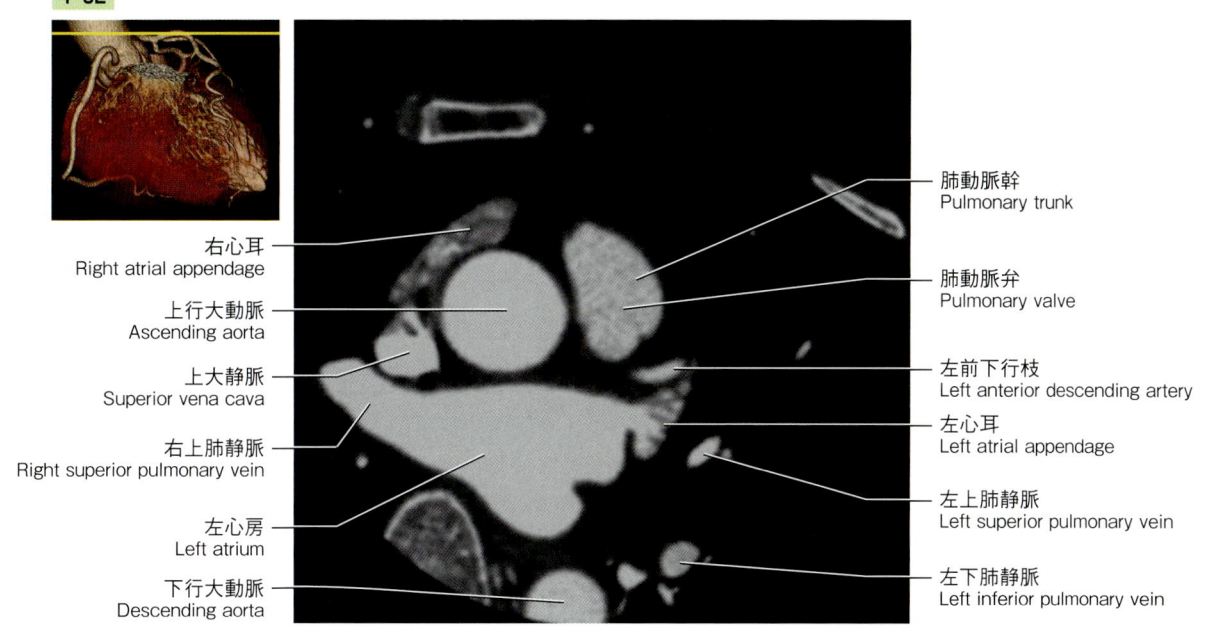

- 肺動脈幹 / Pulmonary trunk
- 右心耳 / Right atrial appendage
- 肺動脈弁 / Pulmonary valve
- 上行大動脈 / Ascending aorta
- 上大静脈 / Superior vena cava
- 左前下行枝 / Left anterior descending artery
- 左心耳 / Left atrial appendage
- 右上肺静脈 / Right superior pulmonary vein
- 左上肺静脈 / Left superior pulmonary vein
- 左心房 / Left atrium
- 左下肺静脈 / Left inferior pulmonary vein
- 下行大動脈 / Descending aorta

4-93

- 右心室（動脈円錐） / Conus arteriosus
- 右心耳 / Right atrial appendage
- 左冠動脈主幹部 / Left main trunk（LMT）
- 上大静脈 / Superior vena cava
- 左前下行枝 / Left anterior descending artery
- 上行大動脈 / Ascending aorta
- 第1対角枝 / D1（First diagonal branch）
- 右上肺静脈 / Right superior pulmonary vein
- 左上肺静脈 / Left superior pulmonary vein
- 左心房 / Left atrium
- 左下肺静脈 / Left inferior pulmonary vein
- 左下肺静脈 / Left inferior pulmonary vein
- 下行大動脈 / Descending aorta

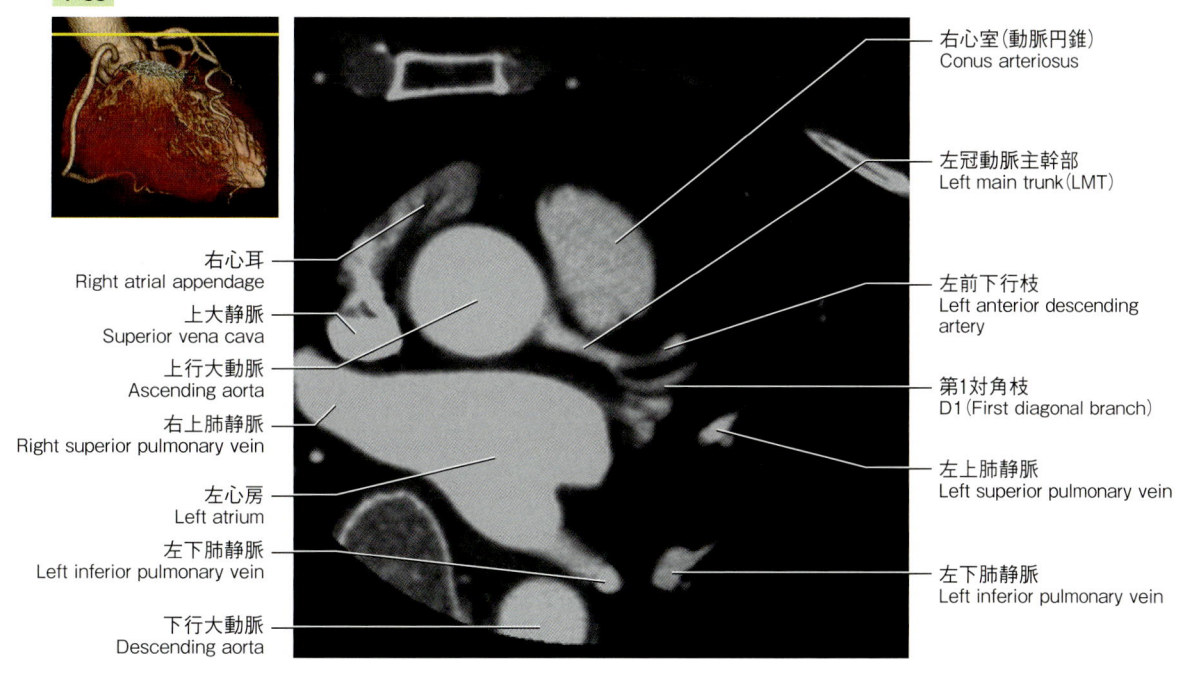

NOTE 右心房の頭側では，最も背側の部分が上大静脈の流入部に相当し，腹側の部分は上行大動脈を巻くような形態を呈し，右心耳とよばれる．一方，左心房から連続し，肺動脈幹の左側で左冠動脈を背側から頭側に覆うように左心耳が存在する．左心耳内面には櫛状筋によってできる多数の筋性隆起が存在する．

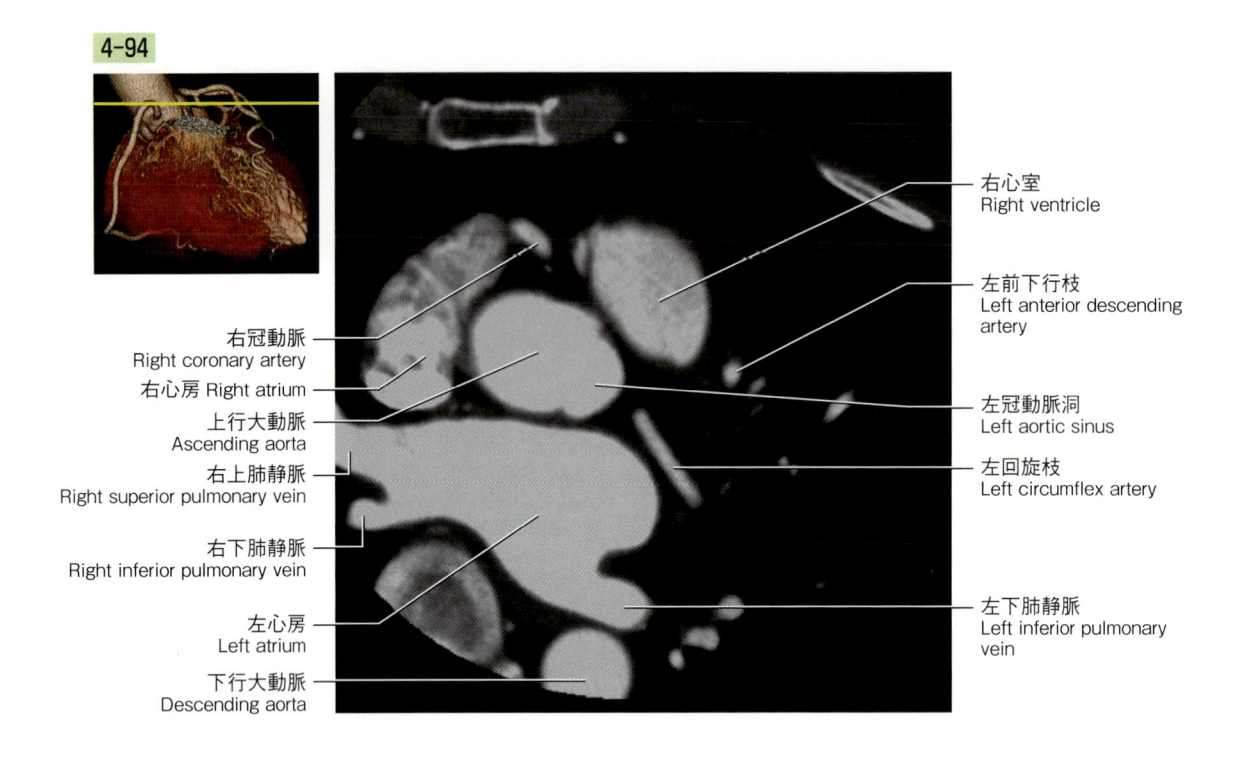

心臓の断層解剖 ［横断像（造影CT）］

4-94

- 右心室 Right ventricle
- 左前下行枝 Left anterior descending artery
- 左冠動脈洞 Left aortic sinus
- 左回旋枝 Left circumflex artery
- 左下肺静脈 Left inferior pulmonary vein
- 右冠動脈 Right coronary artery
- 右心房 Right atrium
- 上行大動脈 Ascending aorta
- 右上肺静脈 Right superior pulmonary vein
- 右下肺静脈 Right inferior pulmonary vein
- 左心房 Left atrium
- 下行大動脈 Descending aorta

4-95

- 右心室 Right ventricle
- 左前下行枝 Left anterior descending artery
- 左冠動脈洞 Left aortic sinus
- 左回旋枝 Left circumflex artery
- 左下肺静脈 Left inferior pulmonary vein
- 右心耳 Right atrial appendage
- 右心房 Right atrium
- 右冠動脈洞 Right aortic sinus
- 上行大動脈 Ascending aorta
- 右下肺静脈 Right inferior pulmonary vein
- 下行大動脈 Descending aorta

> **NOTE** 上行大動脈の起始部は膨隆しており，大動脈球部とよばれ，またその内腔は冠動脈洞あるいはValsalva洞とよばれる．冠動脈洞は右冠動脈洞，左冠動脈洞，および無冠動脈洞の3つからなり，最も腹側に存在するのが右冠動脈洞，左側に存在するのが左冠動脈洞，右背側に存在するのが無冠動脈洞である．

心臓の断層解剖 ［横断像（造影CT）］

4-96

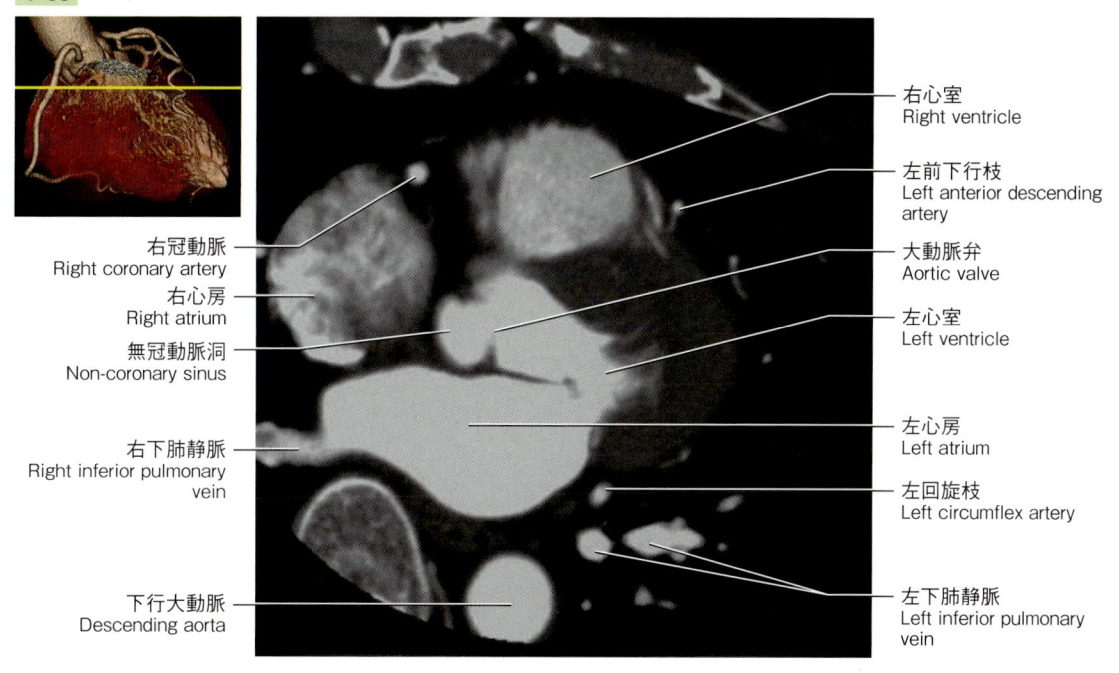

- 右心室 Right ventricle
- 左前下行枝 Left anterior descending artery
- 右冠動脈 Right coronary artery
- 大動脈弁 Aortic valve
- 右心房 Right atrium
- 左心室 Left ventricle
- 無冠動脈洞 Non-coronary sinus
- 左心房 Left atrium
- 右下肺静脈 Right inferior pulmonary vein
- 左回旋枝 Left circumflex artery
- 下行大動脈 Descending aorta
- 左下肺静脈 Left inferior pulmonary vein

4-97

- 心室中隔 Interventricular septum
- 左前下行枝 Left anterior descending artery
- 右冠動脈 Right coronary artery
- 左心室 Left ventricle
- 前乳頭筋 Anterior papillary muscle
- 右心房 Right atrium
- 僧帽弁前尖 Mitral valve anterior leaflet
- 三尖弁 Tricuspid valve
- 僧帽弁後尖 Mitral valve posterior leaflet
- 右心室 Right ventricle
- 左回旋枝 Left circumflex artery
- 左心房 Left atrium
- 下行大動脈 Descending aorta

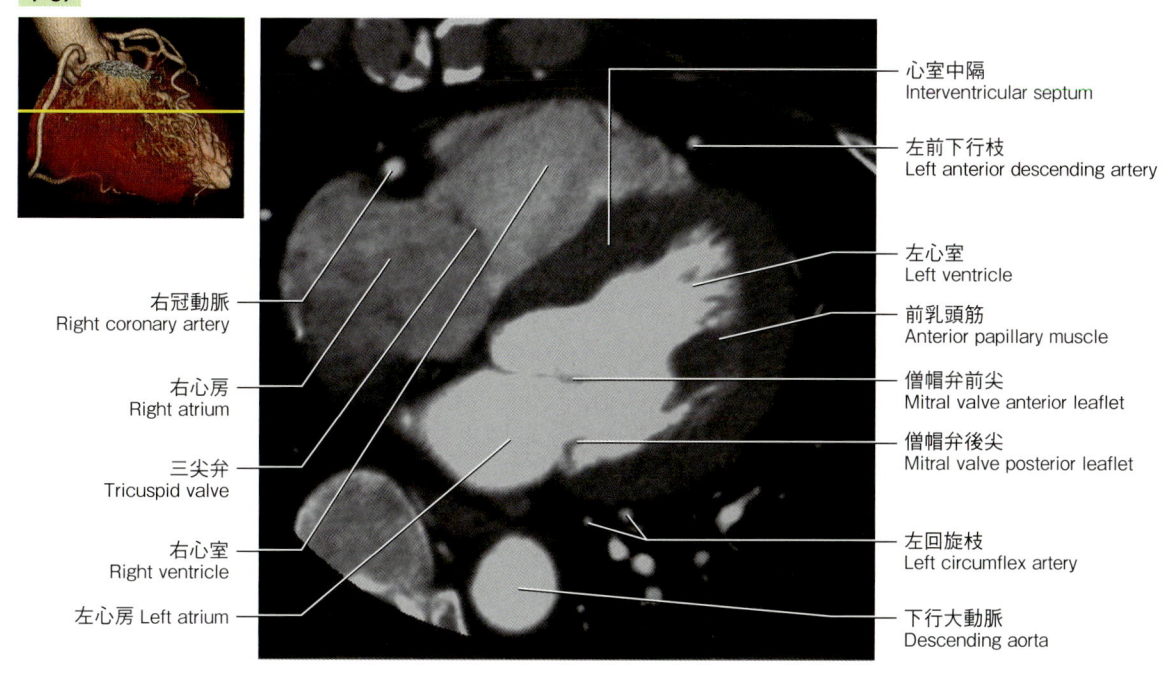

NOTE 僧房弁は，前尖と後尖という2つの弁尖からなる．心臓にある他の3弁（三尖弁，肺動脈弁，大動脈弁）がすべて3つの弁尖から成り立っていることと比較して特徴的であり，別名で二尖弁ともよばれる．先端は左心室側にあり，ヒモ状の腱索を介して乳頭筋につながっている．

心臓の断層解剖 [横断像（造影CT）]

4-98

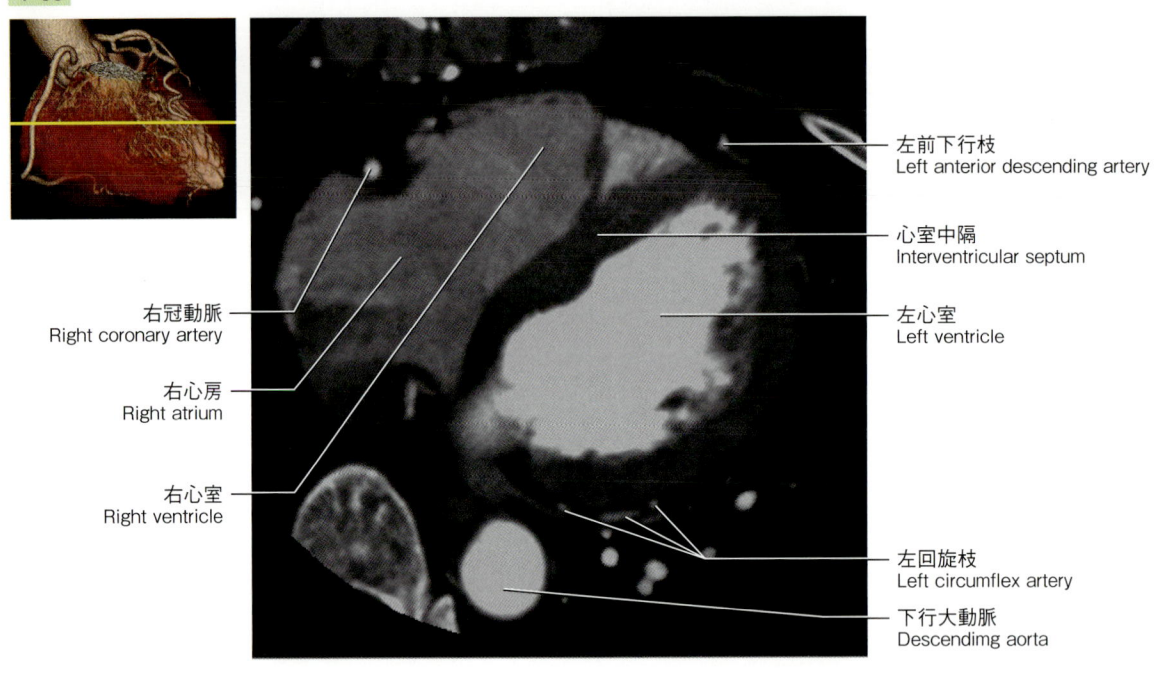

- 右冠動脈 Right coronary artery
- 右心房 Right atrium
- 右心室 Right ventricle
- 左前下行枝 Left anterior descending artery
- 心室中隔 Interventricular septum
- 左心室 Left ventricle
- 左回旋枝 Left circumflex artery
- 下行大動脈 Descendimg aorta

4-99

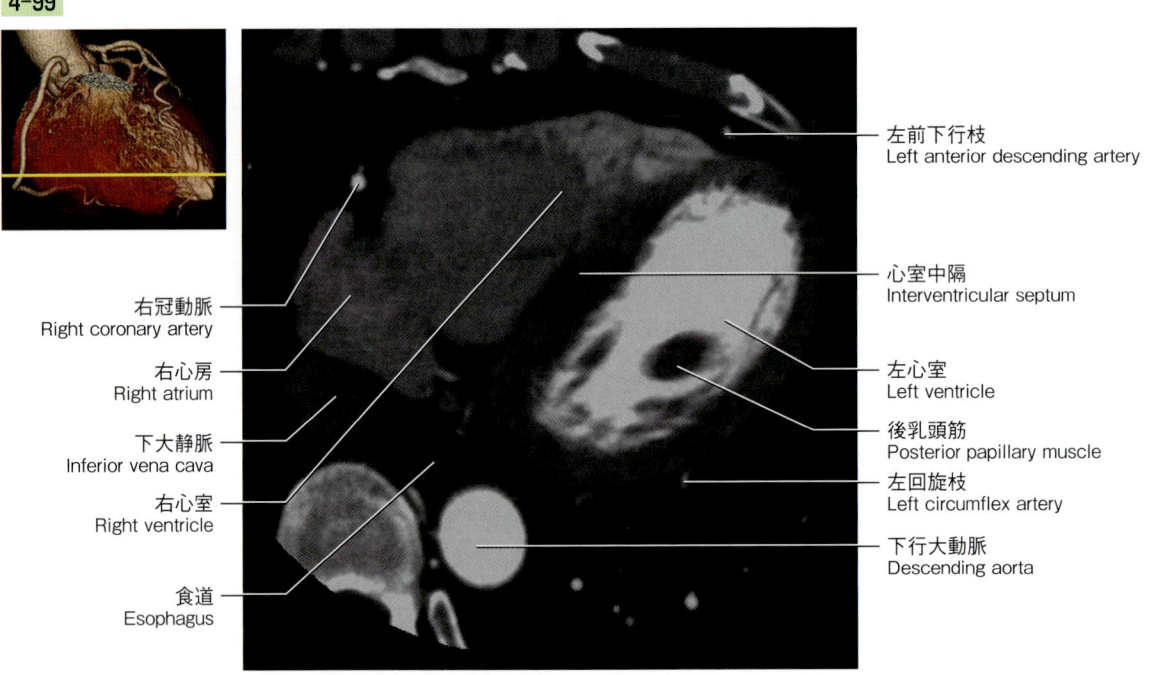

- 右冠動脈 Right coronary artery
- 右心房 Right atrium
- 下大静脈 Inferior vena cava
- 右心室 Right ventricle
- 食道 Esophagus
- 左前下行枝 Left anterior descending artery
- 心室中隔 Interventricular septum
- 左心室 Left ventricle
- 後乳頭筋 Posterior papillary muscle
- 左回旋枝 Left circumflex artery
- 下行大動脈 Descending aorta

心臓の断層解剖 ［横断像（造影CT）］

4-100

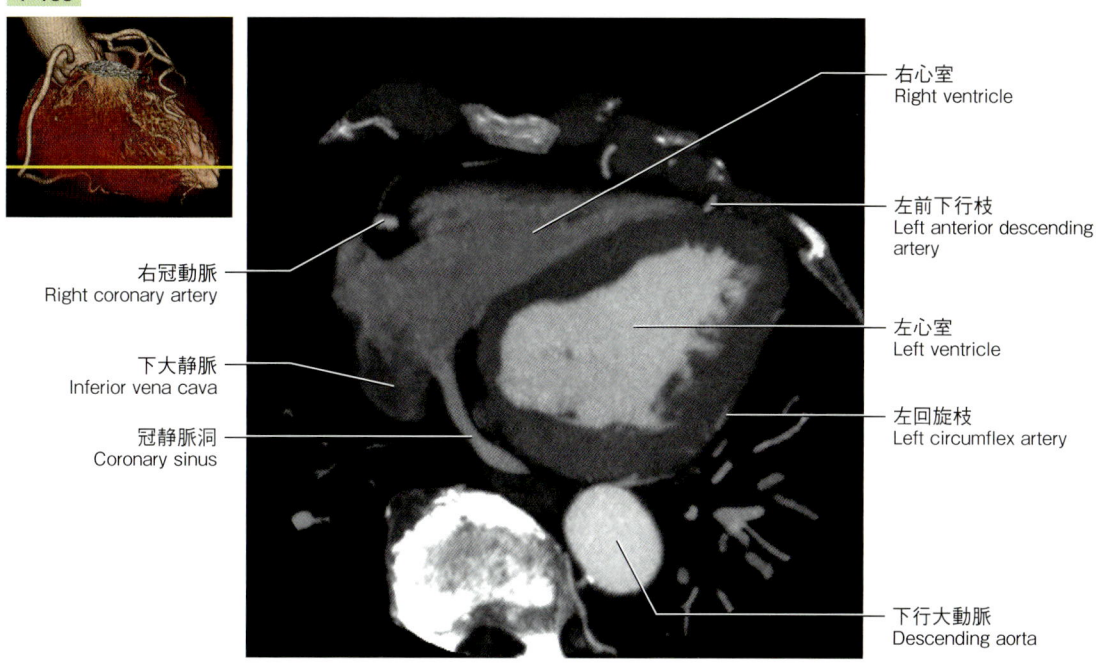

- 右心室 / Right ventricle
- 左前下行枝 / Left anterior descending artery
- 左心室 / Left ventricle
- 左回旋枝 / Left circumflex artery
- 下行大動脈 / Descending aorta
- 右冠動脈 / Right coronary artery
- 下大静脈 / Inferior vena cava
- 冠静脈洞 / Coronary sinus

4-101

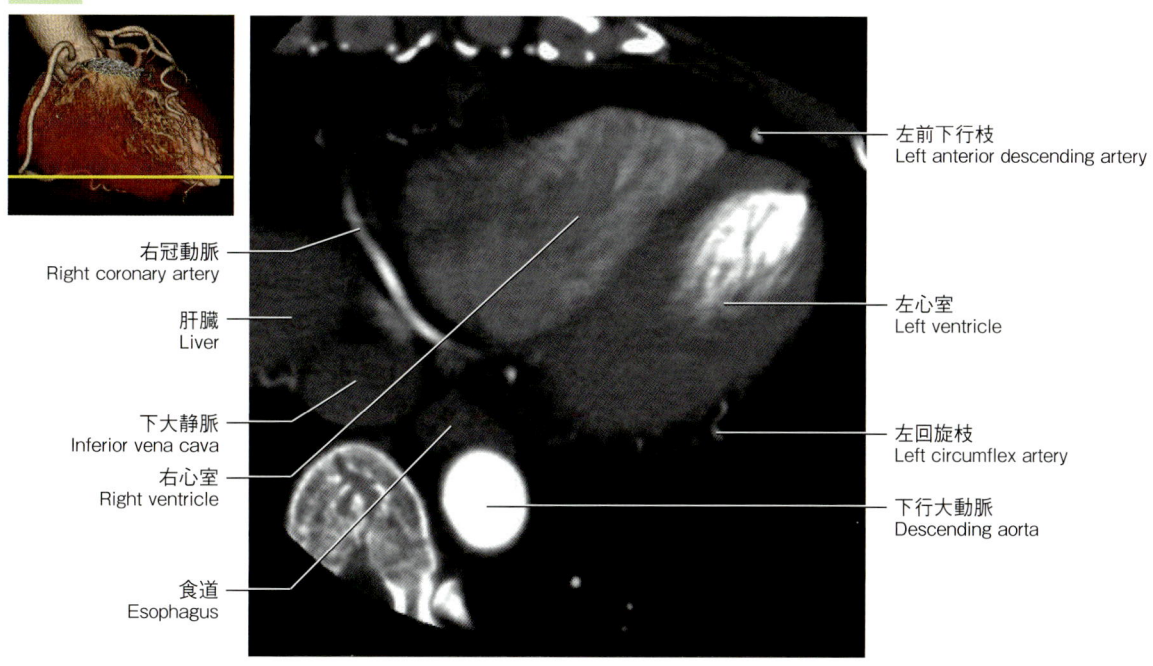

- 左前下行枝 / Left anterior descending artery
- 左心室 / Left ventricle
- 左回旋枝 / Left circumflex artery
- 下行大動脈 / Descending aorta
- 右冠動脈 / Right coronary artery
- 肝臓 / Liver
- 下大静脈 / Inferior vena cava
- 右心室 / Right ventricle
- 食道 / Esophagus

心臓の断層解剖 ［矢状断像（造影CT）］

4-102

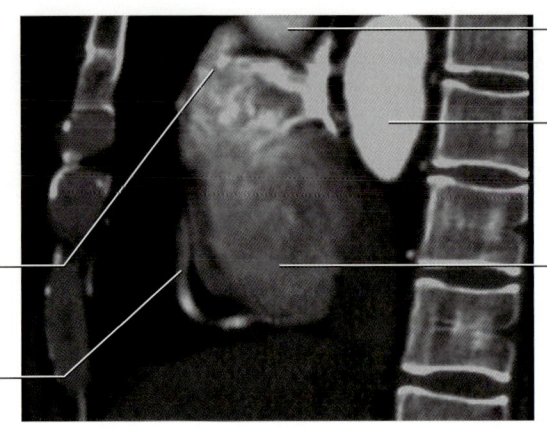

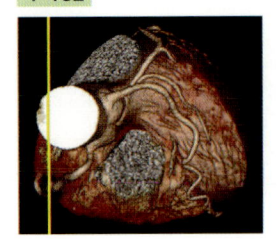

- 上行大動脈 Ascending aorta
- 左心房 Left atrium
- 上大静脈 Superior vena cava
- 右心房 Right atrium
- 右冠動脈 Right coronary artery

4-103

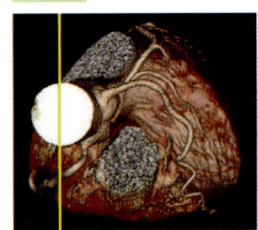

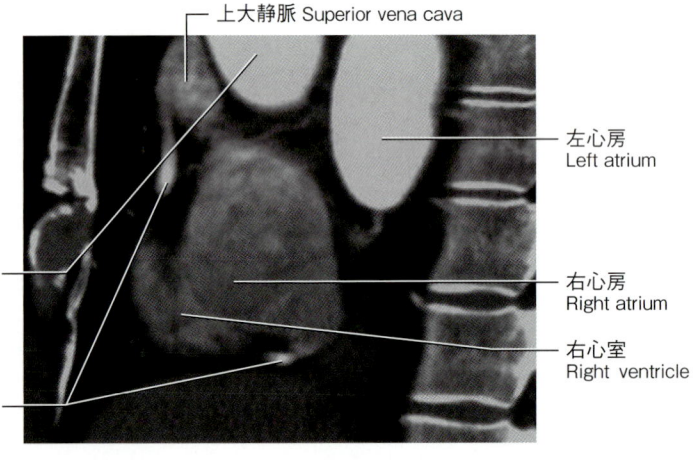

- 上大静脈 Superior vena cava
- 左心房 Left atrium
- 上行大動脈 Ascending aorta
- 右心房 Right atrium
- 右心室 Right ventricle
- 右冠動脈 Right coronary artery

4-104

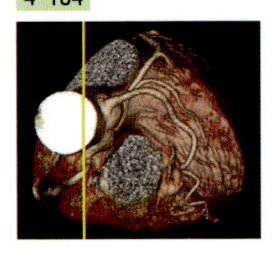

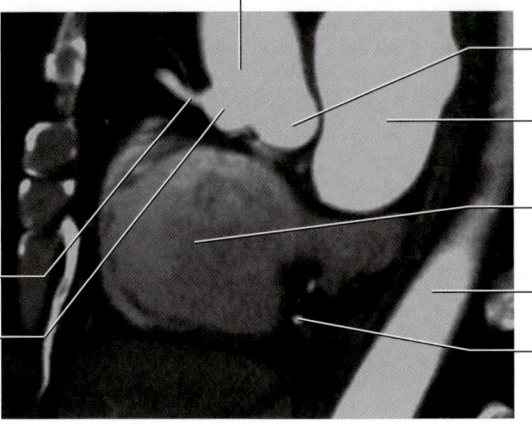

- 上行大動脈 Ascending aorta
- 無冠動脈洞 Non-coronary sinus
- 左心房 Left atrium
- 右心室 Right ventricle
- 右冠動脈 Right coronary artery
- 右冠動脈洞 Right aortic sinus
- 下行大動脈 Descending aorta
- 右冠動脈 Right coronary artery

心臓の断層解剖 ［矢状断像（造影CT）］

4-105

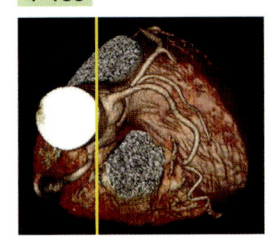

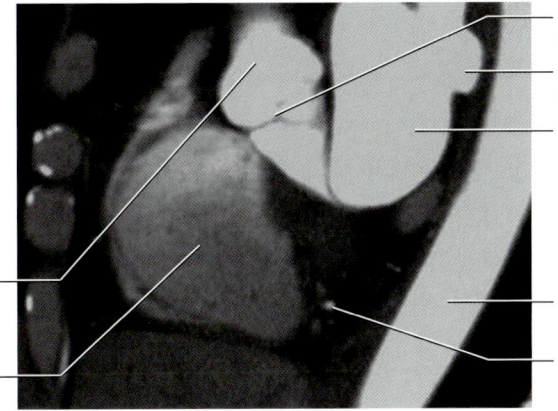

- 大動脈弁 Aortic valve
- 左下肺静脈 Left inferior pulmonary vein
- 左心房 Left atrium
- 上行大動脈 Ascending aorta
- 下行大動脈 Descending aorta
- 右心室 Right ventricle
- 右冠動脈 Right coronary artery

4-106

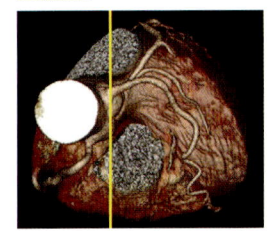

- 肺動脈弁 Pulmonary valve
- 左心房 Left atrium
- 左冠動脈主幹部 Left main trunk（LMT）
- 左冠動脈洞 Left aortic sinus
- 右心室（動脈円錐） Conus arteriosus
- 左心室 Left ventricle
- 大動脈弁 Aortic valve
- 僧帽弁 Mitral valve
- 右心室 Right ventricle
- 右冠動脈 Right coronary artery

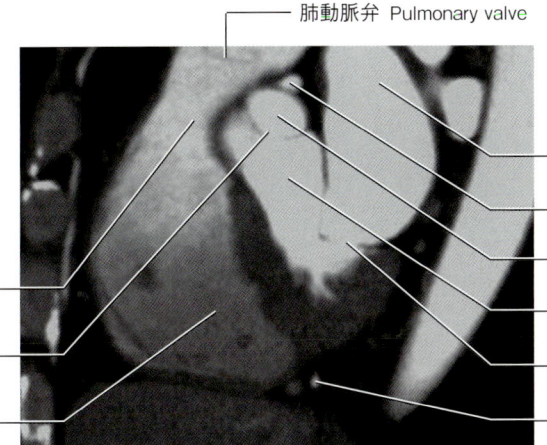

4-107

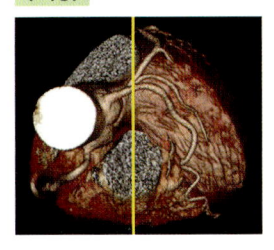

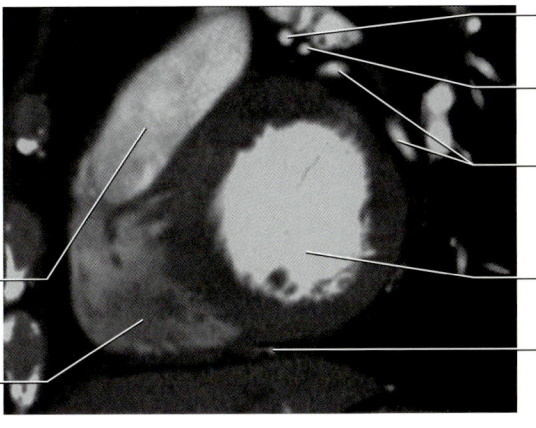

- 左前下行枝 Left anterior descending artery
- 第1対角枝 D1（First diagonal branch）
- 左回旋枝 Left circumflex artery
- 右心室（動脈円錐） Conus arteriosus
- 左心室 Left ventricle
- 右心室 Right ventricle
- 右冠動脈 Light coronary artery

心臓の断層解剖 ［矢状断像（造影CT）］

4-108

- 左前下行枝 Left anterior descending artery
- 第1対角枝 D1 (First diagonal branch)
- 左回旋枝 Left circumflex artery
- 左心室 Left ventricle
- 右冠動脈 Light coronary artery
- 心室中隔 Interventricular septum
- 右心室 Right ventricle

4-109

- 前乳頭筋 Anterior papillary muscle
- 第1対角枝 D1 (First diagonal branch)
- 左前下行枝 Left anterior descending artery
- 左回旋枝 Left circumflex artery
- 後乳頭筋 Posterior papillary muscle
- 心室中隔 Interventricular septum
- 左心室 Left ventricle
- 右心室 Right ventricle

4-110

- 第1対角枝 D1 (First diagonal branch)
- 左前下行枝 Left anterior descending artery
- 左回旋枝 Left circumflex artery
- 前乳頭筋 Anterior papillary muscle
- 後乳頭筋 Posterior papillary muscle
- 心室中隔 Interventricular septum
- 左心室 Left ventricle
- 右心室 Right ventricle

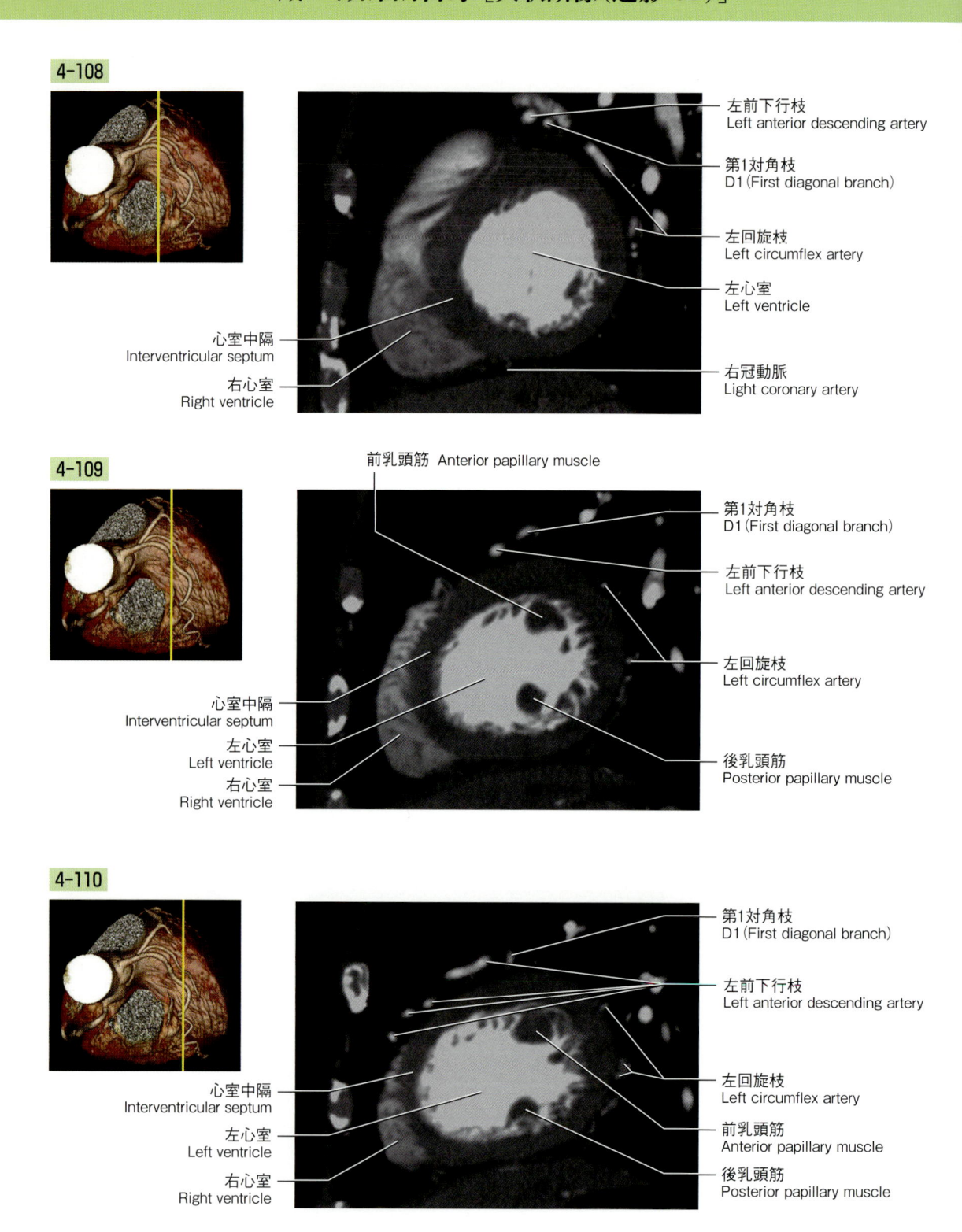

> **NOTE** 乳頭筋は，心室にある円錐形の筋肉で，腱索によって房室弁（三尖弁，僧房弁）と連絡し，弁の開閉機能に重要な役割を果たしている．左心室には前乳頭筋と後乳頭筋があり，おのおのの腱索を介し僧房弁の前尖と後尖を支持している．僧帽弁は左心室側に開くが，閉じる際には弁が左心房側に反転しないように乳頭筋が伸縮し，腱索の緊張を起こす．

心臓の断層解剖 ［冠状断像（造影CT）］

4-111

- 右心房 Right atrium
- 右冠動脈 Right coronary artery
- 右心室 Right ventricle
- 左前下行枝 Left anterior descending artery
- 左心室 Left ventricle
- 左前下行枝 Left anterior descending artery

4-112

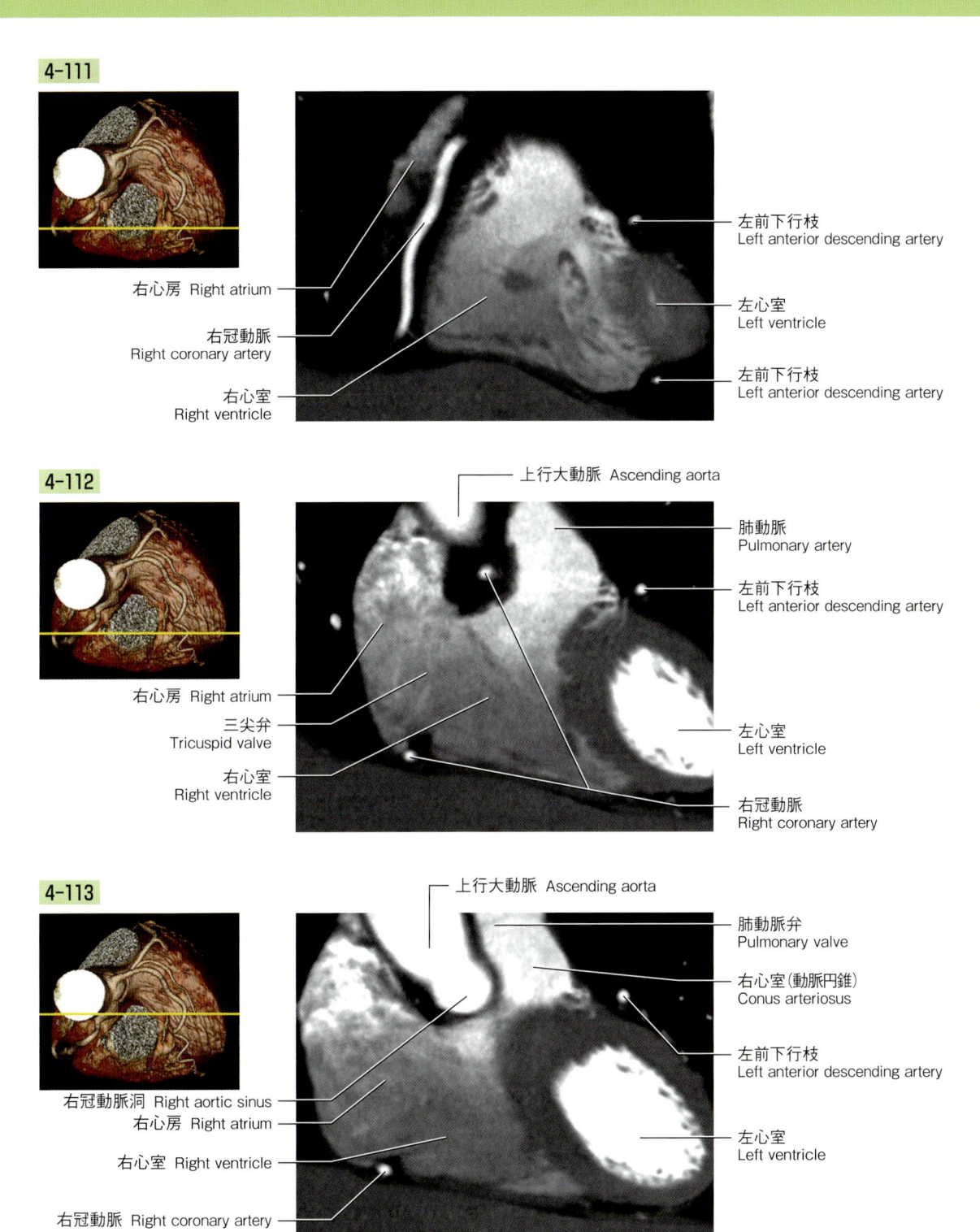

- 右心房 Right atrium
- 三尖弁 Tricuspid valve
- 右心室 Right ventricle
- 上行大動脈 Ascending aorta
- 肺動脈 Pulmonary artery
- 左前下行枝 Left anterior descending artery
- 左心室 Left ventricle
- 右冠動脈 Right coronary artery

4-113

- 右冠動脈洞 Right aortic sinus
- 右心房 Right atrium
- 右心室 Right ventricle
- 右冠動脈 Right coronary artery
- 上行大動脈 Ascending aorta
- 肺動脈弁 Pulmonary valve
- 右心室（動脈円錐） Conus arteriosus
- 左前下行枝 Left anterior descending artery
- 左心室 Left ventricle

心臓の断層解剖 ［冠状断像（造影 CT）］

4-114

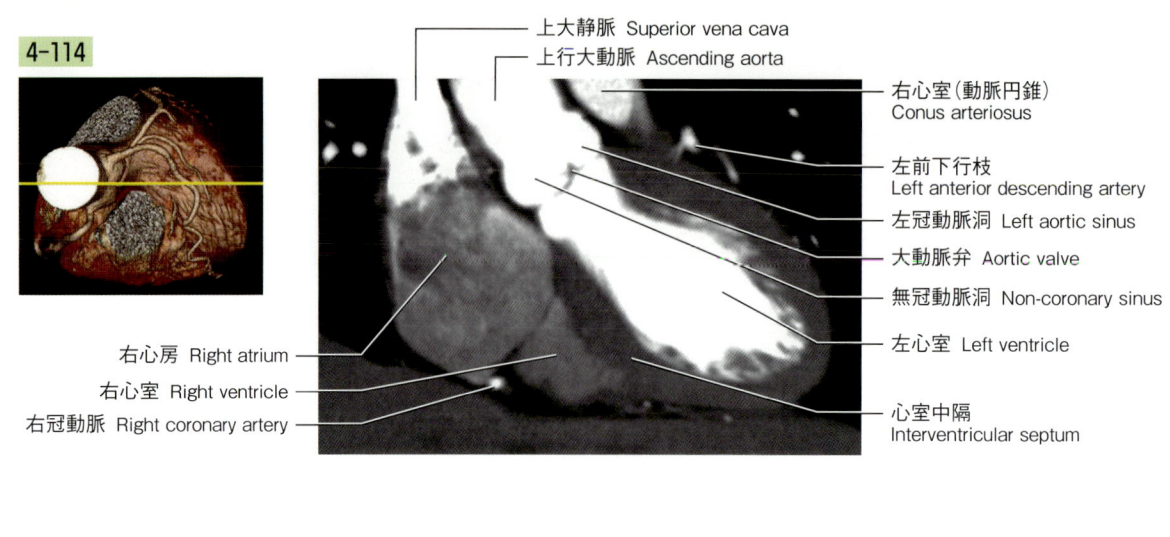

- 上大静脈 Superior vena cava
- 上行大動脈 Ascending aorta
- 右心室（動脈円錐） Conus arteriosus
- 左前下行枝 Left anterior descending artery
- 左冠動脈洞 Left aortic sinus
- 大動脈弁 Aortic valve
- 無冠動脈洞 Non-coronary sinus
- 左心室 Left ventricle
- 心室中隔 Interventricular septum
- 右心房 Right atrium
- 右心室 Right ventricle
- 右冠動脈 Right coronary artery

4-115

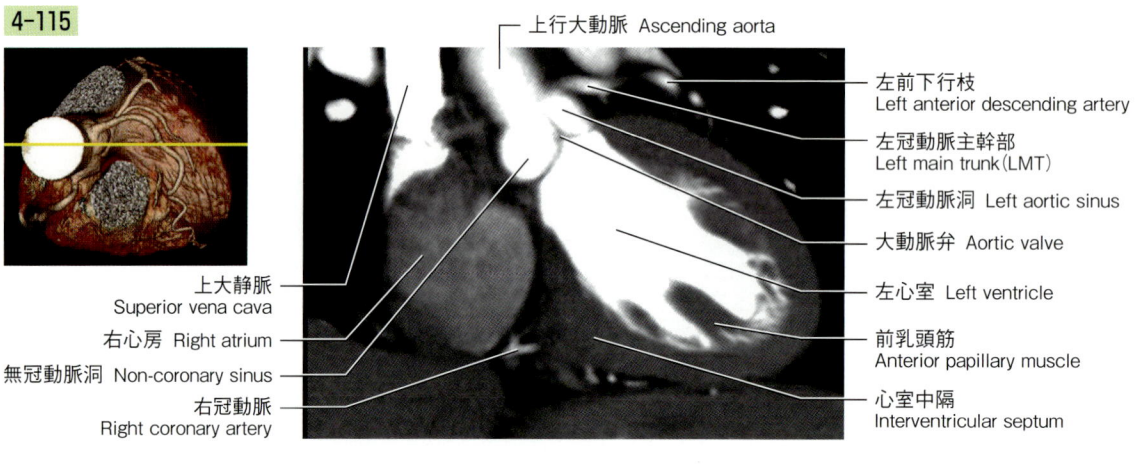

- 上行大動脈 Ascending aorta
- 左前下行枝 Left anterior descending artery
- 左冠動脈主幹部 Left main trunk（LMT）
- 左冠動脈洞 Left aortic sinus
- 大動脈弁 Aortic valve
- 左心室 Left ventricle
- 前乳頭筋 Anterior papillary muscle
- 心室中隔 Interventricular septum
- 上大静脈 Superior vena cava
- 右心房 Right atrium
- 無冠動脈洞 Non-coronary sinus
- 右冠動脈 Right coronary artery

4-116

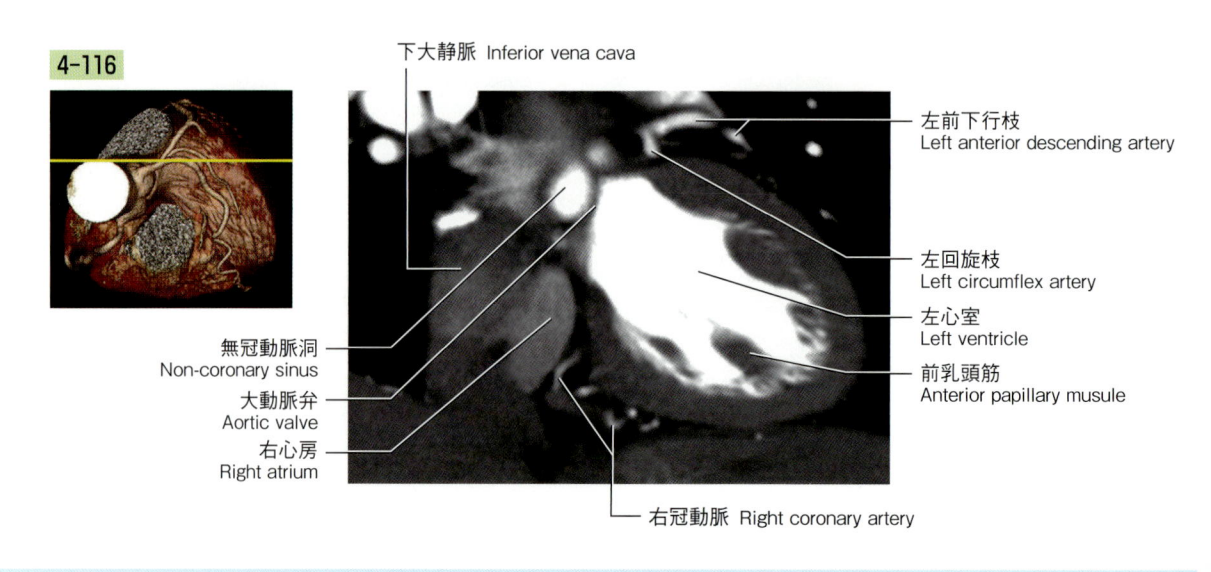

- 下大静脈 Inferior vena cava
- 左前下行枝 Left anterior descending artery
- 左回旋枝 Left circumflex artery
- 左心室 Left ventricle
- 前乳頭筋 Anterior papillary musule
- 無冠動脈洞 Non-coronary sinus
- 大動脈弁 Aortic valve
- 右心房 Right atrium
- 右冠動脈 Right coronary artery

NOTE 冠動脈は冠動脈洞から起始し，通常は右冠動脈洞から右冠動脈が，左冠動脈洞から左冠動脈が起始している．冠動脈が通常とは異なる洞から起始するタイプや，洞を越えて高位（遠位側）に位置するタイプ（高位起始）などの起始異常も経験され，臨床上問題となることがある．

心臓の断層解剖 ［冠状断像（造影 CT）］

4-117

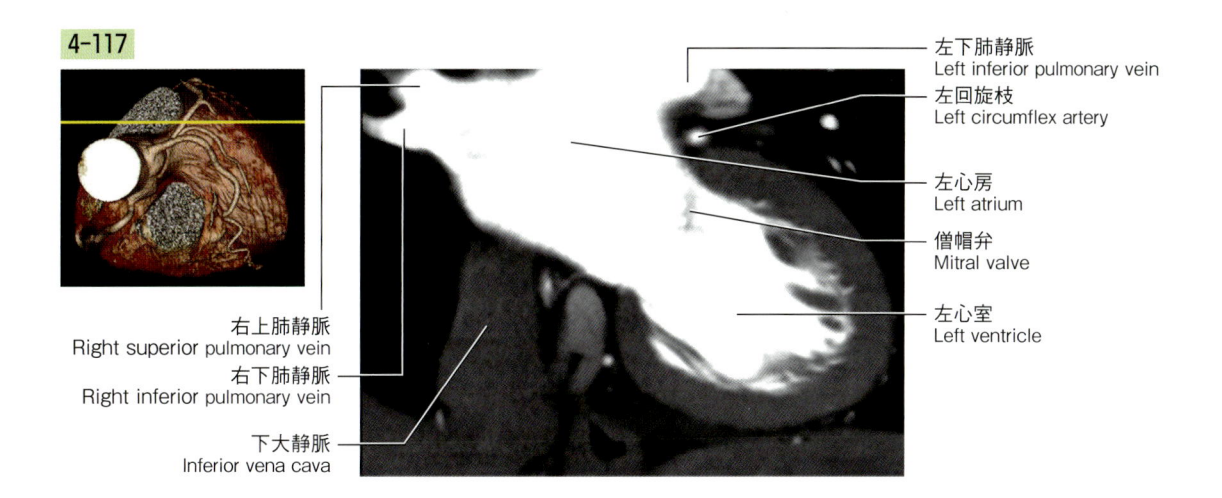

- 左下肺静脈 Left inferior pulmonary vein
- 左回旋枝 Left circumflex artery
- 左心房 Left atrium
- 僧帽弁 Mitral valve
- 左心室 Left ventricle
- 右上肺静脈 Right superior pulmonary vein
- 右下肺静脈 Right inferior pulmonary vein
- 下大静脈 Inferior vena cava

4-118

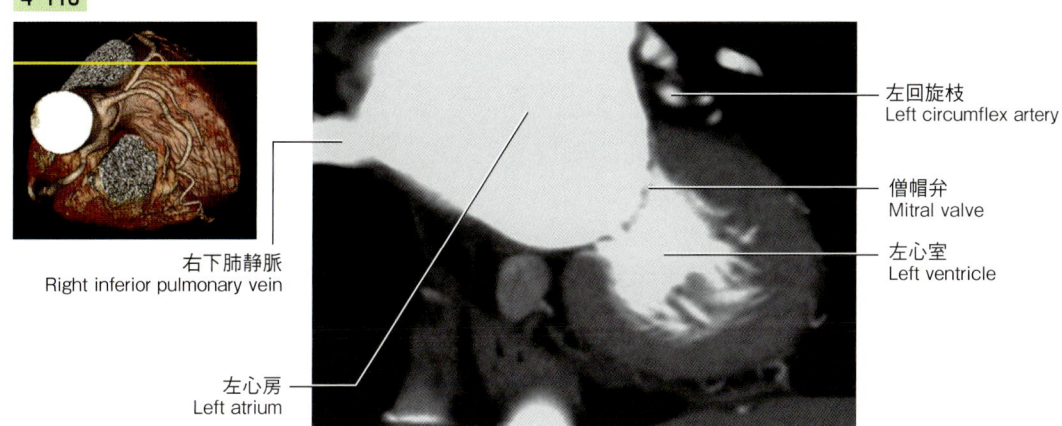

- 左回旋枝 Left circumflex artery
- 僧帽弁 Mitral valve
- 左心室 Left ventricle
- 右下肺静脈 Right inferior pulmonary vein
- 左心房 Left atrium

NOTE 僧帽弁 Mitral valve

Mitral valve は，カトリックの司教冠 "mitra"（ミトラ：ラテン語）からきた語．典礼執行時にかぶる前後に平らな尖頭状の帽子で，左心室と左心房間にある2尖弁によく似る．背壁にある僧帽（筋）(Trapezius muscle) とは，日本名は同じでも語源が異なる(86 頁の NOTE も参照)．

心臓の断層解剖 [左心室短軸像（造影CT）]

4-119 左心室短軸像

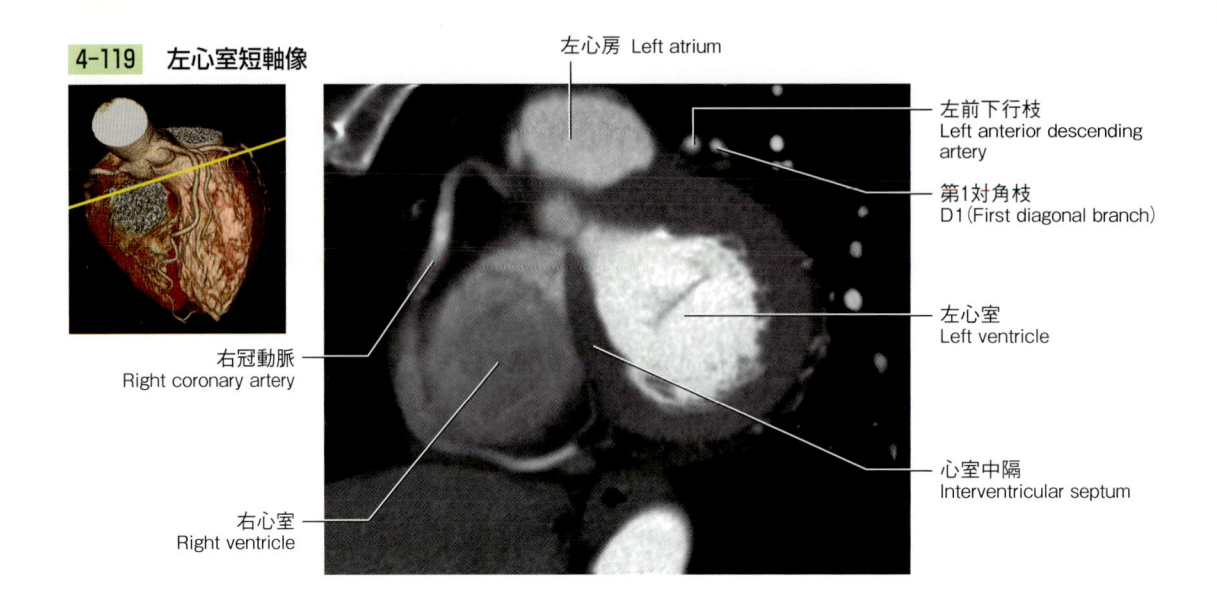

- 左心房 Left atrium
- 左前下行枝 Left anterior descending artery
- 第1対角枝 D1 (First diagonal branch)
- 左心室 Left ventricle
- 心室中隔 Interventricular septum
- 右冠動脈 Right coronary artery
- 右心室 Right ventricle

4-120 左心室短軸像

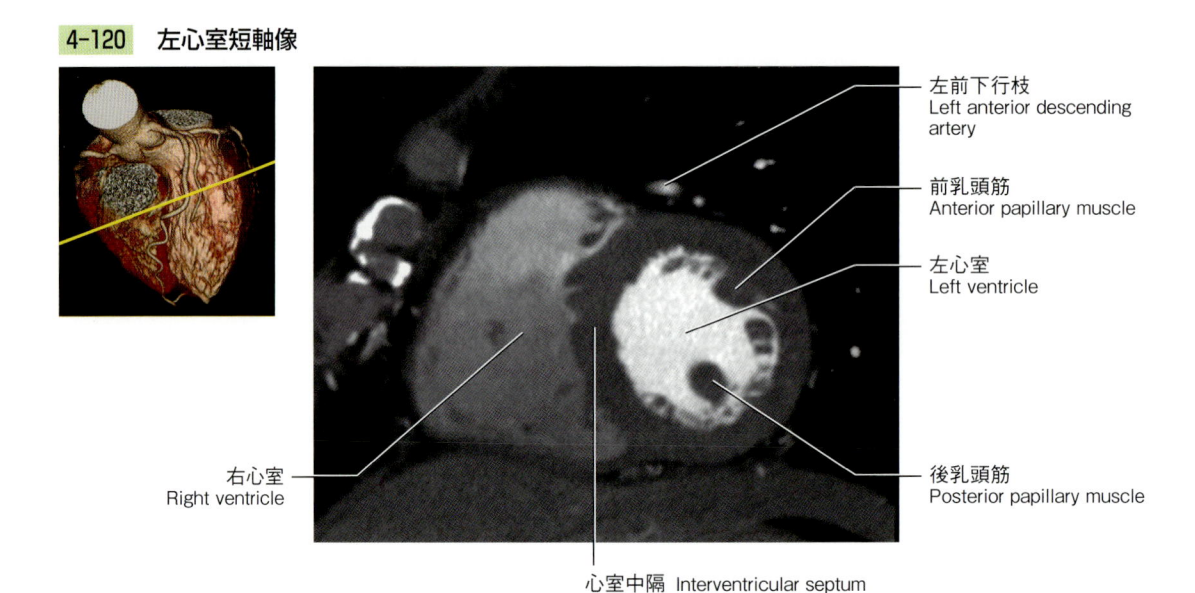

- 左前下行枝 Left anterior descending artery
- 前乳頭筋 Anterior papillary muscle
- 左心室 Left ventricle
- 後乳頭筋 Posterior papillary muscle
- 右心室 Right ventricle
- 心室中隔 Interventricular septum

心臓の断層解剖 ［左心室短軸像，左心室長軸像（造影CT）］

4-121　左心室短軸像

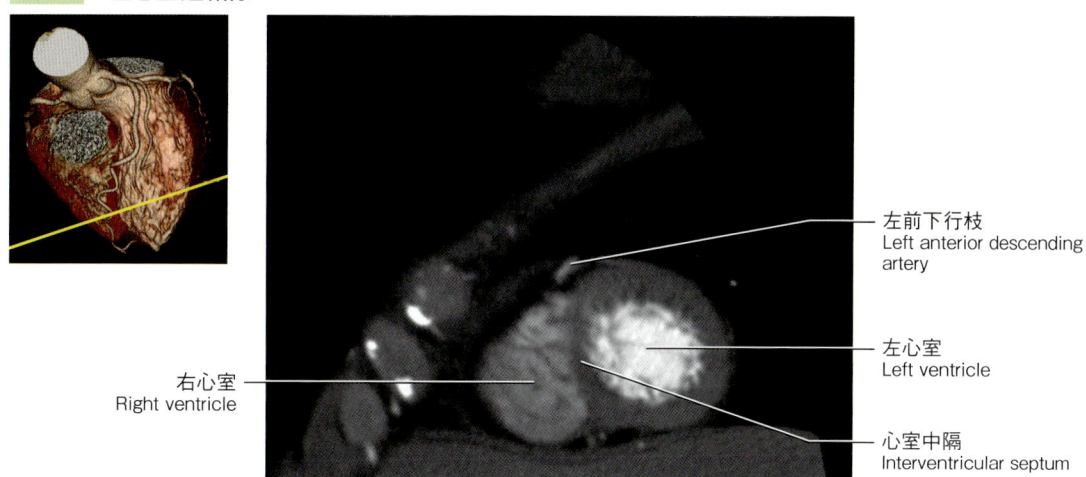

- 左前下行枝　Left anterior descending artery
- 左心室　Left ventricle
- 心室中隔　Interventricular septum
- 右心室　Right ventricle

4-122　左心室長軸像

- 左回旋枝　Left circumflex artery
- 僧帽弁前尖　Mitral valve anterior leaflet
- 左心室　Left ventricle
- 左心房　Left atrium
- 下行大動脈　Descending aorta
- 僧帽弁後尖　Mitral valve posterior leaflet

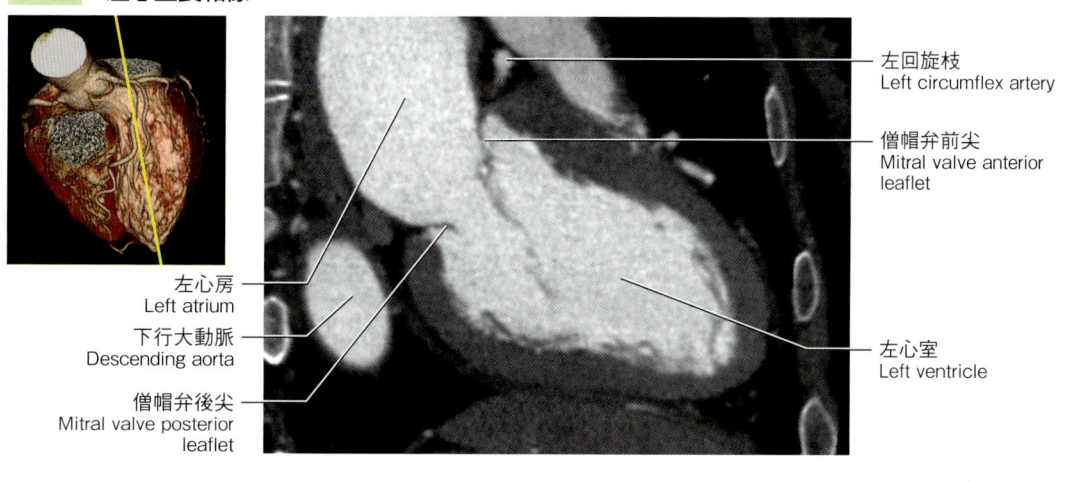

心臓の断層解剖 [四腔断像，三腔断像（造影CT）]

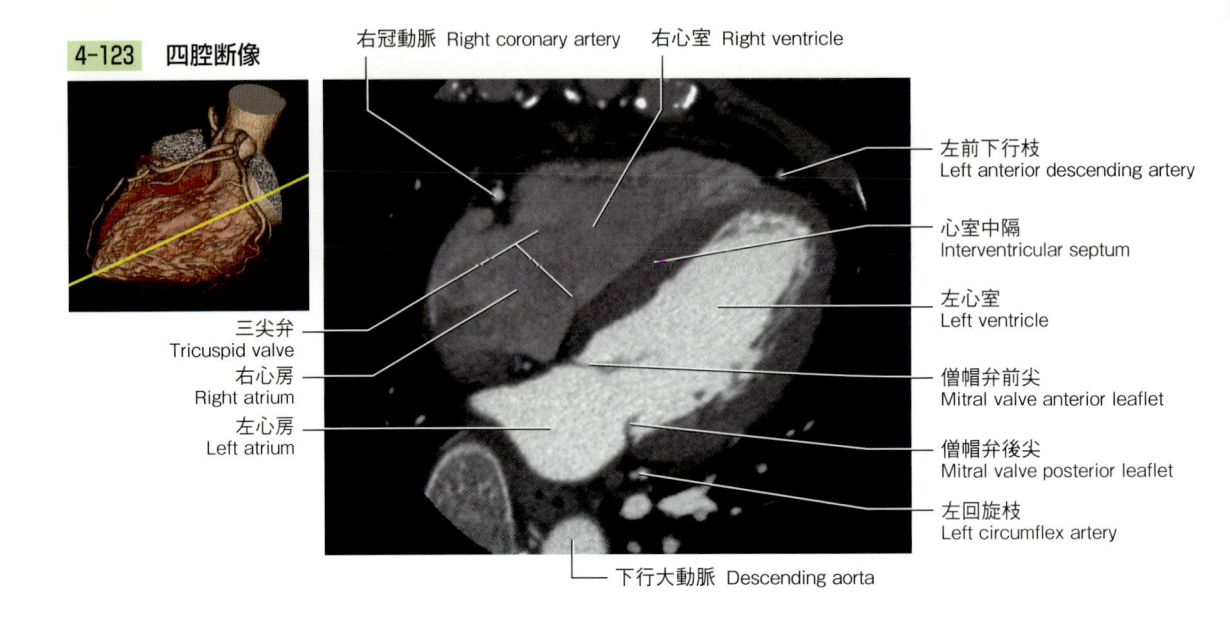

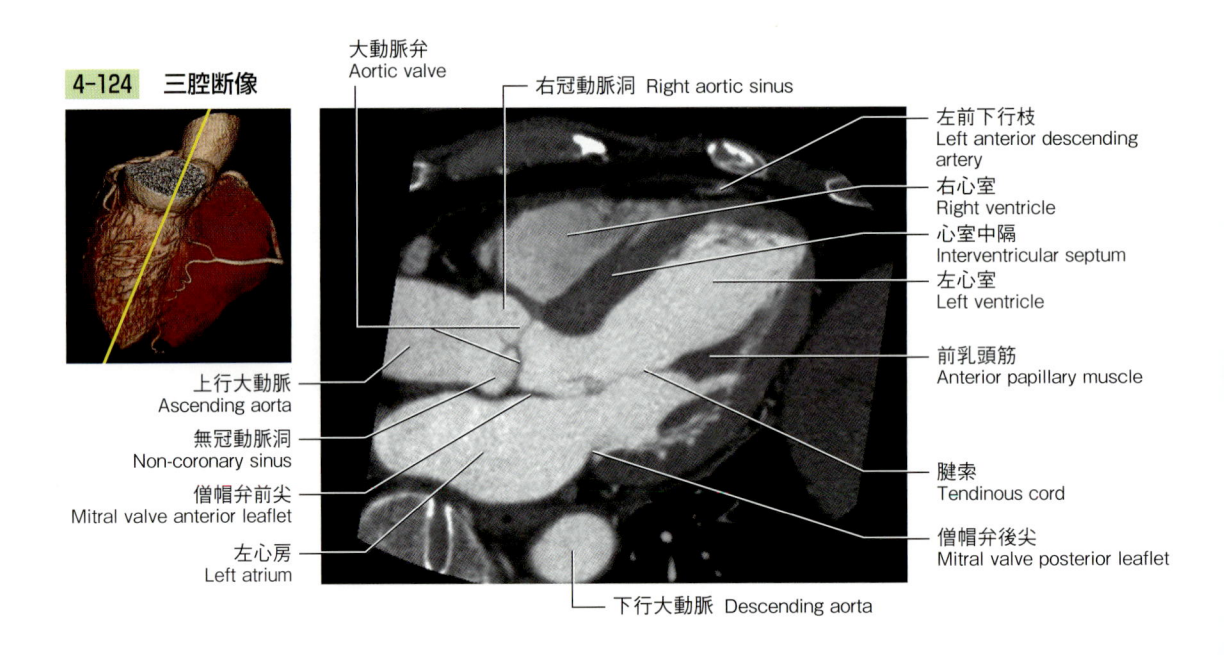

4-123 四腔断像

- 右冠動脈 Right coronary artery
- 右心室 Right ventricle
- 左前下行枝 Left anterior descending artery
- 心室中隔 Interventricular septum
- 左心室 Left ventricle
- 三尖弁 Tricuspid valve
- 僧帽弁前尖 Mitral valve anterior leaflet
- 右心房 Right atrium
- 僧帽弁後尖 Mitral valve posterior leaflet
- 左心房 Left atrium
- 左回旋枝 Left circumflex artery
- 下行大動脈 Descending aorta

4-124 三腔断像

- 大動脈弁 Aortic valve
- 右冠動脈洞 Right aortic sinus
- 左前下行枝 Left anterior descending artery
- 右心室 Right ventricle
- 心室中隔 Interventricular septum
- 左心室 Left ventricle
- 前乳頭筋 Anterior papillary muscle
- 上行大動脈 Ascending aorta
- 無冠動脈洞 Non-coronary sinus
- 腱索 Tendinous cord
- 僧帽弁前尖 Mitral valve anterior leaflet
- 僧帽弁後尖 Mitral valve posterior leaflet
- 左心房 Left atrium
- 下行大動脈 Descending aorta

V

腹 部
Abdomen

腹部の体表解剖（CT, VR像）

5-1 体表解剖と腹部臓器

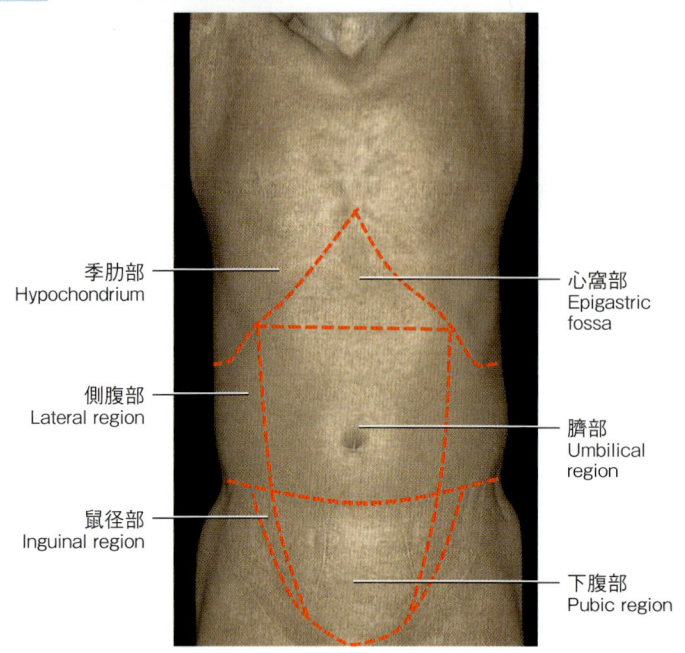

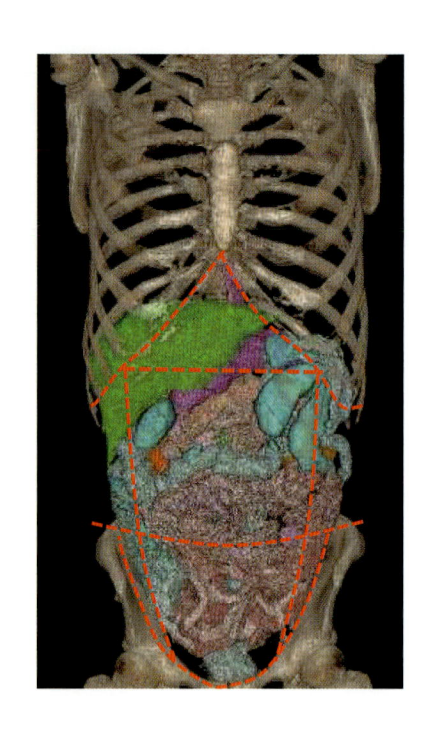

- 季肋部 Hypochondrium
- 側腹部 Lateral region
- 鼠径部 Inguinal region
- 心窩部 Epigastric fossa
- 臍部 Umbilical region
- 下腹部 Pubic region

5-2 腹部の9領域（Nine abdominal regions）と腹部臓器

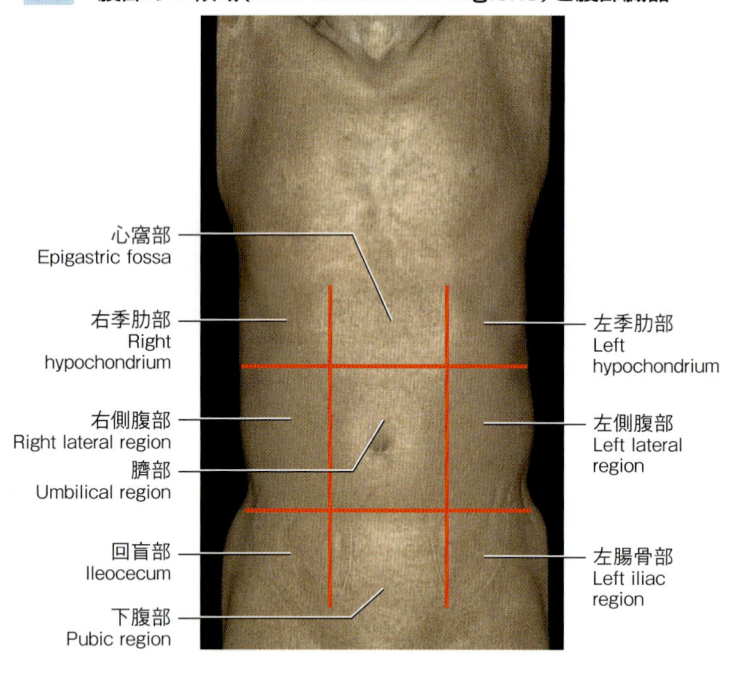

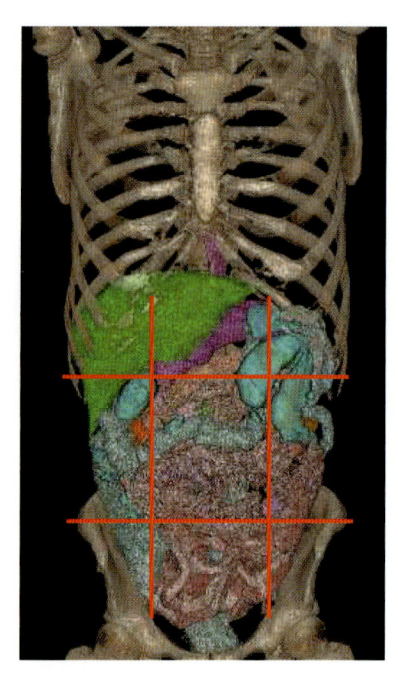

- 心窩部 Epigastric fossa
- 右季肋部 Right hypochondrium
- 右側腹部 Right lateral region
- 臍部 Umbilical region
- 回盲部 Ileocecum
- 下腹部 Pubic region
- 左季肋部 Left hypochondrium
- 左側腹部 Left lateral region
- 左腸骨部 Left iliac region

> **NOTE** 腹部は9つあるいは4つの領域に分けて表現することが多い．いずれも身体所見を表現したり記述したりするときに用いるが，それぞれの領域にどのような臓器が存在するのかを理解することが重要である．

骨格と腹部臓器 (CT, VR 像)

5-3 骨格と腹部臓器

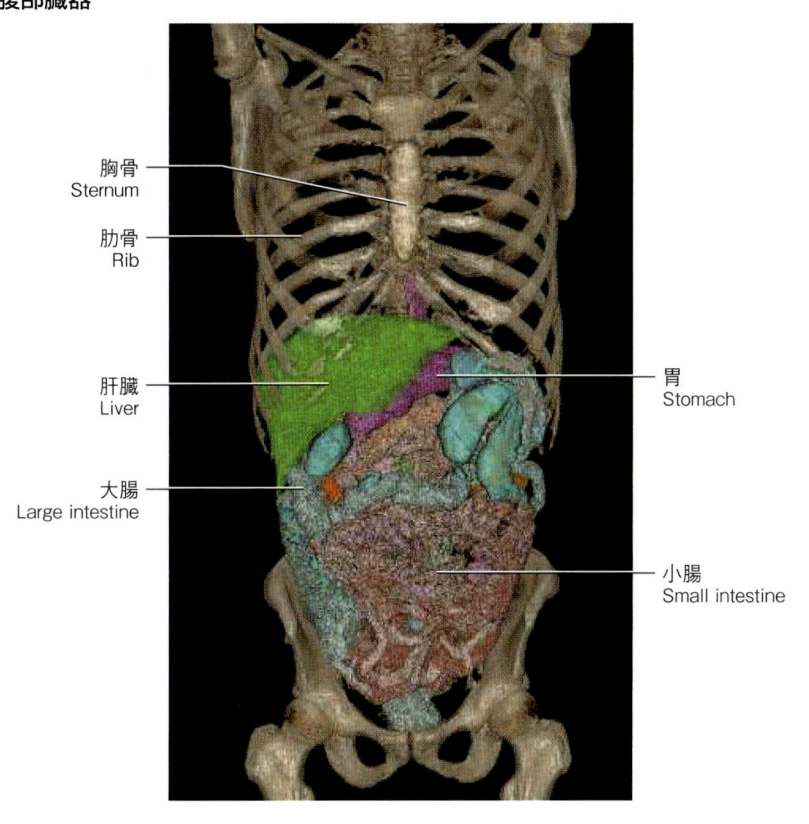

胸骨 Sternum
肋骨 Rib
肝臓 Liver
大腸 Large intestine
胃 Stomach
小腸 Small intestine

5-4 骨格と腹部臓器（消化管を除く）

正面　　背面　　右側面　　左側面

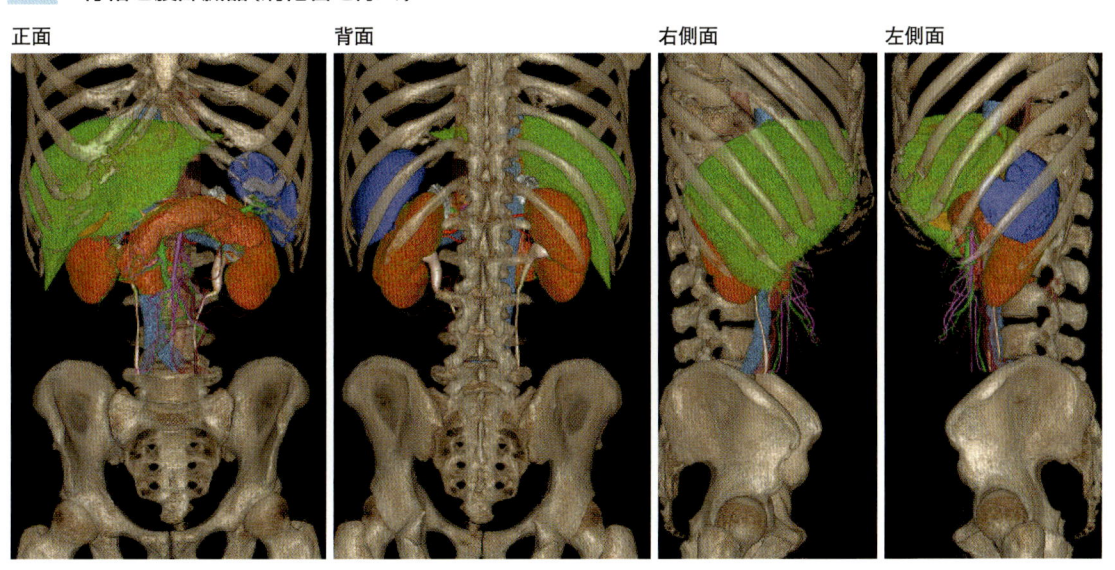

（解剖名は次頁5-5を参照）

NOTE 3次元画像の利用は，それを用いることにより診断がより確実になったり，病変と既存構造との立体関係の把握，上下方向の病変の進展の評価，手術前のシミュレーション，患者や家族へのわかりやすい説明のためなど，明確な目的がなくてはならない．

腹部臓器（消化管を除く）（造影CT, VR像）

5-5 上腹部の臓器（前面から）

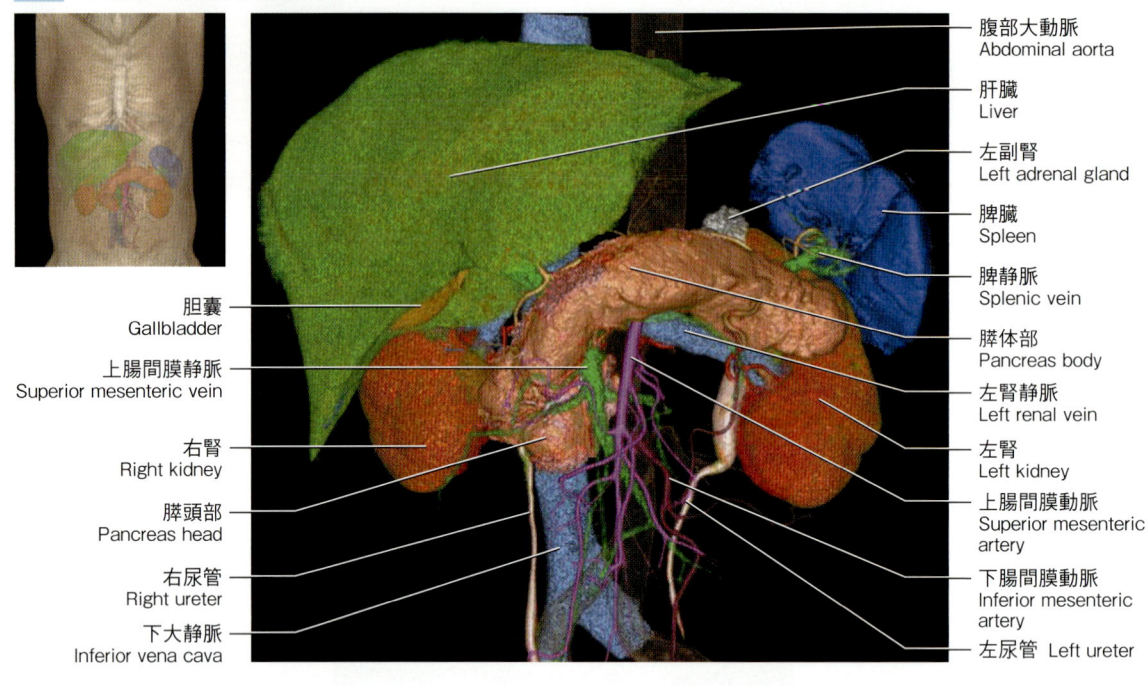

- 腹部大動脈 Abdominal aorta
- 肝臓 Liver
- 左副腎 Left adrenal gland
- 脾臓 Spleen
- 脾静脈 Splenic vein
- 膵体部 Pancreas body
- 左腎静脈 Left renal vein
- 左腎 Left kidney
- 上腸間膜動脈 Superior mesenteric artery
- 下腸間膜動脈 Inferior mesenteric artery
- 左尿管 Left ureter
- 胆嚢 Gallbladder
- 上腸間膜静脈 Superior mesenteric vein
- 右腎 Right kidney
- 膵頭部 Pancreas head
- 右尿管 Right ureter
- 下大静脈 Inferior vena cava

5-6 上腹部の血管（前面から）

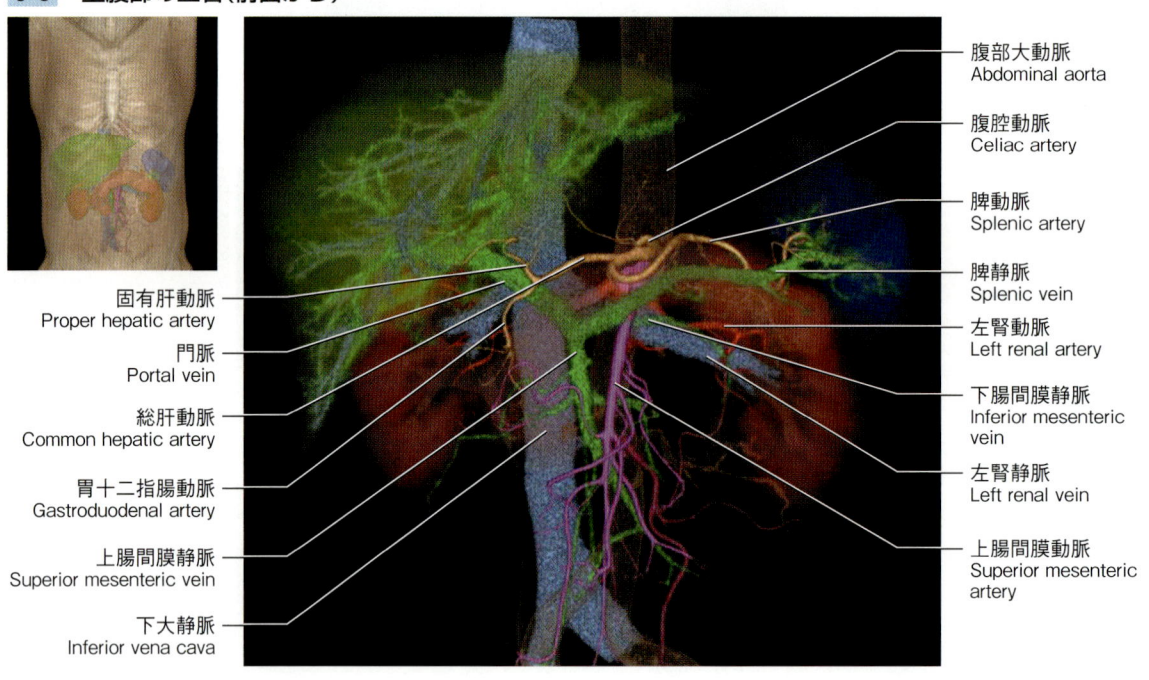

- 腹部大動脈 Abdominal aorta
- 腹腔動脈 Celiac artery
- 脾動脈 Splenic artery
- 脾静脈 Splenic vein
- 左腎動脈 Left renal artery
- 下腸間膜静脈 Inferior mesenteric vein
- 左腎静脈 Left renal vein
- 上腸間膜動脈 Superior mesenteric artery
- 固有肝動脈 Proper hepatic artery
- 門脈 Portal vein
- 総肝動脈 Common hepatic artery
- 胃十二指腸動脈 Gastroduodenal artery
- 上腸間膜静脈 Superior mesenteric vein
- 下大静脈 Inferior vena cava

NOTE 上腸間膜動脈は，空腸・回腸・盲腸・上行結腸・横行結腸を栄養している．下腸間膜動脈は下行結腸・S状結腸・直腸上部を栄養している．これらの分枝血管の吻合にはかなりのバリエーションがある．

腹部臓器（消化管を除く）（造影 CT, VR 像）

5-7 上腹部の臓器（背面から）

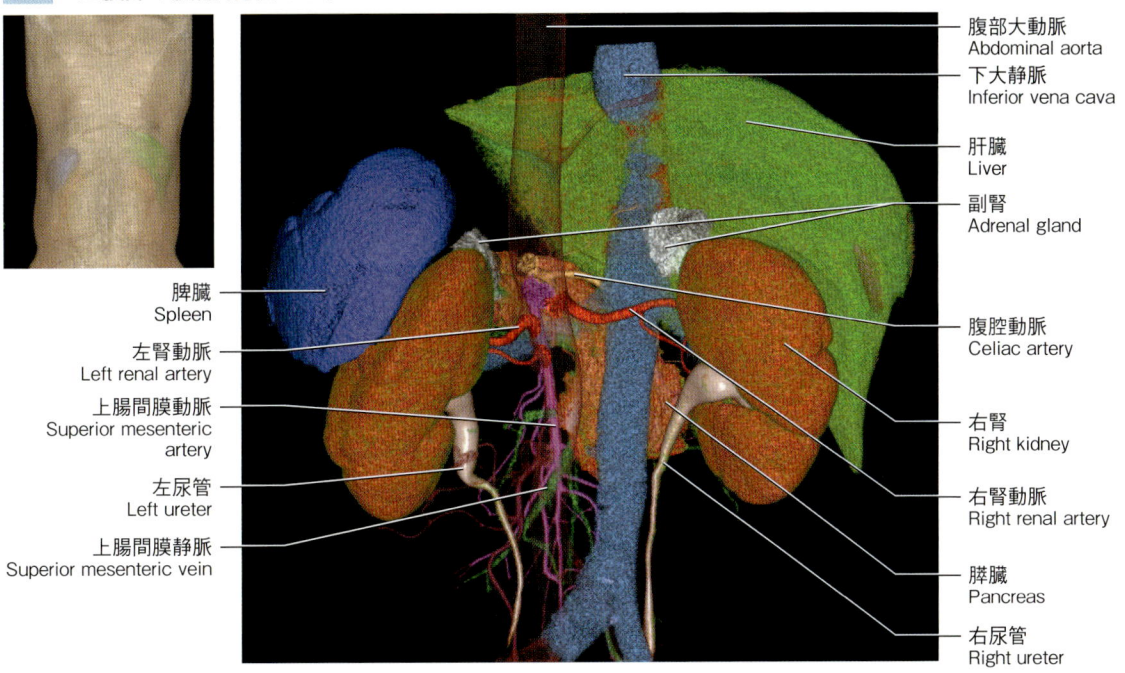

- 腹部大動脈 Abdominal aorta
- 下大静脈 Inferior vena cava
- 肝臓 Liver
- 副腎 Adrenal gland
- 腹腔動脈 Celiac artery
- 右腎 Right kidney
- 右腎動脈 Right renal artery
- 膵臓 Pancreas
- 右尿管 Right ureter
- 脾臓 Spleen
- 左腎動脈 Left renal artery
- 上腸間膜動脈 Superior mesenteric artery
- 左尿管 Left ureter
- 上腸間膜静脈 Superior mesenteric vein

5-8 上腹部の臓器（下面から）

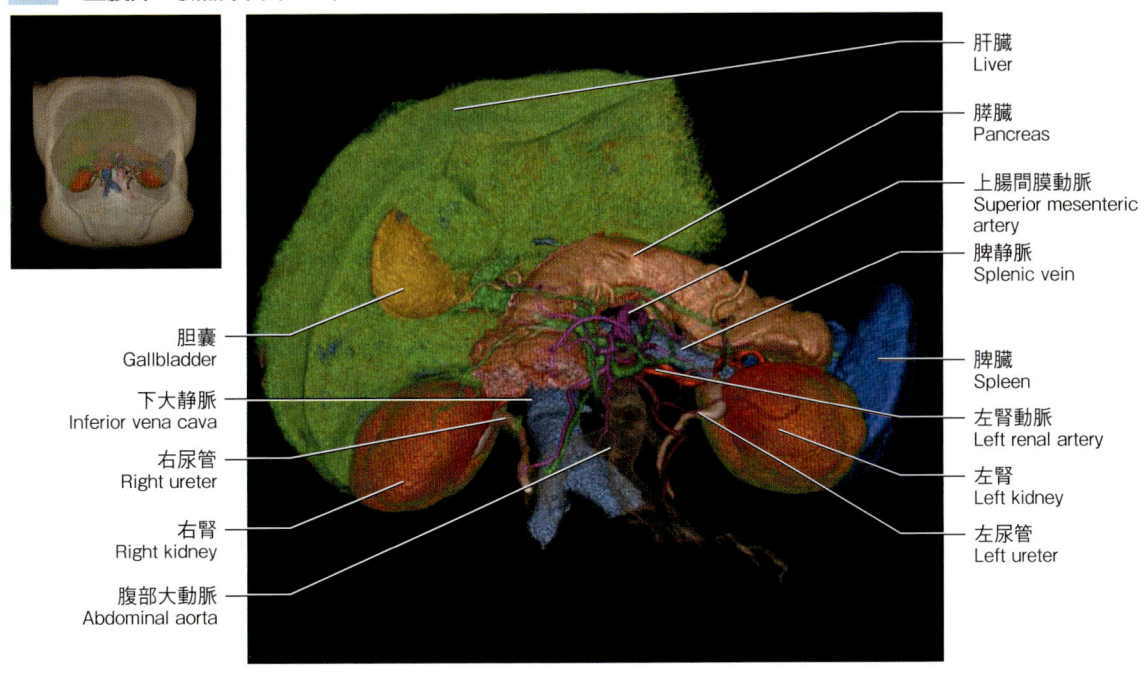

- 肝臓 Liver
- 膵臓 Pancreas
- 上腸間膜動脈 Superior mesenteric artery
- 脾静脈 Splenic vein
- 脾臓 Spleen
- 左腎動脈 Left renal artery
- 左腎 Left kidney
- 左尿管 Left ureter
- 胆嚢 Gallbladder
- 下大静脈 Inferior vena cava
- 右尿管 Right ureter
- 右腎 Right kidney
- 腹部大動脈 Abdominal aorta

肝臓・脾臓と横断面

5-9 肝臓・脾臓（前面から）
（造影 CT 動脈相，VR 像）

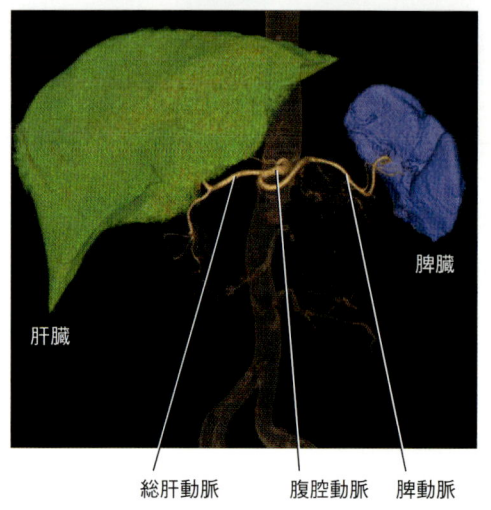

肝臓／脾臓／総肝動脈／腹腔動脈／脾動脈

5-10 肝臓・脾臓（左斜め前）
（造影 CT 動脈相，VR 像）

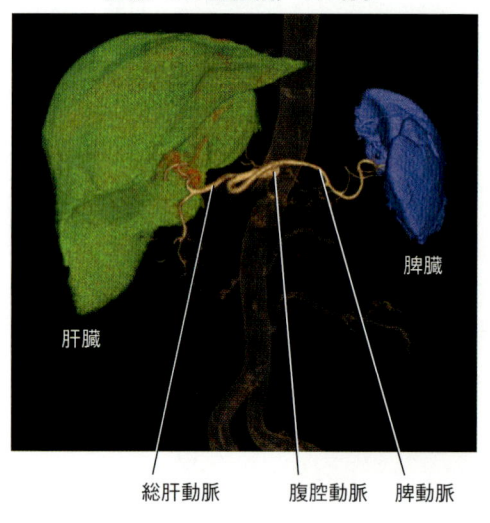

肝臓／脾臓／総肝動脈／腹腔動脈／脾動脈

5-11 肝臓の横断面
（造影 CT 平衡相）

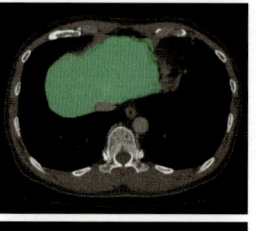

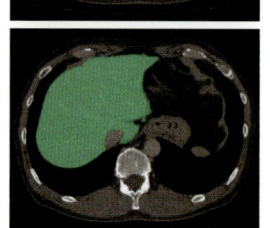

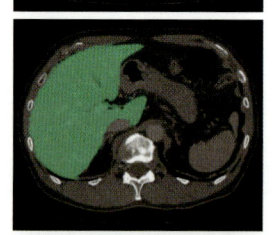

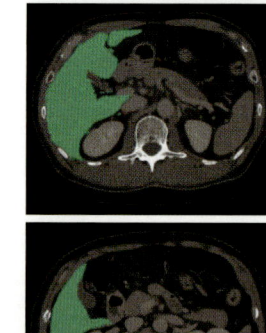

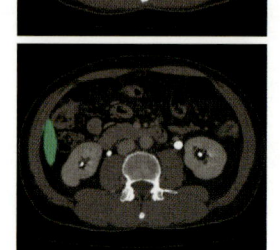

5-12 脾臓の横断面
（造影 CT 平衡相）

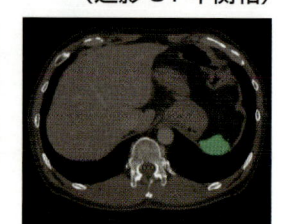

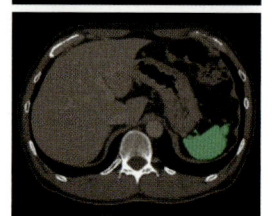

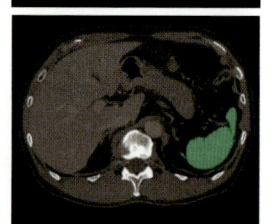

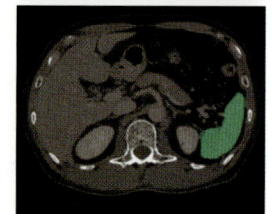

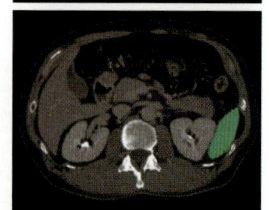

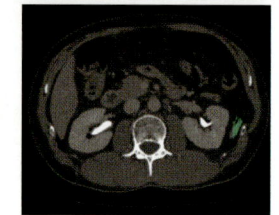

> **NOTE** 脾臓は横隔膜と胃底部の間に位置し，第9～11肋間の高さにある．脾腫の判定基準に確立したものはないが，CTでは頭尾方向に10 cm以上ある場合，最大横断面で，外側縁が4肋間以上にわたって描出される場合などで脾腫と診断される．

胆嚢・膵臓と横断面

5-13 胆嚢・膵臓（前面から）
（造影 CT 動脈相，VR 像）

胆嚢　膵臓
上腸間膜動脈

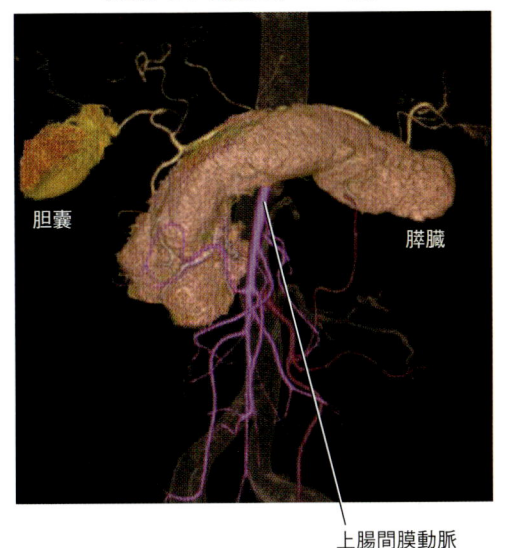

5-14 胆嚢・膵臓（背面から）
（造影 CT 動脈相，VR 像）

膵臓　胆嚢
上腸間膜動脈

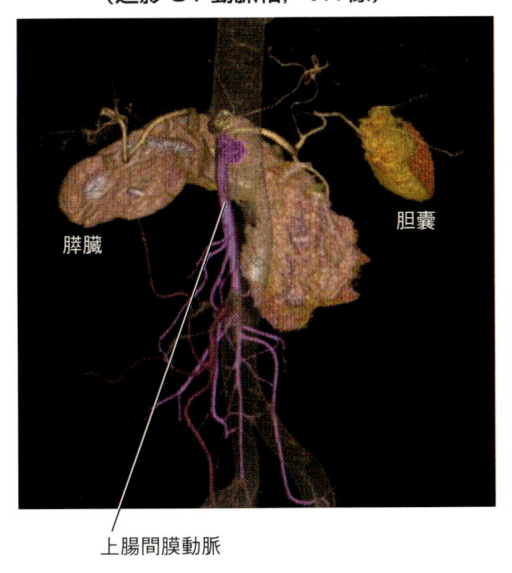

5-15 胆嚢と横断面
（造影 CT 平衡相）

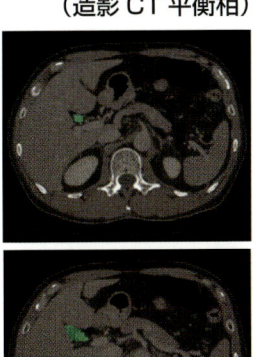

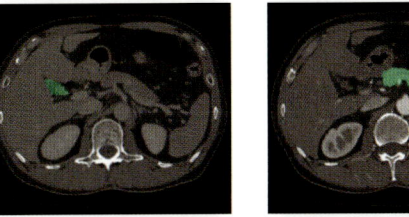

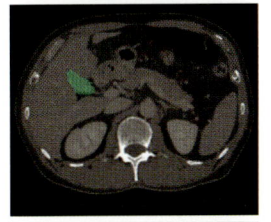

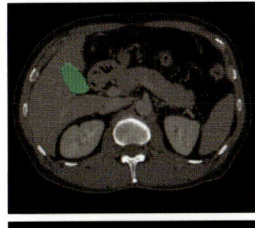

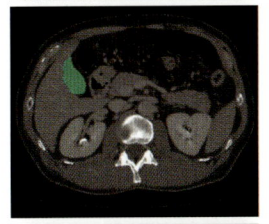

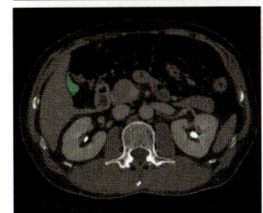

5-16 膵臓と横断面
（造影 CT 平衡相）

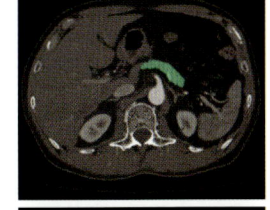

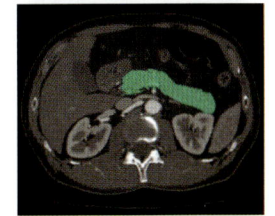

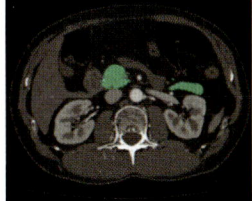

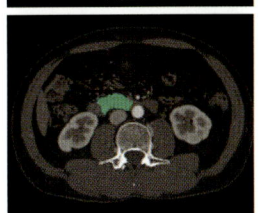

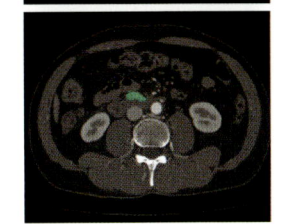

> **NOTE** 胆道とは肝細胞から分泌された胆汁が十二指腸に流出するまでの構造で，肝内胆管系と肝外胆管系に大きく分けられる．肝内胆管は 2 mm 以上になると CT 上描出されるようになり，閉塞機転を考慮しなくてはならない．膵臓の大きさはいろいろ基準値があるが，形，大きさ，実質濃度は年齢を含め，個人差が大きい．全体のバランスが大切である．

腎臓・副腎と横断面

5-17 腎臓・副腎（前面から）（造影CT動脈相，VR像）

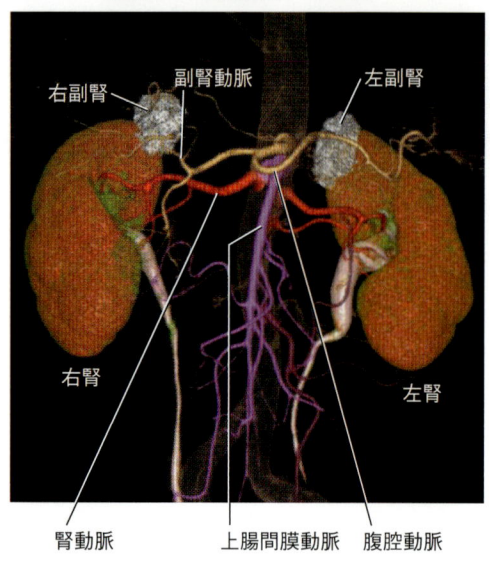

5-18 腎臓・副腎（右斜め後方から）（造影CT動脈相，VR像）

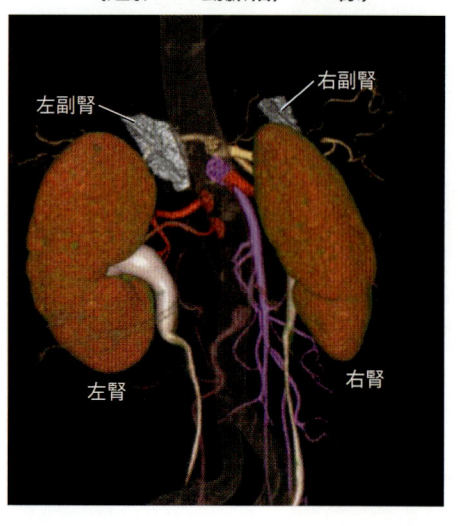

5-19 腎臓と横断面（造影CT平衡相）

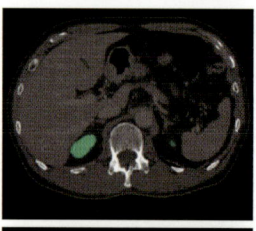

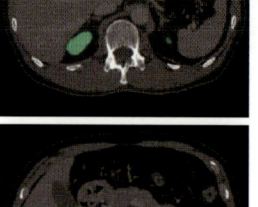

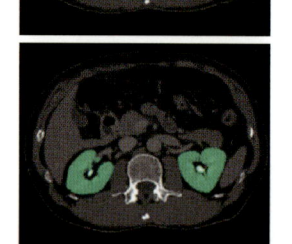

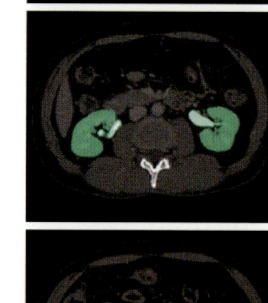

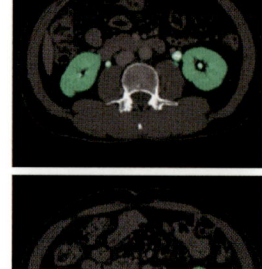

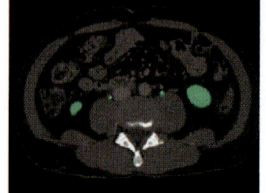

5-20 副腎と横断面（造影CT平衡相）

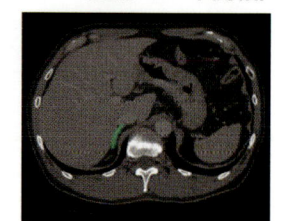

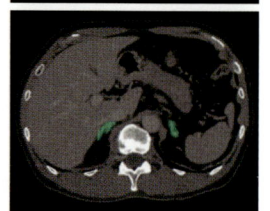

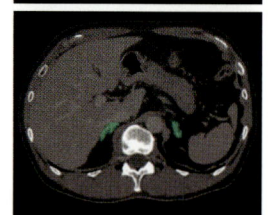

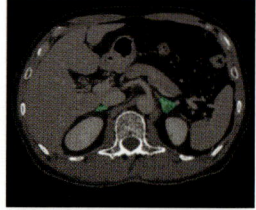

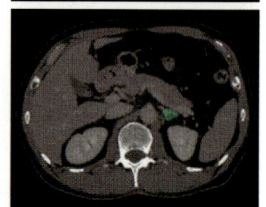

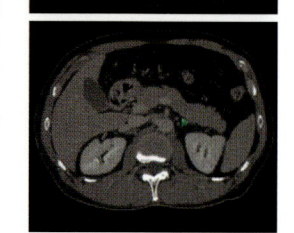

NOTE 副腎は転移の多い臓器である．肺癌・乳癌からの転移が特に多い．しかし，副腎そのものが小さな臓器であり，転移が小さなものであれば見逃しやすい．そのため，特に意識してチェックする必要のある重要な臓器である．転移は両側性であることが多い．

消化管（CT, VR像） 235

5-21 骨格と消化管（前面から）

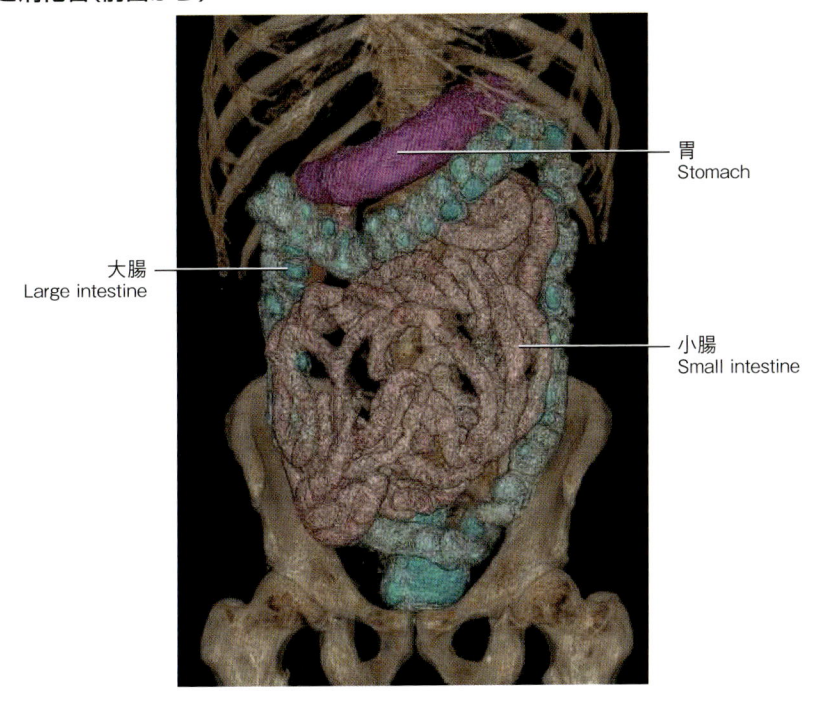

- 胃 Stomach
- 大腸 Large intestine
- 小腸 Small intestine

5-22 消化管（後面から）

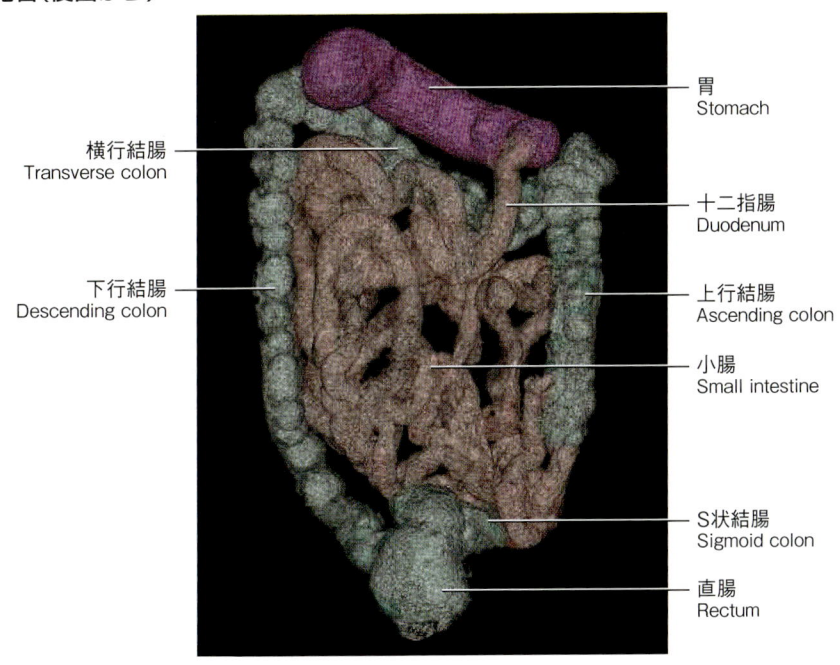

- 横行結腸 Transverse colon
- 下行結腸 Descending colon
- 胃 Stomach
- 十二指腸 Duodenum
- 上行結腸 Ascending colon
- 小腸 Small intestine
- S状結腸 Sigmoid colon
- 直腸 Rectum

> **NOTE** 大腸は，盲腸・上行結腸・横行結腸・下行結腸・S状結腸・直腸・肛門管の7つの領域に分けられる．小腸との違いは，結腸ひも，結腸隆起（ハウストラ：Haustra），これを境する半月ヒダがある．ハウストラの見え方は結腸ひもの緊張により異なる．

消化管 (CT, VR像)

5-23 胃・小腸（前面から）

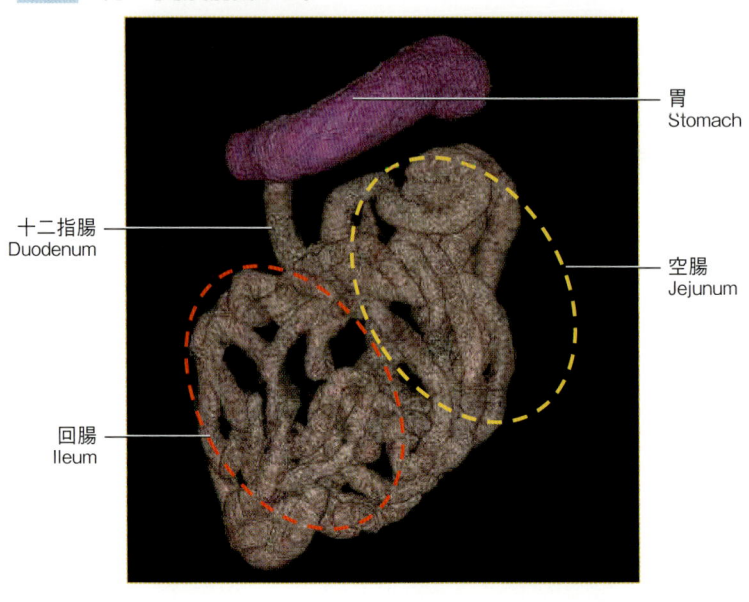

胃 Stomach
十二指腸 Duodenum
空腸 Jejunum
回腸 Ileum

5-24 大腸（前面から）

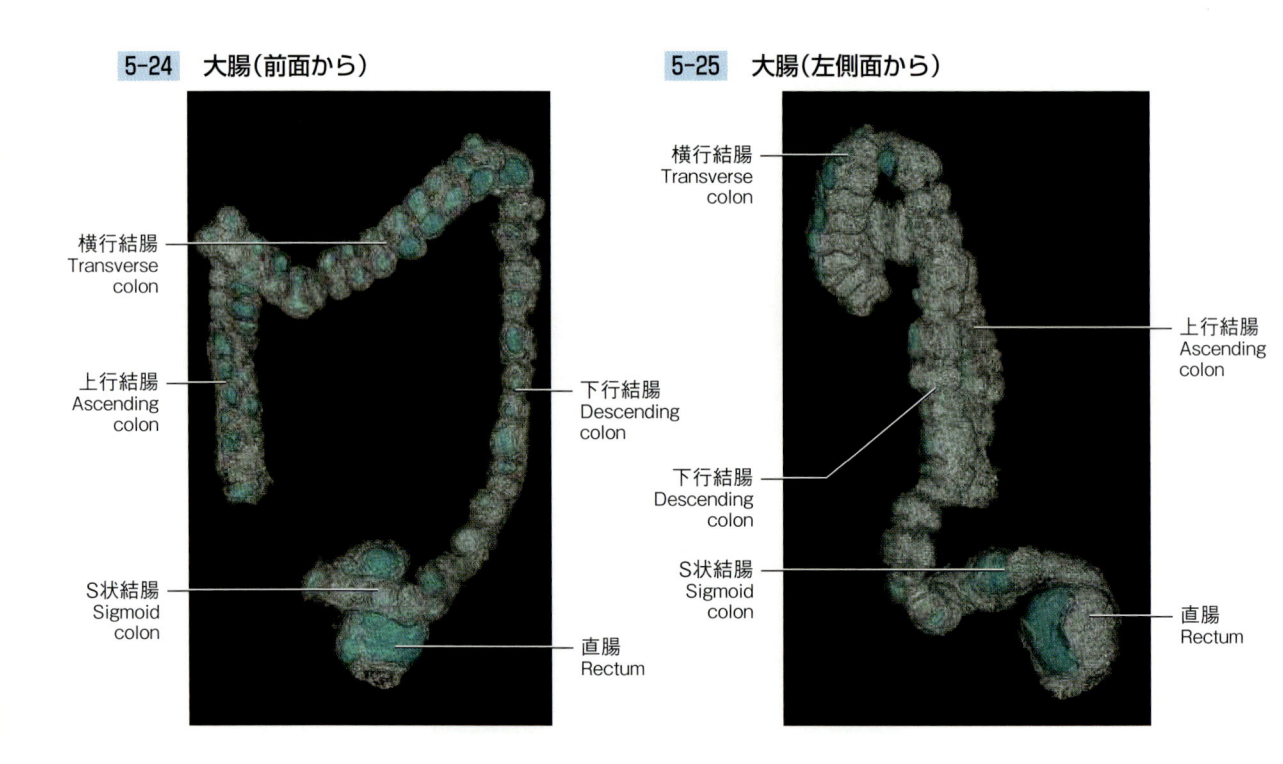

横行結腸 Transverse colon
上行結腸 Ascending colon
S状結腸 Sigmoid colon
下行結腸 Descending colon
直腸 Rectum

5-25 大腸（左側面から）

横行結腸 Transverse colon
上行結腸 Ascending colon
下行結腸 Descending colon
S状結腸 Sigmoid colon
直腸 Rectum

NOTE 小腸ははじめの2/5が空腸，残りの3/5が回腸であるが，両者に明確な境界があるわけではない．横行結腸は背側で横行結腸間膜で牽引されて最腹側を横走するが，その固定は比較的弱く，かなり可動性を有する．下方へ強く垂れ下がるように存在することも多く，注意が必要である．

消化管のバリエーション（S状結腸過長症）（CT, VR 像） 237

5-26 骨格と消化管（前面から）

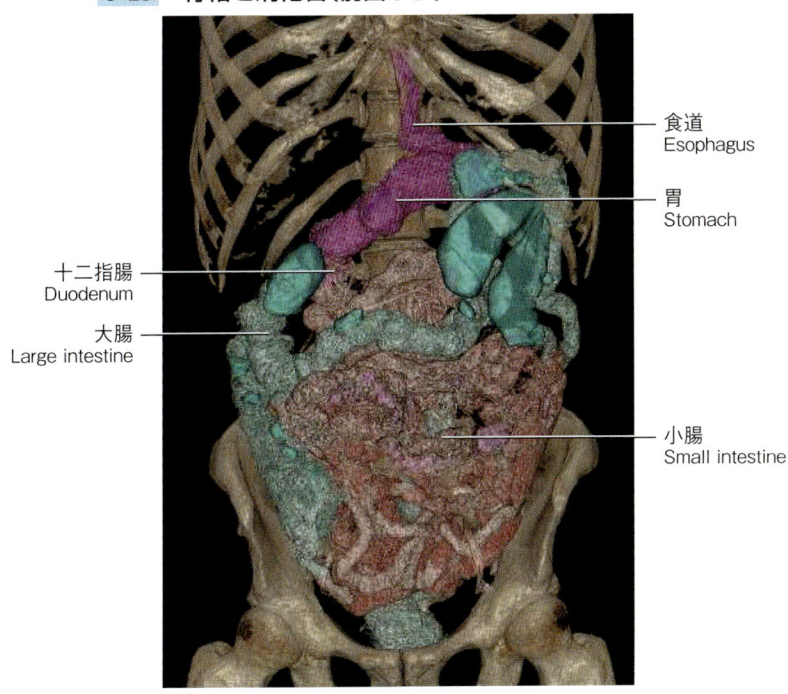

- 食道 Esophagus
- 胃 Stomach
- 十二指腸 Duodenum
- 大腸 Large intestine
- 小腸 Small intestine

5-27 消化管（背面から）

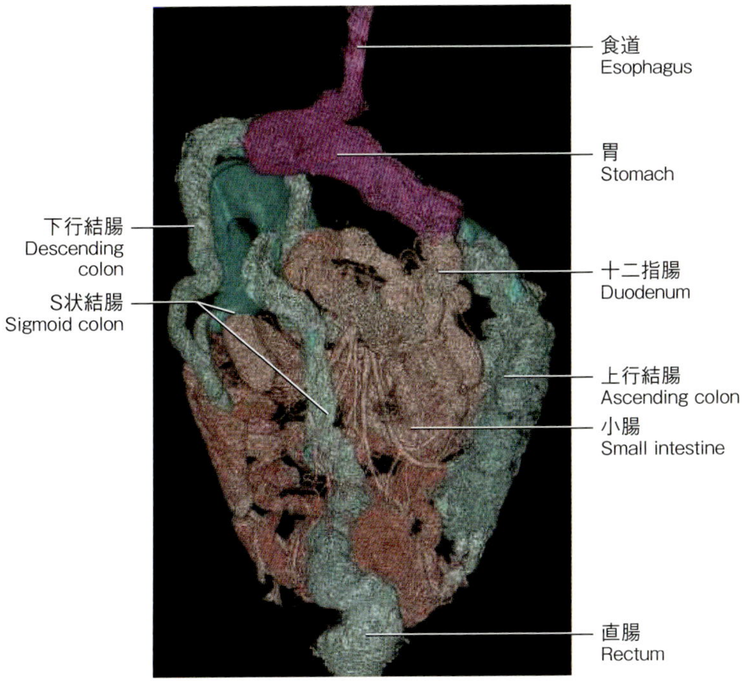

- 食道 Esophagus
- 胃 Stomach
- 下行結腸 Descending colon
- S状結腸 Sigmoid colon
- 十二指腸 Duodenum
- 上行結腸 Ascending colon
- 小腸 Small intestine
- 直腸 Rectum

5-28 大腸（S状結腸過長症）（前面から）

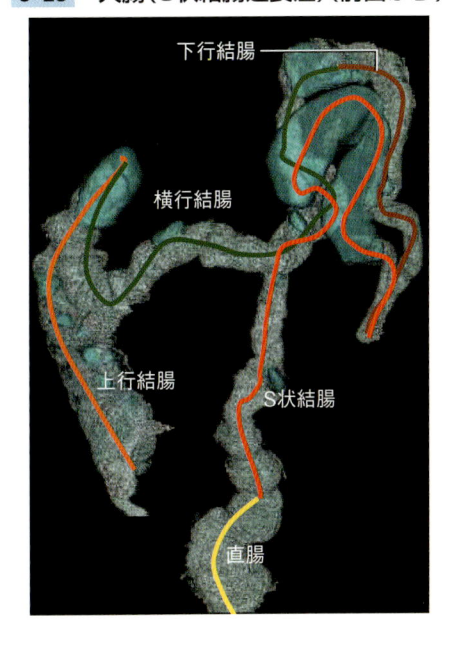

- 下行結腸
- 横行結腸
- 上行結腸
- S状結腸
- 直腸

NOTE 結腸過長症とは，結腸が異常に長く，移動性に富んでいる状態で，S状結腸に最も多く，上行・下行結腸にもみられる．S状結腸過長症は，小児のS状結腸捻転症に関与することがある．

消化管の走行と冠状断面（平衡相 CT MPR + VR 像）

5-29 肝門部冠状断面＋大腸 VR（前面）

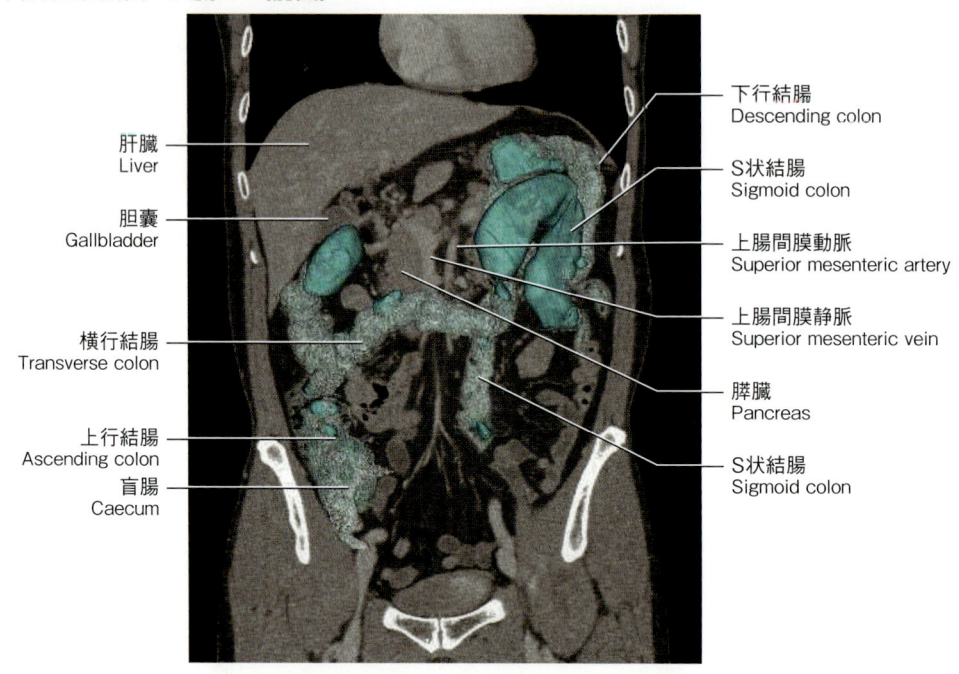

- 肝臓 Liver
- 胆嚢 Gallbladder
- 横行結腸 Transverse colon
- 上行結腸 Ascending colon
- 盲腸 Caecum
- 下行結腸 Descending colon
- S状結腸 Sigmoid colon
- 上腸間膜動脈 Superior mesenteric artery
- 上腸間膜静脈 Superior mesenteric vein
- 膵臓 Pancreas
- S状結腸 Sigmoid colon

5-30 肝門部冠状断面＋大腸 VR（背面）

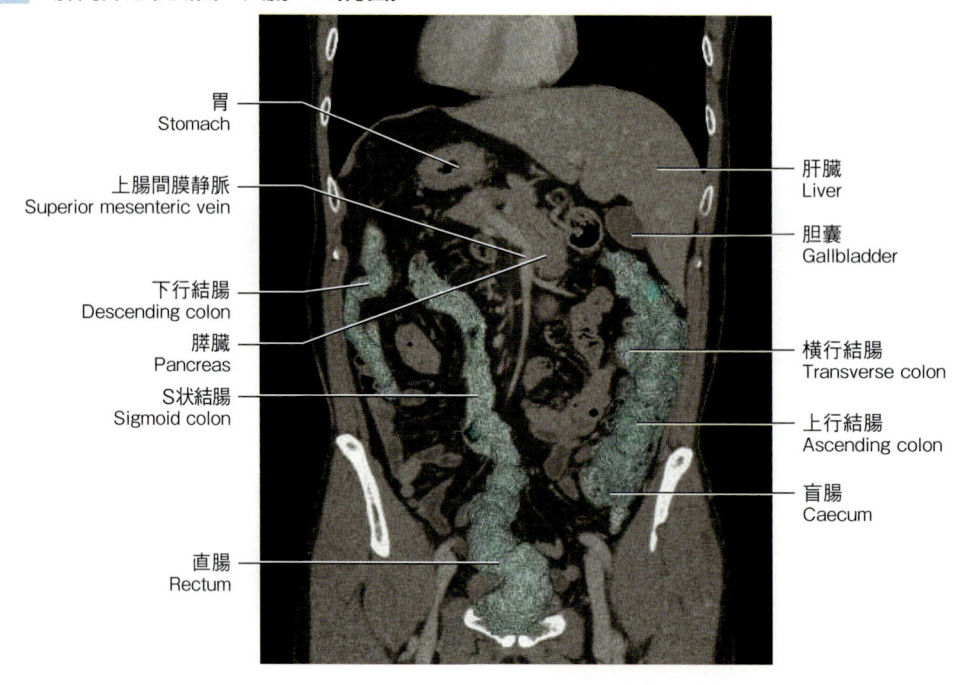

- 胃 Stomach
- 上腸間膜静脈 Superior mesenteric vein
- 下行結腸 Descending colon
- 膵臓 Pancreas
- S状結腸 Sigmoid colon
- 直腸 Rectum
- 肝臓 Liver
- 胆嚢 Gallbladder
- 横行結腸 Transverse colon
- 上行結腸 Ascending colon
- 盲腸 Caecum

上腹部の血管系（造影 CT 動脈相＋門脈相，VR 像） 239

5-31 上腹部の血管系（正面）

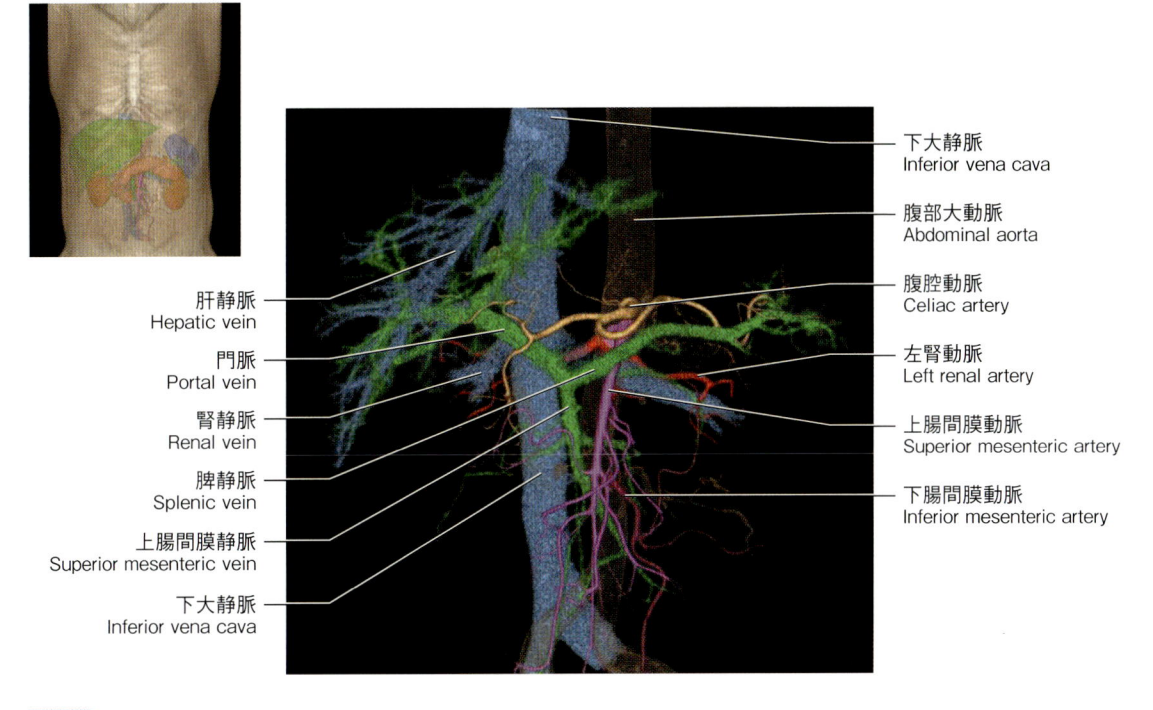

- 下大静脈 Inferior vena cava
- 腹部大動脈 Abdominal aorta
- 腹腔動脈 Celiac artery
- 左腎動脈 Left renal artery
- 上腸間膜動脈 Superior mesenteric artery
- 下腸間膜動脈 Inferior mesenteric artery
- 肝静脈 Hepatic vein
- 門脈 Portal vein
- 腎静脈 Renal vein
- 脾静脈 Splenic vein
- 上腸間膜静脈 Superior mesenteric vein
- 下大静脈 Inferior vena cava

5-32 上腹部の血管系（背面）

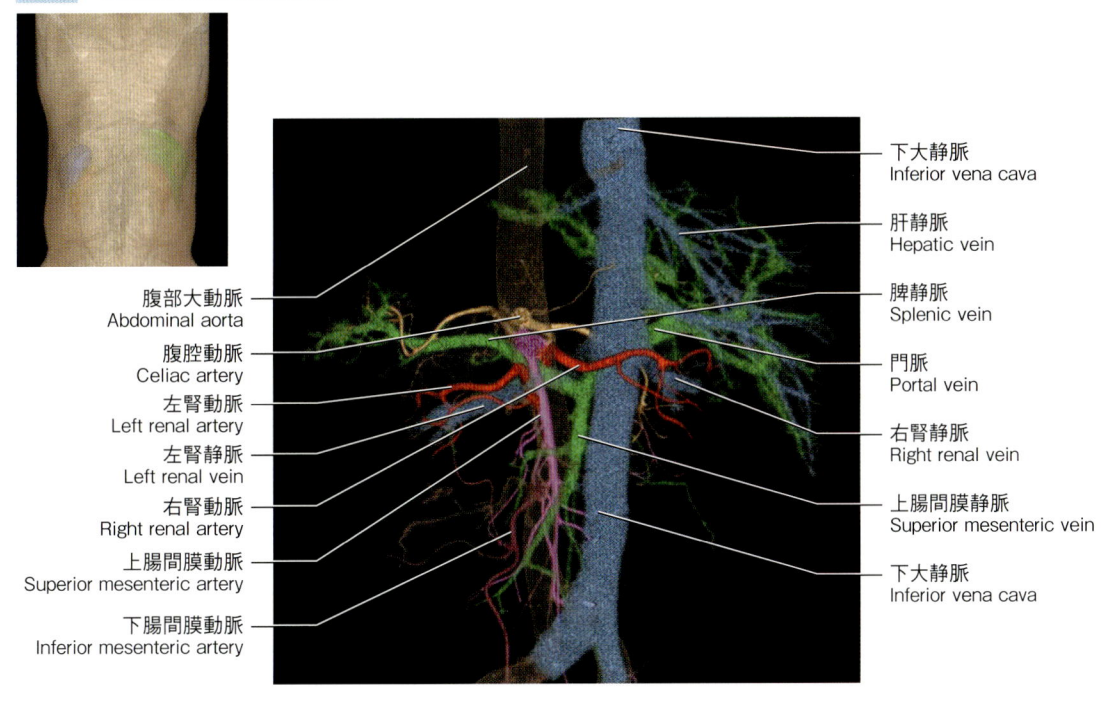

- 腹部大動脈 Abdominal aorta
- 腹腔動脈 Celiac artery
- 左腎動脈 Left renal artery
- 左腎静脈 Left renal vein
- 右腎動脈 Right renal artery
- 上腸間膜動脈 Superior mesenteric artery
- 下腸間膜動脈 Inferior mesenteric artery
- 下大静脈 Inferior vena cava
- 肝静脈 Hepatic vein
- 脾静脈 Splenic vein
- 門脈 Portal vein
- 右腎静脈 Right renal vein
- 上腸間膜静脈 Superior mesenteric vein
- 下大静脈 Inferior vena cava

> **NOTE** 腹腔動脈は，第 12 胸椎から第 1 腰椎の高さで腹部大動脈前面より分岐し，肝臓，膵臓，脾臓，十二指腸，胆嚢などへの血流を支配している．上腸間膜動脈は，腹腔動脈の直下から 20 mm 程度の間で腹部大動脈前面より分岐し，膵の背側を下方へ走行する．

上腹部の動脈（造影CT動脈相，VR像）

5-33 上腹部の動脈（正面）

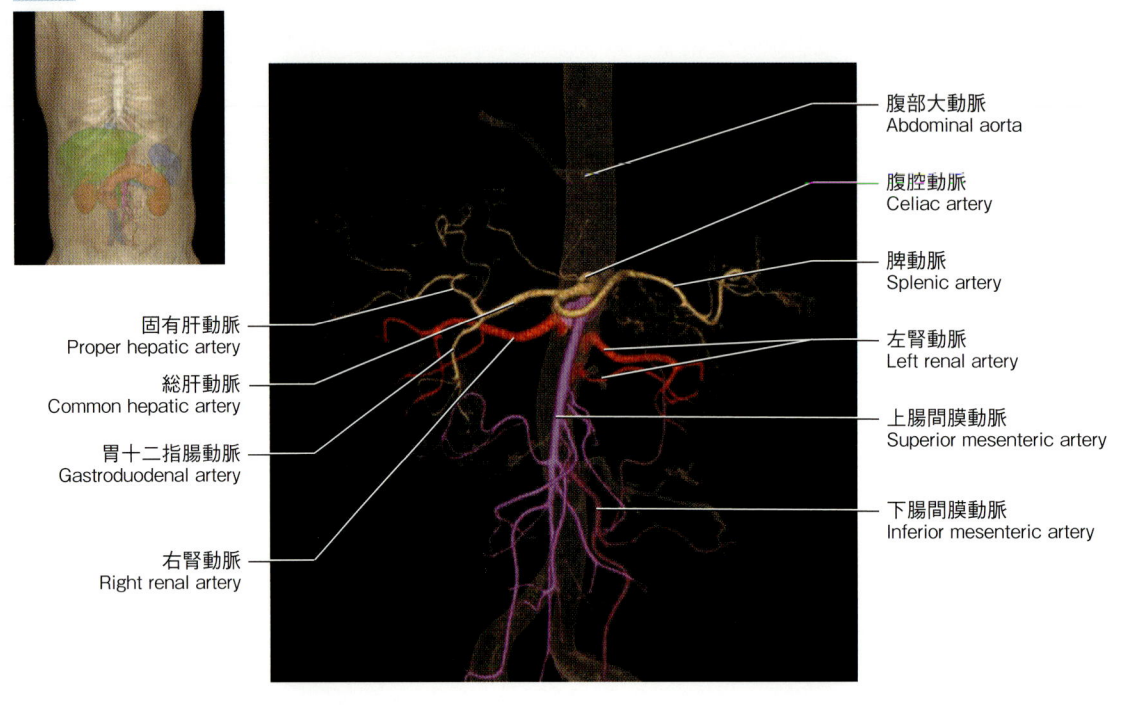

- 腹部大動脈 Abdominal aorta
- 腹腔動脈 Celiac artery
- 脾動脈 Splenic artery
- 左腎動脈 Left renal artery
- 上腸間膜動脈 Superior mesenteric artery
- 下腸間膜動脈 Inferior mesenteric artery
- 固有肝動脈 Proper hepatic artery
- 総肝動脈 Common hepatic artery
- 胃十二指腸動脈 Gastroduodenal artery
- 右腎動脈 Right renal artery

5-34 上腹部の動脈（左斜め前）

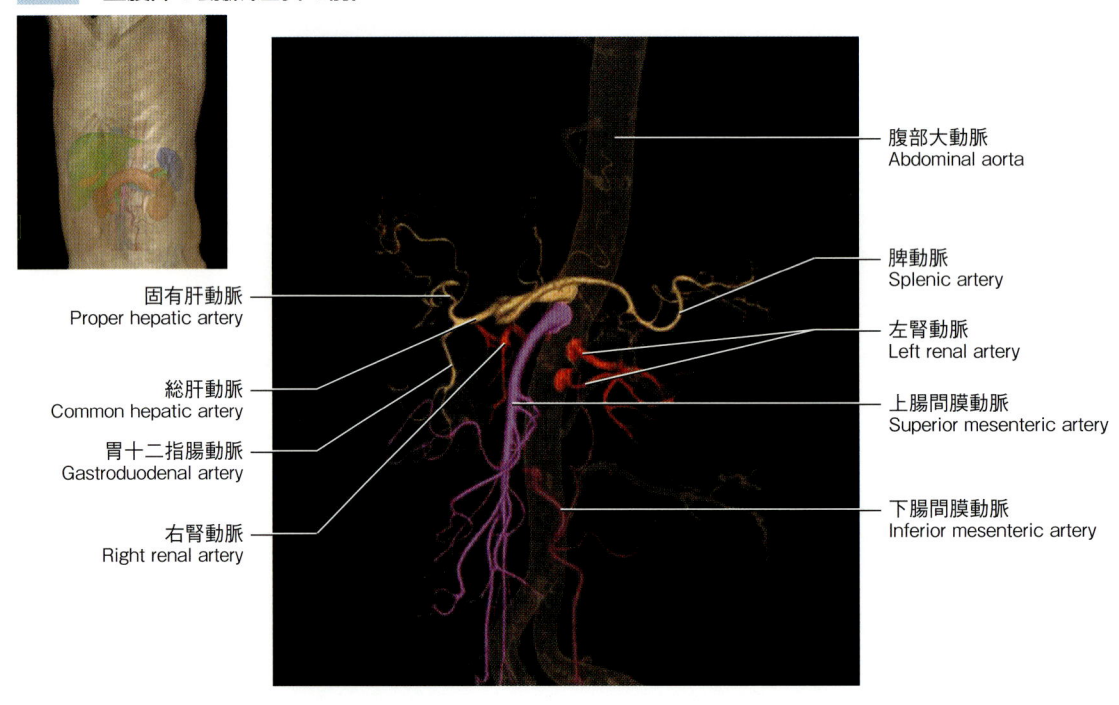

- 腹部大動脈 Abdominal aorta
- 脾動脈 Splenic artery
- 左腎動脈 Left renal artery
- 上腸間膜動脈 Superior mesenteric artery
- 下腸間膜動脈 Inferior mesenteric artery
- 固有肝動脈 Proper hepatic artery
- 総肝動脈 Common hepatic artery
- 胃十二指腸動脈 Gastroduodenal artery
- 右腎動脈 Right renal artery

NOTE 腎動脈は，第1あるいは第2腰椎の高さで大動脈から分岐する．右腎動脈は下大静脈の背側を走行する．腎動脈は腎門部で背側枝，腹側枝に分かれる．5-33では左腎動脈が2本分岐していることがわかる．複数の腎動脈が大動脈から分岐することはまれではなく，片側の腎動脈が2本以上存在する頻度は約25％とされる．

上腹部の静脈（造影CT門脈相, VR像） 241

5-35 上腹部の静脈（正面）

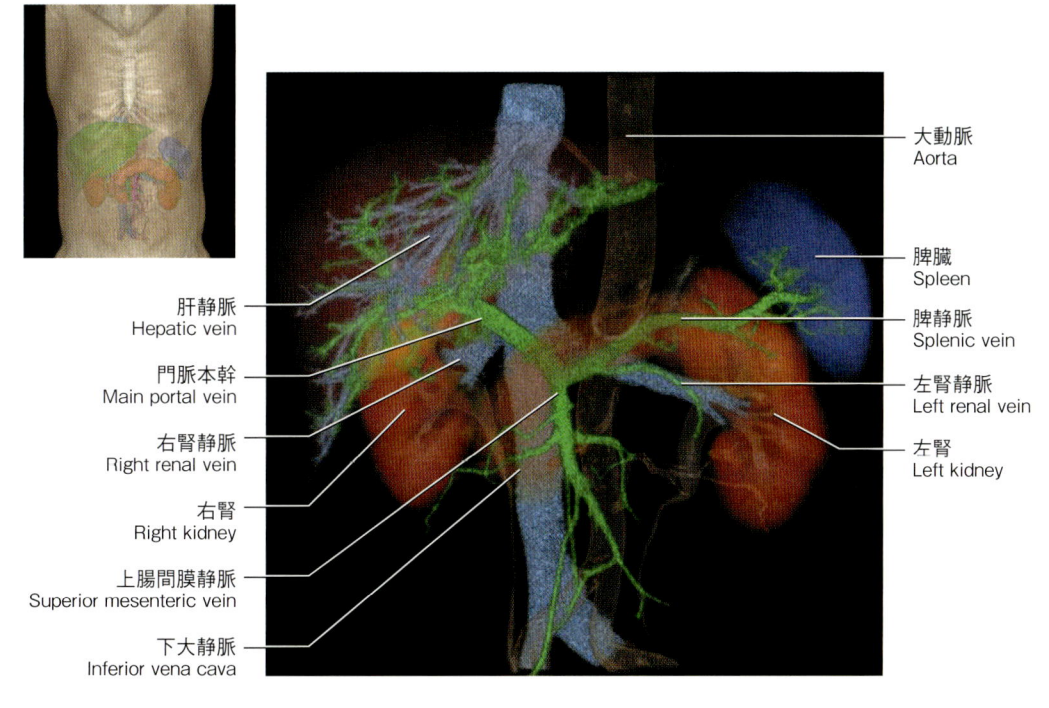

- 肝静脈 Hepatic vein
- 門脈本幹 Main portal vein
- 右腎静脈 Right renal vein
- 右腎 Right kidney
- 上腸間膜静脈 Superior mesenteric vein
- 下大静脈 Inferior vena cava
- 大動脈 Aorta
- 脾臓 Spleen
- 脾静脈 Splenic vein
- 左腎静脈 Left renal vein
- 左腎 Left kidney

5-36 上腹部の静脈（左斜め前）

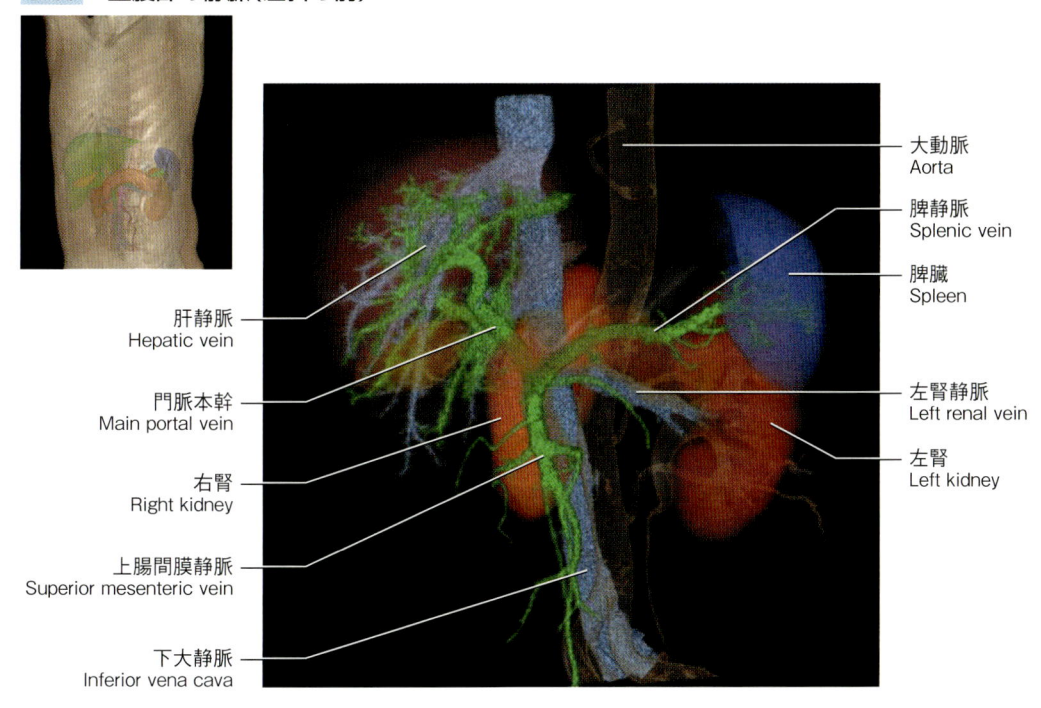

- 肝静脈 Hepatic vein
- 門脈本幹 Main portal vein
- 右腎 Right kidney
- 上腸間膜静脈 Superior mesenteric vein
- 下大静脈 Inferior vena cava
- 大動脈 Aorta
- 脾静脈 Splenic vein
- 脾臓 Spleen
- 左腎静脈 Left renal vein
- 左腎 Left kidney

> **NOTE** 肝静脈は，肝区域間を走行するし，通常，左右肝静脈，中肝静脈に分かれている（5-41〜5-44参照）．これらは斜め方向，頭側に走行し，下大静脈に注ぐ．多くは，左肝静脈と中肝静脈が合流してから下大静脈に注ぎ，右肝静脈は別に独立して下大静脈に注ぐ．

上腹部の動脈と横断面（造影CT動脈相＋VR像）

5-37 腹腔動脈レベル

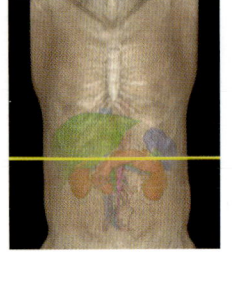

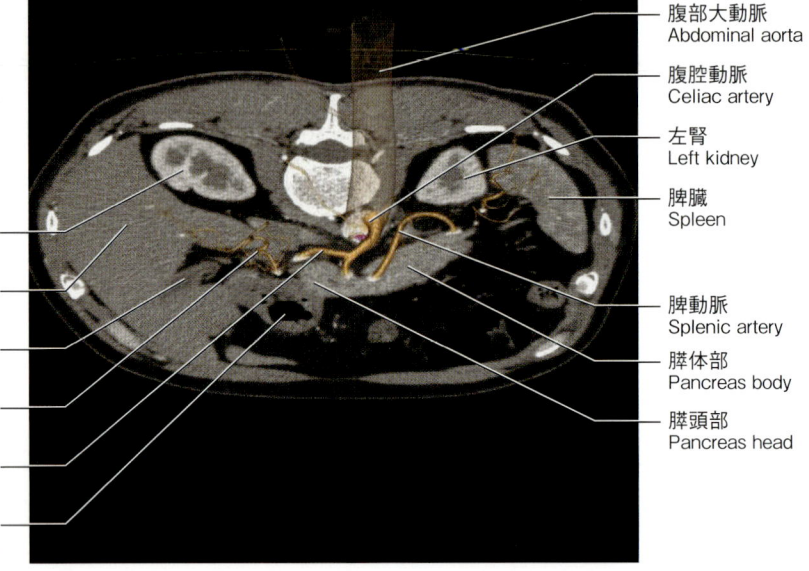

- 腹部大動脈 Abdominal aorta
- 腹腔動脈 Celiac artery
- 左腎 Left kidney
- 脾臓 Spleen
- 脾動脈 Splenic artery
- 膵体部 Pancreas body
- 膵頭部 Pancreas head
- 右腎 Right kidney
- 肝臓 Liver
- 胆嚢 Gallbladder
- 固有肝動脈 Proper hepatic artery
- 総肝動脈 Common hepatic artery
- 十二指腸 Duodenum

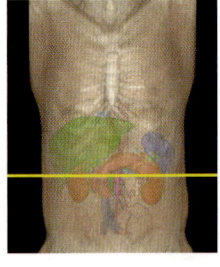

5-38 腎動脈レベル

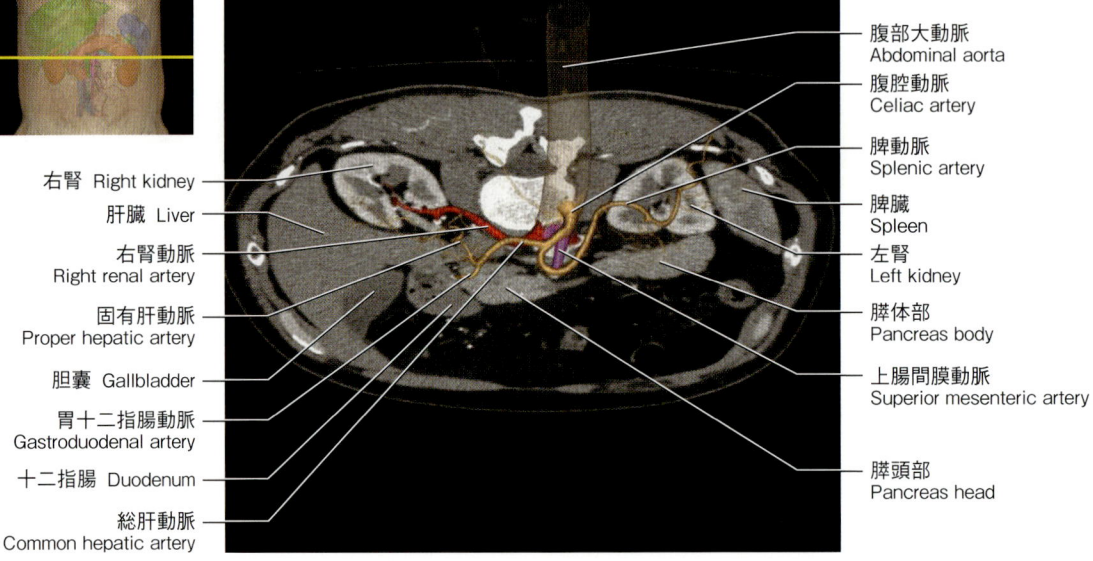

- 腹部大動脈 Abdominal aorta
- 腹腔動脈 Celiac artery
- 脾動脈 Splenic artery
- 脾臓 Spleen
- 左腎 Left kidney
- 膵体部 Pancreas body
- 上腸間膜動脈 Superior mesenteric artery
- 膵頭部 Pancreas head
- 右腎 Right kidney
- 肝臓 Liver
- 右腎動脈 Right renal artery
- 固有肝動脈 Proper hepatic artery
- 胆嚢 Gallbladder
- 胃十二指腸動脈 Gastroduodenal artery
- 十二指腸 Duodenum
- 総肝動脈 Common hepatic artery

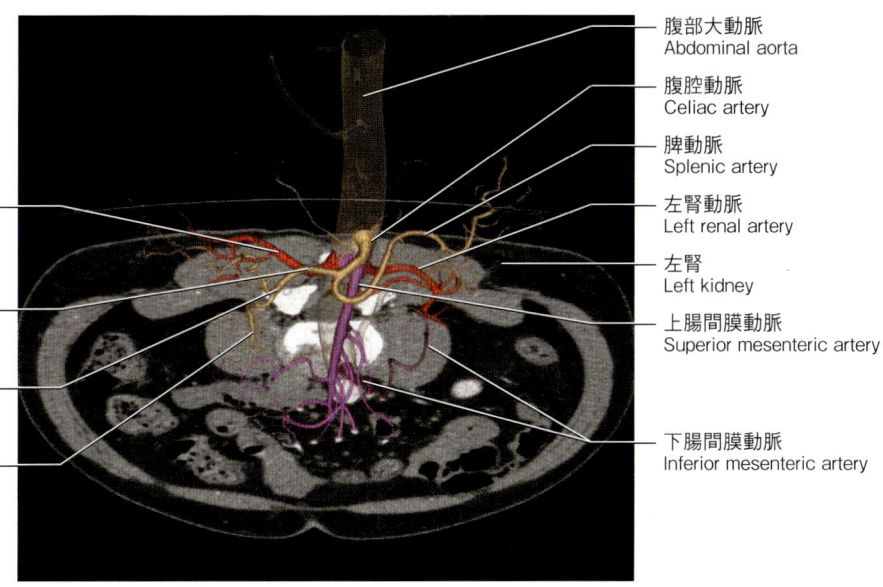

上腹部の動脈と横断面（造影 CT 動脈相＋VR 像）

5-39　膵頭部レベル

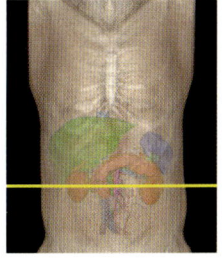

- 腹部大動脈　Abdominal aorta
- 腹腔動脈　Celiac artery
- 脾動脈　Splenic artery
- 左腎動脈　Left renal artery
- 左腎　Left kidney
- 脾臓　Spleen
- 膵体部　Pancreas body
- 上腸間膜動脈　Superior mesenteric artery
- 膵頭部　Pancreas head
- 右腎　Right kidney
- 肝臓　Liver
- 固有肝動脈　Proper hepatic artery
- 右腎動脈　Right renal artery
- 十二指腸　Duodenum
- 胃十二指腸動脈　Gastroduodenal artery
- 総肝動脈　Common hepatic artery

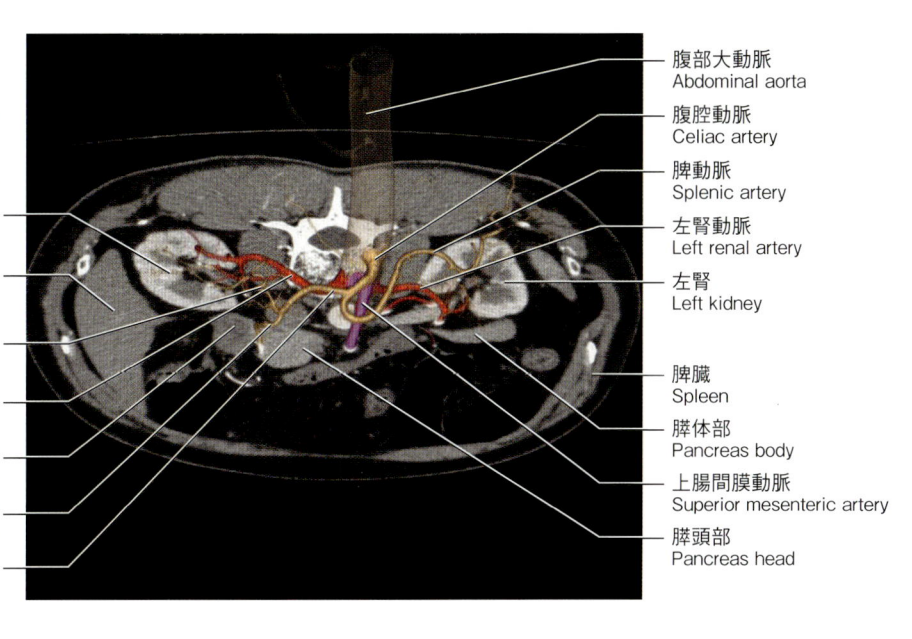

5-40　臍部レベル

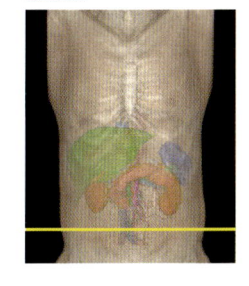

- 腹部大動脈　Abdominal aorta
- 腹腔動脈　Celiac artery
- 脾動脈　Splenic artery
- 左腎動脈　Left renal artery
- 左腎　Left kidney
- 上腸間膜動脈　Superior mesenteric artery
- 下腸間膜動脈　Inferior mesenteric artery
- 右腎動脈　Right renal artery
- 総肝動脈　Common hepatic artery
- 固有肝動脈　Proper hepatic artery
- 胃十二指腸動脈　Gastroduodenal artery

上腹部の静脈と横断面（造影CT門脈相＋VR像）

5-41 腸骨稜レベル

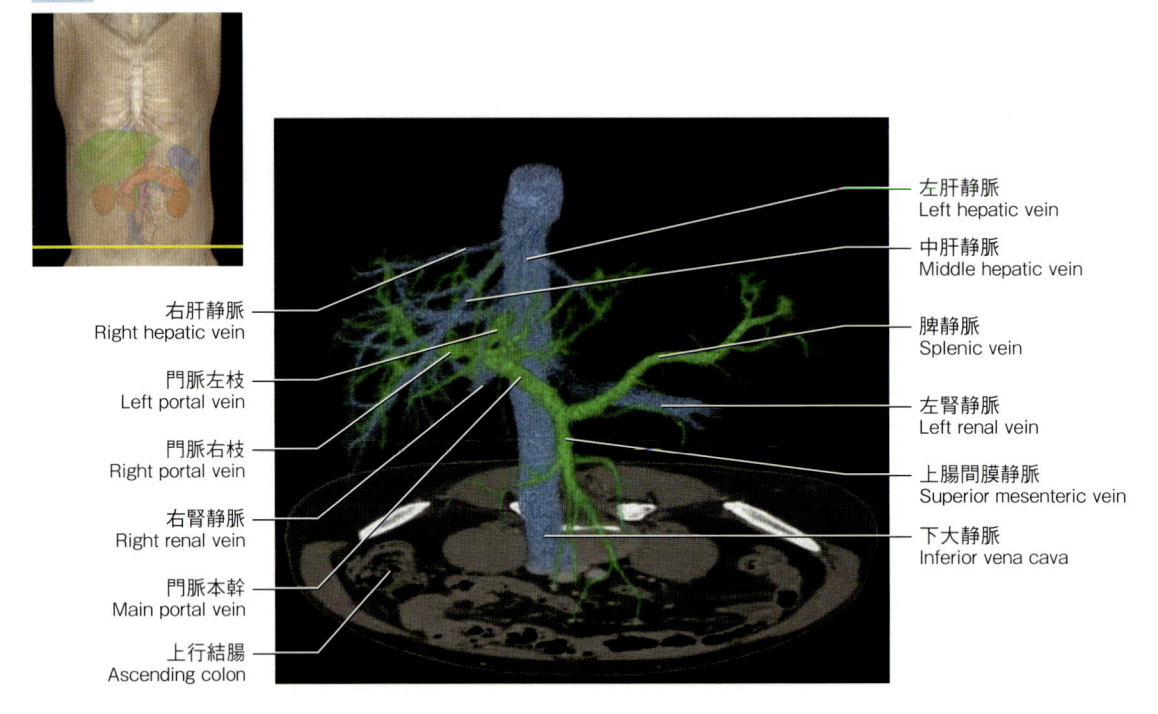

- 右肝静脈 Right hepatic vein
- 門脈左枝 Left portal vein
- 門脈右枝 Right portal vein
- 右腎静脈 Right renal vein
- 門脈本幹 Main portal vein
- 上行結腸 Ascending colon
- 左肝静脈 Left hepatic vein
- 中肝静脈 Middle hepatic vein
- 脾静脈 Splenic vein
- 左腎静脈 Left renal vein
- 上腸間膜静脈 Superior mesenteric vein
- 下大静脈 Inferior vena cava

5-42 腎静脈レベル

- 右肝静脈 Right hepatic vein
- 中肝静脈 Middle hepatic vein
- 門脈左枝 Left portal vein
- 門脈右枝 Right portal vein
- 肝臓 Liver
- 右腎 Right kidney
- 右腎静脈 Right renal vein
- 上行結腸 Ascending colon
- 門脈本幹 Main portal vein
- 膵臓 Pancreas
- 左肝静脈 Left hepatic vein
- 脾静脈 Splenic vein
- 左腎 Left kidney
- 左腎静脈 Left renal vein
- 下行結腸 Descending colon
- 上腸間膜静脈 Superior mesenteric vein

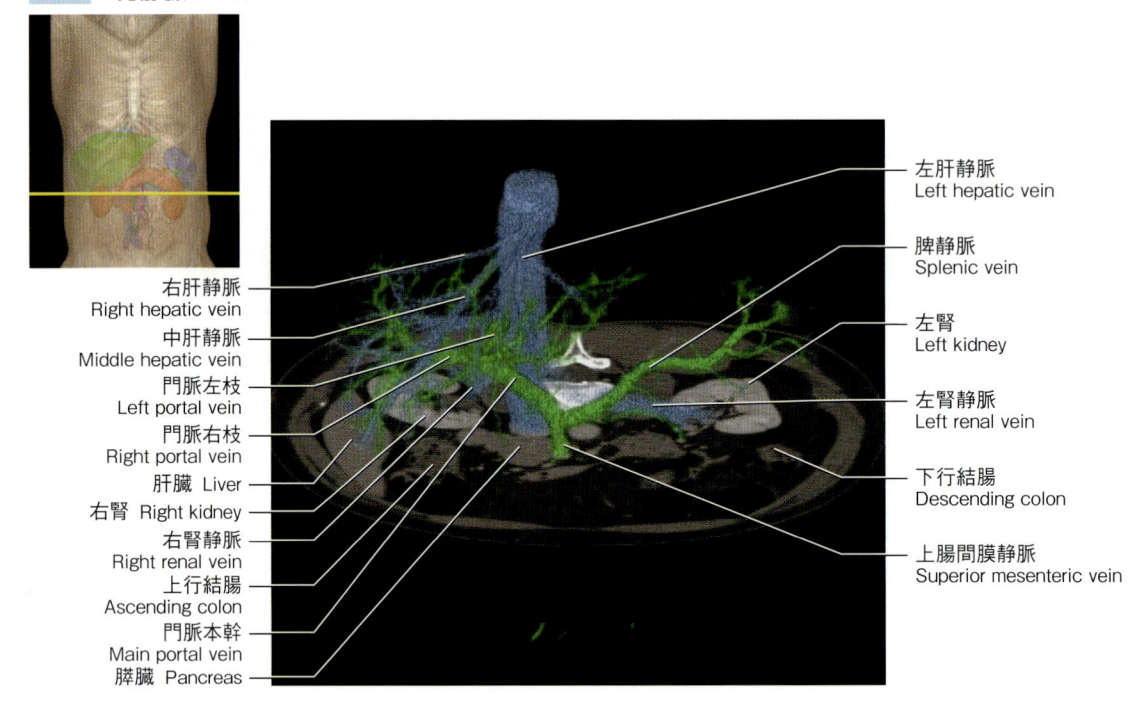

> **NOTE** 門脈は上腸間膜静脈と脾静脈が合流し，門脈本幹となる．肝門部で門脈左枝，門脈右枝に分かれる．門脈左枝は急峻に腹側へ曲がる．肝門部ほど太くなる．

上腹部の静脈と横断面（造影CT門脈相＋VR像） | 245

5-43 膵体部レベル

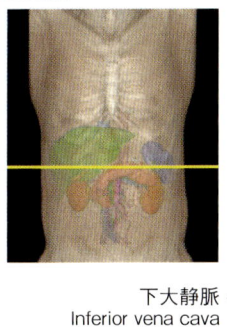

- 下大静脈 Inferior vena cava
- 右肝静脈 Right hepatic vein
- 中肝静脈 Middle hepatic vein
- 肝臓 Liver
- 門脈右枝 Right portal vein
- 胆嚢 Gallbladder
- 門脈左枝 Left portal vein
- 門脈本幹 Main portal vein
- 胃 Stomach
- 左肝静脈 Left hepatic vein
- 脾静脈 Splenic vein
- 右腎 Right kidney
- 膵臓 Pancreas
- 下行結腸 Descending colon

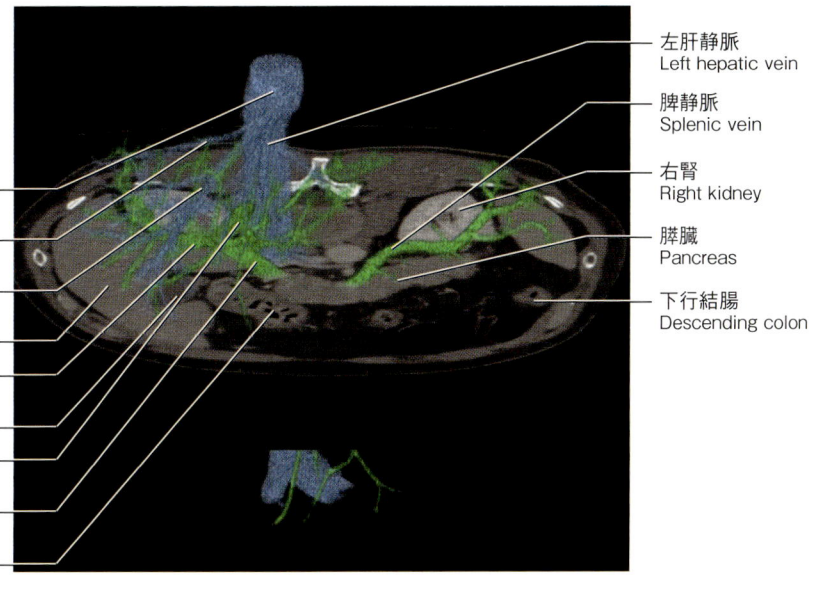

5-44 肝上部レベル

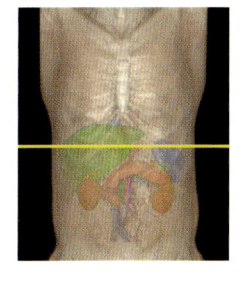

- 右肝静脈 Right hepatic vein
- 中肝静脈 Middle hepatic vein
- 肝臓 Liver
- 左肝静脈 Left hepatic vein
- 脾臓 Spleen
- 胃 Stomach

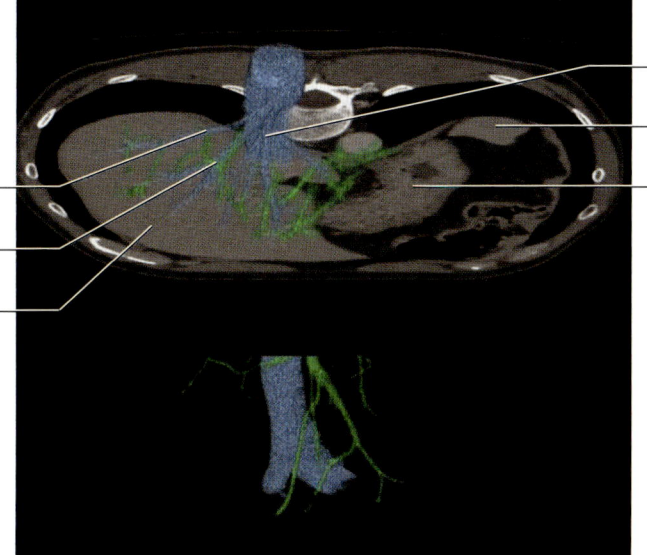

NOTE　肝臓の脈管系は動脈・門脈・静脈からなる．肝臓の静脈は右・中・左の3本が横隔膜直下の下大静脈に流入している．頭側，下大静脈側に行くに従い太くなる．

肝区域

5-45 Couinaud 分類

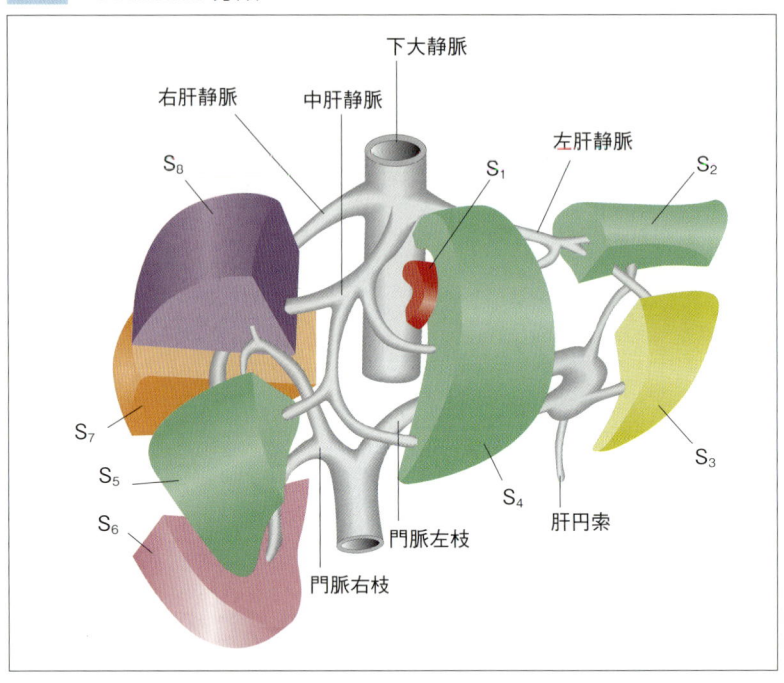

5-46 肝臓の静脈・門脈

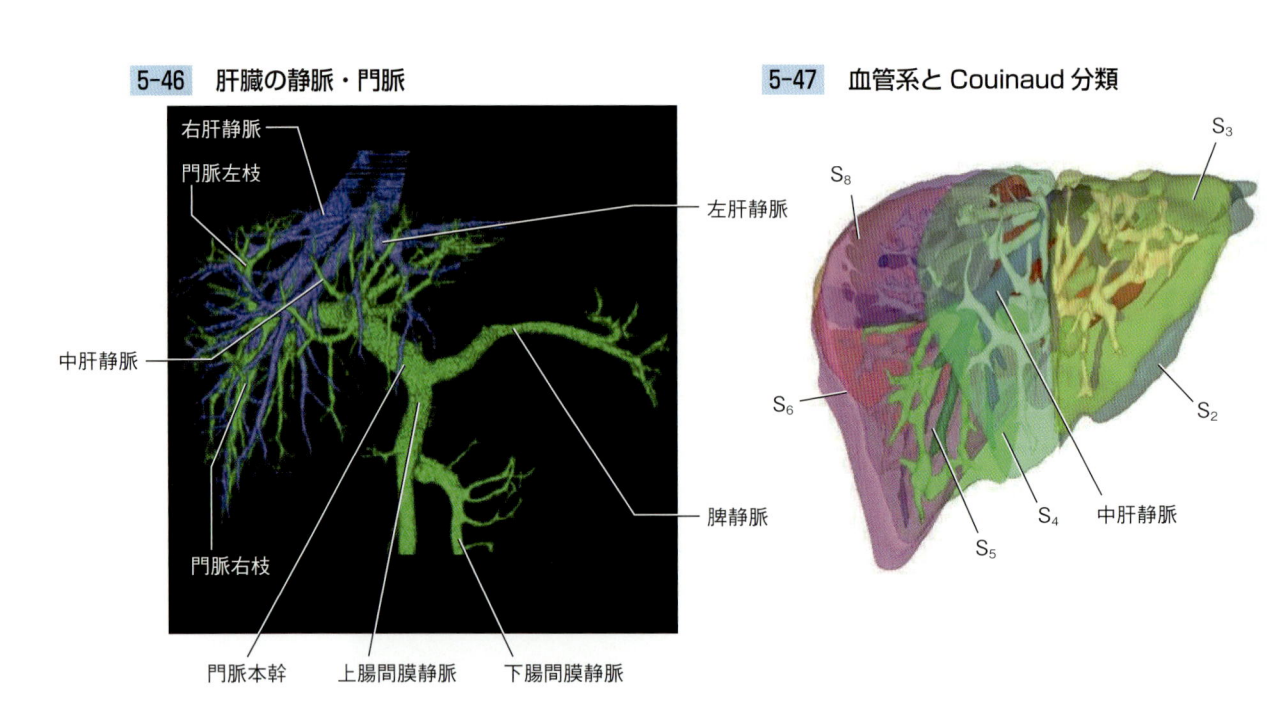

5-47 血管系と Couinaud 分類

> **NOTE** Couinaud（クイノー）の分類は，左・中・右の3本の肝静脈本幹で肝臓をS_1～S_8の8つの区域に分ける．左肝静脈本幹は左葉外側区（S_2, S_3）の中央を走り，外側後区（S_2）と外側前区（S_3）を境界する．中肝静脈本幹は内側区（S_4）と右葉前区（S_5, S_8）を境界する，Cantlie（カントリー）線にほぼ一致する境界線である．右肝静脈本幹は右葉の中央を貫き右葉前区（S_5, S_8）と後区（S_6, S_7）とに分ける．

肝区域 ［造影CT門脈相，静脈相，VR像（肝臓解析ソフトを使用）］

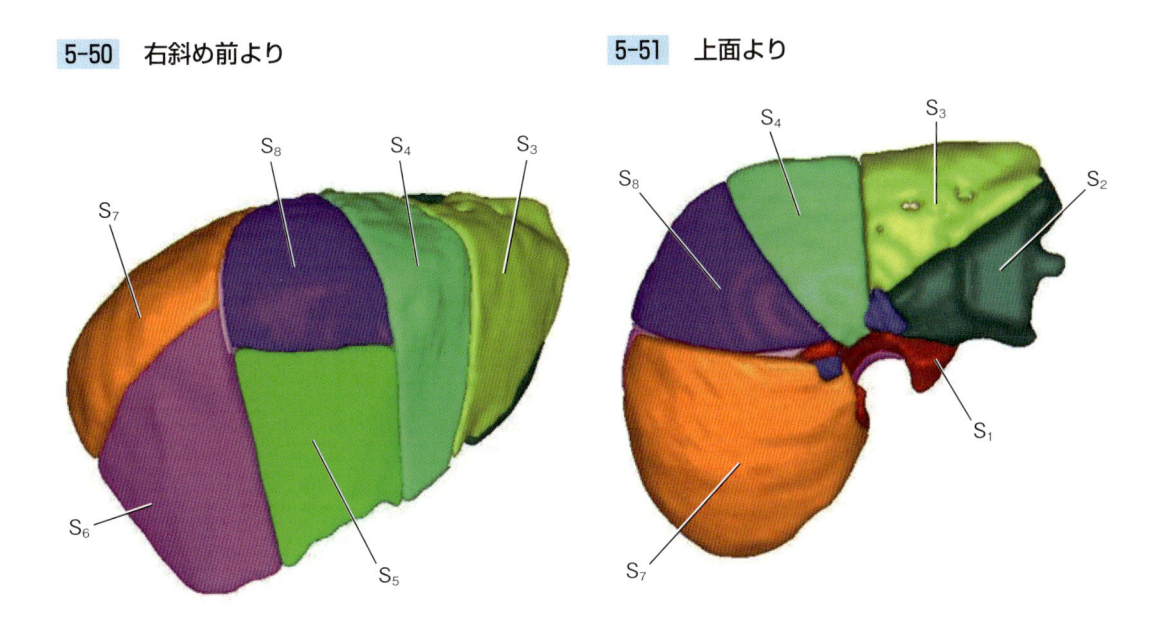

5-48 前面より

S$_8$, S$_4$, S$_3$, S$_2$, S$_6$, S$_5$

5-49 下面より

S$_5$, S$_4$, S$_3$, S$_8$, S$_6$, S$_2$, S$_1$, S$_7$

5-50 右斜め前より

S$_8$, S$_4$, S$_3$, S$_7$, S$_6$, S$_5$

5-51 上面より

S$_4$, S$_3$, S$_8$, S$_2$, S$_7$, S$_1$

NOTE 肝臓は外表面の切痕，分葉により肉眼的に右葉，左葉，方形葉，尾状葉に分けられる．さらに，S$_1$（尾状葉），S$_2$（左葉背外側区），S$_3$（左葉腹外側区），S$_4$（左葉内側区），S$_5$（右葉前下区），S$_6$（右葉後区域），S$_7$（右葉後上区），S$_8$（右葉前上区）の8区域に分けられる．

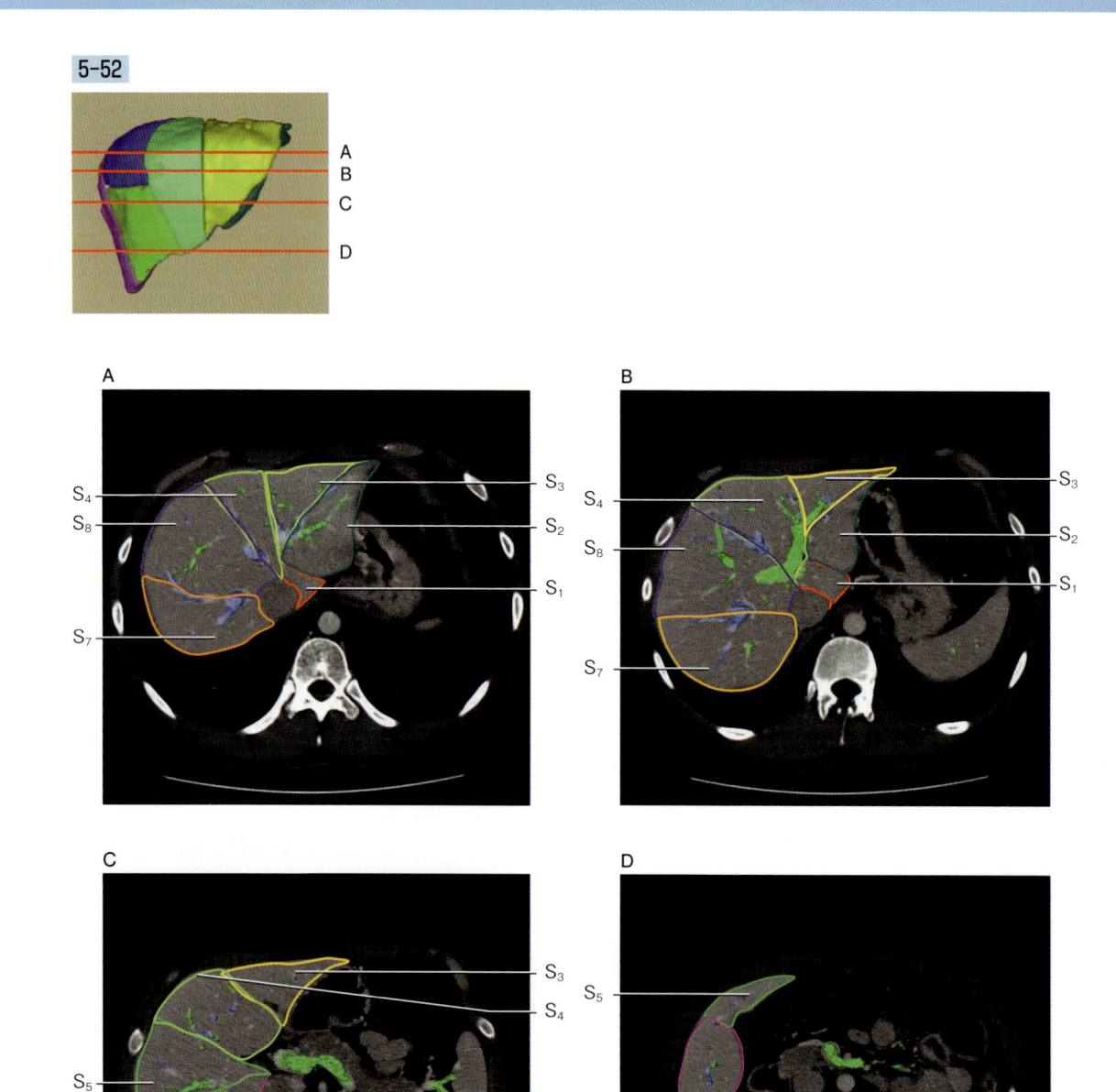

肝区域の横断面（造影CT門脈相）

5-52

A

S4, S8, S7 — S3, S2, S1

B

S4, S8, S7 — S3, S2, S1

C

S5, S6 — S3, S4

D

S6 — S5

> **NOTE** モニター診断では画像を高速にページングできるため，肝門を走行する血管を同定しやすい．門脈・肝静脈を目印に肝区域を知ることは比較的容易である．5-52では，門脈を緑，肝静脈を青で示している．

腹部の断層解剖 ［横断像（造影 CT 平衡相）］

5-53

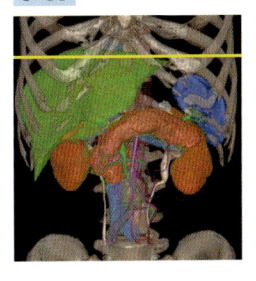

- 肝臓 Liver
- 食道 Esophagus
- 腹部大動脈 Abdominal aorta
- 左肝静脈 Left hepatic vein
- 中肝静脈 Middle hepatic vein
- 下大静脈 Inferior vena cava

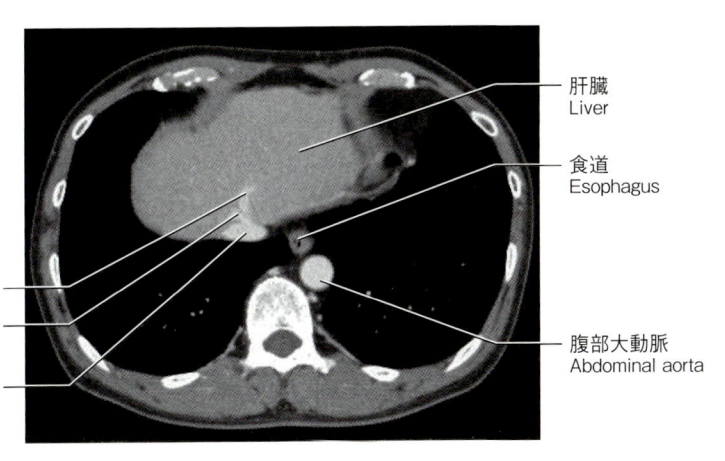

5-54

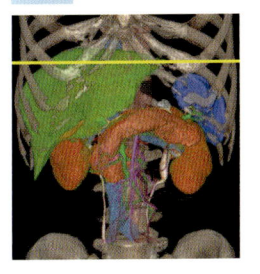

- 横隔膜 Diaphragm
- 食道 Esophagus
- 腹部大動脈 Abdominal aorta
- 下大静脈 Inferior vena cava
- 左肝静脈 Left hepatic vein
- 右肝静脈 Right hepatic vein
- 中肝静脈 Middle hepatic vein

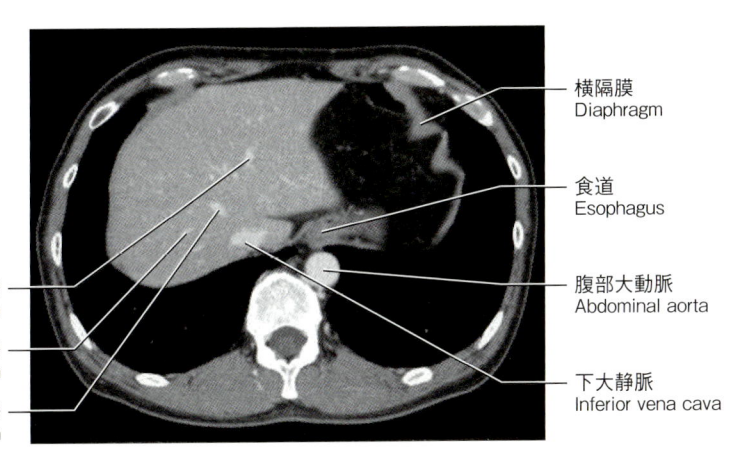

5-55

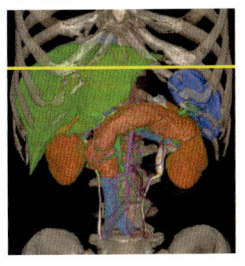

- 門脈左枝 Left portal vein
- 胃 Stomach
- 下大静脈 Inferior vena cava
- 腹部大動脈 Abdominal aorta
- 中肝静脈 Middle hepatic vein
- 右肝静脈 Right hepatic vein
- 左肝静脈 Left hepatic vein

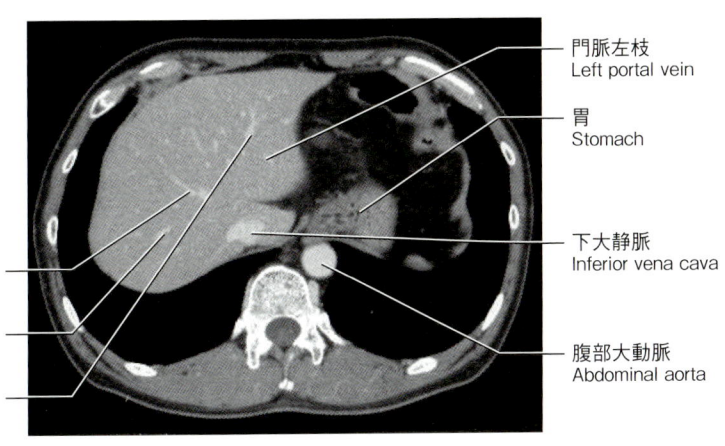

> **NOTE** 門脈 Portal vein
> 肝静脈と門脈は頭側下大静脈方向へ向かうものと，肝門部方向へ向かうもので鑑別可能．porta はラテン語で門の意味で，港の意味をもつ．これから import（輸入），export（輸出）という語へ発展した．

腹部の断層解剖 ［横断像（造影CT平衡相）］

5-56

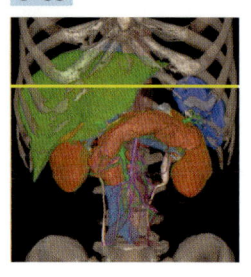

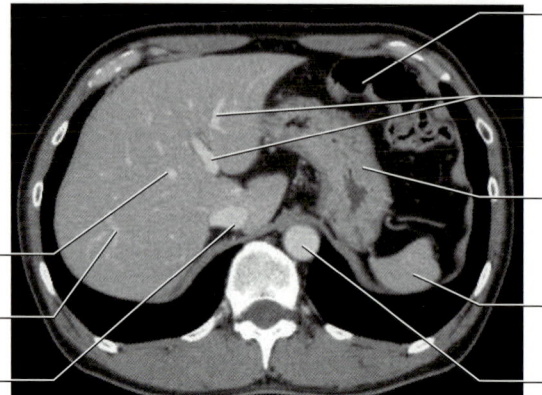

- 横行結腸 Transverse colon
- 門脈左枝 Left portal vein
- 胃 Stomach
- 脾臓 Spleen
- 腹部大動脈 Abdominal aorta
- 中肝静脈 Middle hepatic vein
- 右肝静脈 Right hepatic vein
- 下大静脈 Inferior vena cava

5-57

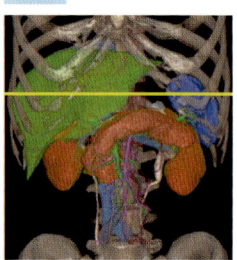

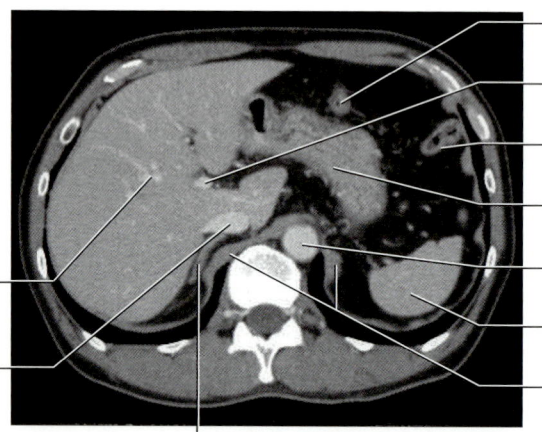

- 横行結腸 Transverse colon
- 門脈左枝 Left portal vein
- 下行結腸 Descending colon
- 胃 Stomach
- 腹部大動脈 Abdominal aorta
- 脾臓 Spleen
- 横隔膜脚 Crus of diaphragm
- 中肝静脈 Middle hepatic vein
- 下大静脈 Inferior vena cava
- 右副腎 Right adrenal gland

5-58

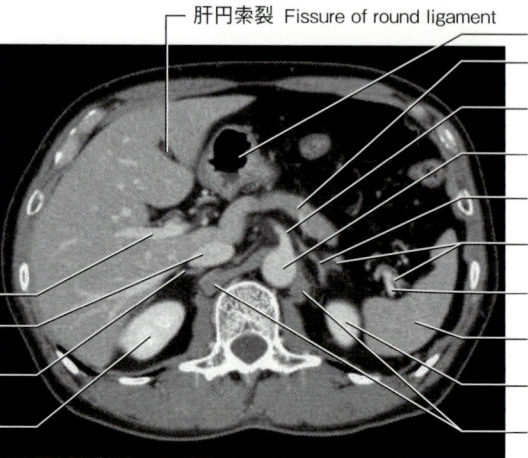

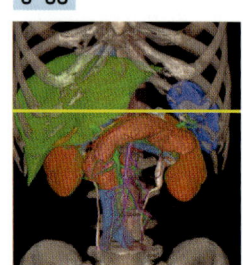

- 肝円索裂 Fissure of round ligament
- 胃 Stomach
- 膵臓 Pancreas
- 腹腔動脈 Celiac artery
- 腹部大動脈 Abdominal aorta
- 左副腎 Left adrenal gland
- 脾動脈 Splenic artery
- 脾静脈 Splenic vein
- 脾臓 Spleen
- 左腎 Left kidney
- 横隔膜脚 Crus of diaphragm
- 門脈右枝 Right portal vein
- 下大静脈 Inferior vena cava
- 右副腎 Right adrenal gland
- 右腎 Right kidney

NOTE 胃は噴門から胃体部にかけて腹腔内を背側から腹側に向かい，胃角部から幽門部は腹壁直下に存在する．幽門部から十二指腸にかけて再び背側へ向かう．胃は空腹時，食後などにより，拡張の程度や形態が異なってくる．

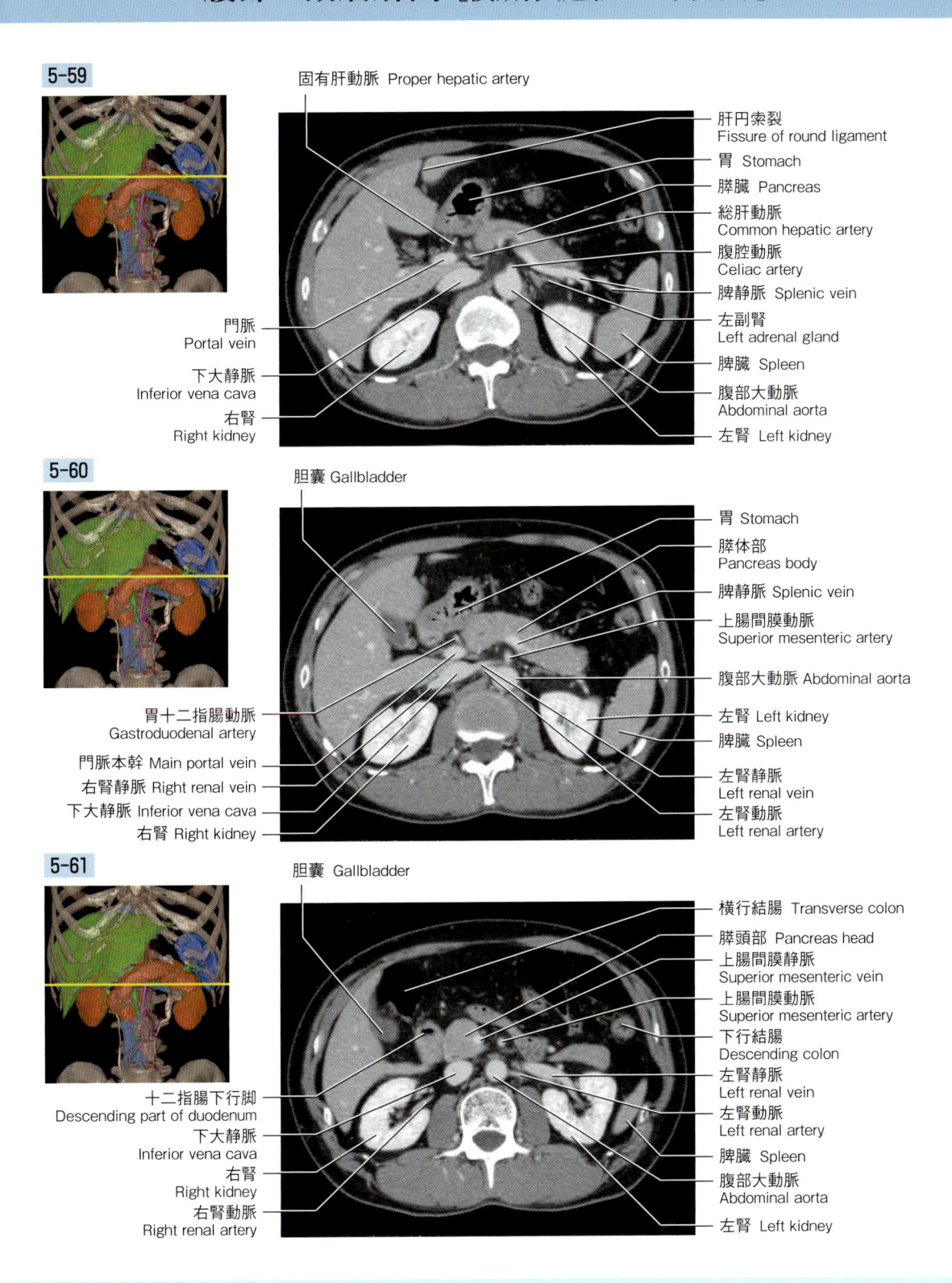

腹部の断層解剖 ［横断像（造影 CT 平衡相）］

5-59

- 固有肝動脈 Proper hepatic artery
- 肝円索裂 Fissure of round ligament
- 胃 Stomach
- 膵臓 Pancreas
- 総肝動脈 Common hepatic artery
- 腹腔動脈 Celiac artery
- 脾静脈 Splenic vein
- 左副腎 Left adrenal gland
- 脾臓 Spleen
- 腹部大動脈 Abdominal aorta
- 左腎 Left kidney
- 門脈 Portal vein
- 下大静脈 Inferior vena cava
- 右腎 Right kidney

5-60

- 胆嚢 Gallbladder
- 胃 Stomach
- 膵体部 Pancreas body
- 脾静脈 Splenic vein
- 上腸間膜動脈 Superior mesenteric artery
- 腹部大動脈 Abdominal aorta
- 左腎 Left kidney
- 脾臓 Spleen
- 左腎静脈 Left renal vein
- 左腎動脈 Left renal artery
- 胃十二指腸動脈 Gastroduodenal artery
- 門脈本幹 Main portal vein
- 右腎静脈 Right renal vein
- 下大静脈 Inferior vena cava
- 右腎 Right kidney

5-61

- 胆嚢 Gallbladder
- 横行結腸 Transverse colon
- 膵頭部 Pancreas head
- 上腸間膜静脈 Superior mesenteric vein
- 上腸間膜動脈 Superior mesenteric artery
- 下行結腸 Descending colon
- 左腎静脈 Left renal vein
- 左腎動脈 Left renal artery
- 脾臓 Spleen
- 腹部大動脈 Abdominal aorta
- 左腎 Left kidney
- 十二指腸下行脚 Descending part of duodenum
- 下大静脈 Inferior vena cava
- 右腎 Right kidney
- 右腎動脈 Right renal artery

> **NOTE** 体軸横断面の背側から腹側に向かって，腹部大動脈，左腎静脈，上腸間膜動脈，脾静脈，膵臓の順である．左腎静脈が腹部大動脈と上腸間膜動脈に圧迫されて血流障害が生じるとナットクラッカー症候群（Nutcracker syndrome）が発生する．断層面が異なると，腹部大動脈と上腸間膜動脈の間には十二指腸水平脚が入るが，十二指腸が挟まれ通過障害が起こると上腸間膜動脈症候群（Superior mesenteric artery syndrome：SMA syndrome）とよばれる．

腹部の断層解剖 ［横断像（造影CT平衡相）］

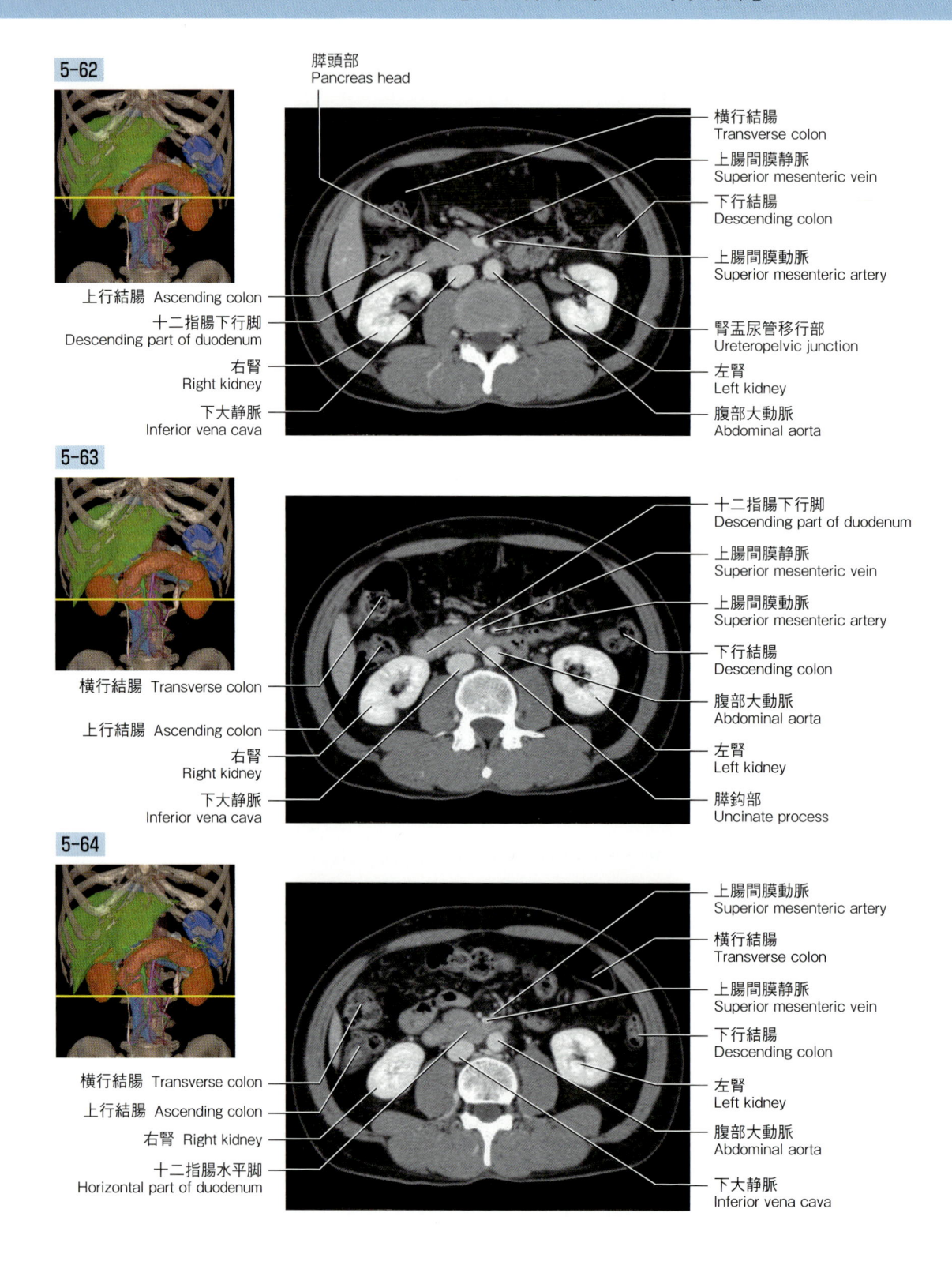

5-62

- 膵頭部 Pancreas head
- 横行結腸 Transverse colon
- 上腸間膜静脈 Superior mesenteric vein
- 下行結腸 Descending colon
- 上腸間膜動脈 Superior mesenteric artery
- 腎盂尿管移行部 Ureteropelvic junction
- 左腎 Left kidney
- 腹部大動脈 Abdominal aorta
- 上行結腸 Ascending colon
- 十二指腸下行脚 Descending part of duodenum
- 右腎 Right kidney
- 下大静脈 Inferior vena cava

5-63

- 十二指腸下行脚 Descending part of duodenum
- 上腸間膜静脈 Superior mesenteric vein
- 上腸間膜動脈 Superior mesenteric artery
- 下行結腸 Descending colon
- 腹部大動脈 Abdominal aorta
- 左腎 Left kidney
- 膵鉤部 Uncinate process
- 横行結腸 Transverse colon
- 上行結腸 Ascending colon
- 右腎 Right kidney
- 下大静脈 Inferior vena cava

5-64

- 上腸間膜動脈 Superior mesenteric artery
- 横行結腸 Transverse colon
- 上腸間膜静脈 Superior mesenteric vein
- 下行結腸 Descending colon
- 左腎 Left kidney
- 腹部大動脈 Abdominal aorta
- 下大静脈 Inferior vena cava
- 横行結腸 Transverse colon
- 上行結腸 Ascending colon
- 右腎 Right kidney
- 十二指腸水平脚 Horizontal part of duodenum

> **NOTE** 上腸間膜静脈（Superior mesenteric vein：SMV）は上腸間膜動脈（Superior mesenteric artery：SMA）の右側にあり，この位置関係の観察が腸間膜の捻転の評価に有用なことがある．SMVは通常SMAより太く，細い場合は"Smaller SMV sign"として上腸間膜動脈閉塞症を疑う所見である．

腹部の断層解剖　[横断像（造影 CT 平衡相）]

5-65

- 横行結腸　Transverse colon
- 十二指腸水平脚　Horizontal part of duodenum
- 白線　Linea alba
- 腹直筋　Rectus abdominis muscle
- 腹部大動脈　Abdominal aorta
- 外腹斜筋　External oblique muscle
- 内腹斜筋　Internal oblique muscle
- 腹横筋　Transverse abdominal muscle
- 上行結腸　Ascending colon
- 下大静脈　Inferior vena cava
- 腰筋　Psoas muscle
- 下行結腸　Descending colon
- 腰方形筋　Quadratus lumborum muscle
- 脊柱起立筋　Erector spinae muscle
- 左腎　Left kidney

5-66

- 横行結腸　Transverse colon
- 腹部大動脈　Abdominal aorta
- 上行結腸　Ascending colon
- 虫垂　Appendix
- 下大静脈　Inferior vena cava
- 下行結腸　Descending colon

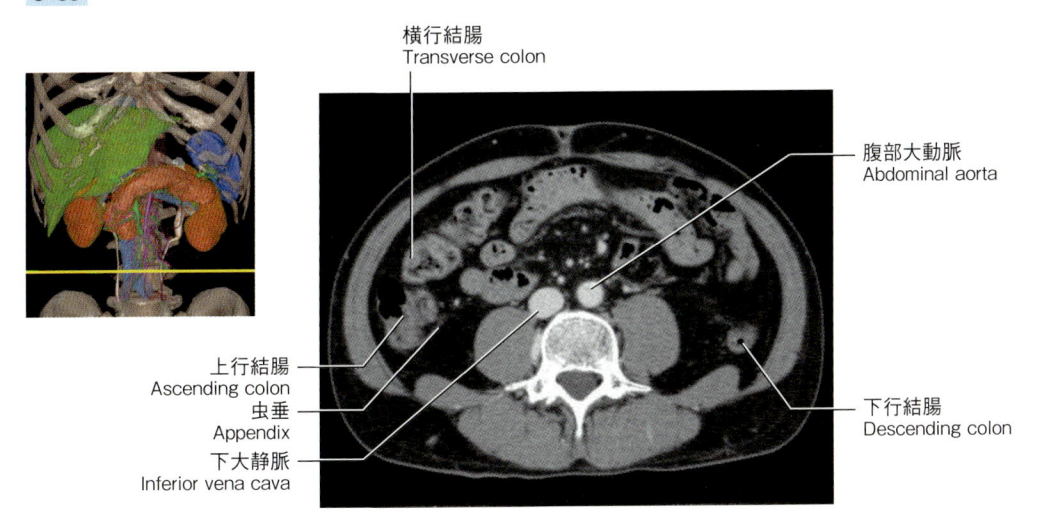

> **NOTE**　横行結腸，S状結腸などと比べ，上行結腸と下行結腸は，後腹膜腔に固定されているので通常移動が少なく，同定しやすい．したがって結腸の同定には，まず右外側の上行結腸，左外側にある下行結腸を同定し，連続性を追っていくことが重要である．

腹部の断層解剖 ［冠状断像（造影CT 平衡相）］

5-67

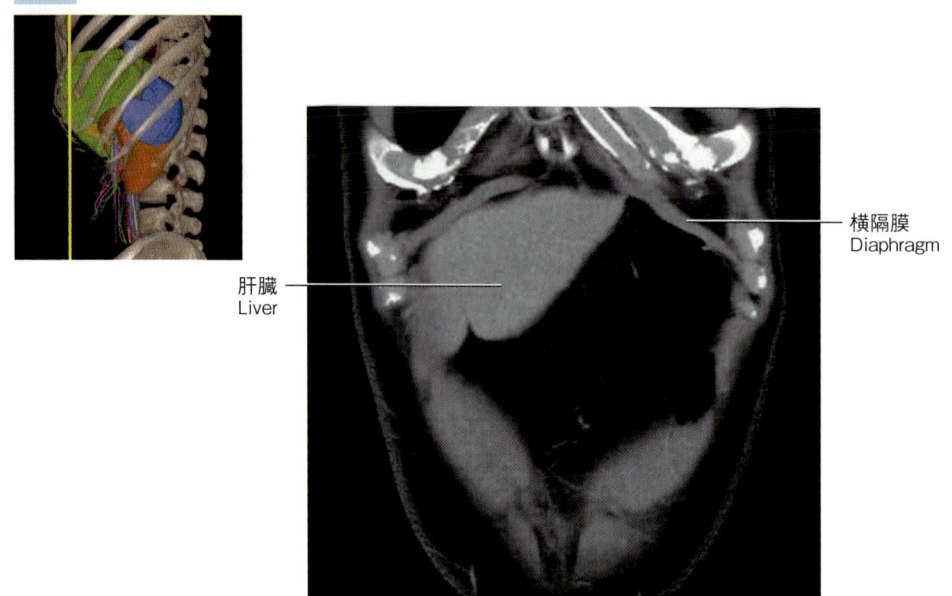

- 横隔膜 Diaphragm
- 肝臓 Liver

5-68

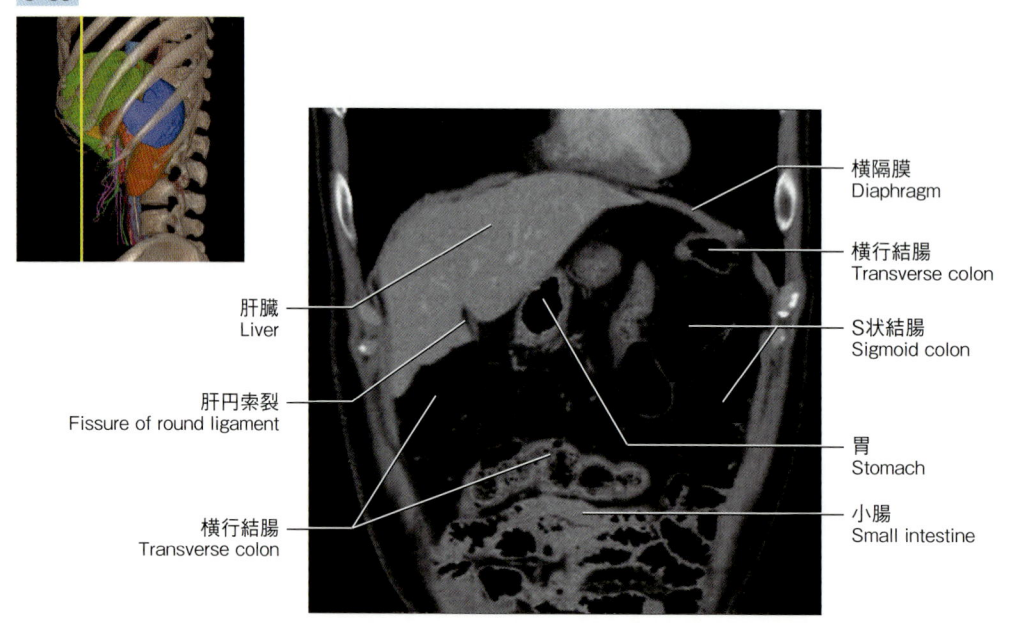

- 横隔膜 Diaphragm
- 横行結腸 Transverse colon
- S状結腸 Sigmoid colon
- 胃 Stomach
- 小腸 Small intestine
- 肝臓 Liver
- 肝円索裂 Fissure of round ligament
- 横行結腸 Transverse colon

> **NOTE** 横隔膜 Diaphragm
> Diaphragmは"dia-［…を経て（through）］"と垣根を表すギリシャ語の"phragma"との合成語である．Diarrhea（下痢）はdia-＋rrhea（漏出，流出），Diabetes（糖尿病）はdia-＋bainein（行く：糖が腎臓を通過するという意味）と，医学用語としてdia-は多数あらわれる．diagnosisはdia-＋gnosis（認識・知識）．ちなみに，Prognosis（予後）はpro-（前）＋gnosisの合成語である．

腹部の断層解剖　[冠状断像（造影 CT 平衡相）]

5-69

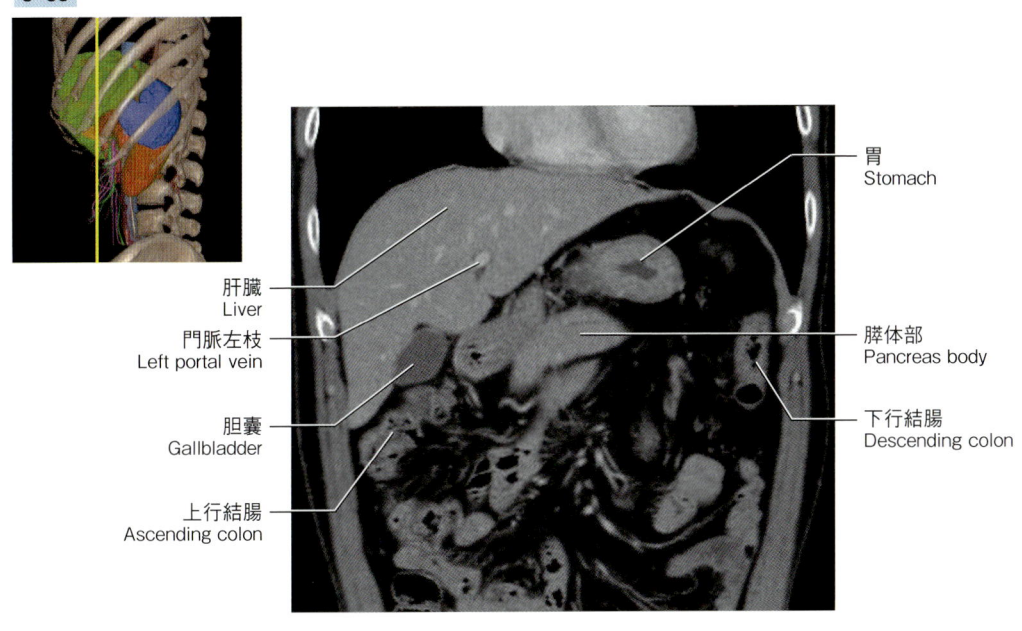

- 肝臓 Liver
- 門脈左枝 Left portal vein
- 胆嚢 Gallbladder
- 上行結腸 Ascending colon
- 胃 Stomach
- 膵体部 Pancreas body
- 下行結腸 Descending colon

5-70

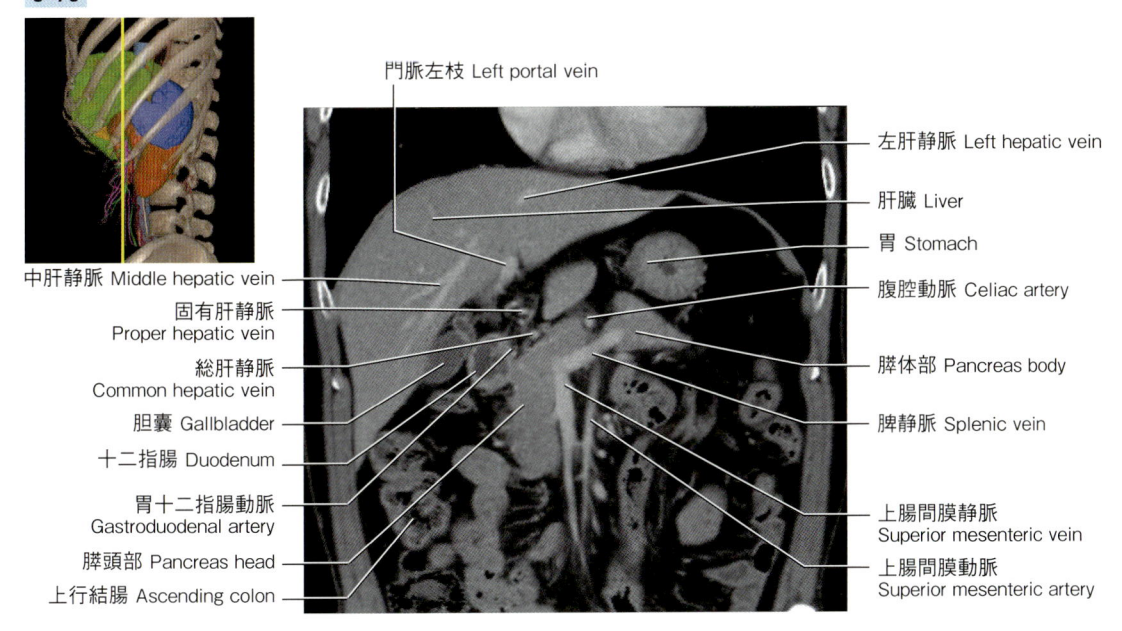

- 中肝静脈 Middle hepatic vein
- 固有肝静脈 Proper hepatic vein
- 総肝静脈 Common hepatic vein
- 胆嚢 Gallbladder
- 十二指腸 Duodenum
- 胃十二指腸動脈 Gastroduodenal artery
- 膵頭部 Pancreas head
- 上行結腸 Ascending colon
- 門脈左枝 Left portal vein
- 左肝静脈 Left hepatic vein
- 肝臓 Liver
- 胃 Stomach
- 腹腔動脈 Celiac artery
- 膵体部 Pancreas body
- 脾静脈 Splenic vein
- 上腸間膜静脈 Superior mesenteric vein
- 上腸間膜動脈 Superior mesenteric artery

NOTE 膵体部の外側に十二指腸，胆嚢が位置する．胆嚢は肝右葉前区域の下面に位置する．胆嚢癌が浸潤をきたしやすい．肝左葉外側区域と内側区域を門脈左葉枝が前後に走行する．上腸間膜静脈が脾静脈と合流して門脈となる．

腹部の断層解剖 ［冠状断像（造影 CT 平衡相）］

5-71

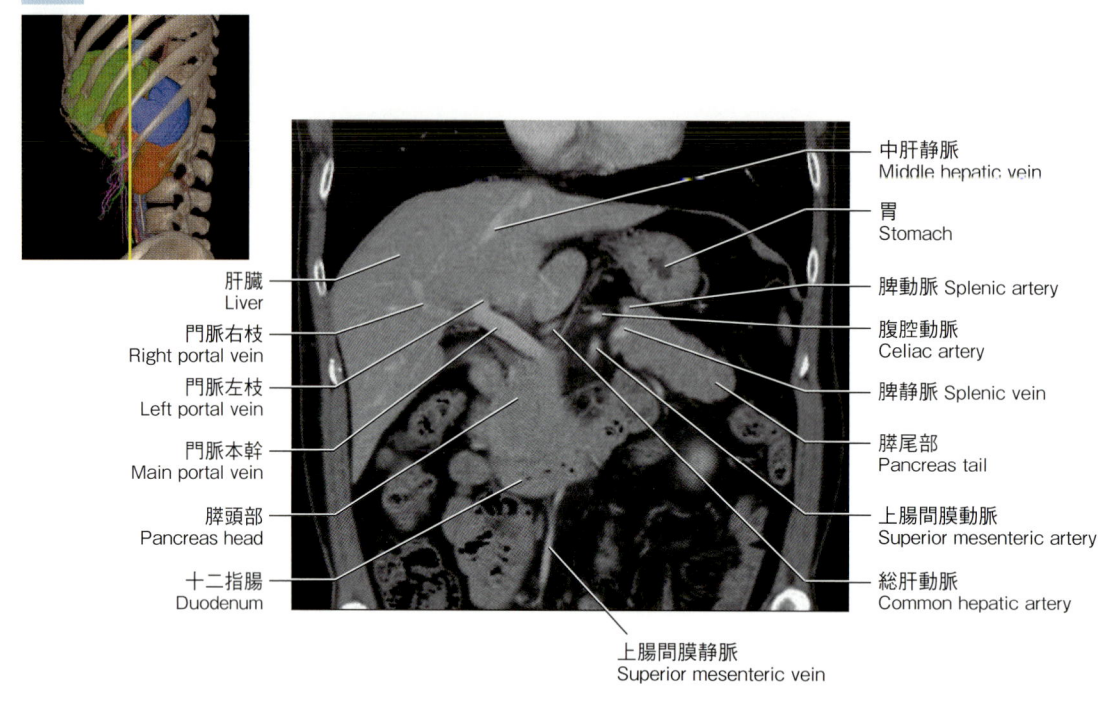

- 中肝静脈 Middle hepatic vein
- 胃 Stomach
- 肝臓 Liver
- 脾動脈 Splenic artery
- 門脈右枝 Right portal vein
- 腹腔動脈 Celiac artery
- 門脈左枝 Left portal vein
- 脾静脈 Splenic vein
- 門脈本幹 Main portal vein
- 膵尾部 Pancreas tail
- 膵頭部 Pancreas head
- 上腸間膜動脈 Superior mesenteric artery
- 十二指腸 Duodenum
- 総肝動脈 Common hepatic artery
- 上腸間膜静脈 Superior mesenteric vein

5-72 造影 CT 動脈相

- 胃 Stomach
- 腹腔動脈 Celiac artery
- 肝臓 Liver
- 脾動脈 Splenic artery
- 脾静脈 Splenic vein
- 門脈 Portal vein
- 膵尾部 Pancreas tail
- 膵頭部 Pancreas head
- 上腸間膜動脈 Superior mesenteric artery
- 十二指腸 Duodenum
- 左腎静脈 Left renal vein
- 上腸間膜静脈 Superior mesenteric vein
- 膵管 Pancreatic duct

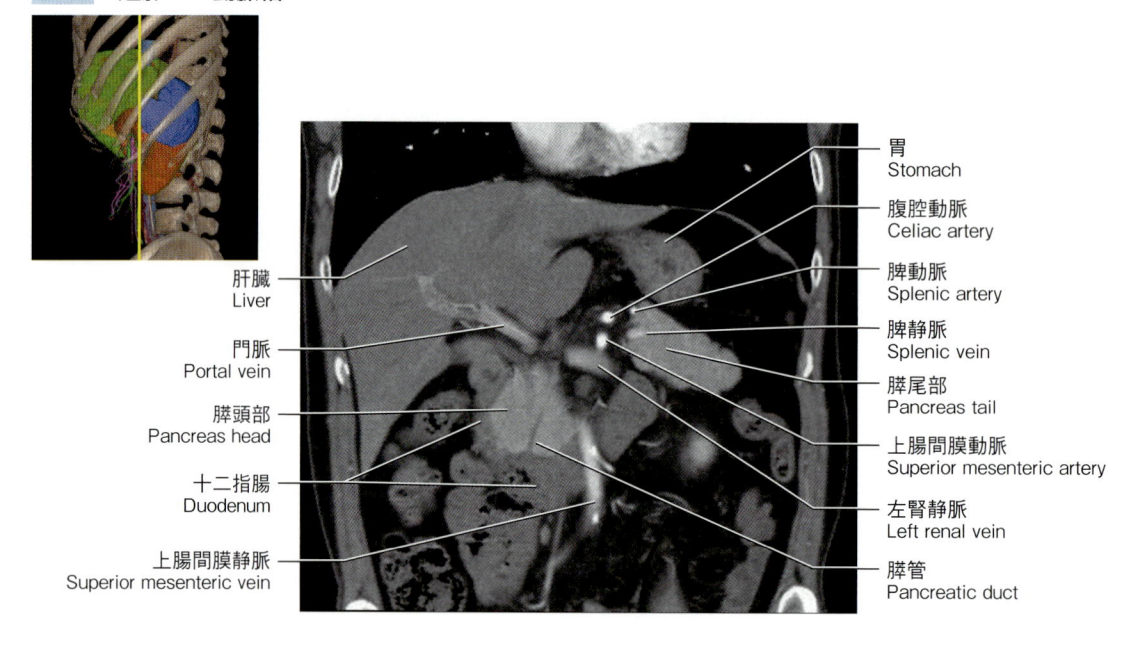

NOTE 膵頭部と体部の境界は，上腸間膜静脈・門脈の左側縁とする．膵体部と尾部の境界は，頭部を除いた尾側膵を二等分する線となる．膵鉤部は頭部に含める．

腹部の断層解剖 ［冠状断像（造影CT 平衡相）］

5-73　MRCP（T2強調冠状断像）

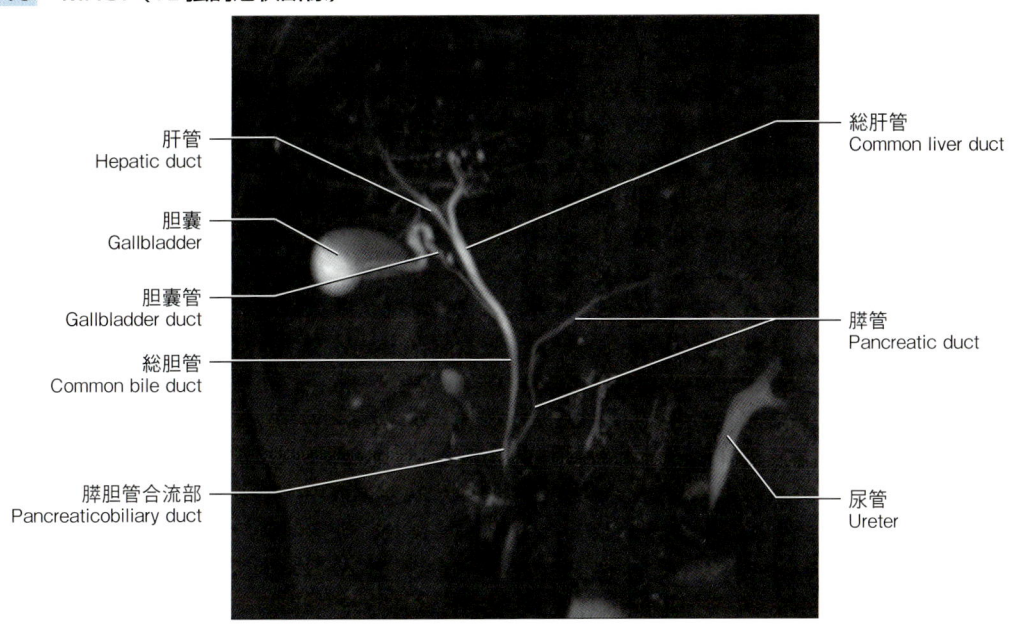

- 肝管 Hepatic duct
- 胆嚢 Gallbladder
- 胆嚢管 Gallbladder duct
- 総胆管 Common bile duct
- 膵胆管合流部 Pancreaticobiliary duct
- 総肝管 Common liver duct
- 膵管 Pancreatic duct
- 尿管 Ureter

5-74

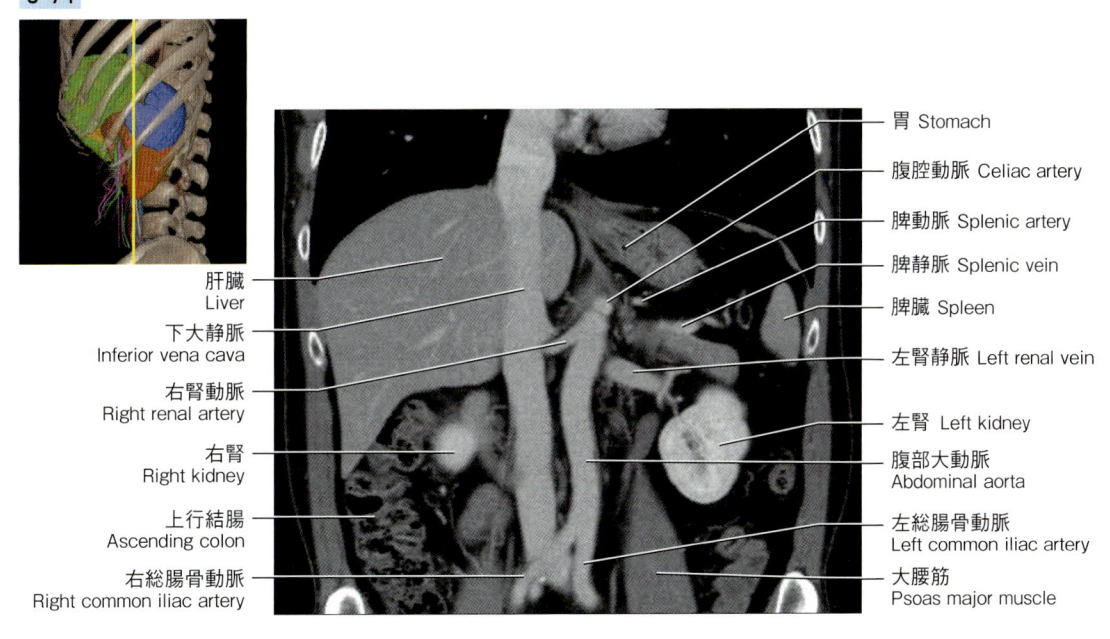

- 肝臓 Liver
- 下大静脈 Inferior vena cava
- 右腎動脈 Right renal artery
- 右腎 Right kidney
- 上行結腸 Ascending colon
- 右総腸骨動脈 Right common iliac artery
- 胃 Stomach
- 腹腔動脈 Celiac artery
- 脾動脈 Splenic artery
- 脾静脈 Splenic vein
- 脾臓 Spleen
- 左腎静脈 Left renal vein
- 左腎 Left kidney
- 腹部大動脈 Abdominal aorta
- 左総腸骨動脈 Left common iliac artery
- 大腰筋 Psoas major muscle

NOTE　MRCP（magnetic resonance cholangiopancreatography）はMR hydrographyのひとつであり，静止あるいは動きの少ない液体成分を強調して画像化する．肝内胆管から肝臓外に出た左右肝管は肝門部で合流し，その後，胆嚢管が合流する（三管合流部）．三管合流部から乳頭部までを総胆管とよぶ．総胆管は乳頭部で膵管と合流する．

腹部の断層解剖 ［冠状断像（造影 CT 平衡相）］

5-75 造影 CT 動脈相

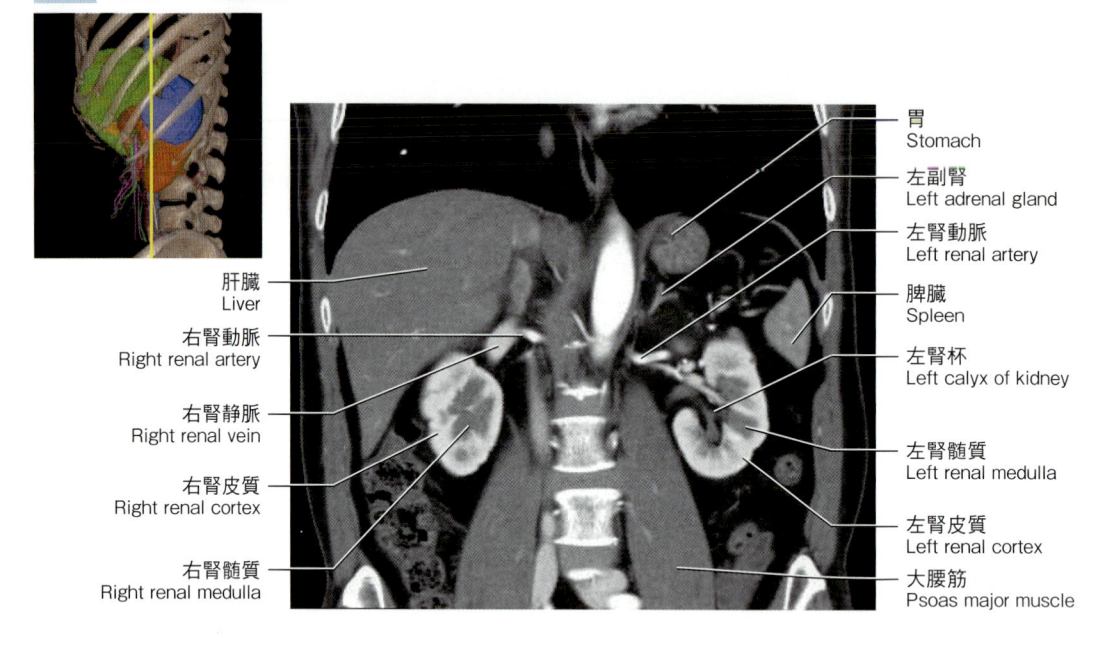

- 肝臓 Liver
- 右腎動脈 Right renal artery
- 右腎静脈 Right renal vein
- 右腎皮質 Right renal cortex
- 右腎髄質 Right renal medulla
- 胃 Stomach
- 左副腎 Left adrenal gland
- 左腎動脈 Left renal artery
- 脾臓 Spleen
- 左腎杯 Left calyx of kidney
- 左腎髄質 Left renal medulla
- 左腎皮質 Left renal cortex
- 大腰筋 Psoas major muscle

5-76

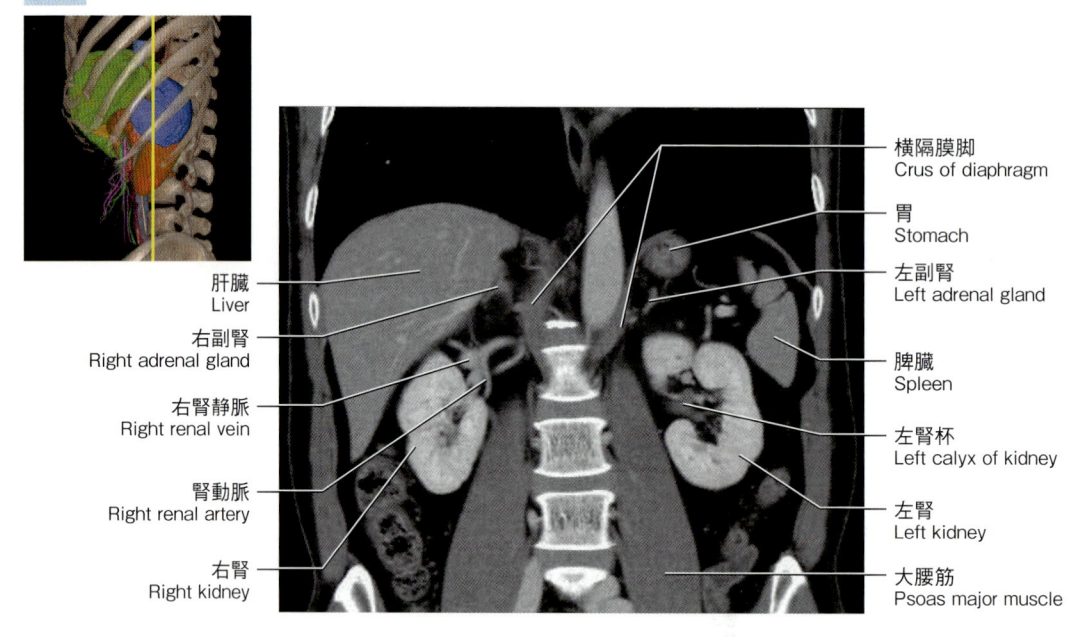

- 肝臓 Liver
- 右副腎 Right adrenal gland
- 右腎静脈 Right renal vein
- 腎動脈 Right renal artery
- 右腎 Right kidney
- 横隔膜脚 Crus of diaphragm
- 胃 Stomach
- 左副腎 Left adrenal gland
- 脾臓 Spleen
- 左腎杯 Left calyx of kidney
- 左腎 Left kidney
- 大腰筋 Psoas major muscle

NOTE 腎臓は後腹膜臓器であり，線維性被膜の中で脂肪に覆われている．第 12 胸椎から第 3 腰椎の高さに位置することが多い．右腎は上方に肝臓があるため，通常，左腎よりやや下方に位置する．

腹部の断層解剖［冠状断像（造影 CT 平衡相）］

5-77

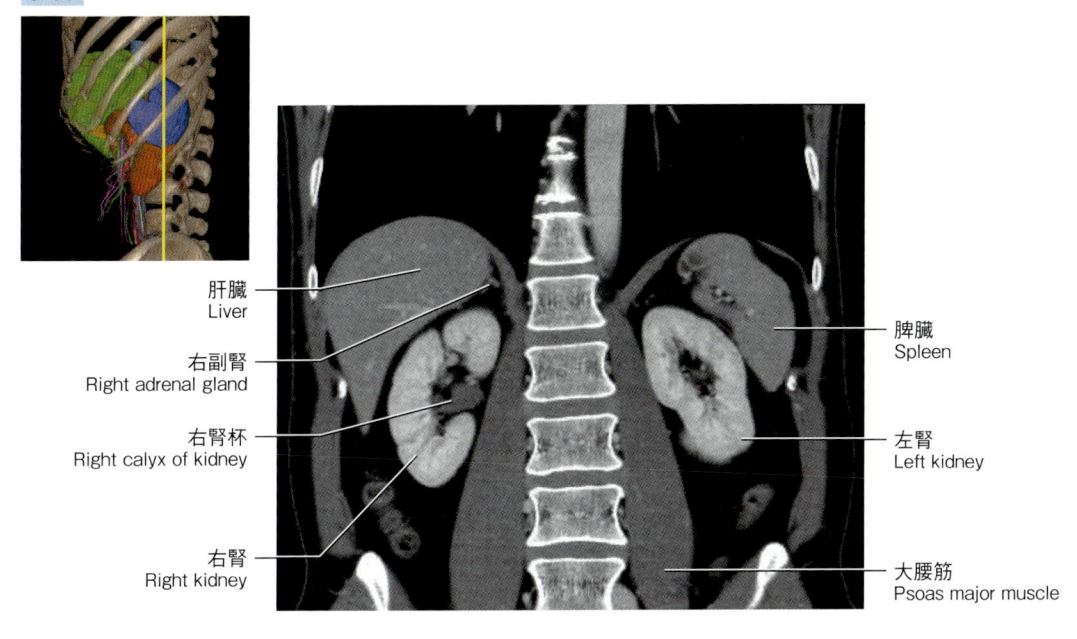

- 肝臓 Liver
- 右副腎 Right adrenal gland
- 右腎杯 Right calyx of kidney
- 右腎 Right kidney
- 脾臓 Spleen
- 左腎 Left kidney
- 大腰筋 Psoas major muscle

5-78

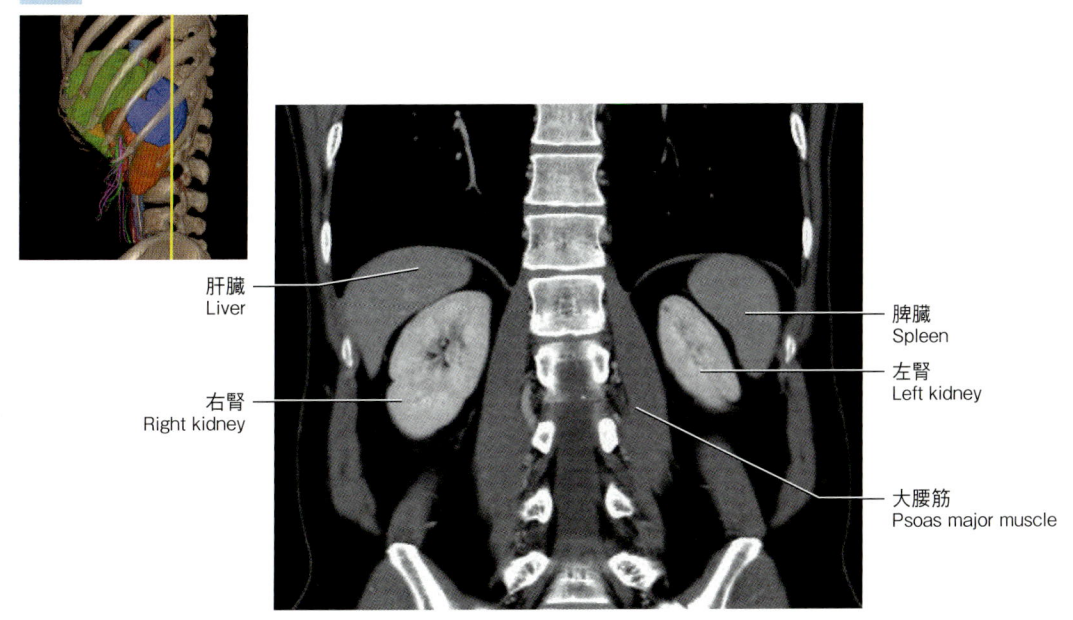

- 肝臓 Liver
- 右腎 Right kidney
- 脾臓 Spleen
- 左腎 Left kidney
- 大腰筋 Psoas major muscle

NOTE　副腎 Adrenal gland

　ad-は，近接の意の接頭語である．Adrenal gland は副腎，Adrenal medulla（副腎髄質）から出るホルモン Adrenalin（アドレナリン）はこの応用である．

腹部の断層解剖 ［矢状断像（造影CT 平衡相）］

5-79

肝臓
Liver

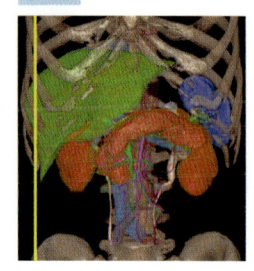

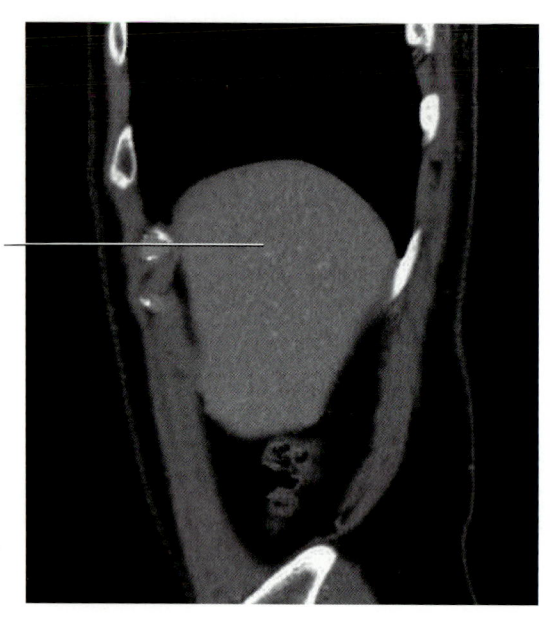

5-80

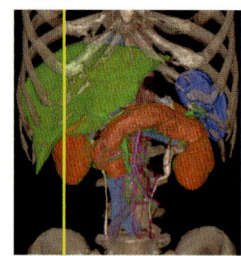

肝臓
Liver

胆嚢
Gallbladder

横行結腸
Transverse colon

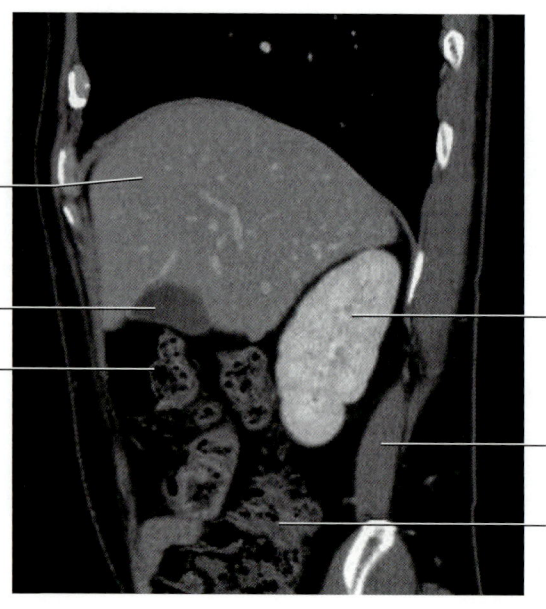

右腎
Right kidney

大腰筋
Psoas major muscle

上行結腸
Ascending colon

NOTE　横隔膜レベルの矢状断像で，背側肺が腎上極レベルまで尾側に深く進展していることがわかる．

腹部の断層解剖 ［矢状断像（造影CT 平衡相）］

5-81

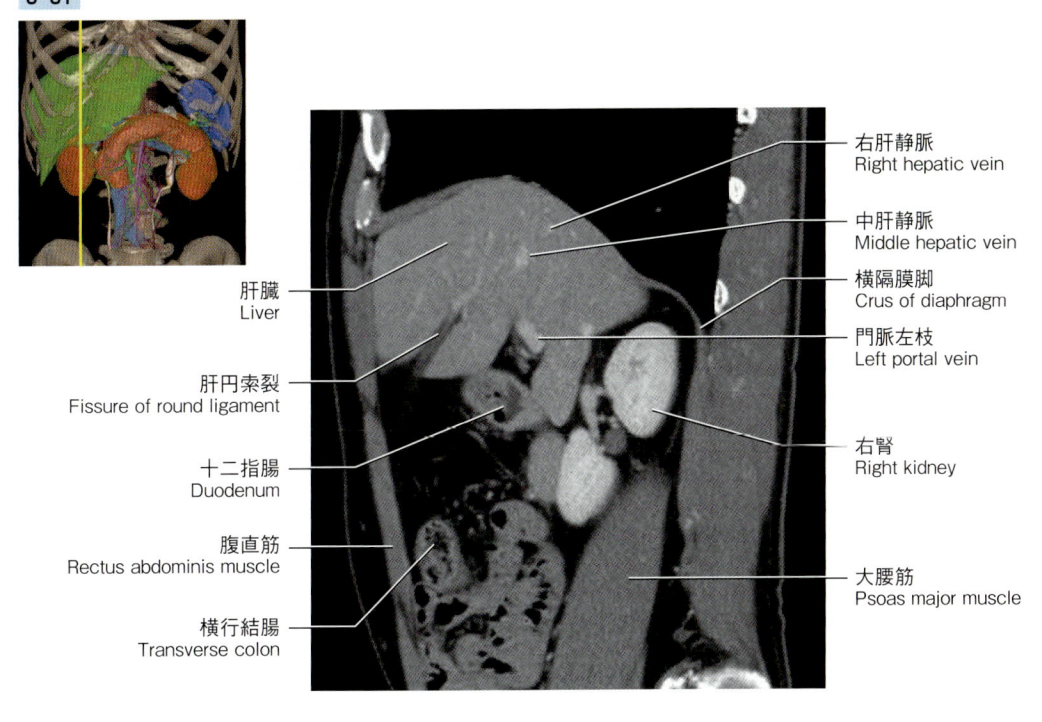

- 肝臓 Liver
- 肝円索裂 Fissure of round ligament
- 十二指腸 Duodenum
- 腹直筋 Rectus abdominis muscle
- 横行結腸 Transverse colon
- 右肝静脈 Right hepatic vein
- 中肝静脈 Middle hepatic vein
- 横隔膜脚 Crus of diaphragm
- 門脈左枝 Left portal vein
- 右腎 Right kidney
- 大腰筋 Psoas major muscle

5-82

- 肝臓 Liver
- 門脈左枝 Left portal vein
- 総胆管 Common bile duct
- 十二指腸 Duodenum
- 腹直筋 Rectus abdominis muscle
- 横行結腸 Transverse colon
- 右肝静脈 Right hepatic vein
- 中肝静脈 Middle hepatic vein
- 門脈左枝 Left portal vein
- 門脈本幹 Main portal vein
- 右腎静脈 Right renal vein
- 右腎動脈 Right renal artery
- 大腰筋 Psoas major muscle

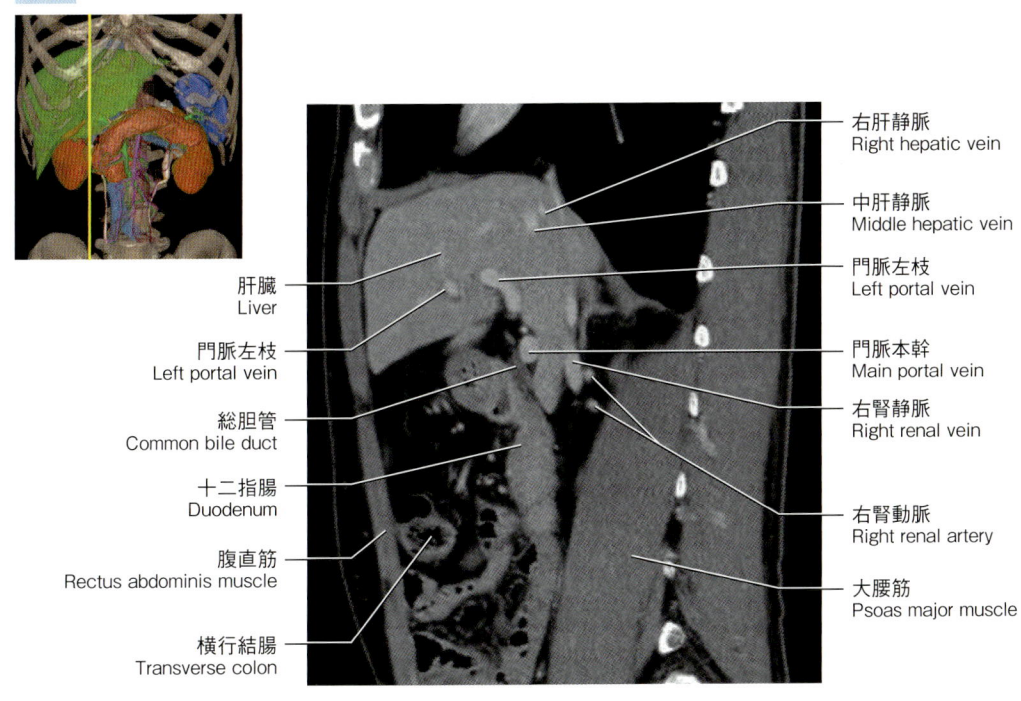

> **NOTE** 横隔膜脚 Crus of diaphragm
> 　横隔膜の尾側は左右の脚（きゃく）により腰椎に付着するが，第1腰椎の上縁で交叉し大動脈裂孔，そのやや左上方で食道裂孔をつくる（5-76を参照）．Crusは脚（あし）の意味で，中脳の腹側で大脳から左右一対の脚が生えているようにみえる（1-72, 73を参照）．

腹部の断層解剖 ［矢状断像（造影CT 平衡相）］

5-83

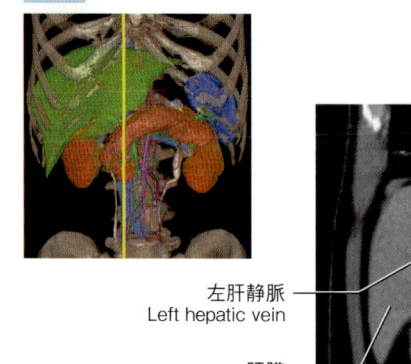

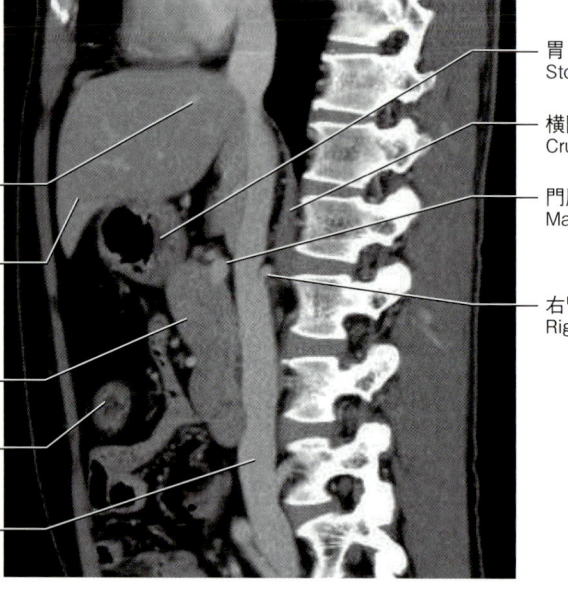

- 左肝静脈 Left hepatic vein
- 肝臓 Liver
- 膵頭部 Pancreas head
- 横行結腸 Transverse colon
- 下大静脈 Inferior vena cava
- 胃 Stomach
- 横隔膜脚 Crus of diaphragm
- 門脈本幹 Main portal vein
- 右腎動脈 Right renal artery

5-84

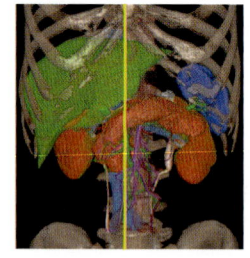

- 肝臓 Liver
- 膵臓 Pancreas
- 上腸間膜静脈 Superior mesenteric vein
- 横行結腸 Transverse colon
- 下大静脈 Inferior vena cava
- 胃 Stomach
- 総肝動脈 Common hepatic artery
- 右腎静脈 Right renal vein
- 右腎動脈 Right renal artery

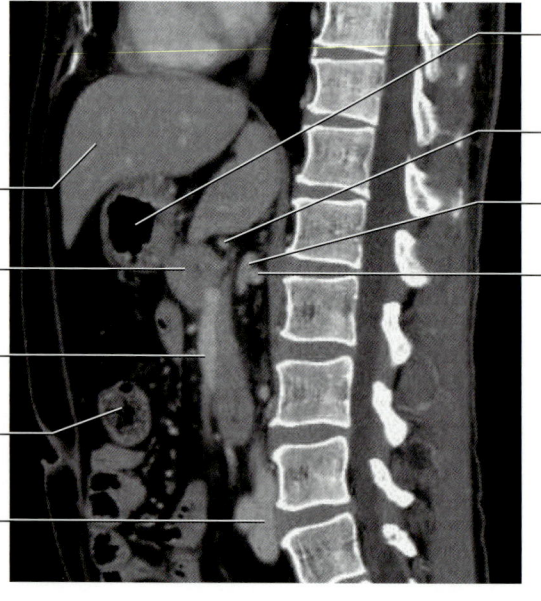

腹部の断層解剖　［矢状断像（造影CT 平衡相）］

5-85

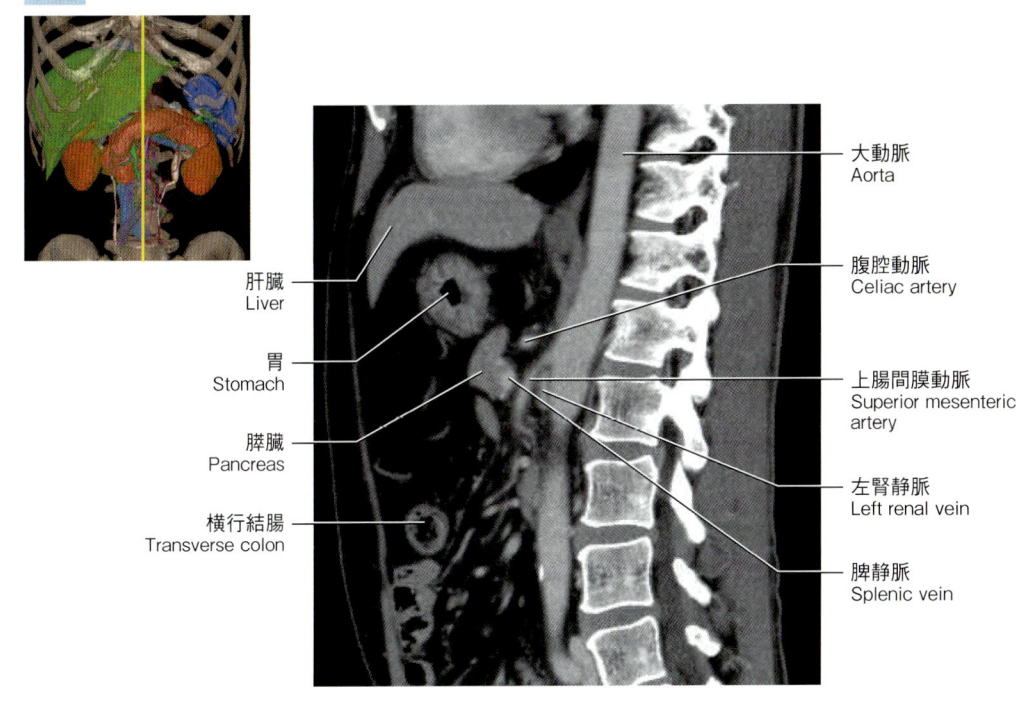

- 肝臓 / Liver
- 胃 / Stomach
- 膵臓 / Pancreas
- 横行結腸 / Transverse colon
- 大動脈 / Aorta
- 腹腔動脈 / Celiac artery
- 上腸間膜動脈 / Superior mesenteric artery
- 左腎静脈 / Left renal vein
- 脾静脈 / Splenic vein

5-86

- 肝臓 / Liver
- 胃 / Stomach
- 脾動脈 / Splenic artery
- 膵臓 / Pancreas
- 横行結腸 / Transverse colon
- 大動脈 / Aorta
- 食道 / Esophagus
- 腹腔動脈 / Celiac artery
- 上腸間膜動脈 / Superior mesenteric artery
- 脾静脈 / Splenic vein
- 左腎静脈 / Left renal vein
- 左腎動脈 / Left renal artery

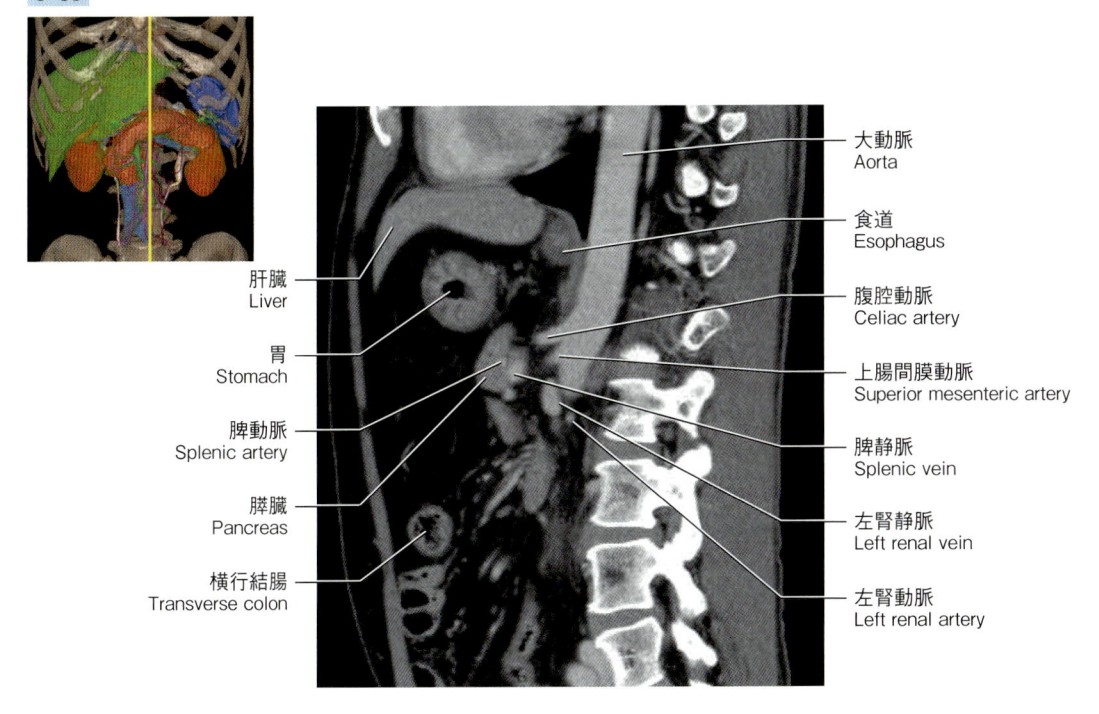

NOTE 左腎静脈が腹部大動脈と上腸間膜動脈起始部がつくる狭い空間を走行することがわかる（5-59～5-61の横断面およびNOTEを参照）．

腹部の断層解剖 ［矢状断像（造影CT 平衡相）］

5-87

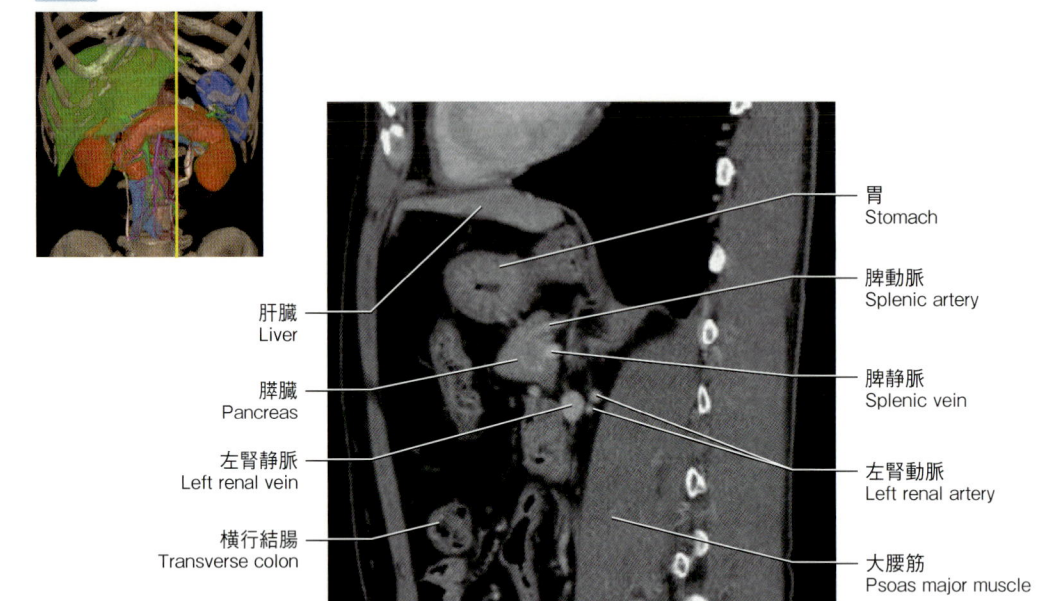

- 肝臓 Liver
- 膵臓 Pancreas
- 左腎静脈 Left renal vein
- 横行結腸 Transverse colon
- 胃 Stomach
- 脾動脈 Splenic artery
- 脾静脈 Splenic vein
- 左腎動脈 Left renal artery
- 大腰筋 Psoas major muscle

5-88

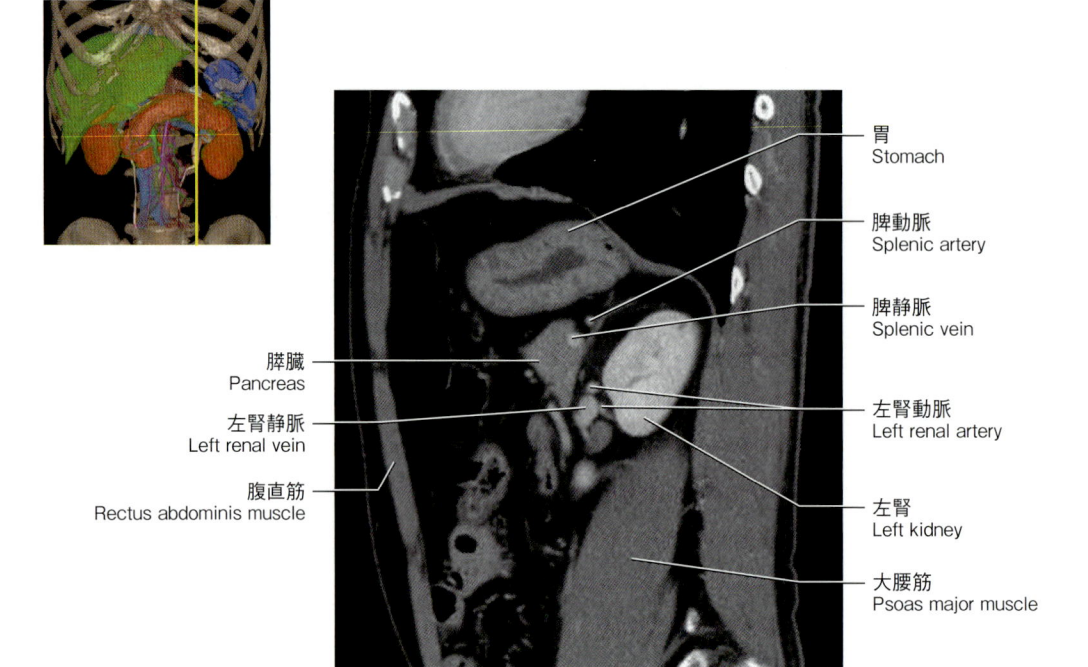

- 膵臓 Pancreas
- 左腎静脈 Left renal vein
- 腹直筋 Rectus abdominis muscle
- 胃 Stomach
- 脾動脈 Splenic artery
- 脾静脈 Splenic vein
- 左腎動脈 Left renal artery
- 左腎 Left kidney
- 大腰筋 Psoas major muscle

NOTE 膵臓の背側に脾静脈，腎動静脈が位置する．

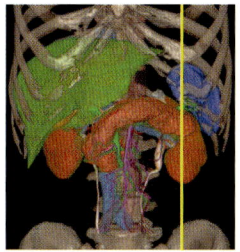

腹部の断層解剖［矢状断像（造影 CT 平衡相）］

5-89

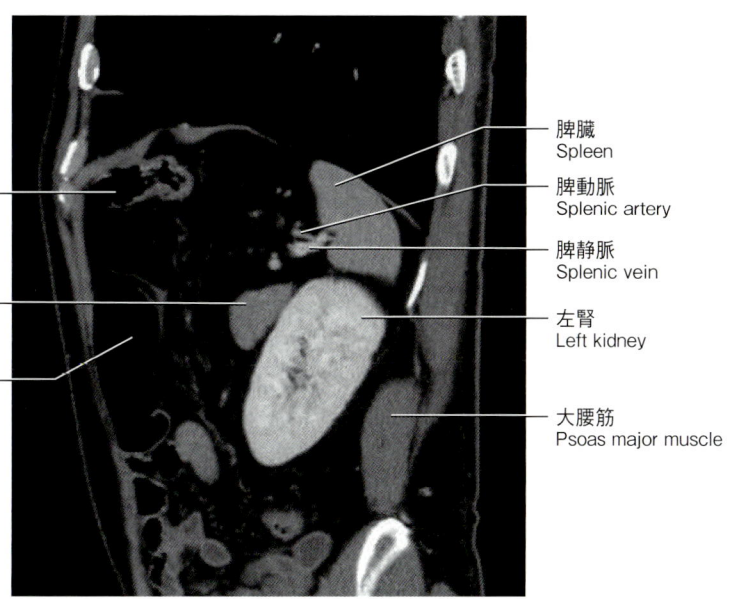

- 横行結腸 Transverse colon
- 膵臓 Pancreas
- S状結腸 Sigmoid colon
- 脾臓 Spleen
- 脾動脈 Splenic artery
- 脾静脈 Splenic vein
- 左腎 Left kidney
- 大腰筋 Psoas major muscle

5-90

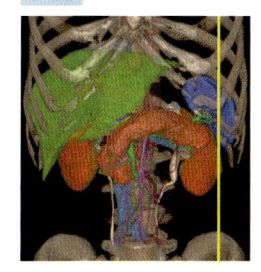

- 下行結腸 Descending colon
- 脾臓 Spleen
- 脾動脈 Splenic artery

NOTE 脾臓は左腎上極に密接する．

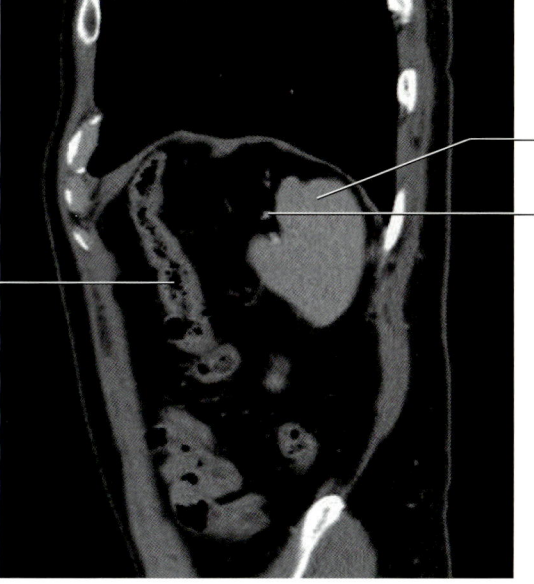

腹部の断層解剖 ［矢状断像（造影 CT 平衡相）］

5-91

脾臓
Spleen

下行結腸
Descending colon

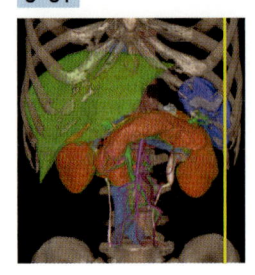

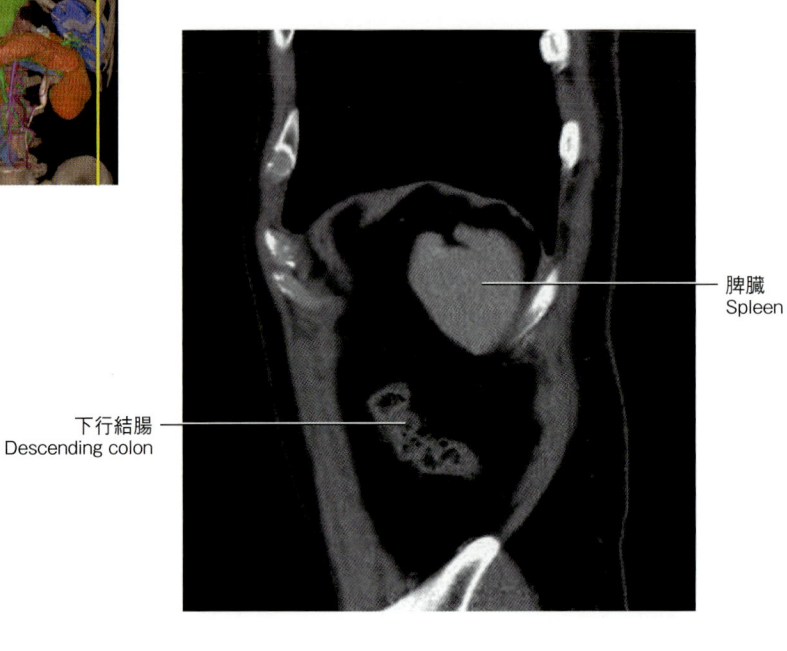

> **NOTE** 解剖 Anatomy
> 　　ana- は「上」，「後ろ」，「広く」など，多くの意味をもつ接頭語．-tome は「切る」を示す．全体に広く切ることより Anatomy という語ができたとされる．脾臓摘出術は，Splenectomy．また a- は「～でない」との接頭語で広く用いられるが，atom はこれ以上切れない最小の物 atomon（原子）の英語で，古代ギリシャの哲学者 Democritus（デモクリトス）は万物の根源と考えた．

VI

骨盤部
Pelvis

男性骨盤部の体表と骨格・泌尿器（CT, VR像）

6-1 体表と骨格・泌尿器

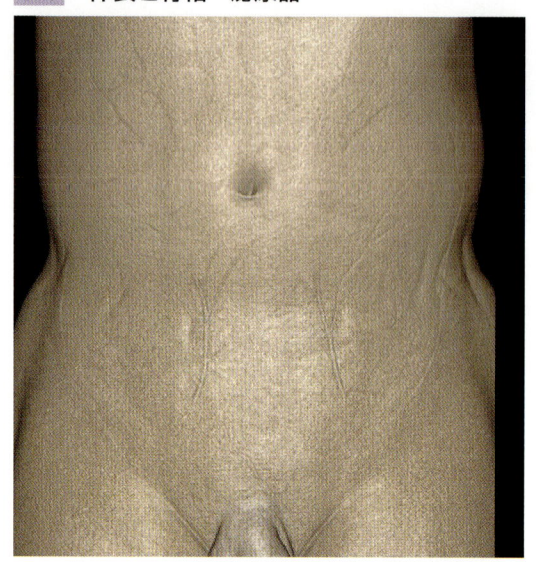

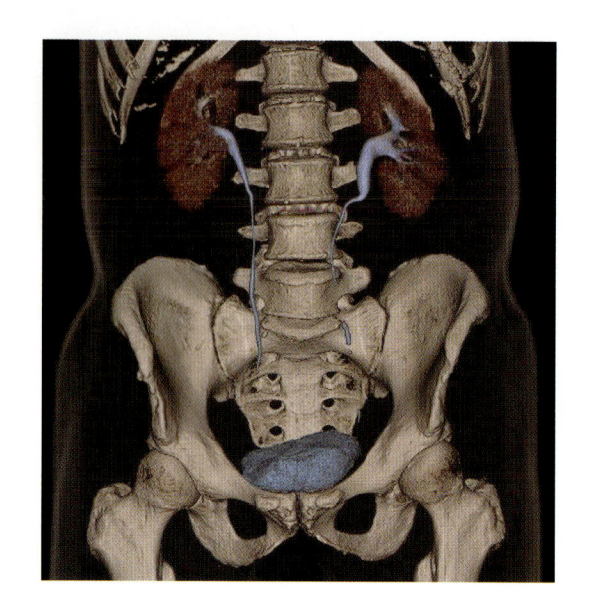

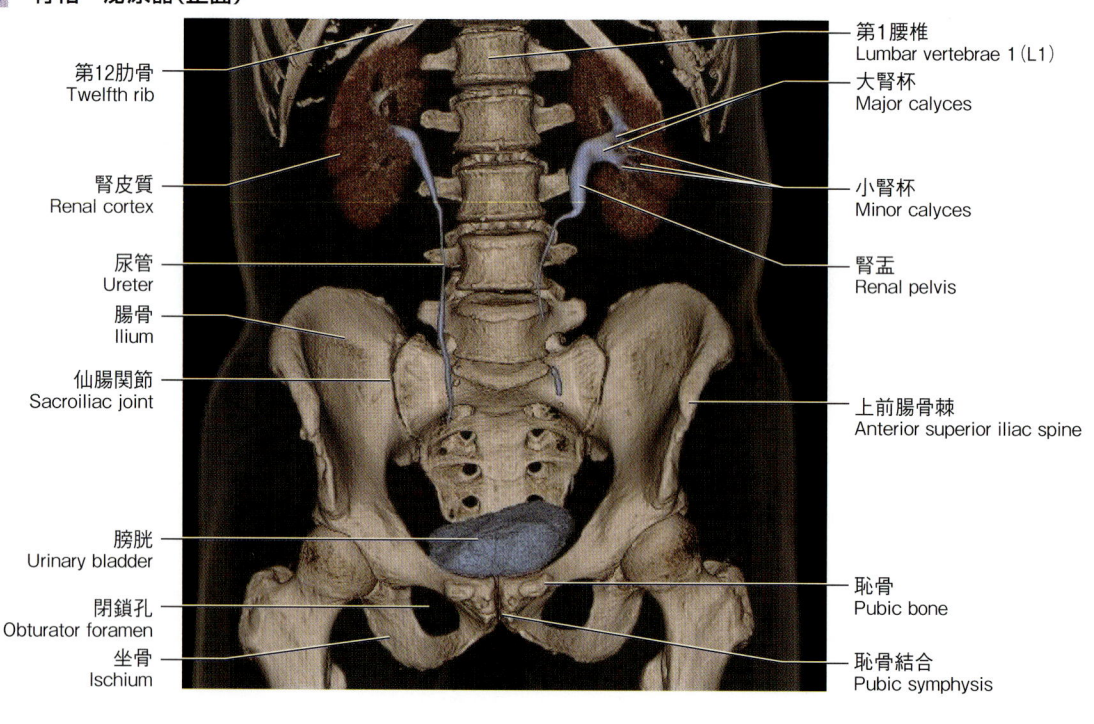

6-2 骨格・泌尿器（正面）

- 第12肋骨 Twelfth rib
- 腎皮質 Renal cortex
- 尿管 Ureter
- 腸骨 Ilium
- 仙腸関節 Sacroiliac joint
- 膀胱 Urinary bladder
- 閉鎖孔 Obturator foramen
- 坐骨 Ischium
- 第1腰椎 Lumbar vertebrae 1 (L1)
- 大腎杯 Major calyces
- 小腎杯 Minor calyces
- 腎盂 Renal pelvis
- 上前腸骨棘 Anterior superior iliac spine
- 恥骨 Pubic bone
- 恥骨結合 Pubic symphysis

NOTE 尿管は，腎盂から起始し，後腹膜区域の中でやや前方を下行し，膀胱の後面に開口する．尿管の生理的狭窄部位は，腎盂からの起始部（腎盂尿管移行部），外腸骨動静脈または総腸骨動静脈を乗り越える部分，膀胱開口部（尿管膀胱移行部）の3か所であり，結石嵌頓の好発部位として知られている．

男性骨盤部の骨格・泌尿器・生殖器(CT, VR像) | 269

6-3 骨格・泌尿器(左側面)

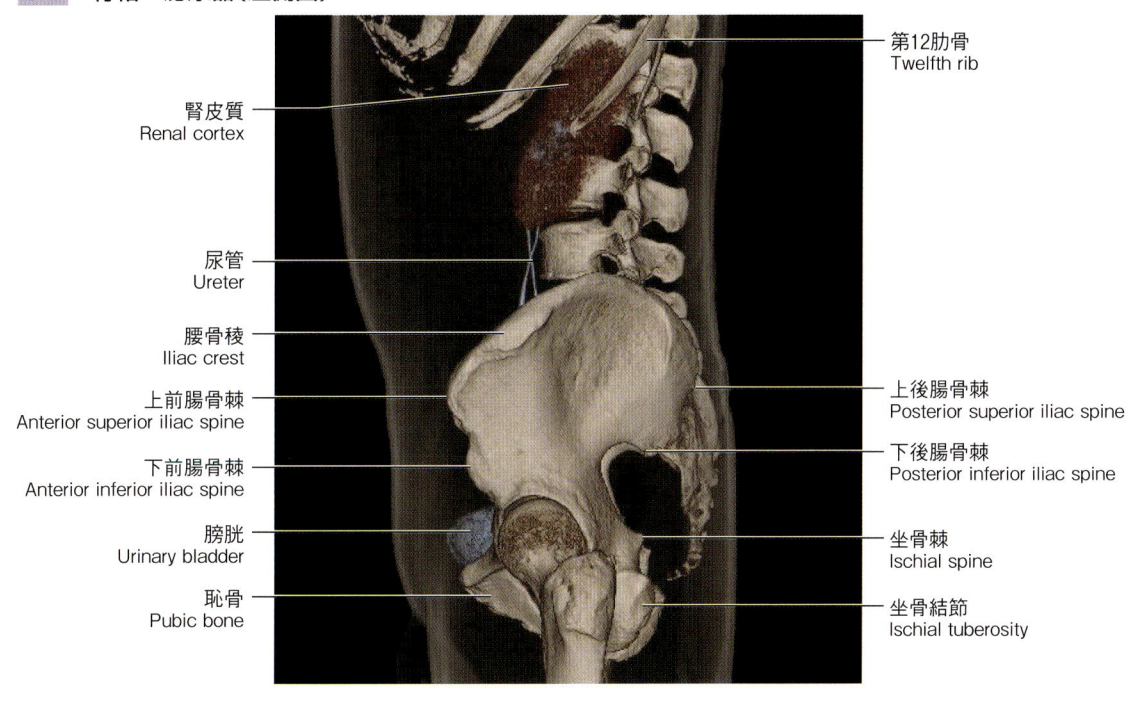

- 腎皮質 Renal cortex
- 尿管 Ureter
- 腸骨稜 Iliac crest
- 上前腸骨棘 Anterior superior iliac spine
- 下前腸骨棘 Anterior inferior iliac spine
- 膀胱 Urinary bladder
- 恥骨 Pubic bone
- 第12肋骨 Twelfth rib
- 上後腸骨棘 Posterior superior iliac spine
- 下後腸骨棘 Posterior inferior iliac spine
- 坐骨棘 Ischial spine
- 坐骨結節 Ischial tuberosity

6-4 骨格・泌尿器・生殖器(左側面)

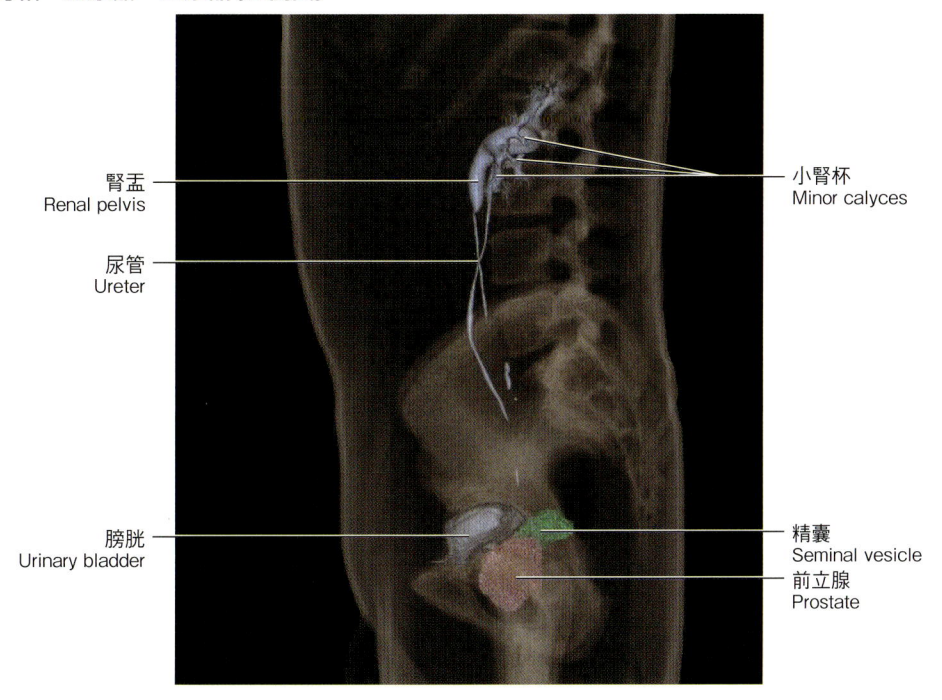

- 腎盂 Renal pelvis
- 尿管 Ureter
- 膀胱 Urinary bladder
- 小腎杯 Minor calyces
- 精嚢 Seminal vesicle
- 前立腺 Prostate

NOTE 左右の尿管の側面像からの把握ができる．腎結石は尿管閉塞のよくある原因のひとつであり，非常に強い痛みを起こすことで知られている．結石が尿管に入ると，尿管壁の平滑筋は結石を排出しようと強く収縮するため，疼痛を引き起こす．副交感神経を抑制する薬物の使用がこの痛みを軽減する．

男性骨盤部 ［冠状断像（3次元画像＋造影CT）］

6-5 左斜め上から（腹壁から 90 mm）

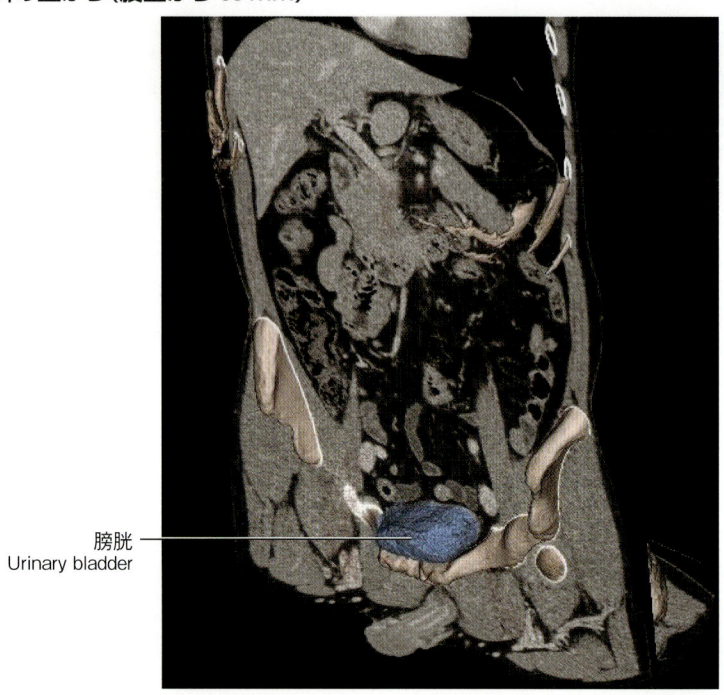

膀胱
Urinary bladder

6-6 左斜め上から（腹壁から 110 mm）

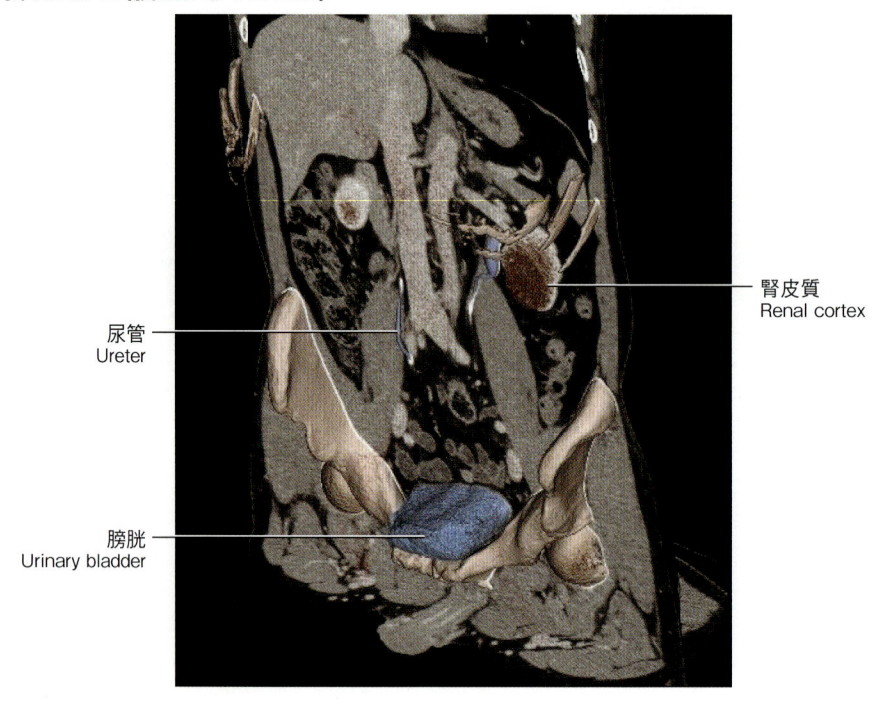

尿管
Ureter

腎皮質
Renal cortex

膀胱
Urinary bladder

> **NOTE** 膀胱は小骨盤内に位置し，骨盤隔壁の上，肛門挙筋とその筋膜の上に乗っている．

男性骨盤部 ［冠状断像（3次元画像＋造影CT）］

6-7 左斜め上から（腹壁から120 mm）

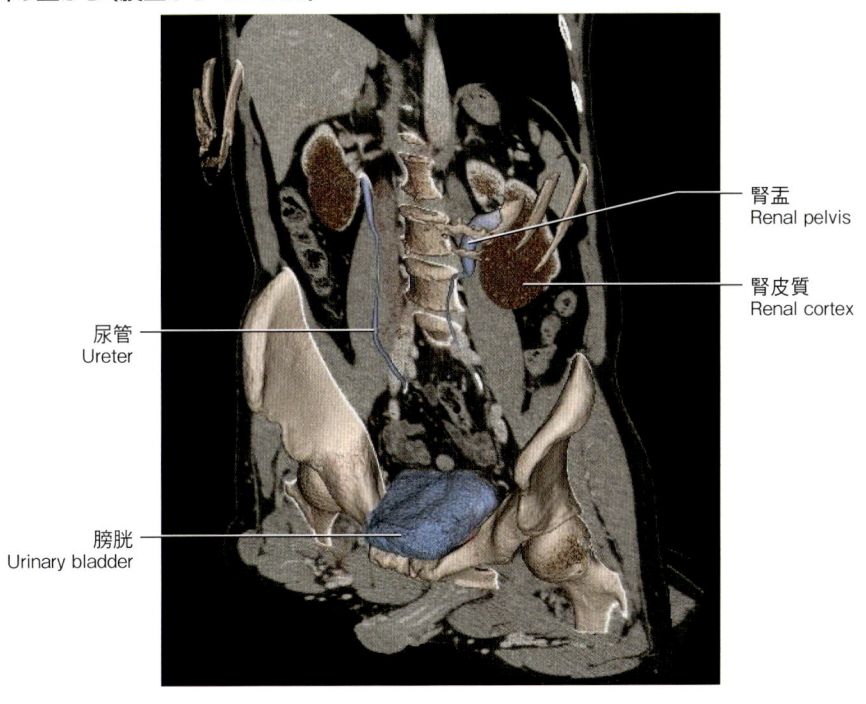

腎盂
Renal pelvis

腎皮質
Renal cortex

尿管
Ureter

膀胱
Urinary bladder

6-8 左斜め上から（腹壁から135 mm）

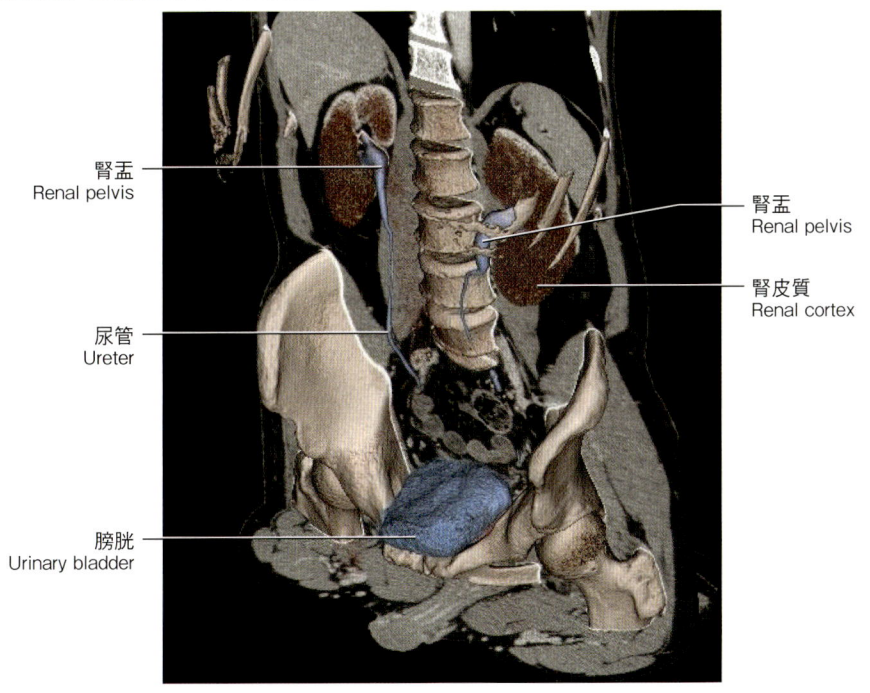

腎盂
Renal pelvis

腎盂
Renal pelvis

腎皮質
Renal cortex

尿管
Ureter

膀胱
Urinary bladder

> **NOTE** 膀胱は尿の貯留の程度により拡張と虚脱をくり返すが，拡張した膀胱はほぼ球形である．正常な膀胱壁の厚みは，拡張していない膀胱で5 mm以下，よく拡張した膀胱で3 mm以下と定義され，壁肥厚がある場合には膀胱炎などの炎症や腫瘍性病変を疑う．拡張不足の膀胱では壁肥厚を過大に評価してしまう傾向があるため注意が必要だが，3次元画像での膀胱の立体的描出はその助けになる．

男性骨盤部 ［冠状断像，矢状断像（3次元画像＋造影CT）］

6-9 左斜め上から（腹壁から 150 mm）

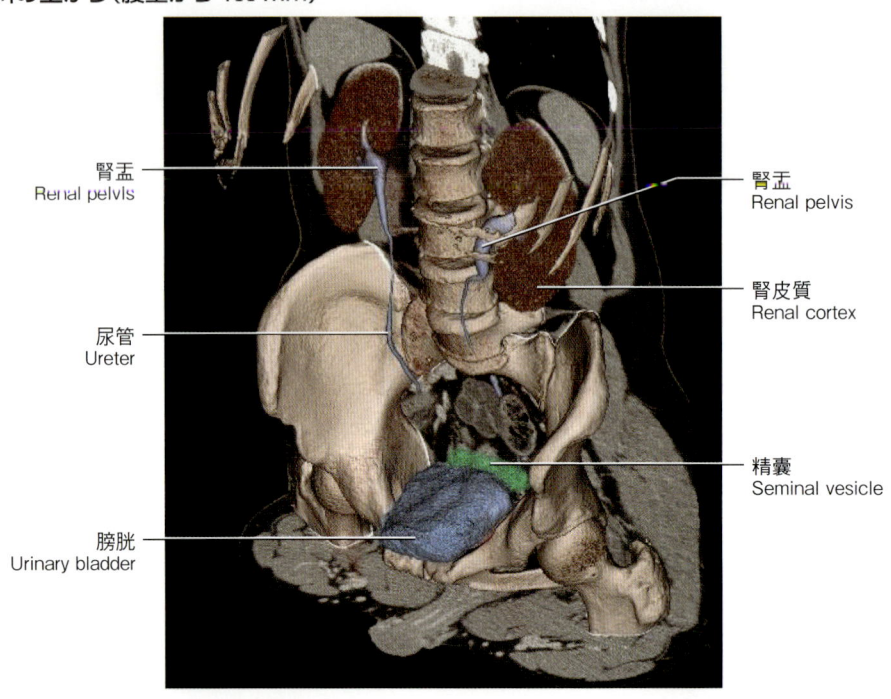

6-10 正中から右へ 20 mm（矢状断像）

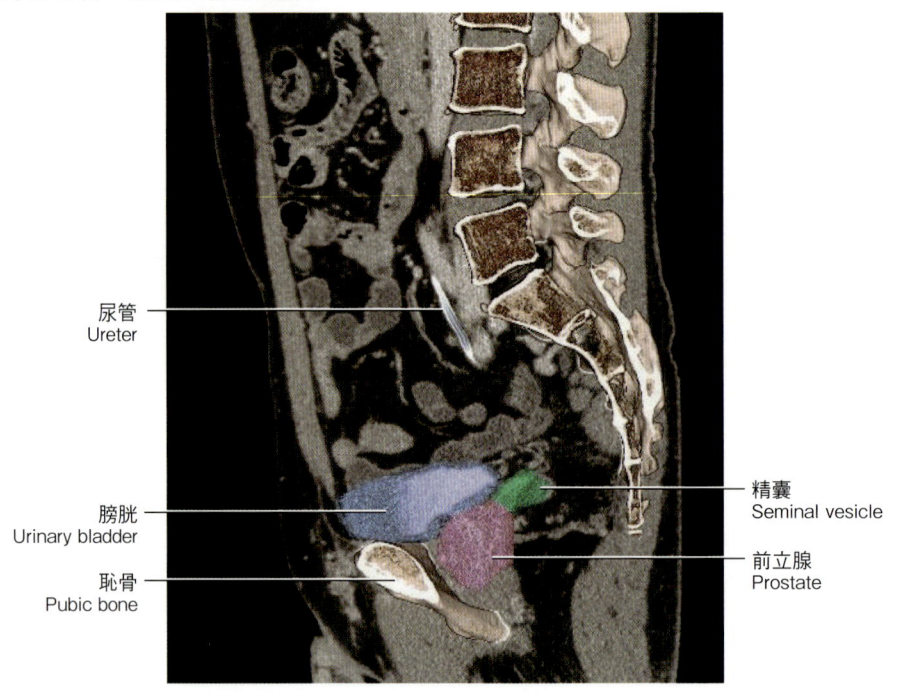

> **NOTE** 矢状断像（6-10）で，膀胱，精囊，前立腺の位置関係が明瞭である．前立腺肥大症は中高齢男性における common disease であるが，画像上の評価法として，前立腺の体積を，前後径，横径，上下径の積に $0.52（\pi/6）$をかけ，40 mL を超える場合は肥大と捉える方法，上下径 3 cm，左右径 4 cm，前後径 2 cm を超える場合に肥大ととる方法がある．

男性骨盤部の動脈（CTA 3 次元表示） 273

6-11 正面

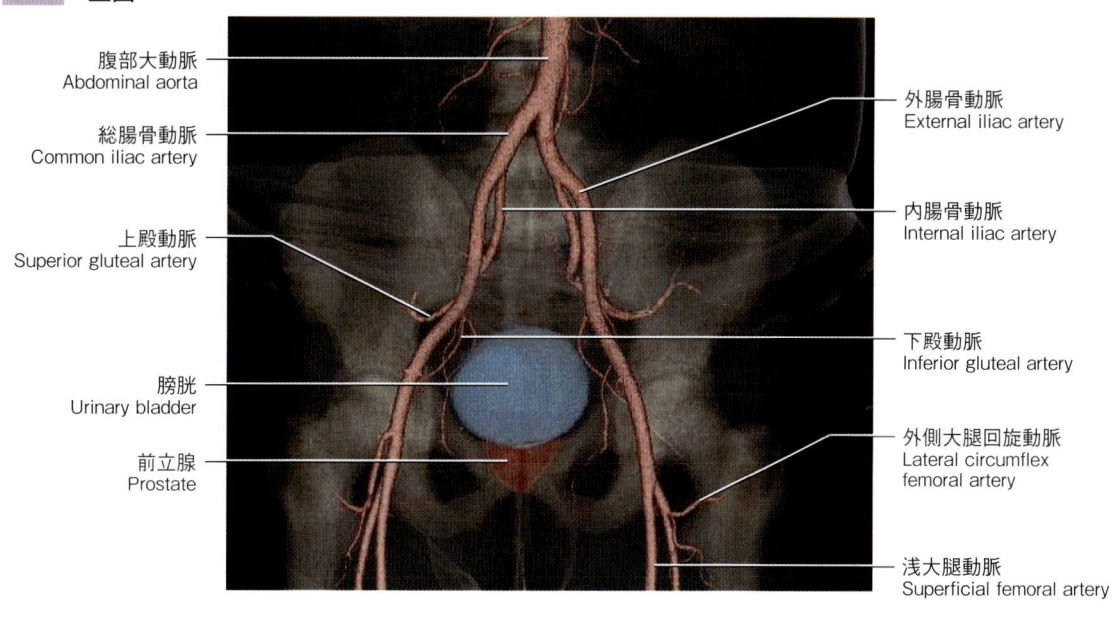

- 腹部大動脈 Abdominal aorta
- 総腸骨動脈 Common iliac artery
- 上殿動脈 Superior gluteal artery
- 膀胱 Urinary bladder
- 前立腺 Prostate
- 外腸骨動脈 External iliac artery
- 内腸骨動脈 Internal iliac artery
- 下殿動脈 Inferior gluteal artery
- 外側大腿回旋動脈 Lateral circumflex femoral artery
- 浅大腿動脈 Superficial femoral artery

6-12 左斜め前から

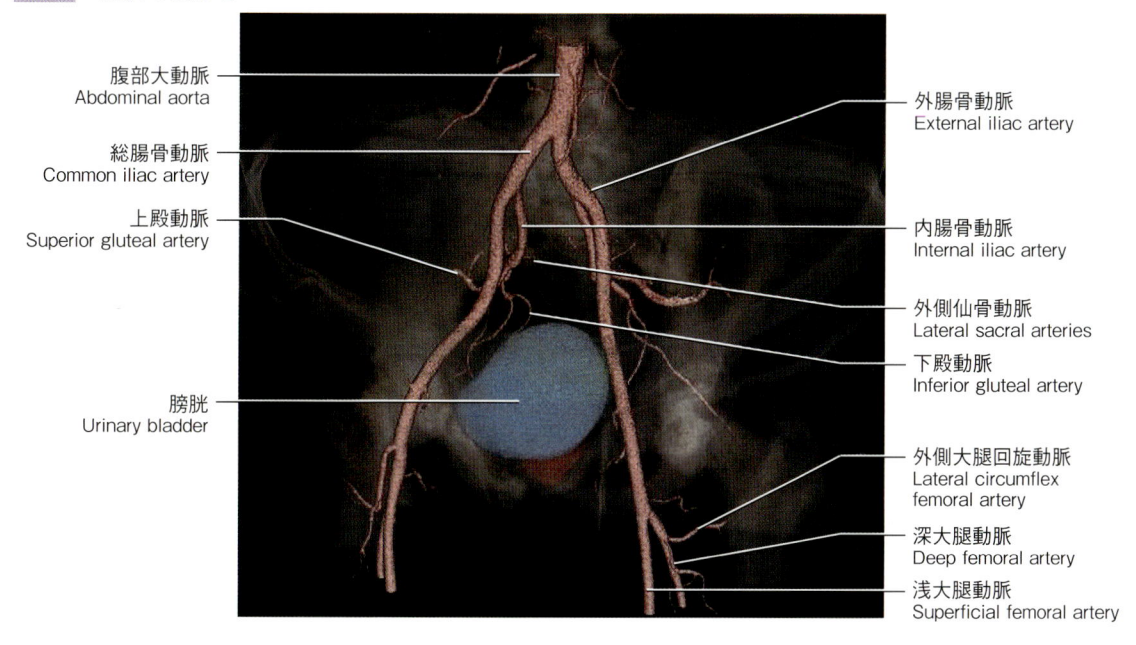

- 腹部大動脈 Abdominal aorta
- 総腸骨動脈 Common iliac artery
- 上殿動脈 Superior gluteal artery
- 膀胱 Urinary bladder
- 外腸骨動脈 External iliac artery
- 内腸骨動脈 Internal iliac artery
- 外側仙骨動脈 Lateral sacral arteries
- 下殿動脈 Inferior gluteal artery
- 外側大腿回旋動脈 Lateral circumflex femoral artery
- 深大腿動脈 Deep femoral artery
- 浅大腿動脈 Superficial femoral artery

NOTE 血管造影の際の穿刺のリスクを最小化するためには，適切な穿刺部位を選択することが不可欠である．大腿動脈穿刺におけるその実際は，目視で鼠径部の皺を確認する，透視で大腿骨頭の内側 1/3 寄りの中心を確認すること，などであるが，本画像のごとく 3 次元画像で個体差のある血管走行を把握しておくことも有用である．

274 女性骨盤部の体表と骨格・泌尿器・生殖器(CT, VR像)

6-13 体表解剖と骨格・泌尿器・生殖器

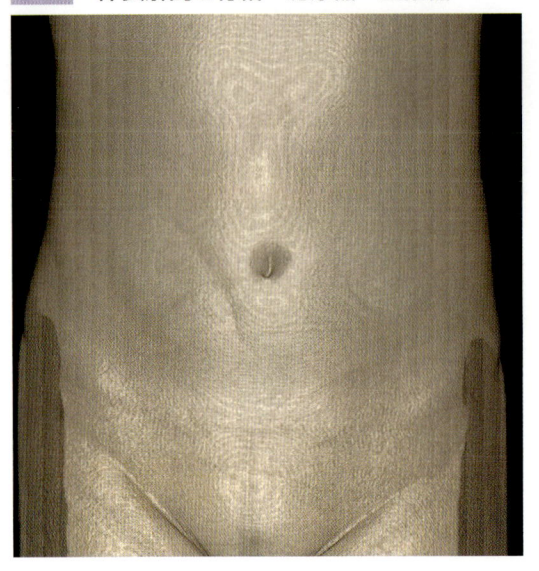

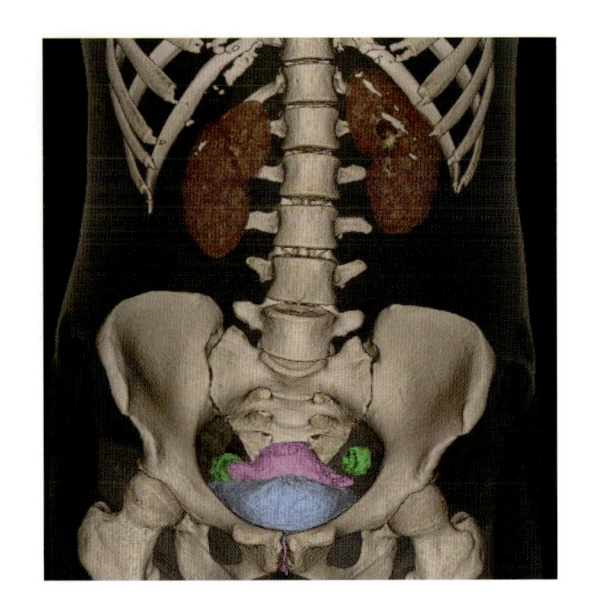

6-14 骨格・泌尿器・生殖器（正面）

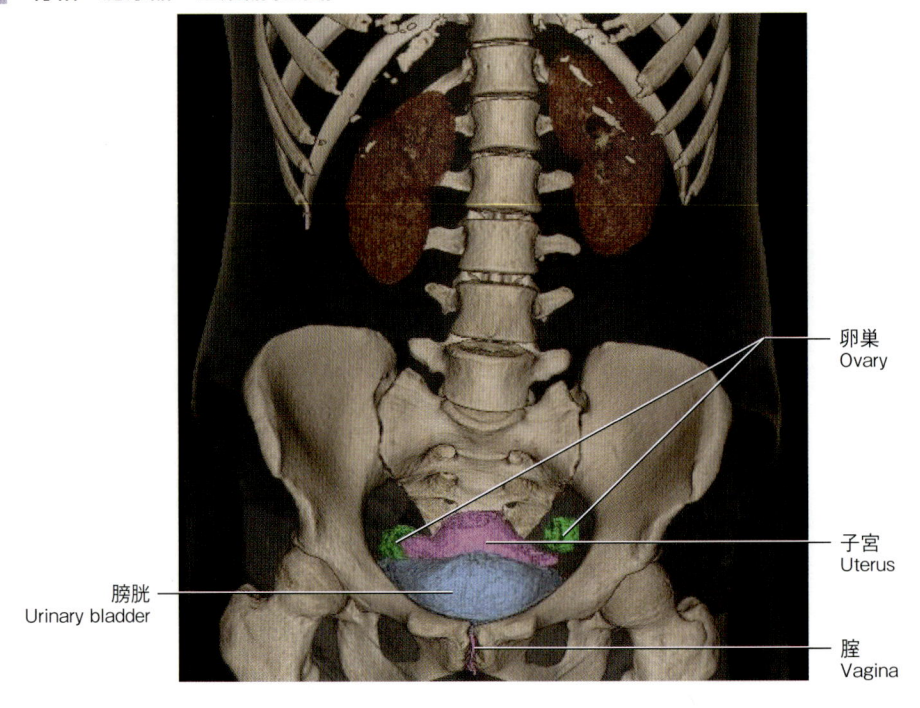

卵巣 Ovary
子宮 Uterus
膀胱 Urinary bladder
腟 Vagina

> **NOTE** 女性生殖器とその画像は，年齢および生理周期により，ダイナミックに変化することが知られている．子宮と両側の卵巣との位置関係の立体的な把握は，3次元画像を用いると容易である．

女性骨盤部の骨格・泌尿器・生殖器(CT, VR像) 275

6-15 骨格・泌尿器・生殖器(正面)

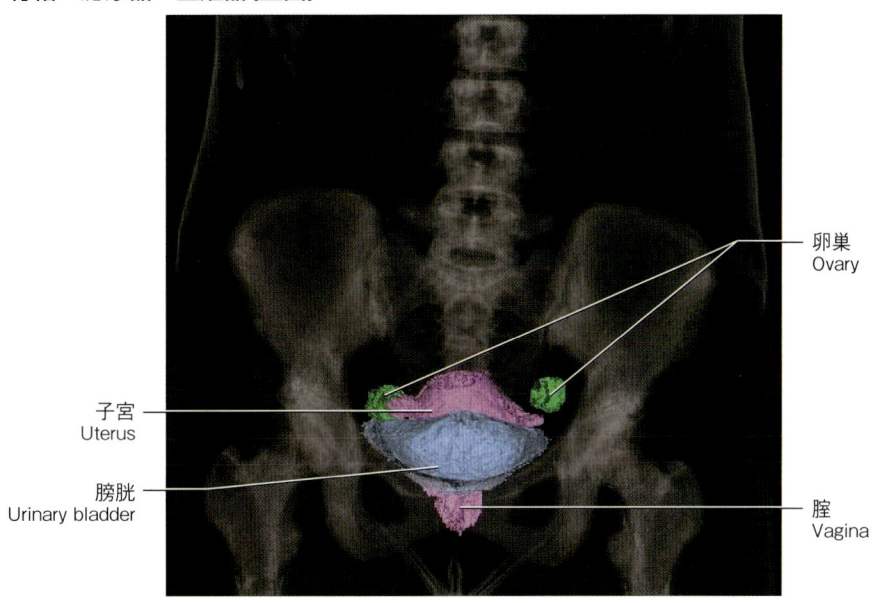

- 卵巣 Ovary
- 子宮 Uterus
- 膀胱 Urinary bladder
- 腟 Vagina

6-16 骨格・泌尿器・生殖器(左側面)

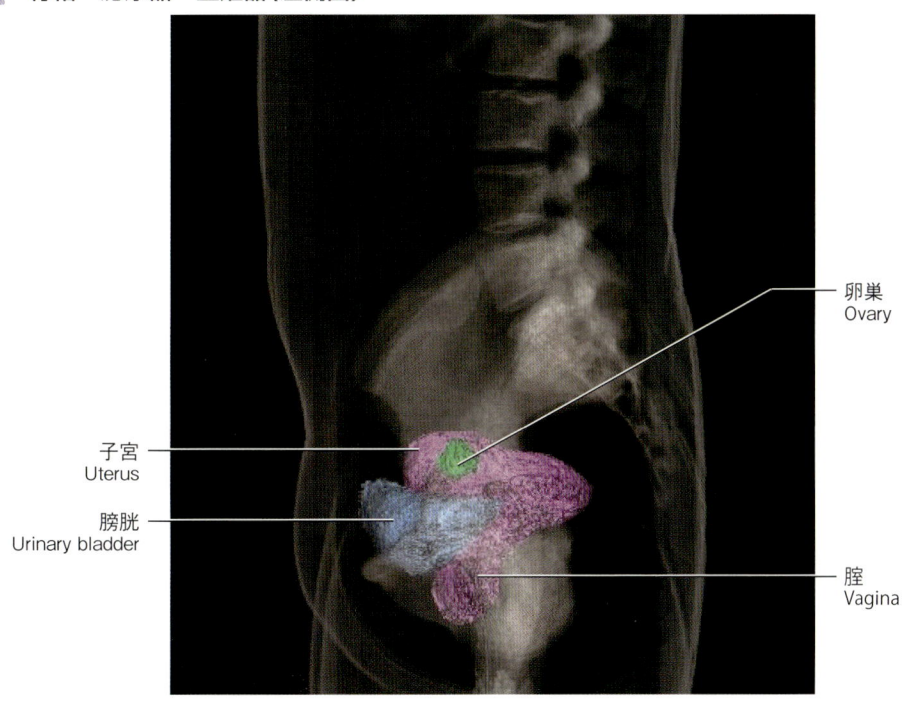

- 卵巣 Ovary
- 子宮 Uterus
- 膀胱 Urinary bladder
- 腟 Vagina

NOTE 骨盤腔における子宮腟部は坐骨棘の高さで骨盤の中心に位置し,正常では前傾前屈を呈する.その位置は,膀胱や直腸の拡張度が変わることにより,生理的に軽度変化する.また,子宮内膜症などによる癒着が存在すると,後屈などの傾き屈曲の変化が生じる.

女性骨盤部 [冠状断像（3次元画像＋造影CT）]

6-17 左斜め上から（腹壁から85 mm）

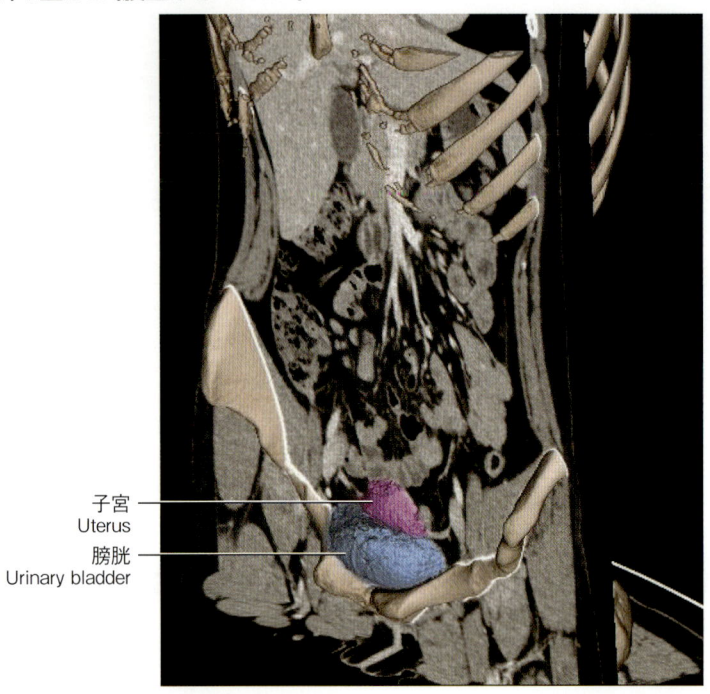

子宮
Uterus
膀胱
Urinary bladder

6-18 左斜め上から（腹壁から100 mm）

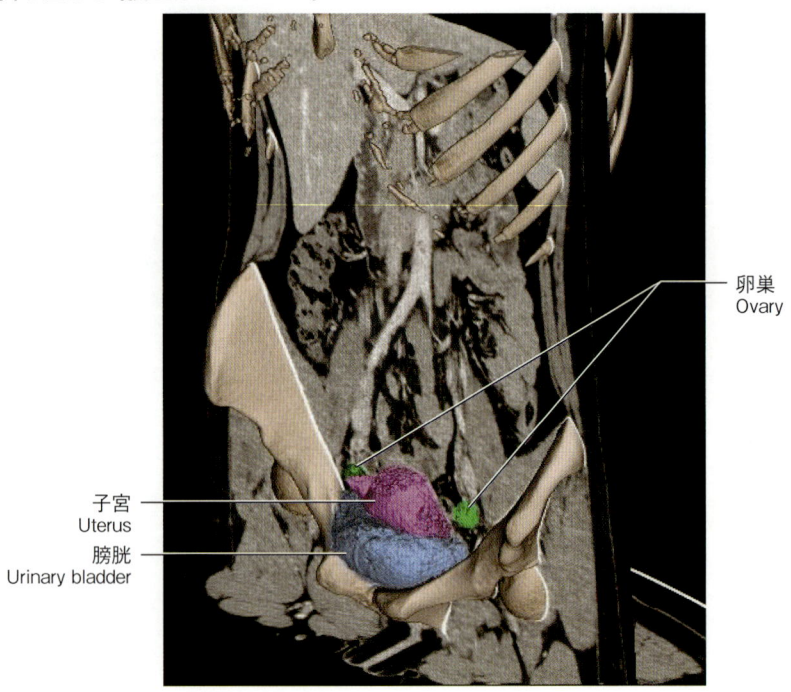

卵巣
Ovary
子宮
Uterus
膀胱
Urinary bladder

> **NOTE** 分娩の際，胎児は母体のさまざまな骨盤面を通る．臨床的に最も大事なのは骨盤の前後径である．最も短い前後径は真結合線で，恥骨結合の後表面と仙骨岬角を結ぶ最短距離をいうが，これが11 cm以下である場合には正常な経腟分娩が困難になることがある．これに対して胎児因子で重要なのは，頭部の最大前後径である．

女性骨盤部 ［冠状断像（3次元画像＋造影CT）］

6-19 左斜め上から（腹壁から115 mm）

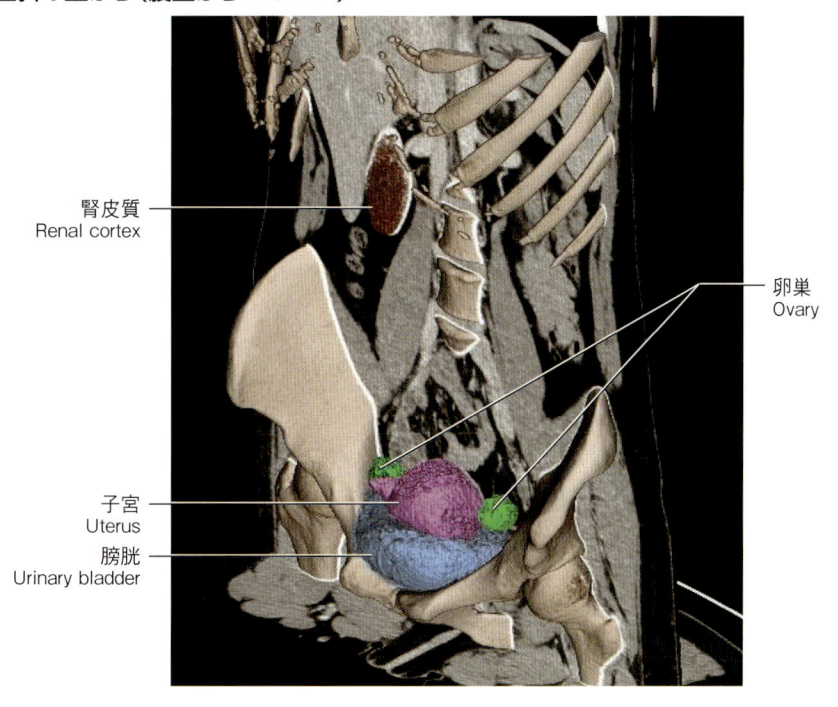

腎皮質
Renal cortex

卵巣
Ovary

子宮
Uterus

膀胱
Urinary bladder

6-20 左斜め上から（腹壁から155 mm）

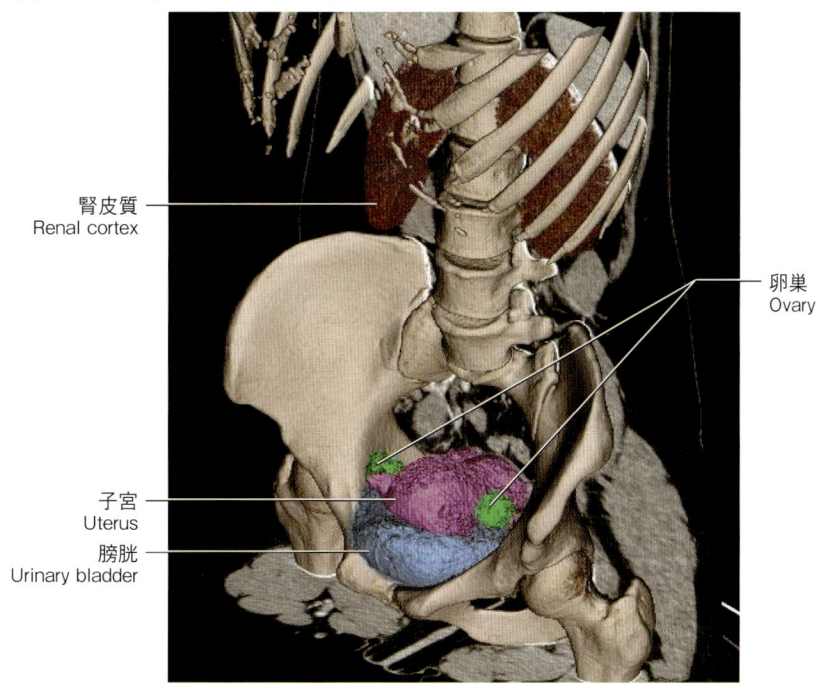

腎皮質
Renal cortex

卵巣
Ovary

子宮
Uterus

膀胱
Urinary bladder

NOTE 卵巣，卵管，および子宮の大部分は腹膜に覆われており，卵巣は卵巣間膜により子宮広間膜の後上表面に接している．これらの腹膜に覆われた結合組織帯は，腸間膜が腸管を緩やかに腹壁に固定するように，それぞれの生殖器を骨盤壁に固定している．3次元画像では，両側の卵巣と子宮の位置関係が明瞭に把握できる．

女性骨盤部 ［冠状断像，矢状断像（3次元画像＋造影CT）］

6-21 左斜め上から（腹壁から170 mm）

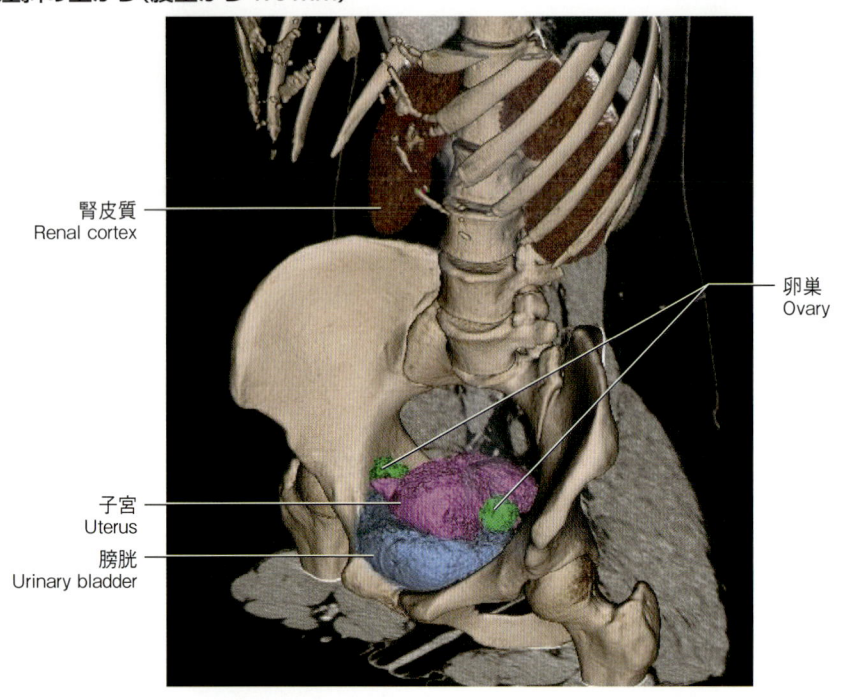

- 腎皮質 Renal cortex
- 卵巣 Ovary
- 子宮 Uterus
- 膀胱 Urinary bladder

6-22 正中から右へ20 mm（矢状断像）

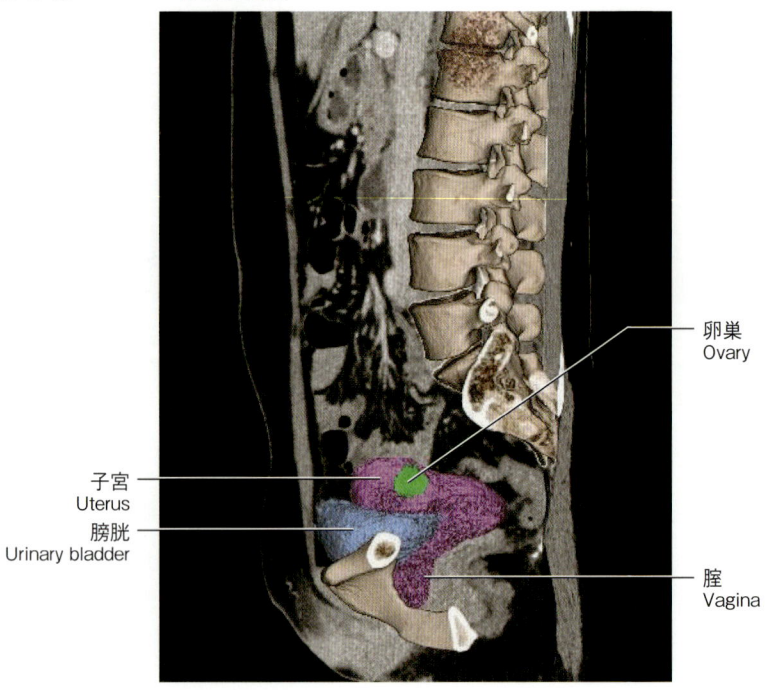

- 卵巣 Ovary
- 子宮 Uterus
- 膀胱 Urinary bladder
- 腟 Vagina

NOTE 子宮の位置は種々の理由で変化する．複数回の経腟分娩後に，骨盤底筋の筋力低下などにより子宮はしばしば下降する．結果，偏位した子宮が隣接する膀胱，尿管などを圧迫し，機能障害や不定愁訴を認めることがある．また，高齢者に認める子宮脱では，子宮の腟部が肛門から脱出し，QOLの改善のために外科的な治療が必要となることがある．

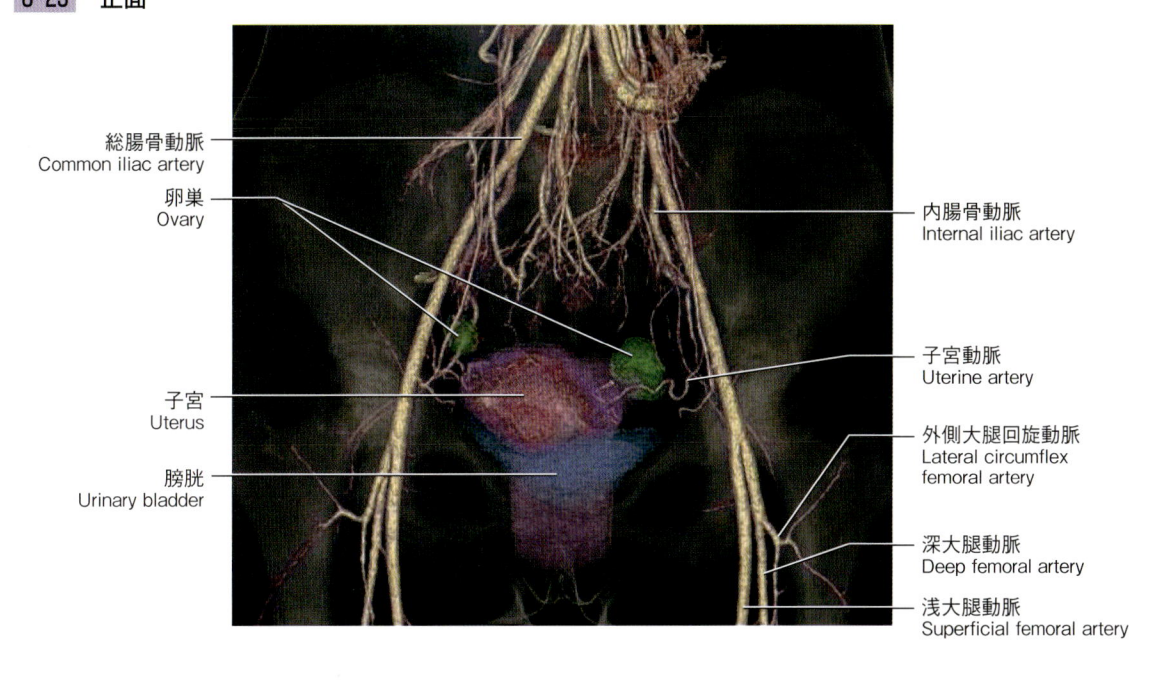

女性骨盤部の動脈（CTA 3次元表示）

6-23 正面

- 総腸骨動脈 Common iliac artery
- 卵巣 Ovary
- 子宮 Uterus
- 膀胱 Urinary bladder
- 内腸骨動脈 Internal iliac artery
- 子宮動脈 Uterine artery
- 外側大腿回旋動脈 Lateral circumflex femoral artery
- 深大腿動脈 Deep femoral artery
- 浅大腿動脈 Superficial femoral artery

6-24 左斜め前から

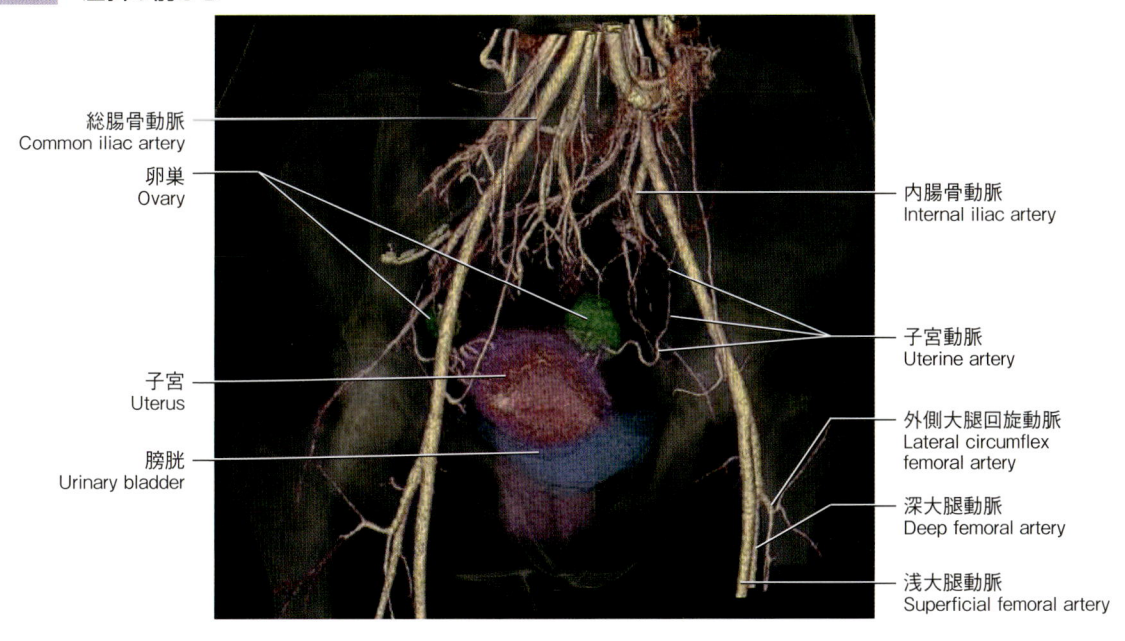

- 総腸骨動脈 Common iliac artery
- 卵巣 Ovary
- 子宮 Uterus
- 膀胱 Urinary bladder
- 内腸骨動脈 Internal iliac artery
- 子宮動脈 Uterine artery
- 外側大腿回旋動脈 Lateral circumflex femoral artery
- 深大腿動脈 Deep femoral artery
- 浅大腿動脈 Superficial femoral artery

> **NOTE** 女性生殖器に関連する IVR（interventional radiology）の適応は，子癇出血などにおける活動性のある動脈性出血の止血，月経過多や骨盤痛を起こす子宮筋腫の治療など，適応が広い．3次元画像での動脈走行の把握は，リスクの最小化に貢献する．

男性骨盤部の断層解剖　[横断像（造影CT）]

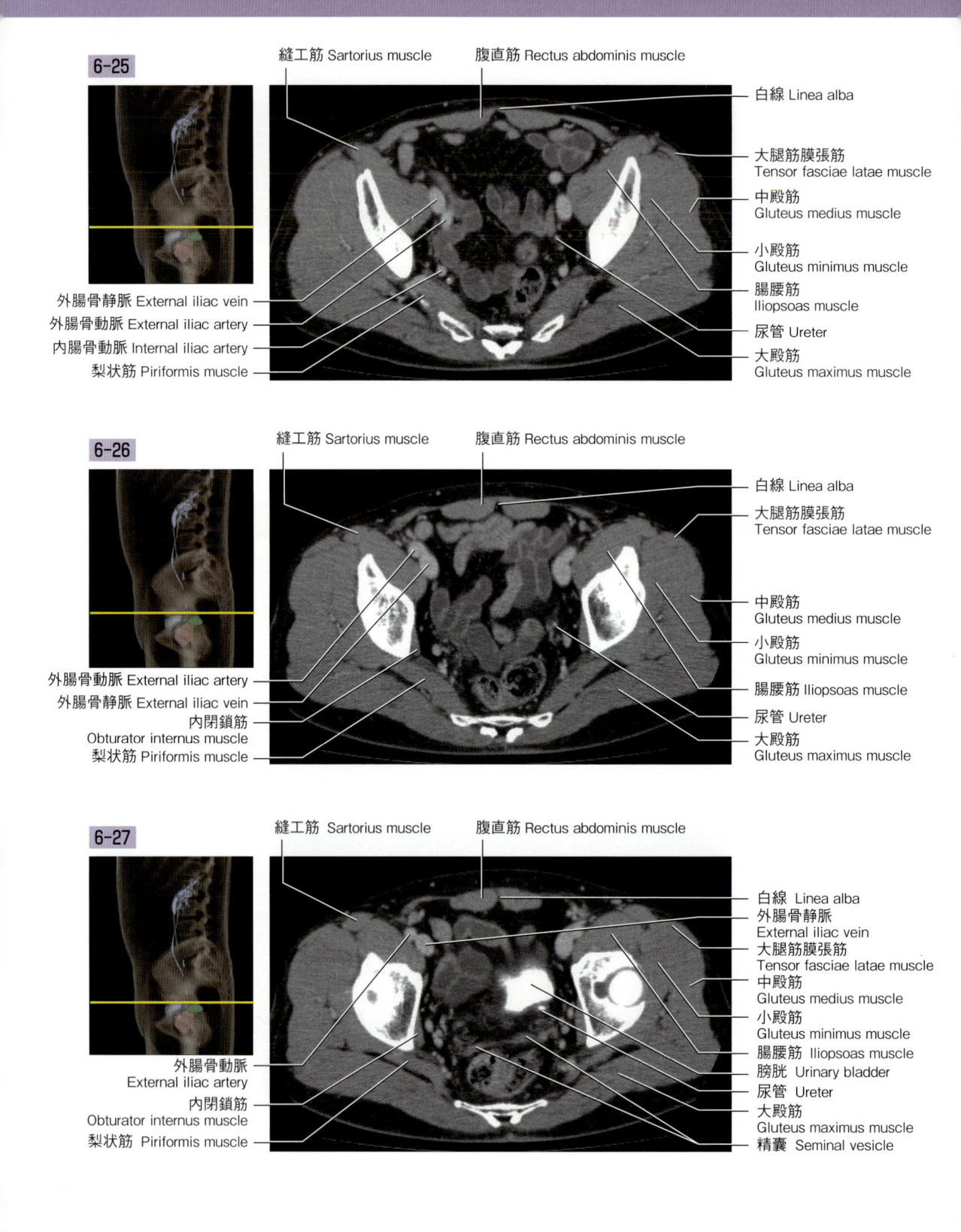

6-25

- 縫工筋 Sartorius muscle
- 腹直筋 Rectus abdominis muscle
- 白線 Linea alba
- 大腿筋膜張筋 Tensor fasciae latae muscle
- 中殿筋 Gluteus medius muscle
- 小殿筋 Gluteus minimus muscle
- 腸腰筋 Iliopsoas muscle
- 尿管 Ureter
- 大殿筋 Gluteus maximus muscle
- 外腸骨静脈 External iliac vein
- 外腸骨動脈 External iliac artery
- 内腸骨動脈 Internal iliac artery
- 梨状筋 Piriformis muscle

6-26

- 縫工筋 Sartorius muscle
- 腹直筋 Rectus abdominis muscle
- 白線 Linea alba
- 大腿筋膜張筋 Tensor fasciae latae muscle
- 中殿筋 Gluteus medius muscle
- 小殿筋 Gluteus minimus muscle
- 腸腰筋 Iliopsoas muscle
- 尿管 Ureter
- 大殿筋 Gluteus maximus muscle
- 外腸骨動脈 External iliac artery
- 外腸骨静脈 External iliac vein
- 内閉鎖筋 Obturator internus muscle
- 梨状筋 Piriformis muscle

6-27

- 縫工筋 Sartorius muscle
- 腹直筋 Rectus abdominis muscle
- 白線 Linea alba
- 外腸骨静脈 External iliac vein
- 大腿筋膜張筋 Tensor fasciae latae muscle
- 中殿筋 Gluteus medius muscle
- 小殿筋 Gluteus minimus muscle
- 腸腰筋 Iliopsoas muscle
- 膀胱 Urinary bladder
- 尿管 Ureter
- 大殿筋 Gluteus maximus muscle
- 精嚢 Seminal vesicle
- 外腸骨動脈 External iliac artery
- 内閉鎖筋 Obturator internus muscle
- 梨状筋 Piriformis muscle

NOTE 総腸骨動脈は，仙腸関節の位置で内外腸骨動脈に分岐する．内腸骨動脈は，壁側枝と臓側枝に分かれ，壁側枝により骨盤壁や殿部を栄養し，臓側枝により子宮や卵巣を主とした内臓を栄養する．

男性骨盤部の断層解剖　[横断像（造影CT）]

6-28

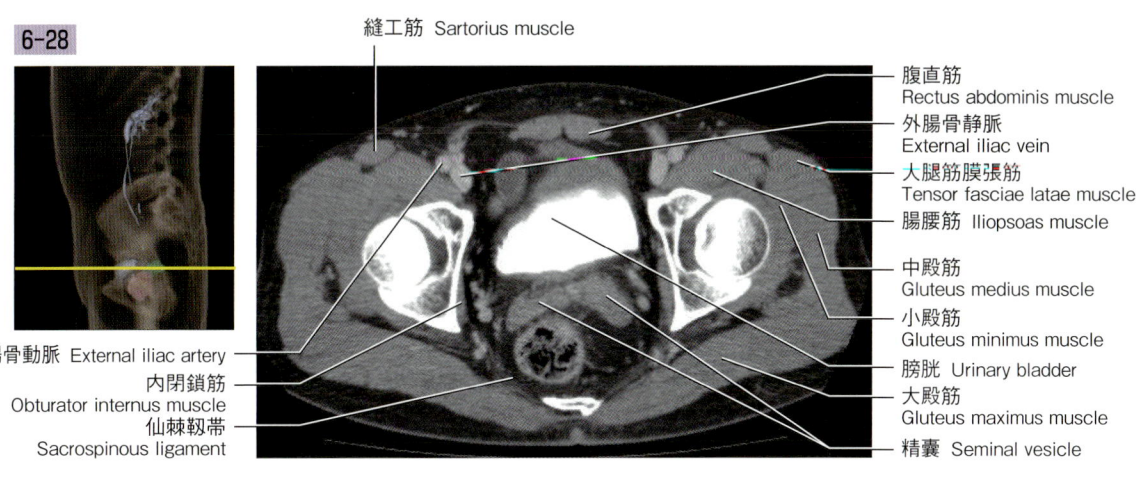

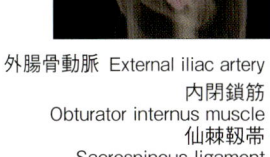

- 縫工筋　Sartorius muscle
- 腹直筋　Rectus abdominis muscle
- 外腸骨静脈　External iliac vein
- 大腿筋膜張筋　Tensor fasciae latae muscle
- 腸腰筋　Iliopsoas muscle
- 中殿筋　Gluteus medius muscle
- 小殿筋　Gluteus minimus muscle
- 膀胱　Urinary bladder
- 大殿筋　Gluteus maximus muscle
- 精嚢　Seminal vesicle
- 外腸骨動脈　External iliac artery
- 内閉鎖筋　Obturator internus muscle
- 仙棘靱帯　Sacrospinous ligament

6-29

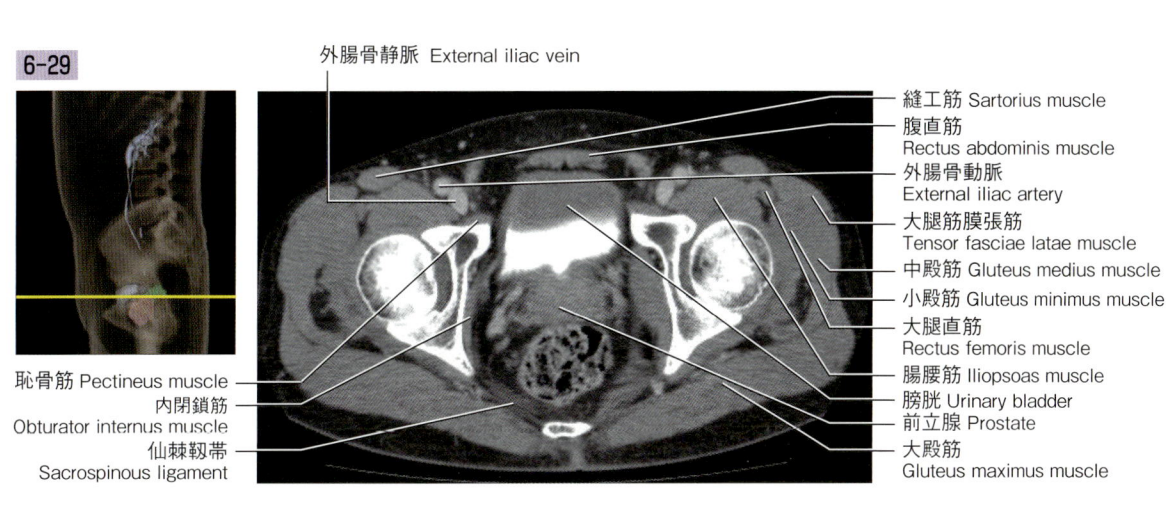

- 外腸骨静脈　External iliac vein
- 縫工筋　Sartorius muscle
- 腹直筋　Rectus abdominis muscle
- 外腸骨動脈　External iliac artery
- 大腿筋膜張筋　Tensor fasciae latae muscle
- 中殿筋　Gluteus medius muscle
- 小殿筋　Gluteus minimus muscle
- 大腿直筋　Rectus femoris muscle
- 腸腰筋　Iliopsoas muscle
- 膀胱　Urinary bladder
- 前立腺　Prostate
- 大殿筋　Gluteus maximus muscle
- 恥骨筋　Pectineus muscle
- 内閉鎖筋　Obturator internus muscle
- 仙棘靱帯　Sacrospinous ligament

6-30

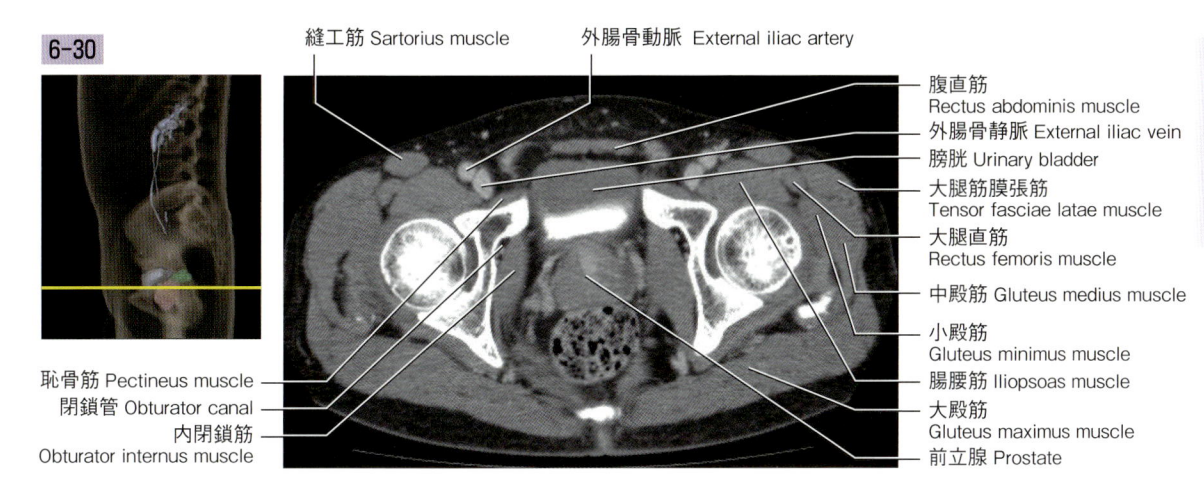

- 縫工筋　Sartorius muscle
- 外腸骨動脈　External iliac artery
- 腹直筋　Rectus abdominis muscle
- 外腸骨静脈　External iliac vein
- 膀胱　Urinary bladder
- 大腿筋膜張筋　Tensor fasciae latae muscle
- 大腿直筋　Rectus femoris muscle
- 中殿筋　Gluteus medius muscle
- 小殿筋　Gluteus minimus muscle
- 腸腰筋　Iliopsoas muscle
- 大殿筋　Gluteus maximus muscle
- 前立腺　Prostate
- 恥骨筋　Pectineus muscle
- 閉鎖管　Obturator canal
- 内閉鎖筋　Obturator internus muscle

NOTE　前立腺の解剖は，1980年代後半に，顕微鏡的な解析によりゾーン（zone：中心域，辺縁域，移行域）が定義された．このことは前立腺癌と良性の前立腺肥大症に対する理解に大きな影響を与えた．辺縁域は，前立腺癌，慢性炎症などの好発部位である．

男性骨盤部の断層解剖　[横断像（造影CT）]

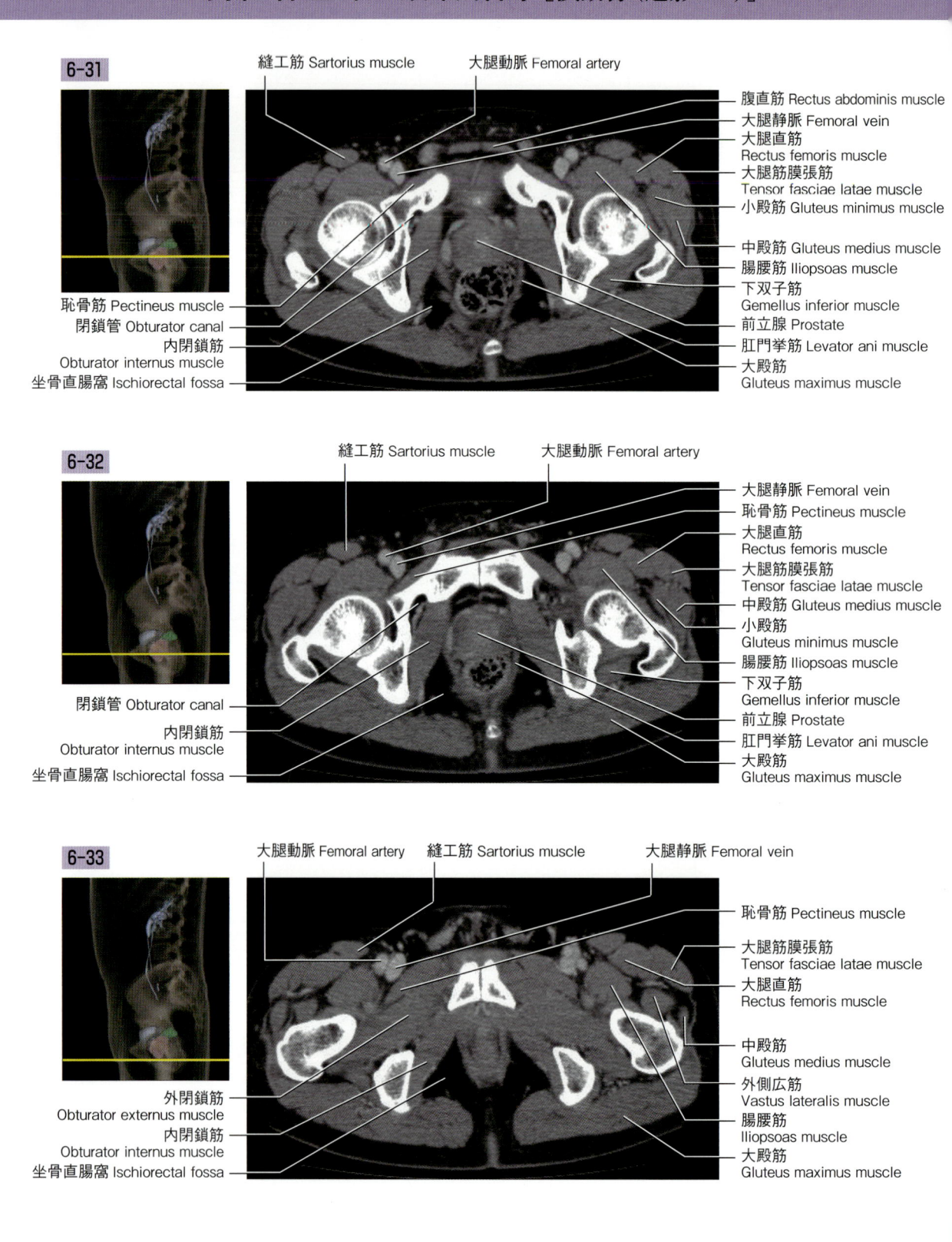

6-31

- 縫工筋 Sartorius muscle
- 大腿動脈 Femoral artery
- 腹直筋 Rectus abdominis muscle
- 大腿静脈 Femoral vein
- 大腿直筋 Rectus femoris muscle
- 大腿筋膜張筋 Tensor fasciae latae muscle
- 小殿筋 Gluteus minimus muscle
- 中殿筋 Gluteus medius muscle
- 腸腰筋 Iliopsoas muscle
- 下双子筋 Gemellus inferior muscle
- 前立腺 Prostate
- 肛門挙筋 Levator ani muscle
- 大殿筋 Gluteus maximus muscle
- 恥骨筋 Pectineus muscle
- 閉鎖管 Obturator canal
- 内閉鎖筋 Obturator internus muscle
- 坐骨直腸窩 Ischiorectal fossa

6-32

- 縫工筋 Sartorius muscle
- 大腿動脈 Femoral artery
- 大腿静脈 Femoral vein
- 恥骨筋 Pectineus muscle
- 大腿直筋 Rectus femoris muscle
- 大腿筋膜張筋 Tensor fasciae latae muscle
- 中殿筋 Gluteus medius muscle
- 小殿筋 Gluteus minimus muscle
- 腸腰筋 Iliopsoas muscle
- 下双子筋 Gemellus inferior muscle
- 前立腺 Prostate
- 肛門挙筋 Levator ani muscle
- 大殿筋 Gluteus maximus muscle
- 閉鎖管 Obturator canal
- 内閉鎖筋 Obturator internus muscle
- 坐骨直腸窩 Ischiorectal fossa

6-33

- 大腿動脈 Femoral artery
- 縫工筋 Sartorius muscle
- 大腿静脈 Femoral vein
- 恥骨筋 Pectineus muscle
- 大腿筋膜張筋 Tensor fasciae latae muscle
- 大腿直筋 Rectus femoris muscle
- 中殿筋 Gluteus medius muscle
- 外側広筋 Vastus lateralis muscle
- 腸腰筋 Iliopsoas muscle
- 大殿筋 Gluteus maximus muscle
- 外閉鎖筋 Obturator externus muscle
- 内閉鎖筋 Obturator internus muscle
- 坐骨直腸窩 Ischiorectal fossa

> **NOTE**　外腸骨動静脈は，腸骨筋の内側縁に沿って骨盤腔を下行し，鼠径靱帯を潜って，大腿動静脈と名前を変える．大腿静脈の内側には大腿輪とよばれる腹壁の薄い部分があり，大腿輪から伏在裂孔に至る潜在腔が大腿管とよばれる．大腿管から伏在裂孔へのルートが，大腿ヘルニアの主な脱出経路である．

男性骨盤部の断層解剖 ［横断像（造影CT）］

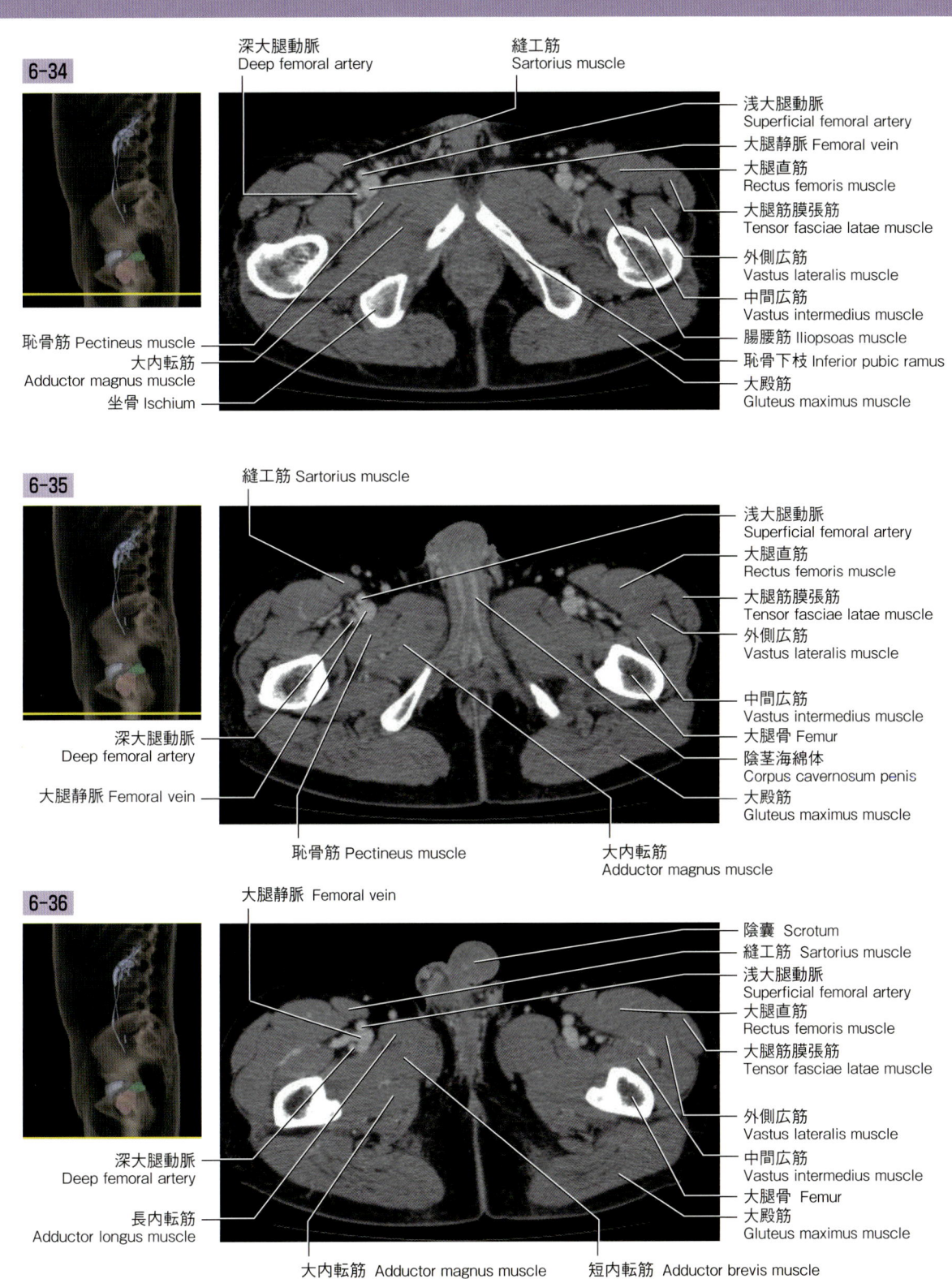

6-34

- 深大腿動脈 Deep femoral artery
- 縫工筋 Sartorius muscle
- 浅大腿動脈 Superficial femoral artery
- 大腿静脈 Femoral vein
- 大腿直筋 Rectus femoris muscle
- 大腿筋膜張筋 Tensor fasciae latae muscle
- 外側広筋 Vastus lateralis muscle
- 中間広筋 Vastus intermedius muscle
- 腸腰筋 Iliopsoas muscle
- 恥骨下枝 Inferior pubic ramus
- 大殿筋 Gluteus maximus muscle
- 恥骨筋 Pectineus muscle
- 大内転筋 Adductor magnus muscle
- 坐骨 Ischium

6-35

- 縫工筋 Sartorius muscle
- 浅大腿動脈 Superficial femoral artery
- 大腿直筋 Rectus femoris muscle
- 大腿筋膜張筋 Tensor fasciae latae muscle
- 外側広筋 Vastus lateralis muscle
- 中間広筋 Vastus intermedius muscle
- 大腿骨 Femur
- 陰茎海綿体 Corpus cavernosum penis
- 大殿筋 Gluteus maximus muscle
- 深大腿動脈 Deep femoral artery
- 大腿静脈 Femoral vein
- 恥骨筋 Pectineus muscle
- 大内転筋 Adductor magnus muscle

6-36

- 大腿静脈 Femoral vein
- 陰嚢 Scrotum
- 縫工筋 Sartorius muscle
- 浅大腿動脈 Superficial femoral artery
- 大腿直筋 Rectus femoris muscle
- 大腿筋膜張筋 Tensor fasciae latae muscle
- 外側広筋 Vastus lateralis muscle
- 中間広筋 Vastus intermedius muscle
- 大腿骨 Femur
- 大殿筋 Gluteus maximus muscle
- 深大腿動脈 Deep femoral artery
- 長内転筋 Adductor longus muscle
- 大内転筋 Adductor magnus muscle
- 短内転筋 Adductor brevis muscle

NOTE 陰茎は，3つの血管に富んだ円柱構造（背側に位置する2つの陰茎海綿体，腹側正中に位置する1つの尿道海綿体）からなる．それぞれの海綿体は，白膜とよばれる膜に覆われている．

男性骨盤部の断層解剖［冠状断像（造影CT）］

6-37

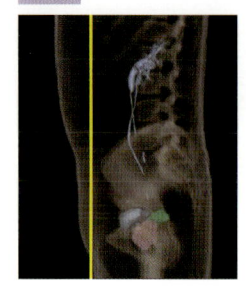

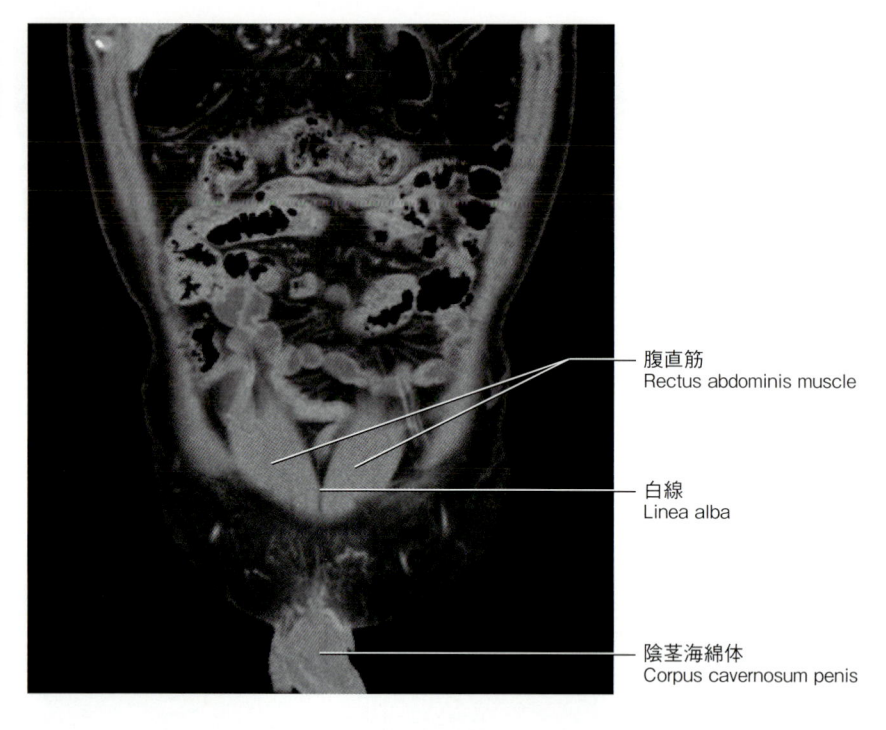

- 腹直筋 Rectus abdominis muscle
- 白線 Linea alba
- 陰茎海綿体 Corpus cavernosum penis

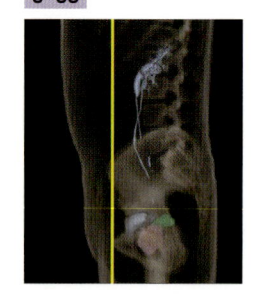

6-38

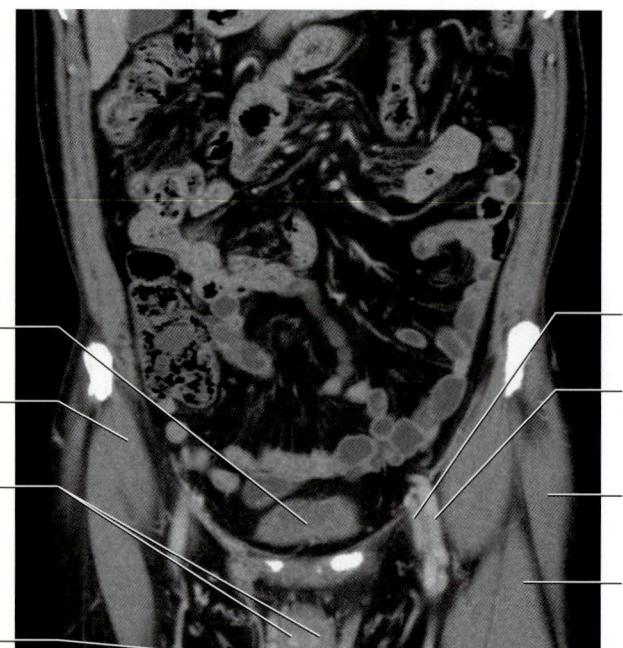

- 膀胱 Urinary bladder
- 腸腰筋 Iliopsoas muscle
- 陰茎海綿体 Corpus cavernosum penis
- 尿道海綿体 Corpus cavernosum urethrae
- 大腿静脈 Femoral vein
- 大腿動脈 Femoral artery
- 大腿筋膜張筋 Tensor fasciae latae muscle
- 大腿直筋 Rectus femoris muscle
- 縫工筋 Sartorius muscle

> **NOTE** 大腿ヘルニアと直接鼠径ヘルニアの鑑別には，鼠径靱帯の同定が重要である．鼠径靱帯は，横断像では同定がしばしば困難であるが，冠状断像において同定が可能な例が多いとの報告がある．

男性骨盤部の断層解剖 ［冠状断像（造影 CT）］

6-39

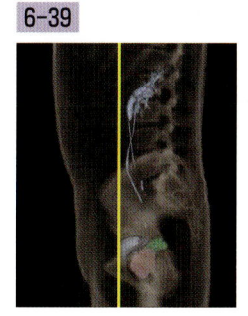

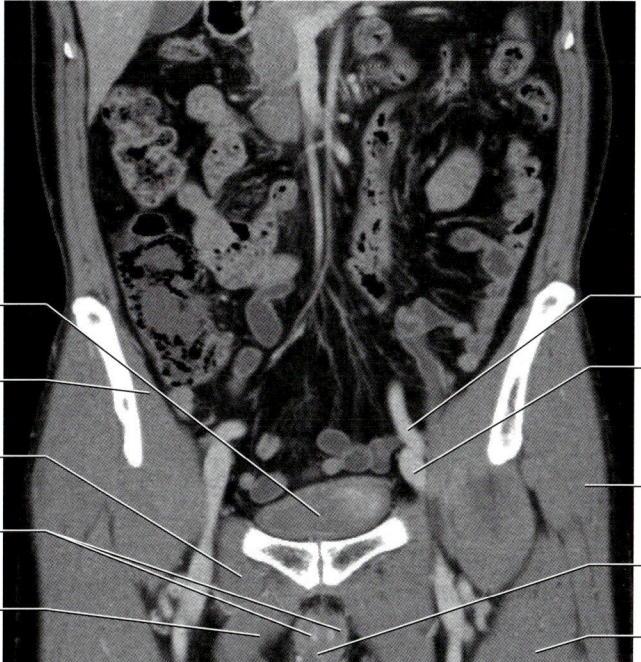

- 膀胱 / Urinary bladder
- 腸骨筋 / Iliacus muscle
- 恥骨筋 / Pectineus muscle
- 陰茎海綿体 / Corpus cavernosum penis
- 長内転筋 / Adductor longus muscle
- 外腸骨動脈 / External iliac artery
- 外腸骨静脈 / External iliac vein
- 大腿筋膜張筋 / Tensor fasciae latae muscle
- 尿道海綿体 / Corpus cavernosum urethrae
- 大腿直筋 / Rectus femoris muscle

6-40

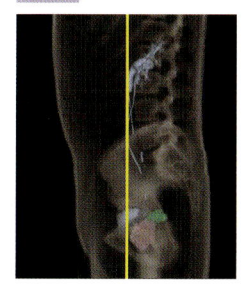

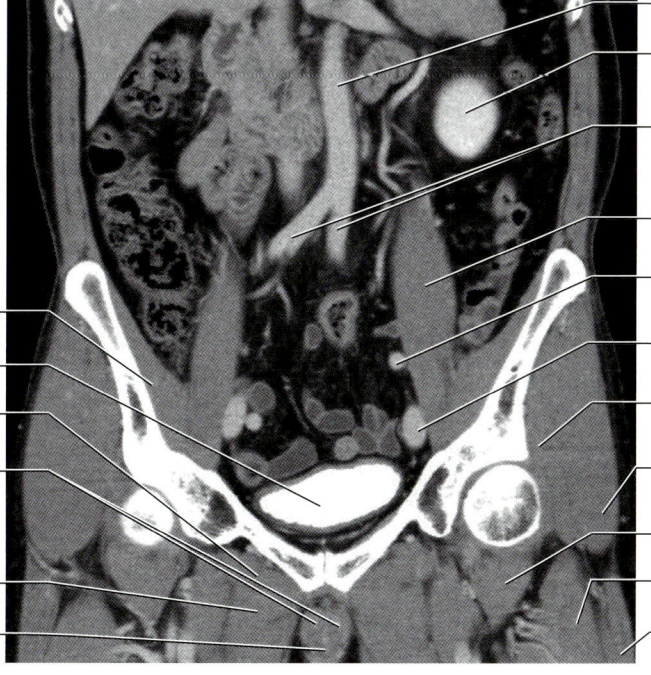

- 腸骨筋 / Iliacus muscle
- 膀胱 / Urinary bladder
- 外閉鎖筋 / Obturator externus muscle
- 陰茎海綿体 / Corpus cavernosum penis
- 恥骨筋 / Pectineus muscle
- 尿道海綿体 / Corpus cavernosum urethrae
- 腹部大動脈 / Abdominal aorta
- 腎皮質 / Renal cortex
- 総腸骨動脈 / Common iliac artery
- 大腰筋 / Psoas major muscle
- 外腸骨動脈 / External iliac artery
- 外腸骨静脈 / External iliac vein
- 小殿筋 / Gluteus minimus muscle
- 中殿筋 / Gluteus medius muscle
- 腸腰筋 / Iliopsoas muscle
- 大腿直筋 / Rectus femoris muscle
- 外側広筋 / Vastus lateralis muscle

> **NOTE** 腹部単純 X 線写真において，肝臓，腎臓のほか，大腰筋の輪郭は，それを囲む後腹膜脂肪組織によりコントラストされて同定される．輪郭が消失している場合には，水濃度を示す構造や炎症の存在などが示唆される．

男性骨盤部の断層解剖　[冠状断像（造影CT）]

6-41

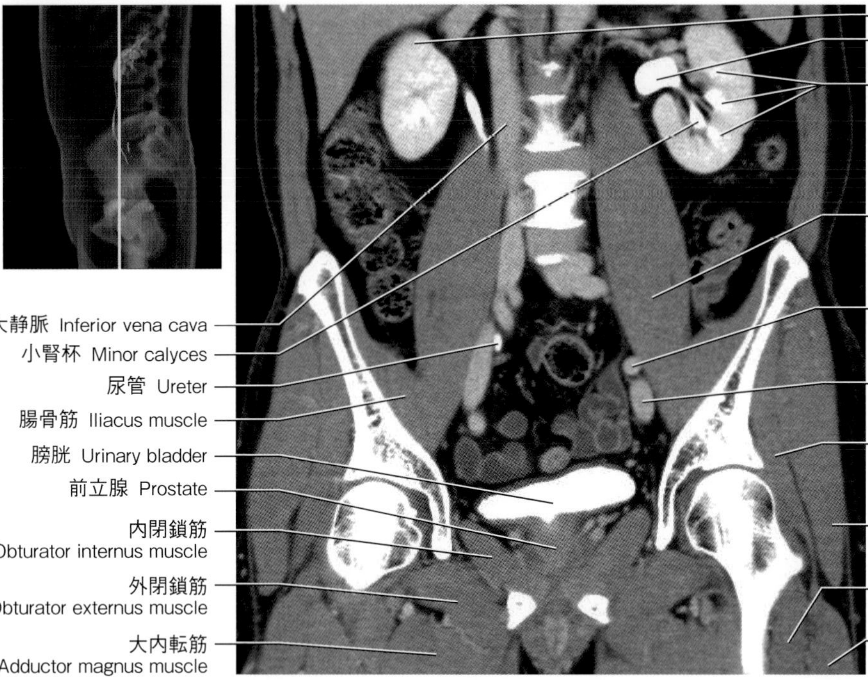

- 腎皮質 Renal cortex
- 腎盂 Renal pelvis
- 腎錐体 Renal pyramids
- 大腰筋 Psoas major muscle
- 外腸骨動脈 External iliac artery
- 外腸骨静脈 External iliac vein
- 小殿筋 Gluteus minimus muscle
- 中殿筋 Gluteus medius muscle
- 中間広筋 Vastus intermedius muscle
- 外側広筋 Vastus lateralis muscle
- 下大静脈 Inferior vena cava
- 小腎杯 Minor calyces
- 尿管 Ureter
- 腸骨筋 Iliacus muscle
- 膀胱 Urinary bladder
- 前立腺 Prostate
- 内閉鎖筋 Obturator internus muscle
- 外閉鎖筋 Obturator externus muscle
- 大内転筋 Adductor magnus muscle

6-42

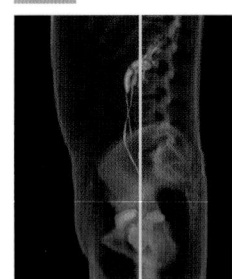

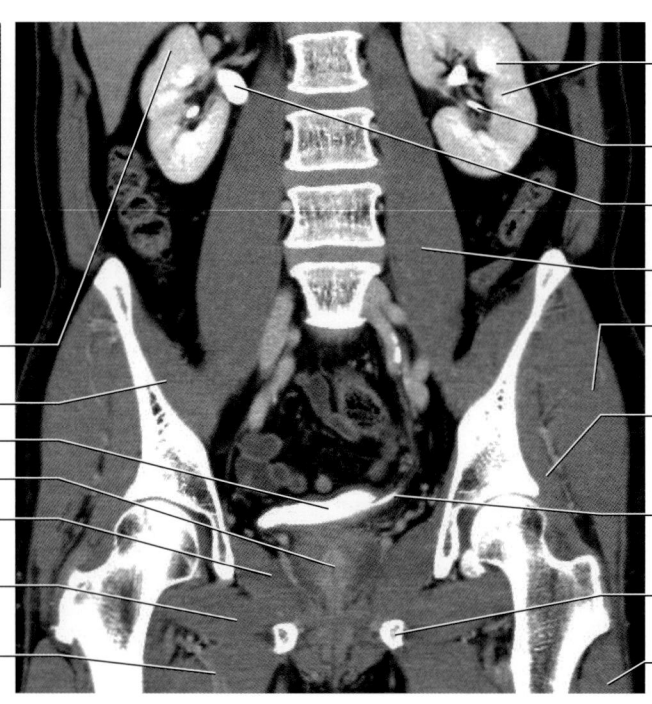

- 腎錐体 Renal pyramids
- 小腎杯 Minor calyces
- 腎盂 Renal pelvis
- 大腰筋 Psoas major muscle
- 中殿筋 Gluteus medius muscle
- 小殿筋 Gluteus minimus muscle
- 尿管 Ureter
- 恥骨 Pubic bone
- 外側広筋 Vastus lateralis muscle
- 腎皮質 Renal cortex
- 腸骨筋 Iliacus muscle
- 膀胱 Urinary bladder
- 前立腺 Prostate
- 内閉鎖筋 Obturator internus muscle
- 外閉鎖筋 Obturator externus muscle
- 大内転筋 Adductor magnus muscle

男性骨盤部の断層解剖 ［冠状断像（造影 CT）］

6-43

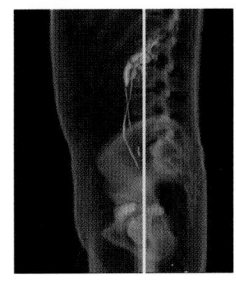

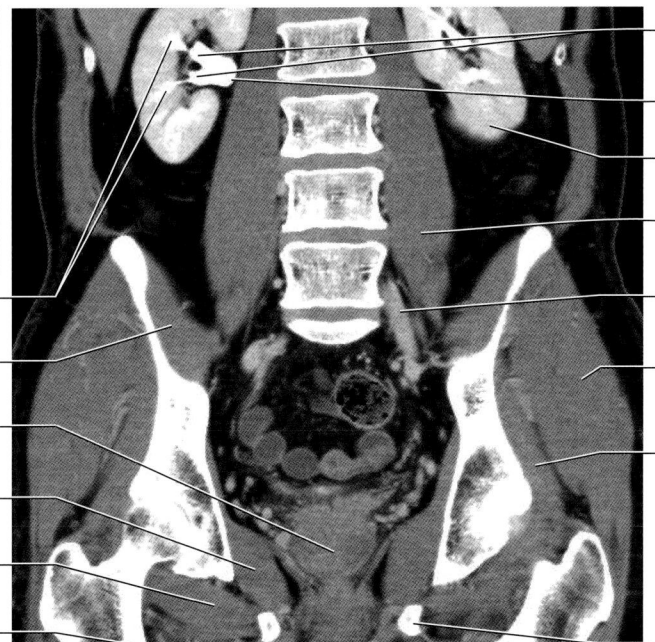

- 大腎杯 Major calyces
- 腎盂 Renal pelvis
- 腎皮質 Renal cortex
- 大腰筋 Psoas major muscle
- 内腸骨動脈 Internal iliac artery
- 中殿筋 Gluteus medius muscle
- 小殿筋 Gluteus minimus muscle
- 恥骨 Pubic bone
- 腎錐体 Renal pyramids
- 腸骨筋 Iliacus muscle
- 前立腺 Prostate
- 内閉鎖筋 Obturator internus muscle
- 外閉鎖筋 Obturator externus muscle
- 大内転筋 Adductor magnus muscle

6-44

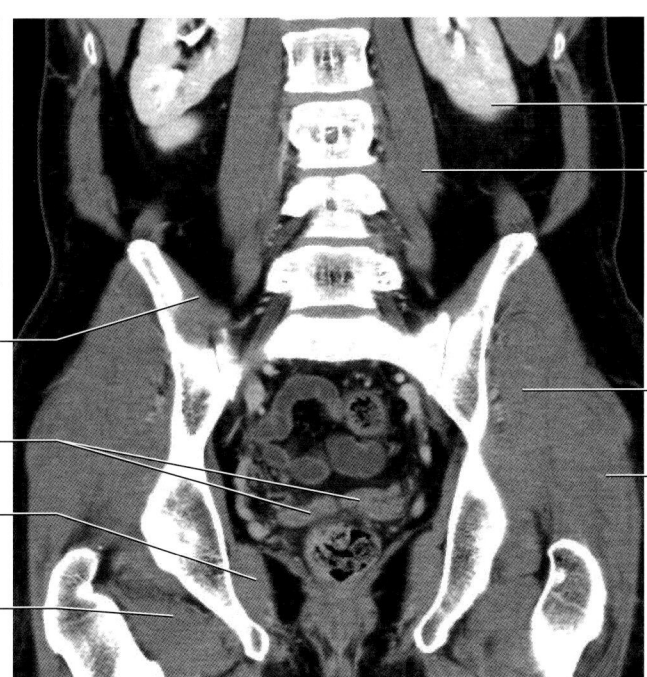

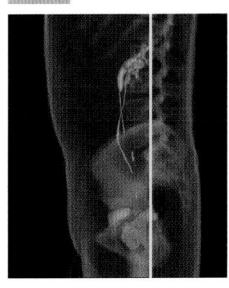

- 腎皮質 Renal cortex
- 大腰筋 Psoas major muscle
- 中殿筋 Gluteus medius muscle
- 大殿筋 Gluteus maximus muscle
- 腸骨筋 Iliacus muscle
- 精嚢 Seminal vesicle
- 内閉鎖筋 Obturator internus muscle
- 外閉鎖筋 Obturator externus muscle

男性骨盤部の断層解剖 ［矢状断像（造影CT）］

6-45

- 脊柱起立筋 Erector spinae muscle
- 下大静脈 Inferior vena cava
- 腹直筋 Rectus abdominis muscle
- 膀胱 Urinary bladder
- 内閉鎖筋 Obturator internus muscle
- 大内転筋 Adductor magnus muscle
- 精嚢 Seminal vesicle
- 大殿筋 Gluteus maximus muscle

6-46

- 脊柱起立筋 Erector spinae muscle
- 下大静脈 Inferior vena cava
- 腹直筋 Rectus abdominis muscle
- 膀胱 Urinary bladder
- 前立腺 Prostate
- 精嚢 Seminal vesicle
- 大殿筋 Gluteus maximus muscle

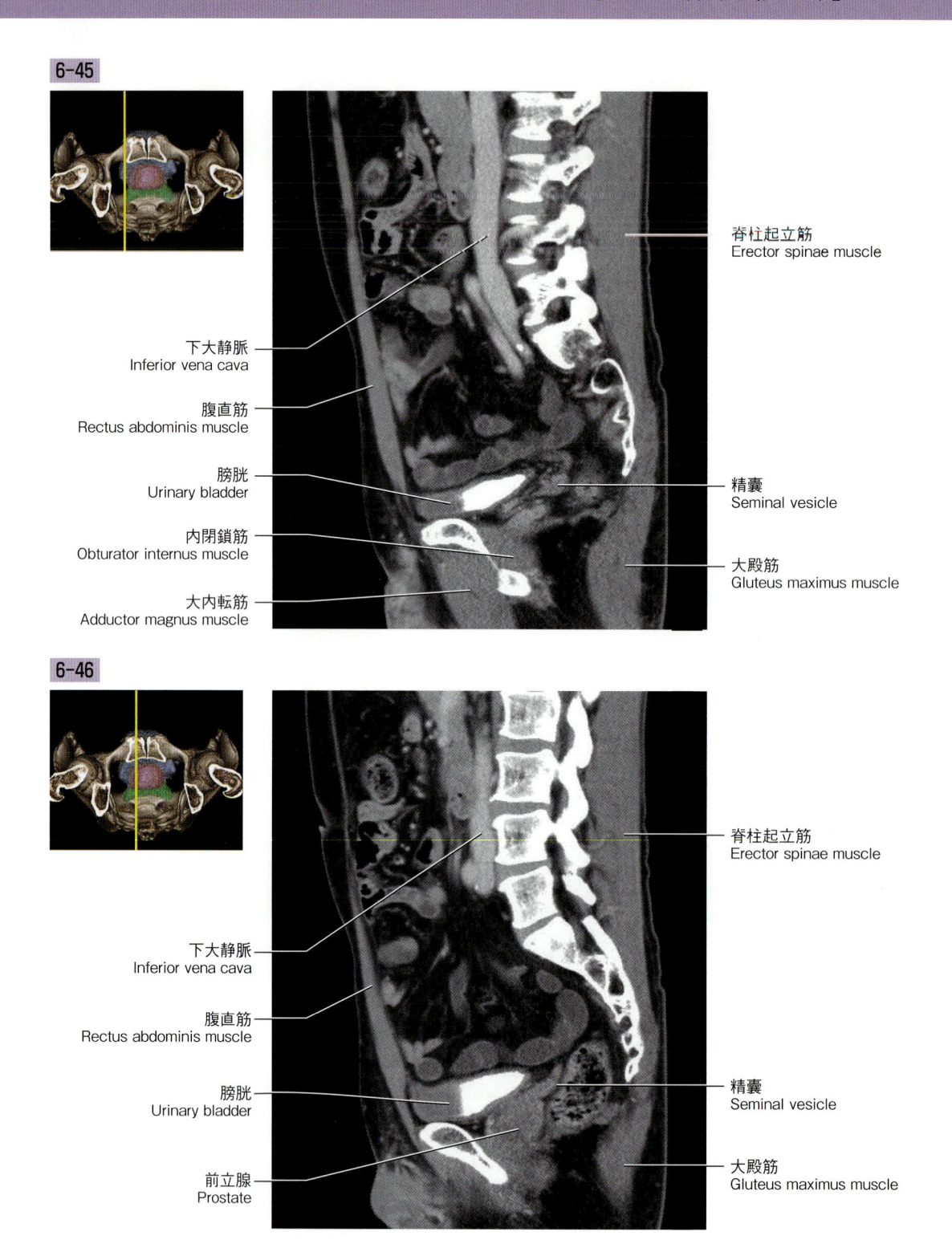

NOTE 第5腰椎の高さにおいて，大動脈分岐部後下方で，左右の総腸骨静脈が合流し，下大静脈となる．その後，下大静脈は腹部大動脈の右側を上行し，第8胸椎の高さにある大静脈孔で横隔膜を貫き，その直後に心膜を貫いて，心臓の下方から右心房の開口部に達する．

男性骨盤部の断層解剖 ［矢状断像（造影CT）］

6-47

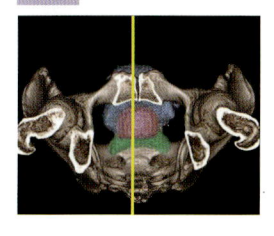

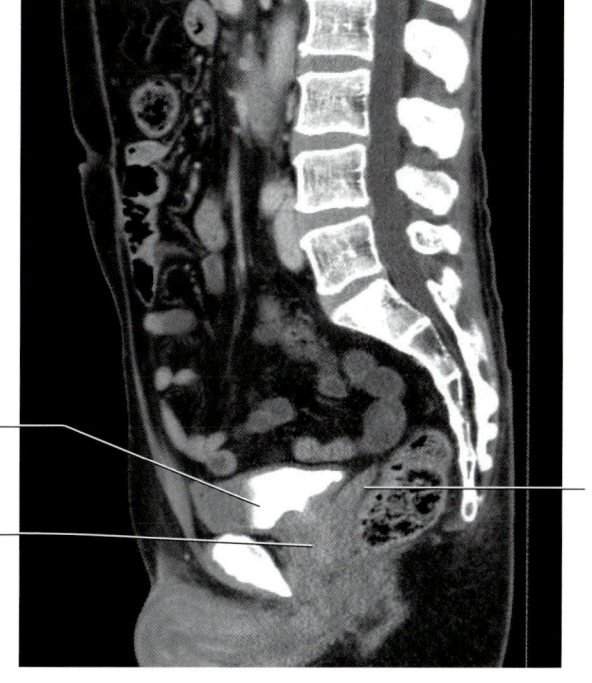

- 膀胱 Urinary bladder
- 前立腺 Prostate
- 精嚢 Seminal vesicle

6-48

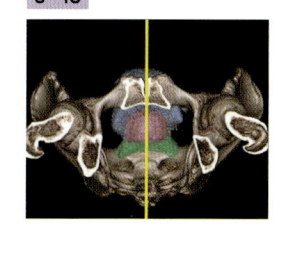

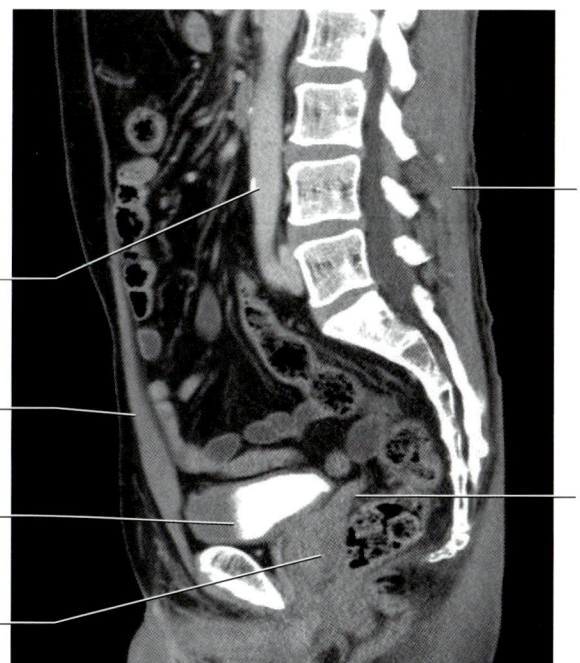

- 脊柱起立筋 Erector spinae muscle
- 腹部大静脈 Abdominal aorta
- 腹直筋 Rectus abdominis muscle
- 膀胱 Urinary bladder
- 前立腺 Prostate
- 精嚢 Seminal vesicle

NOTE 腹部大動脈は，正中線のやや左側をおよそ第4腰椎の高さまで走り，左右の総腸骨動脈に分岐する．腹部大動脈からは，腹部と骨盤部を栄養する多数の枝が分岐し，主な分岐部位は，腹腔動脈は第12胸椎／第1腰椎レベル，上腸間膜動脈は第1腰椎レベル，腎動脈は第1/第2腰椎レベル，下腸間膜動脈は第3腰椎レベルである．

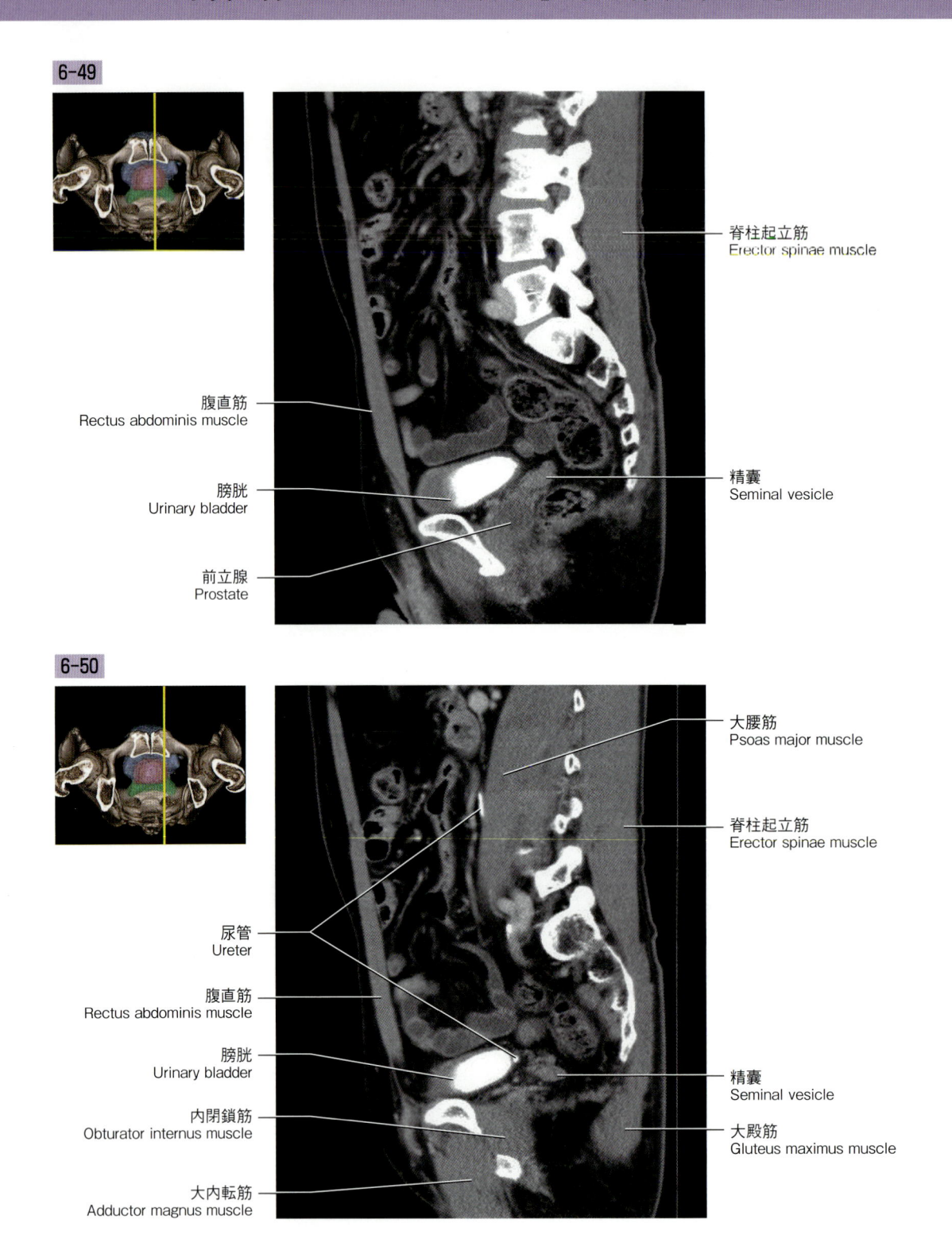

男性骨盤部の断層解剖 ［矢状断像（造影 CT）］

6-49

- 脊柱起立筋 Erector spinae muscle
- 腹直筋 Rectus abdominis muscle
- 膀胱 Urinary bladder
- 前立腺 Prostate
- 精囊 Seminal vesicle

6-50

- 大腰筋 Psoas major muscle
- 脊柱起立筋 Erector spinae muscle
- 尿管 Ureter
- 腹直筋 Rectus abdominis muscle
- 膀胱 Urinary bladder
- 内閉鎖筋 Obturator internus muscle
- 大内転筋 Adductor magnus muscle
- 精囊 Seminal vesicle
- 大殿筋 Gluteus maximus muscle

> **NOTE** 尿管の膀胱移行部が描出されている．尿管は拡張していない場合では，同定が難しいことが多い．尿管拡張の原因は，その遠位部における尿管狭窄であるが，その原因は多岐にわたる．

女性骨盤部の断層解剖 ［横断像（造影CT）］

6-51

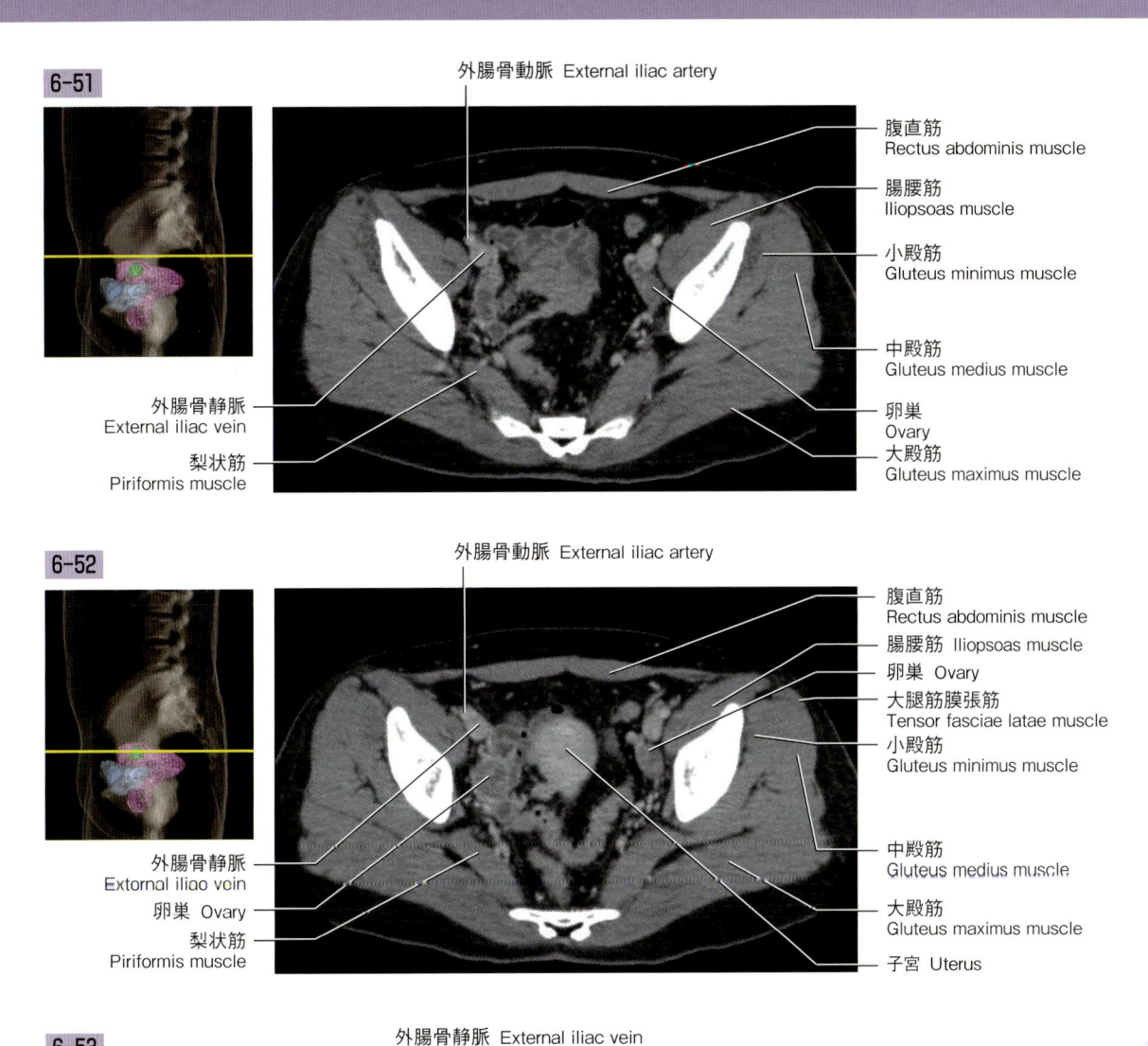

- 外腸骨動脈 External iliac artery
- 腹直筋 Rectus abdominis muscle
- 腸腰筋 Iliopsoas muscle
- 小殿筋 Gluteus minimus muscle
- 中殿筋 Gluteus medius muscle
- 卵巣 Ovary
- 大殿筋 Gluteus maximus muscle
- 外腸骨静脈 External iliac vein
- 梨状筋 Piriformis muscle

6-52

- 外腸骨動脈 External iliac artery
- 腹直筋 Rectus abdominis muscle
- 腸腰筋 Iliopsoas muscle
- 卵巣 Ovary
- 大腿筋膜張筋 Tensor fasciae latae muscle
- 小殿筋 Gluteus minimus muscle
- 中殿筋 Gluteus medius muscle
- 大殿筋 Gluteus maximus muscle
- 子宮 Uterus
- 外腸骨静脈 External iliac vein
- 卵巣 Ovary
- 梨状筋 Piriformis muscle

6-53

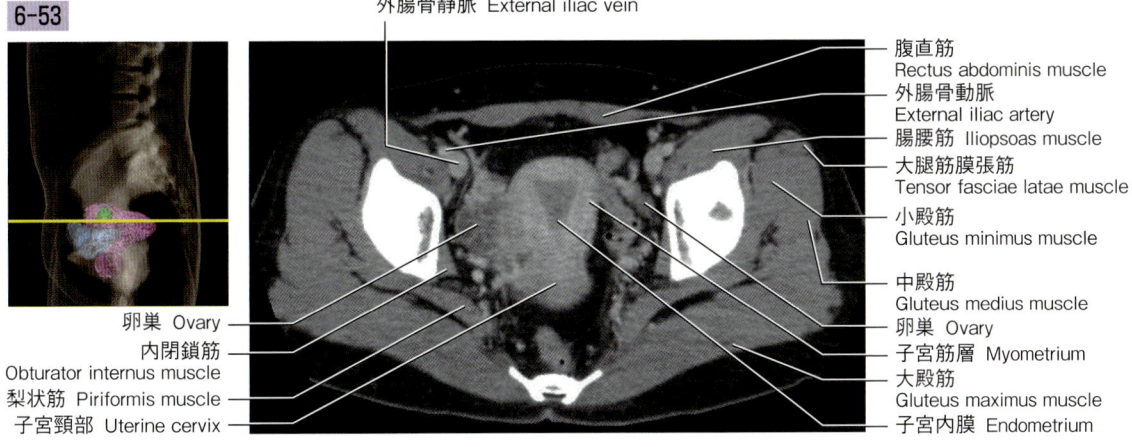

- 外腸骨静脈 External iliac vein
- 腹直筋 Rectus abdominis muscle
- 外腸骨動脈 External iliac artery
- 腸腰筋 Iliopsoas muscle
- 大腿筋膜張筋 Tensor fasciae latae muscle
- 小殿筋 Gluteus minimus muscle
- 中殿筋 Gluteus medius muscle
- 卵巣 Ovary
- 子宮筋層 Myometrium
- 大殿筋 Gluteus maximus muscle
- 子宮内膜 Endometrium
- 卵巣 Ovary
- 内閉鎖筋 Obturator internus muscle
- 梨状筋 Piriformis muscle
- 子宮頸部 Uterine cervix

NOTE 腟の前壁と後壁は近接しているので，横断面では腟の内腔はH型をしている．

NOTE 大腰筋と腸骨筋とを合わせて腸腰筋とよぶ．起始部が異なるが，停止部がともに大腿骨小転子なので，断層面の尾側では分離することが困難である（6-61〜64を参照）．

女性骨盤部の断層解剖 ［横断像（造影CT）］

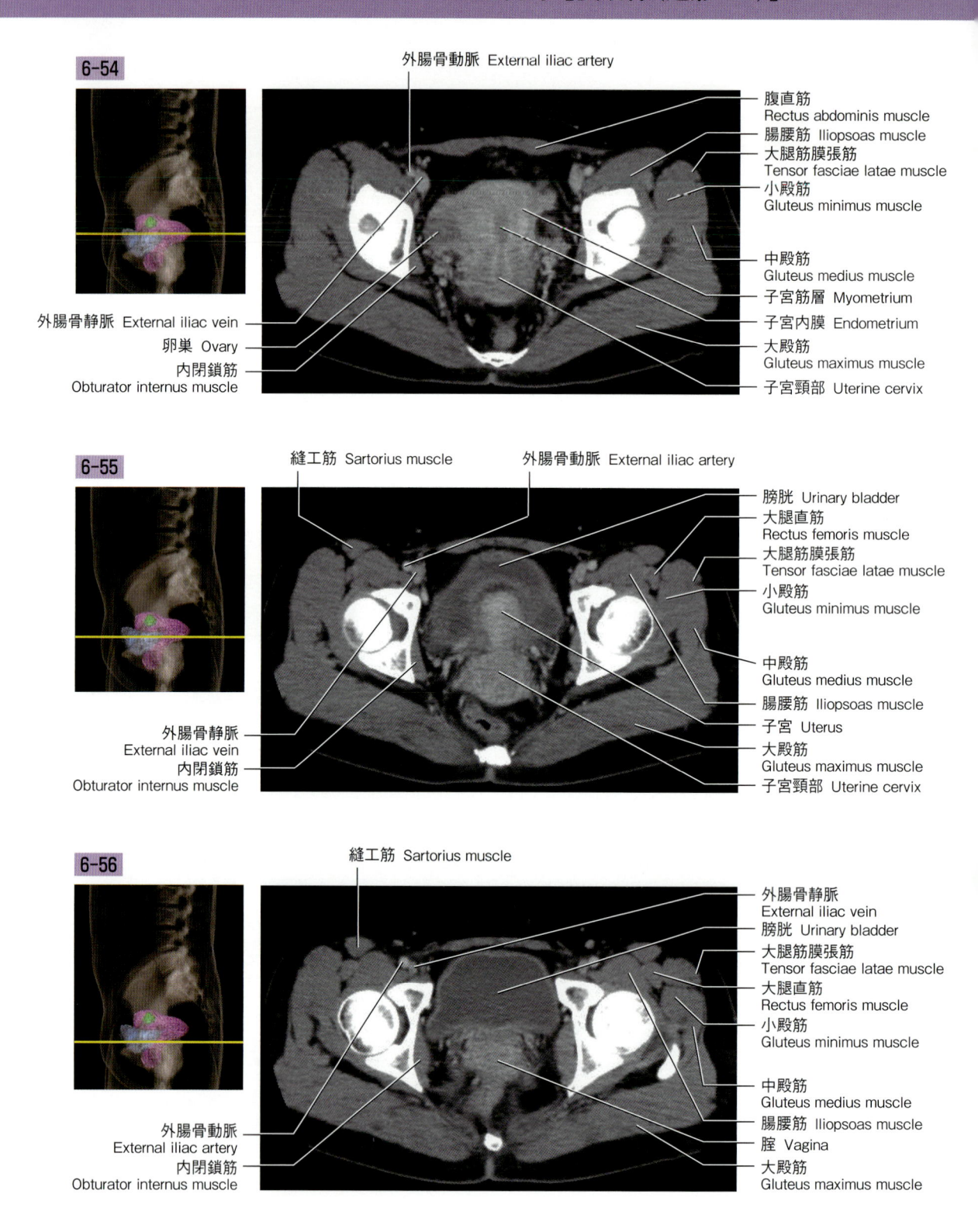

6-54

- 外腸骨動脈 External iliac artery
- 腹直筋 Rectus abdominis muscle
- 腸腰筋 Iliopsoas muscle
- 大腿筋膜張筋 Tensor fasciae latae muscle
- 小殿筋 Gluteus minimus muscle
- 中殿筋 Gluteus medius muscle
- 子宮筋層 Myometrium
- 子宮内膜 Endometrium
- 大殿筋 Gluteus maximus muscle
- 子宮頸部 Uterine cervix
- 外腸骨静脈 External iliac vein
- 卵巣 Ovary
- 内閉鎖筋 Obturator internus muscle

6-55

- 縫工筋 Sartorius muscle
- 外腸骨動脈 External iliac artery
- 膀胱 Urinary bladder
- 大腿直筋 Rectus femoris muscle
- 大腿筋膜張筋 Tensor fasciae latae muscle
- 小殿筋 Gluteus minimus muscle
- 中殿筋 Gluteus medius muscle
- 腸腰筋 Iliopsoas muscle
- 子宮 Uterus
- 大殿筋 Gluteus maximus muscle
- 子宮頸部 Uterine cervix
- 外腸骨静脈 External iliac vein
- 内閉鎖筋 Obturator internus muscle

6-56

- 縫工筋 Sartorius muscle
- 外腸骨静脈 External iliac vein
- 膀胱 Urinary bladder
- 大腿筋膜張筋 Tensor fasciae latae muscle
- 大腿直筋 Rectus femoris muscle
- 小殿筋 Gluteus minimus muscle
- 中殿筋 Gluteus medius muscle
- 腸腰筋 Iliopsoas muscle
- 腟 Vagina
- 大殿筋 Gluteus maximus muscle
- 外腸骨動脈 External iliac artery
- 内閉鎖筋 Obturator internus muscle

> **NOTE** 正常な卵巣は卵巣窩に位置する．卵巣窩は，前方は外腸骨動静脈，後方は内腸骨動静脈および尿管で境される．

女性骨盤部の断層解剖 ［横断像（造影 CT）］

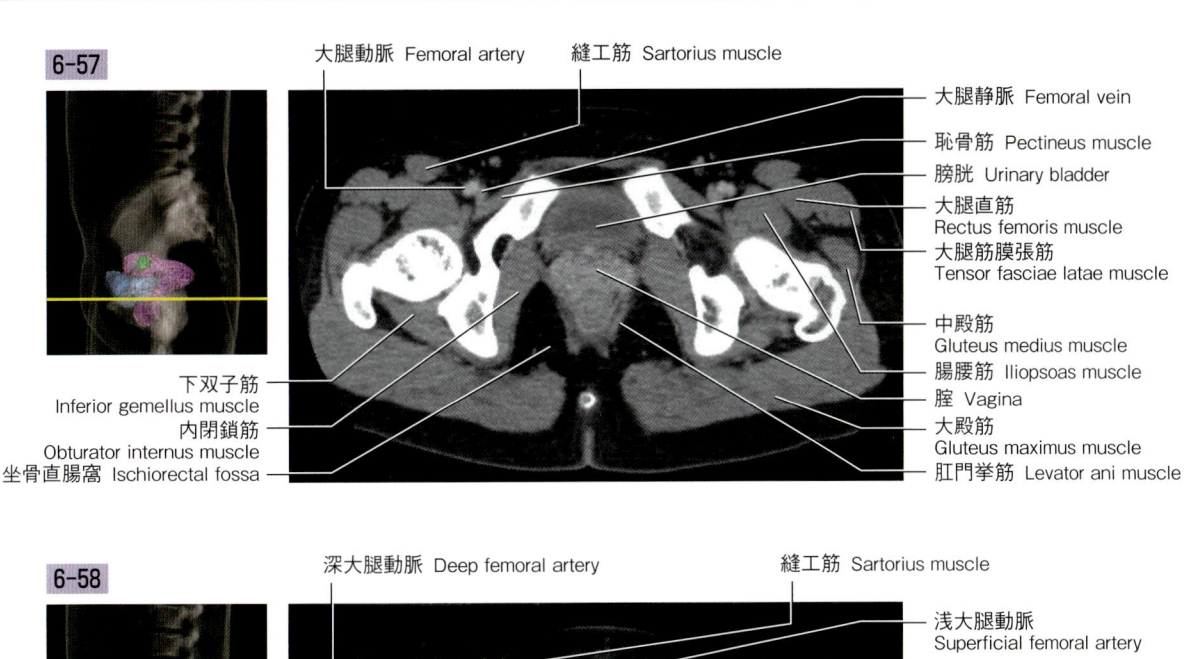

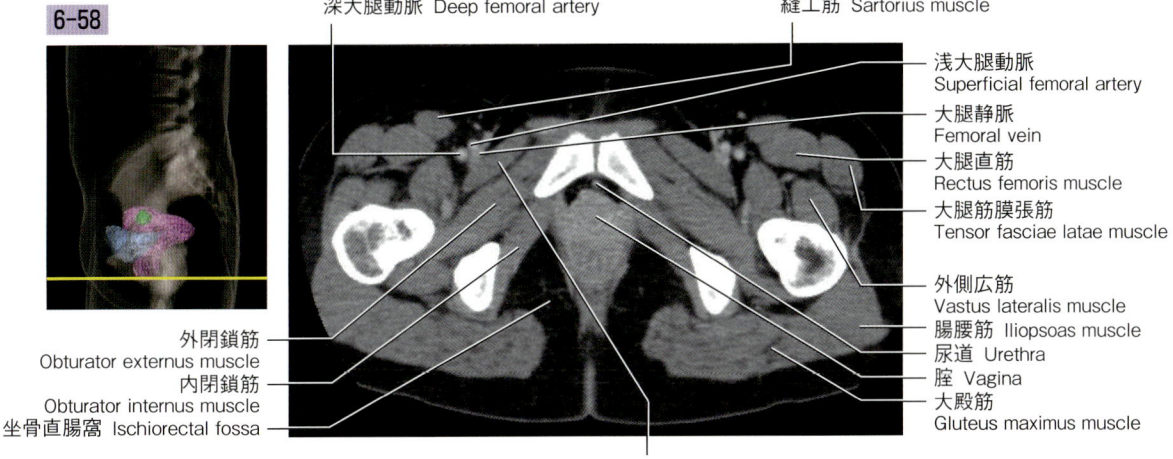

6-57

大腿動脈 Femoral artery
縫工筋 Sartorius muscle
大腿静脈 Femoral vein
恥骨筋 Pectineus muscle
膀胱 Urinary bladder
大腿直筋 Rectus femoris muscle
大腿筋膜張筋 Tensor fasciae latae muscle
中殿筋 Gluteus medius muscle
腸腰筋 Iliopsoas muscle
腟 Vagina
大殿筋 Gluteus maximus muscle
肛門挙筋 Levator ani muscle
下双子筋 Inferior gemellus muscle
内閉鎖筋 Obturator internus muscle
坐骨直腸窩 Ischiorectal fossa

6-58

深大腿動脈 Deep femoral artery
縫工筋 Sartorius muscle
浅大腿動脈 Superficial femoral artery
大腿静脈 Femoral vein
大腿直筋 Rectus femoris muscle
大腿筋膜張筋 Tensor fasciae latae muscle
外側広筋 Vastus lateralis muscle
腸腰筋 Iliopsoas muscle
尿道 Urethra
腟 Vagina
大殿筋 Gluteus maximus muscle
外閉鎖筋 Obturator externus muscle
内閉鎖筋 Obturator internus muscle
坐骨直腸窩 Ischiorectal fossa
恥骨筋 Pectineus muscle

女性骨盤部の断層解剖 ［冠状断像（造影CT）］

6-59

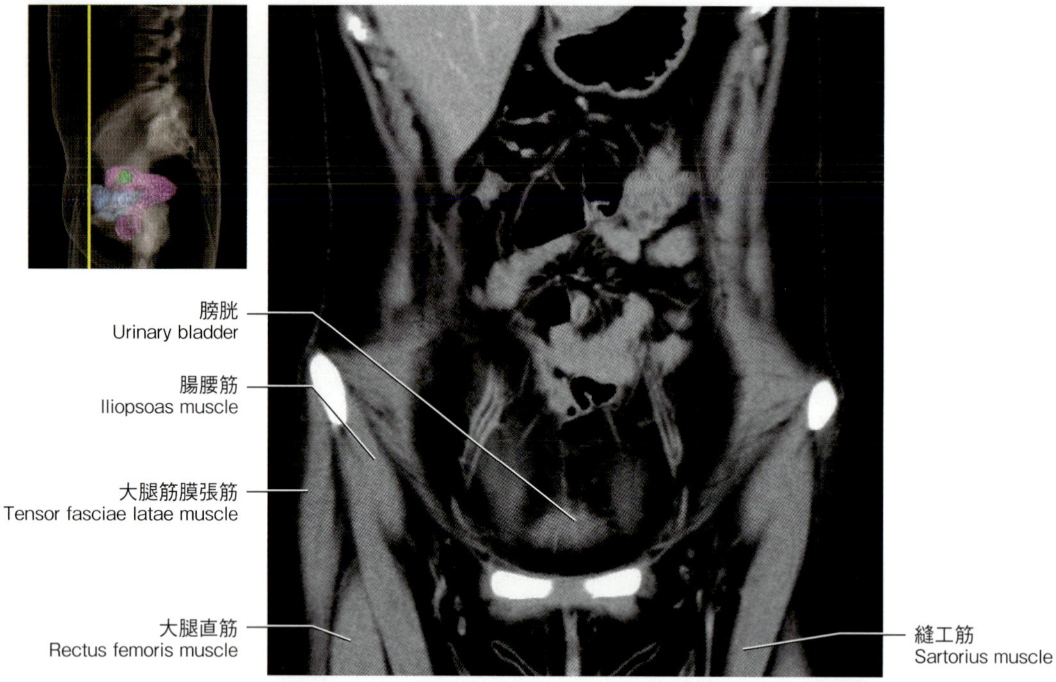

- 膀胱 Urinary bladder
- 腸腰筋 Iliopsoas muscle
- 大腿筋膜張筋 Tensor fasciae latae muscle
- 大腿直筋 Rectus femoris muscle
- 縫工筋 Sartorius muscle

6-60

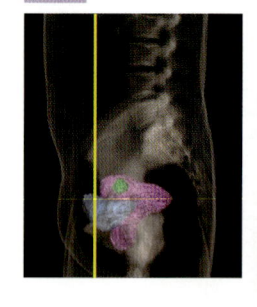

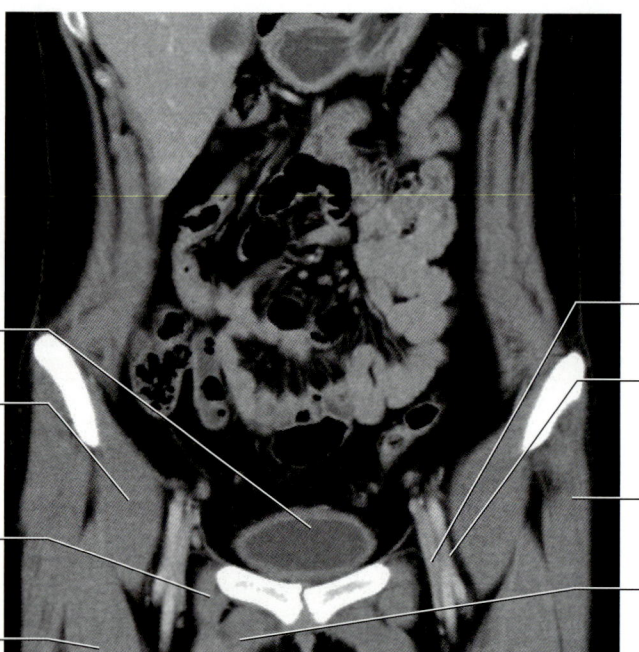

- 膀胱 Urinary bladder
- 腸腰筋 Iliopsoas muscle
- 恥骨筋 Pectineus muscle
- 大腿直筋 Rectus femoris muscle
- 大腿静脈 Femoral vein
- 大腿動脈 Femoral artery
- 大腿筋膜張筋 Tensor fasciae latae muscle
- 長内転筋 Adductor longus muscle

NOTE 女性の膀胱は子宮の下に位置し，膀胱が拡張すると子宮を上へ押し上げる．経腟分娩などによる損傷で骨盤底の構造が弱くなると膀胱が下行し，尿失禁の原因となることが知られている．

女性骨盤部の断層解剖［冠状断像（造影CT）］

6-61

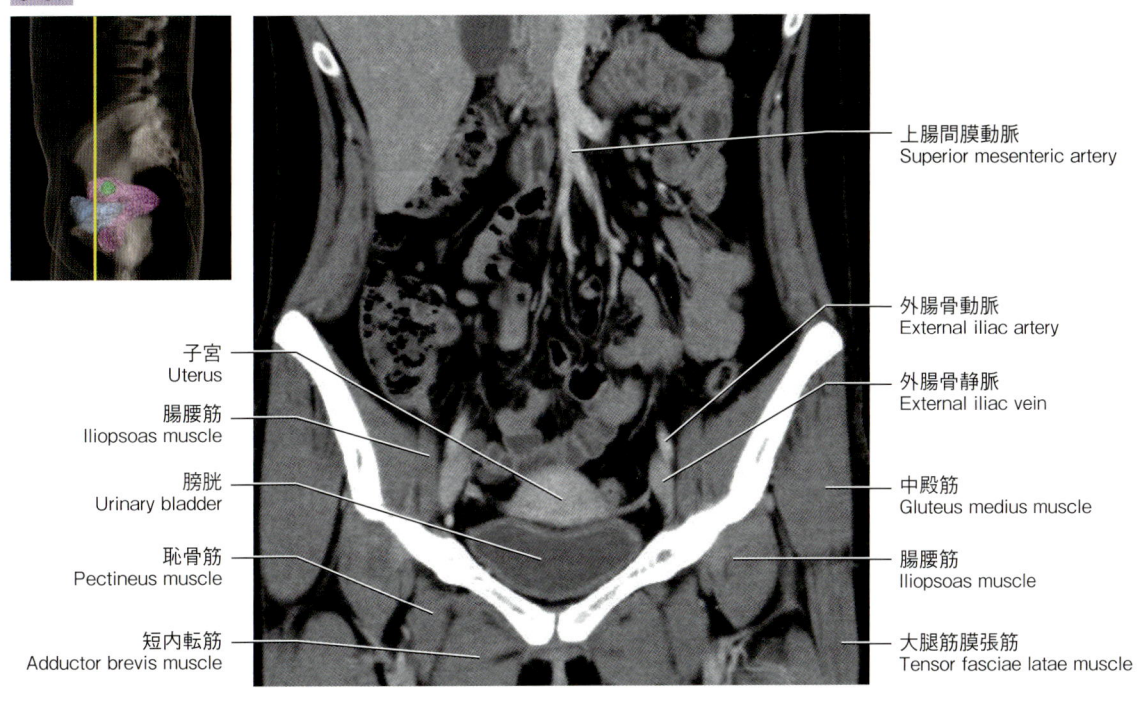

- 上腸間膜動脈 Superior mesenteric artery
- 子宮 Uterus
- 腸腰筋 Iliopsoas muscle
- 膀胱 Urinary bladder
- 恥骨筋 Pectineus muscle
- 短内転筋 Adductor brevis muscle
- 外腸骨動脈 External iliac artery
- 外腸骨静脈 External iliac vein
- 中殿筋 Gluteus medius muscle
- 腸腰筋 Iliopsoas muscle
- 大腿筋膜張筋 Tensor fasciae latae muscle

6-62

- 子宮内膜 Endometrium
- 腸腰筋 Iliopsoas muscle
- 膀胱 Urinary bladder
- 外閉鎖筋 Obturator externus muscle
- 短内転筋 Adductor brevis muscle
- 子宮筋層 Myometrium
- 外腸骨動脈 External iliac artery
- 外腸骨静脈 External iliac vein
- 中殿筋 Gluteus medius muscle
- 外側広筋 Vastus lateralis muscle

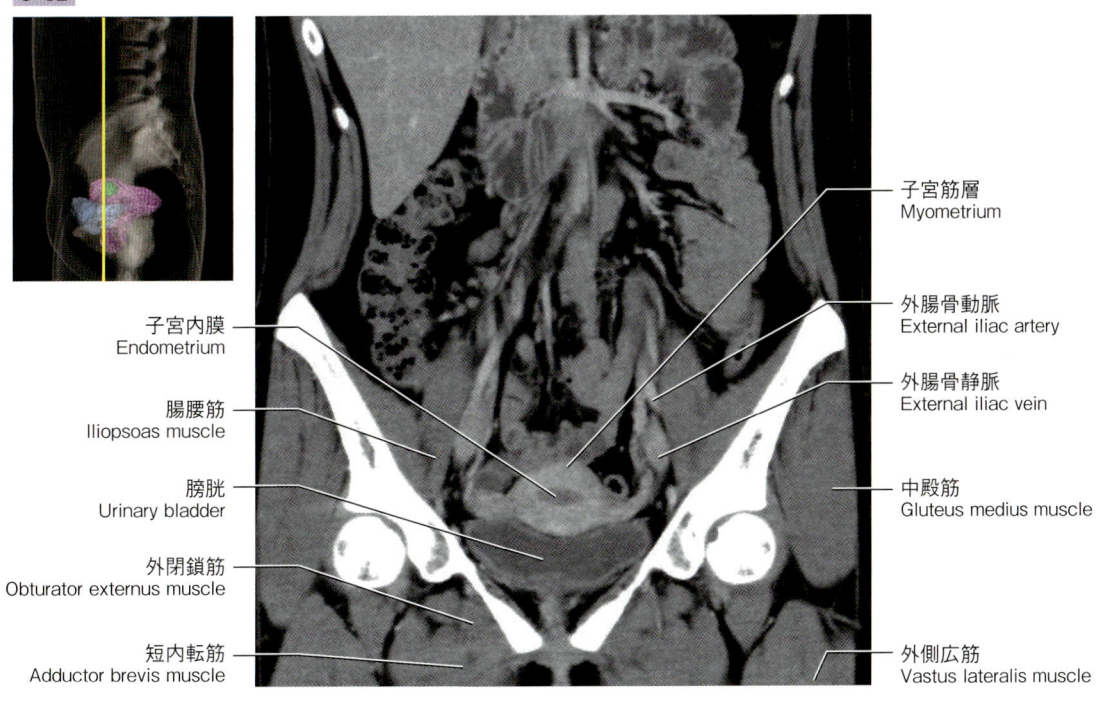

> **NOTE** 上腸間膜動脈は，第1腰椎の高さで腹部大動脈の前面から分岐し，右側に向かう多数の枝を出しながら前下方走行する．上腸間膜動脈とその枝は，小腸（空腸動脈と回腸動脈），膵臓の一部（下膵十二指腸動脈），左結腸曲までの大腸の多く（回結腸動脈・前後盲腸動脈・虫垂動脈・右結腸動脈・中結腸動脈）を栄養している．

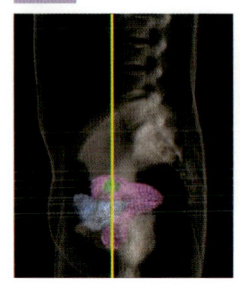

女性骨盤部の断層解剖 ［冠状断像（造影 CT）］

6-63

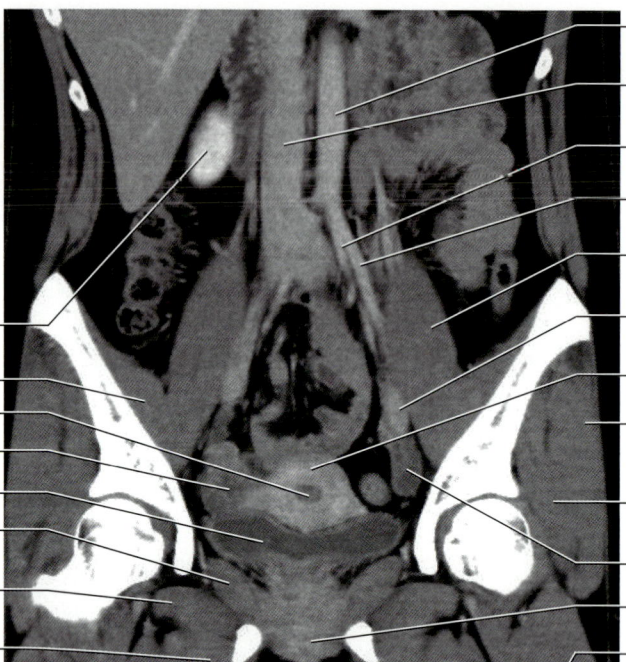

- 腹部大動脈 Abdominal aorta
- 下大静脈 Inferior vena cava
- 内腸骨動脈 Internal iliac artery
- 外腸骨動脈 External iliac artery
- 大腰筋 Psoas major muscle
- 外腸骨静脈 External iliac vein
- 子宮筋層 Myometrium
- 中殿筋 Gluteus medius muscle
- 小殿筋 Gluteus minimus muscle
- 卵巣 Ovary
- 腟 Vagina
- 外側広筋 Vastus lateralis muscle
- 腎皮質 Renal cortex
- 腸骨筋 Iliacus muscle
- 子宮内膜 Endometrium
- 卵巣 Ovary
- 膀胱 Urinary bladder
- 内閉鎖筋 Obturator internus muscle
- 外閉鎖筋 Obturator externus muscle
- 短内転筋 Adductor brevis muscle

6-64

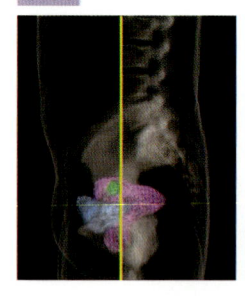

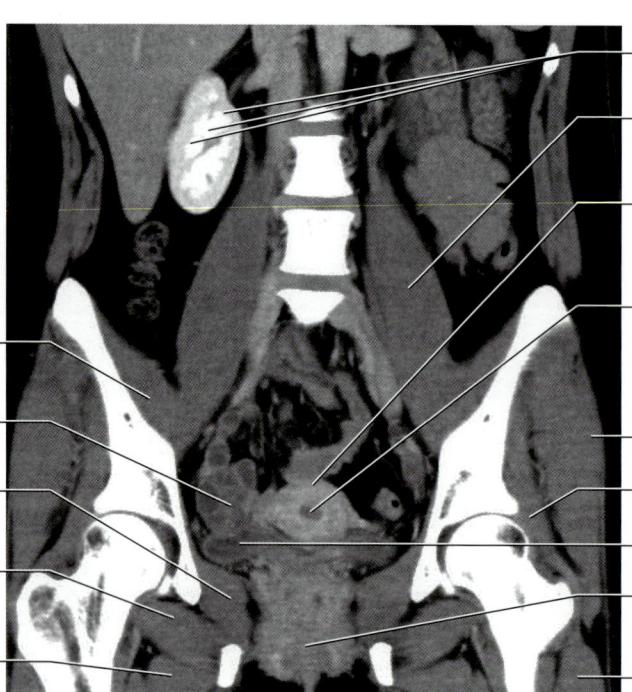

- 腎錐体 Renal pyramids
- 大腰筋 Psoas major muscle
- 子宮筋層 Myometrium
- 子宮内膜 Endometrium
- 中殿筋 Gluteus medius muscle
- 小殿筋 Gluteus minimus muscle
- 膀胱 Urinary bladder
- 腟 Vagina
- 外側広筋 Vastus lateralis muscle
- 腸骨筋 Iliacus muscle
- 卵巣 Ovary
- 内閉鎖筋 Obturator internus muscle
- 外閉鎖筋 Obturator externus muscle
- 短内転筋 Adductor brevis muscle

> **NOTE** 子宮は体部と頸部からなる．子宮体部と頸部の境界部は内子宮口とよばれる．高齢者に頻度の高い子宮内膜癌は子宮内膜の肥厚として描出されることが多く，MRI では体部の傾きに対する直交断面の撮像は，筋層浸潤の評価に有用である．また，筋層浸潤の有無は予後に影響を与えることが知られている．

女性骨盤部の断層解剖 ［冠状断像（造影 CT）］

6-65

- 腎錐体 Renal pyramids
- 腸骨筋 Iliacus muscle
- 内閉鎖筋 Obturator internus muscle
- 外閉鎖筋 Obturator externus muscle
- 大腰筋 Psoas major muscle
- 子宮 Uterus
- 中殿筋 Gluteus medius muscle
- 小殿筋 Gluteus minimus muscle
- 外側広筋 Vastus lateralis muscle

6-66

- 腎錐体 Renal pyramids
- 腸骨筋 Iliacus muscle
- 内閉鎖筋 Obturator internus muscle
- 大腰筋 Psoas major muscle
- 子宮 Uterus
- 中殿筋 Gluteus medius muscle
- 大殿筋 Gluteus maximus muscle

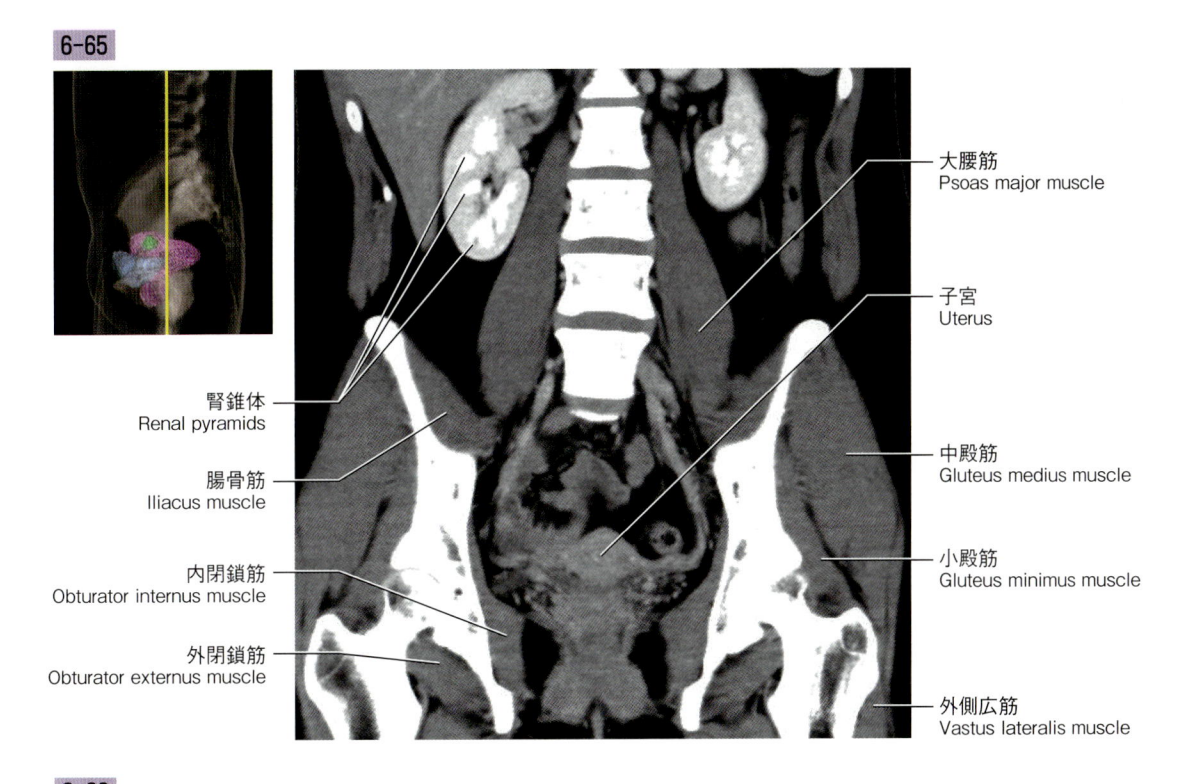

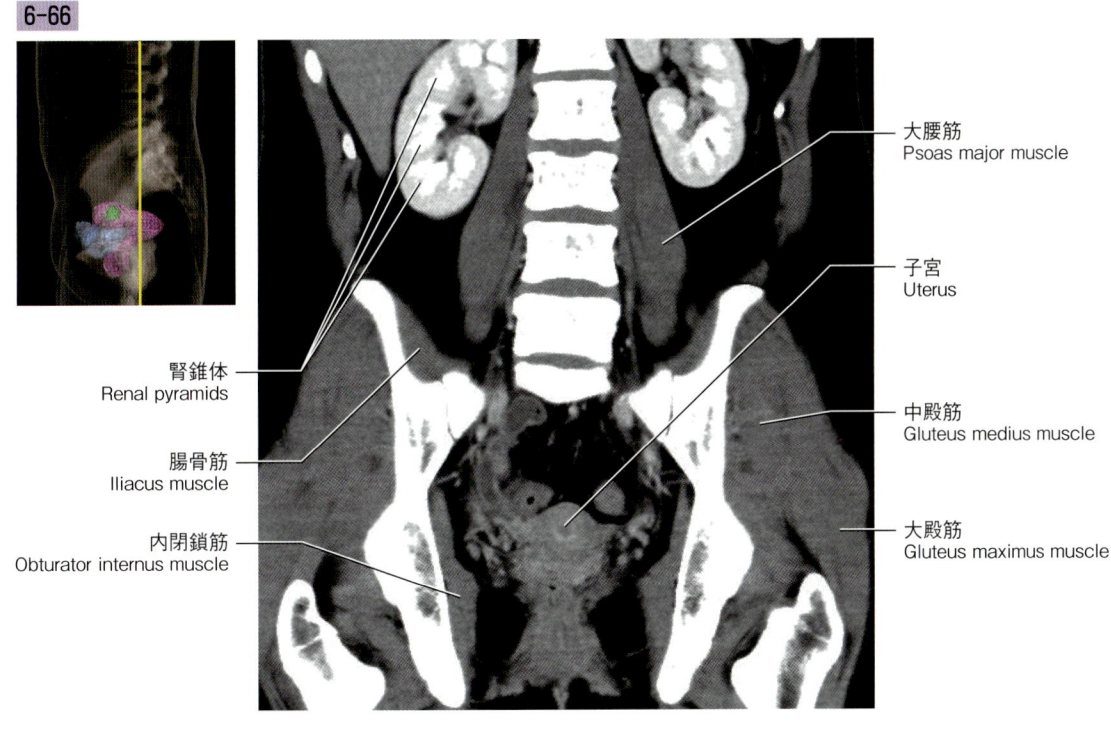

NOTE 子宮体癌と同様に，子宮に発生する悪性疾患として頻度の高い子宮頸癌においても，MRI における病期診断が有用である．頸部間質の信号が保たれているか，子宮傍組織への浸潤があるかが重要である．

女性骨盤部の断層解剖 ［冠状断像（造影CT）］

6-67

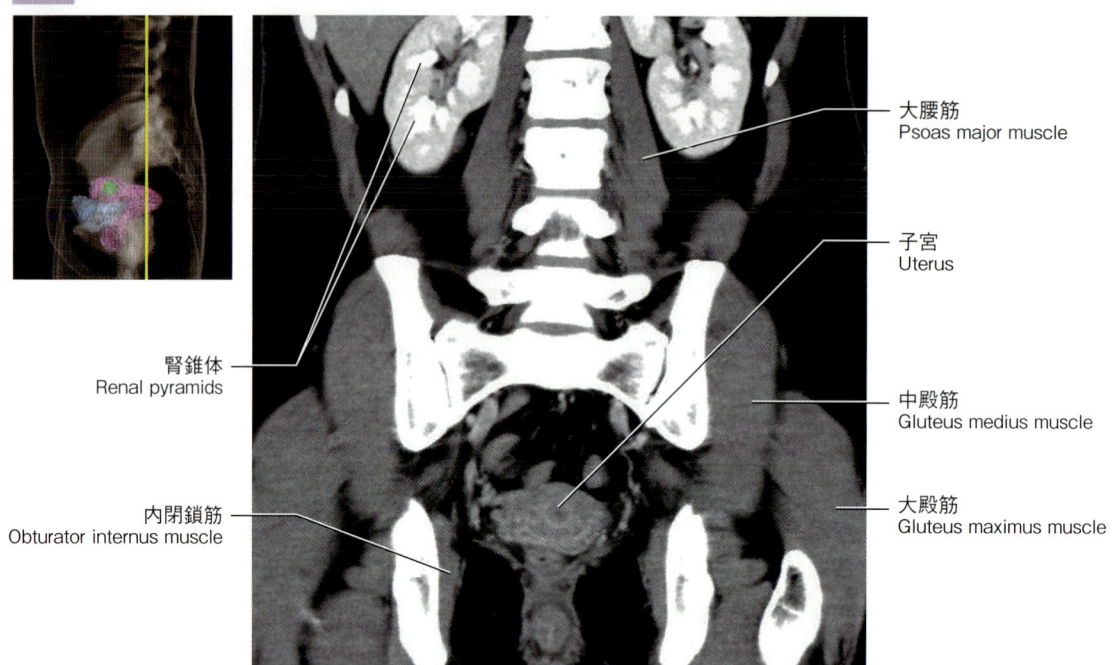

- 腎錐体 Renal pyramids
- 内閉鎖筋 Obturator internus muscle
- 大腰筋 Psoas major muscle
- 子宮 Uterus
- 中殿筋 Gluteus medius muscle
- 大殿筋 Gluteus maximus muscle

6-68

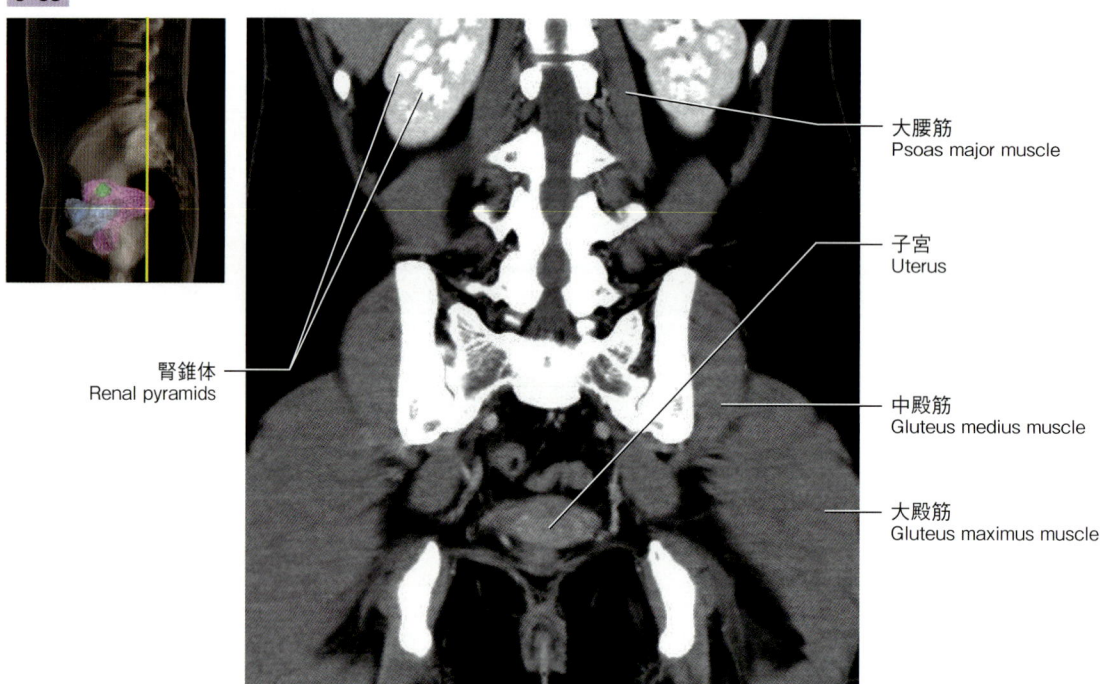

- 腎錐体 Renal pyramids
- 大腰筋 Psoas major muscle
- 子宮 Uterus
- 中殿筋 Gluteus medius muscle
- 大殿筋 Gluteus maximus muscle

> **NOTE** 卵巣 Ovary
> ラテン語 avian は「鳥」の意味で，aviation は英語で「航空術」．a が o に変化して oval（卵形の），Ovary になったとされる．古来，卵といえば鳥のものらしい．

女性骨盤部の断層解剖　[矢状断像（造影CT）]

6-69

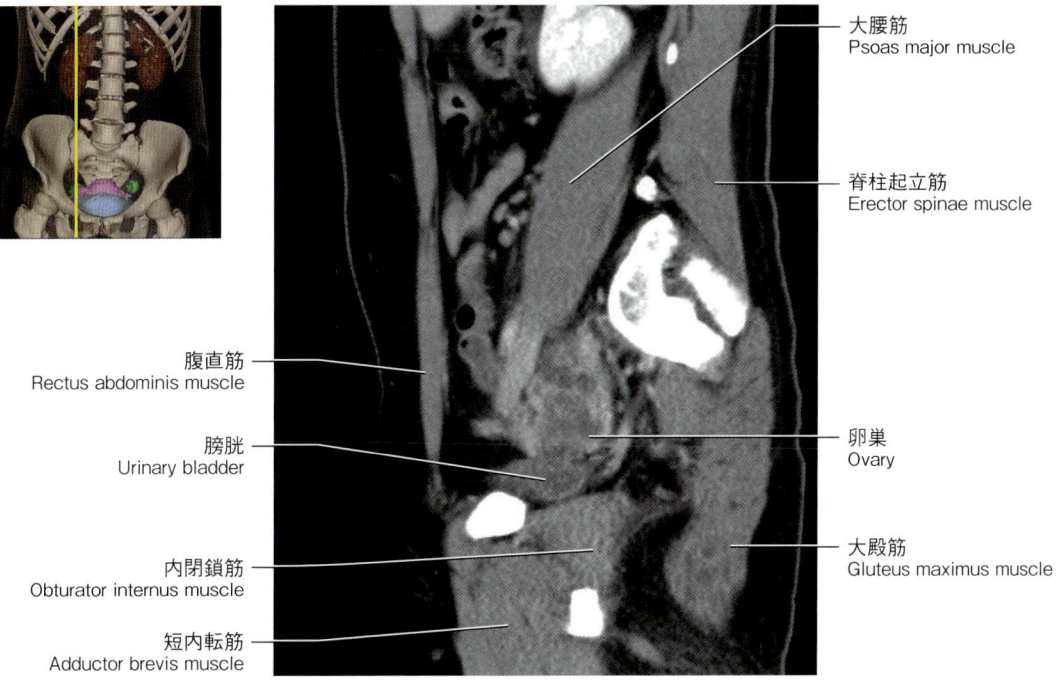

- 大腰筋　Psoas major muscle
- 脊柱起立筋　Erector spinae muscle
- 腹直筋　Rectus abdominis muscle
- 膀胱　Urinary bladder
- 卵巣　Ovary
- 内閉鎖筋　Obturator internus muscle
- 短内転筋　Adductor brevis muscle
- 大殿筋　Gluteus maximus muscle

6-70

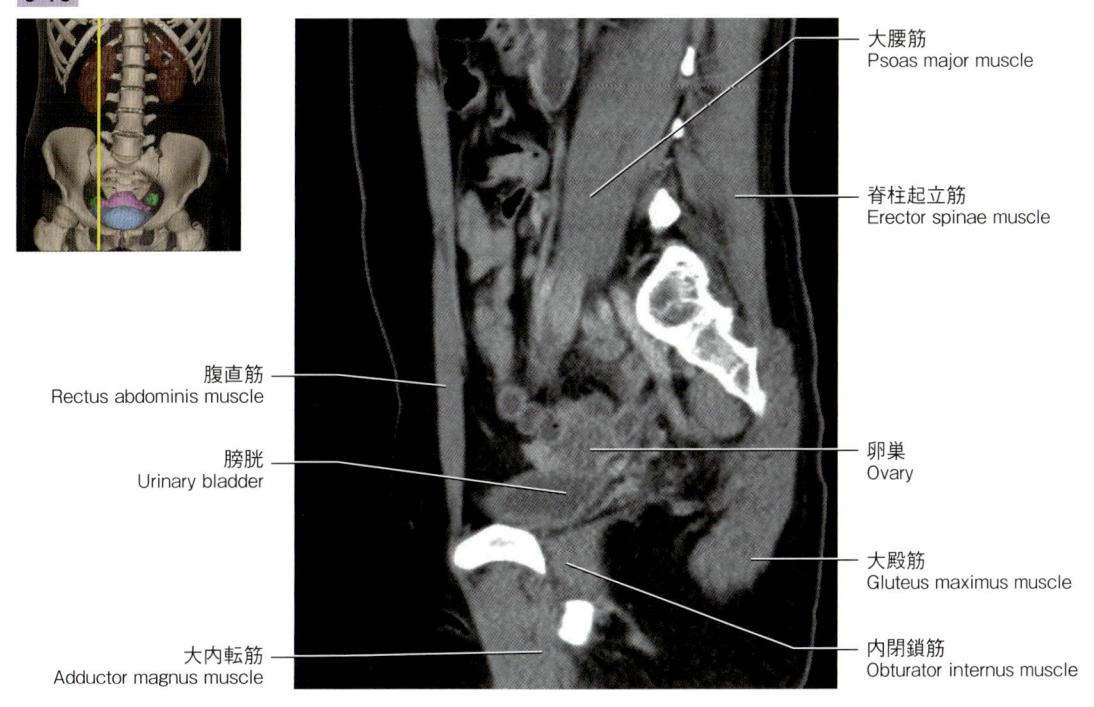

- 大腰筋　Psoas major muscle
- 脊柱起立筋　Erector spinae muscle
- 腹直筋　Rectus abdominis muscle
- 膀胱　Urinary bladder
- 卵巣　Ovary
- 大殿筋　Gluteus maximus muscle
- 内閉鎖筋　Obturator internus muscle
- 大内転筋　Adductor magnus muscle

NOTE　生殖可能な年齢の女性における卵巣の大きさは，約3～5 cm大．被膜（白膜）に覆われ皮質と髄質からなる．皮質にはさまざまな成熟段階の卵胞が含まれている．卵巣の外表面は白膜の周囲を胚上皮が覆っており，この胚上皮から卵巣の悪性腫瘍の多くが発生すると考えられている．

女性骨盤部の断層解剖 ［矢状断像（造影CT）］

6-71

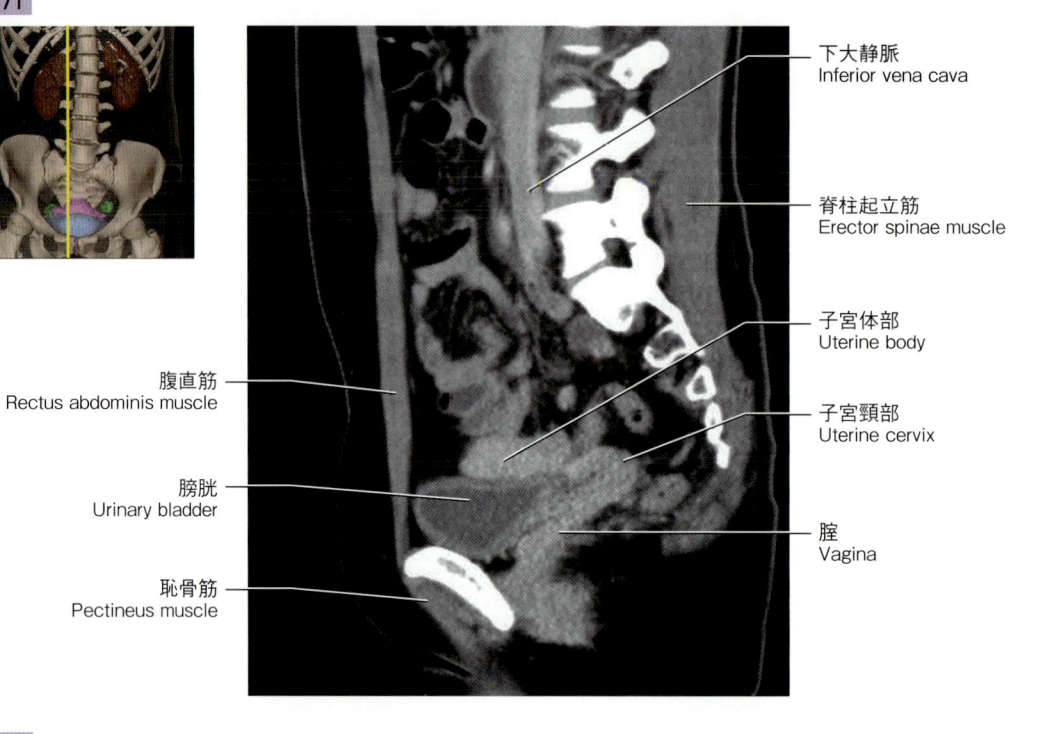

- 下大静脈 Inferior vena cava
- 脊柱起立筋 Erector spinae muscle
- 子宮体部 Uterine body
- 子宮頸部 Uterine cervix
- 腟 Vagina
- 腹直筋 Rectus abdominis muscle
- 膀胱 Urinary bladder
- 恥骨筋 Pectineus muscle

6-72

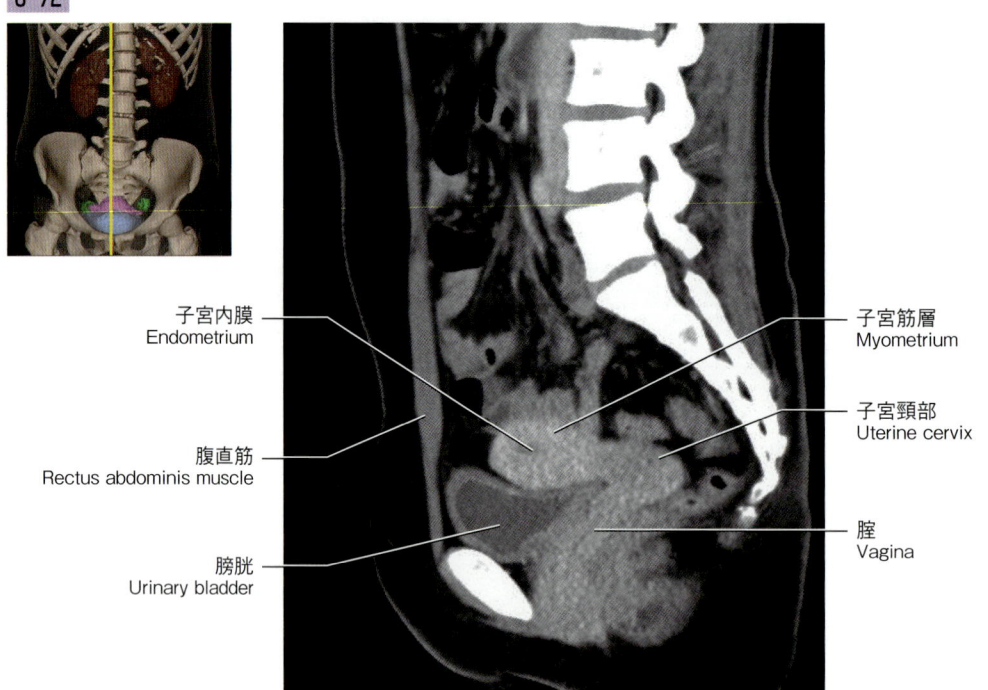

- 子宮内膜 Endometrium
- 子宮筋層 Myometrium
- 子宮頸部 Uterine cervix
- 腟 Vagina
- 腹直筋 Rectus abdominis muscle
- 膀胱 Urinary bladder

NOTE 下大静脈の正常変異のひとつに，重複下大静脈がある．大動脈の左側に，胎生期における主上静脈下部の遺残である左下大静脈を認めるもので，同静脈は左腎静脈の高さまで上行しそこで合流する．

女性骨盤部の断層解剖　[矢状断像（造影 CT）]

6-73

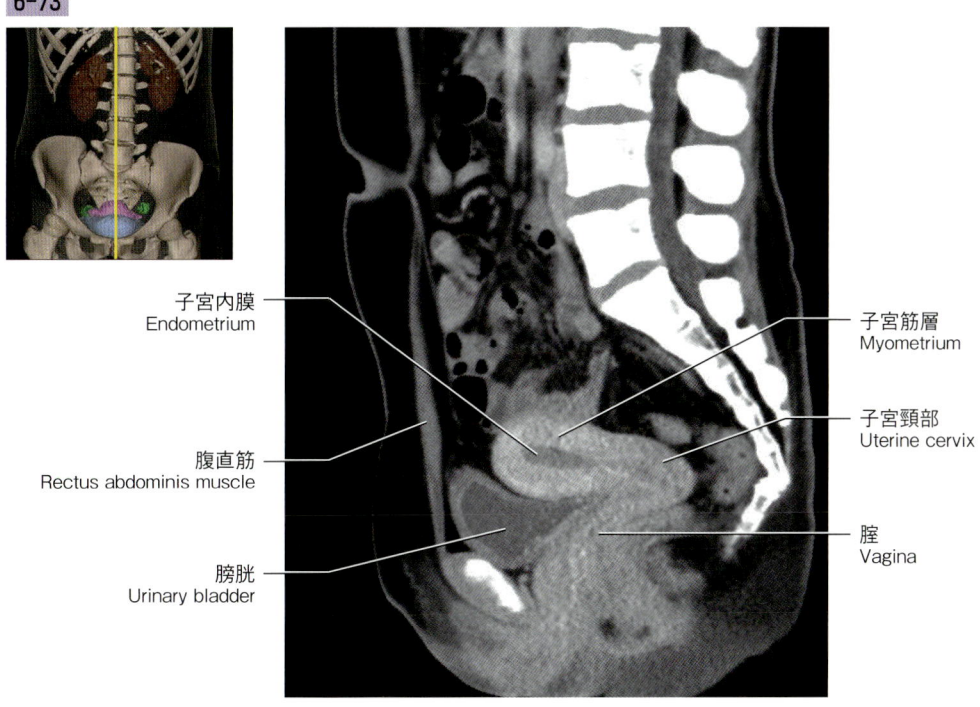

- 子宮内膜　Endometrium
- 腹直筋　Rectus abdominis muscle
- 膀胱　Urinary bladder
- 子宮筋層　Myometrium
- 子宮頸部　Uterine cervix
- 腟　Vagina

6-74

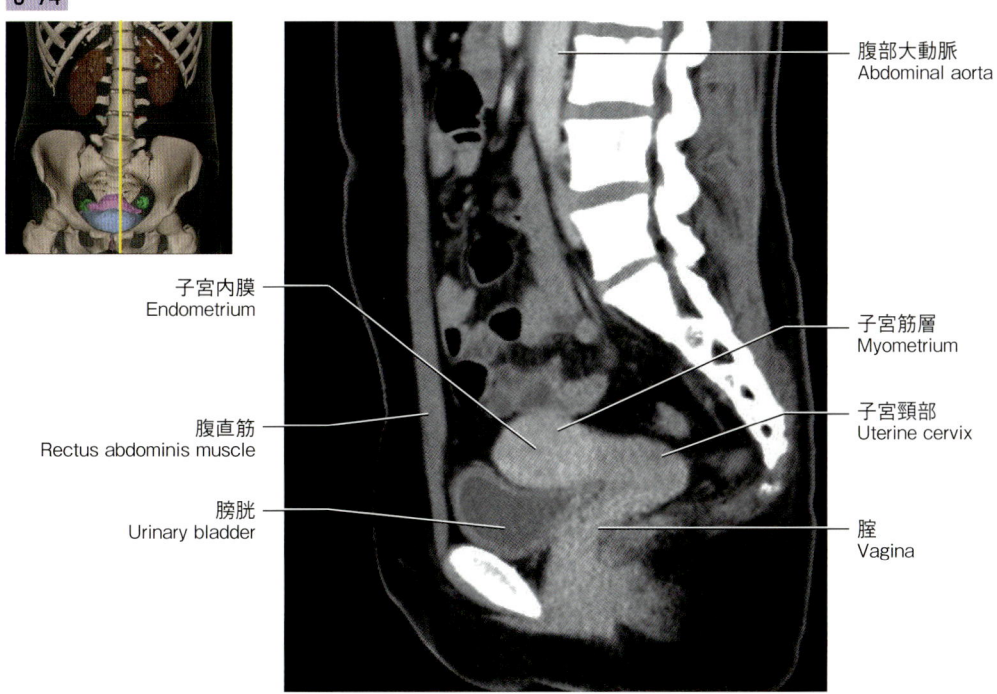

- 子宮内膜　Endometrium
- 腹直筋　Rectus abdominis muscle
- 膀胱　Urinary bladder
- 腹部大動脈　Abdominal aorta
- 子宮筋層　Myometrium
- 子宮頸部　Uterine cervix
- 腟　Vagina

NOTE 子宮は膀胱に被さるように位置し，後方には直腸が位置している．子宮体部および底部は臓側腹膜に覆われている．臓側腹膜は膀胱で折り返して膀胱子宮窩を，直腸で折り返して直腸子宮窩を形成する．

女性骨盤部の断層解剖［矢状断像（造影CT）］

6-75

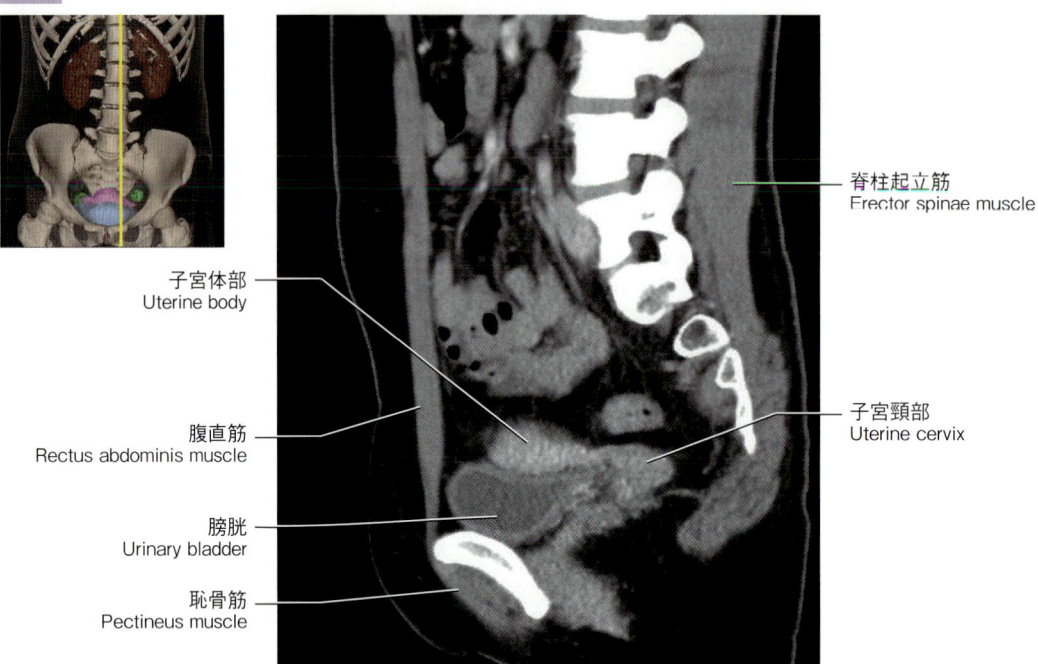

- 子宮体部 Uterine body
- 腹直筋 Rectus abdominis muscle
- 膀胱 Urinary bladder
- 恥骨筋 Pectineus muscle
- 脊柱起立筋 Erector spinae muscle
- 子宮頸部 Uterine cervix

6-76

- 腹直筋 Rectus abdominis muscle
- 膀胱 Urinary bladder
- 大内転筋 Adductor magnus muscle
- 大腰筋 Psoas major muscle
- 脊柱起立筋 Erector spinae muscle
- 大殿筋 Gluteus maximus muscle
- 内閉鎖筋 Obturator internus muscle

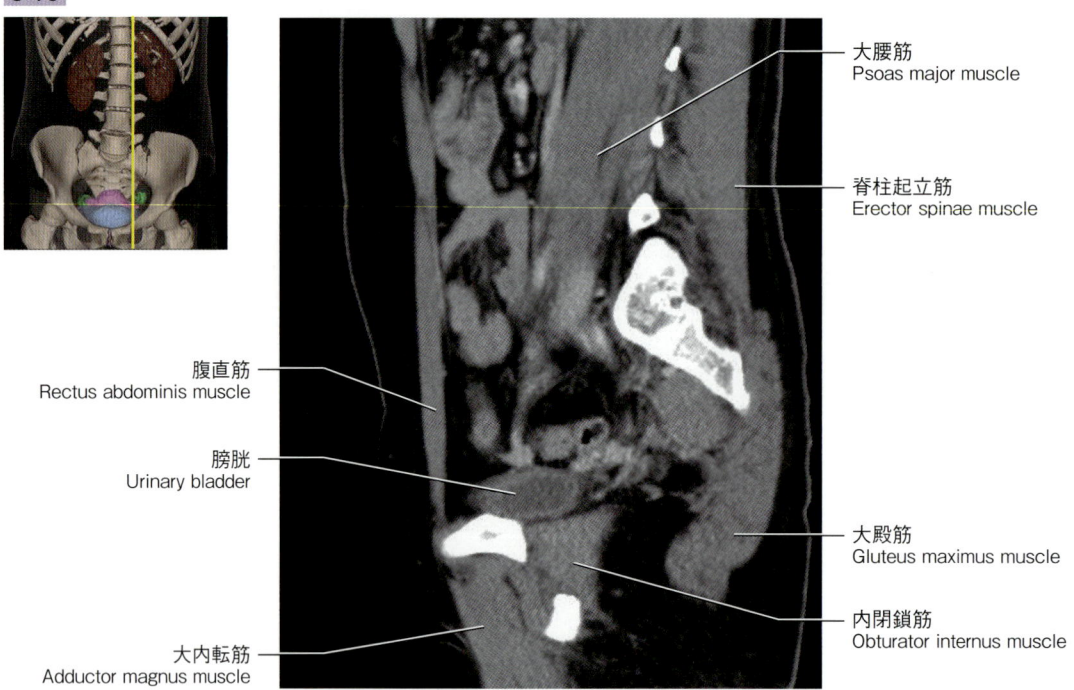

> **NOTE** 正常な子宮は前傾前屈を呈する．後傾した子宮は，腟の長軸に対してより一直線に近くなるので，下降しやすくなる．

女性骨盤部の断層解剖［矢状断像（造影CT）］

6-77

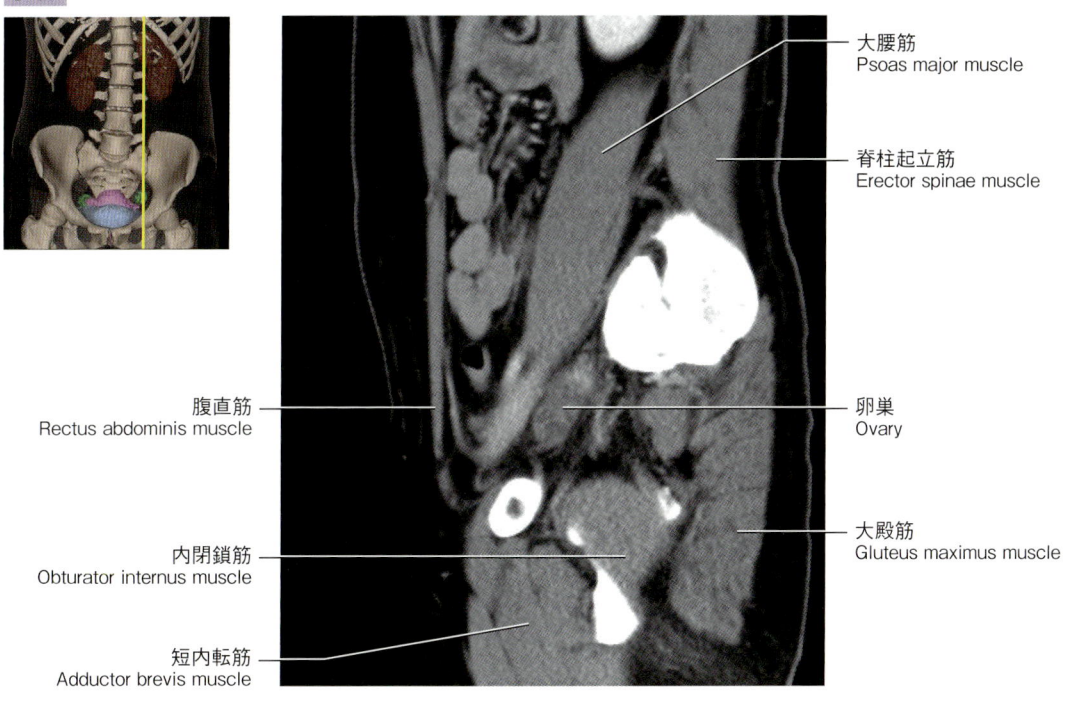

- 大腰筋 Psoas major muscle
- 脊柱起立筋 Erector spinae muscle
- 腹直筋 Rectus abdominis muscle
- 卵巣 Ovary
- 大殿筋 Gluteus maximus muscle
- 内閉鎖筋 Obturator internus muscle
- 短内転筋 Adductor brevis muscle

NOTE 卵巣のいわゆる機能性囊胞は，均一な水濃度を示し，壁は薄く，内部に充実成分や複雑な液体を含まない．機能性囊胞の一部である黄体囊胞は，典型的には虚脱し，ひしゃげた形状の水濃度構造を示し，造影後には壁が濃染して，CTでしばしば同定される．

VII

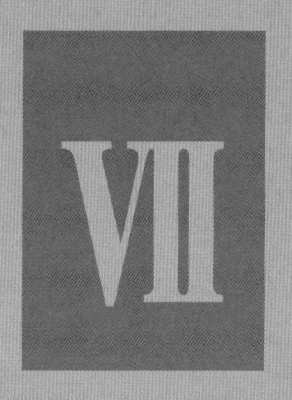

四 肢
Extremities

上肢の主な動脈

7-1 造影 CT, MIP 像(左)と造影 CT, VR 像(右)

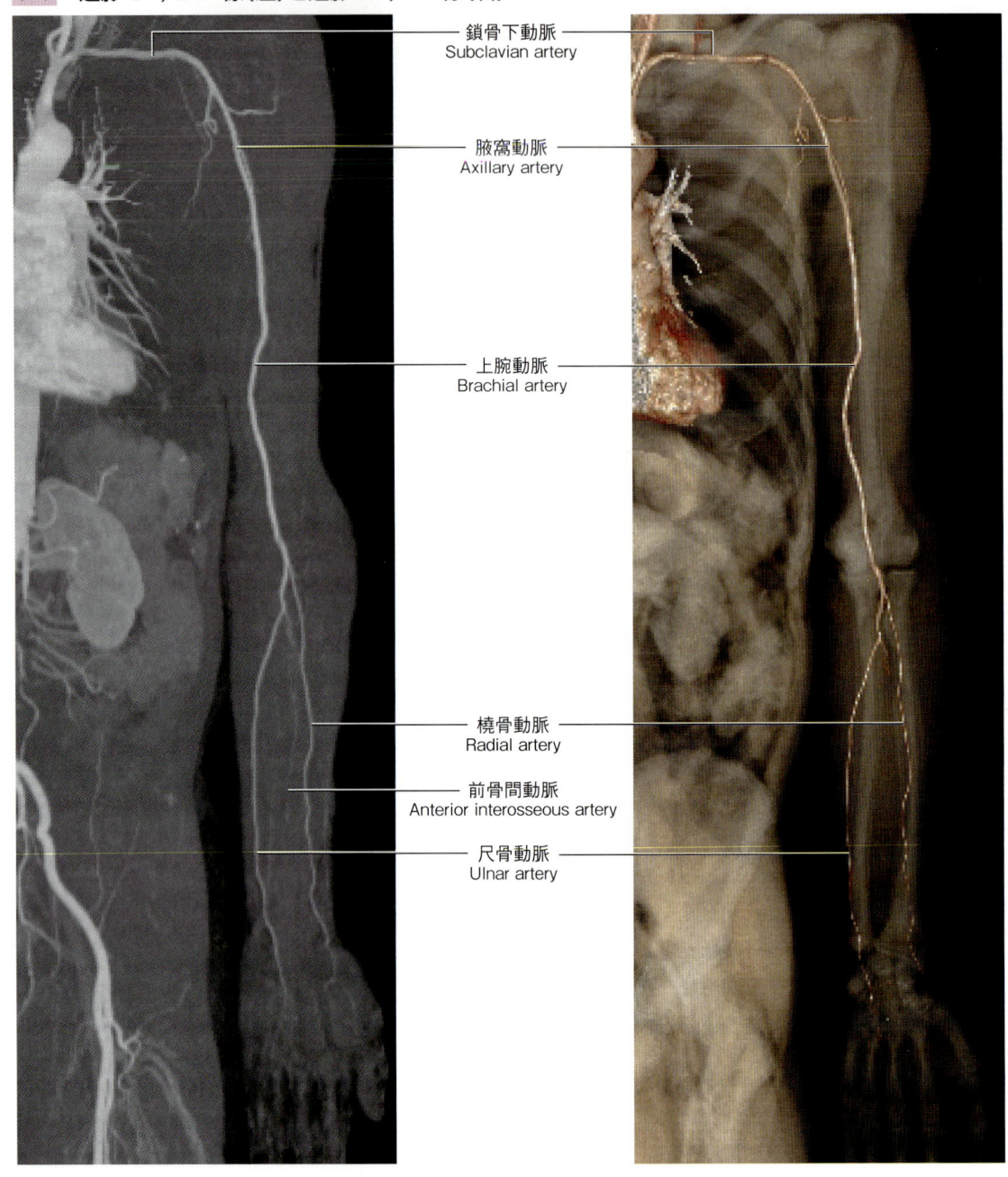

- 鎖骨下動脈 Subclavian artery
- 腋窩動脈 Axillary artery
- 上腕動脈 Brachial artery
- 橈骨動脈 Radial artery
- 前骨間動脈 Anterior interosseous artery
- 尺骨動脈 Ulnar artery

> **NOTE** 冠血管造影・インターベンションの領域では，1989年に橈骨動脈穿刺法が報告されて以降，大腿動脈穿刺法に替わり橈骨動脈穿刺法が急速に普及した．この方法の長所は，①術後の患者安静時間がほとんど必要なく術直後から歩行可能であること，②動脈が体表に位置しているため止血が確実で抗凝固療法併用患者での出血性トラブルが少ないこと，③陰部の剃毛(除毛)が不要，尿道カテーテルの挿入が不要であること，などがある．一方，短所としては，①動脈が細いため穿刺が難しいこと，②太い用具が使用できないこと，③穿刺により動脈の狭小化や閉塞が起こり得ること，④頭部血管に血栓などが飛ぶ恐れがあること，などがある．

上肢の主な静脈

7-2 MRI，2DTOF MIP像

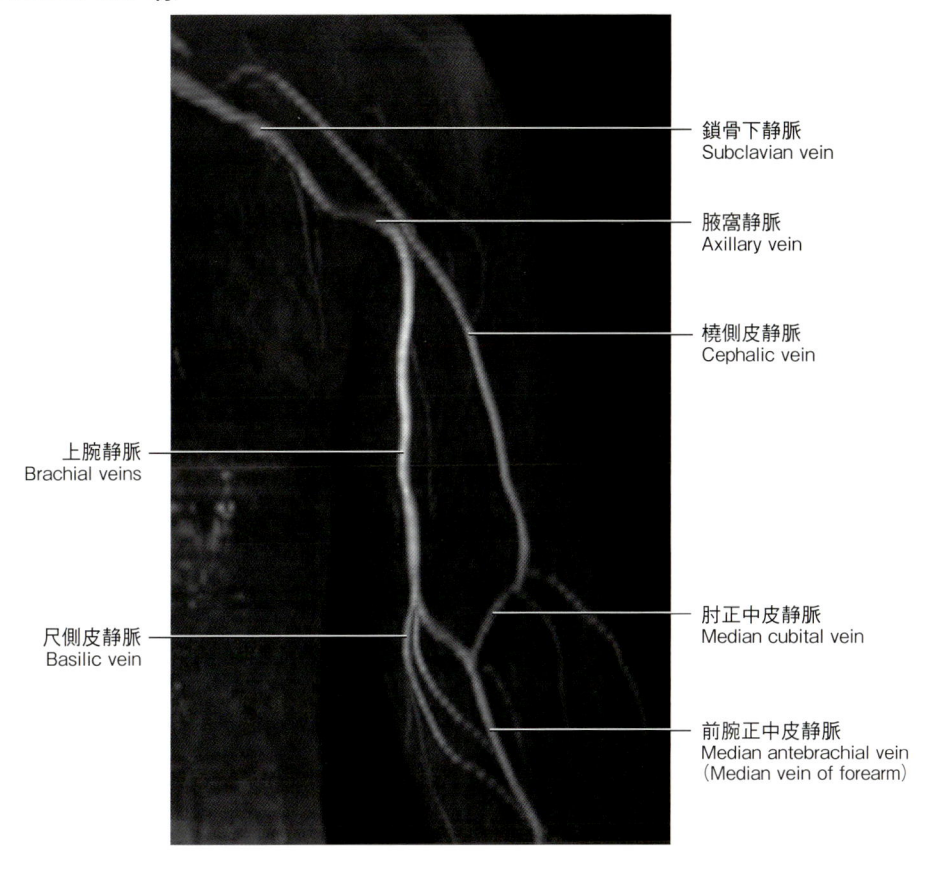

- 鎖骨下静脈 Subclavian vein
- 腋窩静脈 Axillary vein
- 橈側皮静脈 Cephalic vein
- 上腕静脈 Brachial veins
- 尺側皮静脈 Basilic vein
- 肘正中皮静脈 Median cubital vein
- 前腕正中皮静脈 Median antebrachial vein（Median vein of forearm）

NOTE 静脈穿刺に伴う神経損傷を100％防ぐことは現状では困難であり，ある確率で起こりうる合併症と考えられる．神経の分布は個人によって異なり，その走行を体表から判断することは困難で，完全に神経を避けて穿刺することは不可能であるからである．深部の神経は技術的に穿刺を避けることは可能でも，表層を走行する皮神経は適切な方法で穿刺しても損傷を起こす可能性がある．

しかし，神経損傷の発生率を低下させることは可能である．ペインクリニック学会での発表では，神経損傷を生じた症例では，刺入部位のほとんどは手関節部橈側皮静脈もしくは肘関節部尺側正中皮静脈である．手関節の親指側には橈骨神経浅枝が走行しており，特に手関節から10cm中枢側（肘より）までは注意が必要である．肘の小指側では，表面に内側前腕皮神経が，深部には正中神経が走行し，深く刺しすぎなくても危険性がある．

比較的安全に穿刺できる部位は，肘の親指側である．

肩関節 (CT, VR 像)

7-3 肩関節の体表解剖

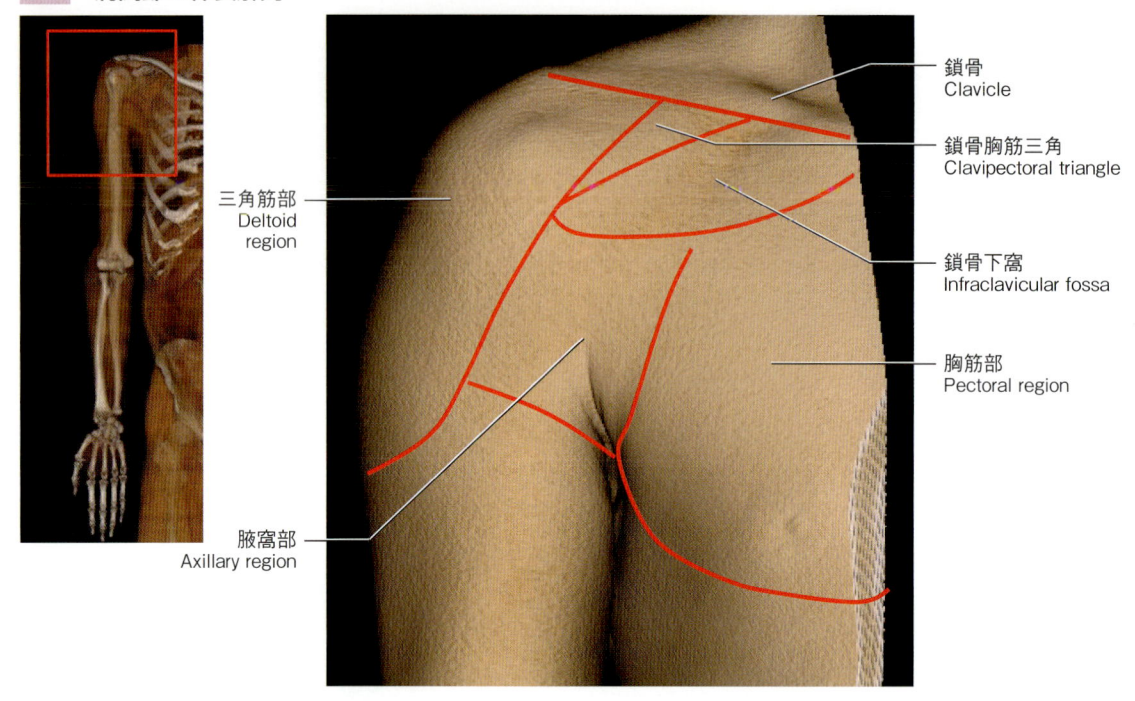

- 鎖骨 Clavicle
- 鎖骨胸筋三角 Clavipectoral triangle
- 鎖骨下窩 Infraclavicular fossa
- 胸筋部 Pectoral region
- 三角筋部 Deltoid region
- 腋窩部 Axillary region

NOTE 肩関節は人間で最大の可動域を有している．その引き替えとして最も脱臼する可能性が高い関節となっている．

肩関節（CT, VR 像）

7-4 肩関節の筋（前面）

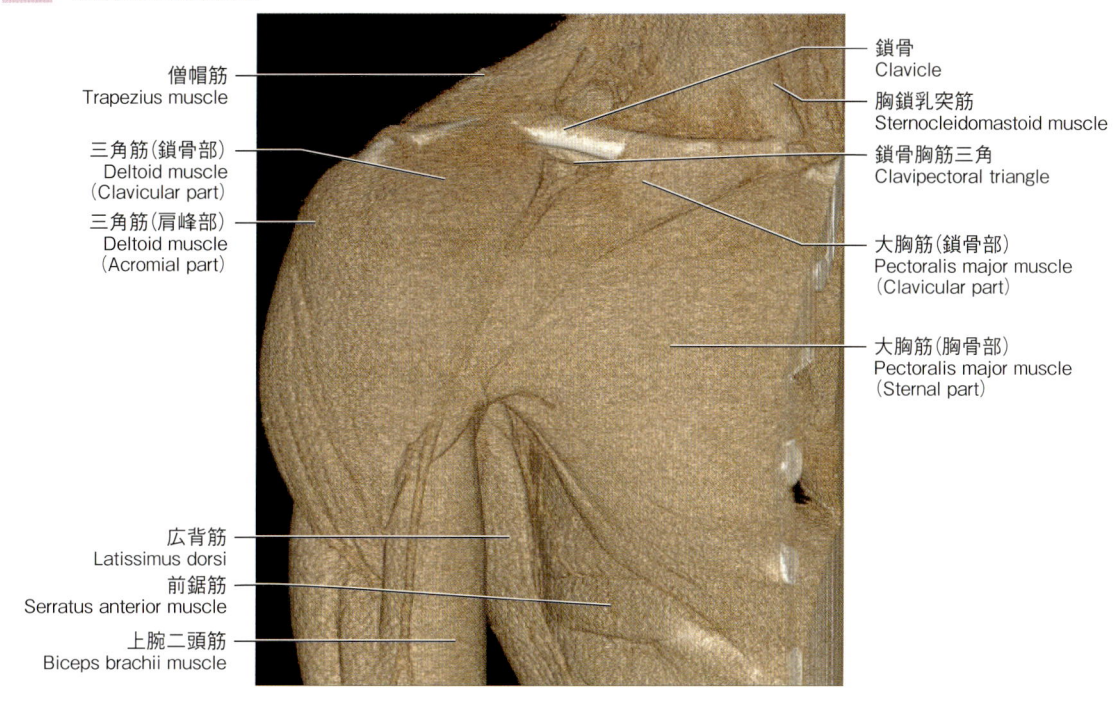

- 僧帽筋 Trapezius muscle
- 三角筋（鎖骨部） Deltoid muscle (Clavicular part)
- 三角筋（肩峰部） Deltoid muscle (Acromial part)
- 鎖骨 Clavicle
- 胸鎖乳突筋 Sternocleidomastoid muscle
- 鎖骨胸筋三角 Clavipectoral triangle
- 大胸筋（鎖骨部） Pectoralis major muscle (Clavicular part)
- 大胸筋（胸骨部） Pectoralis major muscle (Sternal part)
- 広背筋 Latissimus dorsi
- 前鋸筋 Serratus anterior muscle
- 上腕二頭筋 Biceps brachii muscle

7-5 肩関節の筋（右斜め後面）

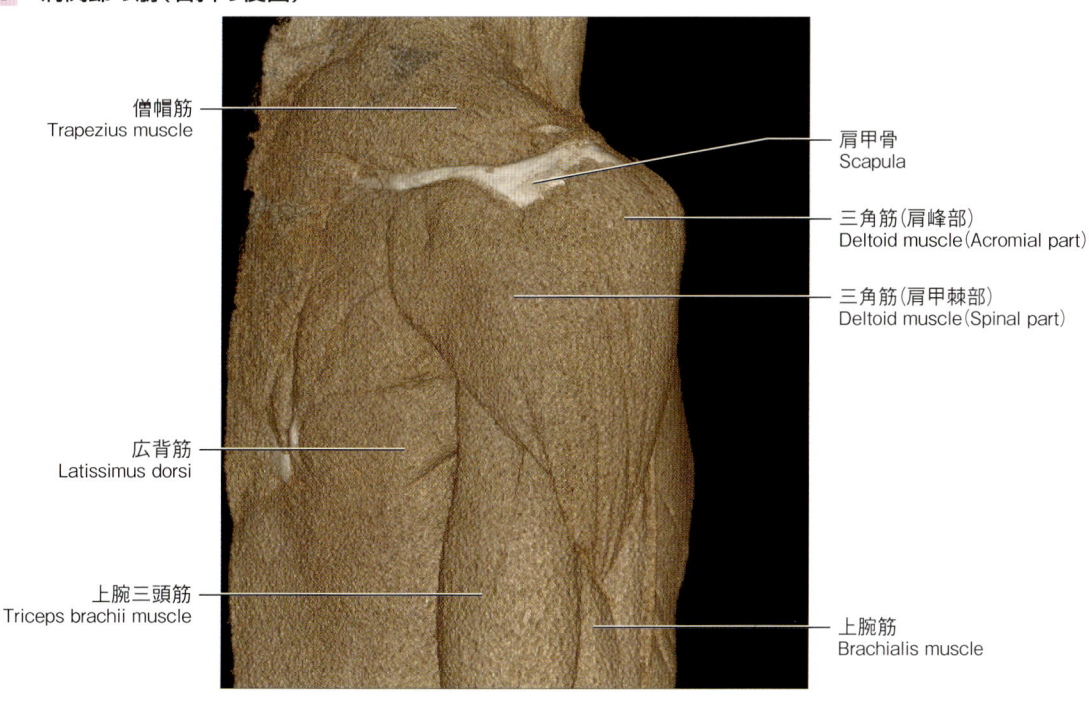

- 僧帽筋 Trapezius muscle
- 肩甲骨 Scapula
- 三角筋（肩峰部） Deltoid muscle (Acromial part)
- 三角筋（肩甲棘部） Deltoid muscle (Spinal part)
- 広背筋 Latissimus dorsi
- 上腕三頭筋 Triceps brachii muscle
- 上腕筋 Brachialis muscle

NOTE 肩関節は17の筋肉で覆われている．肩を構成する筋肉の大部分が肩甲骨に付着部をもつ．肩の筋群は肩関節内側のインナーマッスル（Inner muscles）と肩関節外側のアウターマッスル（Outer muscles）に分類される．

肩関節（CT, VR 像）

7-6 肩関節の骨（前面）

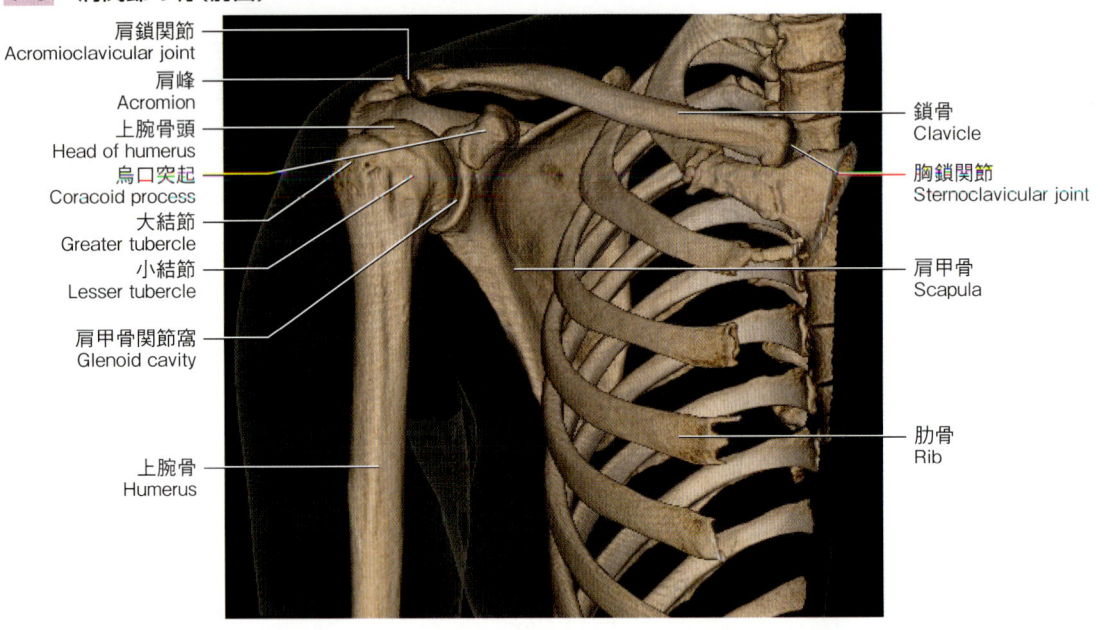

- 肩鎖関節 Acromioclavicular joint
- 肩峰 Acromion
- 上腕骨頭 Head of humerus
- 烏口突起 Coracoid process
- 大結節 Greater tubercle
- 小結節 Lesser tubercle
- 肩甲骨関節窩 Glenoid cavity
- 上腕骨 Humerus
- 鎖骨 Clavicle
- 胸鎖関節 Sternoclavicular joint
- 肩甲骨 Scapula
- 肋骨 Rib

7-7 肩関節の骨（前面）

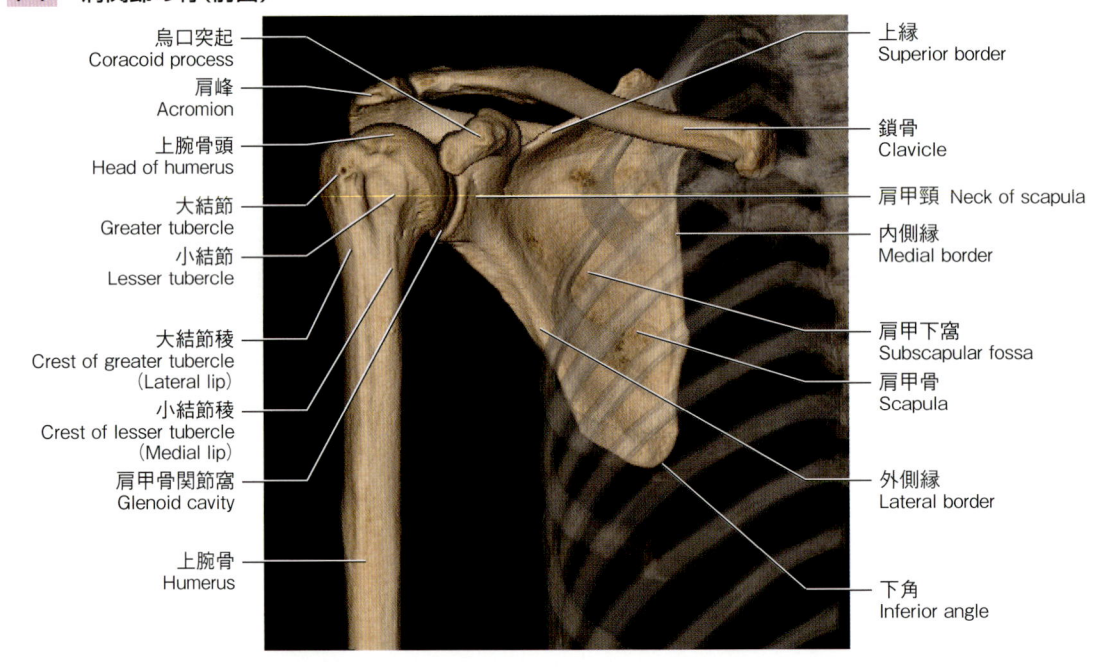

- 烏口突起 Coracoid process
- 肩峰 Acromion
- 上腕骨頭 Head of humerus
- 大結節 Greater tubercle
- 小結節 Lesser tubercle
- 大結節稜 Crest of greater tubercle（Lateral lip）
- 小結節稜 Crest of lesser tubercle（Medial lip）
- 肩甲骨関節窩 Glenoid cavity
- 上腕骨 Humerus
- 上縁 Superior border
- 鎖骨 Clavicle
- 肩甲頸 Neck of scapula
- 内側縁 Medial border
- 肩甲下窩 Subscapular fossa
- 肩甲骨 Scapula
- 外側縁 Lateral border
- 下角 Inferior angle

NOTE 肩関節は上腕骨頭と肩甲骨関節窩からなる狭義の肩関節（Glenohumeral joint）と胸鎖関節，肩鎖関節の3つの関節から構成される．肩は広義の肩関節と肩甲胸郭関節により構成される．

肩関節（CT, VR 像）

7-8　肩関節の骨（右側面）

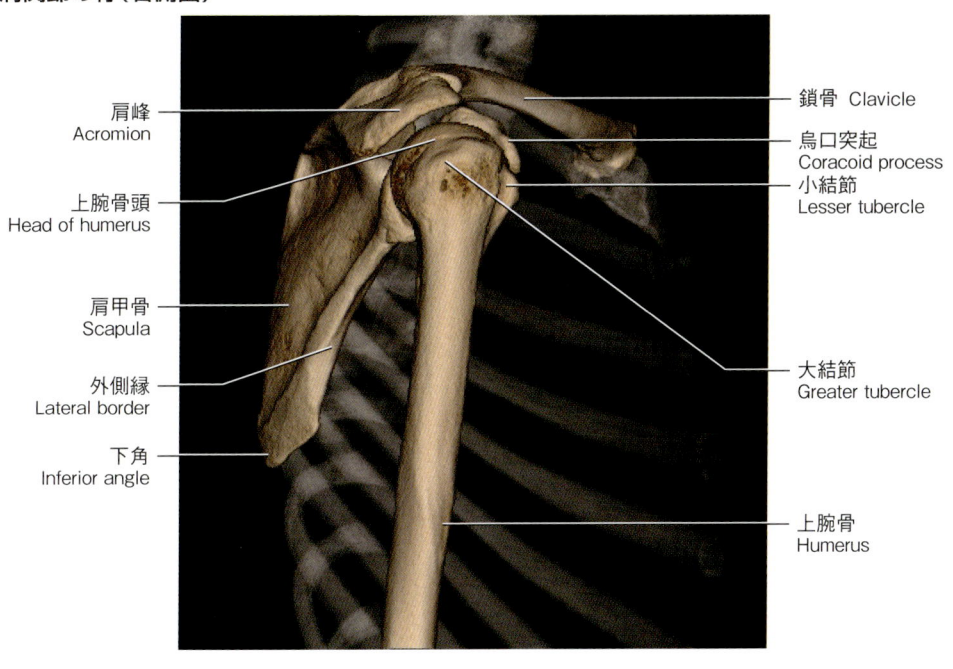

- 肩峰　Acromion
- 上腕骨頭　Head of humerus
- 肩甲骨　Scapula
- 外側縁　Lateral border
- 下角　Inferior angle
- 鎖骨　Clavicle
- 烏口突起　Coracoid process
- 小結節　Lesser tubercle
- 大結節　Greater tubercle
- 上腕骨　Humerus

7-9　肩関節の骨（後面）

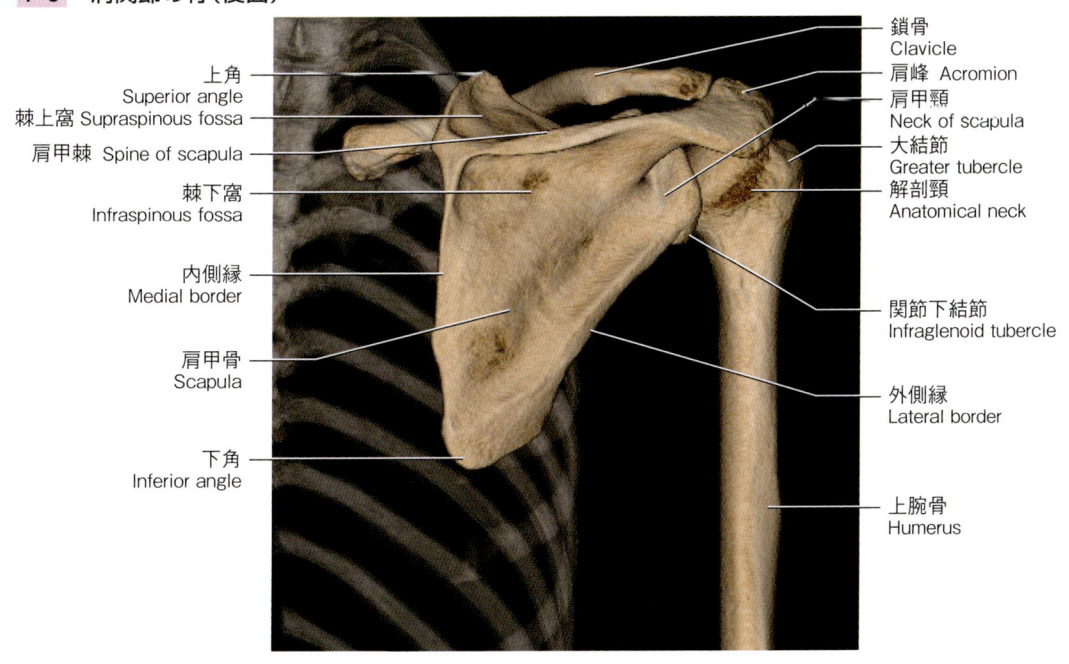

- 上角　Superior angle
- 棘上窩　Supraspinous fossa
- 肩甲棘　Spine of scapula
- 棘下窩　Infraspinous fossa
- 内側縁　Medial border
- 肩甲骨　Scapula
- 下角　Inferior angle
- 鎖骨　Clavicle
- 肩峰　Acromion
- 肩甲頸　Neck of scapula
- 大結節　Greater tubercle
- 解剖頸　Anatomical neck
- 関節下結節　Infraglenoid tubercle
- 外側縁　Lateral border
- 上腕骨　Humerus

> **NOTE**　肩関節の特徴は，上腕骨頭に対応する肩甲骨関節窩が小さいことであり，これを補強するために種々の支持組織が存在する．

312 肩関節の断層解剖 ［横断像（MRI, プロトン密度強調像）］

7-10

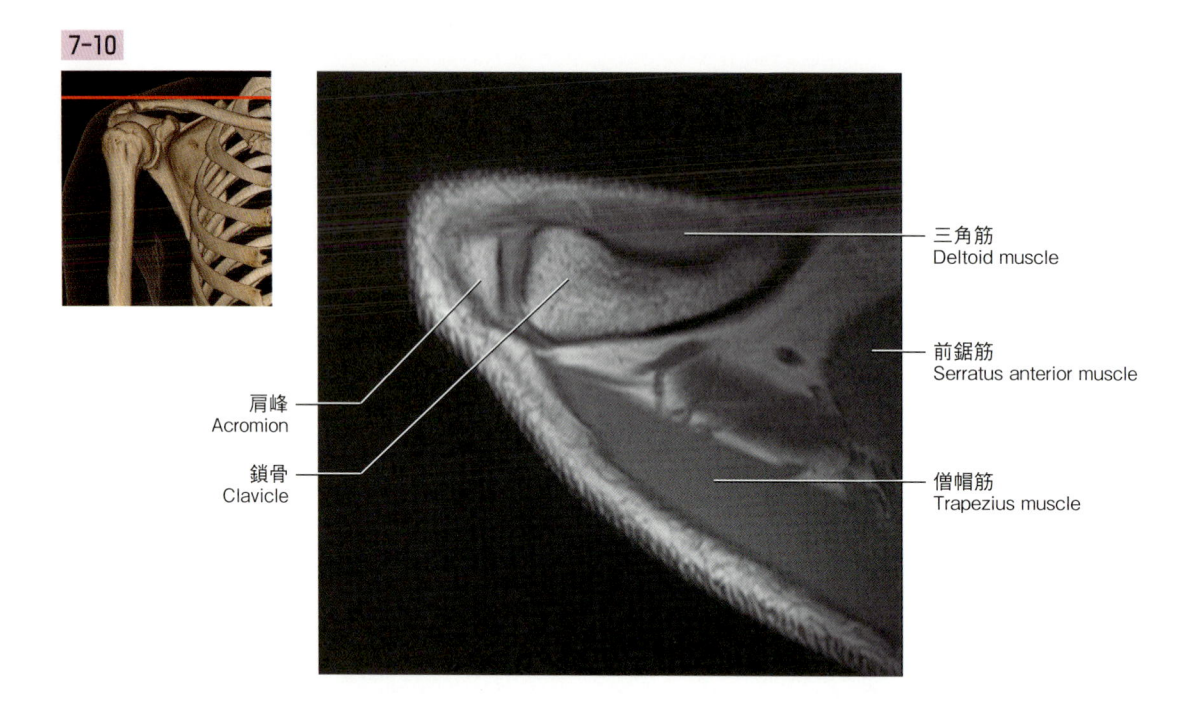

- 肩峰 Acromion
- 鎖骨 Clavicle
- 三角筋 Deltoid muscle
- 前鋸筋 Serratus anterior muscle
- 僧帽筋 Trapezius muscle

7-11

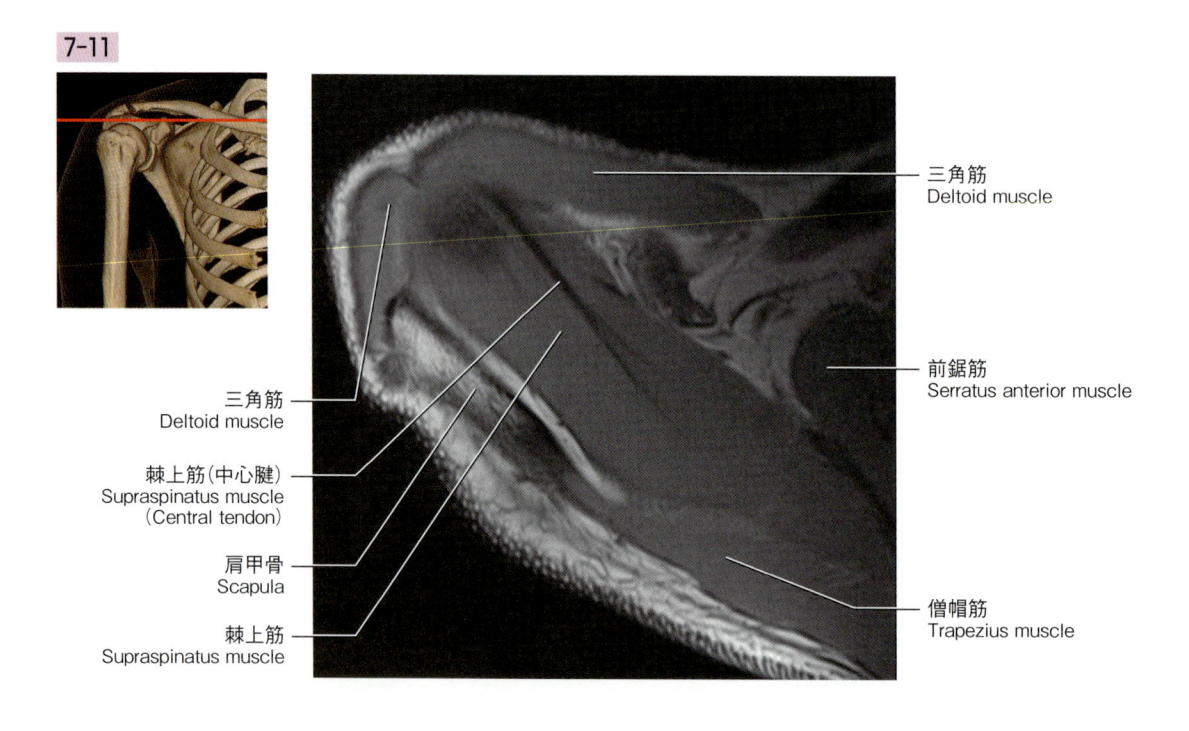

- 三角筋 Deltoid muscle
- 棘上筋（中心腱） Supraspinatus muscle (Central tendon)
- 肩甲骨 Scapula
- 棘上筋 Supraspinatus muscle
- 三角筋 Deltoid muscle
- 前鋸筋 Serratus anterior muscle
- 僧帽筋 Trapezius muscle

NOTE 関節包は肩甲骨では肩甲頸と関節唇に，上腕骨では解剖頸，大結節，小結節に付着する．関節包を外から補強する最も重要な筋腱構成体が腱板である．

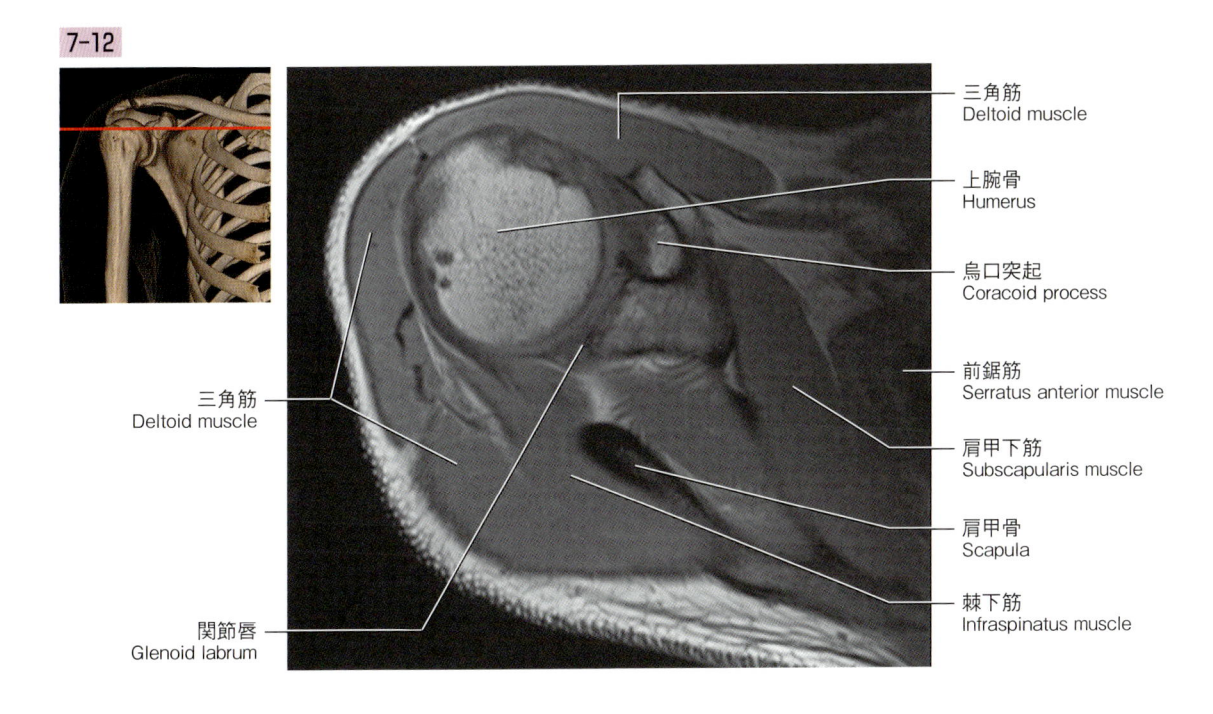

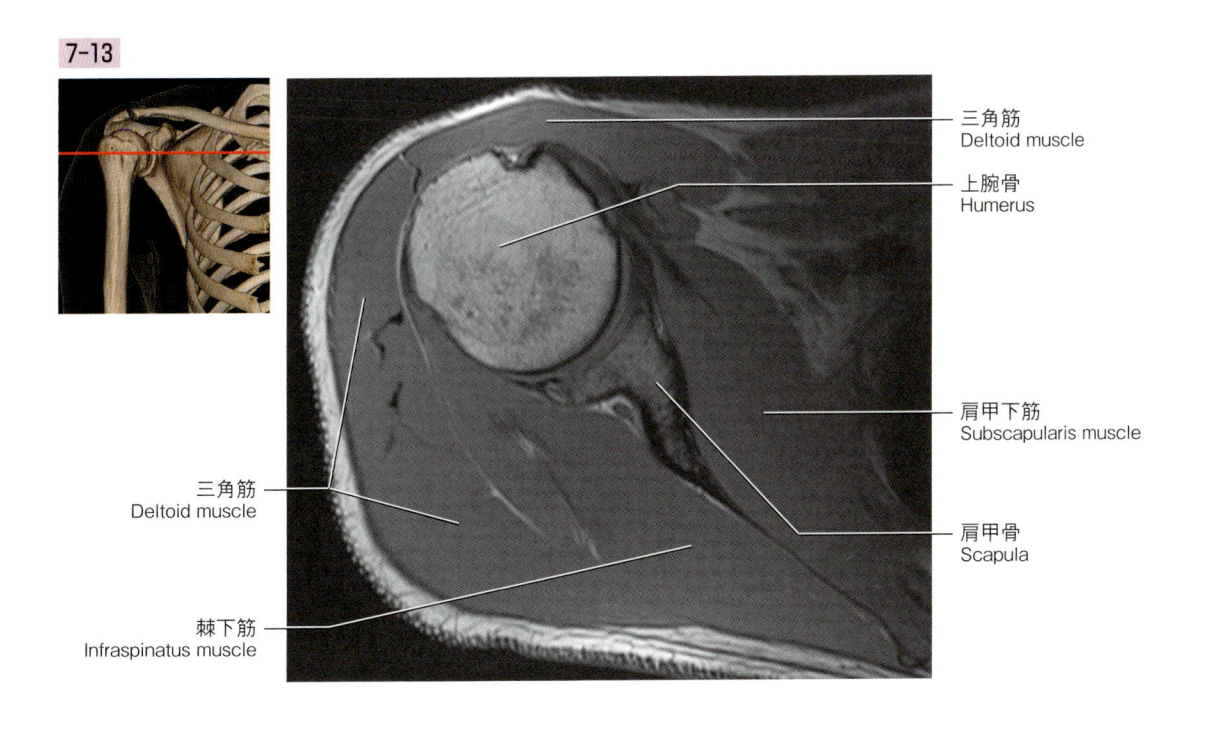

肩関節の断層解剖 ［横断像（MRI，プロトン密度強調像）］

7-12

- 三角筋 Deltoid muscle
- 上腕骨 Humerus
- 烏口突起 Coracoid process
- 前鋸筋 Serratus anterior muscle
- 肩甲下筋 Subscapularis muscle
- 肩甲骨 Scapula
- 棘下筋 Infraspinatus muscle
- 三角筋 Deltoid muscle
- 関節唇 Glenoid labrum

7-13

- 三角筋 Deltoid muscle
- 上腕骨 Humerus
- 肩甲下筋 Subscapularis muscle
- 肩甲骨 Scapula
- 三角筋 Deltoid muscle
- 棘下筋 Infraspinatus muscle

NOTE 腱板は肩甲骨に起始し，上腕骨頭周囲を取り巻いて大結節と小結節に停止する4つの回旋筋腱（棘上筋，棘下筋，小円筋，肩甲下筋）の総称である．

肩関節の断層解剖 ［横断像（MRI，プロトン密度強調像）］

7-14

- 三角筋 Deltoid muscle
- 大胸筋 Pectoralis major muscle
- 上腕骨 Humerus
- 烏口腕筋 Coracobrachialis muscle
- 下方関節唇 Inferior glenoid labrum
- 肩甲下筋 Subscapularis muscle
- 三角筋 Deltoid muscle
- 棘下筋 Infraspinatus muscle
- 肩甲骨 Scapula

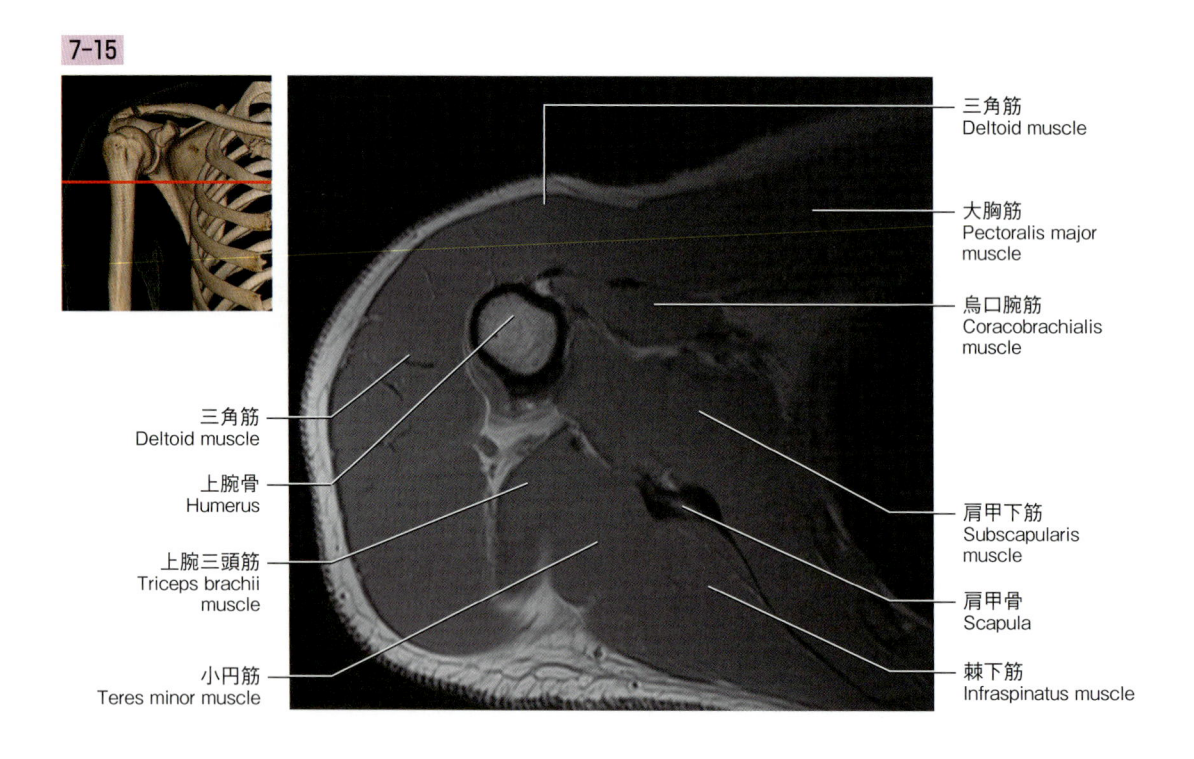

7-15

- 三角筋 Deltoid muscle
- 大胸筋 Pectoralis major muscle
- 烏口腕筋 Coracobrachialis muscle
- 三角筋 Deltoid muscle
- 上腕骨 Humerus
- 上腕三頭筋 Triceps brachii muscle
- 小円筋 Teres minor muscle
- 肩甲下筋 Subscapularis muscle
- 肩甲骨 Scapula
- 棘下筋 Infraspinatus muscle

> **NOTE** 棘上筋，棘下筋，小円筋腱は大結節の上面〜後面に停止し，肩甲下筋腱は小結節の前面に停止する．棘上筋腱と棘下筋腱の間は薄い膜様構造をしており，腱板疎部（Rotator interval）とよばれ，その直下にある結節間溝を関節上結節と関節唇に起始する上腕二頭筋長頭腱が通過する．

肩関節の断層解剖 ［冠状断像（MRI，プロトン密度強調像）］

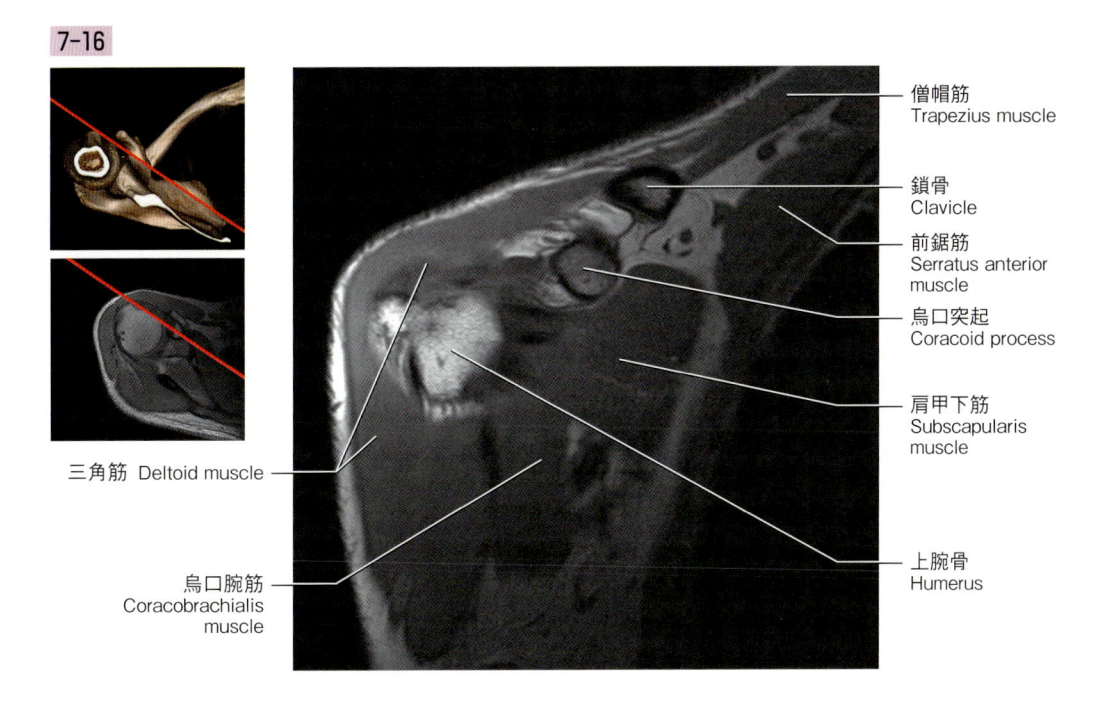

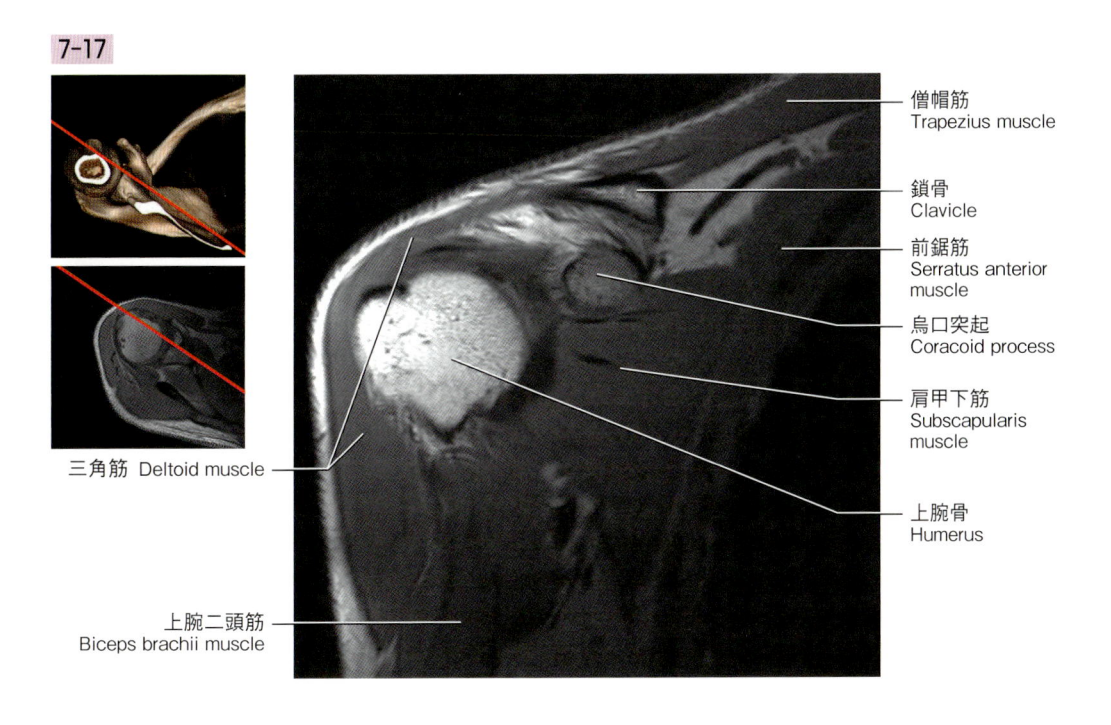

7-16

- 僧帽筋 Trapezius muscle
- 鎖骨 Clavicle
- 前鋸筋 Serratus anterior muscle
- 烏口突起 Coracoid process
- 肩甲下筋 Subscapularis muscle
- 上腕骨 Humerus
- 三角筋 Deltoid muscle
- 烏口腕筋 Coracobrachialis muscle

7-17

- 僧帽筋 Trapezius muscle
- 鎖骨 Clavicle
- 前鋸筋 Serratus anterior muscle
- 烏口突起 Coracoid process
- 肩甲下筋 Subscapularis muscle
- 上腕骨 Humerus
- 三角筋 Deltoid muscle
- 上腕二頭筋 Biceps brachii muscle

肩関節の断層解剖 ［冠状断像（MRI, プロトン密度強調像）］

7-18

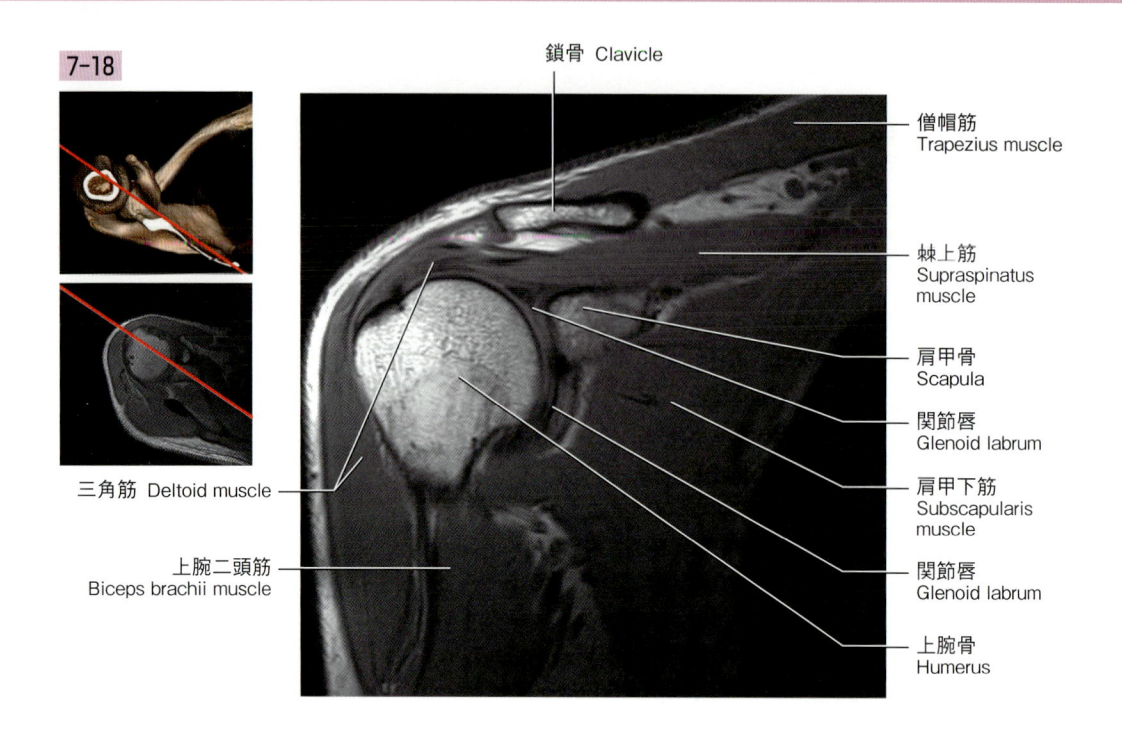

- 鎖骨 Clavicle
- 僧帽筋 Trapezius muscle
- 棘上筋 Supraspinatus muscle
- 肩甲骨 Scapula
- 関節唇 Glenoid labrum
- 肩甲下筋 Subscapularis muscle
- 関節唇 Glenoid labrum
- 上腕骨 Humerus
- 三角筋 Deltoid muscle
- 上腕二頭筋 Biceps brachii muscle

7-19

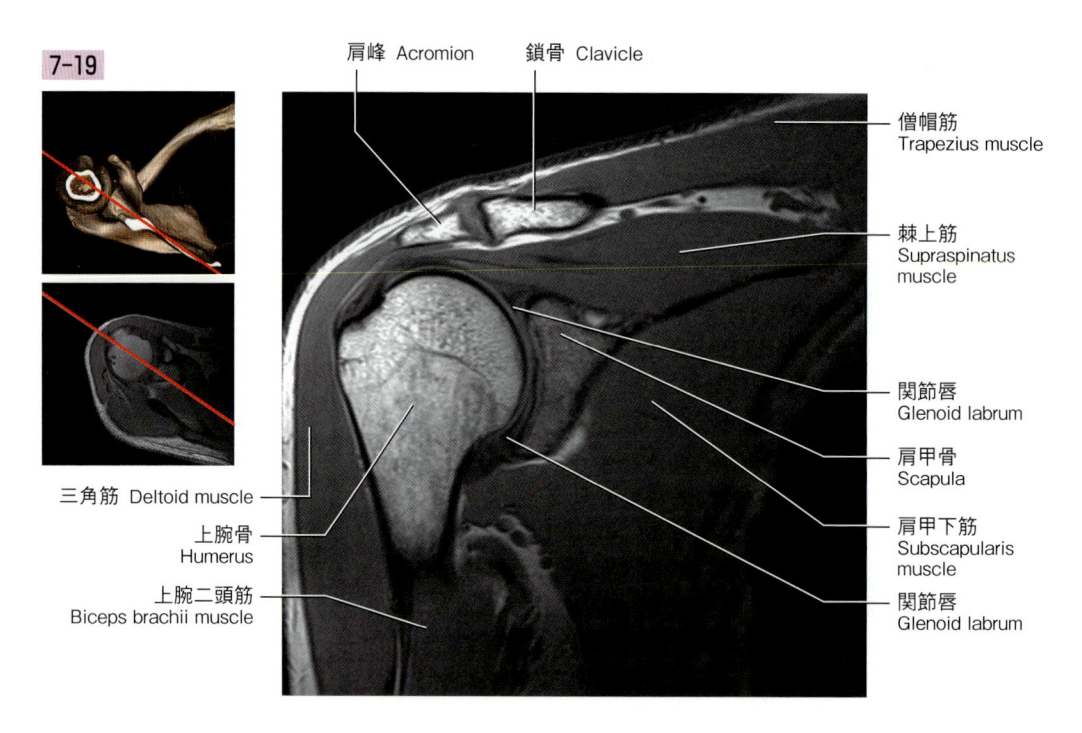

- 肩峰 Acromion
- 鎖骨 Clavicle
- 僧帽筋 Trapezius muscle
- 棘上筋 Supraspinatus muscle
- 関節唇 Glenoid labrum
- 肩甲骨 Scapula
- 肩甲下筋 Subscapularis muscle
- 関節唇 Glenoid labrum
- 三角筋 Deltoid muscle
- 上腕骨 Humerus
- 上腕二頭筋 Biceps brachii muscle

NOTE 関節窩辺縁に付着する線維軟骨性の関節唇は，関節窩を広く深くしている．

NOTE 肩峰 Acromion
acro はギリシャ語の「高み」，「先端」の意．acropolis（アクロポリス）はギリシャの都市にある神殿の丘．acrobat（アクロバット）の bat は「歩行」の意味で，acrophobia（高所恐怖症）の人には勤まらない．

肩関節の断層解剖　[冠状断像（MRI，プロトン密度強調像）]

7-20

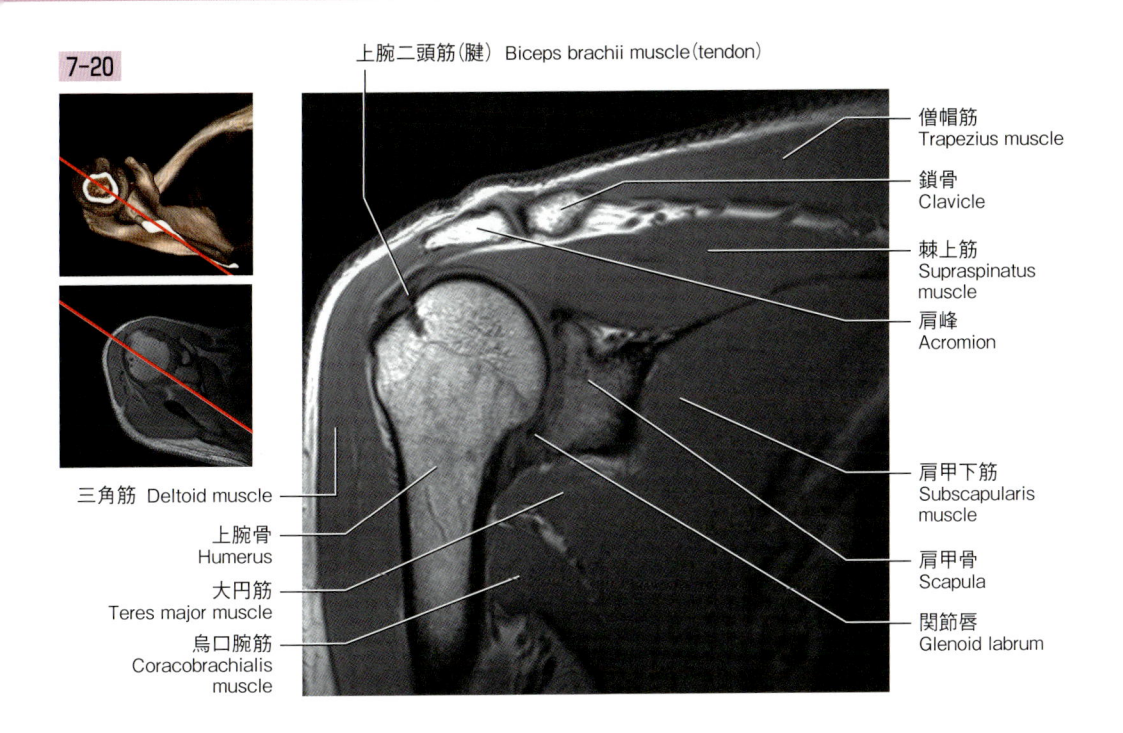

- 上腕二頭筋（腱）Biceps brachii muscle（tendon）
- 僧帽筋 Trapezius muscle
- 鎖骨 Clavicle
- 棘上筋 Supraspinatus muscle
- 肩峰 Acromion
- 肩甲下筋 Subscapularis muscle
- 肩甲骨 Scapula
- 関節唇 Glenoid labrum
- 三角筋 Deltoid muscle
- 上腕骨 Humerus
- 大円筋 Teres major muscle
- 烏口腕筋 Coracobrachialis muscle

7-21

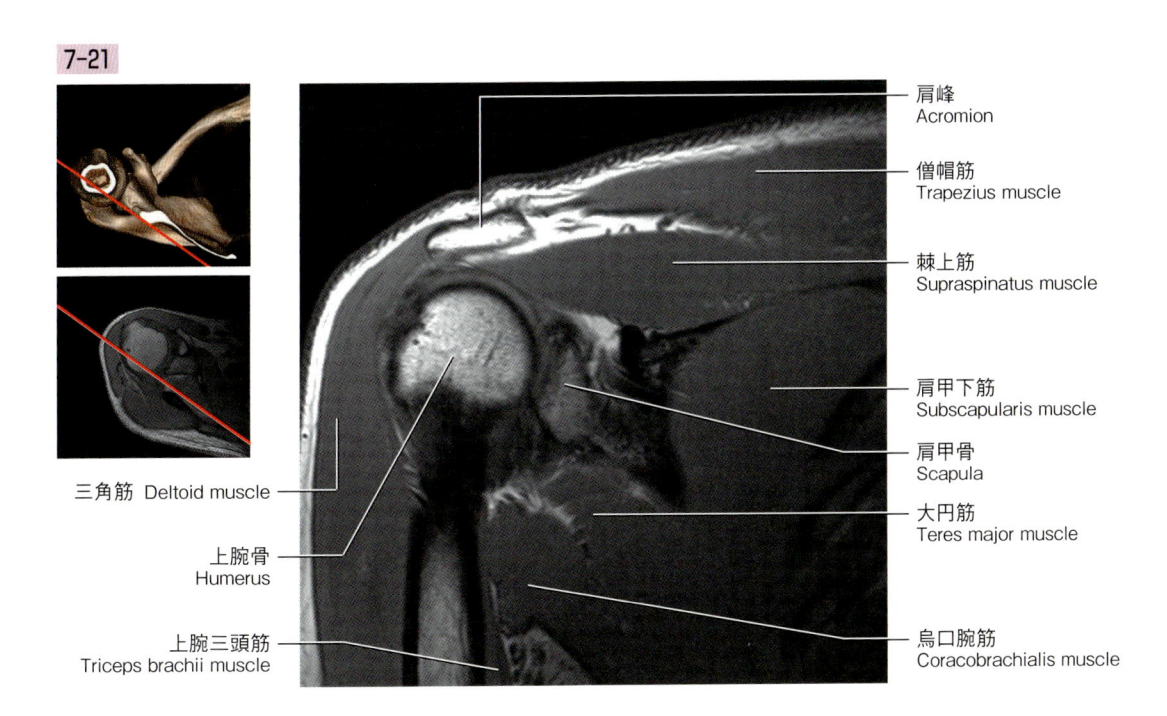

- 肩峰 Acromion
- 僧帽筋 Trapezius muscle
- 棘上筋 Supraspinatus muscle
- 肩甲下筋 Subscapularis muscle
- 肩甲骨 Scapula
- 大円筋 Teres major muscle
- 烏口腕筋 Coracobrachialis muscle
- 三角筋 Deltoid muscle
- 上腕骨 Humerus
- 上腕三頭筋 Triceps brachii muscle

NOTE 肩関節周囲には複数の滑液包が存在する．肩峰下滑液包は，肩鎖関節と三角筋の下方に位置する人体最大の滑液包で，肩関節腔とは腱板によって隔離される．腱板の完全断裂を生じると両者は交通する．

318 肩関節の断層解剖 ［矢状断像（MRI, プロトン密度強調像）］

7-22

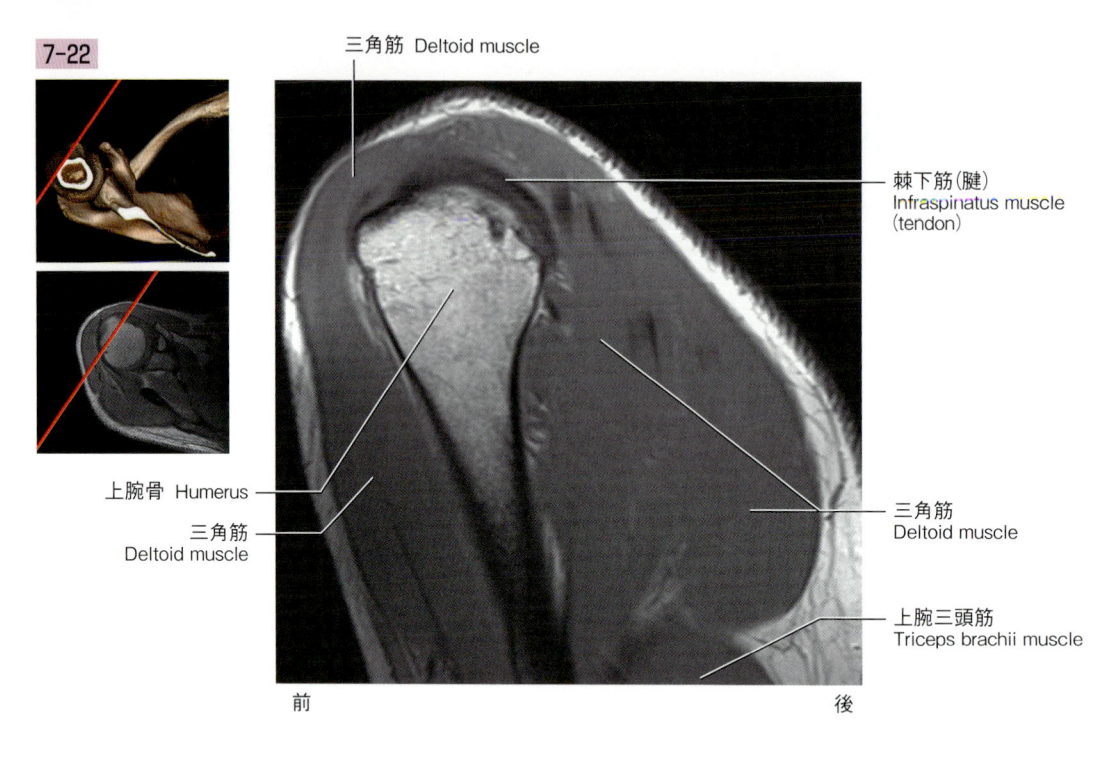

- 三角筋 Deltoid muscle
- 棘下筋（腱） Infraspinatus muscle (tendon)
- 上腕骨 Humerus
- 三角筋 Deltoid muscle
- 三角筋 Deltoid muscle
- 上腕三頭筋 Triceps brachii muscle

前　　後

7-23

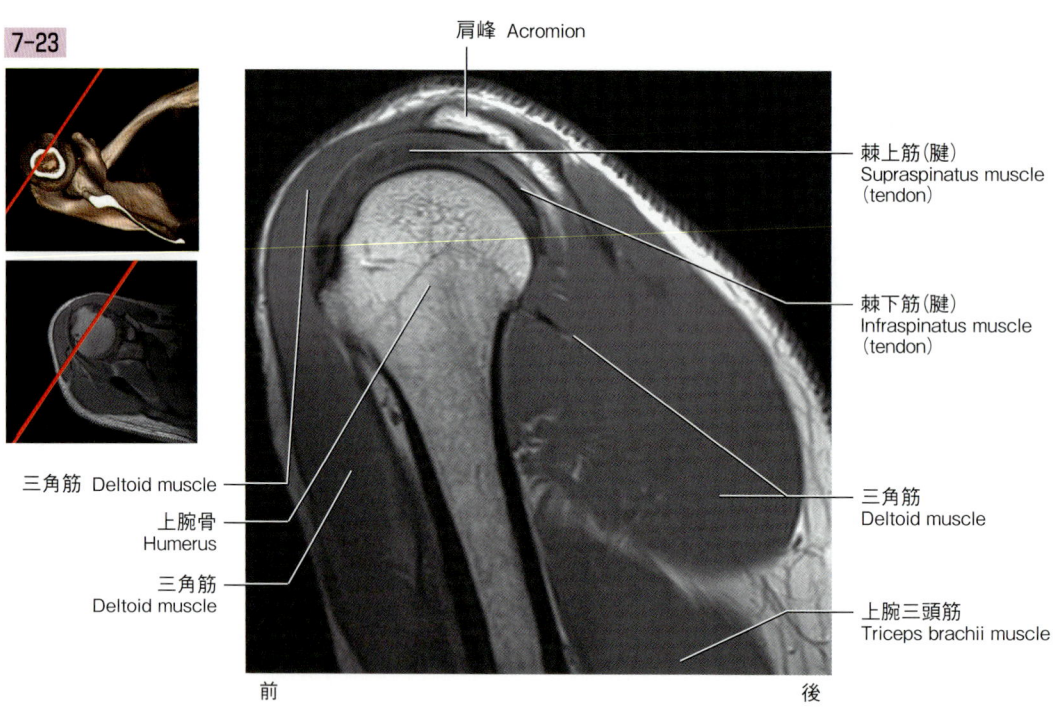

- 肩峰 Acromion
- 棘上筋（腱） Supraspinatus muscle (tendon)
- 棘下筋（腱） Infraspinatus muscle (tendon)
- 三角筋 Deltoid muscle
- 上腕骨 Humerus
- 三角筋 Deltoid muscle
- 三角筋 Deltoid muscle
- 上腕三頭筋 Triceps brachii muscle

前　　後

NOTE 肩関節脱臼の多くは前方脱臼であり，上腕骨の内側前下方に偏位する．

肩関節の断層解剖 ［矢状断像（MRI, プロトン密度強調像）］

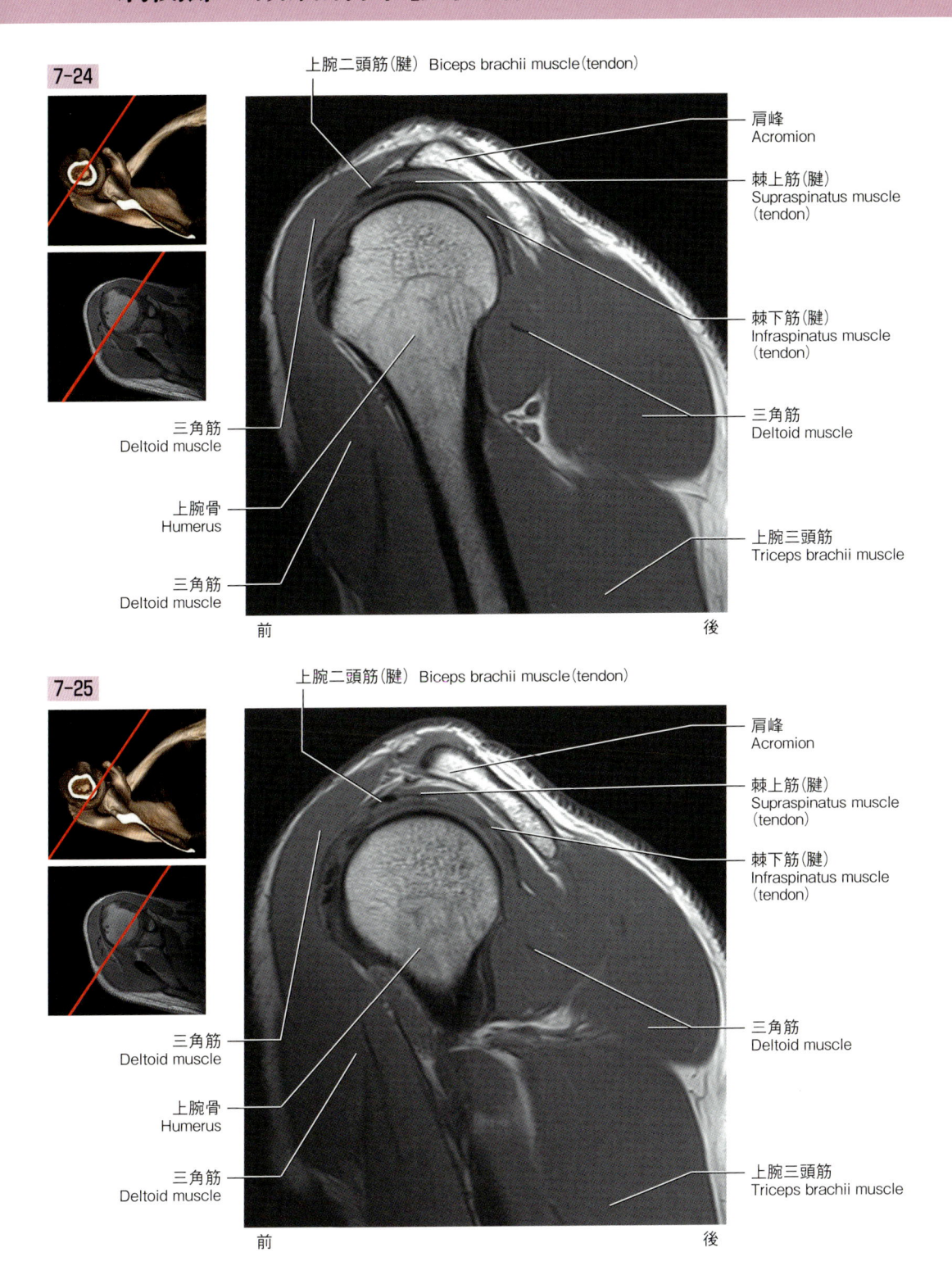

7-24

- 上腕二頭筋（腱） Biceps brachii muscle (tendon)
- 肩峰 Acromion
- 棘上筋（腱） Supraspinatus muscle (tendon)
- 棘下筋（腱） Infraspinatus muscle (tendon)
- 三角筋 Deltoid muscle
- 三角筋 Deltoid muscle
- 上腕骨 Humerus
- 三角筋 Deltoid muscle
- 上腕三頭筋 Triceps brachii muscle

前　後

7-25

- 上腕二頭筋（腱） Biceps brachii muscle (tendon)
- 肩峰 Acromion
- 棘上筋（腱） Supraspinatus muscle (tendon)
- 棘下筋（腱） Infraspinatus muscle (tendon)
- 三角筋 Deltoid muscle
- 三角筋 Deltoid muscle
- 上腕骨 Humerus
- 三角筋 Deltoid muscle
- 上腕三頭筋 Triceps brachii muscle

前　後

> **NOTE** 肩関節脱臼の合併症として上腕骨頭の後外側面の陥没骨折（または骨髄浮腫）を生じる．これを"Hill-Sachs lesion"とよぶ．脱臼の際に関節窩の前縁と衝突するのが原因であり，関節窩の損傷は"Bankart lesion"とよぶ．

肩関節の断層解剖 ［矢状断像（MRI，プロトン密度強調像）］

7-26

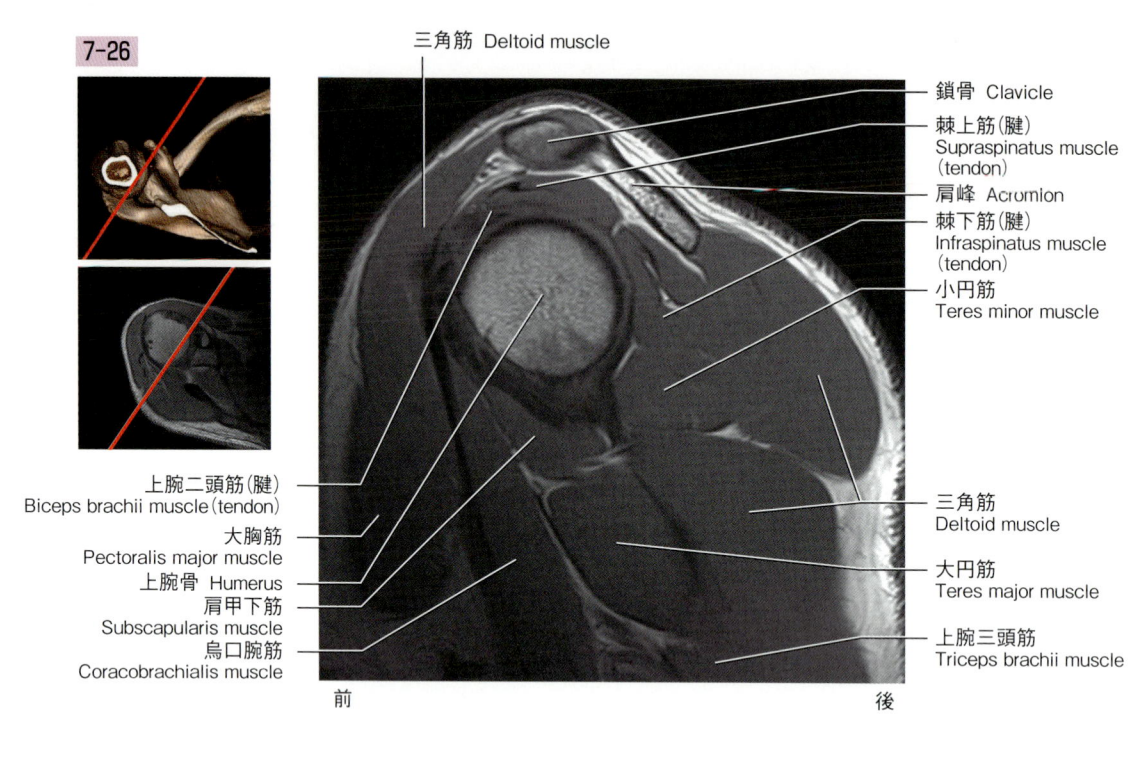

- 三角筋 Deltoid muscle
- 鎖骨 Clavicle
- 棘上筋（腱）Supraspinatus muscle (tendon)
- 肩峰 Acromion
- 棘下筋（腱）Infraspinatus muscle (tendon)
- 小円筋 Teres minor muscle
- 三角筋 Deltoid muscle
- 大円筋 Teres major muscle
- 上腕三頭筋 Triceps brachii muscle
- 上腕二頭筋（腱）Biceps brachii muscle (tendon)
- 大胸筋 Pectoralis major muscle
- 上腕骨 Humerus
- 肩甲下筋 Subscapularis muscle
- 烏口腕筋 Coracobrachialis muscle

前　　後

7-27

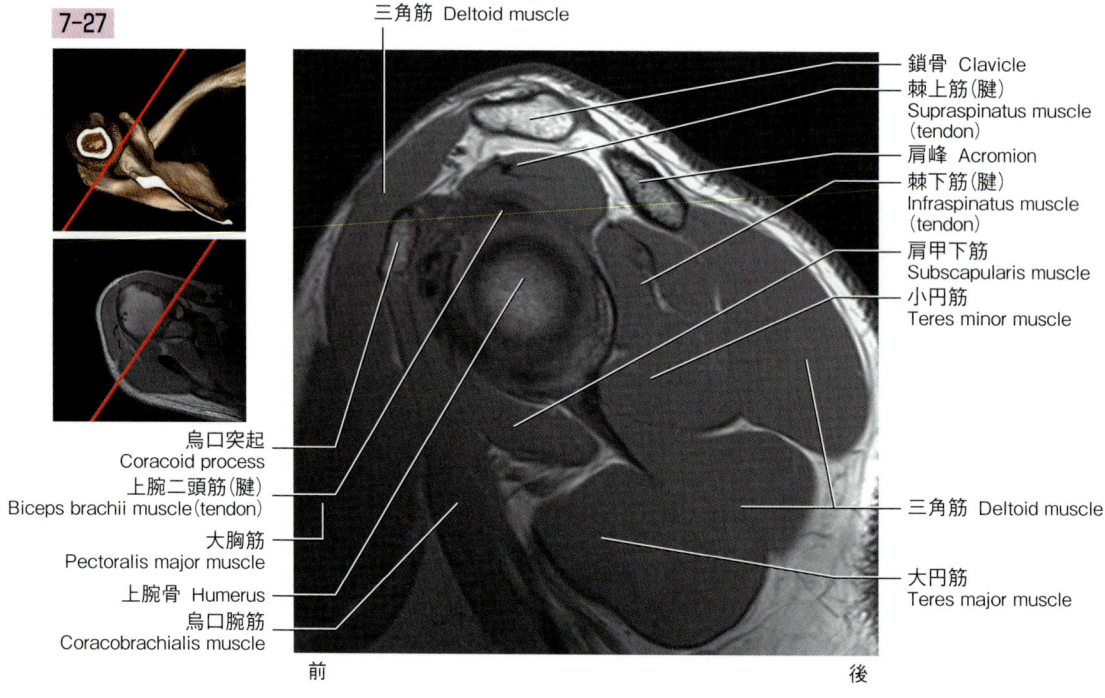

- 三角筋 Deltoid muscle
- 鎖骨 Clavicle
- 棘上筋（腱）Supraspinatus muscle (tendon)
- 肩峰 Acromion
- 棘下筋（腱）Infraspinatus muscle (tendon)
- 肩甲下筋 Subscapularis muscle
- 小円筋 Teres minor muscle
- 三角筋 Deltoid muscle
- 大円筋 Teres major muscle
- 烏口突起 Coracoid process
- 上腕二頭筋（腱）Biceps brachii muscle (tendon)
- 大胸筋 Pectoralis major muscle
- 上腕骨 Humerus
- 烏口腕筋 Coracobrachialis muscle

前　　後

> **NOTE** 烏口肩峰アーチ（Coracoacromial arch）は，肩峰・烏口肩峰靱帯・烏口突起・肩鎖関節を総称した名称である．腱板・肩峰下滑液包・上腕二頭筋長頭腱が，上腕骨頭と烏口肩峰アーチとの間に挟まれて肩の疼痛を引き起こす病態を"インピンジメント症候群"とよぶ．

肩関節の断層解剖 ［矢状断像（MRI, プロトン密度強調像）］

7-28

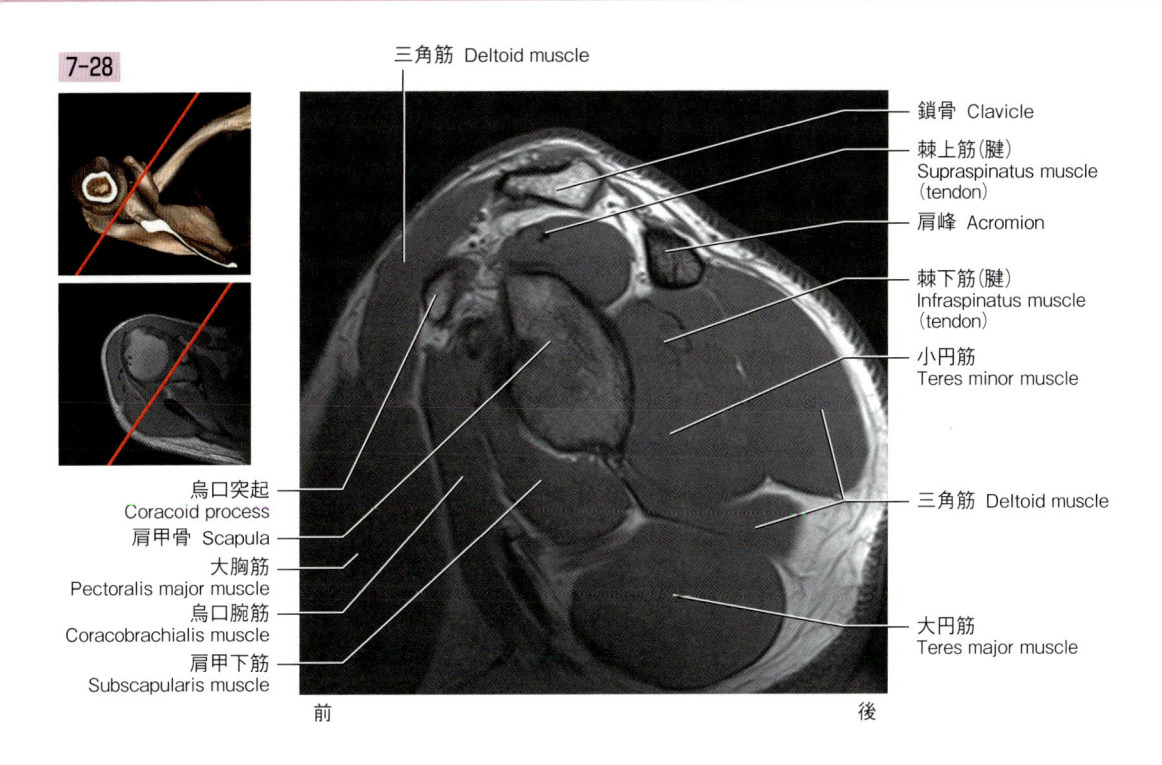

- 三角筋 Deltoid muscle
- 鎖骨 Clavicle
- 棘上筋（腱） Supraspinatus muscle (tendon)
- 肩峰 Acromion
- 棘下筋（腱） Infraspinatus muscle (tendon)
- 小円筋 Teres minor muscle
- 三角筋 Deltoid muscle
- 大円筋 Teres major muscle
- 烏口突起 Coracoid process
- 肩甲骨 Scapula
- 大胸筋 Pectoralis major muscle
- 烏口腕筋 Coracobrachialis muscle
- 肩甲下筋 Subscapularis muscle

前　　後

7-29

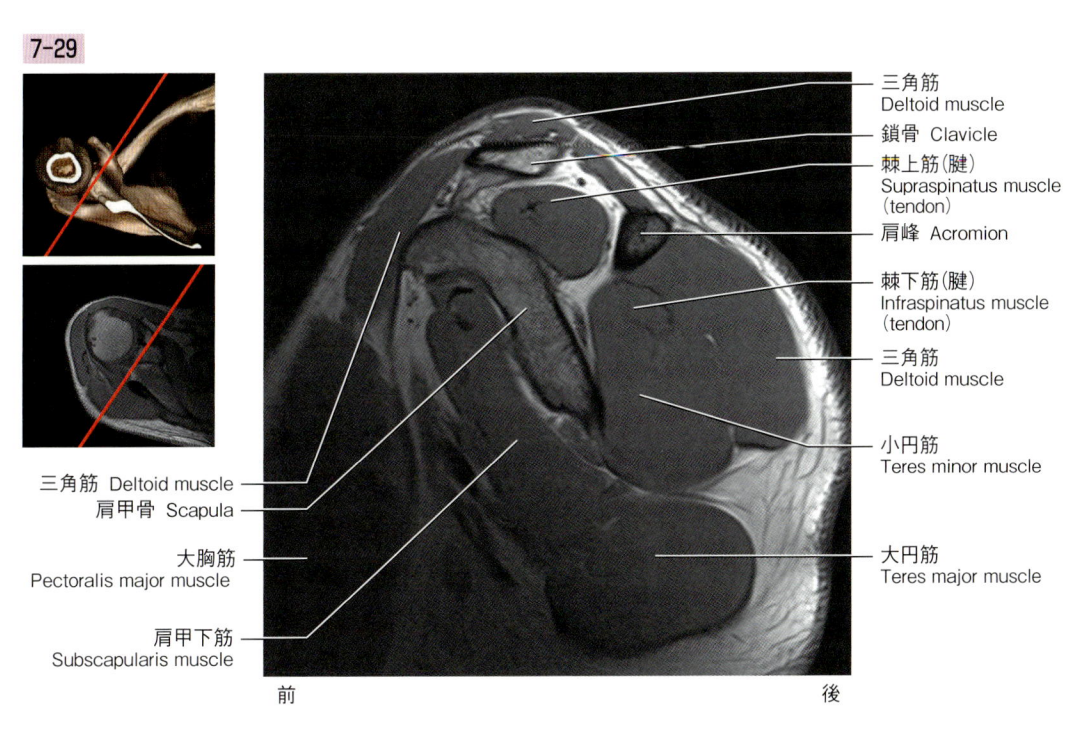

- 三角筋 Deltoid muscle
- 鎖骨 Clavicle
- 棘上筋（腱） Supraspinatus muscle (tendon)
- 肩峰 Acromion
- 棘下筋（腱） Infraspinatus muscle (tendon)
- 三角筋 Deltoid muscle
- 小円筋 Teres minor muscle
- 大円筋 Teres major muscle
- 三角筋 Deltoid muscle
- 肩甲骨 Scapula
- 大胸筋 Pectoralis major muscle
- 肩甲下筋 Subscapularis muscle

前　　後

> **NOTE** 腱板の大結節付着部の約1cm近位部でほぼ1cm径の領域は血流が乏しく、断裂をきたしやすいことからクリティカルゾーン（Critical zone）として知られる．腱板の断裂は、このクリティカルゾーンにおける虚血、経年的変性、インピンジメントによる反復性外傷などにより引き起こされると考えられている．

肩関節の断層解剖 ［矢状断像（MRI，プロトン密度強調像）］

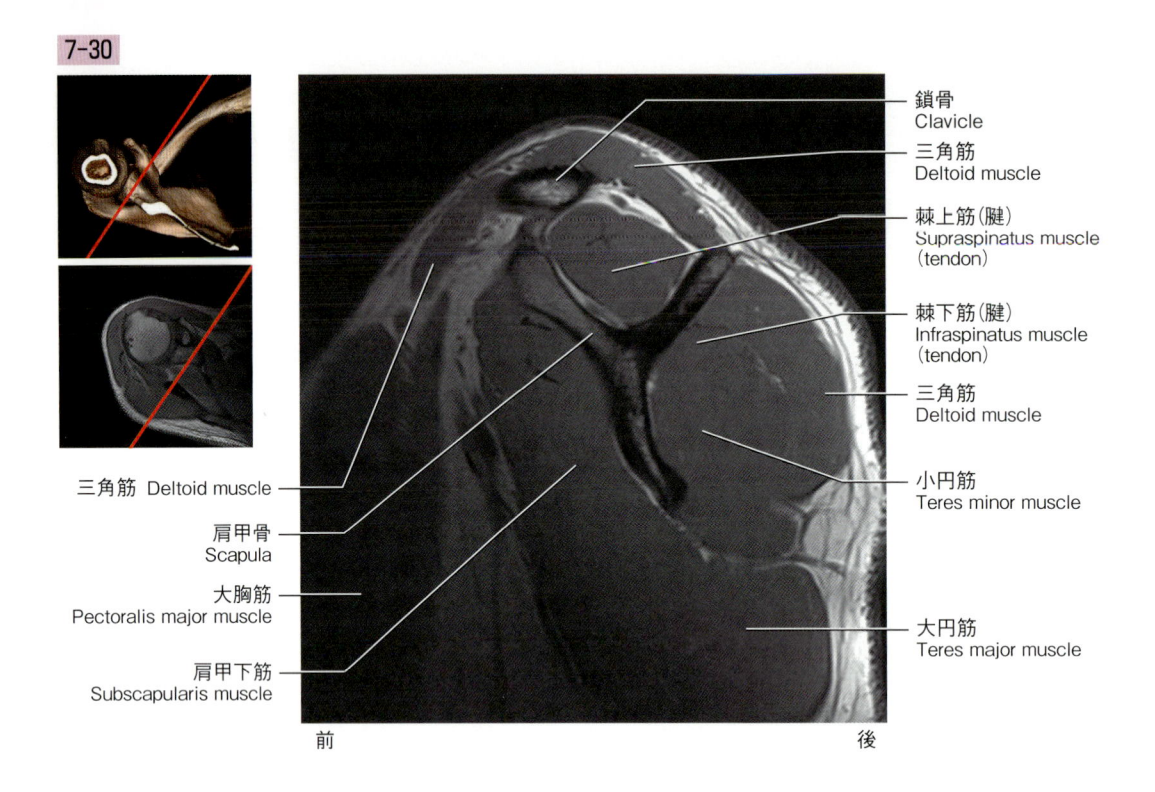

7-30

- 鎖骨 Clavicle
- 三角筋 Deltoid muscle
- 棘上筋（腱）Supraspinatus muscle (tendon)
- 棘下筋（腱）Infraspinatus muscle (tendon)
- 三角筋 Deltoid muscle
- 小円筋 Teres minor muscle
- 大円筋 Teres major muscle
- 三角筋 Deltoid muscle
- 肩甲骨 Scapula
- 大胸筋 Pectoralis major muscle
- 肩甲下筋 Subscapularis muscle

前　　後

NOTE 単純X線写真でのScapula Y撮影は，肩甲胸郭関節，肩峰下・烏口突起と上腕骨頭のスペース，関節窩と上腕骨頭の前後の位置関係を確認するのに有効である．

肘関節 (CT, VR 像)

7-31 肘関節の体表解剖（前面）

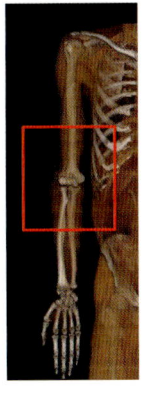

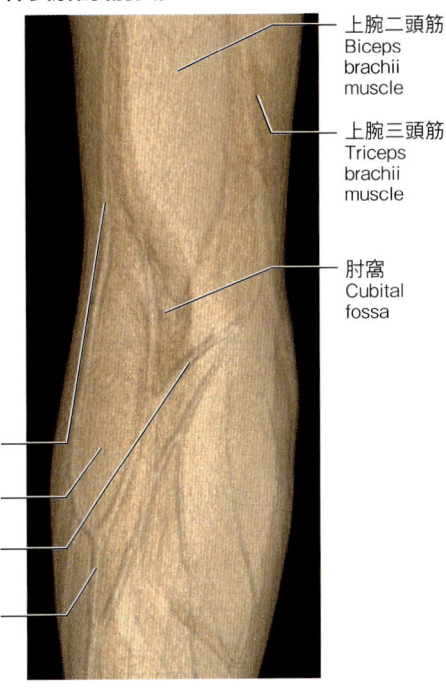

- 上腕二頭筋 Biceps brachii muscle
- 上腕三頭筋 Triceps brachii muscle
- 肘窩 Cubital fossa
- 橈側皮静脈 Cephalic vein
- 腕橈骨筋 Brachioradialis muscle
- 肘正中皮静脈 Median cubital vein
- 前腕正中皮静脈 Median antebrachial vein（Median vein of forearm）

7-32 肘関節の筋（前面）

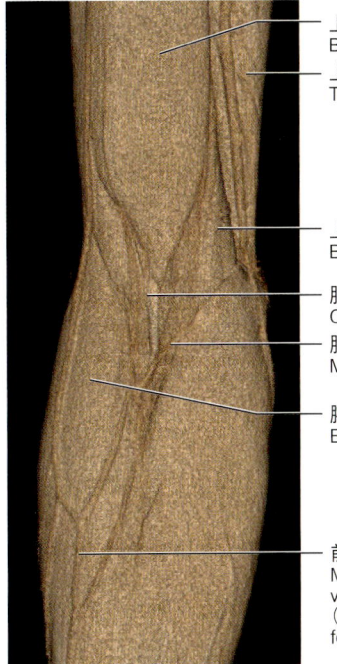

- 上腕二頭筋 Biceps brachii muscle
- 上腕三頭筋 Triceps brachii muscle
- 上腕筋 Brachialis muscle
- 肘窩 Cubital fossa
- 肘正中皮静脈 Median cubital vein
- 腕橈骨筋 Brachioradialis muscle
- 前腕正中皮静脈 Median antebrachial vein（Median vein of forearm）

7-33 肘関節の体表解剖（後面）

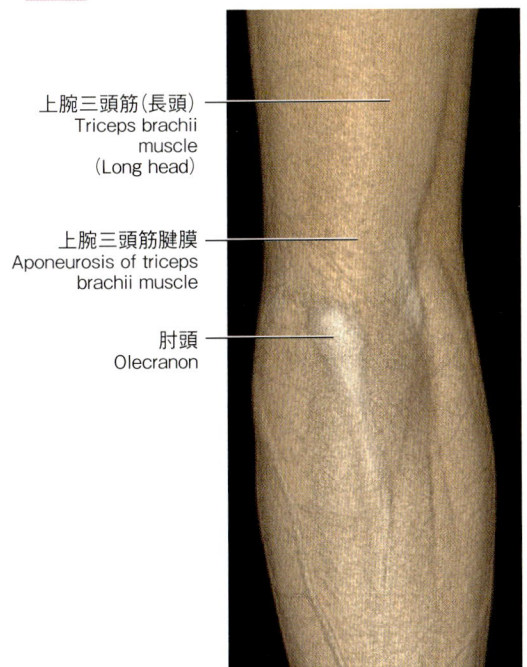

- 上腕三頭筋（長頭） Triceps brachii muscle（Long head）
- 上腕三頭筋腱膜 Aponeurosis of triceps brachii muscle
- 肘頭 Olecranon

7-34 肘関節の筋（後面）

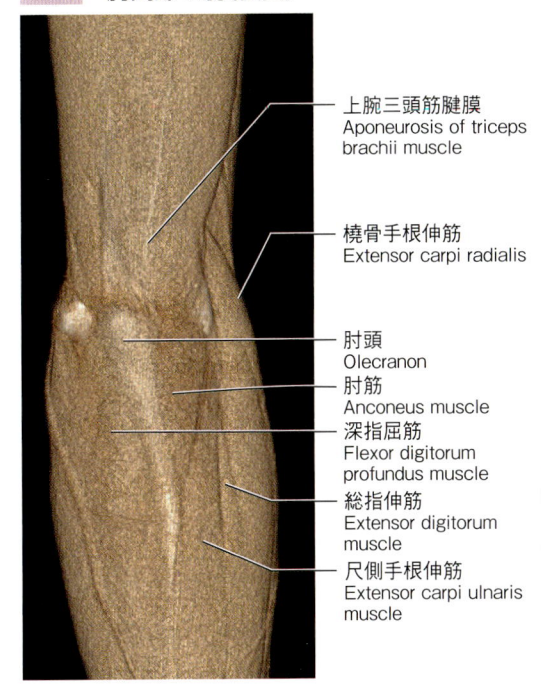

- 上腕三頭筋腱膜 Aponeurosis of triceps brachii muscle
- 橈骨手根伸筋 Extensor carpi radialis
- 肘頭 Olecranon
- 肘筋 Anconeus muscle
- 深指屈筋 Flexor digitorum profundus muscle
- 総指伸筋 Extensor digitorum muscle
- 尺側手根伸筋 Extensor carpi ulnaris muscle

NOTE 肘関節は右上腕骨，尺骨，橈骨により構成される．共通の関節包内に腕橈関節，腕尺関節，上橈尺関節を有している．上腕において上腕動脈，尺骨神経，正中神経は，上腕二頭筋と上腕三頭筋（内側上腕筋間中隔）の間の内側二頭筋溝（Medial bicipital sulcus）の中を通過する．

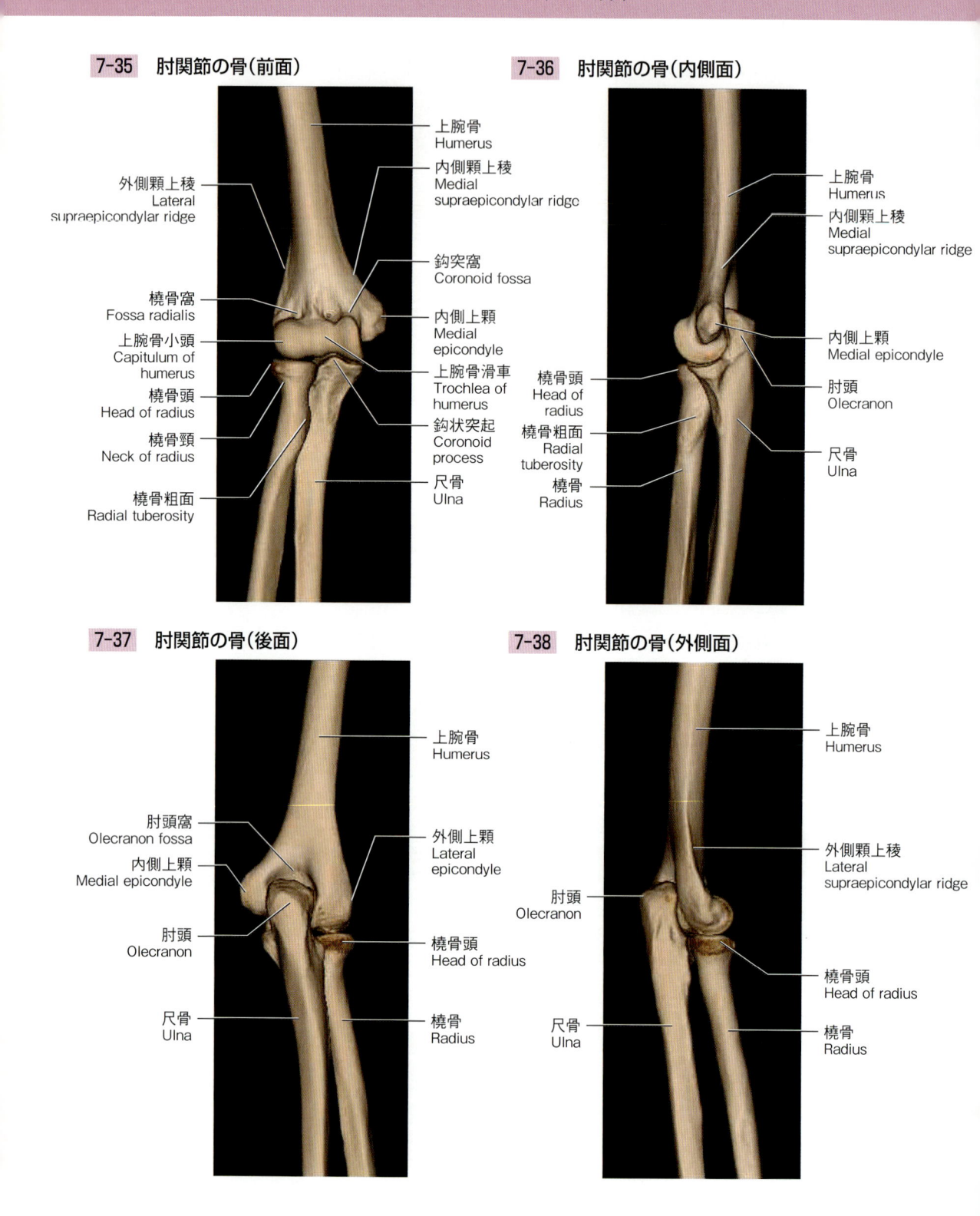

肘関節（CT, VR像）

7-35 肘関節の骨（前面）

- 上腕骨 Humerus
- 内側顆上稜 Medial supraepicondylar ridge
- 外側顆上稜 Lateral supraepicondylar ridge
- 鉤突窩 Coronoid fossa
- 橈骨窩 Fossa radialis
- 上腕骨小頭 Capitulum of humerus
- 内側上顆 Medial epicondyle
- 橈骨頭 Head of radius
- 上腕骨滑車 Trochlea of humerus
- 橈骨頸 Neck of radius
- 鉤状突起 Coronoid process
- 橈骨粗面 Radial tuberosity
- 尺骨 Ulna

7-36 肘関節の骨（内側面）

- 上腕骨 Humerus
- 内側顆上稜 Medial supraepicondylar ridge
- 内側上顆 Medial epicondyle
- 橈骨頭 Head of radius
- 肘頭 Olecranon
- 橈骨粗面 Radial tuberosity
- 尺骨 Ulna
- 橈骨 Radius

7-37 肘関節の骨（後面）

- 上腕骨 Humerus
- 肘頭窩 Olecranon fossa
- 内側上顆 Medial epicondyle
- 外側上顆 Lateral epicondyle
- 肘頭 Olecranon
- 橈骨頭 Head of radius
- 尺骨 Ulna
- 橈骨 Radius

7-38 肘関節の骨（外側面）

- 上腕骨 Humerus
- 外側顆上稜 Lateral supraepicondylar ridge
- 肘頭 Olecranon
- 橈骨頭 Head of radius
- 尺骨 Ulna
- 橈骨 Radius

> **NOTE** 肘関節の腕橈関節，腕尺関節，上橈尺関節の3つの関節の中で，腕橈関節と腕尺関節が肘関節の屈伸運動を行い，上橈尺関節と腕橈関節が前腕遠位端の下橈尺関節と協調して前腕の回旋運動を行う．

肘関節の断層解剖 ［横断像（MRI，プロトン密度強調像）］

7-39

- 上腕二頭筋 Biceps brachii muscle
- 上腕筋 Brachialis muscle
- 腕橈骨筋 Brachioradialis muscle
- 橈側手根伸筋 Extensor carpi radialis muscle
- 上腕骨 Humerus
- 上腕三頭筋 Triceps brachii muscle
- 上腕三頭筋（腱） Triceps brachii muscle (tendon)

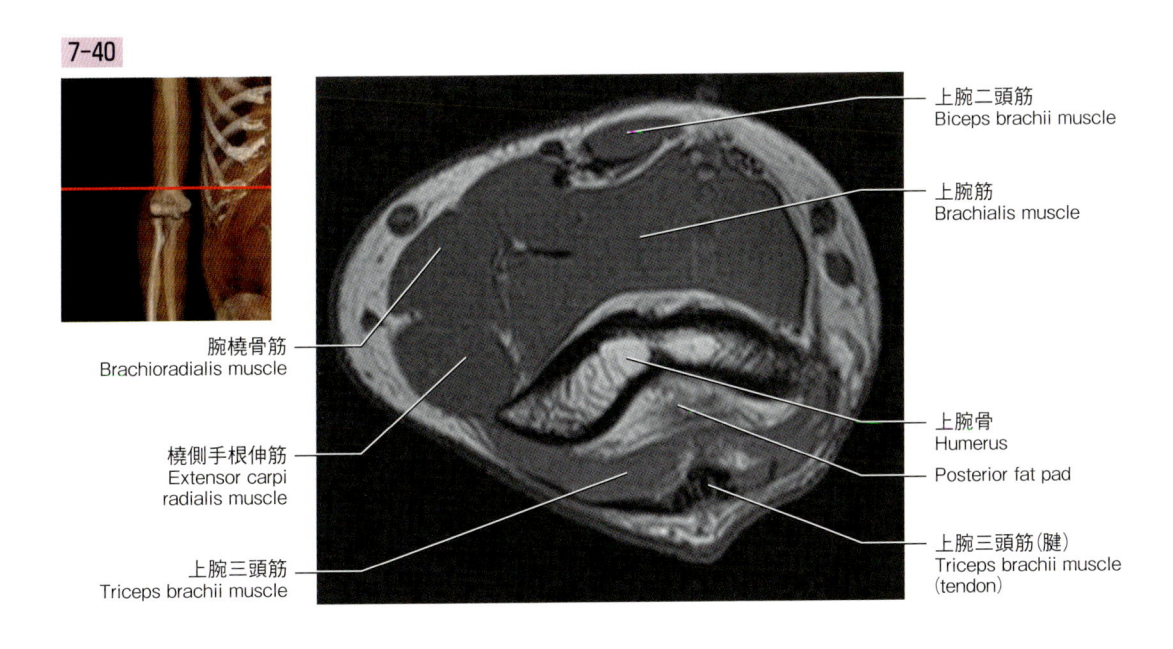

7-40

- 上腕二頭筋 Biceps brachii muscle
- 上腕筋 Brachialis muscle
- 腕橈骨筋 Brachioradialis muscle
- 橈側手根伸筋 Extensor carpi radialis muscle
- 上腕骨 Humerus
- Posterior fat pad
- 上腕三頭筋 Triceps brachii muscle
- 上腕三頭筋（腱） Triceps brachii muscle (tendon)

> **NOTE** 上腕動脈は上腕遠位部で上腕筋の前方を通り肘窩に至る．肘関節辺縁の外傷の合併症のひとつにVolkmann（フォルクマン）拘縮がある．これは，小児の上腕骨顆上骨折に続発して起こることが多く，主に上腕動脈の損傷や閉塞により前腕屈筋群の急性阻血性壊死を生じさせて惹起される拘縮である．

肘関節の断層解剖　[横断像（MRI, プロトン密度強調像）]

7-41

- 上腕二頭筋　Biceps brachii muscle
- 上腕筋　Brachialis muscle
- 円回内筋　Pronator teres muscle
- 上腕骨内側上顆　Medial epicondyle of humerus
- 尺骨神経　Ulnar nerve
- 肘頭　Olecranon
- 腕橈骨筋　Brachioradialis muscle
- 橈側手根伸筋　Extensor carpi radialis muscle
- 上腕骨外側上顆　Lateral epicondyle
- 肘筋　Anconeus muscle

7-42

- 上腕二頭筋（腱）　Biceps brachii muscle (tendon)
- 上腕筋　Brachialis muscle
- 円回内筋　Pronator teres muscle
- 上腕骨　Humerus
- 肘頭　Olecranon
- 腕橈骨筋　Brachioradialis muscle
- 橈側手根伸筋　Extensor carpi radialis muscle
- 肘筋　Anconeus muscle

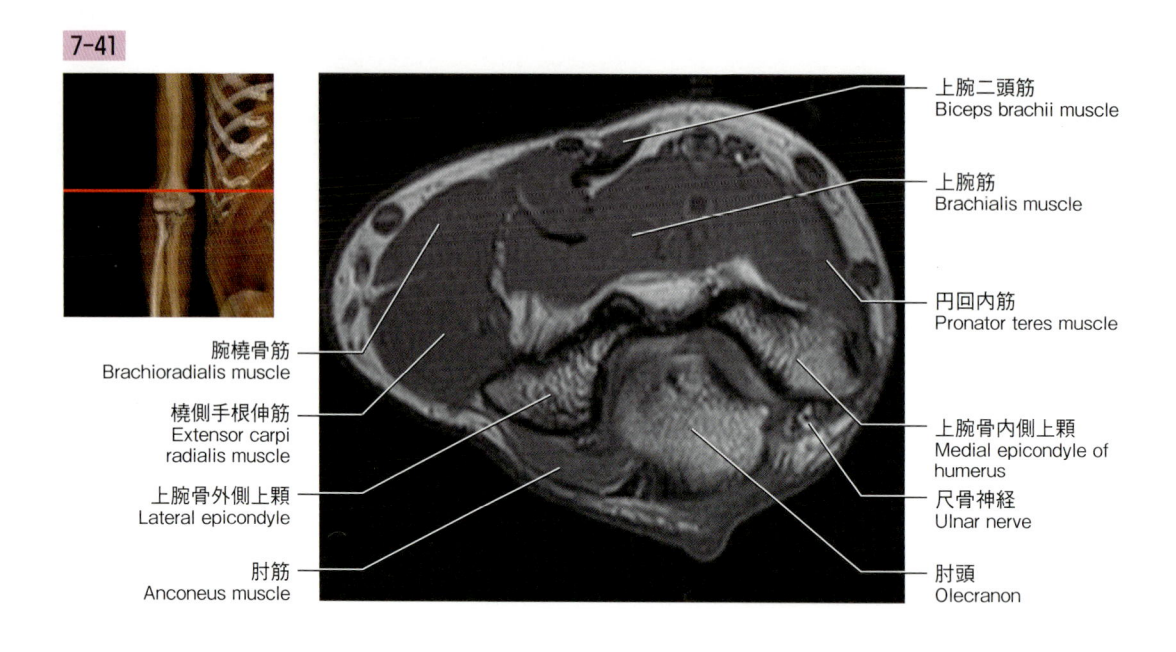

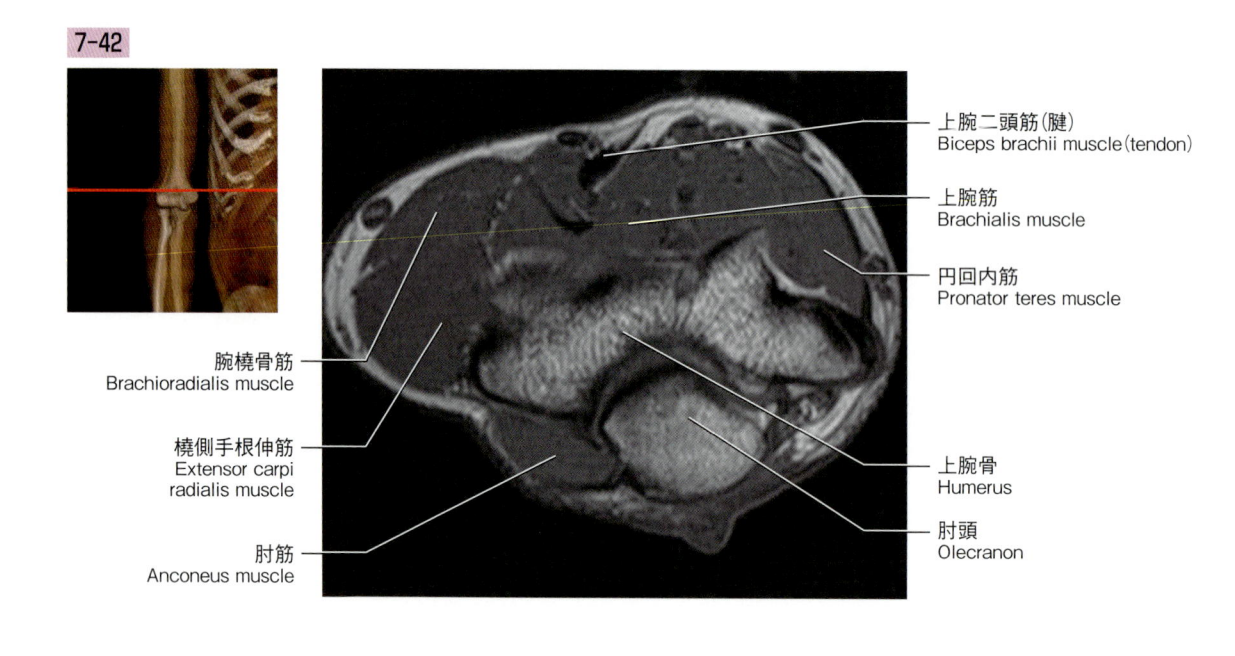

NOTE　尺骨神経は内側上顆レベルで肘部管（Cubital tunnel）内を通過する．このレベルの横断像で尺骨神経は明瞭に描出される．肘部管はその前方を内側上顆後面の尺骨神経溝，内側を内側側副靱帯，後方を尺側手根屈筋の上腕頭と尺骨頭の両頭間の靱帯（Arcuate ligament）で形成される．

肘関節の断層解剖 ［横断像（MRI，プロトン密度強調像）］

7-43

- 上腕二頭筋（腱） Biceps brachii muscle (tendon)
- 上腕筋 Brachialis muscle
- 円回内筋 Pronator teres muscle
- 尺骨神経 Ulnar nerve
- 上腕三頭筋（腱） Triceps brachii muscle (tendon)
- 肘頭 Olecranon
- 腕橈骨筋 Brachioradialis muscle
- 橈側手根伸筋 Extensor carpi radialis muscle
- 上腕骨 Humerus
- 肘筋 Anconeus muscle

7-44

- 上腕二頭筋（腱） Biceps brachii muscle (tendon)
- 上腕筋 Brachialis muscle
- 円回内筋 Pronator teres muscle
- 上腕三頭筋 Triceps brachii muscle
- 肘頭 Olecranon
- 腕橈骨筋 Brachioradialis muscle
- 橈側手根伸筋 Extensor carpi radialis muscle
- 上腕骨 Humerus
- 肘筋 Anconeus muscle

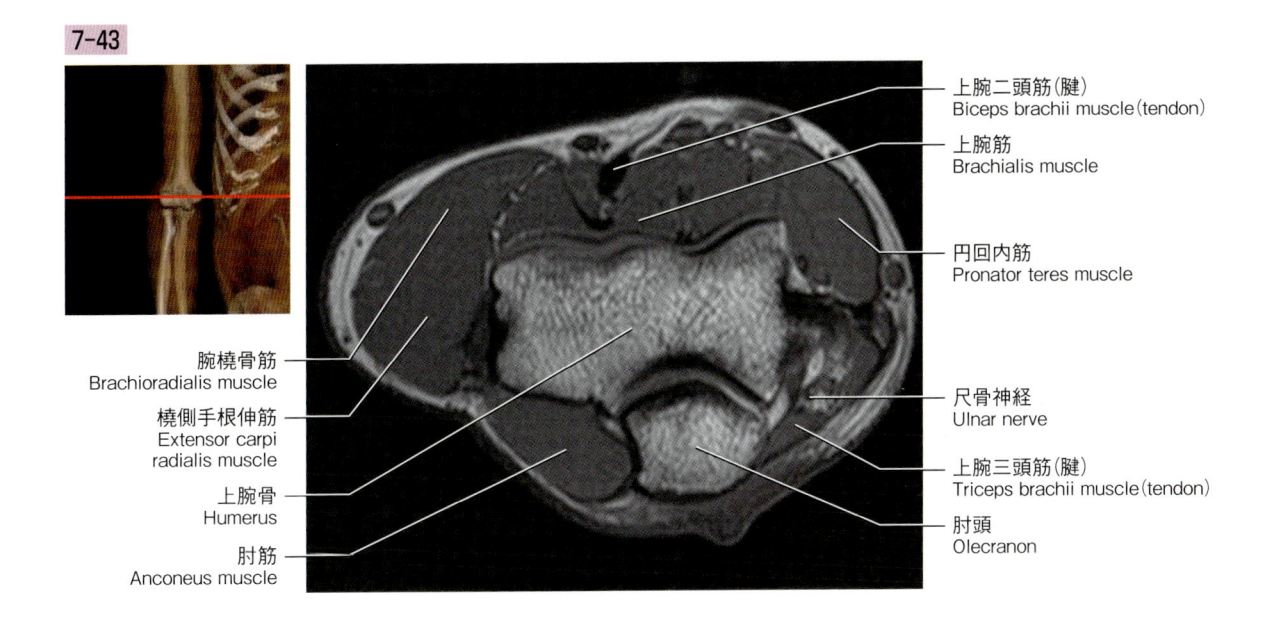

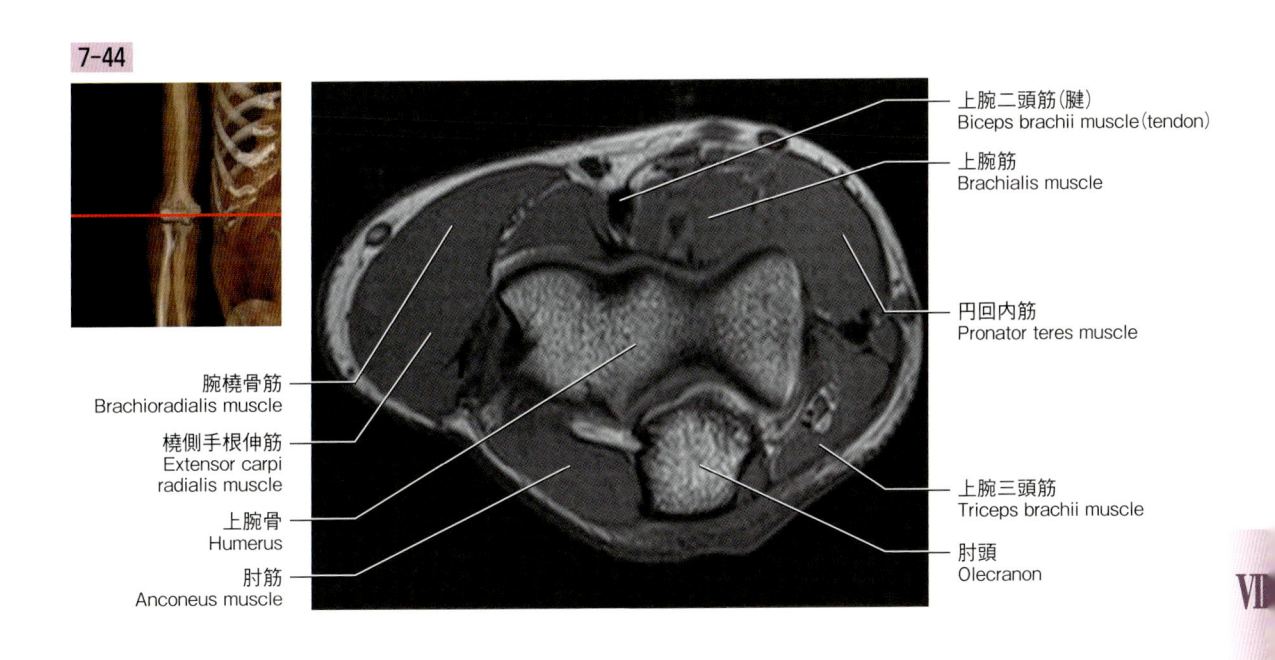

> **NOTE** 肘部管症候群（Cubital tunnel syndrome）は，肘部管で尺骨神経が障害されて生じる尺骨神経麻痺の総称である．初期の症状は，第4および第5指のしびれ感や知覚鈍麻であるが，徐々に進行し，鷲指変形や小指球萎縮，母指球萎縮をきたす．その原因には，幼児期の上腕骨外顆骨折や顆上骨折後の外反肘に続発する遅発性尺骨神経麻痺，浅い尺骨神経溝のために，肘の屈曲時に尺骨神経が滑脱する摩擦性尺骨神経炎，変形性肘関節症，ガングリオン（Ganglion）などがある．尺骨神経は肘部管を離れた後，尺側手根屈筋の上腕頭と尺骨頭の間を走行する．

肘関節の断層解剖 ［横断像（MRI，プロトン密度強調像）］

7-45

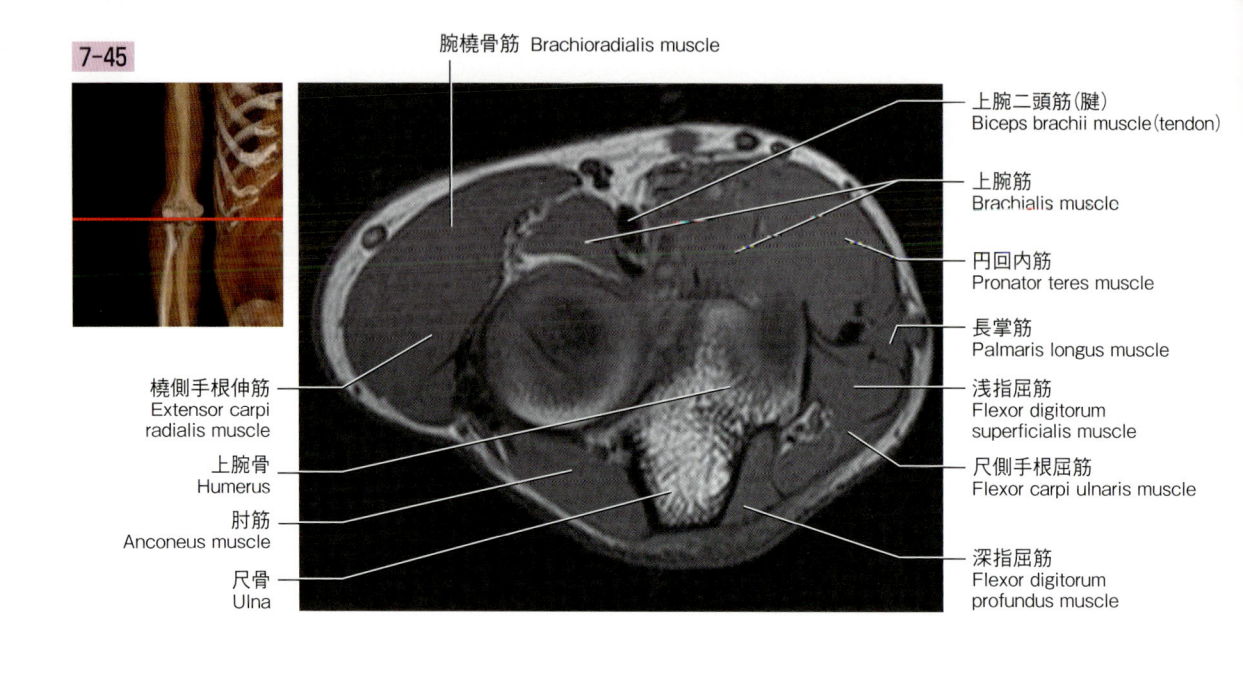

- 腕橈骨筋 Brachioradialis muscle
- 上腕二頭筋（腱） Biceps brachii muscle（tendon）
- 上腕筋 Brachialis muscle
- 円回内筋 Pronator teres muscle
- 長掌筋 Palmaris longus muscle
- 浅指屈筋 Flexor digitorum superficialis muscle
- 尺側手根屈筋 Flexor carpi ulnaris muscle
- 深指屈筋 Flexor digitorum profundus muscle
- 橈側手根伸筋 Extensor carpi radialis muscle
- 上腕骨 Humerus
- 肘筋 Anconeus muscle
- 尺骨 Ulna

7-46

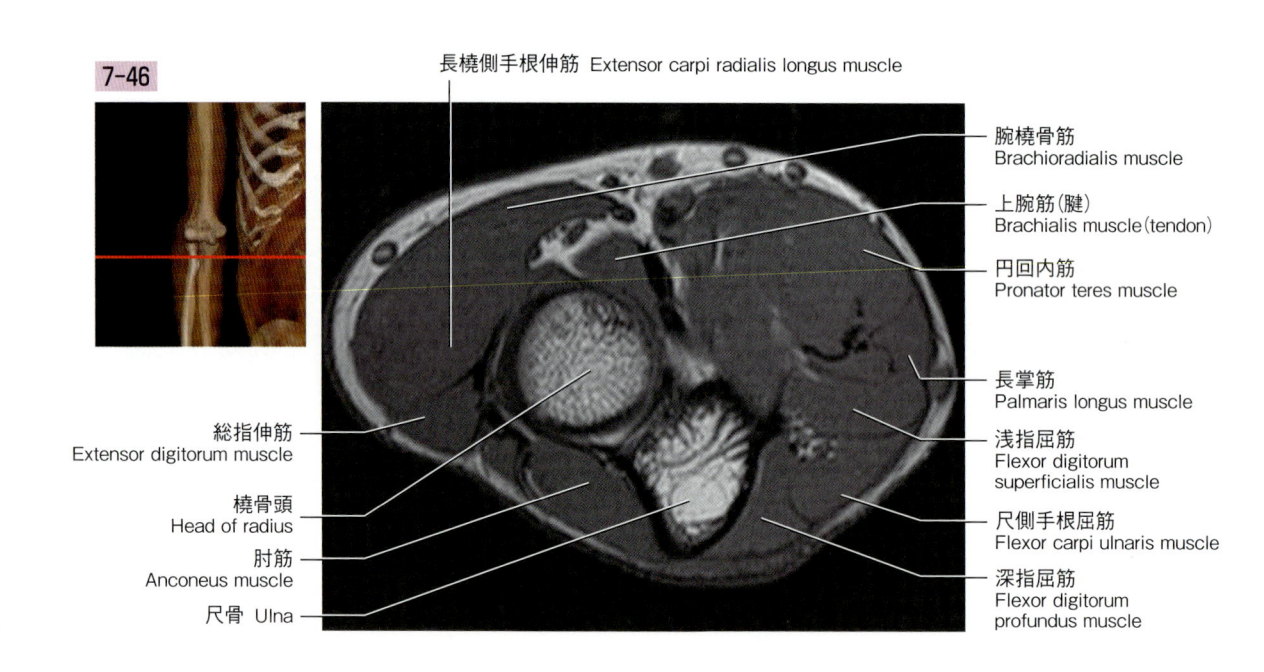

- 長橈側手根伸筋 Extensor carpi radialis longus muscle
- 腕橈骨筋 Brachioradialis muscle
- 上腕筋（腱） Brachialis muscle（tendon）
- 円回内筋 Pronator teres muscle
- 長掌筋 Palmaris longus muscle
- 浅指屈筋 Flexor digitorum superficialis muscle
- 尺側手根屈筋 Flexor carpi ulnaris muscle
- 深指屈筋 Flexor digitorum profundus muscle
- 総指伸筋 Extensor digitorum muscle
- 橈骨頭 Head of radius
- 肘筋 Anconeus muscle
- 尺骨 Ulna

> **NOTE** 正中神経は上腕動脈とともに上腕筋の前を通り肘窩に至る．円回内筋の上腕頭と尺骨頭の間を通り抜けたのち，浅指屈筋と深指屈筋に挟まれて下行しながら最大の運動枝である前骨間神経を分岐する．肘関節レベルにおける正中神経障害には，回内筋症候群（Pronator syndrome）と前骨間神経症候群（Anterior interosseous nerve syndrome）がある．回内筋症候群では，広範な前腕部の疼痛と正中神経支配領域の知覚異常をきたす．前骨間神経症候群では，長母指屈筋，示指の深指屈筋の麻痺により物をつまむのに著しい障害をきたすが，一般的に知覚障害は伴わない．

肘関節の断層解剖［横断像（MRI, プロトン密度強調像）］

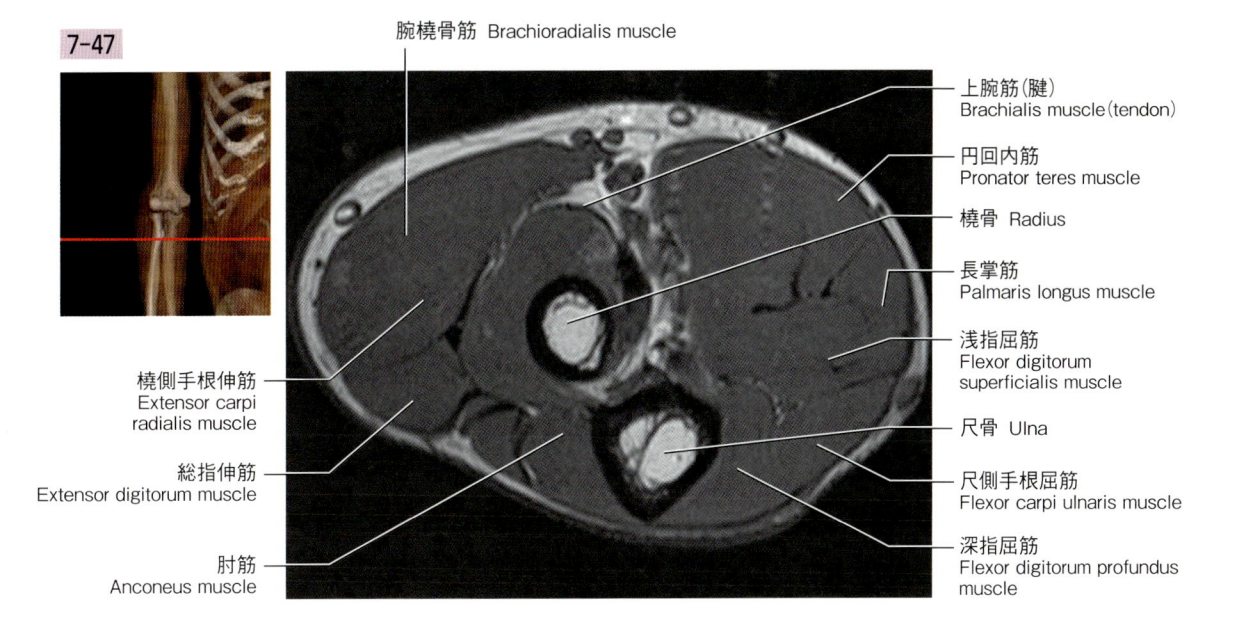

7-47

- 腕橈骨筋 Brachioradialis muscle
- 上腕筋（腱）Brachialis muscle（tendon）
- 円回内筋 Pronator teres muscle
- 橈骨 Radius
- 長掌筋 Palmaris longus muscle
- 浅指屈筋 Flexor digitorum superficialis muscle
- 尺骨 Ulna
- 尺側手根屈筋 Flexor carpi ulnaris muscle
- 深指屈筋 Flexor digitorum profundus muscle
- 橈側手根伸筋 Extensor carpi radialis muscle
- 総指伸筋 Extensor digitorum muscle
- 肘筋 Anconeus muscle

NOTE 橈骨神経は，上腕骨後面の橈骨神経溝に沿って迂回し，上腕の外側に達する．ここで外側上腕筋間中隔を貫いて上腕の前面に至る．さらに上腕遠位部で上腕筋と腕橈骨の間を通って肘窩に至り，浅枝と深枝（後骨間神経）に分岐する．浅枝は回外筋の前面を通る細い知覚神経で，後骨間神経は手関節と手指の伸筋を支配する運動神経である．後骨間神経は，フローゼのアーケードとよばれる結合組織性アーチより，回外筋の浅頭（Superficial head）と深頭（Deep head）の間に進入する．後骨間神経症候群（Posterior interosseous nerve syndrome）は，後骨間神経が圧排や損傷を受けて生じる母指や示指の伸展障害である．後骨間神経がフローゼのアーケードより回外筋の中に進入する部位で絞扼されることが多い．

330 肘関節の断層解剖 [冠状断像（MRI, プロトン密度強調像）]

7-48

- 上腕筋 Brachialis muscle
- 腕橈骨筋 Brachioradialis muscle
- （長・短）橈側手根伸筋 Extensor carpi radialis (Longus and brevis) muscles

外　　内

7-49

- 上腕筋 Brachialis muscle
- 上腕二頭筋（腱） Biceps brachii muscle (tendon)
- 円回内筋 Pronator teres muscle
- 腕橈骨筋 Brachioradialis muscle
- （長・短）橈側手根伸筋 Extensor carpi radialis (Longus and brevis) muscles

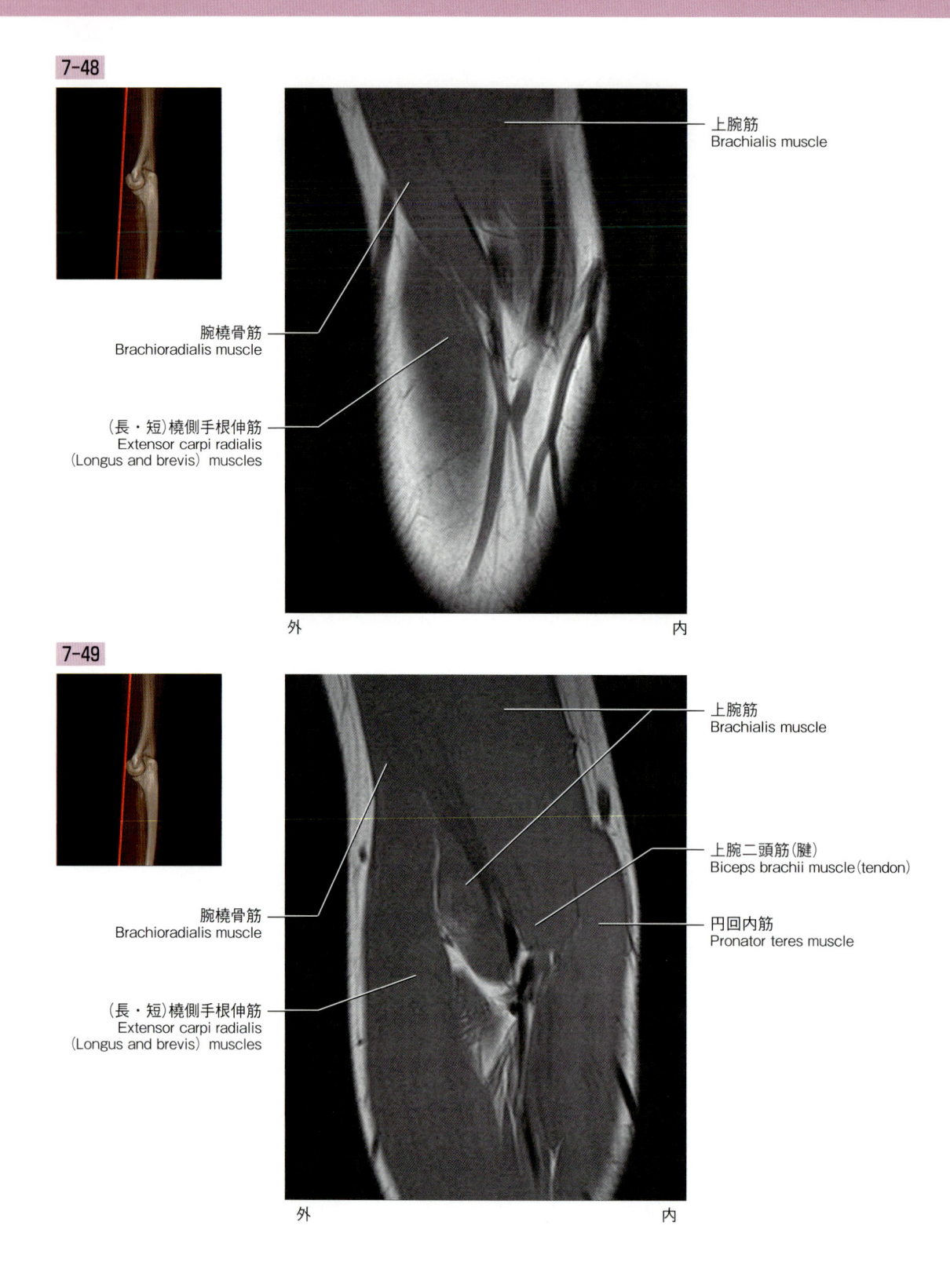

外　　内

肘関節の断層解剖 ［冠状断像（MRI，プロトン密度強調像）］

7-50

- 腕橈骨筋 Brachioradialis muscle
- 上腕骨小頭 Capitulum of humerus
- 上腕骨滑車 Trochlea of humerus
- （長・短）橈側手根伸筋 Extensor carpi radialis (Longus and brevis) muscles
- 橈骨 Radius
- 上腕筋 Brachialis muscle
- 円回内筋 Pronator teres muscle
- 内側上顆 Medial epicondyle
- 回外筋 Supinator muscle
- 深指屈筋 Flexor digitorum profundus muscle

外 / 内

7-51

上腕骨 Humerus

- 腕橈骨筋 Brachioradialis muscle
- 上腕骨小頭 Capitulum of humerus
- 内側上顆 Medial epicondyle
- 橈骨 Radius
- （長・短）橈側手根伸筋 Extensor carpi radialis (Longus and brevis) muscles
- 回外筋 Supinator muscle
- 上腕筋 Brachialis muscle
- 円回内筋 Pronator teres muscle
- 上腕二頭筋（腱） Biceps brachii muscle (tendon)
- 長掌筋 Palmaris longus muscle
- 浅指屈筋 Flexor digitorum superficialis muscle

外 / 内

NOTE 肘関節の内側では，上腕骨内側上顆に手関節屈筋群（橈側手根屈筋，尺側手根屈筋，長掌筋，浅・深手根屈筋）や円回内筋が起始する．外側では，上腕骨外側上顆に手関節伸筋群（長・短橈側手根伸筋，尺側手根伸筋，指伸筋）や回外筋が起始する．これらの筋はいずれも，肘関節近傍において独立した筋腹をもたないため，MRIにおいて個々の筋を独立して同定することは不可能である．

肘関節の断層解剖 ［冠状断像（MRI，プロトン密度強調像）］

7-52

- 上腕骨 Humerus
- 上腕筋 Brachialis muscle
- 円回内筋 Pronator teres muscle
- 腕橈骨筋 Brachioradialis muscle
- 上腕骨小頭 Capitulum of humerus
- 内側上顆 Medial epicondyle
- 上腕二頭筋（腱） Biceps brachii muscle (tendon)
- 橈骨 Radius
- 総指伸筋 Extensor digitorum muscle
- 長掌筋 Palmaris longus muscle
- 回外筋 Supinator muscle
- 浅指屈筋 Flexor digitorum superficialis muscle

外　内

7-53

- 上腕三頭筋 Triceps brachii muscle
- 腕橈骨筋 Brachioradialis muscle
- 上腕筋 Brachialis muscle
- 円回内筋 Pronator teres muscle
- 鈎突窩 Coronoid fossa
- 上腕骨小頭 Capitulum of humerus
- 橈骨 Radius
- 長掌筋 Palmaris longus muscle
- 総指伸筋 Extensor digitorum muscle
- 浅指屈筋 Flexor digitorum superficialis muscle
- 回外筋 Supinator muscle
- 深指屈筋 Flexor digitorum profundus muscle

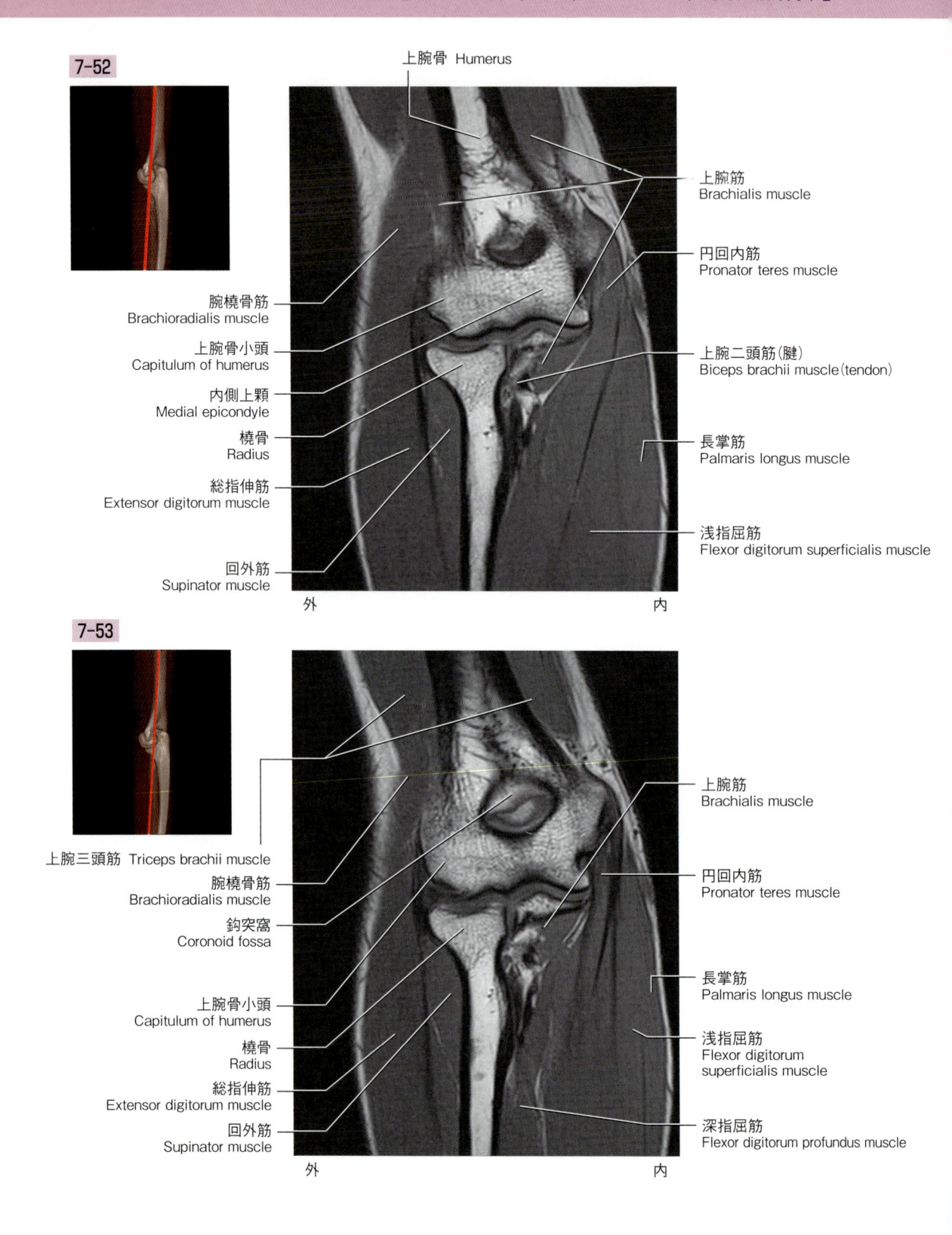

外　内

> **NOTE** 肘関節の使いすぎによる腱の障害，いわゆる"使いすぎ症候群（Overuse syndrome）"は，ラケットスポーツで引き起こされることが多いが，なかでもテニス肘（Tennis elbow）が最もよく知られている．

肘関節の断層解剖 ［冠状断像（MRI，プロトン密度強調像）］

7-54

上腕三頭筋 Triceps brachii muscle
上腕骨小頭 Capitulum of humerus
橈骨 Radius
回外筋 Supinator muscle
総指伸筋 Extensor digitorum muscle

鈎突窩 Coronoid fossa
円回内筋 Pronator teres muscle
長掌筋 Palmaris longus muscle
浅指屈筋 Flexor digitorum superficialis muscle
橈側手根伸筋 Extensor carpi radialis muscle
深指屈筋 Flexor digitorum profundus muscle

外　内

7-55

上腕三頭筋 Triceps brachii muscle
上腕骨小頭 Capitulum of humerus
橈骨 Radius
回外筋 Supinator muscle
総指伸筋 Extensor digitorum muscle

肘頭 Olecranon
内側上顆 Medial epicondyle
尺側手根屈筋 Flexor carpi ulnaris muscle
浅指屈筋 Flexor digitorum superficialis muscle
深指屈筋 Flexor digitorum profundus muscle

外　内

> **NOTE** テニス肘で，外側上顆周辺に疼痛を訴えるものは，外側型テニス肘とよばれ，バックハンドストロークにより痛みが出現する傾向がある．外側上顆に起始する手関節伸筋群，特に短橈側手根伸筋起始部の微小断裂によるものとされている．上腕骨の内側上顆周辺の疼痛を訴えるものは，内側型テニス肘とよばれ，上級テニスプレイヤーに多く，肘関節に強い牽引ストレスと手関節屈筋群の収縮が加わるフォアハンドストロークやサービスにより痛みが出現する傾向がある．

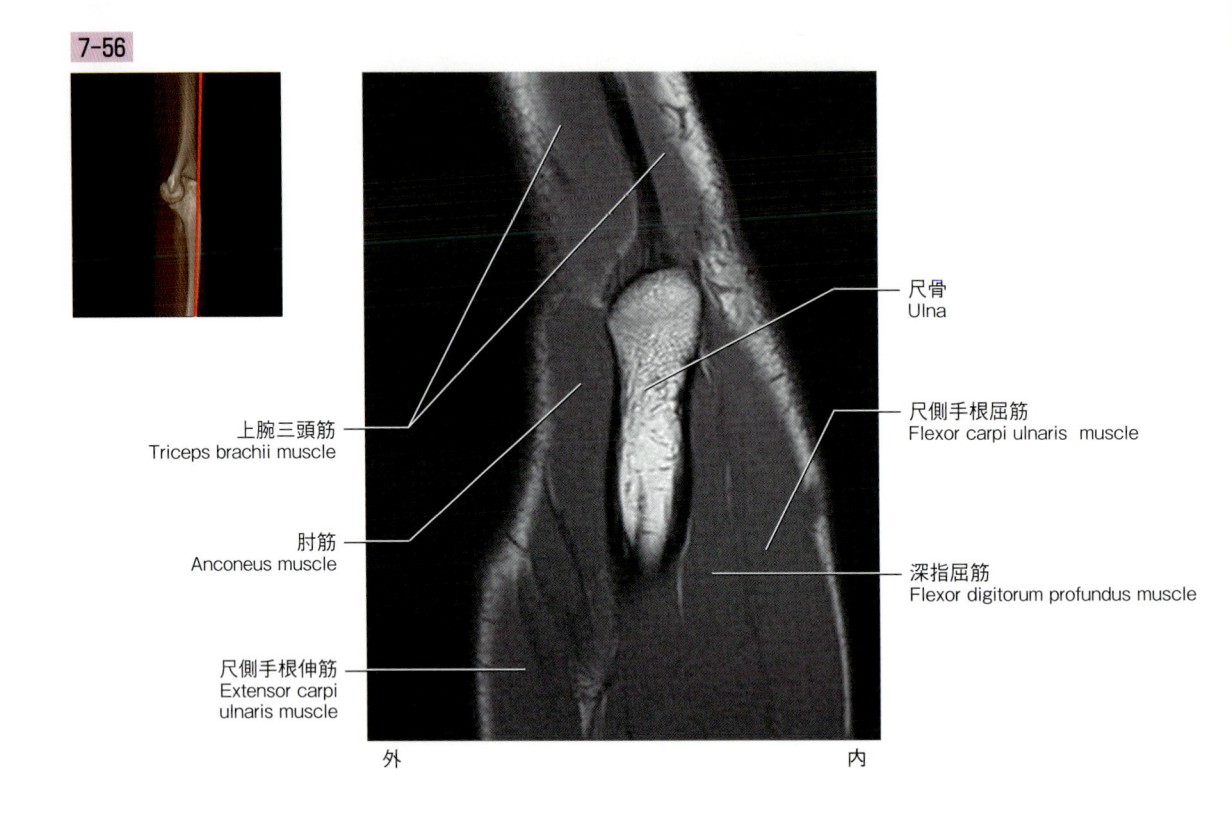

334　肘関節の断層解剖 ［冠状断像（MRI, プロトン密度強調像）］

7-56

- 上腕三頭筋 Triceps brachii muscle
- 肘筋 Anconeus muscle
- 尺側手根伸筋 Extensor carpi ulnaris muscle
- 尺骨 Ulna
- 尺側手根屈筋 Flexor carpi ulnaris muscle
- 深指屈筋 Flexor digitorum profundus muscle

外　　　内

NOTE 尺骨 Ulna と橈骨 Radius

　尺骨とは一尺（30.3 cm）に相当する骨の意味．Ulna はギリシャ語 olene（肘）から派生した語．橈骨の和名は撓（たわ）んだ形に由来する．Radius とはラテン語で尖った棒や杖を表し，この骨の解剖名につながるが，ほかに車輪の輻（spoke）の意味をもつ，円の半径は radius で表す．輻が周囲に散る様子から放射の radiation，そして radiology に発展する．

肘関節の断層解剖 ［矢状断像（MRI，プロトン密度強調像）］

7-57

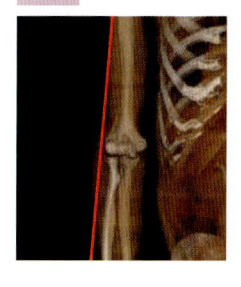

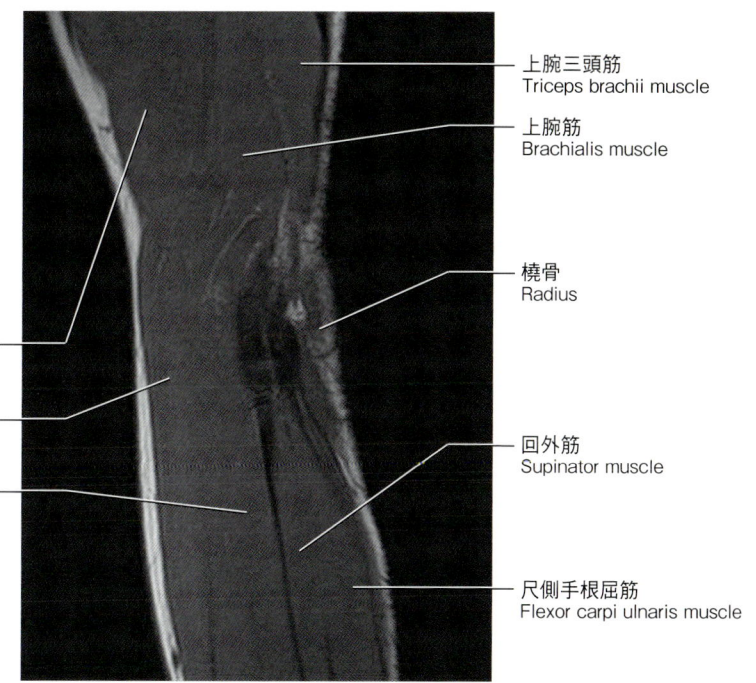

- 上腕三頭筋 Triceps brachii muscle
- 上腕筋 Brachialis muscle
- 橈骨 Radius
- 回外筋 Supinator muscle
- 尺側手根屈筋 Flexor carpi ulnaris muscle
- 上腕二頭筋 Biceps brachii muscle
- 腕橈骨筋 Brachioradialis muscle
- 橈側手根伸筋 Extensor carpi radialis muscle

7-58

- 上腕三頭筋 Triceps brachii muscle
- 上腕筋 Brachialis muscle
- 肘筋 Anconeus muscle
- 回外筋 Supinator muscle
- 尺側手根屈筋 Flexor carpi ulnaris muscle
- 上腕二頭筋 Biceps brachii muscle
- 上腕骨小頭 Capitulum of humerus
- 腕橈骨筋 Brachioradialis muscle
- 橈骨 Radius
- 長橈側手根伸筋 Extensor carpi radialis longus muscle

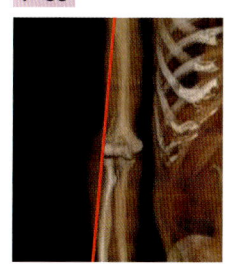

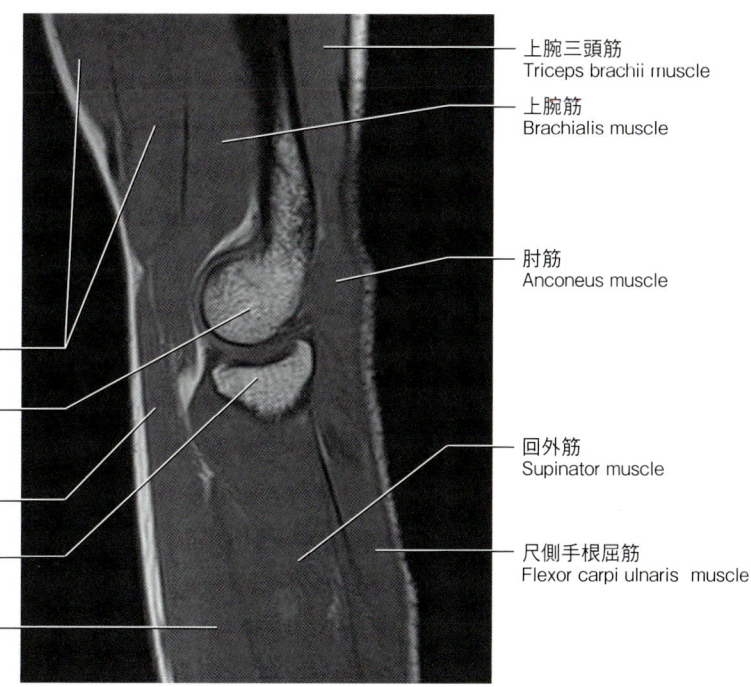

NOTE 屈伸運動には3つの屈筋（上腕筋，上腕二頭筋，腕橈骨筋）と，2つの伸筋（上腕三頭筋，肘筋）が関与する．

肘関節の断層解剖 ［矢状断像（MRI, プロトン密度強調像）］

7-59

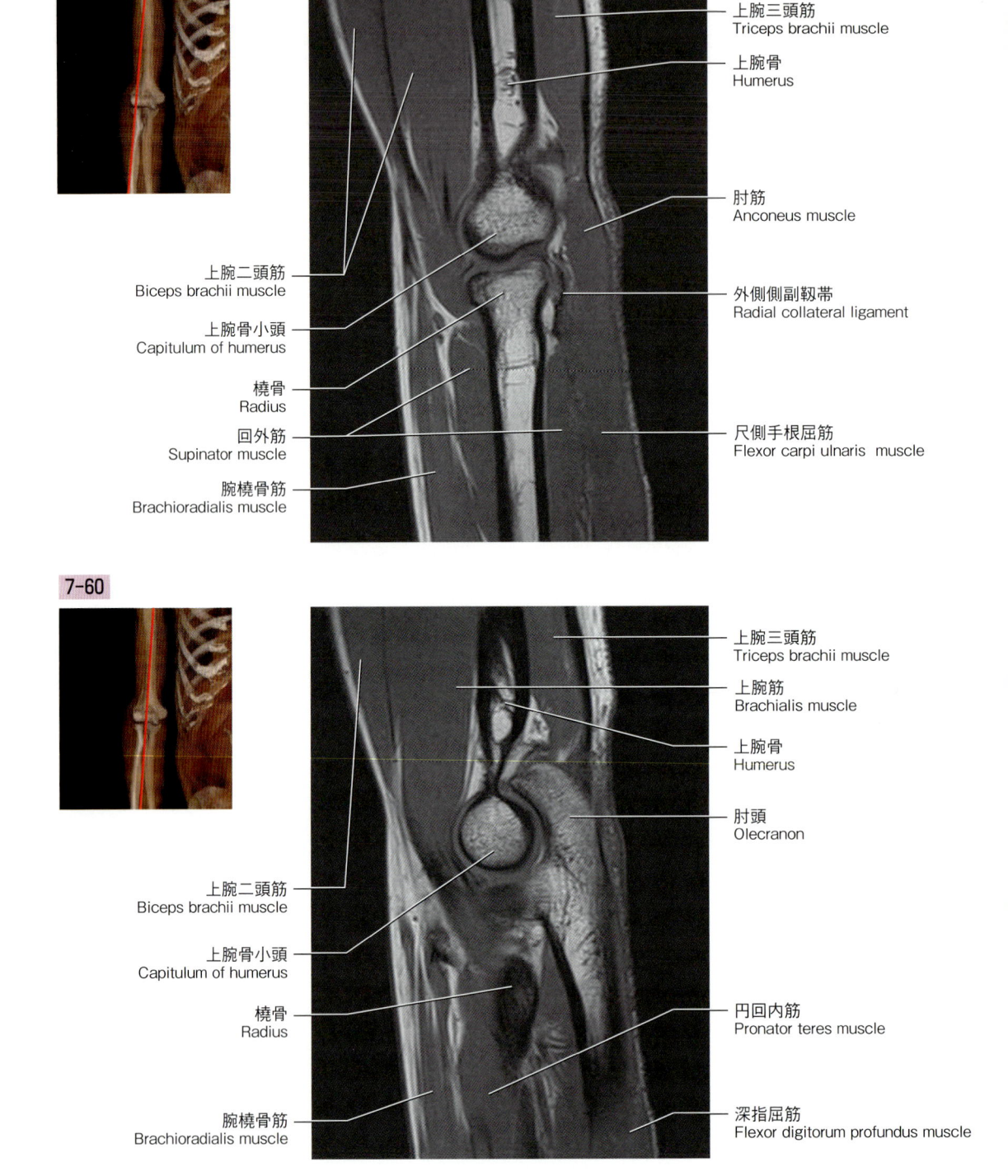

- 上腕三頭筋 Triceps brachii muscle
- 上腕骨 Humerus
- 肘筋 Anconeus muscle
- 外側側副靭帯 Radial collateral ligament
- 尺側手根屈筋 Flexor carpi ulnaris muscle
- 上腕二頭筋 Biceps brachii muscle
- 上腕骨小頭 Capitulum of humerus
- 橈骨 Radius
- 回外筋 Supinator muscle
- 腕橈骨筋 Brachioradialis muscle

7-60

- 上腕三頭筋 Triceps brachii muscle
- 上腕筋 Brachialis muscle
- 上腕骨 Humerus
- 肘頭 Olecranon
- 円回内筋 Pronator teres muscle
- 深指屈筋 Flexor digitorum profundus muscle
- 上腕二頭筋 Biceps brachii muscle
- 上腕骨小頭 Capitulum of humerus
- 橈骨 Radius
- 腕橈骨筋 Brachioradialis muscle

> **NOTE** 屈筋群は肘関節の前方に存在する．上腕筋は肘関節の前方で最も大きな筋として描出され，上腕二頭筋の深部に存在する．上腕筋腱は上腕二頭筋腱よりも細いが，筋腹に囲まれており外傷から保護されている．上腕二頭筋腱は上腕筋の前面で肘窩の表層を通るため，外傷にさらされやすい．腕橈骨筋は前腕が中間位にある時に強力な屈曲運動を行う．

肘関節の断層解剖 ［矢状断像（MRI，プロトン密度強調像）］

7-61

- 上腕三頭筋 Triceps brachii muscle
- 上腕筋 Brachialis muscle
- 上腕骨 Humerus
- 肘頭 Olecranon
- 尺骨 Ulna
- 深指屈筋 Flexor digitorum profundus muscle
- 上腕二頭筋 Biceps brachii muscle
- 上腕骨小頭 Capitulum of humerus
- 橈骨 Radius
- 円回内筋 Pronator teres muscle
- 腕橈骨筋 Brachioradialis muscle

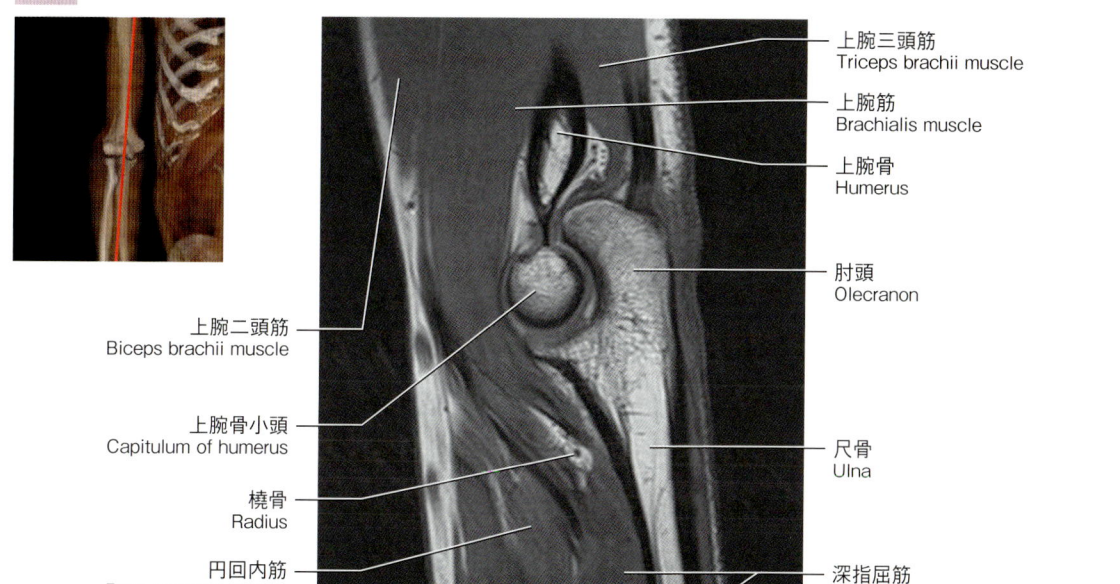

7-62

- 上腕三頭筋 Triceps brachii muscle
- 上腕筋 Brachialis muscle
- 上腕骨 Humerus
- 肘頭 Olecranon
- 深指屈筋 Flexor digitorum profundus muscle
- 上腕二頭筋 Biceps brachii muscle
- 上腕骨小頭 Capitulum of humerus
- 浅指屈筋 Flexor digitorum superficialis muscle
- 円回内筋 Pronator teres muscle

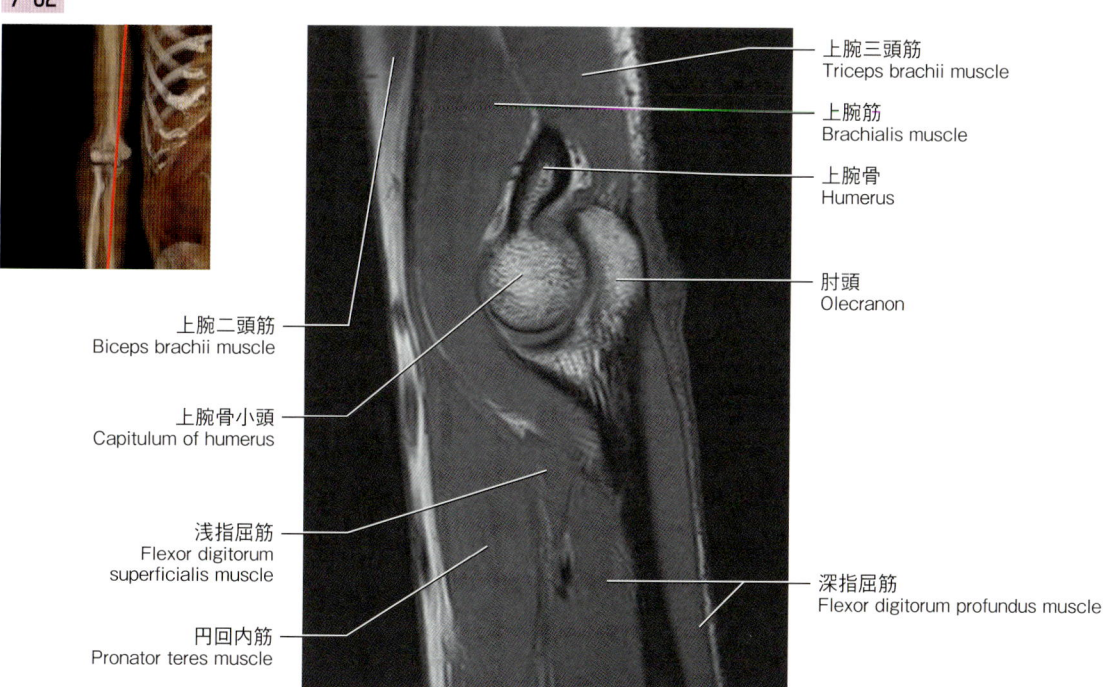

> **NOTE** 伸筋群は肘関節の後方に存在する．上腕三頭筋は腱板を形成して肘頭に停止するが，大腿四頭筋腱と同様に，膠原線維間に索状の信号をもつことがある．これらの索状信号は，健常人においても認められることがあり，腱板損傷と誤る可能性がある．

肘関節の断層解剖 ［矢状断像（MRI, プロトン密度強調像）］

7-63

- 上腕三頭筋 Triceps brachii muscle
- 肘頭 Olecranon
- 浅指屈筋 Flexor digitorum superficialis muscle
- 深指屈筋 Flexor digitorum profundus muscle
- 上腕筋 Brachialis muscle
- 上腕骨滑車 Trochlea of humerus
- 長橈側手根伸筋 Extensor carpi radialis longus muscle

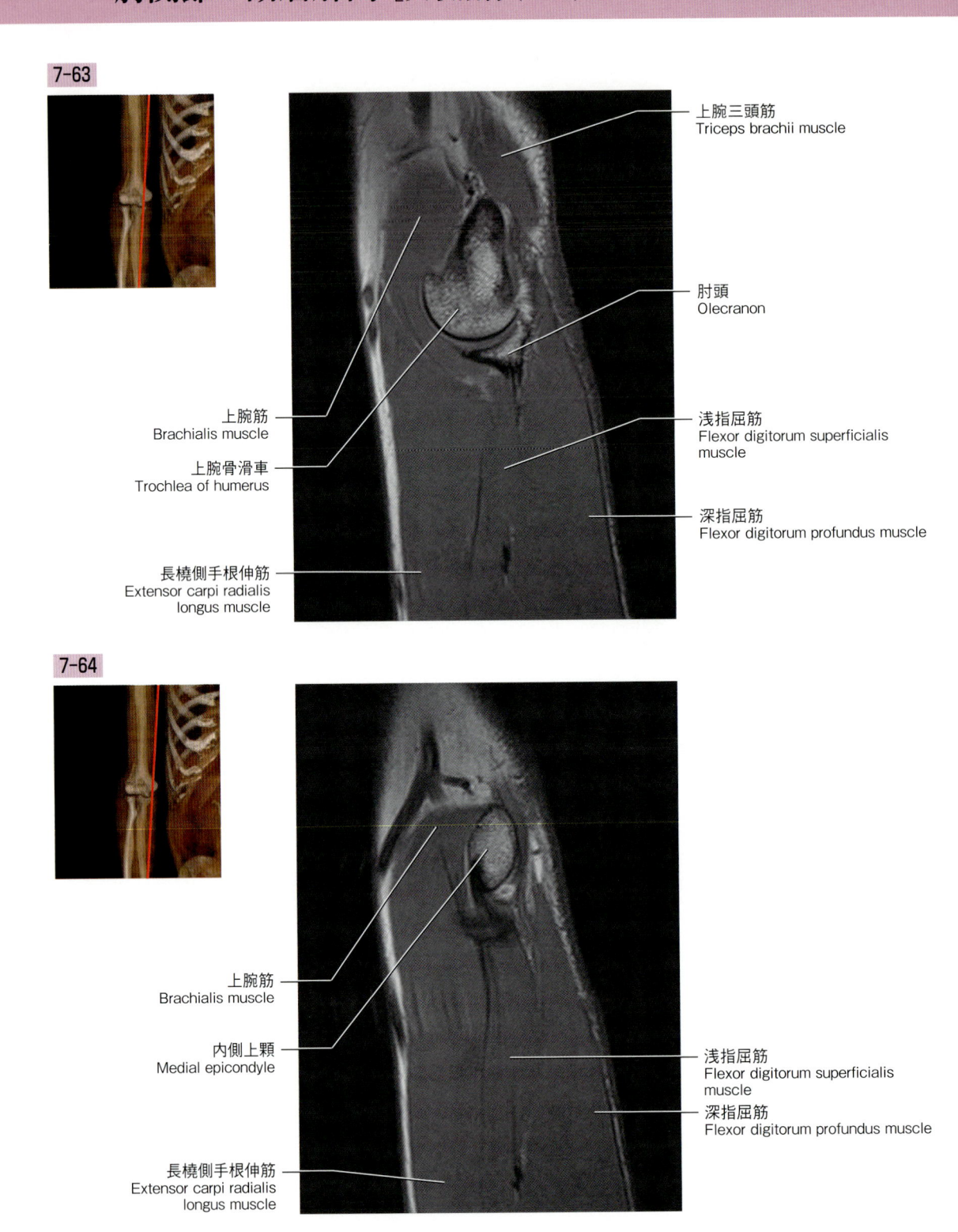

7-64

- 上腕筋 Brachialis muscle
- 内側上顆 Medial epicondyle
- 長橈側手根伸筋 Extensor carpi radialis longus muscle
- 浅指屈筋 Flexor digitorum superficialis muscle
- 深指屈筋 Flexor digitorum profundus muscle

NOTE 回旋運動には2つの回内筋（円回内筋，方形回内筋）と，2つの回外筋（上腕二頭筋，回外筋）が関与する．

肘関節の断層解剖 ［矢状断像（MRI, プロトン密度強調像）］

7-65

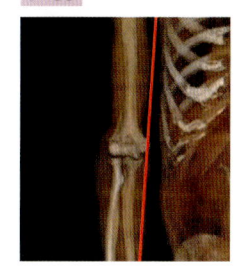

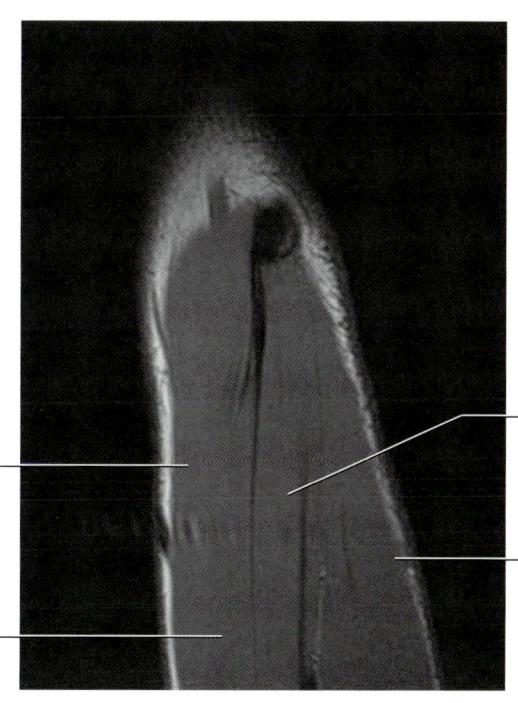

- 円回内筋 Pronator teres muscle
- 長橈側手根伸筋 Extensor carpi radialis longus muscle
- 浅指屈筋 Flexor digitorum superficialis muscle
- 深指屈筋 Flexor digitorum profundus muscle

手関節と手 (CT, VR 像)

7-66 手関節と手の体表解剖（前面）

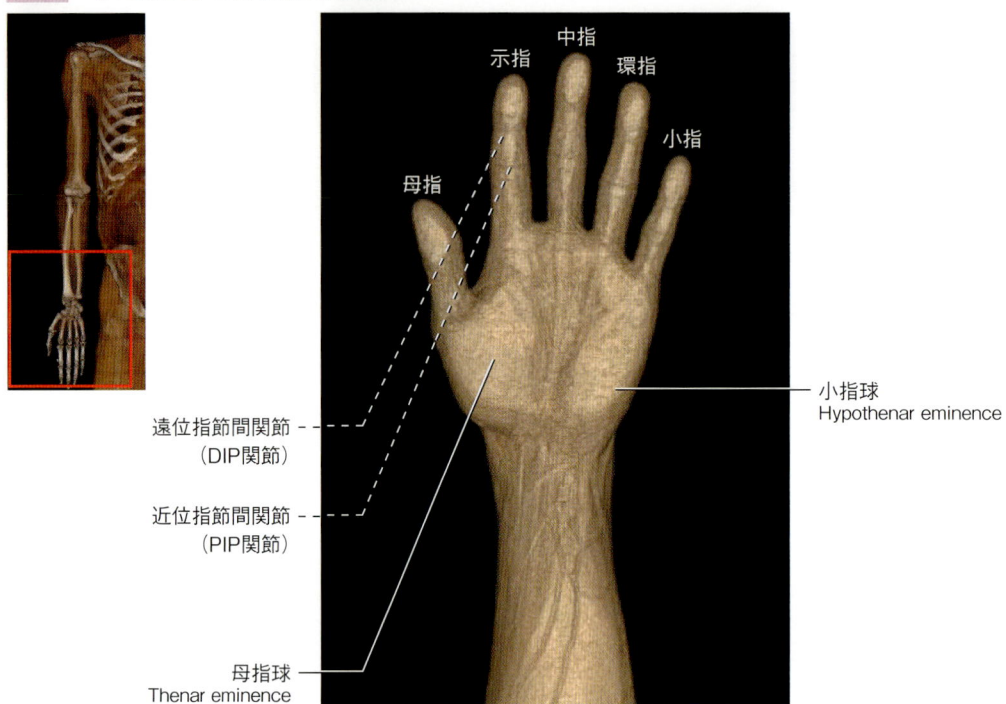

- 示指
- 中指
- 環指
- 小指
- 母指
- 遠位指節間関節（DIP関節）
- 近位指節間関節（PIP関節）
- 小指球 Hypothenar eminence
- 母指球 Thenar eminence

7-67 手関節と手の体表解剖（背面）

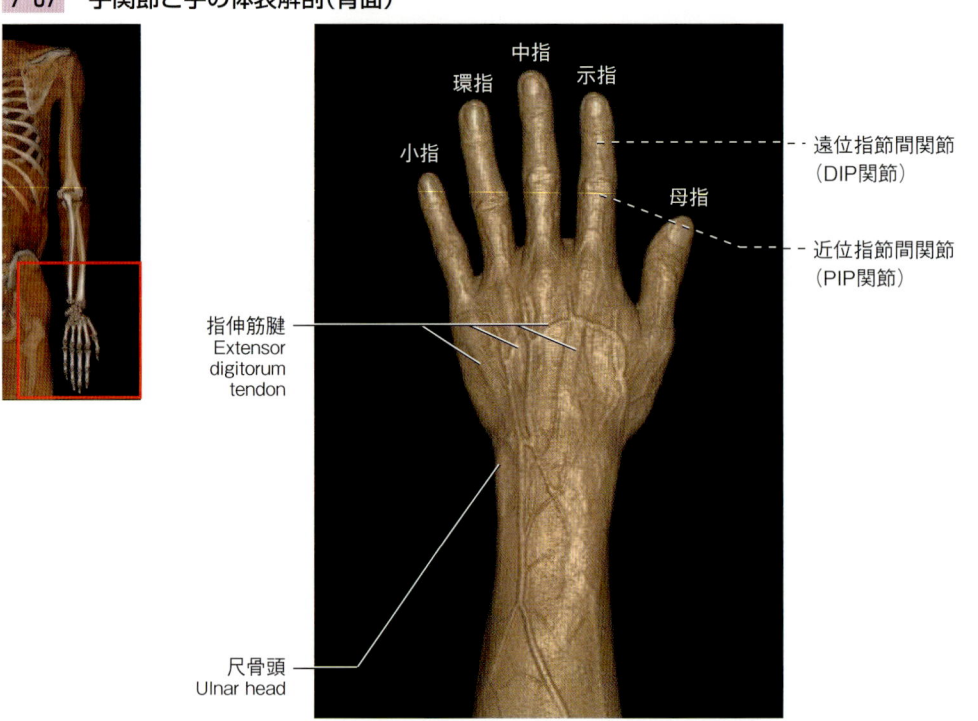

- 小指
- 環指
- 中指
- 示指
- 母指
- 遠位指節間関節（DIP関節）
- 近位指節間関節（PIP関節）
- 指伸筋腱 Extensor digitorum tendon
- 尺骨頭 Ulnar head

手関節と手（CT, VR像）

7-68 手関節と手の骨・腱（前面）

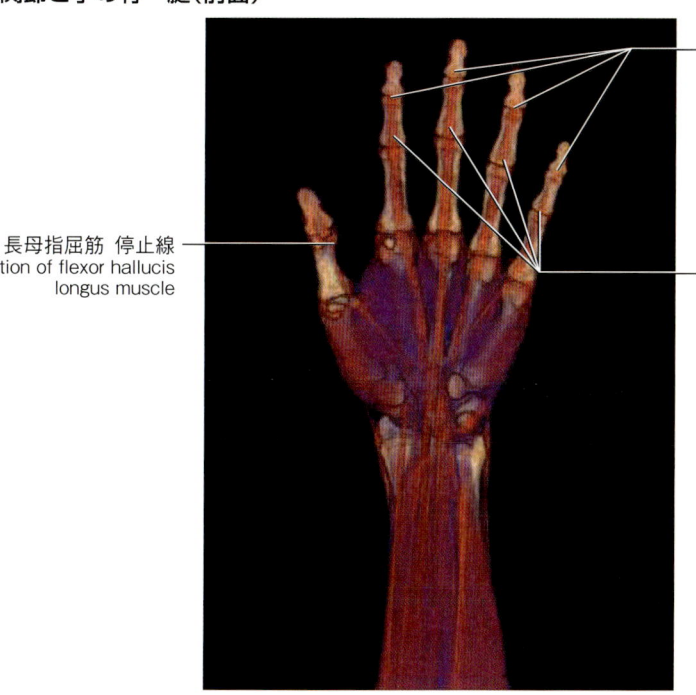

- 深指屈筋 停止線
  Insertion of flexor digitorum superficialis muscle
- 長母指屈筋 停止線
  Insertion of flexor hallucis longus muscle
- 浅指屈筋 停止線
  Insertion of flexor digitorum superficialis muscle

7-69 手関節と手の骨・腱（背面）

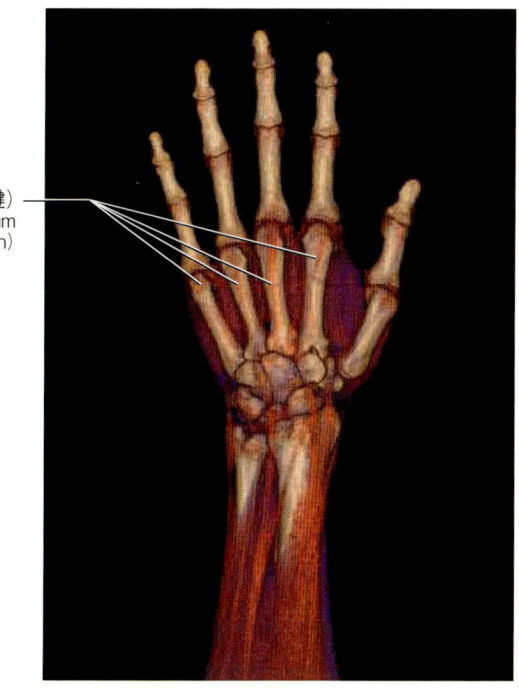

- 指伸筋（腱）
  Extensor digitorum muscle（tendon）

NOTE 手関節（Wrist joint）は，橈骨手根関節，手根間関節，豆状三角骨関節の3つの関節の総称で，橈骨手根関節よりも遠位にあるすべての関節を包括する手の関節（Joints of hand）とは区別される．

手関節と手（CT, VR 像）

7-70 手関節と手の骨（前面）

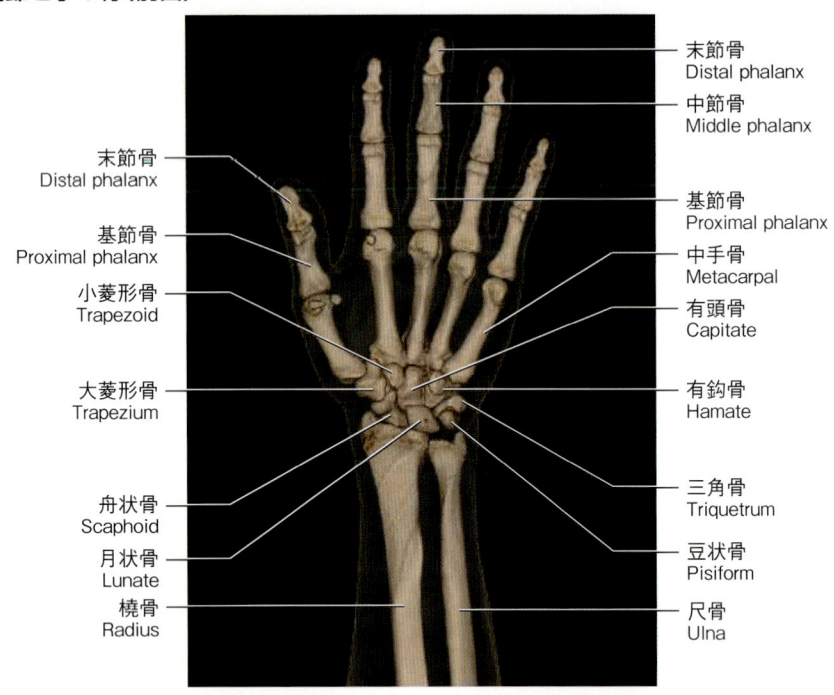

末節骨 Distal phalanx
中節骨 Middle phalanx
基節骨 Proximal phalanx
中手骨 Metacarpal
有頭骨 Capitate
有鈎骨 Hamate
三角骨 Triquetrum
豆状骨 Pisiform
尺骨 Ulna

末節骨 Distal phalanx
基節骨 Proximal phalanx
小菱形骨 Trapezoid
大菱形骨 Trapezium
舟状骨 Scaphoid
月状骨 Lunate
橈骨 Radius

7-71 手関節と手の骨（背面）

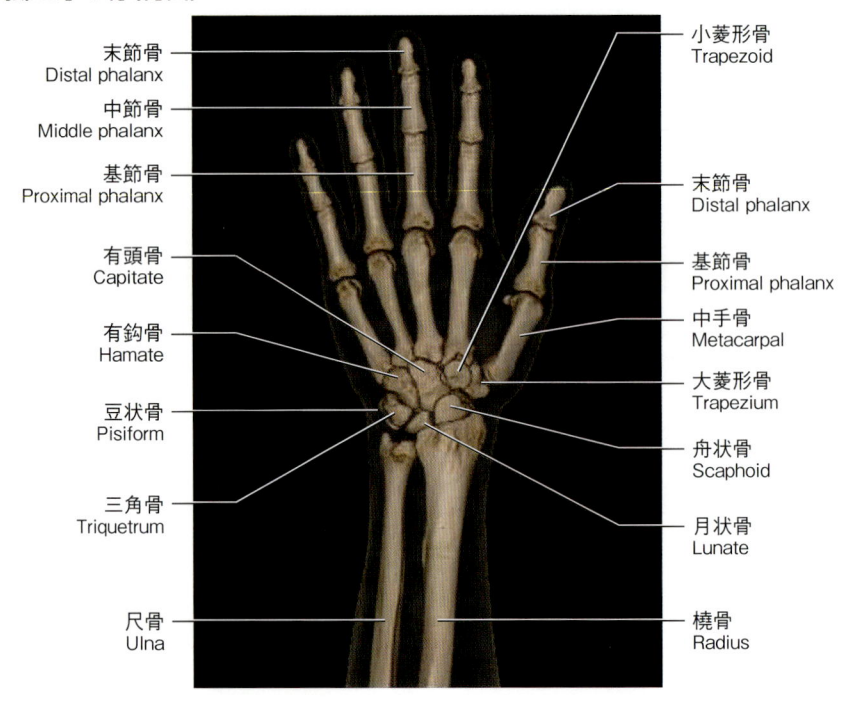

末節骨 Distal phalanx
中節骨 Middle phalanx
基節骨 Proximal phalanx
有頭骨 Capitate
有鈎骨 Hamate
豆状骨 Pisiform
三角骨 Triquetrum
尺骨 Ulna

小菱形骨 Trapezoid
末節骨 Distal phalanx
基節骨 Proximal phalanx
中手骨 Metacarpal
大菱形骨 Trapezium
舟状骨 Scaphoid
月状骨 Lunate
橈骨 Radius

> **NOTE** 手関節を構成する骨は，橈骨と尺骨の遠位端，8個の手根骨，および中手骨である．手根骨は手根骨近位列（Proximal carpal row）と手根骨遠位列（Distal carpal row）とからなり，手根骨近位列は橈骨より舟状骨，月状骨，三角骨，豆状骨，手根骨遠位列は大菱形骨，小菱形骨，有頭骨，有鈎骨である．

手関節と手の断層解剖 [横断像（MRI，プロトン密度強調像）]

7-72

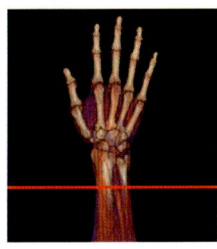

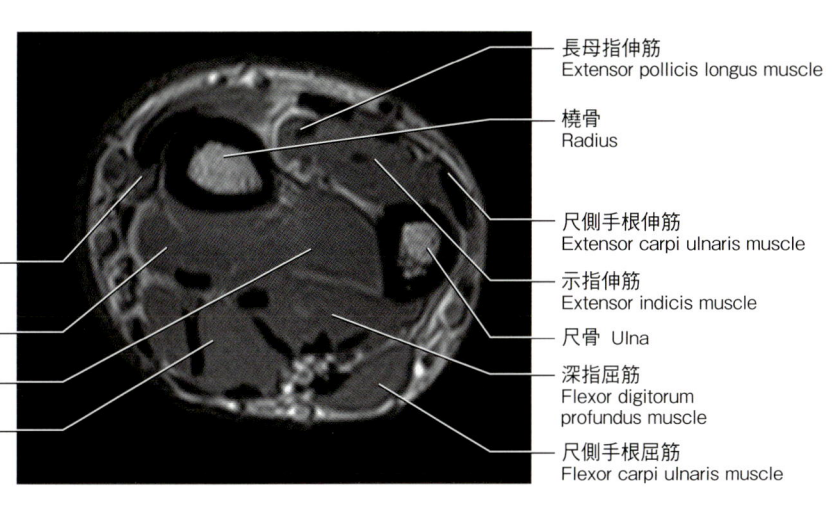

- 長母指伸筋 Extensor pollicis longus muscle
- 橈骨 Radius
- 尺側手根伸筋 Extensor carpi ulnaris muscle
- 示指伸筋 Extensor indicis muscle
- 尺骨 Ulna
- 深指屈筋 Flexor digitorum profundus muscle
- 尺側手根屈筋 Flexor carpi ulnaris muscle
- 長母指外転筋 Abductor pollicis longus muscle
- 長母指屈筋 Flexor pollicis longus muscle
- 方形回内筋 Pronator quadratus muscle
- 浅指屈筋 Flexor digitorum superficialis muscle

7-73

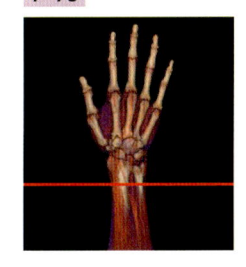

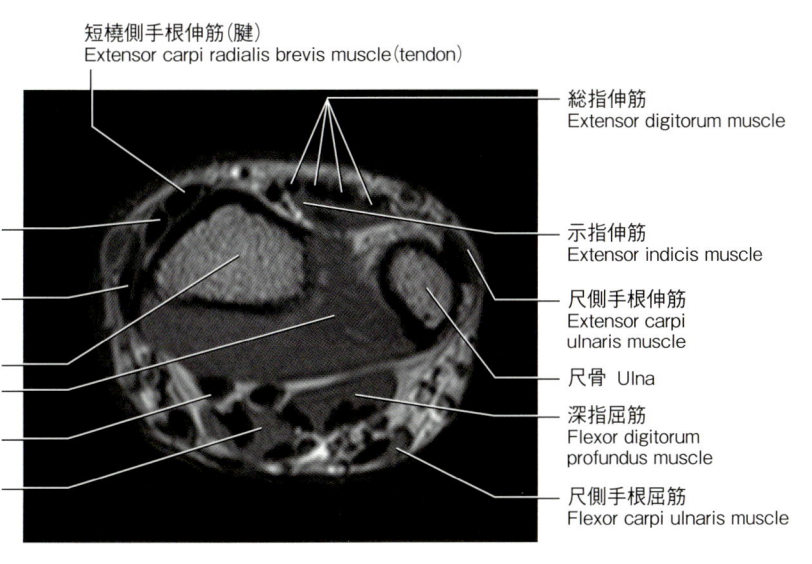

- 短橈側手根伸筋（腱）Extensor carpi radialis brevis muscle (tendon)
- 総指伸筋 Extensor digitorum muscle
- 示指伸筋 Extensor indicis muscle
- 尺側手根伸筋 Extensor carpi ulnaris muscle
- 尺骨 Ulna
- 深指屈筋 Flexor digitorum profundus muscle
- 尺側手根屈筋 Flexor carpi ulnaris muscle
- 長橈側手根伸筋（腱）Extensor carpi radialis longus muscle (tendon)
- 長母指外転筋（腱）Abductor pollicis longus muscle (tendon)
- 橈骨 Radius
- 方形回内筋 Pronator quadratus muscle
- 長母指屈筋 Flexor pollicis longus muscle
- 浅指屈筋 Flexor digitorum superficialis muscle

NOTE 長母指外転筋腱や短母指伸筋腱が，橈骨茎状突起との摩擦などにより腱炎や腱鞘炎を起こしやすく，de Quervain（ドゥ・ケルヴァン）病として知られる．

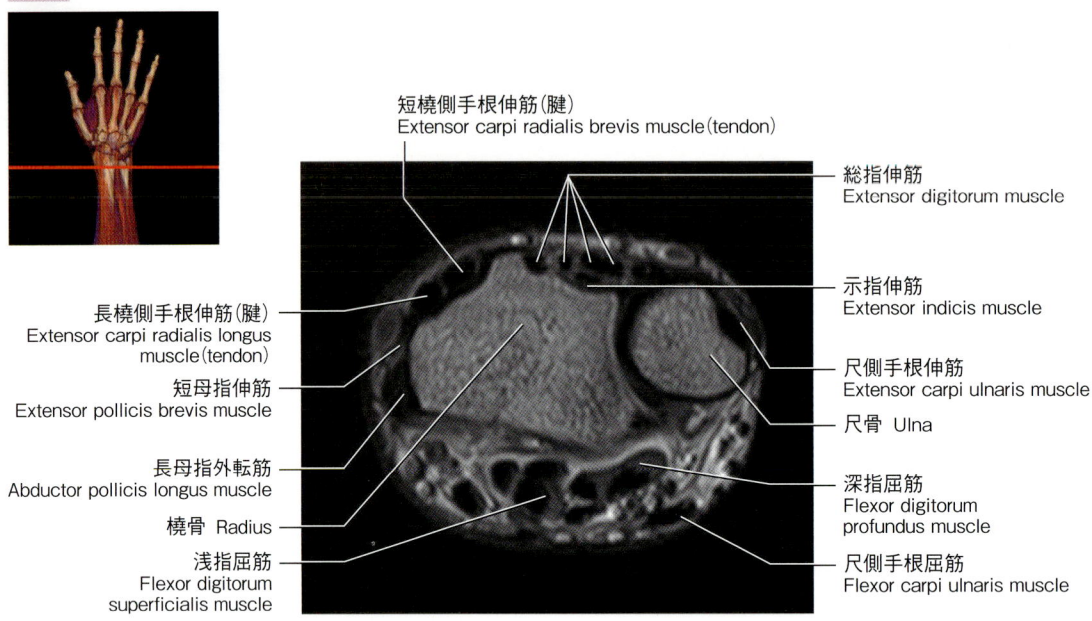

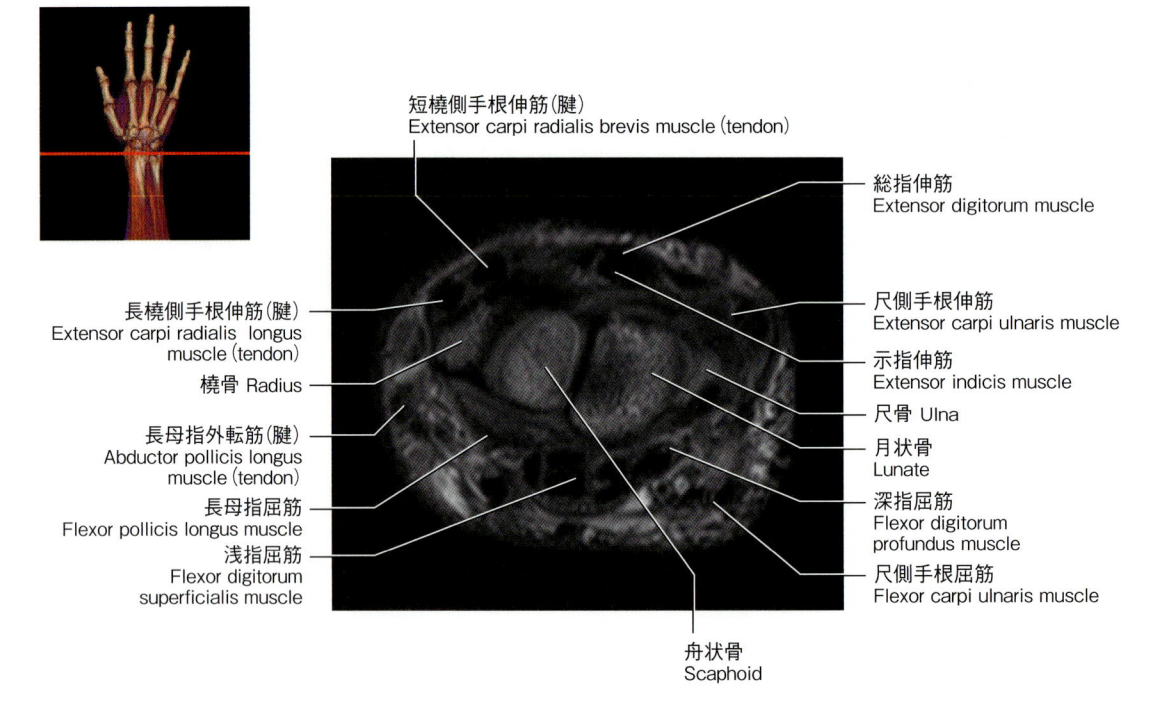

344 手関節と手の断層解剖 ［横断像（MRI, プロトン密度強調像）］

7-74

- 短橈側手根伸筋（腱） Extensor carpi radialis brevis muscle (tendon)
- 総指伸筋 Extensor digitorum muscle
- 示指伸筋 Extensor indicis muscle
- 長橈側手根伸筋（腱） Extensor carpi radialis longus muscle (tendon)
- 短母指伸筋 Extensor pollicis brevis muscle
- 尺側手根伸筋 Extensor carpi ulnaris muscle
- 長母指外転筋 Abductor pollicis longus muscle
- 尺骨 Ulna
- 橈骨 Radius
- 深指屈筋 Flexor digitorum profundus muscle
- 浅指屈筋 Flexor digitorum superficialis muscle
- 尺側手根屈筋 Flexor carpi ulnaris muscle

7-75

- 短橈側手根伸筋（腱） Extensor carpi radialis brevis muscle (tendon)
- 総指伸筋 Extensor digitorum muscle
- 尺側手根伸筋 Extensor carpi ulnaris muscle
- 長橈側手根伸筋（腱） Extensor carpi radialis longus muscle (tendon)
- 示指伸筋 Extensor indicis muscle
- 橈骨 Radius
- 尺骨 Ulna
- 長母指外転筋（腱） Abductor pollicis longus muscle (tendon)
- 月状骨 Lunate
- 長母指屈筋 Flexor pollicis longus muscle
- 深指屈筋 Flexor digitorum profundus muscle
- 浅指屈筋 Flexor digitorum superficialis muscle
- 尺側手根屈筋 Flexor carpi ulnaris muscle
- 舟状骨 Scaphoid

手関節と手の断層解剖 [横断像（MRI，プロトン密度強調像）]

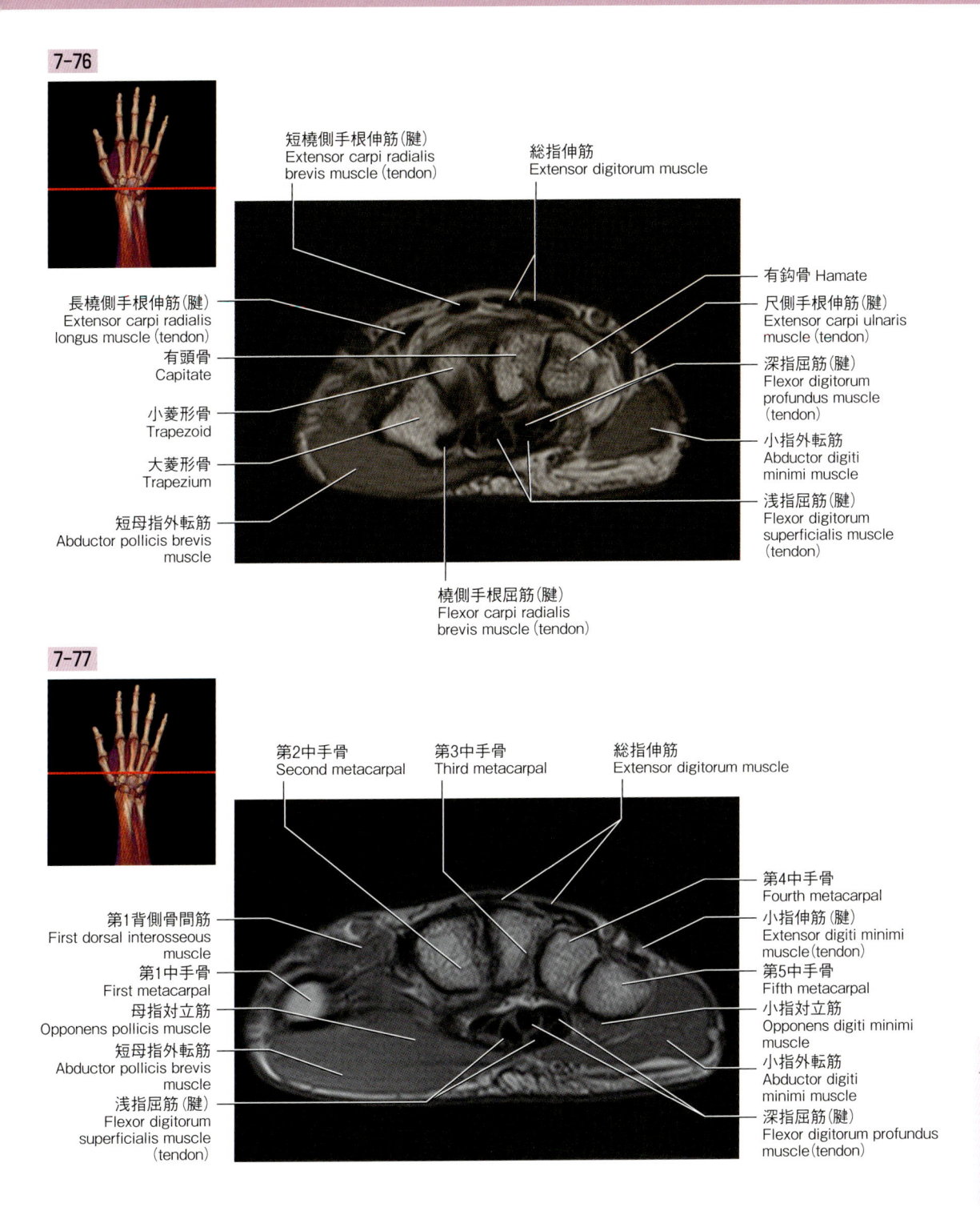

7-76

- 短橈側手根伸筋（腱） Extensor carpi radialis brevis muscle (tendon)
- 総指伸筋 Extensor digitorum muscle
- 有鈎骨 Hamate
- 尺側手根伸筋（腱） Extensor carpi ulnaris muscle (tendon)
- 深指屈筋（腱） Flexor digitorum profundus muscle (tendon)
- 小指外転筋 Abductor digiti minimi muscle
- 浅指屈筋（腱） Flexor digitorum superficialis muscle (tendon)
- 橈側手根屈筋（腱） Flexor carpi radialis brevis muscle (tendon)
- 長橈側手根伸筋（腱） Extensor carpi radialis longus muscle (tendon)
- 有頭骨 Capitate
- 小菱形骨 Trapezoid
- 大菱形骨 Trapezium
- 短母指外転筋 Abductor pollicis brevis muscle

7-77

- 第2中手骨 Second metacarpal
- 第3中手骨 Third metacarpal
- 総指伸筋 Extensor digitorum muscle
- 第4中手骨 Fourth metacarpal
- 小指伸筋（腱） Extensor digiti minimi muscle (tendon)
- 第5中手骨 Fifth metacarpal
- 小指対立筋 Opponens digiti minimi muscle
- 小指外転筋 Abductor digiti minimi muscle
- 深指屈筋（腱） Flexor digitorum profundus muscle (tendon)
- 第1背側骨間筋 First dorsal interosseous muscle
- 第1中手骨 First metacarpal
- 母指対立筋 Opponens pollicis muscle
- 短母指外転筋 Abductor pollicis brevis muscle
- 浅指屈筋（腱） Flexor digitorum superficialis muscle (tendon)

> **NOTE** 手根管(Carpal tunnel)は内側，背側，外側壁を手根骨で，掌側壁を屈筋支帯適正される管腔構造である．その中を合計8本の深枝および浅指屈筋腱と腱鞘，長母指屈筋腱と腱鞘，正中神経が通る．限られた管腔内を多くの腱・腱鞘および正中神経が通過するため，手根管内の腱鞘炎やガングリオンなどにより圧迫性に正中神経障害を生じ，手根管症候群をきたすことがある．ギオン管(Guyon's canal)は，前壁を掌側手根靱帯，後壁を屈筋支帯，尺側壁を豆状骨により形成される管腔構造である．この管腔の中の尺側を尺骨神経が，橈側を尺骨動静脈が通る．

手関節と手の断層解剖 ［横断像（MRI, プロトン密度強調像）］

7-78

- 第3中手骨 Third metacarpal
- 第2中手骨 Second metacarpal
- 背側骨間筋 Dorsal interosseous muscle
- 第1中手骨 First metacarpal
- 長母指屈筋（腱） Flexor pollicis longus muscle (tendon)
- 総指伸筋 Extensor digitorum muscle
- 第4中手骨 Fourth metacarpal
- 掌側骨間筋 Palmar interosseous muscle
- 小指対立筋（腱） Opponens digiti minimi muscle (tendon)
- 小指外転筋 Abductor digiti minimi muscle
- 深指屈筋（腱） Flexor digitorum profundus muscle (tendon)
- 母指内転筋 Adductor pollicis muscle
- 浅指屈筋（腱） Flexor digitorum superficialis muscle (tendon)

7-79

- 第2基節骨 Second proximal phalanx
- 第1末節骨 First distal phalanx
- 指屈筋（腱） Flexor digitorum muscle (tendon)
- 第3基節骨 Third proximal phalanx
- 第5中節骨 Fifth middle phalanx
- 第4基節骨 Fourth proximal phalanx

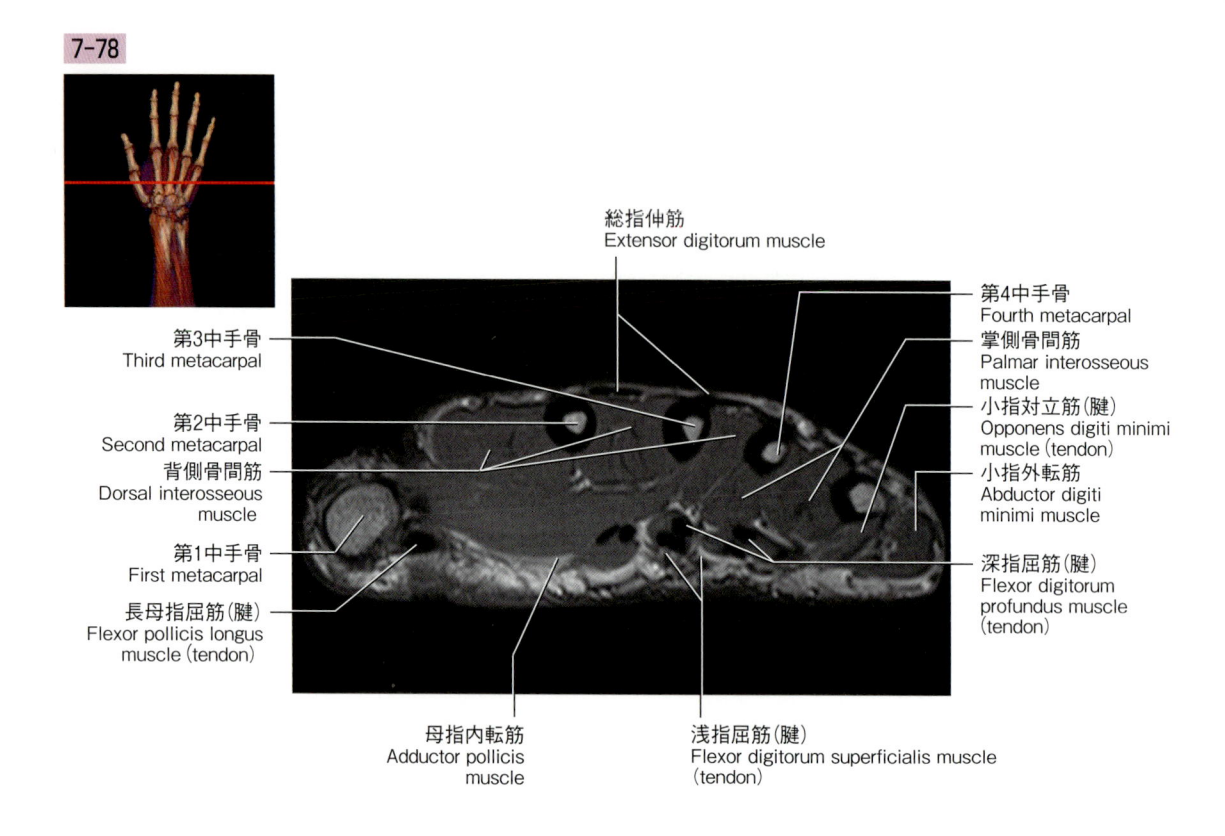

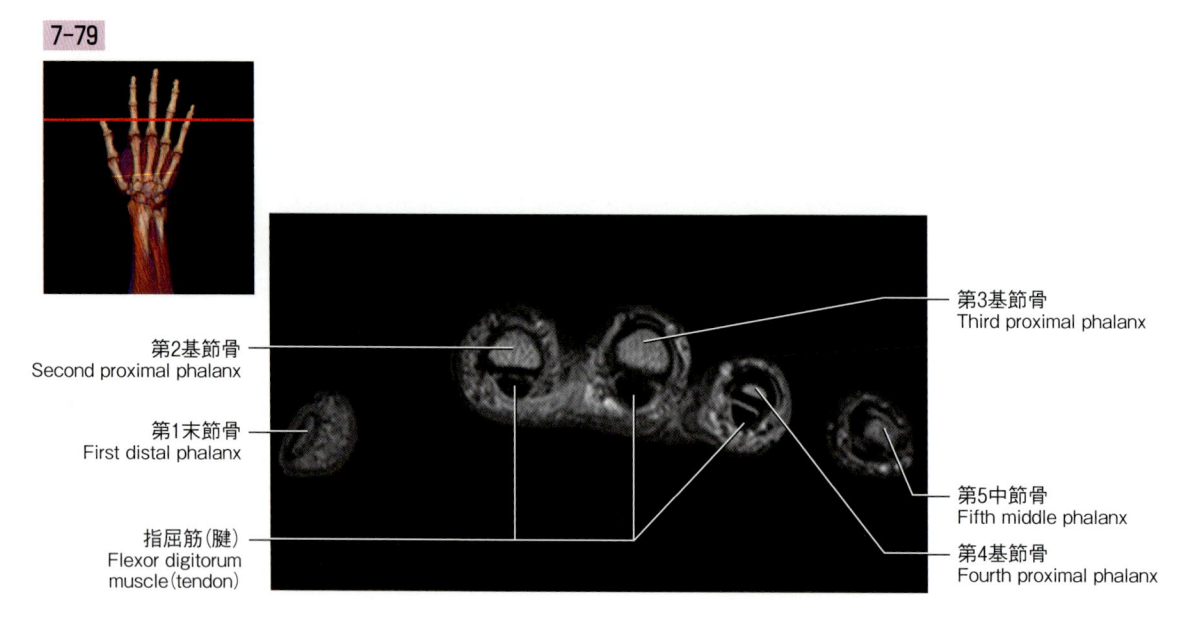

> **NOTE** 手掌腱膜は，長掌筋腱の線維が延長し手掌中央部で扇状に広がったもので，手根部では屈筋支帯の掌側に存在する．手掌腱膜の進行性拘縮はDupuytren（デュピュイトラン）拘縮とよばれ，小指や尺側環指に屈曲拘縮をきたす．

第3指の断層解剖 [横断像（MRI, プロトン密度強調像）]

7-80

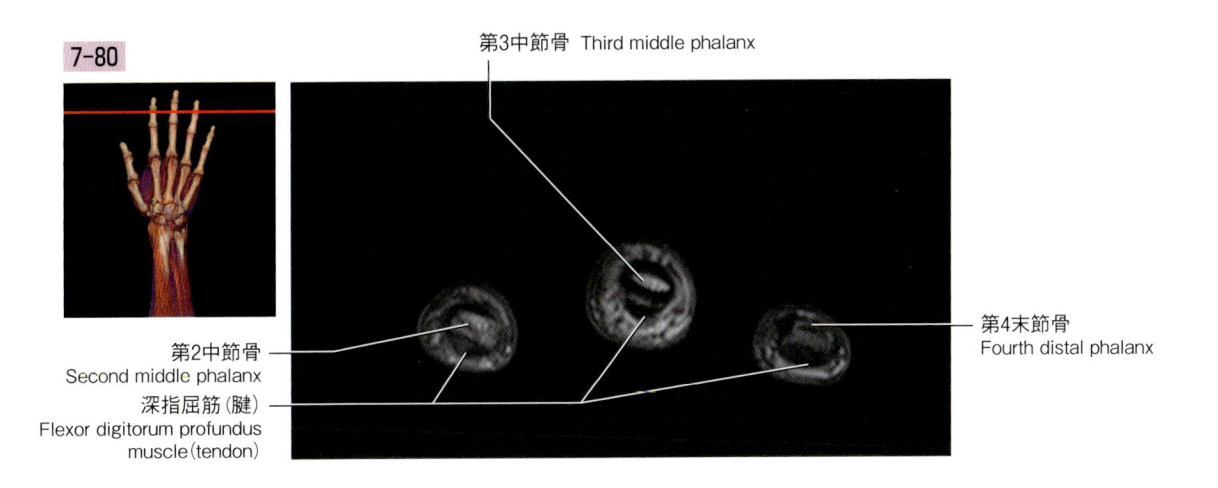

第3中節骨 Third middle phalanx

第2中節骨 Second middle phalanx

深指屈筋（腱） Flexor digitorum profundus muscle（tendon）

第4末節骨 Fourth distal phalanx

7-81

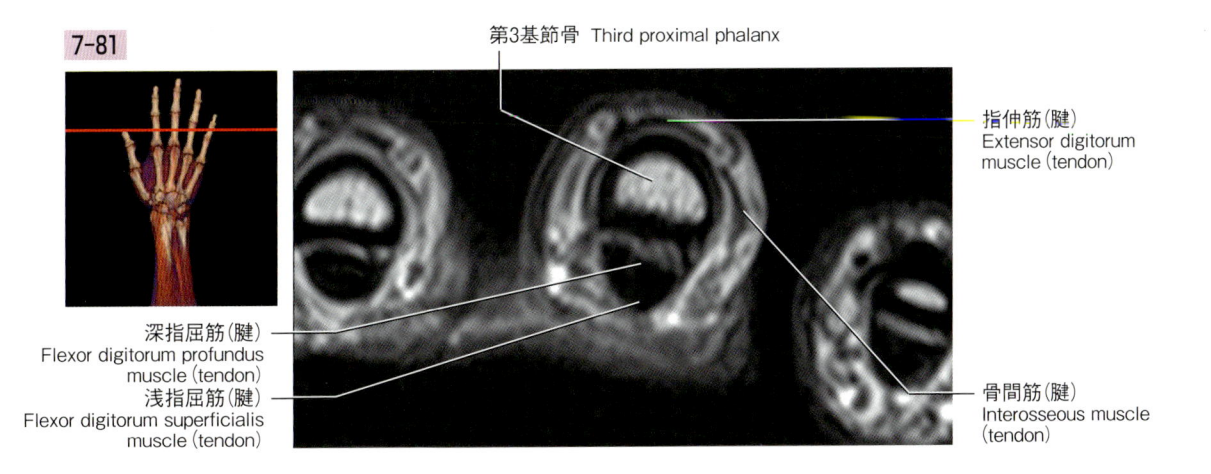

第3基節骨 Third proximal phalanx

指伸筋（腱） Extensor digitorum muscle（tendon）

深指屈筋（腱） Flexor digitorum profundus muscle（tendon）

浅指屈筋（腱） Flexor digitorum superficialis muscle（tendon）

骨間筋（腱） Interosseous muscle（tendon）

第3指の断層解剖 ［横断像（MRI, プロトン密度強調像）］

7-82

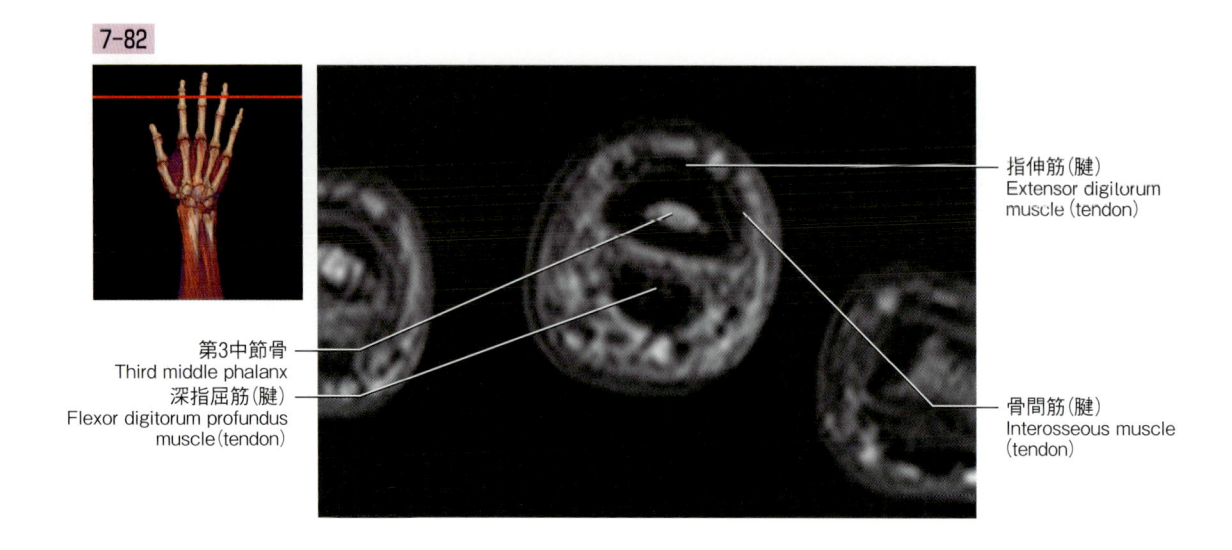

- 第3中節骨 Third middle phalanx
- 深指屈筋（腱） Flexor digitorum profundus muscle (tendon)
- 指伸筋（腱） Extensor digitorum muscle (tendon)
- 骨間筋（腱） Interosseous muscle (tendon)

7-83

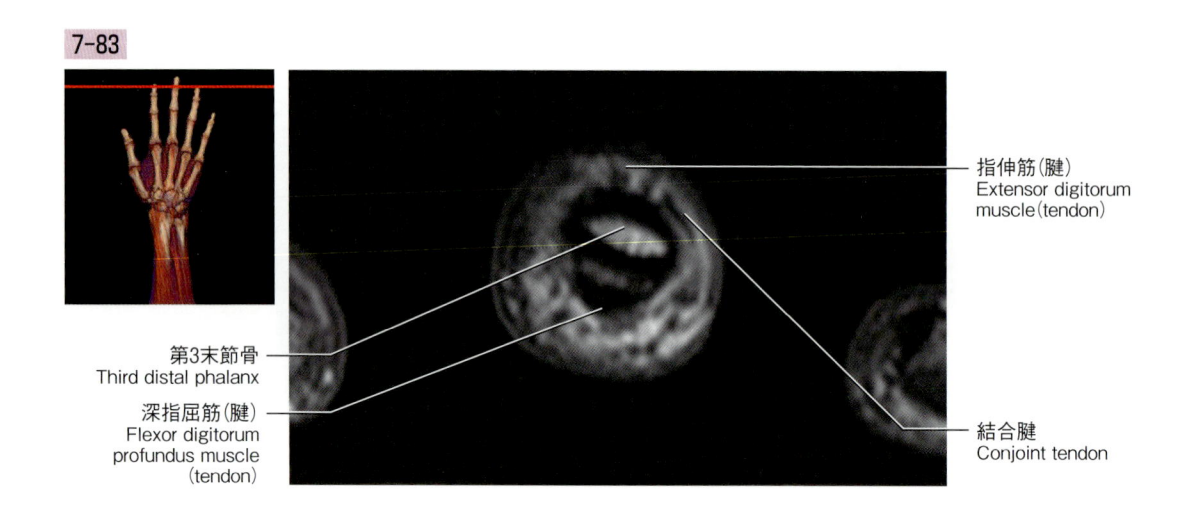

- 第3末節骨 Third distal phalanx
- 深指屈筋（腱） Flexor digitorum profundus muscle (tendon)
- 指伸筋（腱） Extensor digitorum muscle (tendon)
- 結合腱 Conjoint tendon

手関節と手の断層解剖 [冠状断像（MRI, プロトン密度強調像）]

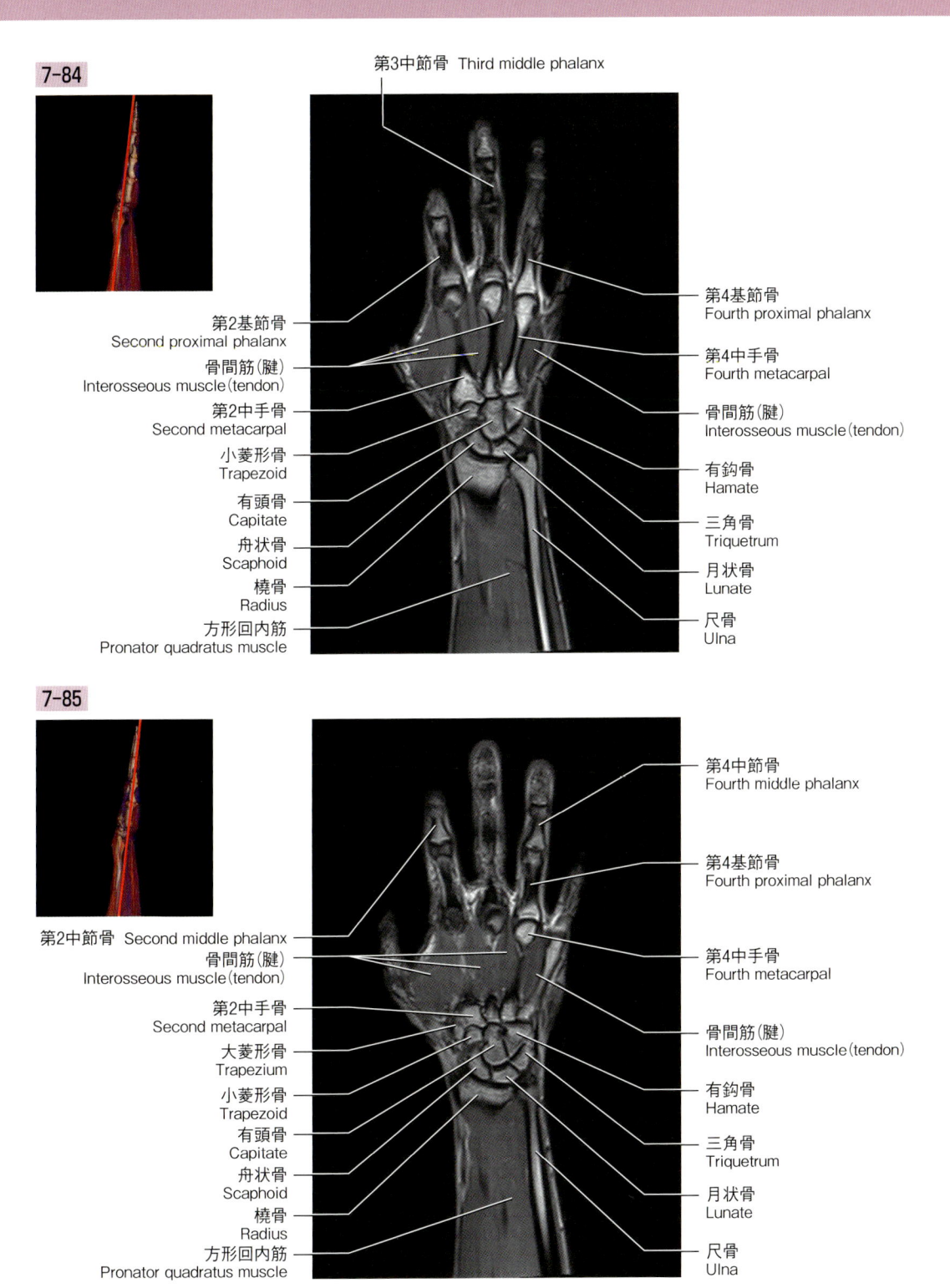

7-84

- 第3中節骨 Third middle phalanx
- 第2基節骨 Second proximal phalanx
- 骨間筋（腱）Interosseous muscle (tendon)
- 第2中手骨 Second metacarpal
- 小菱形骨 Trapezoid
- 有頭骨 Capitate
- 舟状骨 Scaphoid
- 橈骨 Radius
- 方形回内筋 Pronator quadratus muscle
- 第4基節骨 Fourth proximal phalanx
- 第4中手骨 Fourth metacarpal
- 骨間筋（腱）Interosseous muscle (tendon)
- 有鈎骨 Hamate
- 三角骨 Triquetrum
- 月状骨 Lunate
- 尺骨 Ulna

7-85

- 第2中節骨 Second middle phalanx
- 骨間筋（腱）Interosseous muscle (tendon)
- 第2中手骨 Second metacarpal
- 大菱形骨 Trapezium
- 小菱形骨 Trapezoid
- 有頭骨 Capitate
- 舟状骨 Scaphoid
- 橈骨 Radius
- 方形回内筋 Pronator quadratus muscle
- 第4中節骨 Fourth middle phalanx
- 第4基節骨 Fourth proximal phalanx
- 第4中手骨 Fourth metacarpal
- 骨間筋（腱）Interosseous muscle (tendon)
- 有鈎骨 Hamate
- 三角骨 Triquetrum
- 月状骨 Lunate
- 尺骨 Ulna

> **NOTE** 三角線維軟骨複合体（Triangular fibrocartilage complex）には、三角線維軟骨、メニスカス類似体、尺側側副靱帯、背側橈尺靱帯、掌側橈尺靱帯、尺側手根伸筋腱鞘、掌側尺骨手根靱帯（尺骨月状靱帯と尺骨三角靱帯）により構成される。三角線維軟骨複合体は手関節尺側の安定性を保つ。

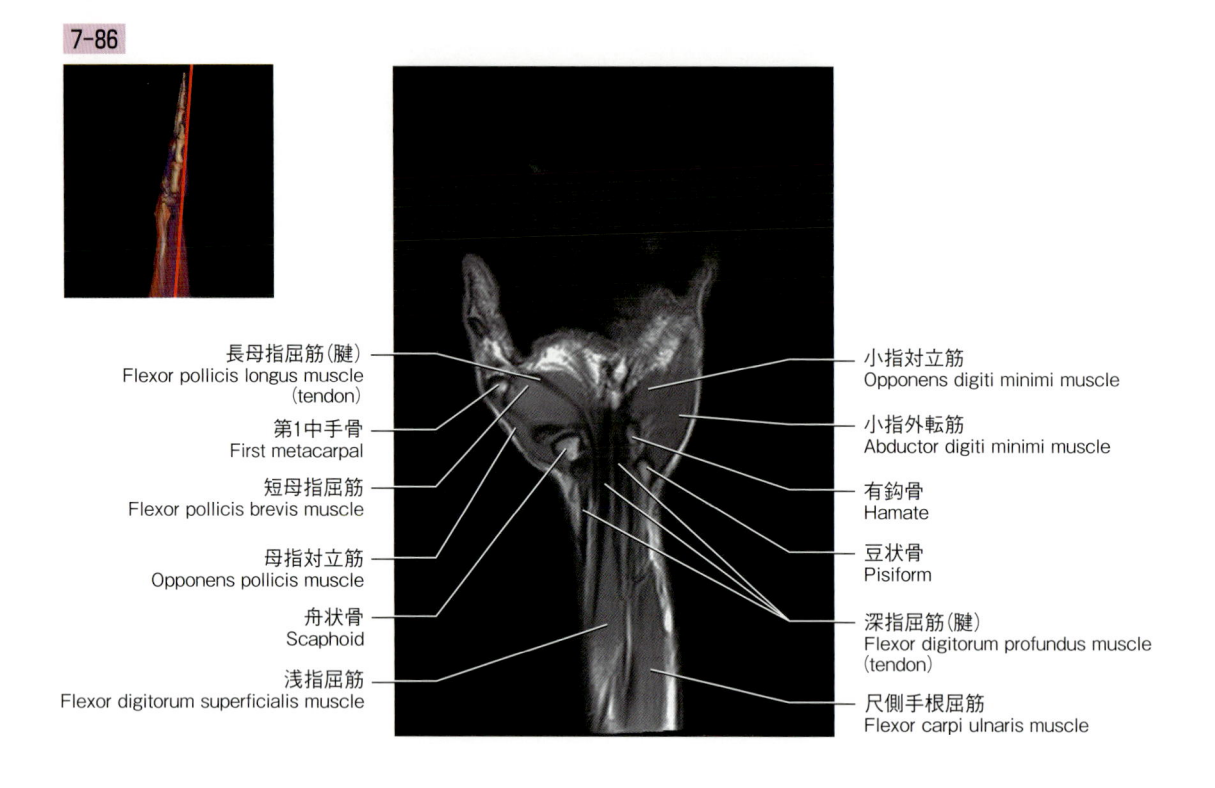

手関節と手の断層解剖 ［冠状断像（MRI，プロトン密度強調像）］

7-86

- 長母指屈筋（腱） Flexor pollicis longus muscle (tendon)
- 第1中手骨 First metacarpal
- 短母指屈筋 Flexor pollicis brevis muscle
- 母指対立筋 Opponens pollicis muscle
- 舟状骨 Scaphoid
- 浅指屈筋 Flexor digitorum superficialis muscle
- 小指対立筋 Opponens digiti minimi muscle
- 小指外転筋 Abductor digiti minimi muscle
- 有鈎骨 Hamate
- 豆状骨 Pisiform
- 深指屈筋（腱） Flexor digitorum profundus muscle (tendon)
- 尺側手根屈筋 Flexor carpi ulnaris muscle

第3指の断層解剖 [矢状断像（MRI，プロトン密度強調像）]

7-87

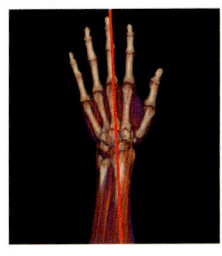

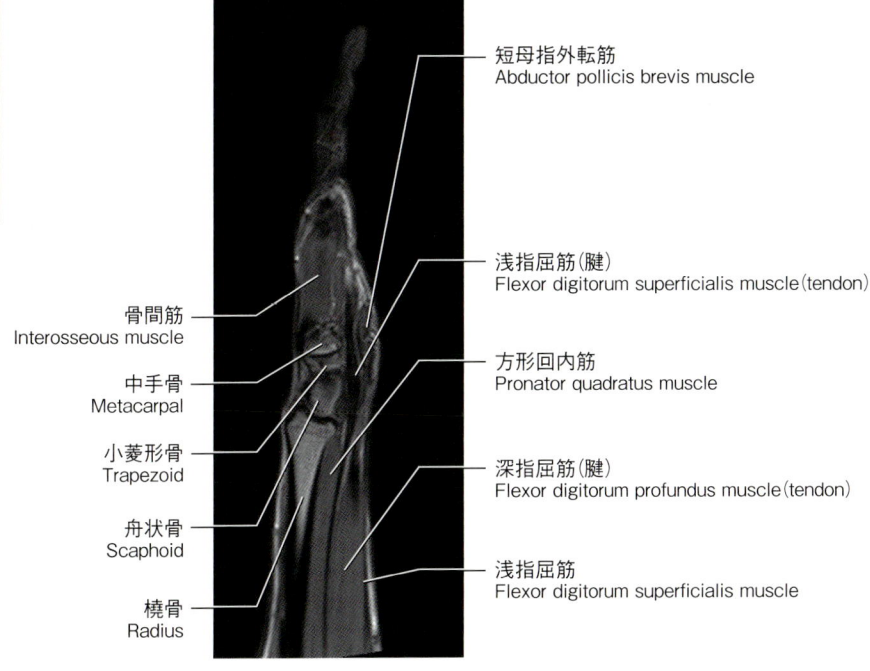

- 短母指外転筋　Abductor pollicis brevis muscle
- 浅指屈筋（腱）　Flexor digitorum superficialis muscle（tendon）
- 方形回内筋　Pronator quadratus muscle
- 深指屈筋（腱）　Flexor digitorum profundus muscle（tendon）
- 浅指屈筋　Flexor digitorum superficialis muscle
- 骨間筋　Interosseous muscle
- 中手骨　Metacarpal
- 小菱形骨　Trapezoid
- 舟状骨　Scaphoid
- 橈骨　Radius

7-88

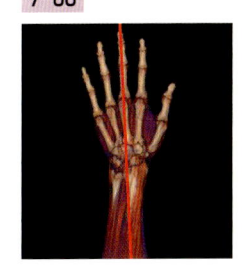

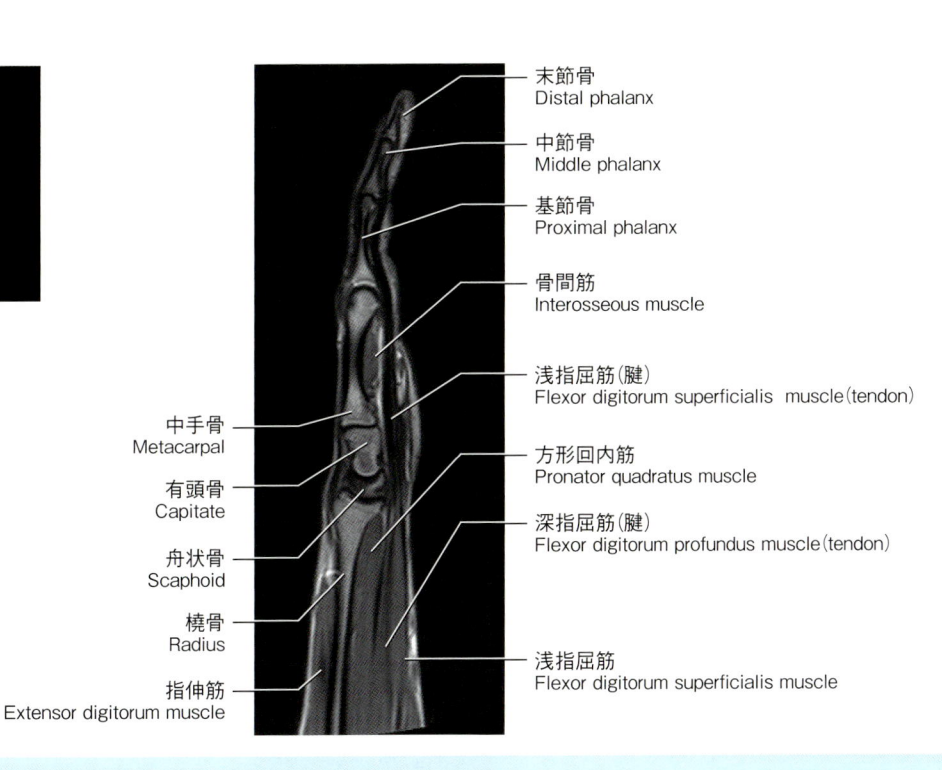

- 末節骨　Distal phalanx
- 中節骨　Middle phalanx
- 基節骨　Proximal phalanx
- 骨間筋　Interosseous muscle
- 浅指屈筋（腱）　Flexor digitorum superficialis muscle（tendon）
- 方形回内筋　Pronator quadratus muscle
- 深指屈筋（腱）　Flexor digitorum profundus muscle（tendon）
- 浅指屈筋　Flexor digitorum superficialis muscle
- 中手骨　Metacarpal
- 有頭骨　Capitate
- 舟状骨　Scaphoid
- 橈骨　Radius
- 指伸筋　Extensor digitorum muscle

NOTE 浅指屈筋腱は手根管を通り抜けたあと，第2～5指の中手指節関節（Metacarpophalangeal joint：MCP関節）レベルで2本に分離し，深指屈筋腱の両側を回ってその背側に向かい，中節骨掌側面に腱交叉を形成しながら停止する．浅指屈筋の主な機能は近位指節間関節（Proximal interphalangeal joint：PIP関節）の屈曲運動である．深指屈筋腱は分離した浅指屈筋腱の間を通り抜け，末節骨の掌側面に停止する．深指屈筋腱の主な機能は遠位指節間関節（Distal interphalangeal joint：DIP関節）の屈曲運動である．

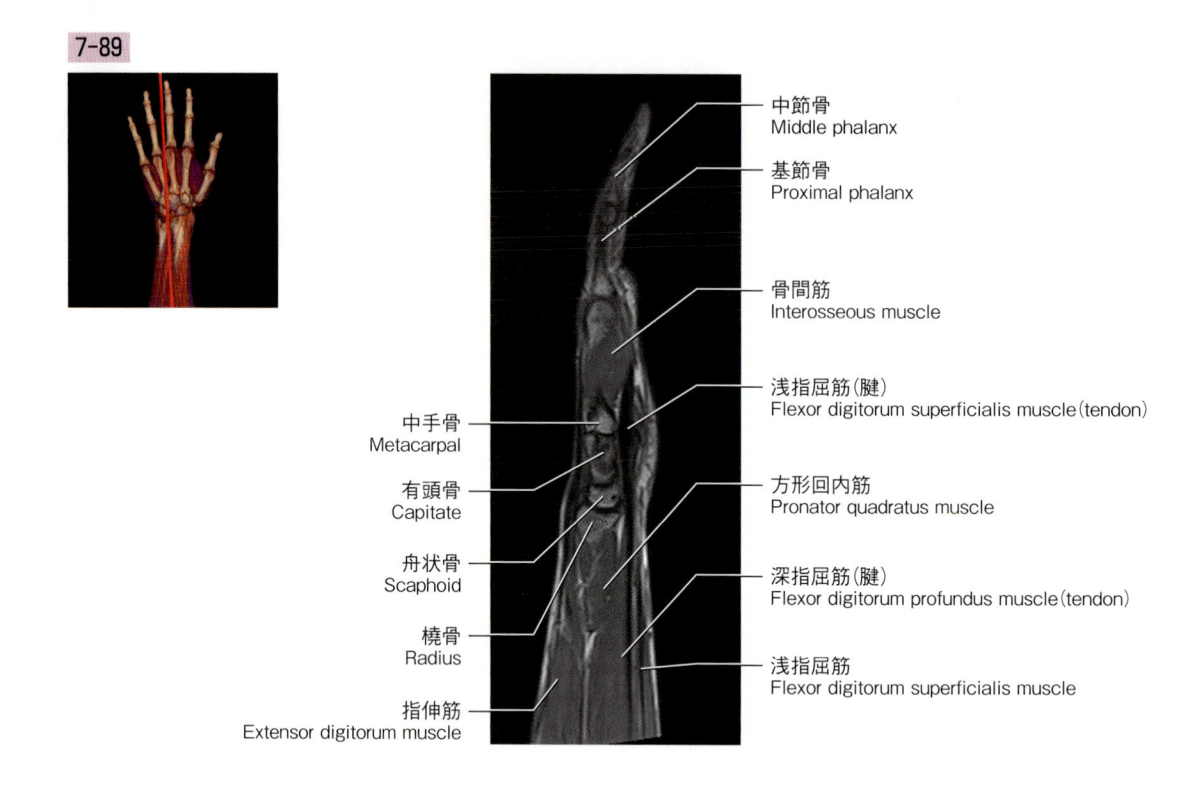

第3指の断層解剖 ［矢状断像（MRI，プロトン密度強調像）］

7-89

中節骨	Middle phalanx
基節骨	Proximal phalanx
骨間筋	Interosseous muscle
浅指屈筋（腱）	Flexor digitorum superficialis muscle (tendon)
中手骨	Metacarpal
方形回内筋	Pronator quadratus muscle
有頭骨	Capitate
舟状骨	Scaphoid
深指屈筋（腱）	Flexor digitorum profundus muscle (tendon)
橈骨	Radius
浅指屈筋	Flexor digitorum superficialis muscle
指伸筋	Extensor digitorum muscle

NOTE 長母指屈筋腱は手根管を出たあと，母指に向かって斜走し，短母指屈筋の浅頭と深頭の間を通って母指の掌側に達し，末梢骨掌側面に停止する．

下肢の主な動脈

7-90 造影CT，MIP像(左)と造影CT，VR像(右)

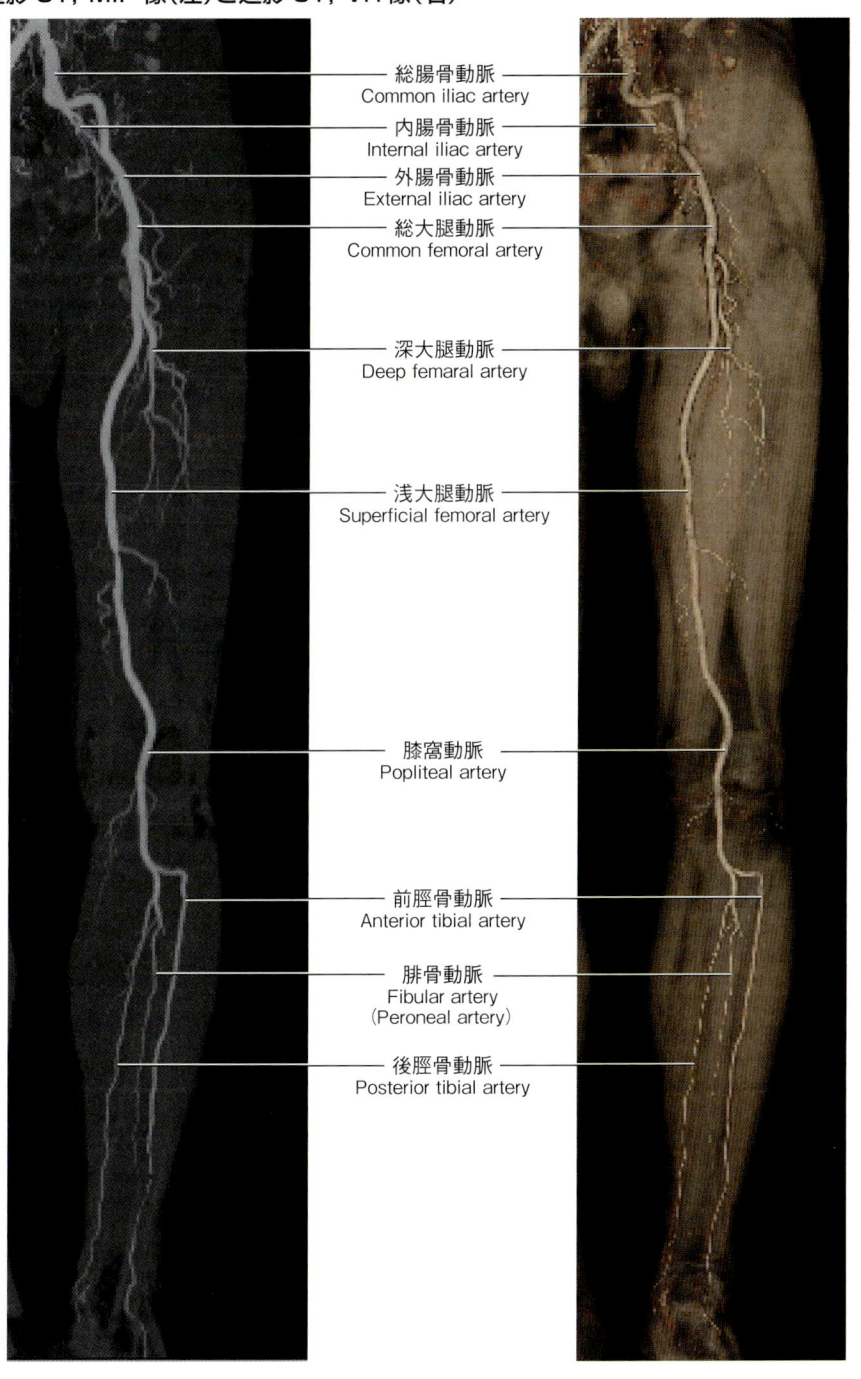

- 総腸骨動脈 Common iliac artery
- 内腸骨動脈 Internal iliac artery
- 外腸骨動脈 External iliac artery
- 総大腿動脈 Common femoral artery
- 深大腿動脈 Deep femoral artery
- 浅大腿動脈 Superficial femoral artery
- 膝窩動脈 Popliteal artery
- 前脛骨動脈 Anterior tibial artery
- 腓骨動脈 Fibular artery（Peroneal artery）
- 後脛骨動脈 Posterior tibial artery

NOTE 坐骨動脈は臍動脈から発生し，胎生期初期には下肢血行路の主幹をなす動脈であるが，大腿動脈系の発達とともに胎生3か月までに退化し消失することが一般的である．遺残坐骨動脈として成人に認められることは非常にまれである．遺残坐骨動脈の多くは間歇跛行，安静時痛，壊死などの症状より発見されることが多く，全体の半数以上に動脈瘤，動脈狭搾や閉塞などの病変を伴うとされている．

下肢の主な静脈

7-91 MRI, 2DTOF MIP 像

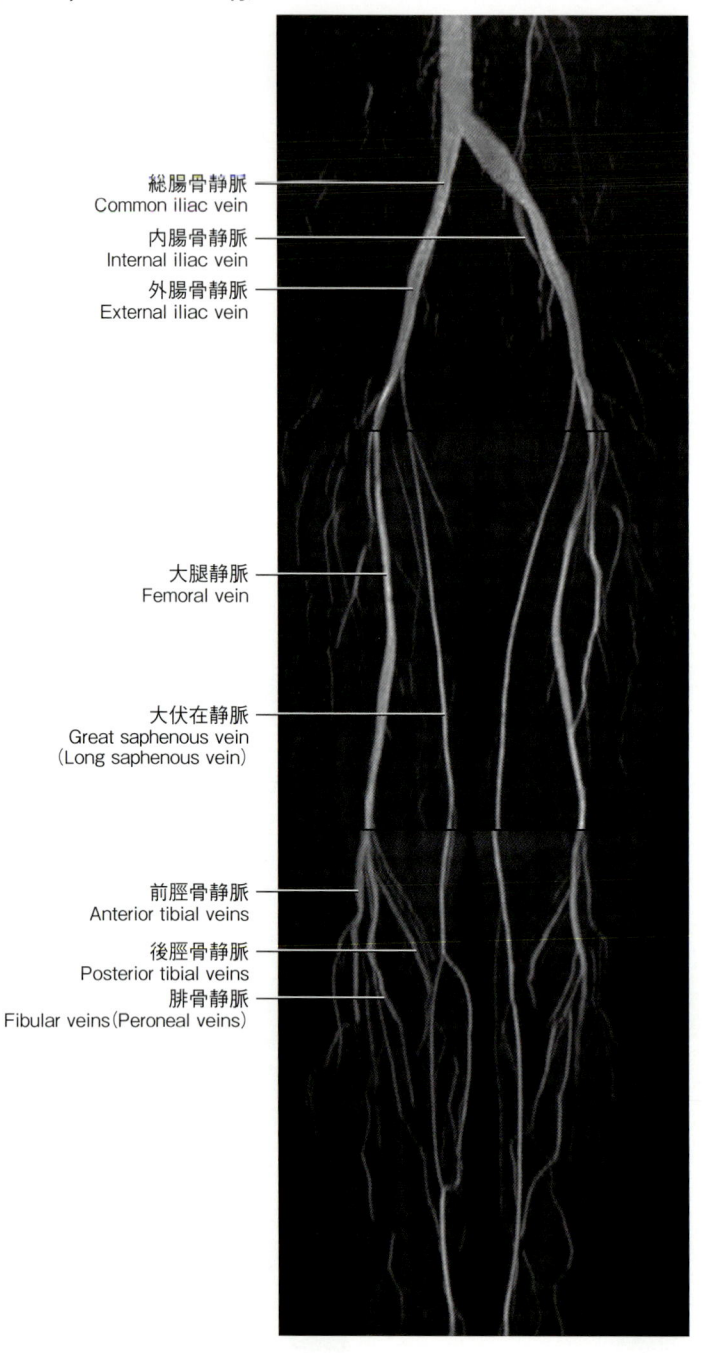

- 総腸骨静脈 Common iliac vein
- 内腸骨静脈 Internal iliac vein
- 外腸骨静脈 External iliac vein
- 大腿静脈 Femoral vein
- 大伏在静脈 Great saphenous vein (Long saphenous vein)
- 前脛骨静脈 Anterior tibial veins
- 後脛骨静脈 Posterior tibial veins
- 腓骨静脈 Fibular veins (Peroneal veins)

> **NOTE** 深部静脈血栓症の発生部位は前脛骨静脈へ合流するヒラメ静脈が重要である．ヒラメ静脈はほかの静脈に比べて静脈環流を筋ポンプ作用に依存しているにもかかわらず，ヒラメ筋自体は足関節運動時にしか動かないため，臥床の状態ではヒラメ筋灌流は減少する．もともとヒラメ筋は血流を貯留する静脈としても機能をもち静脈弁が未発達なため，血流うっ滞により静脈拡張が生じると容易に弁機能不全となる特徴もある．

股関節（CT, VR像）

7-92 下肢の筋（前面）

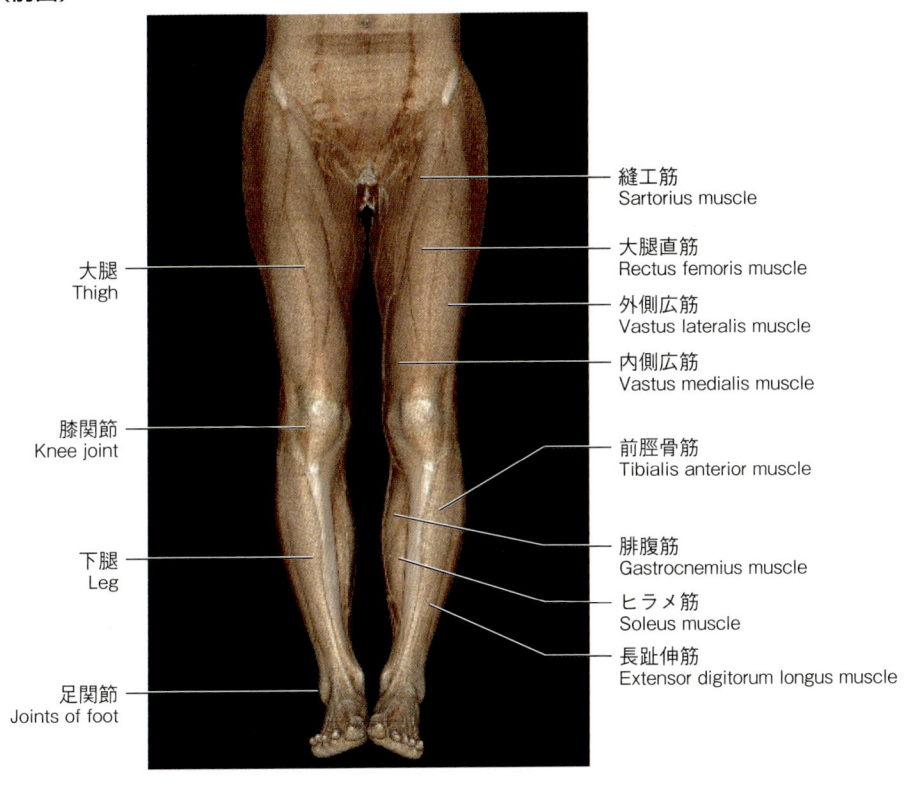

- 大腿 Thigh
- 膝関節 Knee joint
- 下腿 Leg
- 足関節 Joints of foot
- 縫工筋 Sartorius muscle
- 大腿直筋 Rectus femoris muscle
- 外側広筋 Vastus lateralis muscle
- 内側広筋 Vastus medialis muscle
- 前脛骨筋 Tibialis anterior muscle
- 腓腹筋 Gastrocnemius muscle
- ヒラメ筋 Soleus muscle
- 長趾伸筋 Extensor digitorum longus muscle

7-93 骨盤の筋（前面）

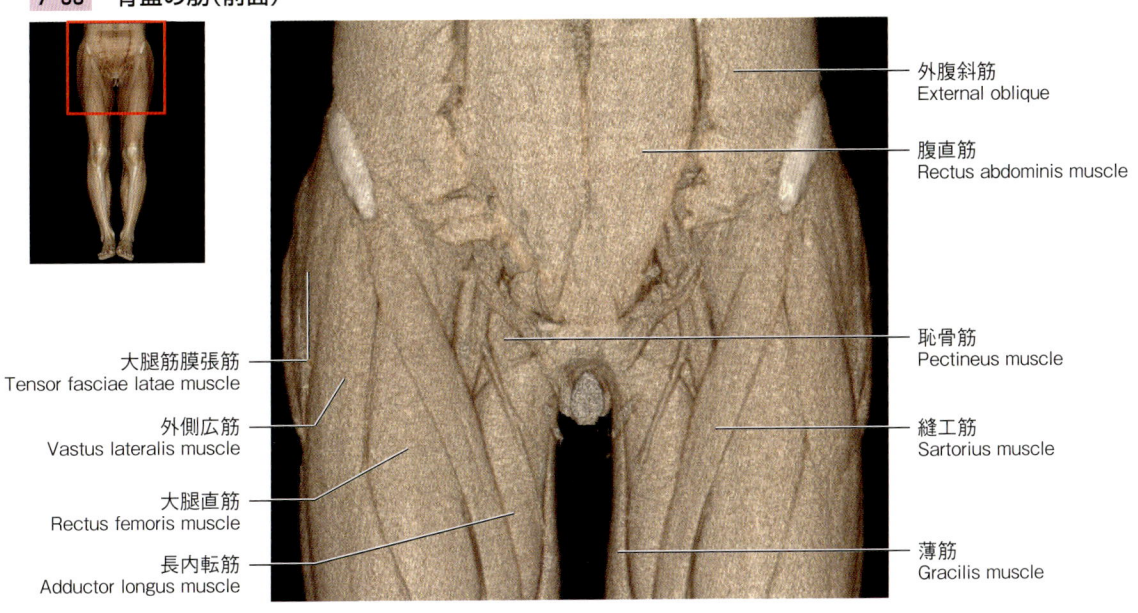

- 大腿筋膜張筋 Tensor fasciae latae muscle
- 外側広筋 Vastus lateralis muscle
- 大腿直筋 Rectus femoris muscle
- 長内転筋 Adductor longus muscle
- 外腹斜筋 External oblique
- 腹直筋 Rectus abdominis muscle
- 恥骨筋 Pectineus muscle
- 縫工筋 Sartorius muscle
- 薄筋 Gracilis muscle

NOTE 股関節の筋肉はその部位から腸骨部，殿部，大腿の3つに分類される．大腿神経，大腿動脈，大腿静脈は，底辺を鼠径靱帯，外側辺を縫工筋の内側縁，内側辺を長内転筋の外側縁で境界された大腿三角を通る．

股関節（CT，VR像）

7-94 骨盤の筋（後面）

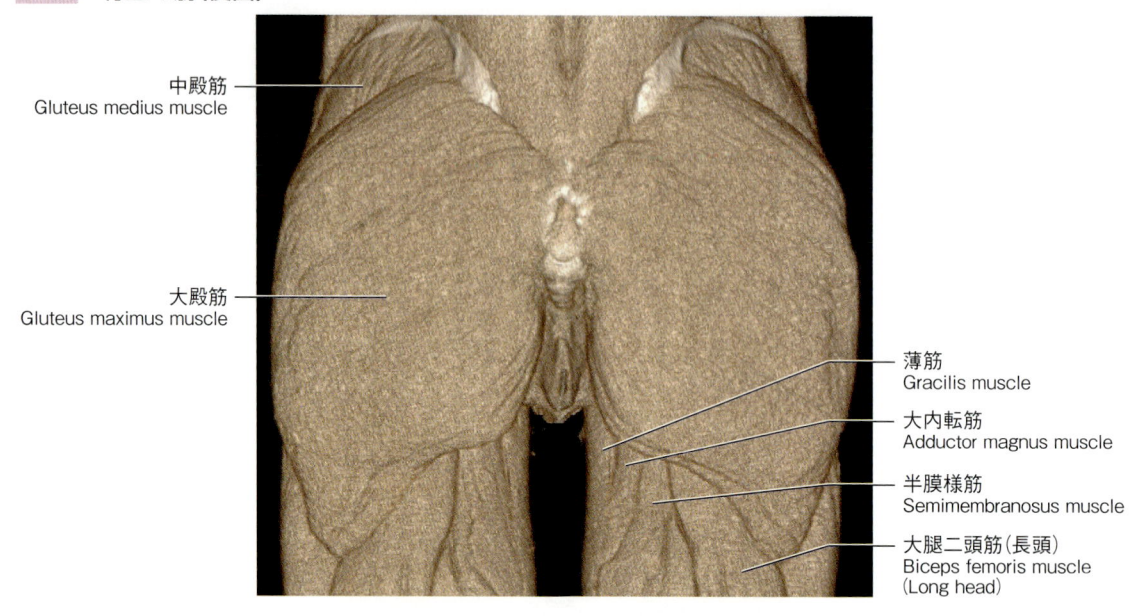

- 中殿筋 Gluteus medius muscle
- 大殿筋 Gluteus maximus muscle
- 薄筋 Gracilis muscle
- 大内転筋 Adductor magnus muscle
- 半膜様筋 Semimembranosus muscle
- 大腿二頭筋（長頭） Biceps femoris muscle (Long head)

7-95 骨盤の骨（前面）

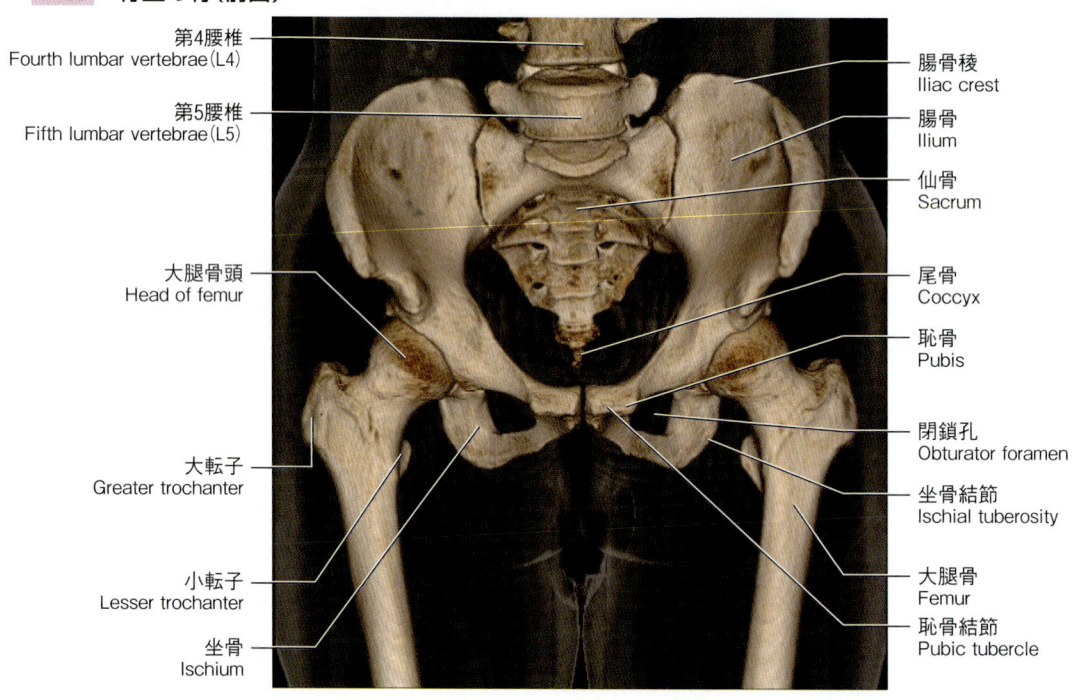

- 第4腰椎 Fourth lumbar vertebrae (L4)
- 第5腰椎 Fifth lumbar vertebrae (L5)
- 大腿骨頭 Head of femur
- 大転子 Greater trochanter
- 小転子 Lesser trochanter
- 坐骨 Ischium
- 腸骨稜 Iliac crest
- 腸骨 Ilium
- 仙骨 Sacrum
- 尾骨 Coccyx
- 恥骨 Pubis
- 閉鎖孔 Obturator foramen
- 坐骨結節 Ischial tuberosity
- 大腿骨 Femur
- 恥骨結節 Pubic tubercle

> **NOTE** 骨端線閉鎖前には，筋腱構成体が骨端線よりも強靱であるために，腱，靱帯，関節包の介達力により骨端裂離骨折が起こる．骨盤骨の骨端（Apophysis）と大腿骨の小転子は，長管骨の骨端（Epiphysis）に比べて出現も骨端線の閉鎖も遅いため，長管骨の骨端外傷が思春期以前に好発するのに対し，骨盤骨の骨端裂離骨折は思春期，ないしそれ以降に好発する．骨端裂離骨折を生じるほどの介達力が成人に加わると，骨端裂離骨折までは至らない"筋（腱）ストレイン"とよばれる筋（腱）組織の弱い部位の損傷をきたすことがある．

股関節（CT, VR 像）

7-96 骨盤の骨（左前面）

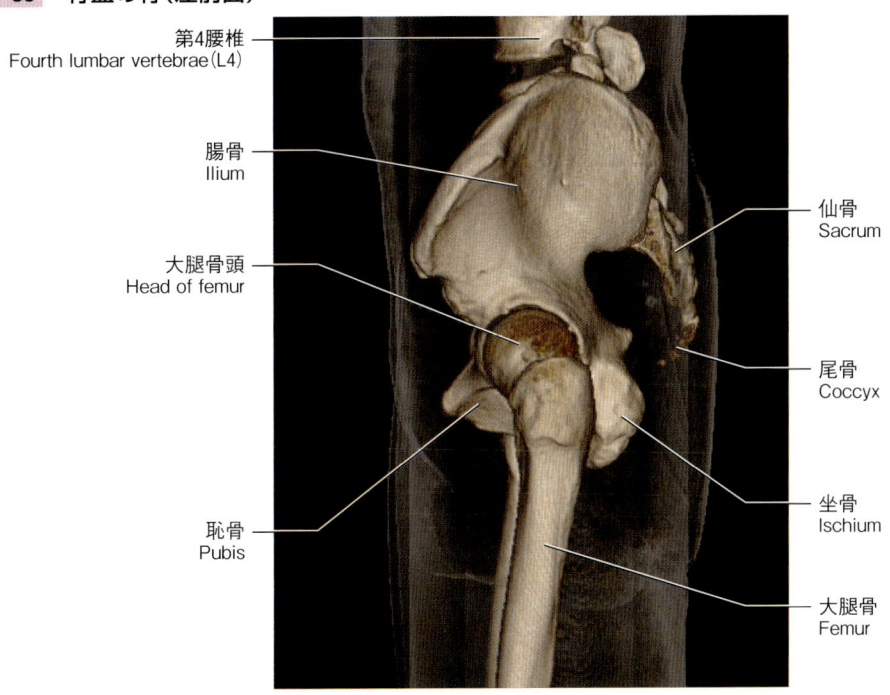

- 第4腰椎 Fourth lumbar vertebrae (L4)
- 腸骨 Ilium
- 大腿骨頭 Head of femur
- 恥骨 Pubis
- 仙骨 Sacrum
- 尾骨 Coccyx
- 坐骨 Ischium
- 大腿骨 Femur

7-97 骨盤の骨（後面）

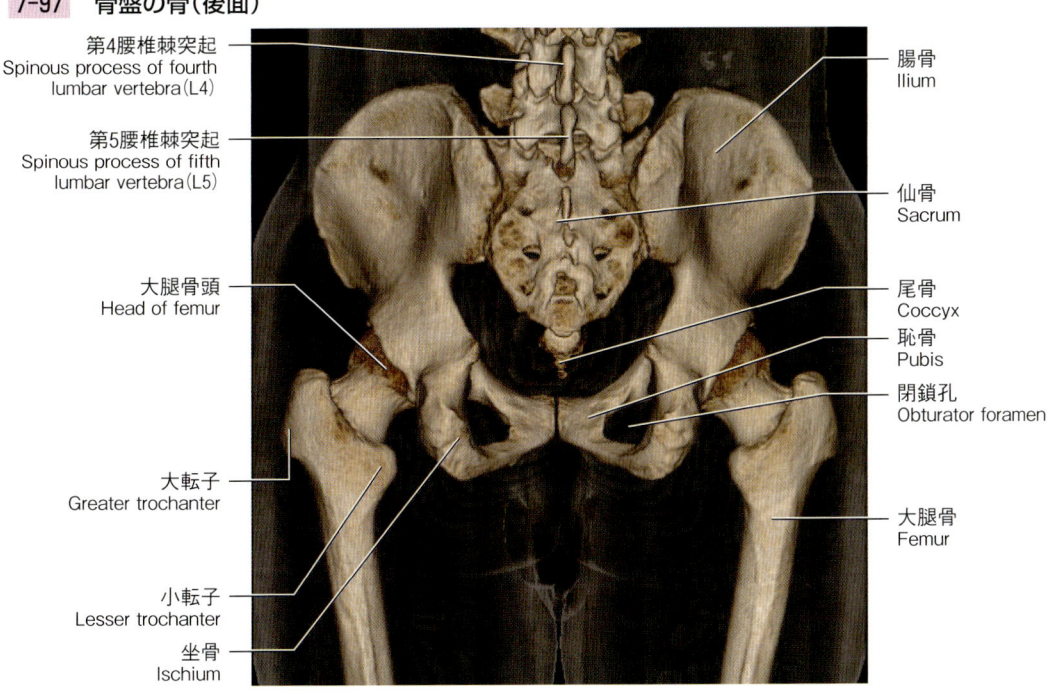

- 第4腰椎棘突起 Spinous process of fourth lumbar vertebra (L4)
- 第5腰椎棘突起 Spinous process of fifth lumbar vertebra (L5)
- 大腿骨頭 Head of femur
- 大転子 Greater trochanter
- 小転子 Lesser trochanter
- 坐骨 Ischium
- 腸骨 Ilium
- 仙骨 Sacrum
- 尾骨 Coccyx
- 恥骨 Pubis
- 閉鎖孔 Obturator foramen
- 大腿骨 Femur

NOTE 骨盤骨の骨端の部位と付着する筋および骨融合をきたす年齢
1. 上前腸骨棘−縫工筋および大腿筋膜張筋　16〜20歳
2. 下前腸骨棘−大腿直筋　25歳
3. 坐骨結節−後大腿筋群（大腿二頭筋長頭，半膜様筋，半腱様筋）　20〜25歳
4. 恥骨結合下部−内側大腿筋群（恥骨筋，薄筋，長・短内転筋，大内転筋，外閉鎖筋）　20〜25歳
5. 腸骨稜−腹筋群（内・外腹斜筋，腰方形筋）　17〜18歳

股関節（CT, VR 像）

7-98 骨盤の骨（右前面）

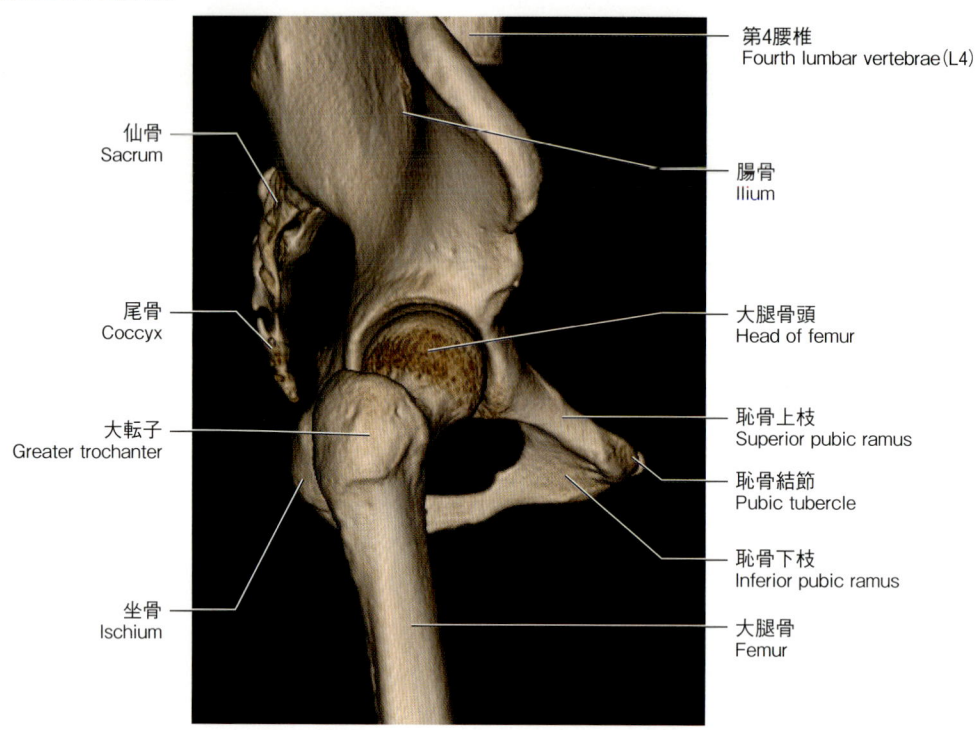

- 第4腰椎 Fourth lumbar vertebrae (L4)
- 仙骨 Sacrum
- 腸骨 Ilium
- 尾骨 Coccyx
- 大腿骨頭 Head of femur
- 大転子 Greater trochanter
- 恥骨上枝 Superior pubic ramus
- 恥骨結節 Pubic tubercle
- 恥骨下枝 Inferior pubic ramus
- 坐骨 Ischium
- 大腿骨 Femur

7-99 骨盤の骨［右前面（大腿部を除く）］

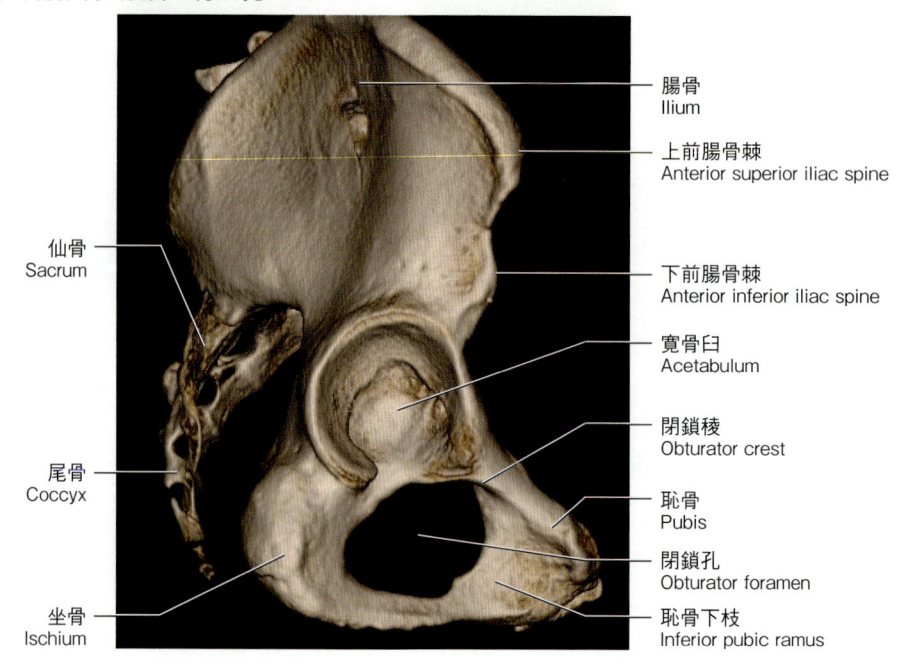

- 腸骨 Ilium
- 上前腸骨棘 Anterior superior iliac spine
- 仙骨 Sacrum
- 下前腸骨棘 Anterior inferior iliac spine
- 寛骨臼 Acetabulum
- 閉鎖稜 Obturator crest
- 尾骨 Coccyx
- 恥骨 Pubis
- 閉鎖孔 Obturator foramen
- 恥骨下枝 Inferior pubic ramus
- 坐骨 Ischium

> **NOTE** 股関節は寛骨臼の月状面と大腿骨頭でつくられる．月状面とは三日月形の関節軟骨に覆われた関節面．寛骨臼は腸骨，恥骨，坐骨の骨端により形成されるが，成長期にはこれらの骨端線は寛骨臼の底部でY字型を形成し，Y軟骨結合とよばれる．Y字軟骨の成長とともに寛骨臼の形と深さは増大する．

股関節（CT, VR像）

7-100 右大腿骨頭（前面）

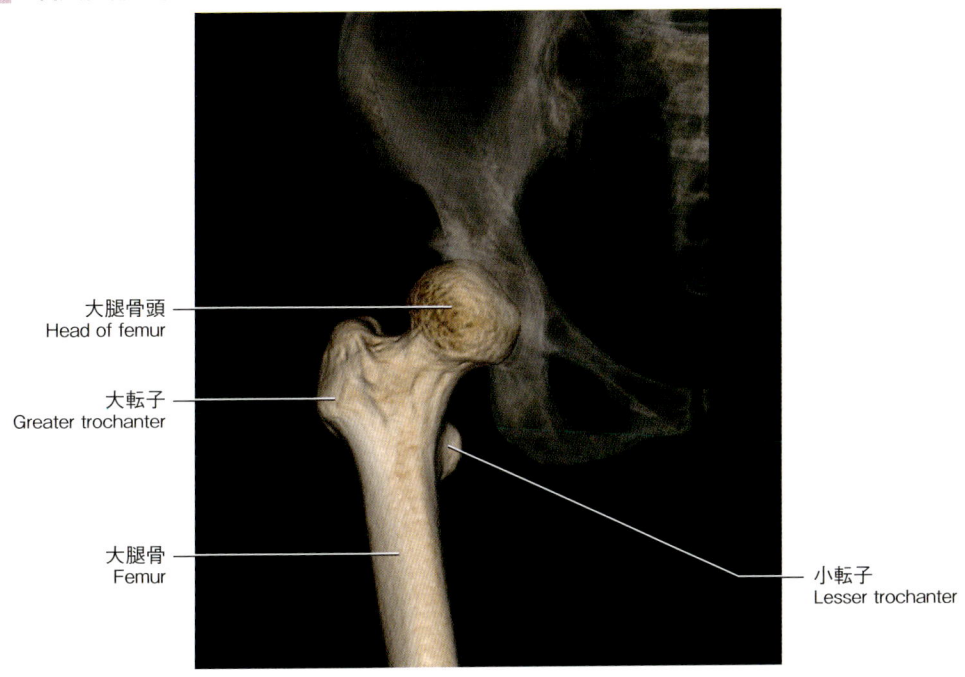

- 大腿骨頭 Head of femur
- 大転子 Greater trochanter
- 大腿骨 Femur
- 小転子 Lesser trochanter

7-101 右大腿骨頭（側面）

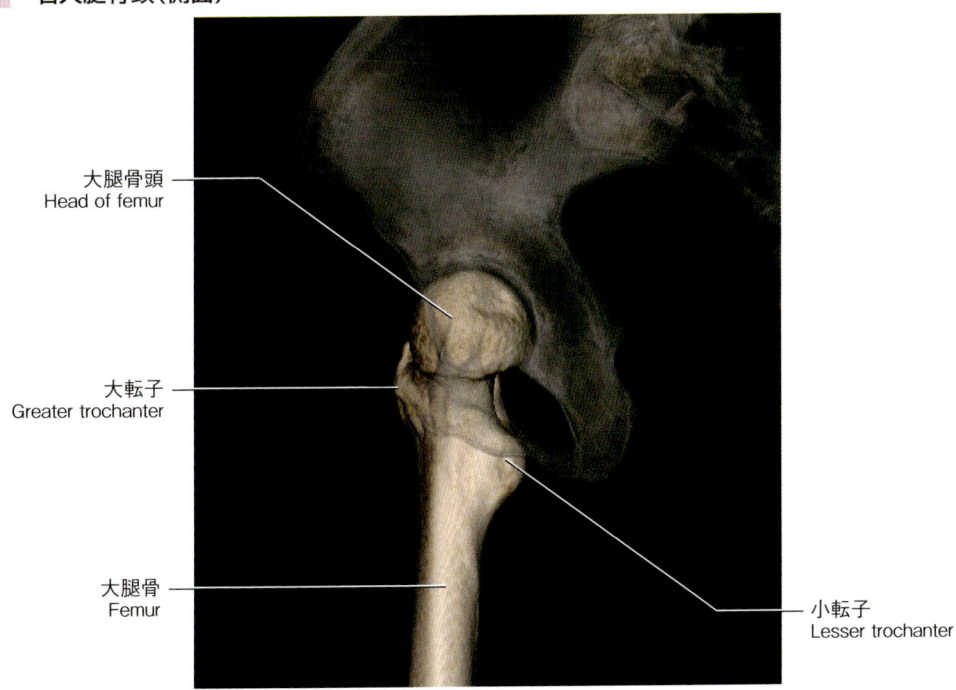

- 大腿骨頭 Head of femur
- 大転子 Greater trochanter
- 大腿骨 Femur
- 小転子 Lesser trochanter

股関節の断層解剖 ［横断像（MRI，プロトン密度強調像）］

7-102

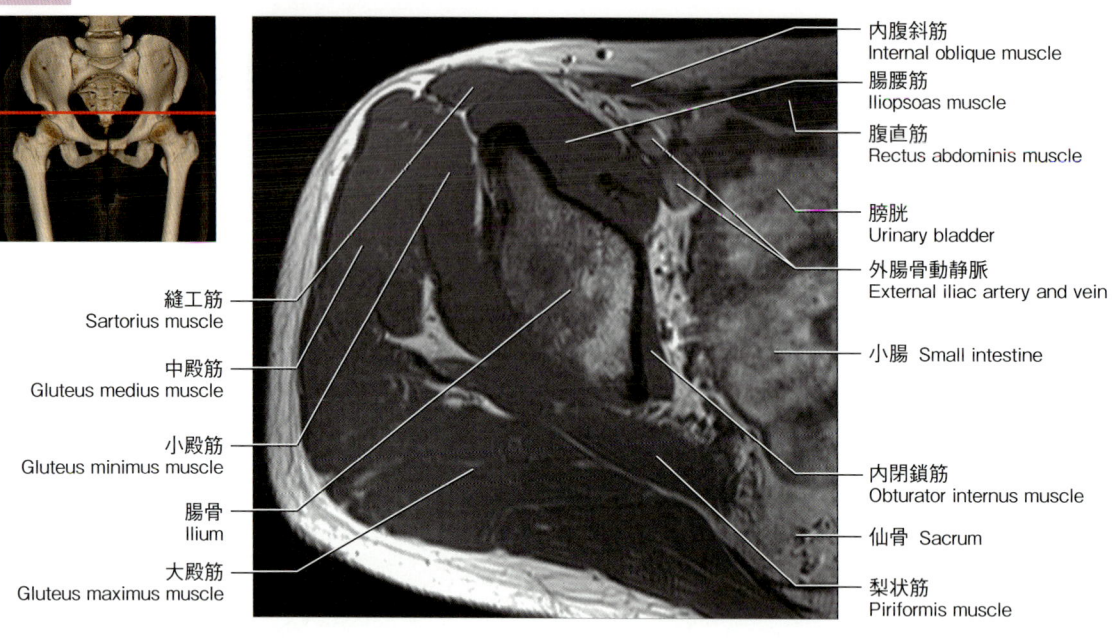

- 内腹斜筋 Internal oblique muscle
- 腸腰筋 Iliopsoas muscle
- 腹直筋 Rectus abdominis muscle
- 膀胱 Urinary bladder
- 外腸骨動静脈 External iliac artery and vein
- 小腸 Small intestine
- 内閉鎖筋 Obturator internus muscle
- 仙骨 Sacrum
- 梨状筋 Piriformis muscle
- 縫工筋 Sartorius muscle
- 中殿筋 Gluteus medius muscle
- 小殿筋 Gluteus minimus muscle
- 腸骨 Ilium
- 大殿筋 Gluteus maximus muscle

7-103

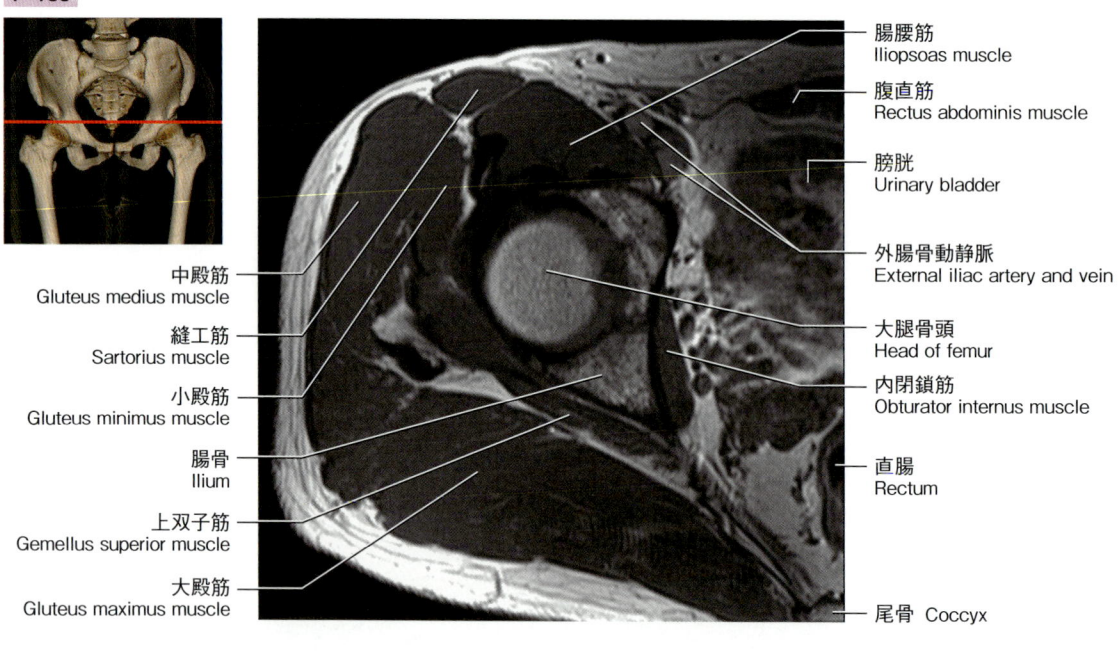

- 腸腰筋 Iliopsoas muscle
- 腹直筋 Rectus abdominis muscle
- 膀胱 Urinary bladder
- 外腸骨動静脈 External iliac artery and vein
- 大腿骨頭 Head of femur
- 内閉鎖筋 Obturator internus muscle
- 直腸 Rectum
- 尾骨 Coccyx
- 中殿筋 Gluteus medius muscle
- 縫工筋 Sartorius muscle
- 小殿筋 Gluteus minimus muscle
- 腸骨 Ilium
- 上双子筋 Gemellus superior muscle
- 大殿筋 Gluteus maximus muscle

NOTE 股関節の屈曲運動は，大腿骨小転子に停止する腸骨部の筋肉である腸腰筋が行う．腸腰筋は大腰筋と腸骨筋の合体したもので，股関節の前方を走り小転子に停止する．さらに，大腿前面の筋肉である下前腸骨棘に起始する大腿直筋と，上前腸骨棘に起始する縫工筋と大腿筋膜張筋も股関節の屈曲運動に関与する．大腿四頭筋の中で，股関節部にみられるものは大腿直筋のみである．縫工筋は大腿三角の外側縁をつくりながら，大腿の外側前面寄りの内側下方に向かう．

股関節の断層解剖　[横断像（MRI，プロトン密度強調像）]

7-104

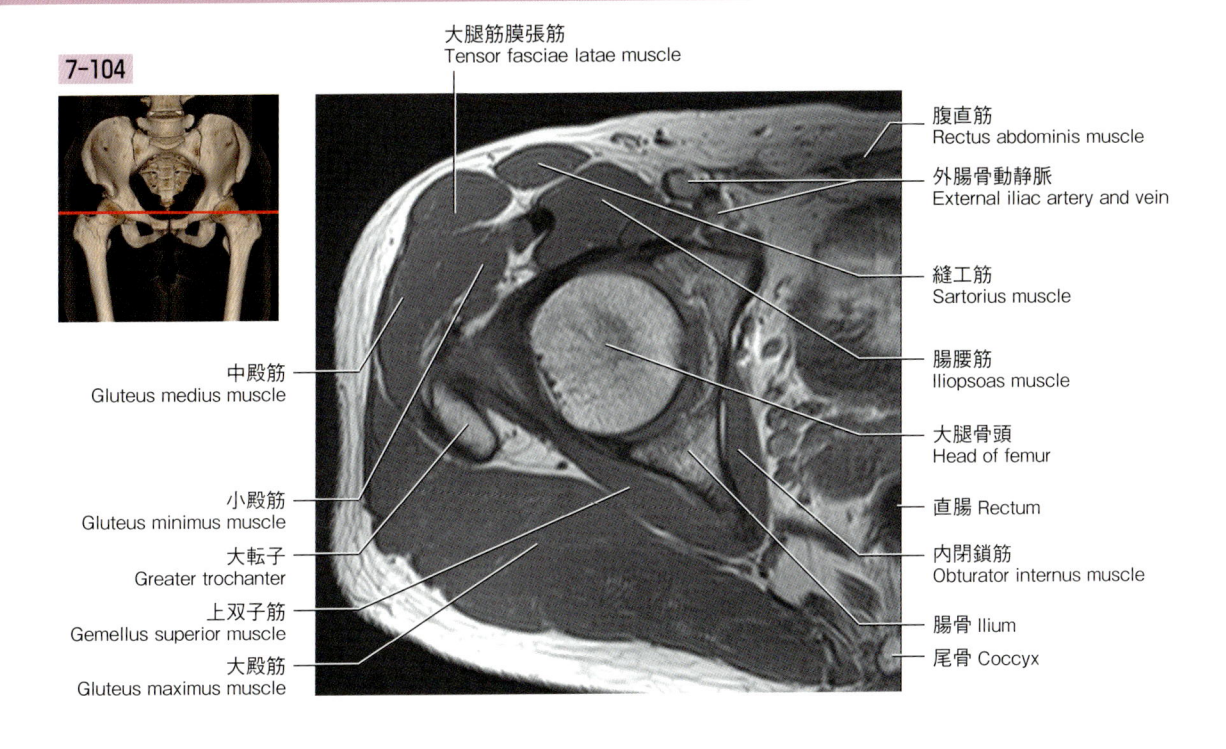

- 大腿筋膜張筋　Tensor fasciae latae muscle
- 腹直筋　Rectus abdominis muscle
- 外腸骨動静脈　External iliac artery and vein
- 縫工筋　Sartorius muscle
- 腸腰筋　Iliopsoas muscle
- 大腿骨頭　Head of femur
- 直腸　Rectum
- 内閉鎖筋　Obturator internus muscle
- 腸骨　Ilium
- 尾骨　Coccyx
- 中殿筋　Gluteus medius muscle
- 小殿筋　Gluteus minimus muscle
- 大転子　Greater trochanter
- 上双子筋　Gemellus superior muscle
- 大殿筋　Gluteus maximus muscle

7-105

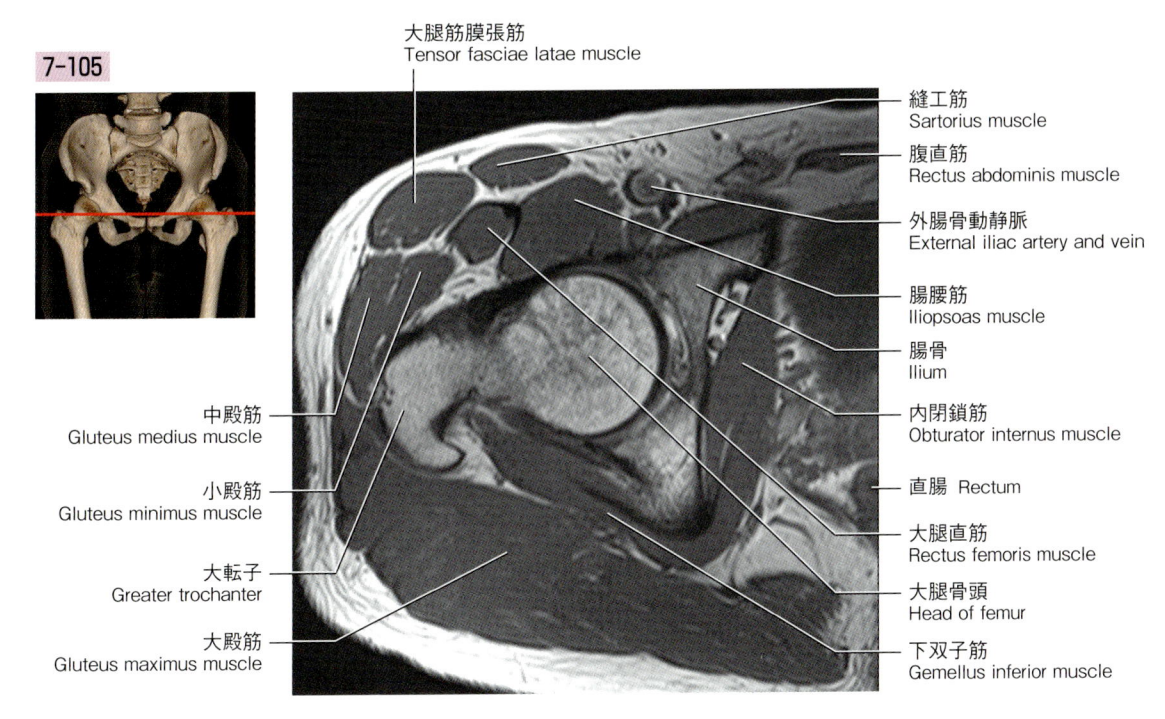

- 大腿筋膜張筋　Tensor fasciae latae muscle
- 縫工筋　Sartorius muscle
- 腹直筋　Rectus abdominis muscle
- 外腸骨動静脈　External iliac artery and vein
- 腸腰筋　Iliopsoas muscle
- 腸骨　Ilium
- 内閉鎖筋　Obturator internus muscle
- 直腸　Rectum
- 大腿直筋　Rectus femoris muscle
- 大腿骨頭　Head of femur
- 下双子筋　Gemellus inferior muscle
- 中殿筋　Gluteus medius muscle
- 小殿筋　Gluteus minimus muscle
- 大転子　Greater trochanter
- 大殿筋　Gluteus maximus muscle

> **NOTE** 外転および外旋は，大腿骨大転子とその近傍に停止する殿筋群および回旋筋群で行われる．主な外転筋は小殿筋と中殿筋で，これに大腿筋膜張筋，梨状筋，大殿筋も関与する．大腿筋膜張筋と大殿筋の筋膜は合体して，大転子の下方で腸脛靱帯となる．主な外旋筋は深部にある梨状筋，内・外閉鎖筋，上・下双子筋，大腿方形筋である．

股関節の断層解剖［横断像（MRI，プロトン密度強調像）］

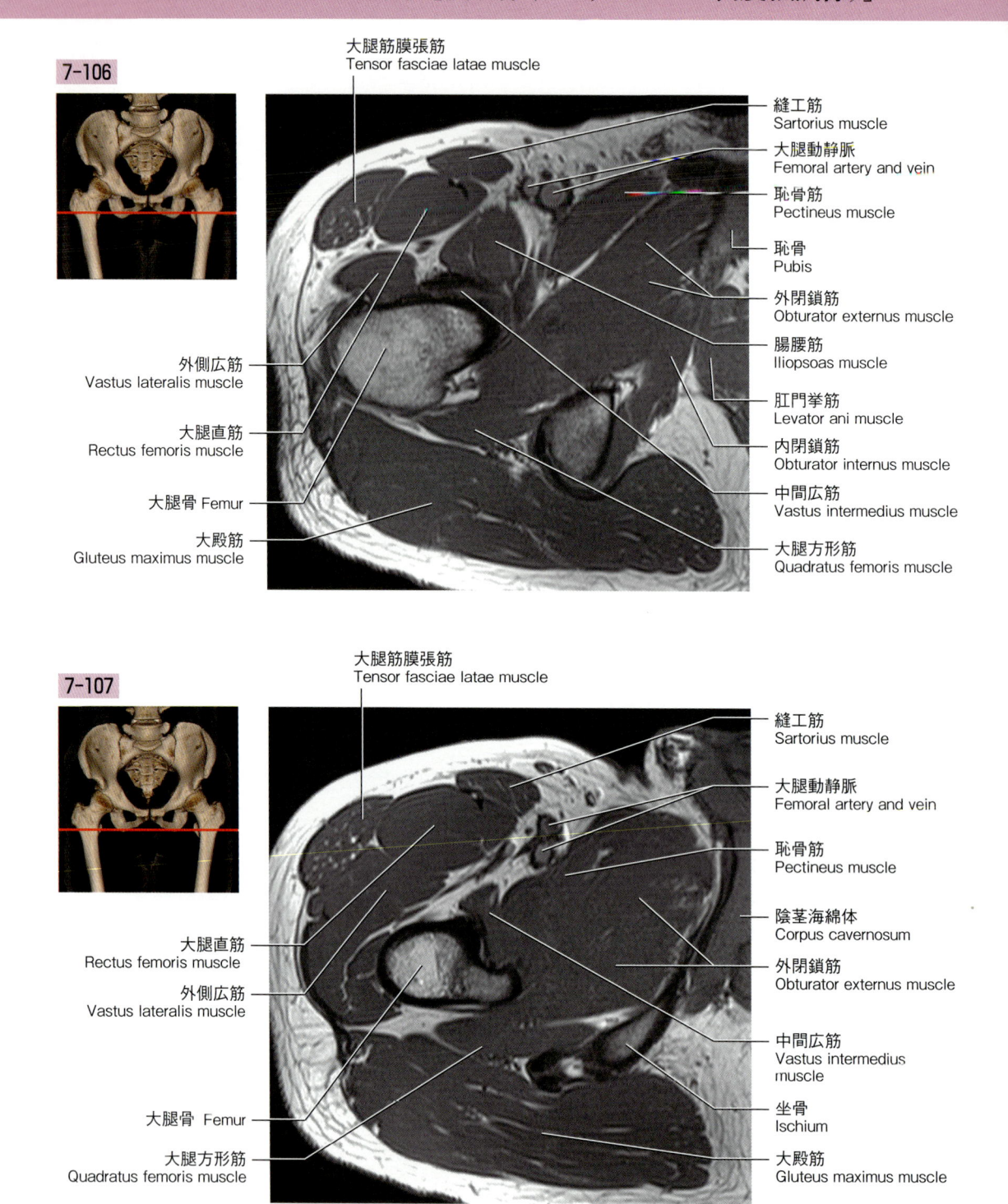

7-106

- 大腿筋膜張筋 Tensor fasciae latae muscle
- 縫工筋 Sartorius muscle
- 大腿動静脈 Femoral artery and vein
- 恥骨筋 Pectineus muscle
- 恥骨 Pubis
- 外閉鎖筋 Obturator externus muscle
- 腸腰筋 Iliopsoas muscle
- 肛門挙筋 Levator ani muscle
- 内閉鎖筋 Obturator internus muscle
- 中間広筋 Vastus intermedius muscle
- 大腿方形筋 Quadratus femoris muscle
- 外側広筋 Vastus lateralis muscle
- 大腿直筋 Rectus femoris muscle
- 大腿骨 Femur
- 大殿筋 Gluteus maximus muscle

7-107

- 大腿筋膜張筋 Tensor fasciae latae muscle
- 縫工筋 Sartorius muscle
- 大腿動静脈 Femoral artery and vein
- 恥骨筋 Pectineus muscle
- 陰茎海綿体 Corpus cavernosum
- 外閉鎖筋 Obturator externus muscle
- 中間広筋 Vastus intermedius muscle
- 坐骨 Ischium
- 大殿筋 Gluteus maximus muscle
- 大腿直筋 Rectus femoris muscle
- 外側広筋 Vastus lateralis muscle
- 大腿骨 Femur
- 大腿方形筋 Quadratus femoris muscle

NOTE 伸展運動は坐骨結節に起始する大腿後面の筋で行われる．これには大腿二頭筋長頭，半膜様筋，半腱様筋がある．これらの筋肉は膝関節の屈曲機能を有する．これら3つの筋肉を総称してハムストリング（Hamstring）とよぶ．大殿筋も股関節の伸展に関与する．内転・内旋運動は，恥骨近傍に起始する大腿内側の筋肉が行う．これには，薄筋，恥骨筋，短・長内転筋，大内転筋がある．

股関節の断層解剖 [冠状断像（MRI，プロトン密度強調像）]

7-108

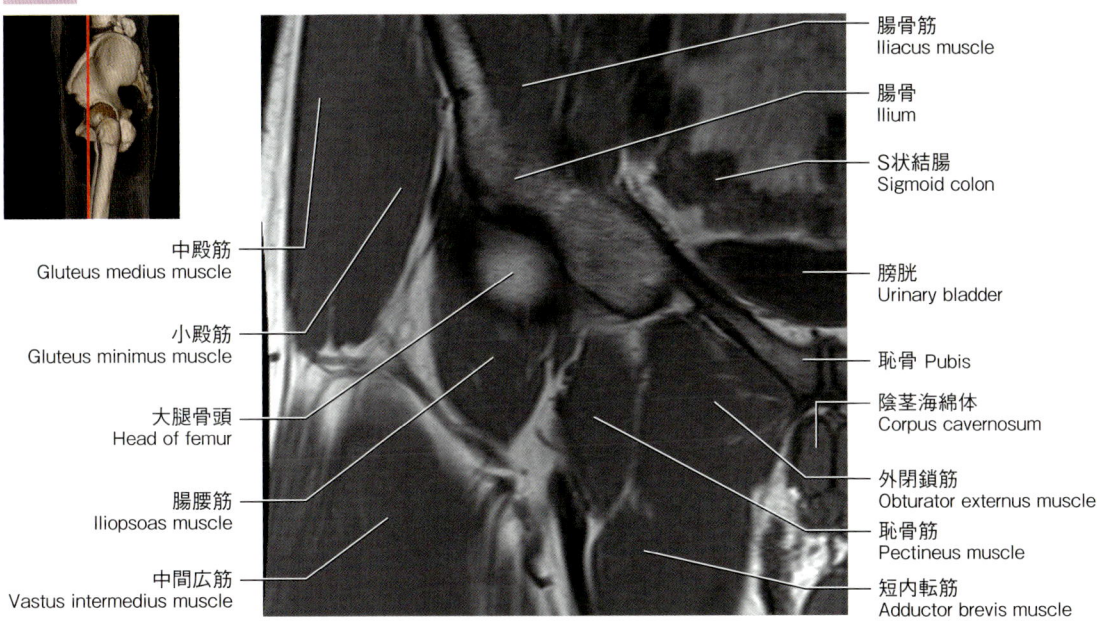

- 腸骨筋 Iliacus muscle
- 腸骨 Ilium
- S状結腸 Sigmoid colon
- 膀胱 Urinary bladder
- 恥骨 Pubis
- 陰茎海綿体 Corpus cavernosum
- 外閉鎖筋 Obturator externus muscle
- 恥骨筋 Pectineus muscle
- 短内転筋 Adductor brevis muscle
- 中殿筋 Gluteus medius muscle
- 小殿筋 Gluteus minimus muscle
- 大腿骨頭 Head of femur
- 腸腰筋 Iliopsoas muscle
- 中間広筋 Vastus intermedius muscle

7-109

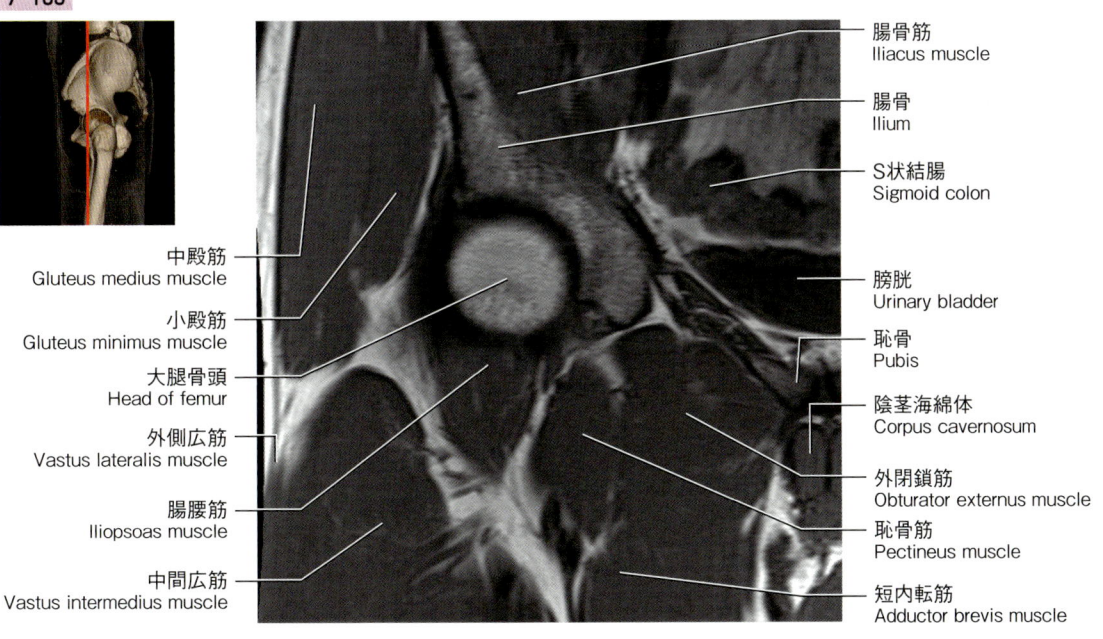

- 腸骨筋 Iliacus muscle
- 腸骨 Ilium
- S状結腸 Sigmoid colon
- 膀胱 Urinary bladder
- 恥骨 Pubis
- 陰茎海綿体 Corpus cavernosum
- 外閉鎖筋 Obturator externus muscle
- 恥骨筋 Pectineus muscle
- 短内転筋 Adductor brevis muscle
- 中殿筋 Gluteus medius muscle
- 小殿筋 Gluteus minimus muscle
- 大腿骨頭 Head of femur
- 外側広筋 Vastus lateralis muscle
- 腸腰筋 Iliopsoas muscle
- 中間広筋 Vastus intermedius muscle

> **NOTE** 大腿骨頭荷重面は骨壊死を生じやすい部位のひとつである．原因のはっきりしている症候性骨壊死と明らかな原因がわからない特発性骨壊死に大別される．特発性骨壊死の誘因としてはステロイド薬の投与やアルコールの多飲が知られている．この2つを除外して狭義の特発性大腿骨頭壊死とよぶこともある．大腿骨頭の血流障害をきたすメカニズムとして，動脈の損傷，塞栓，骨髄内圧の上昇，血管炎，静脈還流の障害などいくつもの説が提唱されているが確立されたものはない．

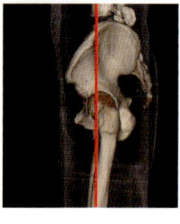

股関節の断層解剖 ［冠状断像（MRI, プロトン密度強調像）］

7-110

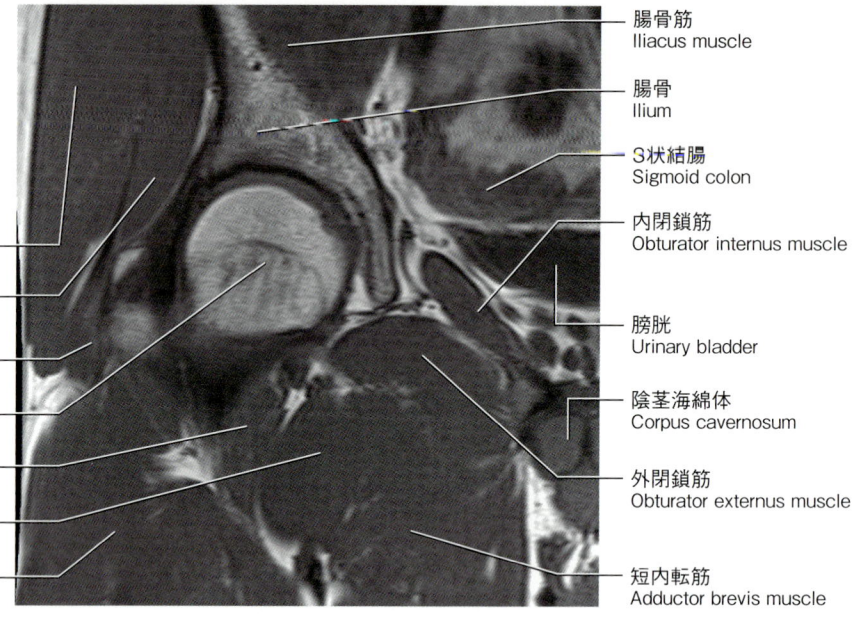

- 腸骨筋 Iliacus muscle
- 腸骨 Ilium
- S状結腸 Sigmoid colon
- 内閉鎖筋 Obturator internus muscle
- 膀胱 Urinary bladder
- 陰茎海綿体 Corpus cavernosum
- 外閉鎖筋 Obturator externus muscle
- 短内転筋 Adductor brevis muscle
- 中殿筋 Gluteus medius muscle
- 小殿筋 Gluteus minimus muscle
- 外側広筋 Vastus lateralis muscle
- 大腿骨頭 Head of femur
- 腸腰筋 Iliopsoas muscle
- 恥骨筋 Pectineus muscle
- 中間広筋 Vastus intermedius muscle

7-111

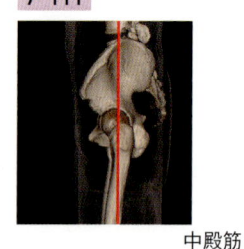

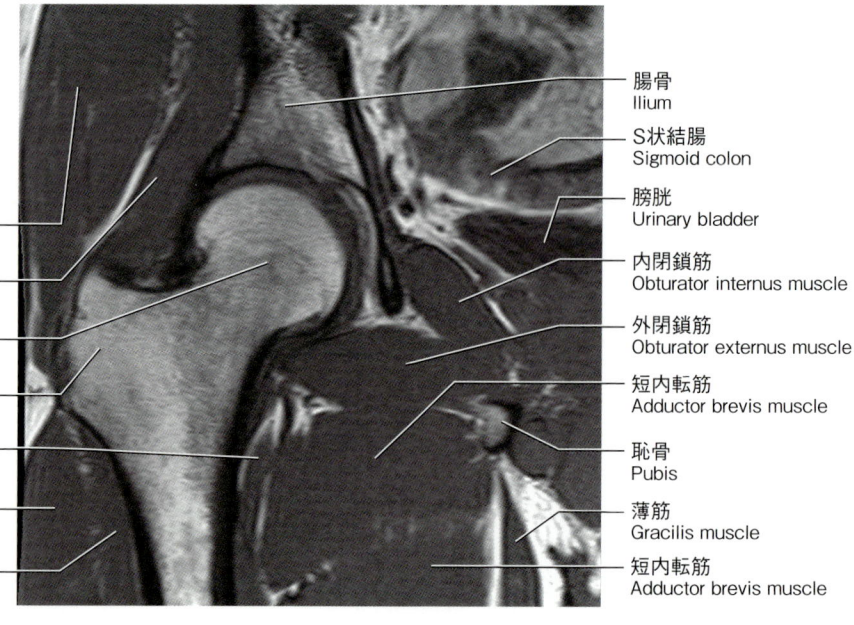

- 腸骨 Ilium
- S状結腸 Sigmoid colon
- 膀胱 Urinary bladder
- 内閉鎖筋 Obturator internus muscle
- 外閉鎖筋 Obturator externus muscle
- 短内転筋 Adductor brevis muscle
- 恥骨 Pubis
- 薄筋 Gracilis muscle
- 短内転筋 Adductor brevis muscle
- 中殿筋 Gluteus medius muscle
- 小殿筋 Gluteus minimus muscle
- 大腿骨頭 Head of femur
- 大転子 Greater trochanter
- 腸腰筋 Iliopsoas muscle
- 外側広筋 Vastus lateralis muscle
- 中間広筋 Vastus intermedius muscle

> **NOTE** 大腿骨頭頸部は高齢者，特に女性で骨折が起こりやすい部位のひとつである．関節包内に骨膜性骨新生がないため難治性であることが多く，大腿骨頭の特殊な血流支配のため骨頭壊死に陥りやすい．単純 X 線写真では骨折線が不明瞭なことが多く，偏位の少ないものでは診断がしばしば困難である．診断困難な症例には MRI が有効とされている．

股関節の断層解剖 ［冠状断像（MRI，プロトン密度強調像）］

7-112

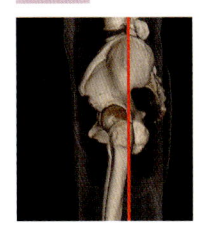

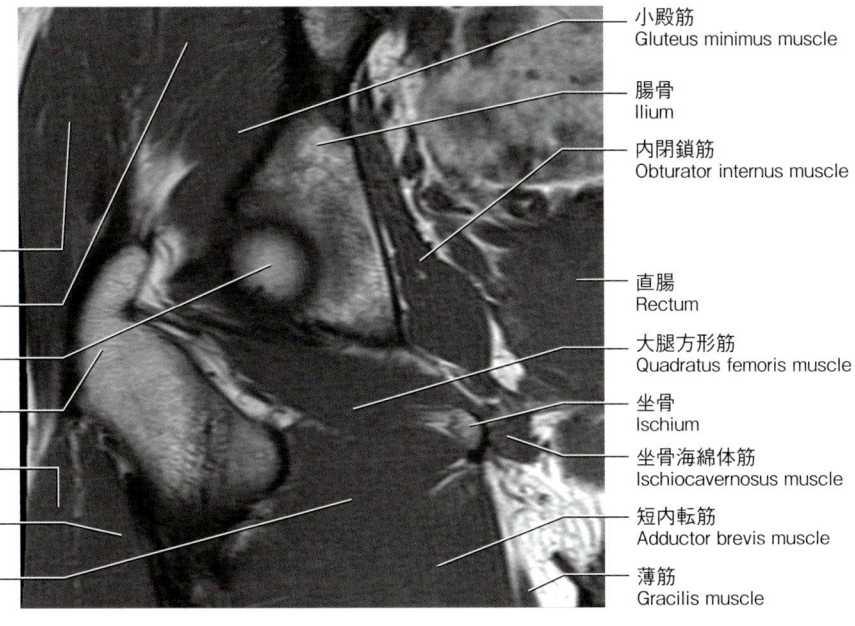

- 小殿筋 Gluteus minimus muscle
- 腸骨 Ilium
- 内閉鎖筋 Obturator internus muscle
- 直腸 Rectum
- 大腿方形筋 Quadratus femoris muscle
- 坐骨 Ischium
- 坐骨海綿体筋 Ischiocavernosus muscle
- 短内転筋 Adductor brevis muscle
- 薄筋 Gracilis muscle

- 大殿筋 Gluteus maximus muscle
- 中殿筋 Gluteus medius muscle
- 大腿骨頭 Head of femur
- 大転子 Greater trochanter
- 外側広筋 Vastus lateralis muscle
- 中間広筋 Vastus intermedius muscle
- 大内転筋 Adductor magnus muscle

7-113

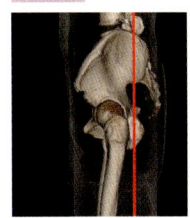

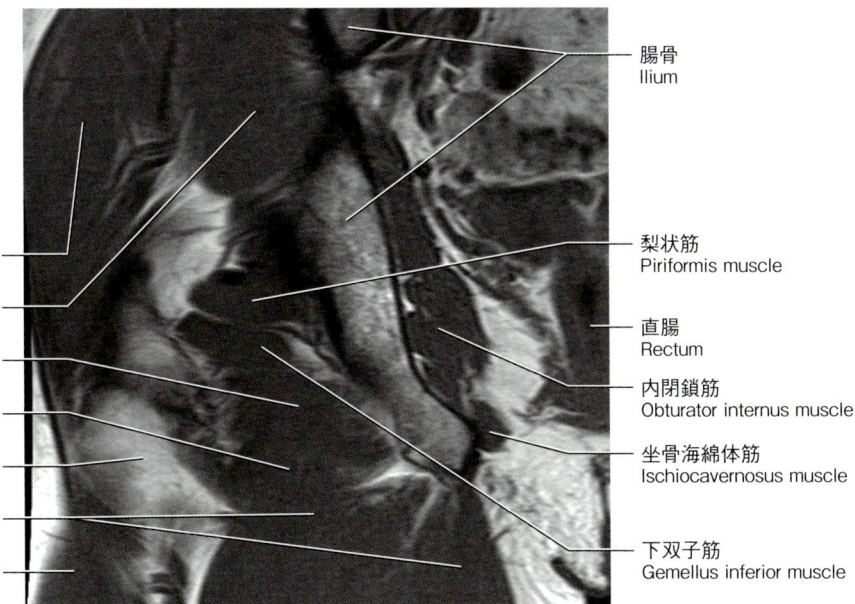

- 腸骨 Ilium
- 梨状筋 Piriformis muscle
- 直腸 Rectum
- 内閉鎖筋 Obturator internus muscle
- 坐骨海綿体筋 Ischiocavernosus muscle
- 下双子筋 Gemellus inferior muscle

- 大殿筋 Gluteus maximus muscle
- 中殿筋 Gluteus medius muscle
- 大腿方形筋 Quadratus femoris muscle
- 小内転筋 Adductor minimus muscle
- 大腿骨 Femur
- 大内転筋 Adductor magnus muscle
- 外側広筋 Vastus lateralis muscle

NOTE 短内転筋 Adductor brevis muscle

brevis は "短い" の意のギリシャ語．"Ars longa, vita brevis" は，ヒポクラテスの格言「学芸は長し，生涯は短し，時期は速し，経験は危うし，判断は難し」の冒頭２句である．

366 股関節の断層解剖 [矢状断像（MRI，プロトン密度強調像）]

7-114

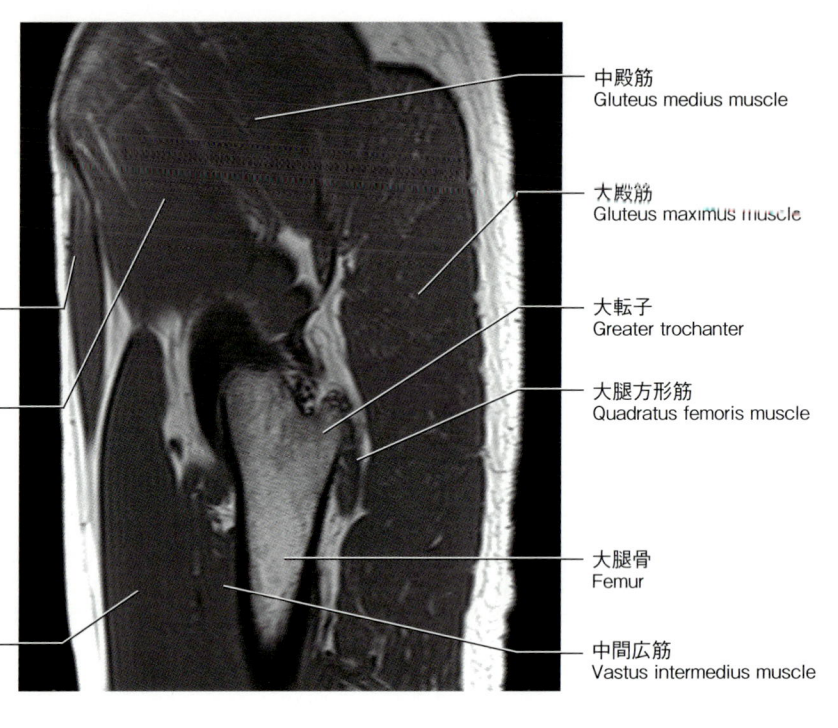

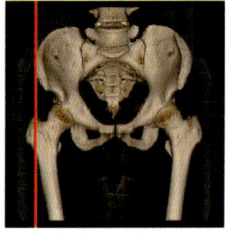

- 縫工筋 Sartorius muscle
- 小殿筋 Gluteus minimus muscle
- 大腿直筋 Rectus femoris muscle
- 中殿筋 Gluteus medius muscle
- 大殿筋 Gluteus maximus muscle
- 大転子 Greater trochanter
- 大腿方形筋 Quadratus femoris muscle
- 大腿骨 Femur
- 中間広筋 Vastus intermedius muscle

7-115

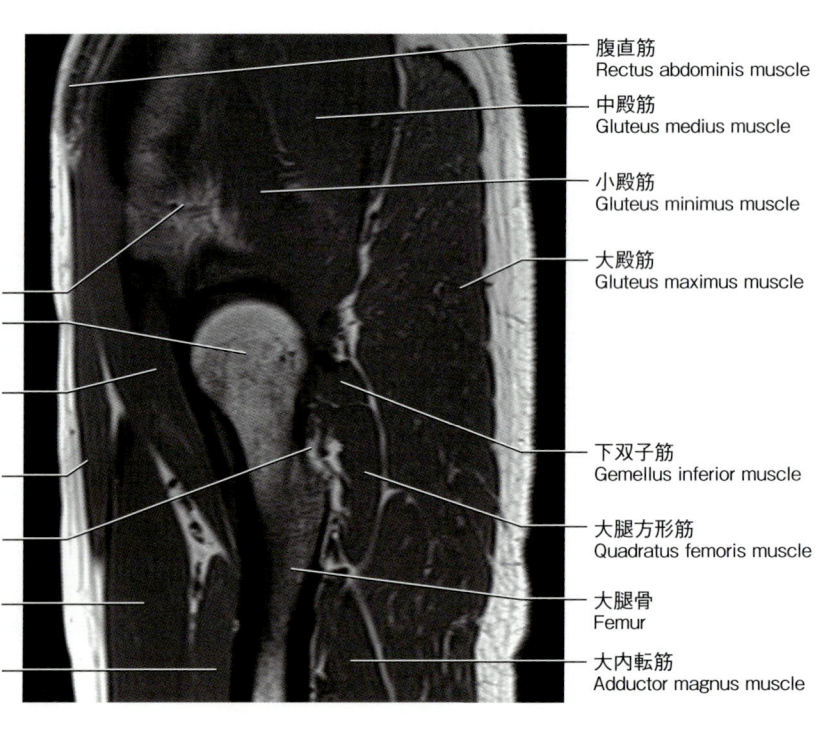

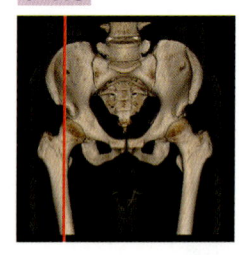

- 腸骨 Ilium
- 大腿骨頭 Head of femur
- 腸腰筋 Iliopsoas muscle
- 縫工筋 Sartorius muscle
- 外閉鎖筋 Obturator externus muscle
- 大腿直筋 Rectus femoris muscle
- 中間広筋 Vastus intermedius muscle
- 腹直筋 Rectus abdominis muscle
- 中殿筋 Gluteus medius muscle
- 小殿筋 Gluteus minimus muscle
- 大殿筋 Gluteus maximus muscle
- 下双子筋 Gemellus inferior muscle
- 大腿方形筋 Quadratus femoris muscle
- 大腿骨 Femur
- 大内転筋 Adductor magnus muscle

> **NOTE** ハムストリング Hamstring
> ハムは豚のもも肉の意味のham（英語），ストリングはひもの意味のstring（英語），ハムストリングとは「もも肉のひも」の意で，肉屋が店頭で豚肉をぶら下げるときにもも裏の筋肉の腱を使ったことに由来する．

股関節の断層解剖 ［矢状断像（MRI，プロトン密度強調像）］

7-116

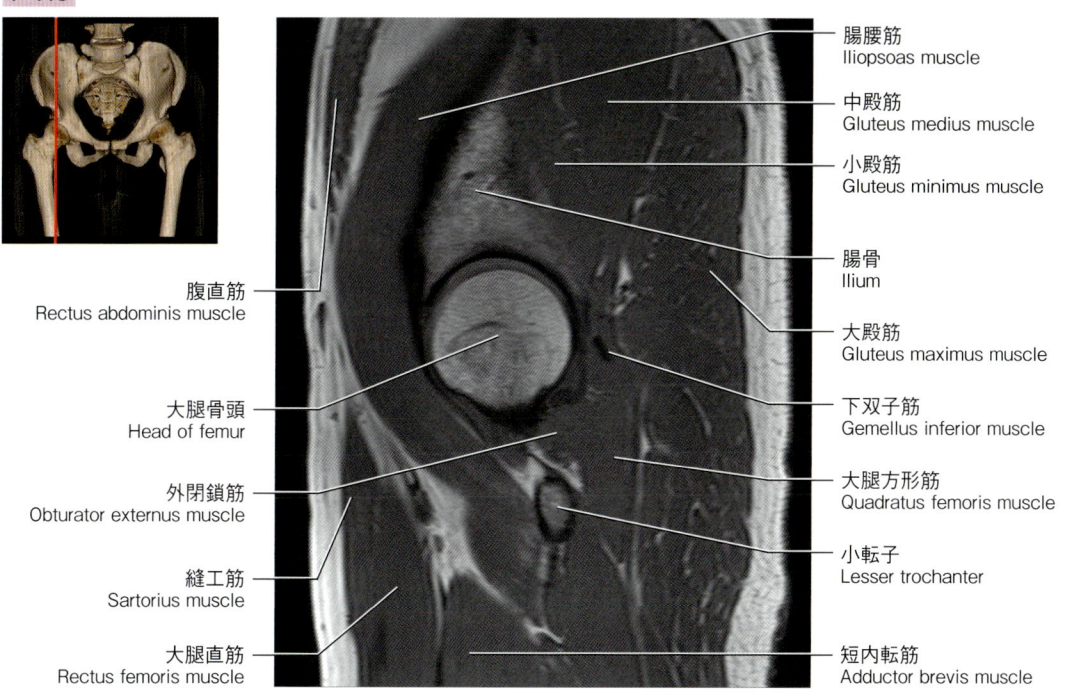

- 腹直筋 Rectus abdominis muscle
- 大腿骨頭 Head of femur
- 外閉鎖筋 Obturator externus muscle
- 縫工筋 Sartorius muscle
- 大腿直筋 Rectus femoris muscle
- 腸腰筋 Iliopsoas muscle
- 中殿筋 Gluteus medius muscle
- 小殿筋 Gluteus minimus muscle
- 腸骨 Ilium
- 大殿筋 Gluteus maximus muscle
- 下双子筋 Gemellus inferior muscle
- 大腿方形筋 Quadratus femoris muscle
- 小転子 Lesser trochanter
- 短内転筋 Adductor brevis muscle

7-117

- 腹直筋 Rectus abdominis muscle
- 大腿骨頭 Head of femur
- 外閉鎖筋 Obturator externus muscle
- 大内転筋 Adductor magnus muscle
- 大腿直筋 Rectus femoris muscle
- 腸腰筋 Iliopsoas muscle
- 腸骨 Ilium
- 中殿筋 Gluteus medius muscle
- 大殿筋 Gluteus maximus muscle
- 下双子筋 Gemellus inferior muscle
- 坐骨 Ischium
- 短内転筋 Adductor brevis muscle

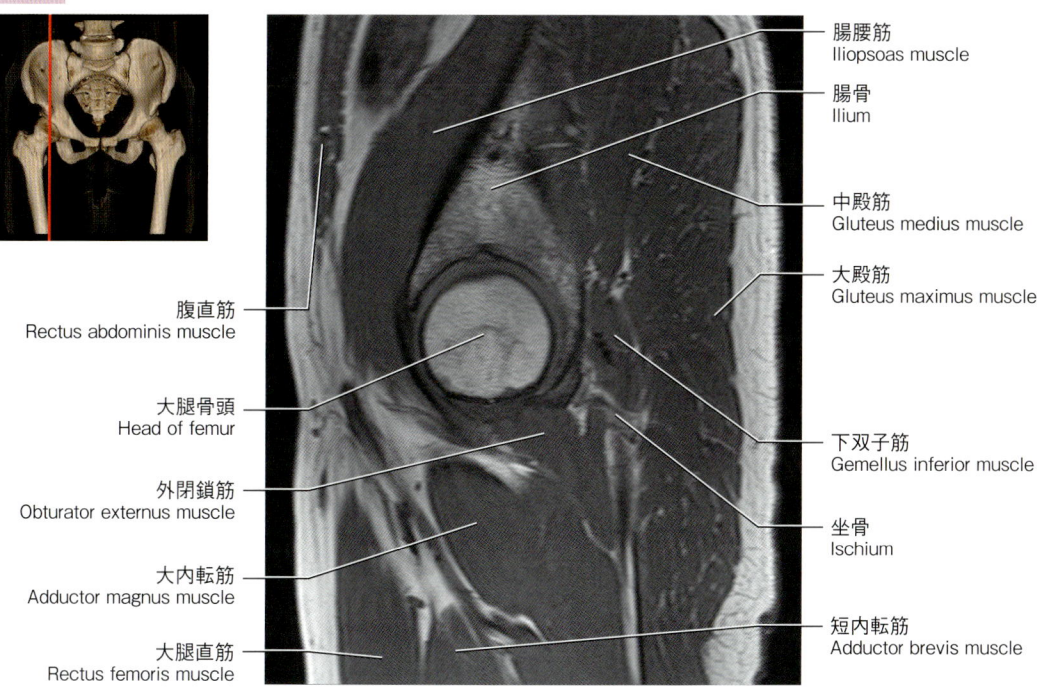

NOTE 大腿神経は腰神経叢最大の神経で，L2〜L4神経根より形成される．大腰筋と腸骨筋の間の前面を腸骨筋膜に包まれて下行し，腸腰筋とともに鼠径靱帯の下の筋裂孔を通って大腿前面に出る．

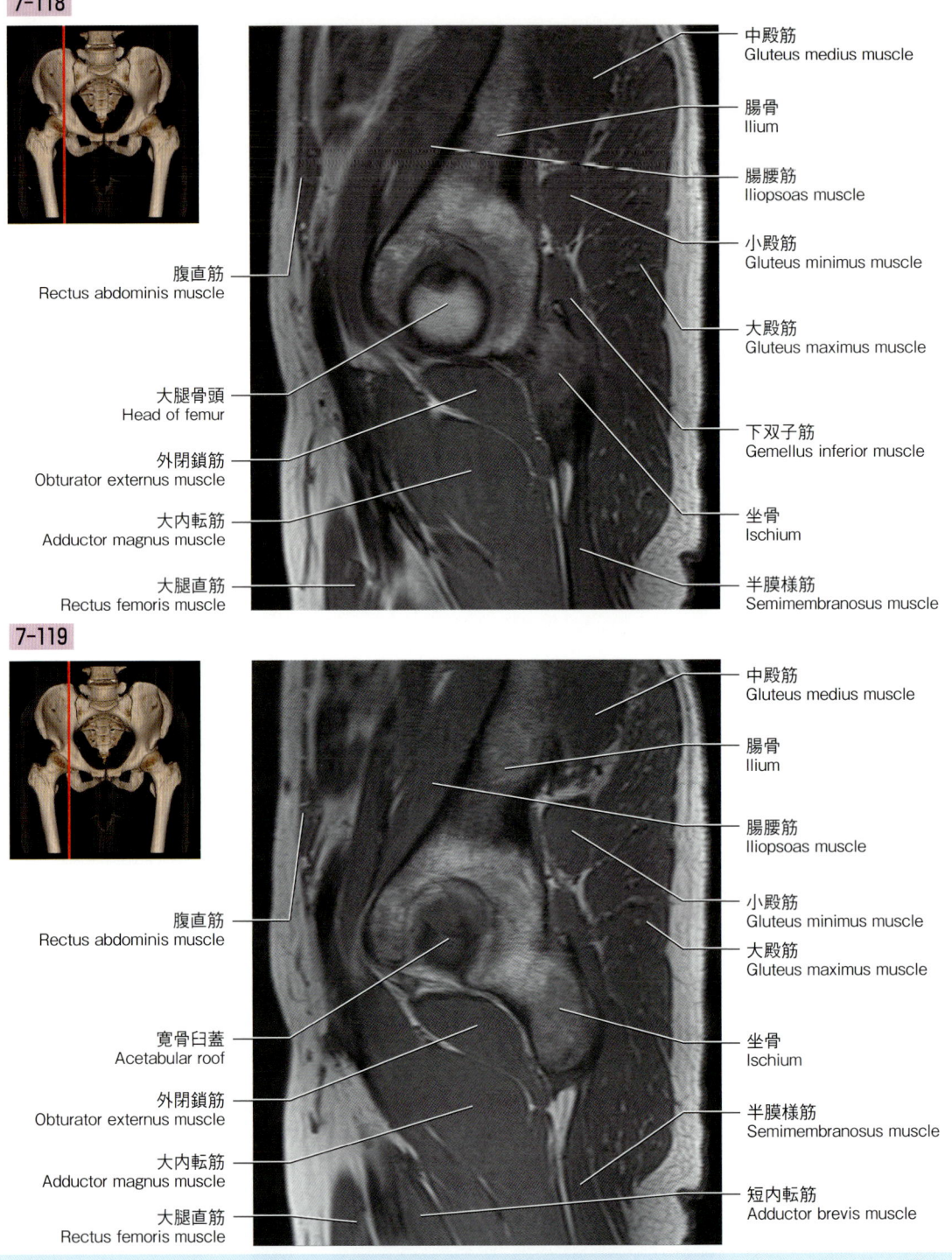

股関節の断層解剖 ［矢状断像（MRI，プロトン密度強調像）］

7-118

- 中殿筋 Gluteus medius muscle
- 腸骨 Ilium
- 腸腰筋 Iliopsoas muscle
- 小殿筋 Gluteus minimus muscle
- 大殿筋 Gluteus maximus muscle
- 下双子筋 Gemellus inferior muscle
- 坐骨 Ischium
- 半膜様筋 Semimembranosus muscle
- 腹直筋 Rectus abdominis muscle
- 大腿骨頭 Head of femur
- 外閉鎖筋 Obturator externus muscle
- 大内転筋 Adductor magnus muscle
- 大腿直筋 Rectus femoris muscle

7-119

- 中殿筋 Gluteus medius muscle
- 腸骨 Ilium
- 腸腰筋 Iliopsoas muscle
- 小殿筋 Gluteus minimus muscle
- 大殿筋 Gluteus maximus muscle
- 坐骨 Ischium
- 半膜様筋 Semimembranosus muscle
- 短内転筋 Adductor brevis muscle
- 腹直筋 Rectus abdominis muscle
- 寛骨臼蓋 Acetabular roof
- 外閉鎖筋 Obturator externus muscle
- 大内転筋 Adductor magnus muscle
- 大腿直筋 Rectus femoris muscle

NOTE 坐骨神経は腰仙神経叢のL4～S3神経根より形成される人体最大の神経で，大坐骨孔を後方に抜けたのち，梨状筋の下縁より殿部に出る．上双子筋，内閉鎖筋，下双子筋，大腿方形筋の背側で大殿筋の腹側を通り，大腿後面を下行し，大内転筋，半膜様筋，半腱様筋，大腿二頭筋に分布する．坐骨神経は膝窩上部でさらに脛骨神経と総腓骨神経に分岐する．坐骨神経あるいはその一部が，梨状筋の筋腹間を貫通するなどの正常変異を認める（10％前後）．このような症例では長距離走のような股関節の反復駆使によって，神経の摩擦や絞扼を生じ坐骨神経炎をきたすことがある．その結果，坐骨神経に沿った放散痛をきたすものは，梨状筋症候群として知られている．

膝関節（CT, VR 像）

7-120 膝部の体表解剖（前面）

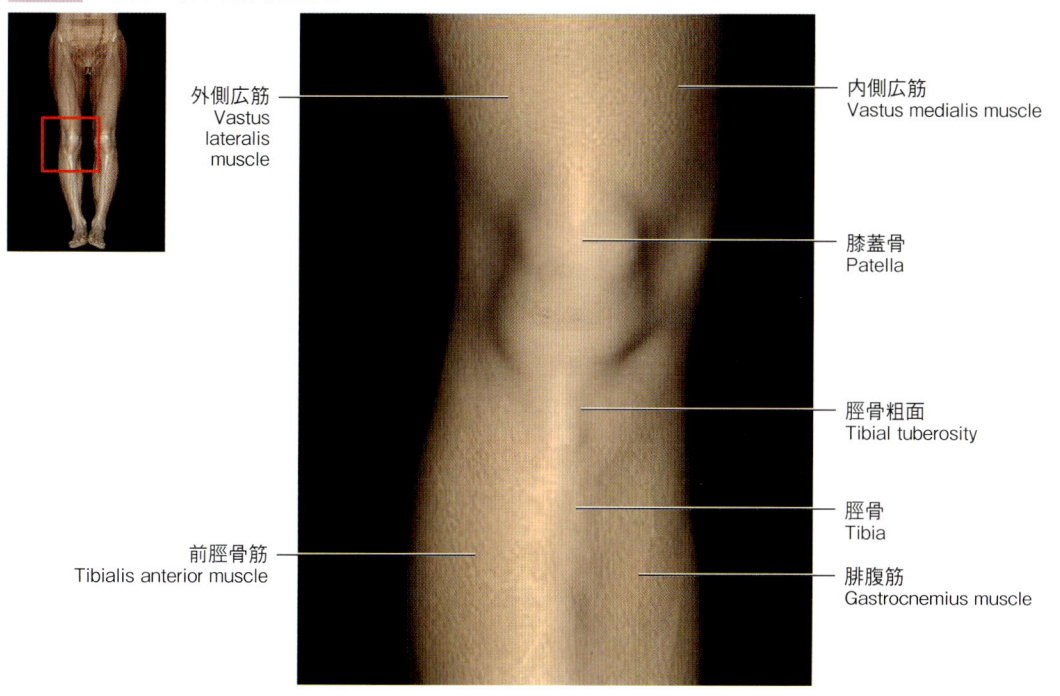

- 外側広筋 Vastus lateralis muscle
- 内側広筋 Vastus medialis muscle
- 膝蓋骨 Patella
- 脛骨粗面 Tibial tuberosity
- 脛骨 Tibia
- 前脛骨筋 Tibialis anterior muscle
- 腓腹筋 Gastrocnemius muscle

NOTE 膝関節は大腿骨，脛骨，および膝蓋骨により構成される．共通の関節包内に大腿脛骨関節と膝蓋大腿関節を有する．膝関節の主な運動は屈伸運動であるが，軽度の回旋運動も行う．

膝関節（CT, VR像）

7-121　膝関節の筋（前面）

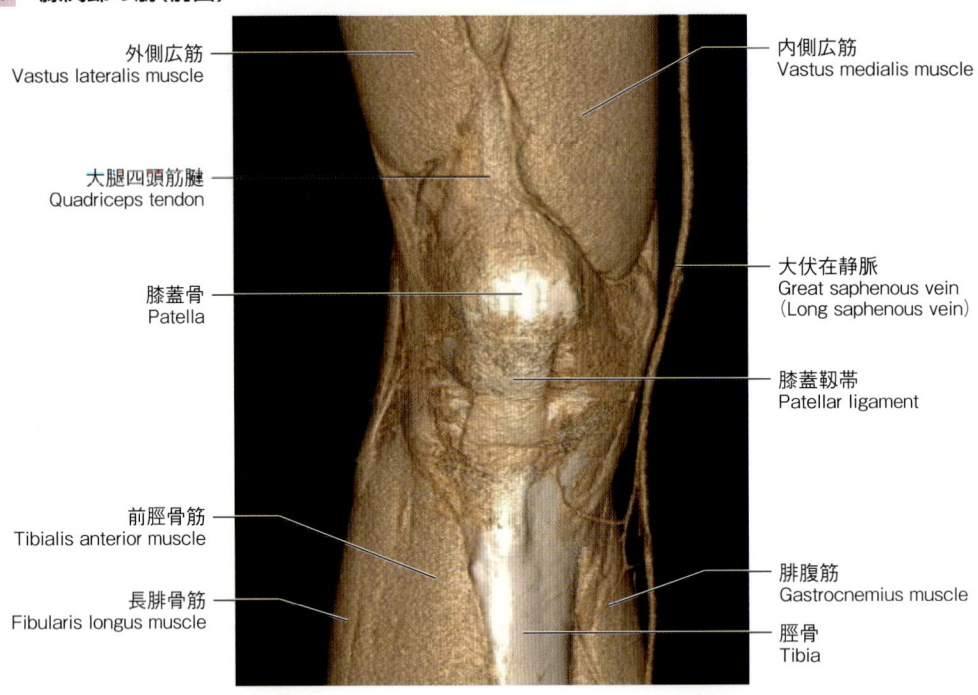

- 外側広筋 Vastus lateralis muscle
- 大腿四頭筋腱 Quadriceps tendon
- 膝蓋骨 Patella
- 前脛骨筋 Tibialis anterior muscle
- 長腓骨筋 Fibularis longus muscle
- 内側広筋 Vastus medialis muscle
- 大伏在静脈 Great saphenous vein（Long saphenous vein）
- 膝蓋靱帯 Patellar ligament
- 腓腹筋 Gastrocnemius muscle
- 脛骨 Tibia

7-122　膝関節の筋（後面）

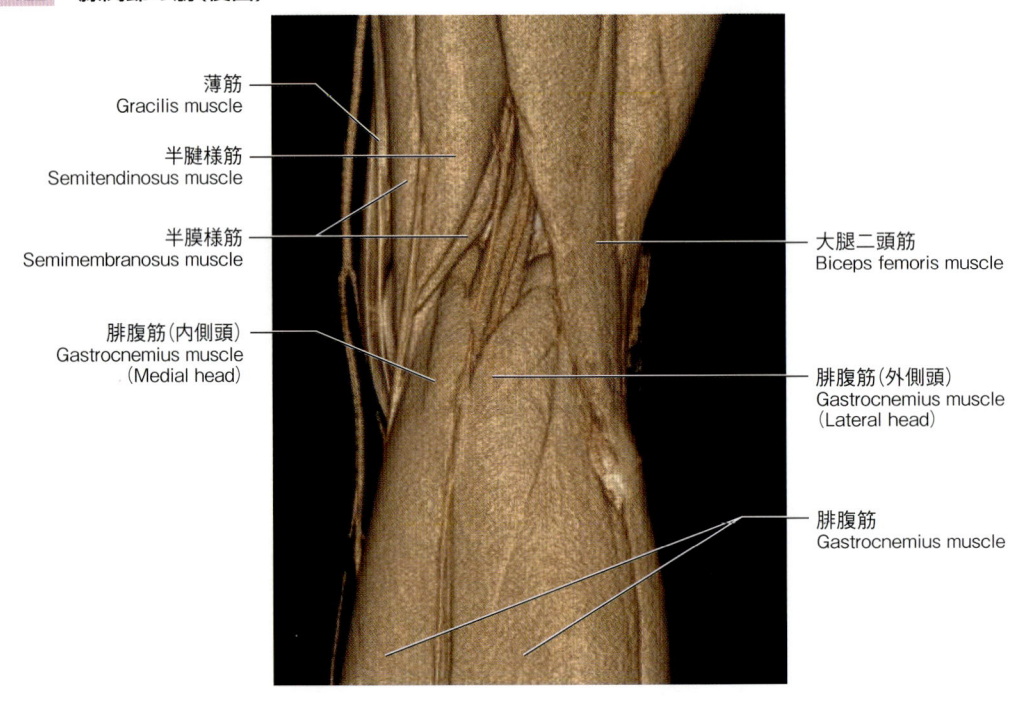

- 薄筋 Gracilis muscle
- 半腱様筋 Semitendinosus muscle
- 半膜様筋 Semimembranosus muscle
- 腓腹筋（内側頭）Gastrocnemius muscle（Medial head）
- 大腿二頭筋 Biceps femoris muscle
- 腓腹筋（外側頭）Gastrocnemius muscle（Lateral head）
- 腓腹筋 Gastrocnemius muscle

> **NOTE**　膝関節の屈伸運動には膝蓋大腿関節が大きな役割を果たすが，その運動と支持には大腿四頭筋・腱，膝蓋骨，内・外側支帯，膝蓋靱帯が関与する．屈曲は大腿部膝屈筋群（Hamstring muscle group：大腿二頭筋，半膜様筋，半腱様筋），縫工筋，薄筋によって行われ，非荷重時には腓腹筋も関与する．

膝関節（CT, VR 像）

7-123 膝関節の筋・靱帯（前面）

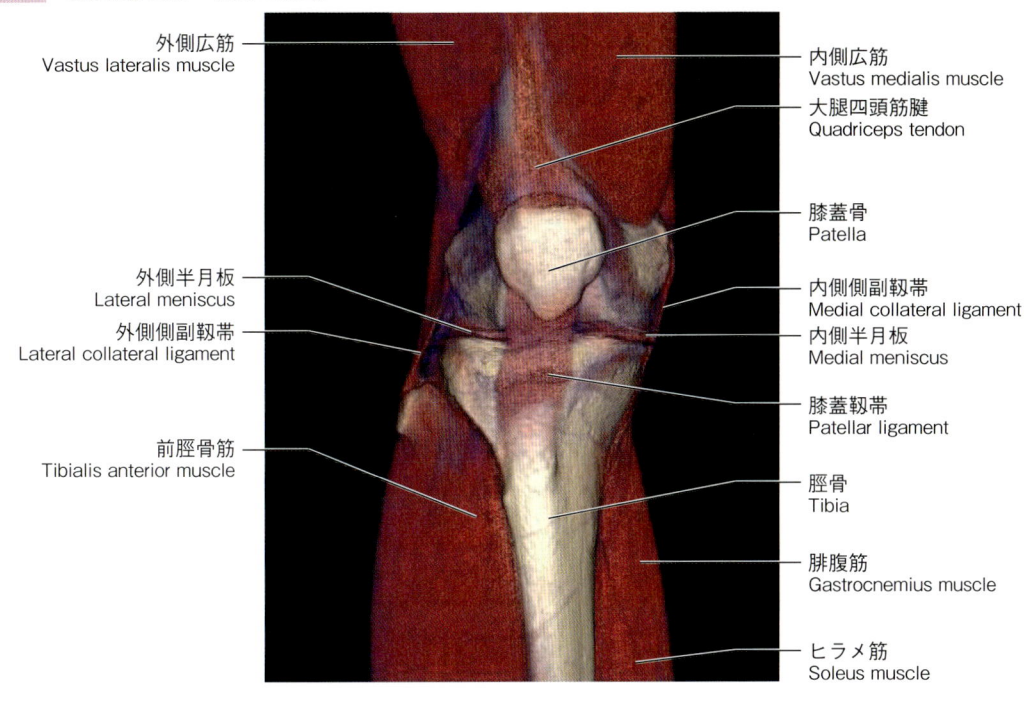

- 外側広筋 Vastus lateralis muscle
- 外側半月板 Lateral meniscus
- 外側側副靱帯 Lateral collateral ligament
- 前脛骨筋 Tibialis anterior muscle
- 内側広筋 Vastus medialis muscle
- 大腿四頭筋腱 Quadriceps tendon
- 膝蓋骨 Patella
- 内側側副靱帯 Medial collateral ligament
- 内側半月板 Medial meniscus
- 膝蓋靱帯 Patellar ligament
- 脛骨 Tibia
- 腓腹筋 Gastrocnemius muscle
- ヒラメ筋 Soleus muscle

7-124 外側側副靱帯（外側側面）

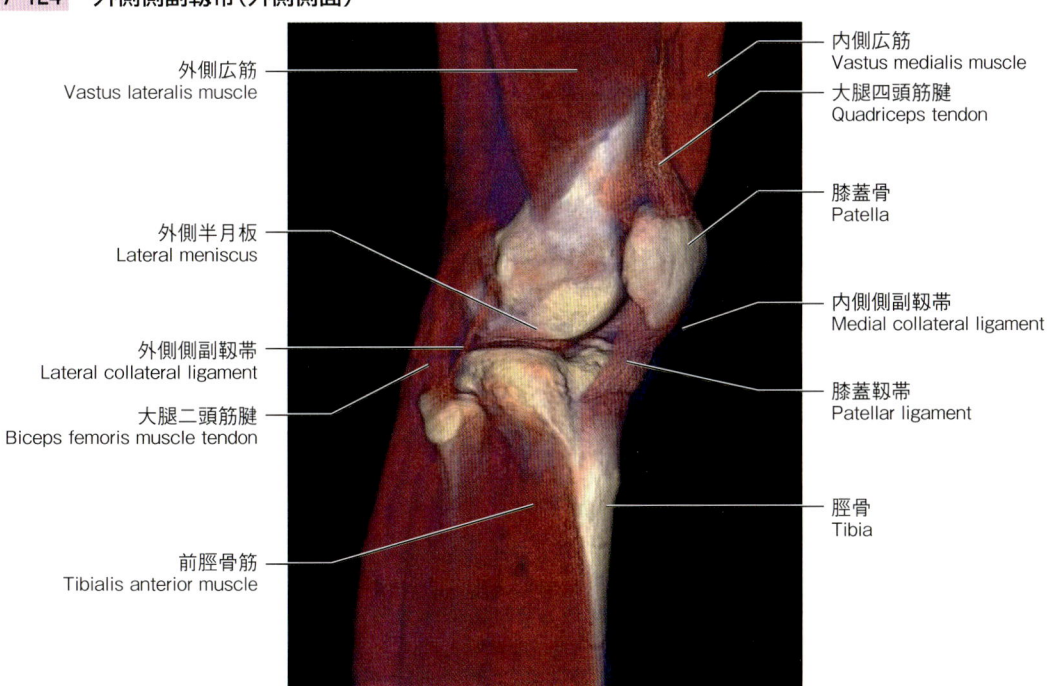

- 外側広筋 Vastus lateralis muscle
- 外側半月板 Lateral meniscus
- 外側側副靱帯 Lateral collateral ligament
- 大腿二頭筋腱 Biceps femoris muscle tendon
- 前脛骨筋 Tibialis anterior muscle
- 内側広筋 Vastus medialis muscle
- 大腿四頭筋腱 Quadriceps tendon
- 膝蓋骨 Patella
- 内側側副靱帯 Medial collateral ligament
- 膝蓋靱帯 Patellar ligament
- 脛骨 Tibia

NOTE 大腿四頭筋は，大腿直筋・内側広筋・外側広筋・中間広筋より構成される．3つの広筋の線維は大腿直筋の腱に癒合して大腿四頭筋腱を形成する．このとき，線維束が異なる深さを走るため，MRIの矢状断像において大腿四頭筋は2層または3層構造を呈する．大腿四頭筋腱の深部は膝蓋骨に停止するが，表層に存在するものは膝蓋骨を越えて，膝蓋靱帯となり脛骨粗面に停止する．

膝関節（CT, VR像）

7-125 内側側副靱帯（内側側面）

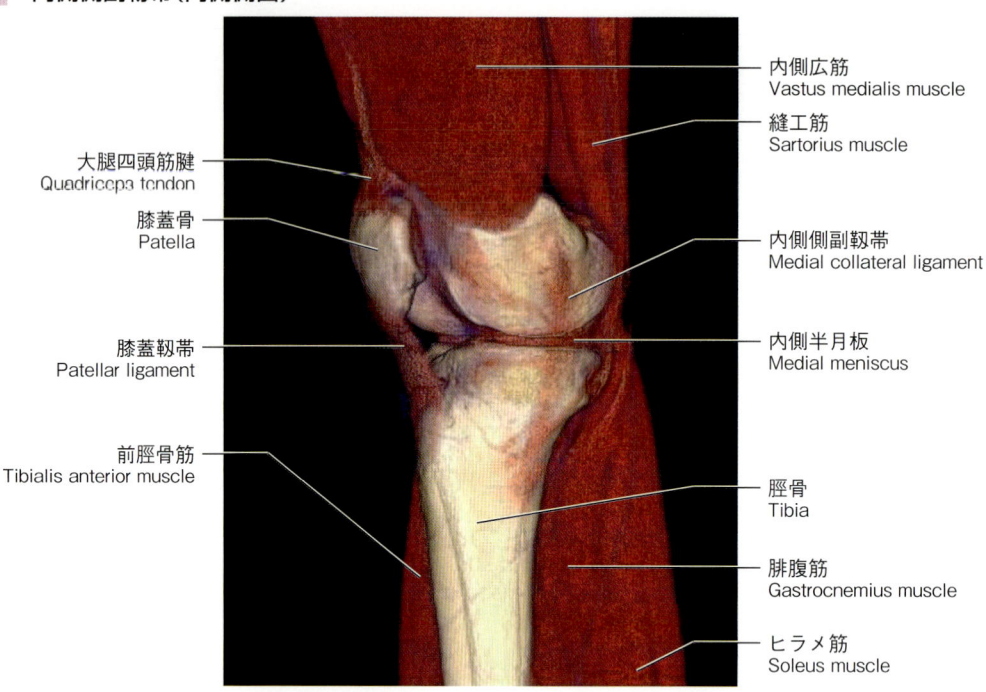

- 大腿四頭筋腱 Quadriceps tendon
- 膝蓋骨 Patella
- 膝蓋靱帯 Patellar ligament
- 前脛骨筋 Tibialis anterior muscle
- 内側広筋 Vastus medialis muscle
- 縫工筋 Sartorius muscle
- 内側側副靱帯 Medial collateral ligament
- 内側半月板 Medial meniscus
- 脛骨 Tibia
- 腓腹筋 Gastrocnemius muscle
- ヒラメ筋 Soleus muscle

7-126 靱帯・半月板

- 後十字靱帯 Posterior cruciate ligament
- 外側半月板 Lateral meniscus
- 脛骨 Tibia
- 大腿骨 Femur
- 前十字靱帯 Anterior cruciate ligament
- 内側半月板 Medial meniscus
- 腓骨 Fibula

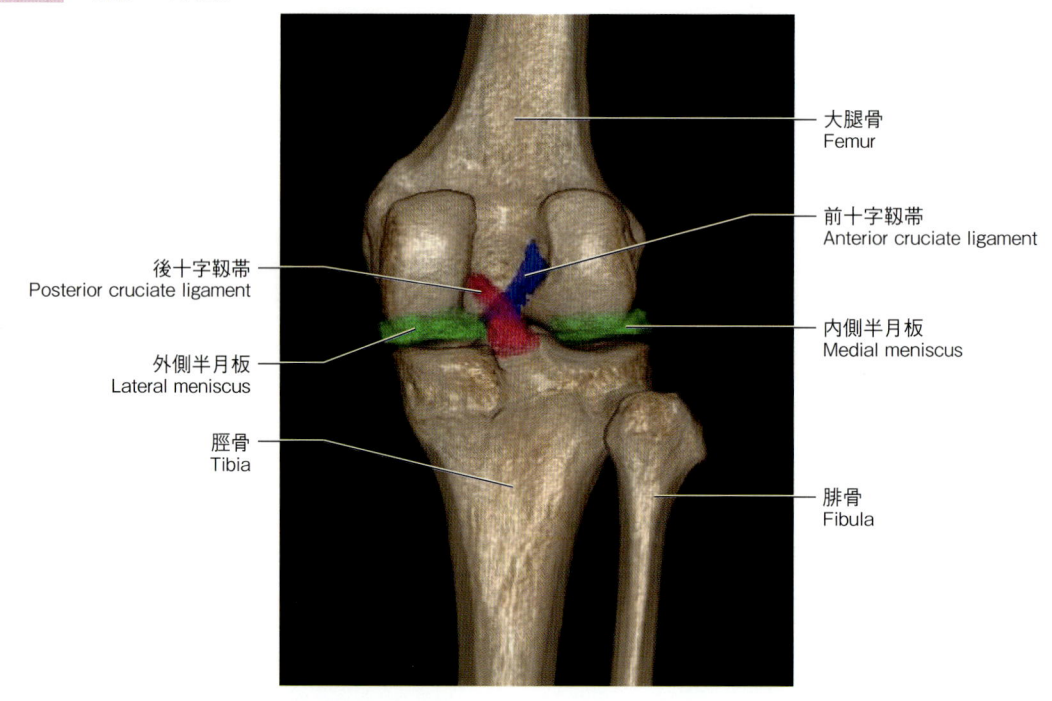

> **NOTE** 前十字靱帯と後十字靱帯はともに関節包内，滑膜外の構造物であり，膝関節の前後方向の安定に貢献する．前十字靱帯は大腿骨外側顆の顆間窩側より起始し，脛骨の前顆間区に停止する．後十字靱帯は大腿骨内側顆の顆間窩側より起始し，後顆間区と外側半月板の後角に停止する．前十字靱帯は2本の線維束すなわち，前内側線維束（Anteromedial bundle）と後外側線維束（Posterolateral bundle）より構成される．屈曲位では前者が緊張し，伸展位では後者が緊張する．後十字靱帯は，前十字靱帯よりも太く強力である．

半月板（CT，VR像）

7-127 半月板（正面）

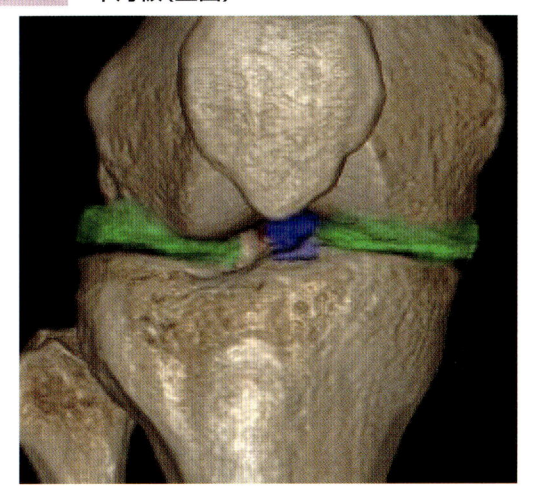

7-128 半月板（内側側面）

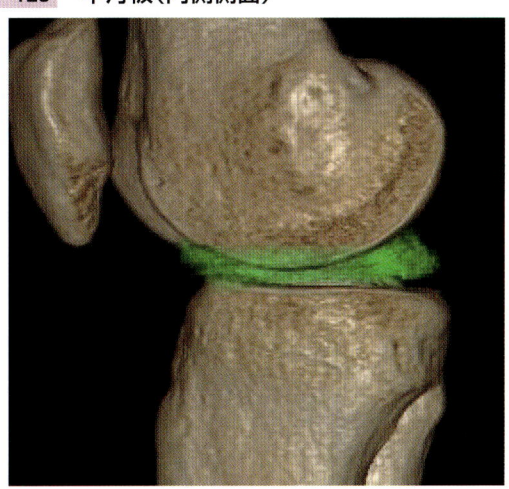

7-129 半月板（頭側から脛骨関節面を観察）

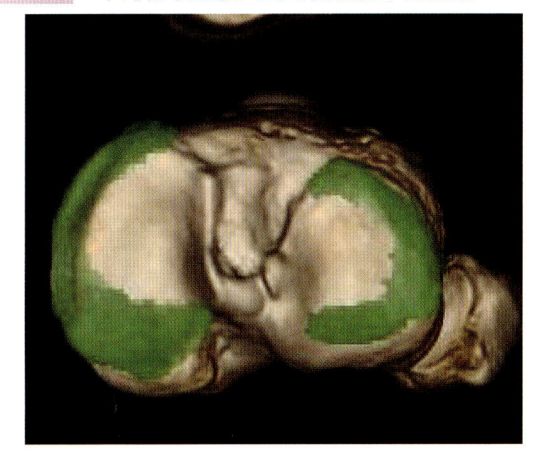

7-130 半月板（尾側から大腿骨関節面を観察）

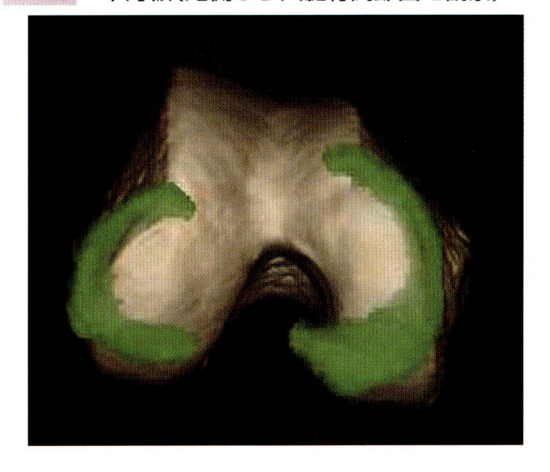

> **NOTE** 内側側副靱帯と外側側副靱帯は，膝関節の側方向の安定に貢献する．それぞれ浅層と深層から構成される．内側側副靱帯の深層は関節包そのものである．深層には内側半月板の体部が付着する．外側側副靱帯の深層も関節包そのもので，外側半月板の体部が付着する．半月大腿靱帯は，外側半月板の後角より起始し，2本に分かれて後十字靱帯の前方と後方を通り，大腿骨内側顆の顆間窩側に付着する．前方のものは Humphry（ハンフリー）靱帯，後方のものは Wrisberg（リスバーグ）靱帯とよぶ．

半月板（CT, VR像およびMRI, プロトン密度強調画像）

7-131 矢状断

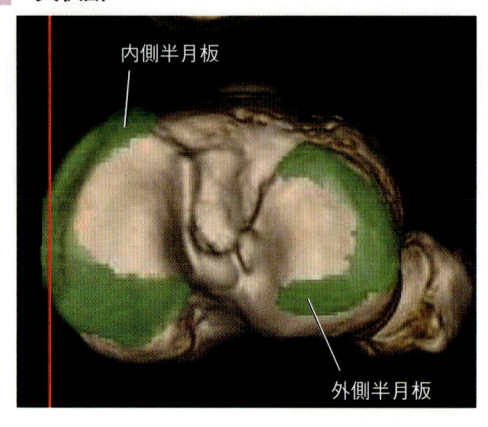

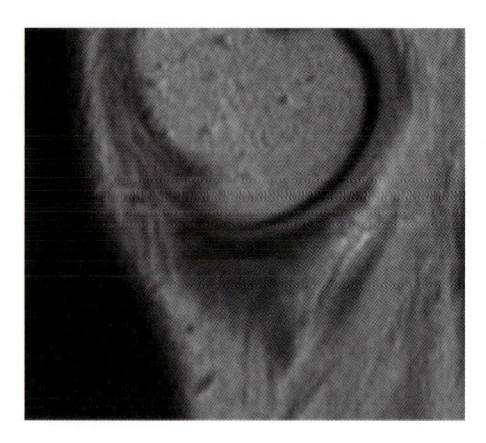

内側半月板
外側半月板

7-132 矢状断

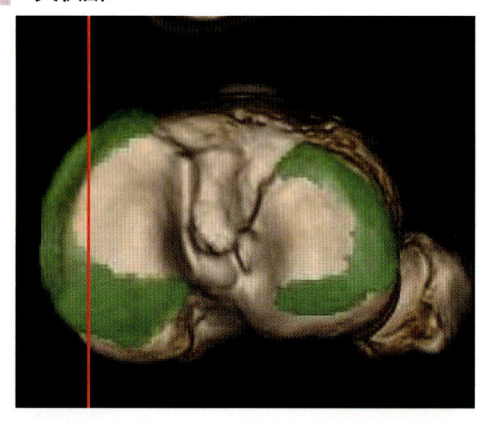

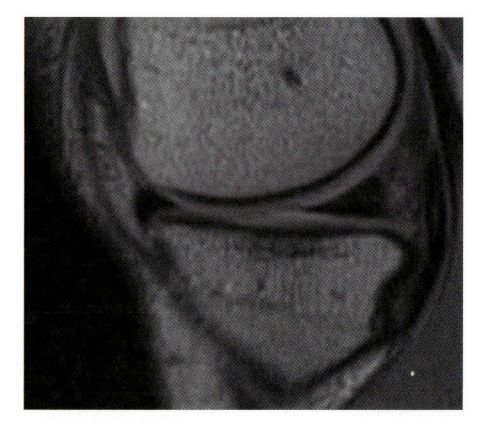

7-133 冠状断

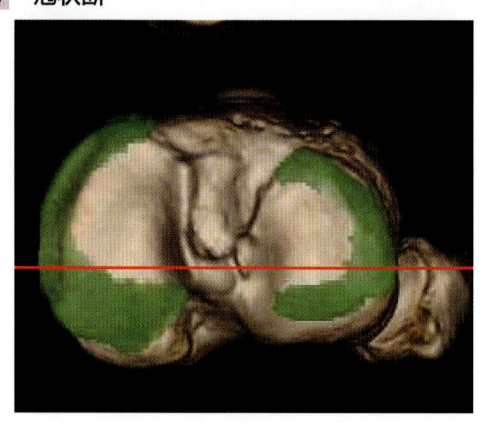

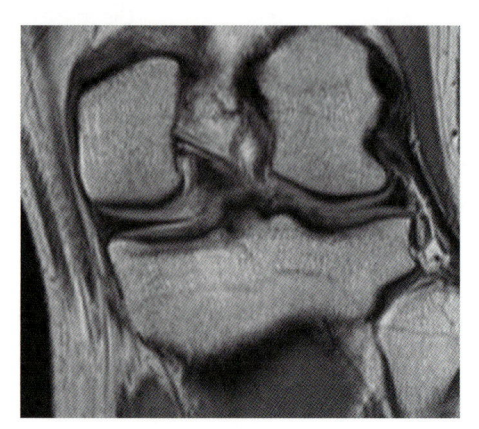

> **NOTE** 半月板は線維軟骨で構成される．内側半月板は半月状に開いたC型をしており，外側半月板は環状に近いC型をしている．内側半月板の脛骨への付着は，前角と後角において線維性組織により行われる．外側半月板は前角から体部まで関節包と密着しているが，後角では膝窩筋腱が半月板関節包接合部を貫通する．膝窩筋腱は大腿骨外顆に起始し，内側下方に向かい，その前内側部を関節滑膜に包まれて外側半月板の後角を貫通する．内側に向かうに従い，膝窩筋腱は半月板の中に埋没し，半月板と関節包が接合する．さらに内側では膝窩筋腱は半月板および関節包の外に出る．

膝関節（CT, VR 像）

7-134 膝関節の骨（前面）

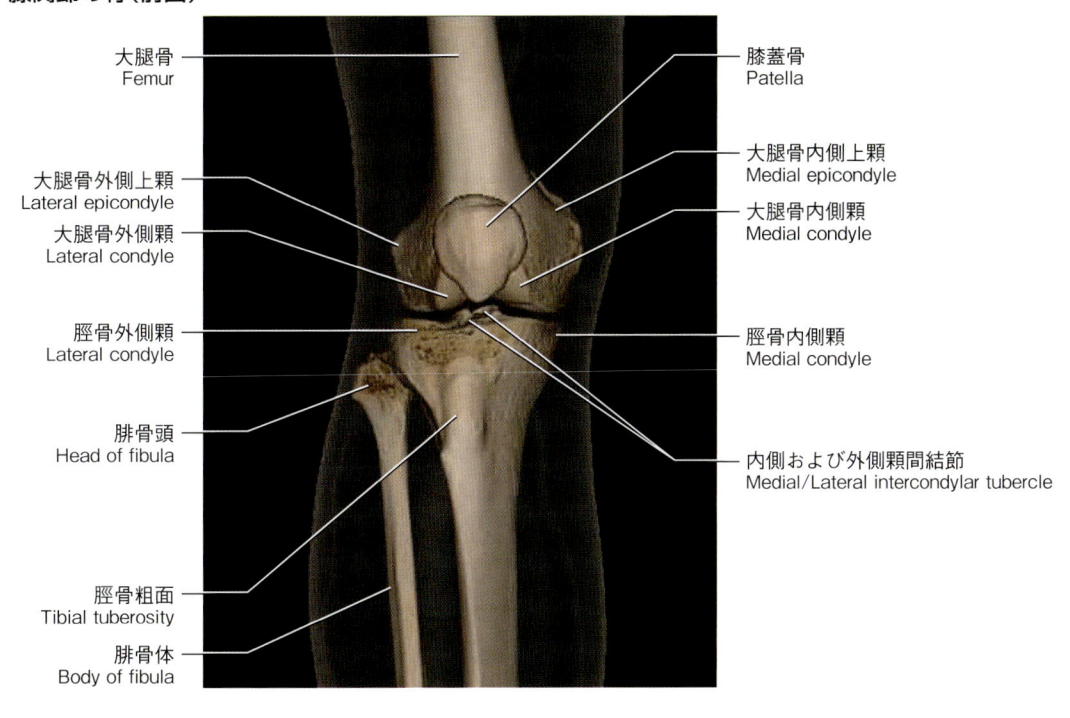

- 大腿骨 Femur
- 膝蓋骨 Patella
- 大腿骨外側上顆 Lateral epicondyle
- 大腿骨内側上顆 Medial epicondyle
- 大腿骨外側顆 Lateral condyle
- 大腿骨内側顆 Medial condyle
- 脛骨外側顆 Lateral condyle
- 脛骨内側顆 Medial condyle
- 腓骨頭 Head of fibula
- 内側および外側顆間結節 Medial/Lateral intercondylar tubercle
- 脛骨粗面 Tibial tuberosity
- 腓骨体 Body of fibula

7-135 膝関節の骨（後面）

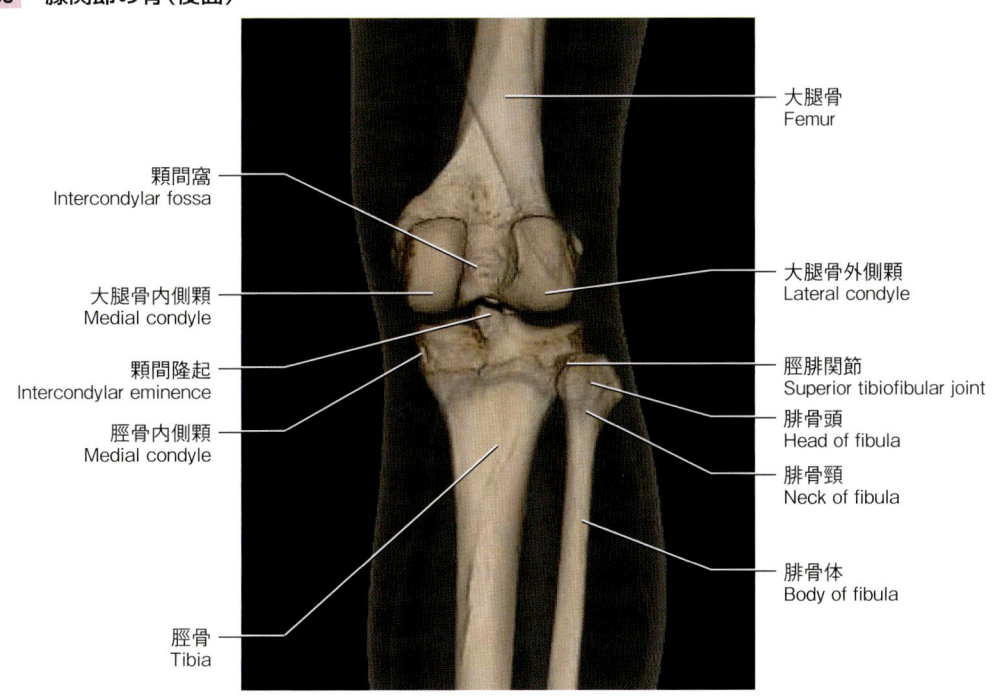

- 大腿骨 Femur
- 顆間窩 Intercondylar fossa
- 大腿骨内側顆 Medial condyle
- 大腿骨外側顆 Lateral condyle
- 顆間隆起 Intercondylar eminence
- 脛腓関節 Superior tibiofibular joint
- 脛骨内側顆 Medial condyle
- 腓骨頭 Head of fibula
- 腓骨頸 Neck of fibula
- 腓骨体 Body of fibula
- 脛骨 Tibia

> **NOTE** 膝蓋骨は人体最大の種子骨である．膝蓋靱帯は膝蓋骨が大腿四頭筋の種子骨であることから，厳密には膝蓋腱であるが，通常，膝蓋靱帯として知られる．この内外側には，主に内側広筋の線維により形成される内側膝蓋支帯と，外側広筋の線維により形成される外側膝蓋支帯が存在する．膝蓋骨は人体の中で最も厚い関節軟骨をもつため，関節軟骨の研究対象として用いられることが多い．

膝関節の断層解剖 [横断像（MRI，プロトン密度強調像）]

7-136

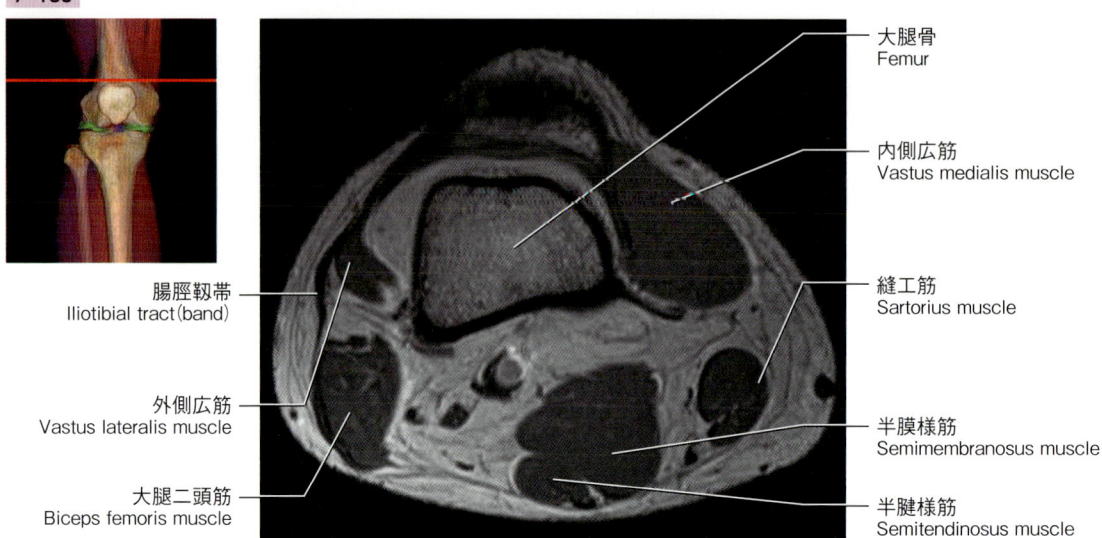

- 大腿骨 Femur
- 内側広筋 Vastus medialis muscle
- 縫工筋 Sartorius muscle
- 半膜様筋 Semimembranosus muscle
- 半腱様筋 Semitendinosus muscle
- 腸脛靱帯 Iliotibial tract (band)
- 外側広筋 Vastus lateralis muscle
- 大腿二頭筋 Biceps femoris muscle

7-137

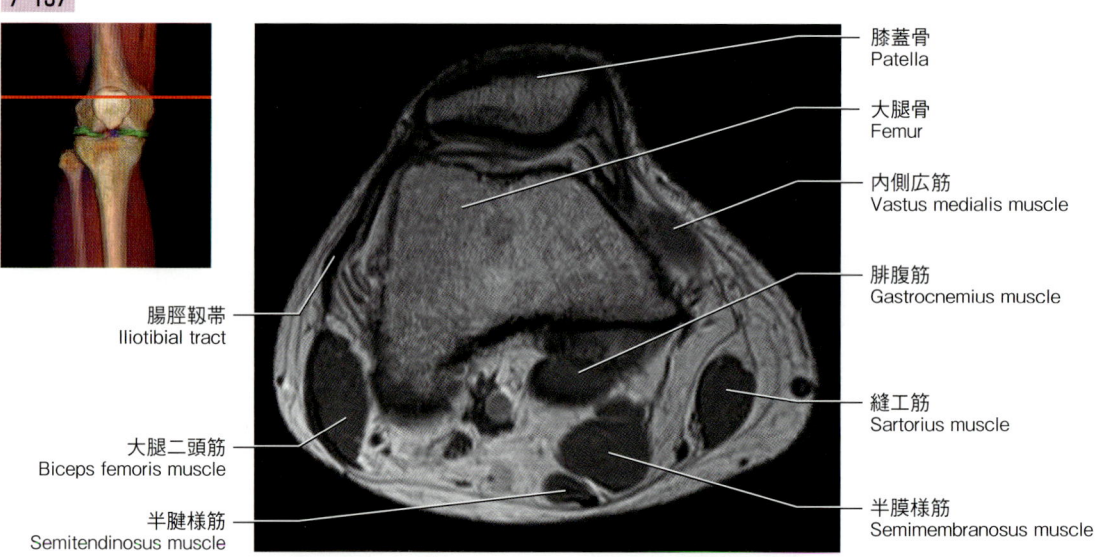

- 膝蓋骨 Patella
- 大腿骨 Femur
- 内側広筋 Vastus medialis muscle
- 腓腹筋 Gastrocnemius muscle
- 縫工筋 Sartorius muscle
- 半膜様筋 Semimembranosus muscle
- 腸脛靱帯 Iliotibial tract
- 大腿二頭筋 Biceps femoris muscle
- 半腱様筋 Semitendinosus muscle

> **NOTE** 内側広筋と一部大腿直筋由来の線維結合組織が内側支帯を形成し，外側広筋と一部大腿直筋由来の線維結合組織が外側支帯を形成する．これらの支帯は膝蓋骨の両側をそれぞれ脛骨の内側顆と外側顆に向かい停止する．

> **NOTE** 内側広筋 Vastus medialis muscle
> 大腿四頭筋は，内側広筋(Vastus medialis muscle)などの四筋よりなるが，"vastus"とは「荒れた，何もない，途方もなく広い」という意味で，解剖名ではこの筋に用いられるのみである．英語の "vast(広漠とした)"，"waste(荒廃させる，無駄にする)" の語源となる．

膝関節の断層解剖　[横断像（MRI, プロトン密度強調像）]

7-138

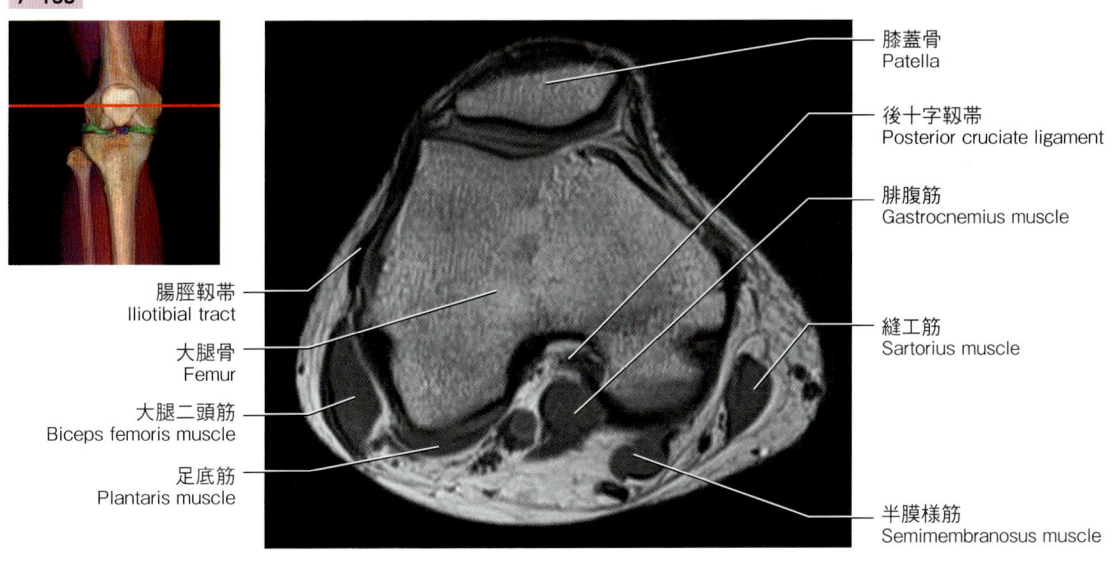

- 膝蓋骨 Patella
- 後十字靱帯 Posterior cruciate ligament
- 腓腹筋 Gastrocnemius muscle
- 縫工筋 Sartorius muscle
- 腸脛靱帯 Iliotibial tract
- 大腿骨 Femur
- 大腿二頭筋 Biceps femoris muscle
- 足底筋 Plantaris muscle
- 半膜様筋 Semimembranosus muscle

7-139

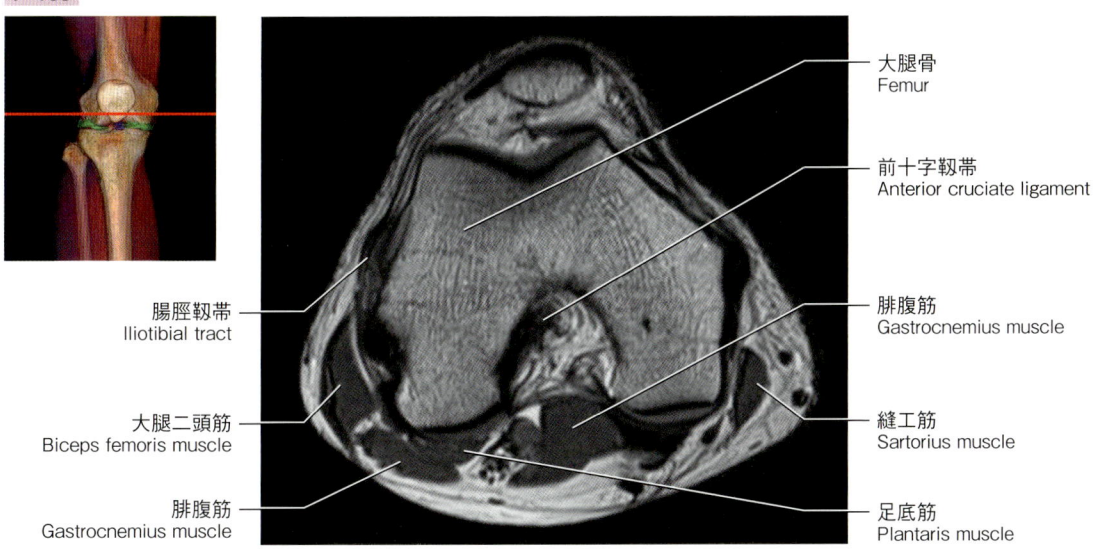

- 大腿骨 Femur
- 前十字靱帯 Anterior cruciate ligament
- 腓腹筋 Gastrocnemius muscle
- 腸脛靱帯 Iliotibial tract
- 大腿二頭筋 Biceps femoris muscle
- 縫工筋 Sartorius muscle
- 腓腹筋 Gastrocnemius muscle
- 足底筋 Plantaris muscle

> **NOTE** 腓腹筋内側頭と半膜様筋腱の間にある滑液包に液体貯留をきたしたものを Baker（ベイカー）嚢胞または膝窩嚢胞とよぶ．多くは中年以降にみられるが，小児や若年者にみられることもある．臨床的に静脈血栓症と誤られることがある．

膝関節の断層解剖 ［横断像（MRI, プロトン密度強調像）］

7-140

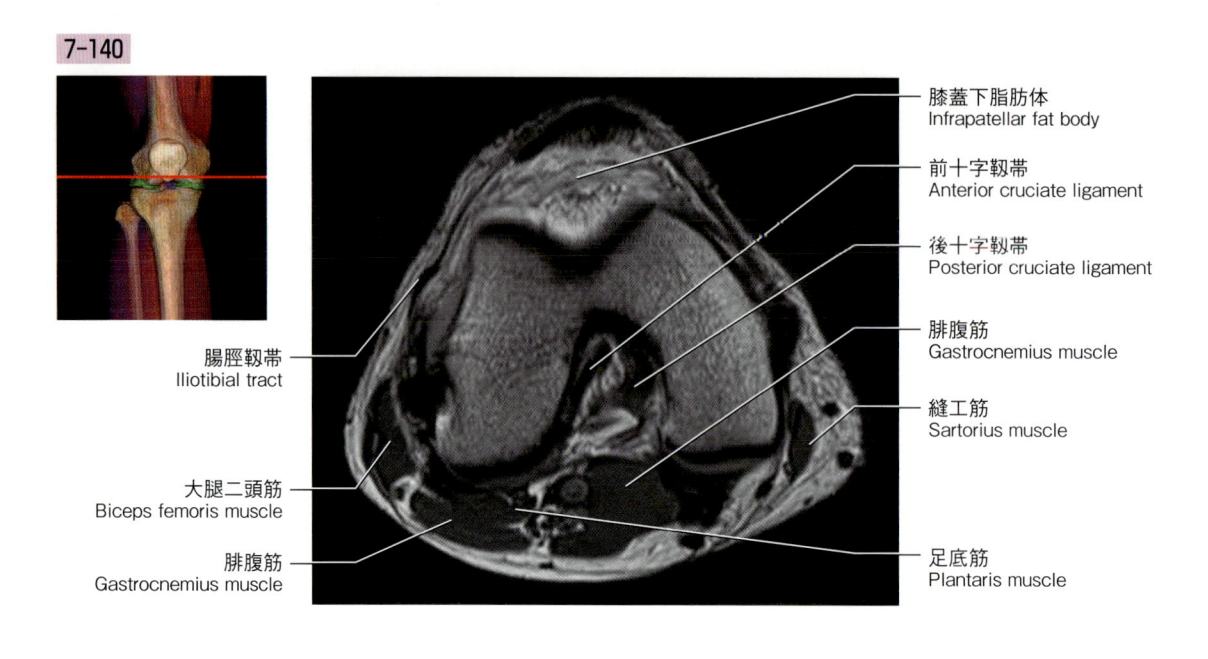

- 膝蓋下脂肪体 Infrapatellar fat body
- 前十字靱帯 Anterior cruciate ligament
- 後十字靱帯 Posterior cruciate ligament
- 腓腹筋 Gastrocnemius muscle
- 縫工筋 Sartorius muscle
- 足底筋 Plantaris muscle
- 腸脛靱帯 Iliotibial tract
- 大腿二頭筋 Biceps femoris muscle
- 腓腹筋 Gastrocnemius muscle

7-141

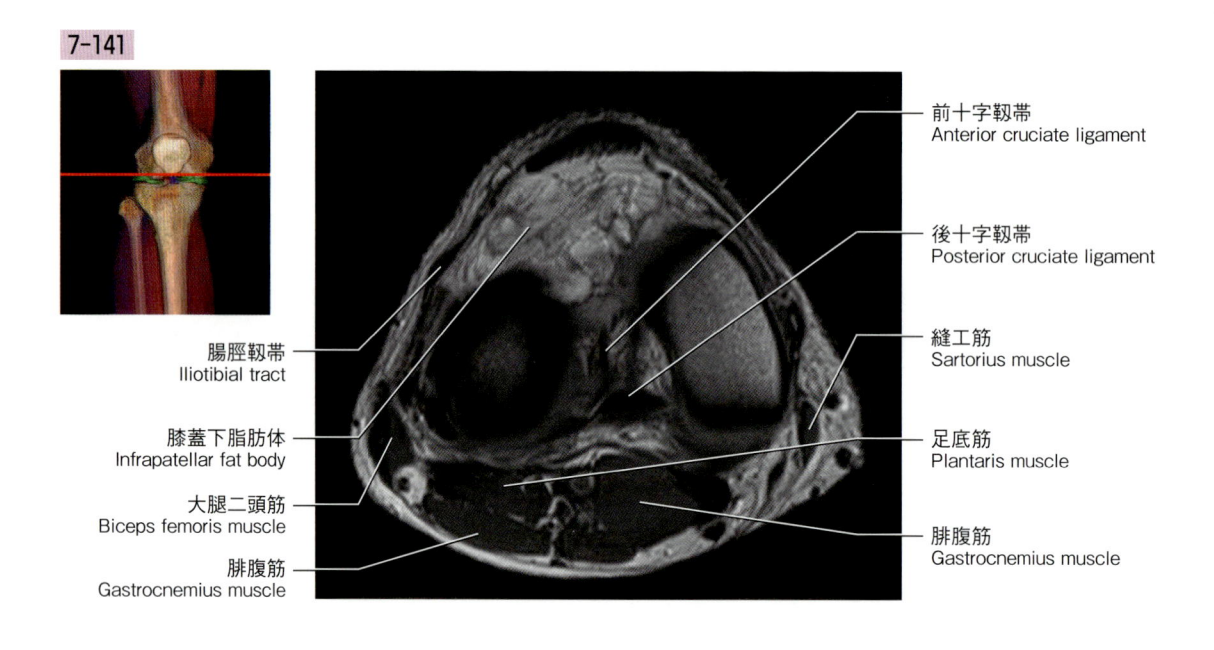

- 前十字靱帯 Anterior cruciate ligament
- 後十字靱帯 Posterior cruciate ligament
- 縫工筋 Sartorius muscle
- 足底筋 Plantaris muscle
- 腓腹筋 Gastrocnemius muscle
- 腸脛靱帯 Iliotibial tract
- 膝蓋下脂肪体 Infrapatellar fat body
- 大腿二頭筋 Biceps femoris muscle
- 腓腹筋 Gastrocnemius muscle

> **NOTE** 腸脛靱帯症候群は，腸脛靱帯摩擦症候群ともよばれ，膝内側の痛みの原因となる．陸上競技の長距離走や競輪，バスケットボール，重量挙げなどの膝の屈伸をくり返すスポーツでみられる．膝の屈伸において腸脛靱帯と大腿骨外側顆の間に摩擦がくり返され，炎症性変化を生じると考えられる．

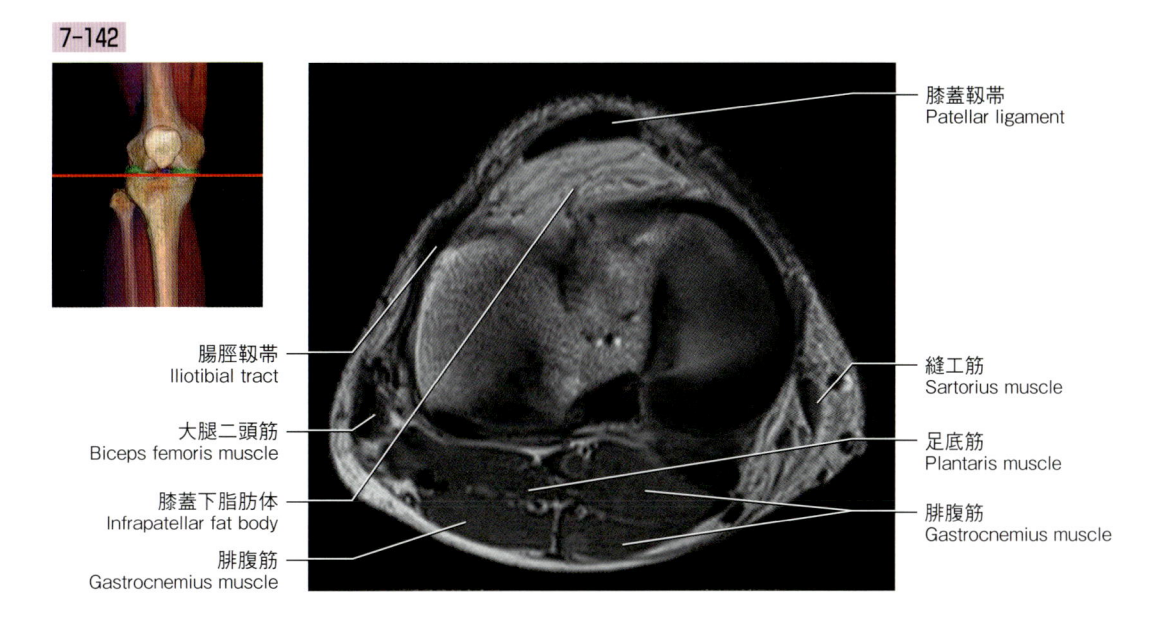

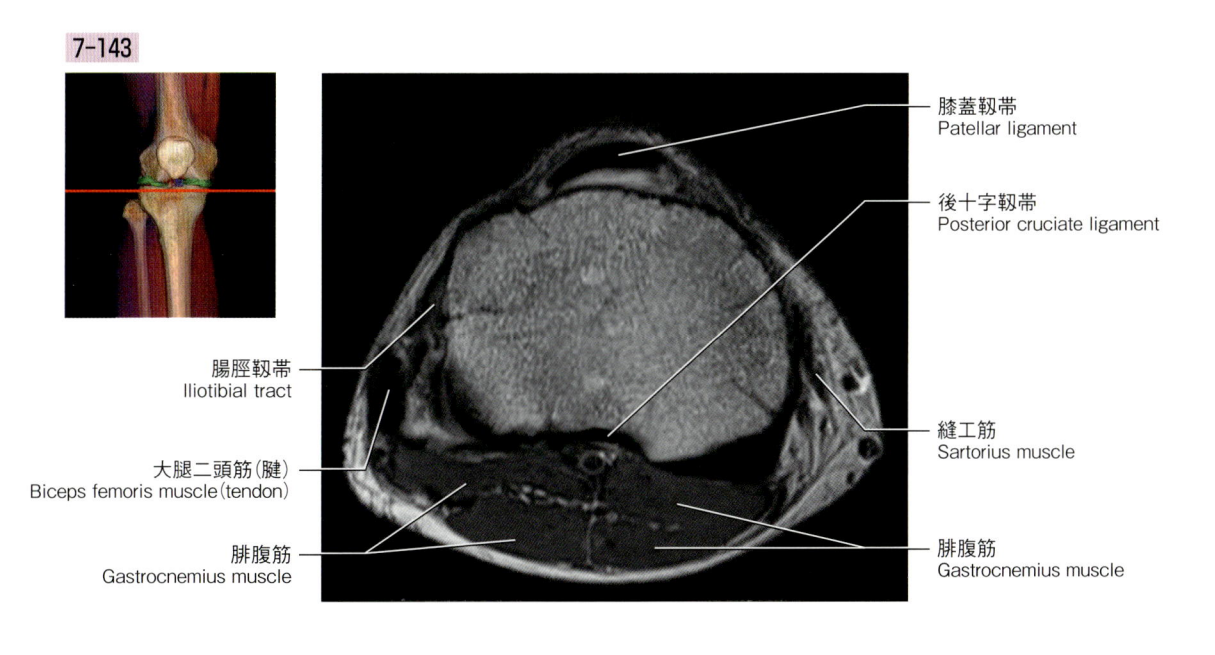

膝関節の断層解剖 ［横断像（MRI, プロトン密度強調像）］

7-142

- 膝蓋靱帯 Patellar ligament
- 腸脛靱帯 Iliotibial tract
- 大腿二頭筋 Biceps femoris muscle
- 膝蓋下脂肪体 Infrapatellar fat body
- 腓腹筋 Gastrocnemius muscle
- 縫工筋 Sartorius muscle
- 足底筋 Plantaris muscle
- 腓腹筋 Gastrocnemius muscle

7-143

- 膝蓋靱帯 Patellar ligament
- 腸脛靱帯 Iliotibial tract
- 大腿二頭筋(腱) Biceps femoris muscle(tendon)
- 腓腹筋 Gastrocnemius muscle
- 後十字靱帯 Posterior cruciate ligament
- 縫工筋 Sartorius muscle
- 腓腹筋 Gastrocnemius muscle

NOTE 縫工筋，薄筋，半腱様筋は共通腱となって脛骨近位部内側に停止するが，これらの腱の停止部の形態が鵞鳥（ガチョウ）の水かきに似ていることから鵞足とよばれる．

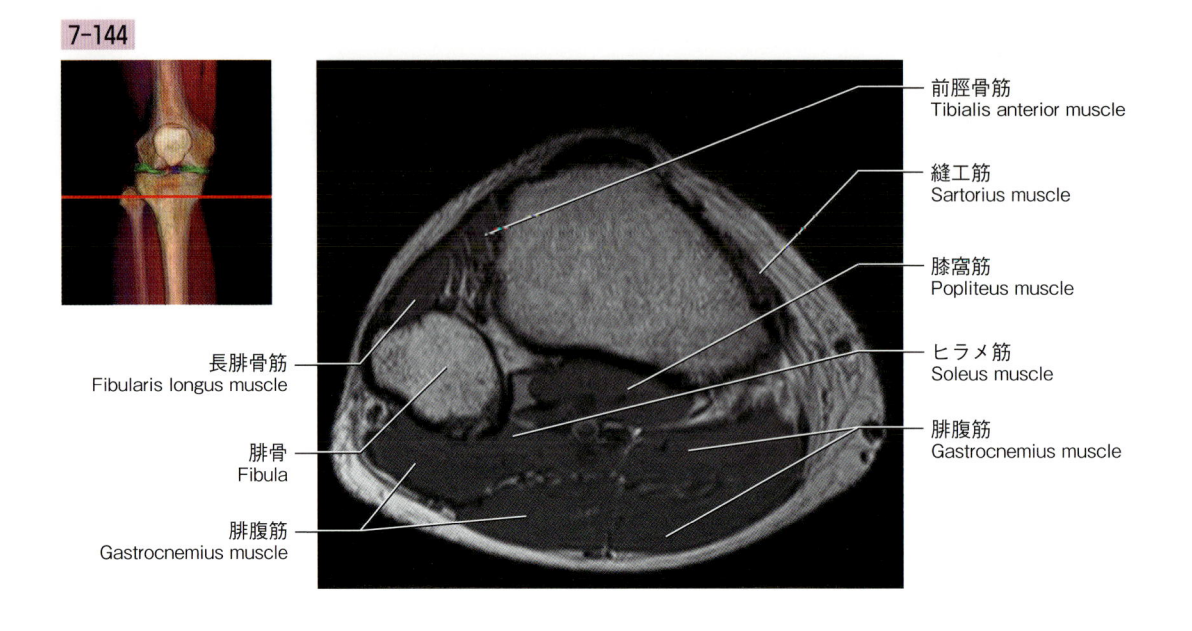

膝関節の断層解剖［横断像（MRI，プロトン密度強調像）］

7-144

- 前脛骨筋 Tibialis anterior muscle
- 縫工筋 Sartorius muscle
- 膝窩筋 Popliteus muscle
- ヒラメ筋 Soleus muscle
- 腓腹筋 Gastrocnemius muscle
- 長腓骨筋 Fibularis longus muscle
- 腓骨 Fibula
- 腓腹筋 Gastrocnemius muscle

NOTE 鵞足部には縫工筋下滑液包，鵞足滑液包の2つの滑液包がある．鵞足炎は肥満，変形性膝関節症で合併することが多く，鵞足部の圧痛や運動痛を特徴とする．

膝関節の断層解剖 ［冠状断像（MRI，プロトン密度強調像）］

7-145

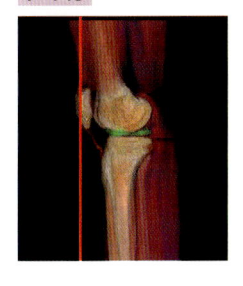

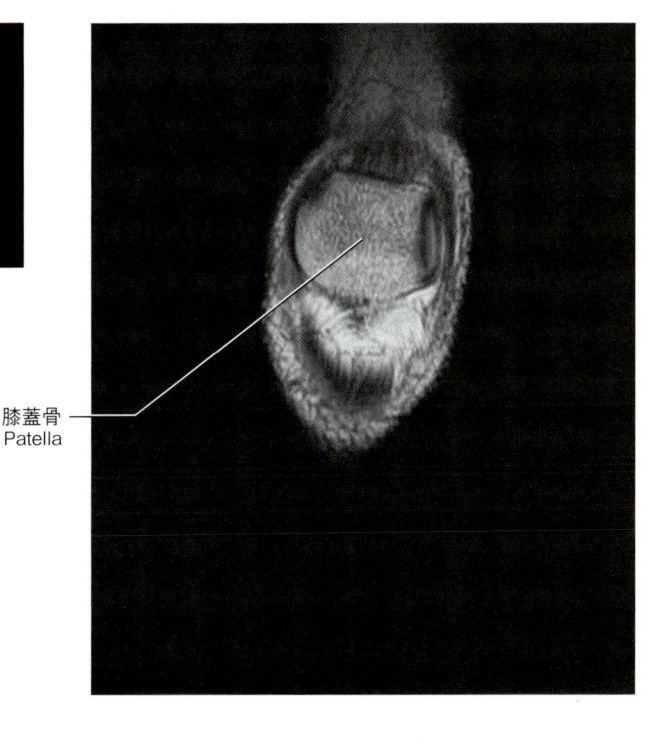

膝蓋骨
Patella

7-146

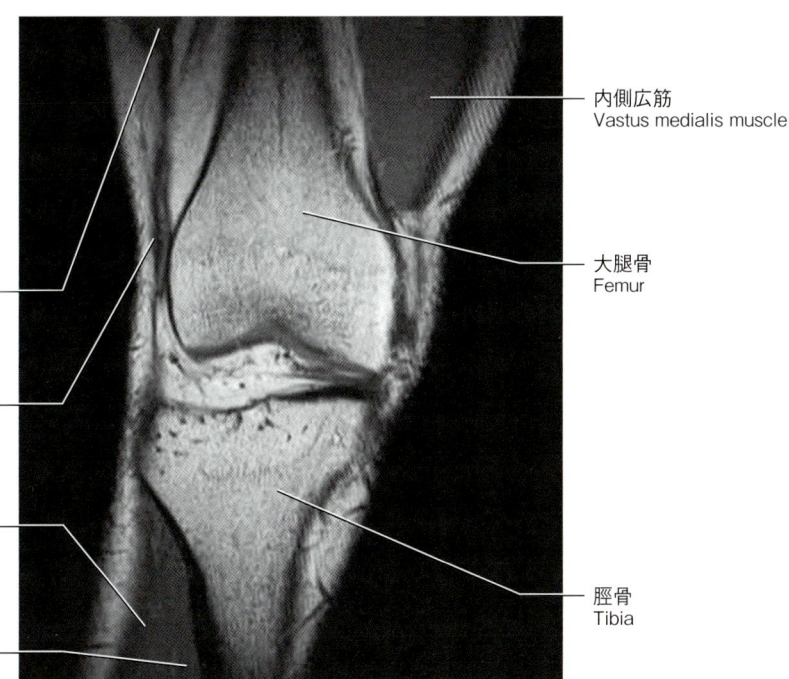

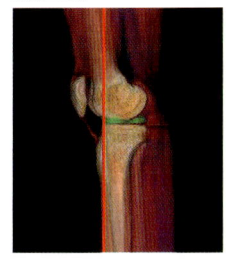

内側広筋
Vastus medialis muscle

大腿骨
Femur

外側広筋
Vastus lateralis muscle

腸脛靱帯
Iliotibial band

長趾伸筋
Extensor digitorum longus muscle

脛骨
Tibia

前脛骨筋
Tibialis anterior muscle

NOTE 膝関節の外側には腸骨稜より脛骨外側顆に至る長い腸脛靱帯が存在する．腸脛靱帯は，人類にのみ存在する靱帯で二足立位動物の膝の安定機構のひとつと考えられている．腸脛靱帯は，膝関節の30°以上の屈曲位で大腿骨外側顆の後方に位置するが，伸展位では前方に位置を変える．腸脛靱帯炎の本態は膝の反復性屈伸運動により，腸脛靱帯が大腿骨外側顆の上を前後に移動することで機械的刺激を受けて生じると考えられている．

膝関節の断層解剖 ［冠状断像（MRI, プロトン密度強調像）］

7-147

- 外側広筋 Vastus lateralis muscle
- 腸脛靱帯 Iliotibial band
- 外側半月板 Lateral meniscus
- 長腓骨筋 Fibularis longus muscle
- 長趾伸筋 Extensor digitorum longus muscle
- 内側広筋 Vastus medialis muscle
- 大腿骨 Femur
- 内側半月板 Medial meniscus
- 脛骨 Tibia
- 前脛骨筋 Tibialis anterior muscle

7-148

- 腸脛靱帯 Iliotibial band
- 膝窩筋（腱）Popliteus muscle (tendon)
- 外側半月板 Lateral meniscus
- 長腓骨筋 Fibularis longus muscle
- 長趾伸筋 Extensor digitorum longus muscle
- 外側広筋 Vastus lateralis muscle
- 内側広筋 Vastus medialis muscle
- 大腿骨 Femur
- 後十字靱帯 Posterior cruciate ligament
- 内側側副靱帯 Medial collateral ligament
- 内側半月板 Medial meniscus
- 脛骨 Tibia
- 前脛骨筋 Tibialis anterior muscle

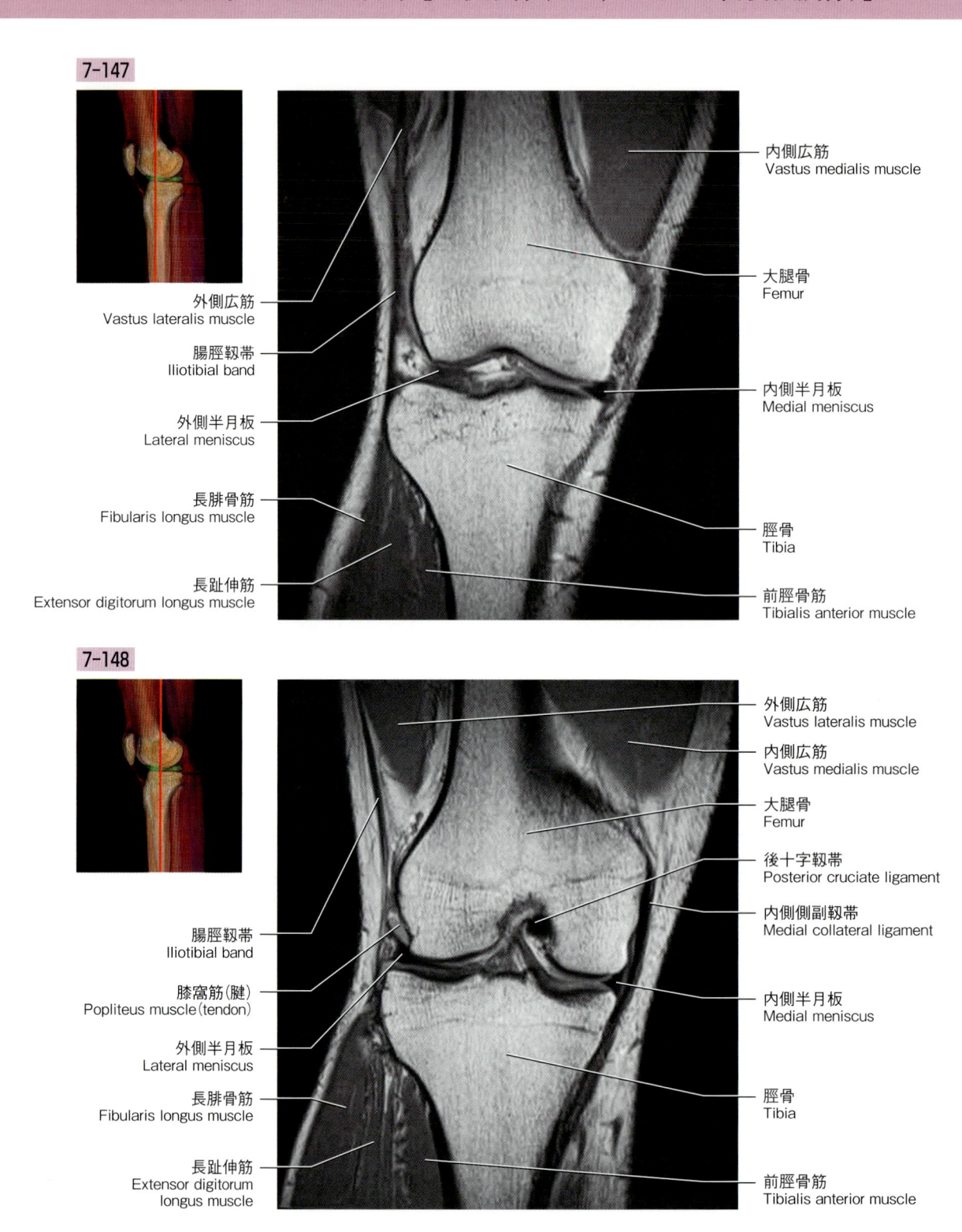

> **NOTE** Segond（セゴン）骨折は脛骨外側顆外側面の裂離骨折で，屈曲した膝に対する内旋および内反負荷により起こる．従来は外側関節包靱帯の付着部に起こると考えられていたが，最近では腸脛靱帯の後方線維および腓側副靱帯の前斜方線維の関与が大きいと考えられている．この骨折がある場合，前十字靱帯断裂が75～100％で，半月板損傷が66～75％で合併することが知られている．

膝関節の断層解剖 ［冠状断像（MRI, プロトン密度強調像）］

7-149

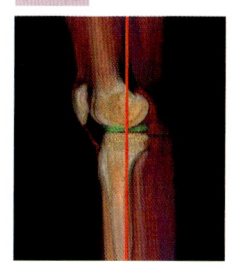

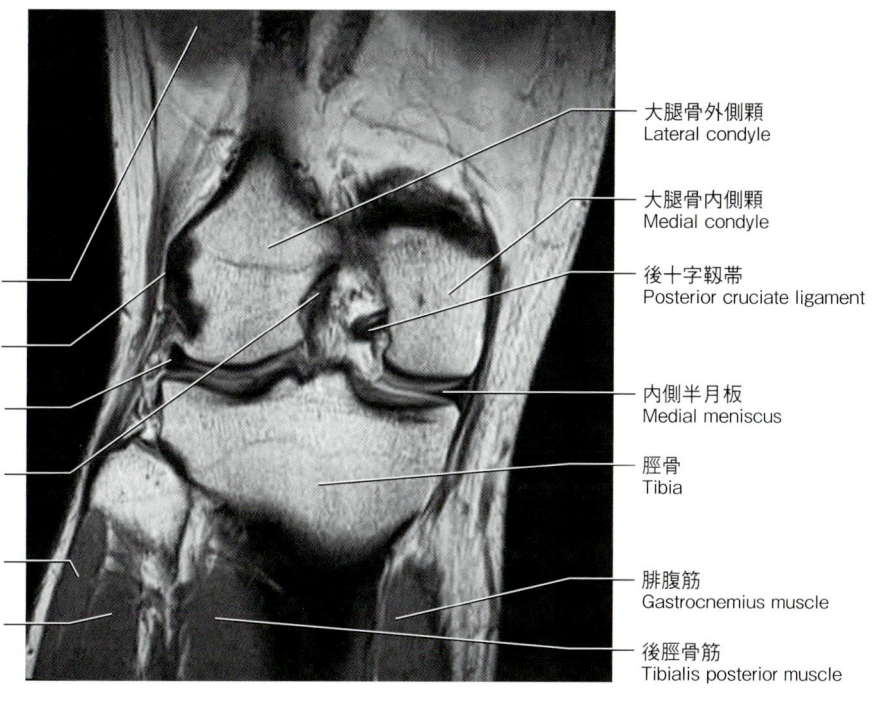

- 外側広筋 Vastus lateralis muscle
- 膝窩筋（腱） Popliteus muscle (tendon)
- 外側半月板 Lateral meniscus
- 前十字靱帯 Anterior cruciate ligament
- 長腓骨筋 Fibularis longus muscle
- 長趾伸筋 Extensor digitorum longus muscle
- 大腿骨外側顆 Lateral condyle
- 大腿骨内側顆 Medial condyle
- 後十字靱帯 Posterior cruciate ligament
- 内側半月板 Medial meniscus
- 脛骨 Tibia
- 腓腹筋 Gastrocnemius muscle
- 後脛骨筋 Tibialis posterior muscle

7-150

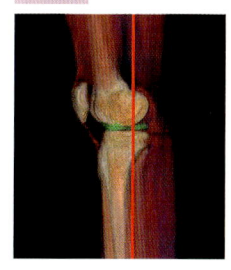

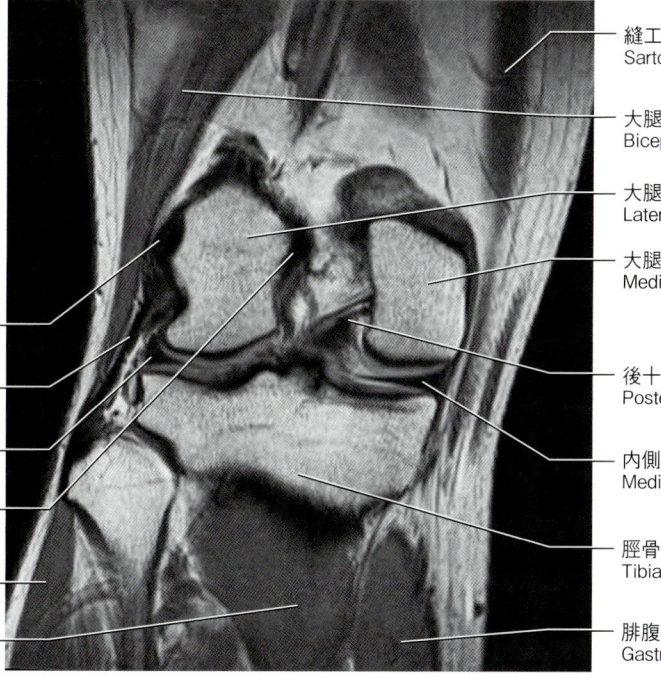

- 膝窩筋（腱） Popliteus muscle (tendon)
- 外側側副靱帯 Lateral collateral ligament
- 外側半月板 Lateral meniscus
- 前十字靱帯 Anterior cruciate ligament
- 長腓骨筋 Fibularis longus muscle
- 膝窩筋 Popliteus muscle
- 縫工筋 Sartorius muscle
- 大腿二頭筋 Biceps femoris muscle
- 大腿骨外側顆 Lateral condyle
- 大腿骨内側顆 Medial condyle
- 後十字靱帯 Posterior cruciate ligament
- 内側半月板 Medial meniscus
- 脛骨 Tibia
- 腓腹筋 Gastrocnemius muscle

膝関節の断層解剖 ［冠状断像（MRI，プロトン密度強調像）］

7-151

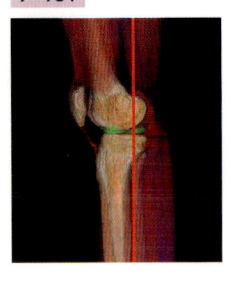

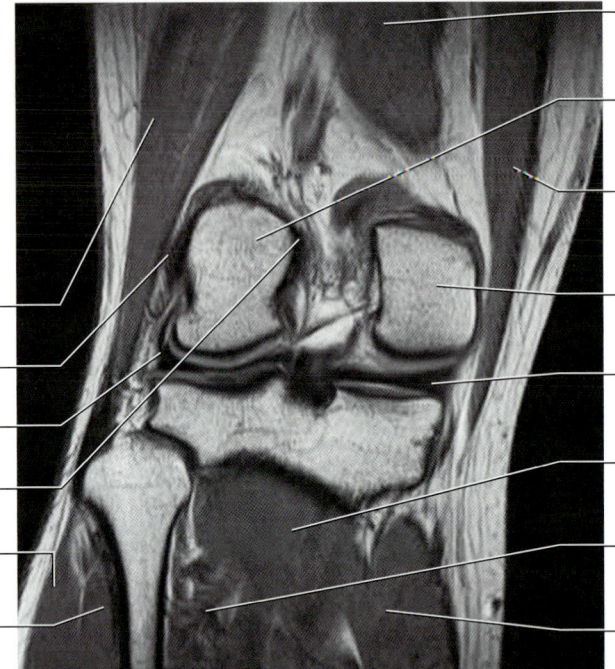

- 内側広筋 Vastus medialis muscle
- 大腿骨外側顆 Lateral condyle
- 縫工筋 Sartorius muscle
- 大腿骨内側顆 Medial condyle
- 内側半月板 Medial meniscus
- ヒラメ筋 Soleus muscle
- 後脛骨筋 Tibialis posterior muscle
- 腓腹筋 Gastrocnemius muscle
- 大腿二頭筋 Biceps femoris muscle
- 膝窩筋（腱） Popliteus muscle (tendon)
- 外側半月板 Lateral meniscus
- 前十字靱帯 Anterior cruciate ligament
- 長腓骨筋 Fibularis longus muscle
- 短腓骨筋 Fibularis brevis muscle

7-152

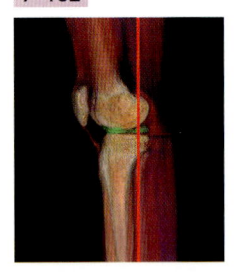

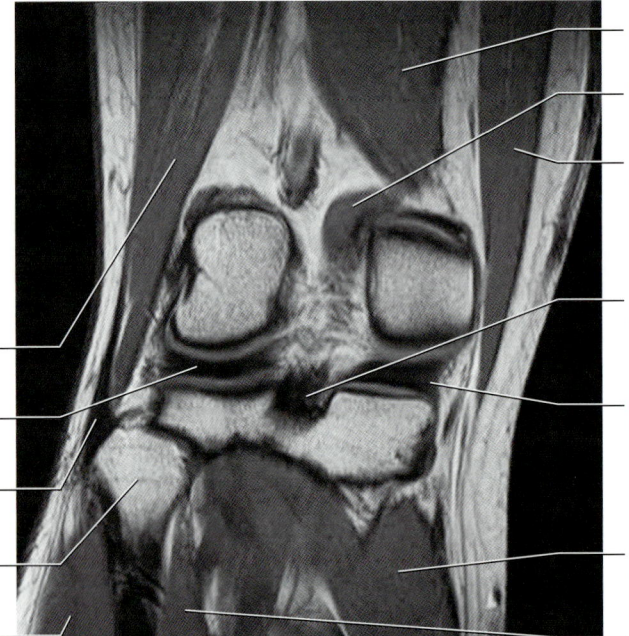

- 内側広筋 Vastus medialis muscle
- 腓腹筋 Gastrocnemius muscle
- 縫工筋 Sartorius muscle
- 後十字靱帯 Posterior cruciate ligament
- 内側半月板 Medial meniscus
- 腓腹筋 Gastrocnemius muscle
- 長母趾屈筋 Flexor hallucis longus muscle
- 大腿二頭筋 Biceps femoris muscle
- 外側半月板 Lateral meniscus
- 外側側副靱帯 Lateral collateral ligament
- 腓骨 Fibula
- ヒラメ筋 Soleus muscle

> **NOTE** 十字靱帯 Cruciate ligament
> Cruciate は動詞 cruciare（拷問にかける＝十字架をかける）の変化形である．crus は脚の意味で，大脳脚 Crus cerebri，横隔膜脚 Crus of diaphragm に用いられるが，V 型や X 型の構造に用いられ，十字架との関連があるとされるのが興味深い（261 頁の NOTE を参照）．

膝関節の断層解剖　[冠状断像（MRI，プロトン密度強調像）]

7-153

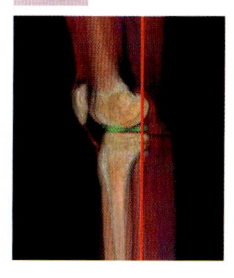

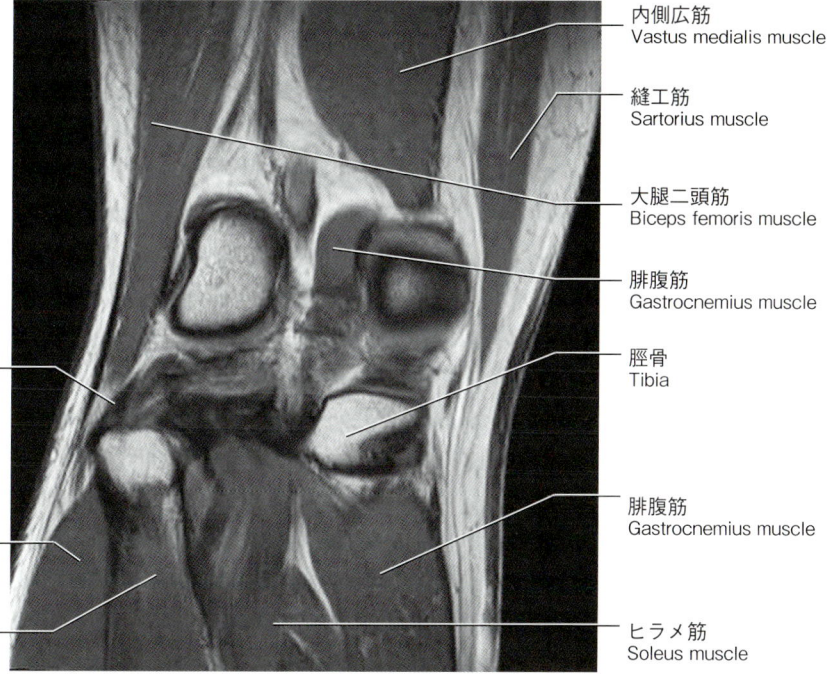

- 内側広筋 Vastus medialis muscle
- 縫工筋 Sartorius muscle
- 大腿二頭筋 Biceps femoris muscle
- 腓腹筋 Gastrocnemius muscle
- 脛骨 Tibia
- 外側側副靱帯 Lateral collateral ligament
- 腓腹筋 Gastrocnemius muscle
- ヒラメ筋 Soleus muscle
- 長母趾屈筋 Flexor hallucis longus muscle
- ヒラメ筋 Soleus muscle

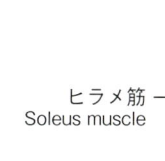

膝関節の断層解剖 [矢状断像（MRI，プロトン密度強調像）]

7-154

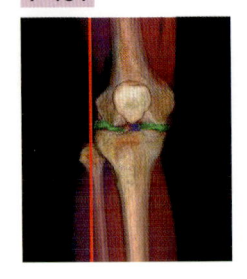

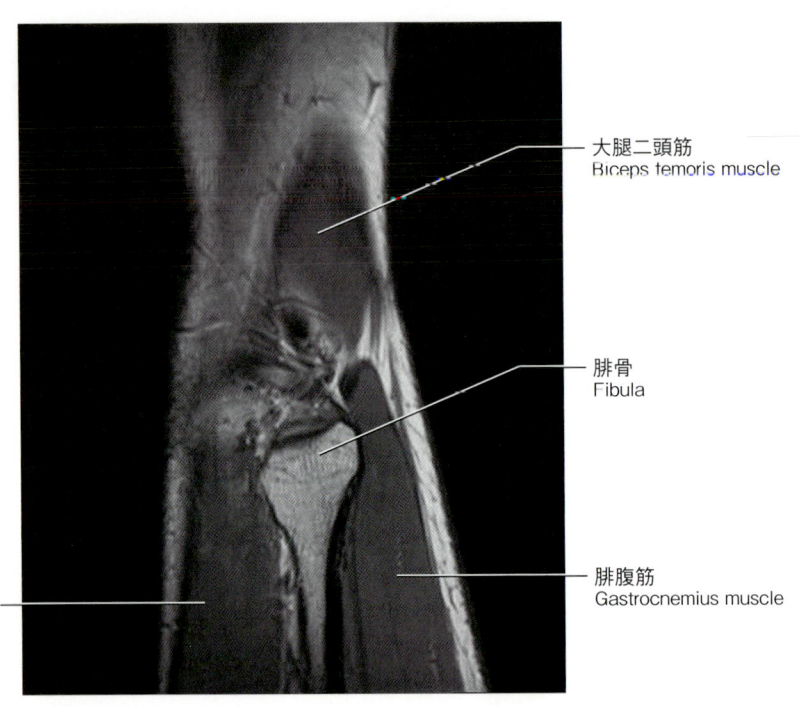

- 大腿二頭筋 Biceps femoris muscle
- 腓骨 Fibula
- 腓腹筋 Gastrocnemius muscle
- 前脛骨筋 Tibialis anterior muscle

7-155

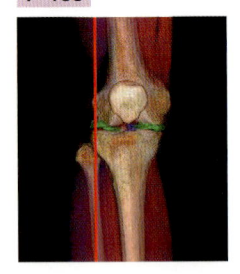

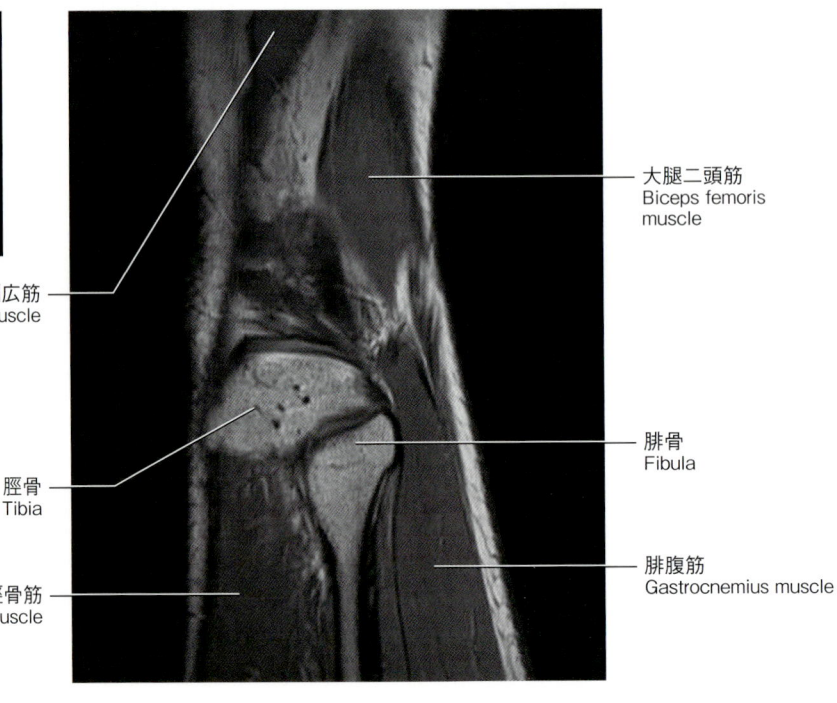

- 外側広筋 Vastus lateralis muscle
- 脛骨 Tibia
- 前脛骨筋 Tibialis anterior muscle
- 大腿二頭筋 Biceps femoris muscle
- 腓骨 Fibula
- 腓腹筋 Gastrocnemius muscle

膝関節の断層解剖［矢状断像（MRI，プロトン密度強調像）］

7-156

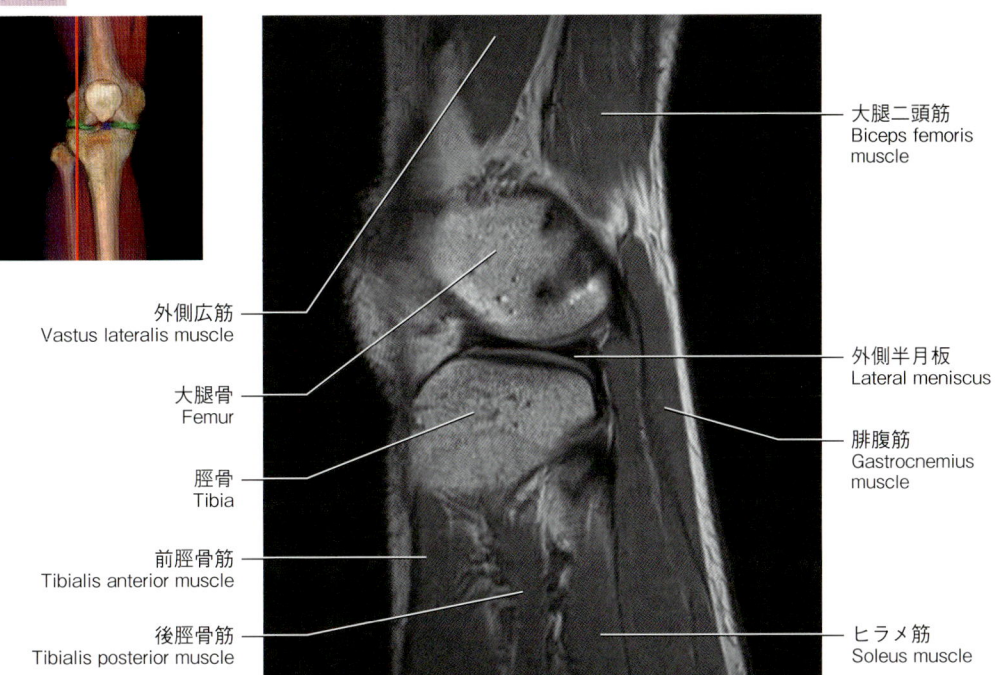

- 外側広筋 Vastus lateralis muscle
- 大腿骨 Femur
- 脛骨 Tibia
- 前脛骨筋 Tibialis anterior muscle
- 後脛骨筋 Tibialis posterior muscle
- 大腿二頭筋 Biceps femoris muscle
- 外側半月板 Lateral meniscus
- 腓腹筋 Gastrocnemius muscle
- ヒラメ筋 Soleus muscle

7-157

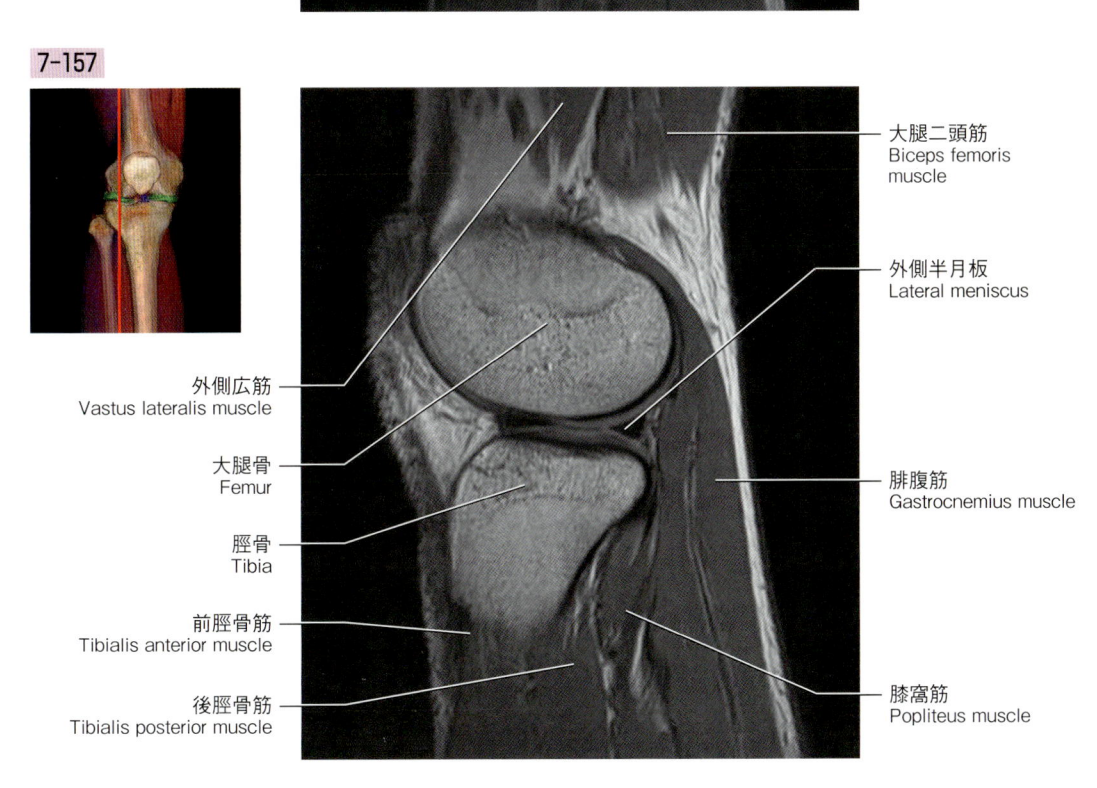

- 外側広筋 Vastus lateralis muscle
- 大腿骨 Femur
- 脛骨 Tibia
- 前脛骨筋 Tibialis anterior muscle
- 後脛骨筋 Tibialis posterior muscle
- 大腿二頭筋 Biceps femoris muscle
- 外側半月板 Lateral meniscus
- 腓腹筋 Gastrocnemius muscle
- 膝窩筋 Popliteus muscle

膝関節の断層解剖［矢状断像（MRI，プロトン密度強調像）］

7-158

- 大腿二頭筋 Biceps femoris muscle
- 大腿骨 Femur
- 外側半月板 Lateral meniscus
- 腓腹筋 Gastrocnemius muscle
- ヒラメ筋 Soleus muscle
- 膝蓋骨 Patella
- 膝蓋下脂肪体 Infrapatellar fat body
- 脛骨 Tibia
- 後脛骨筋 Tibialis posterior muscle

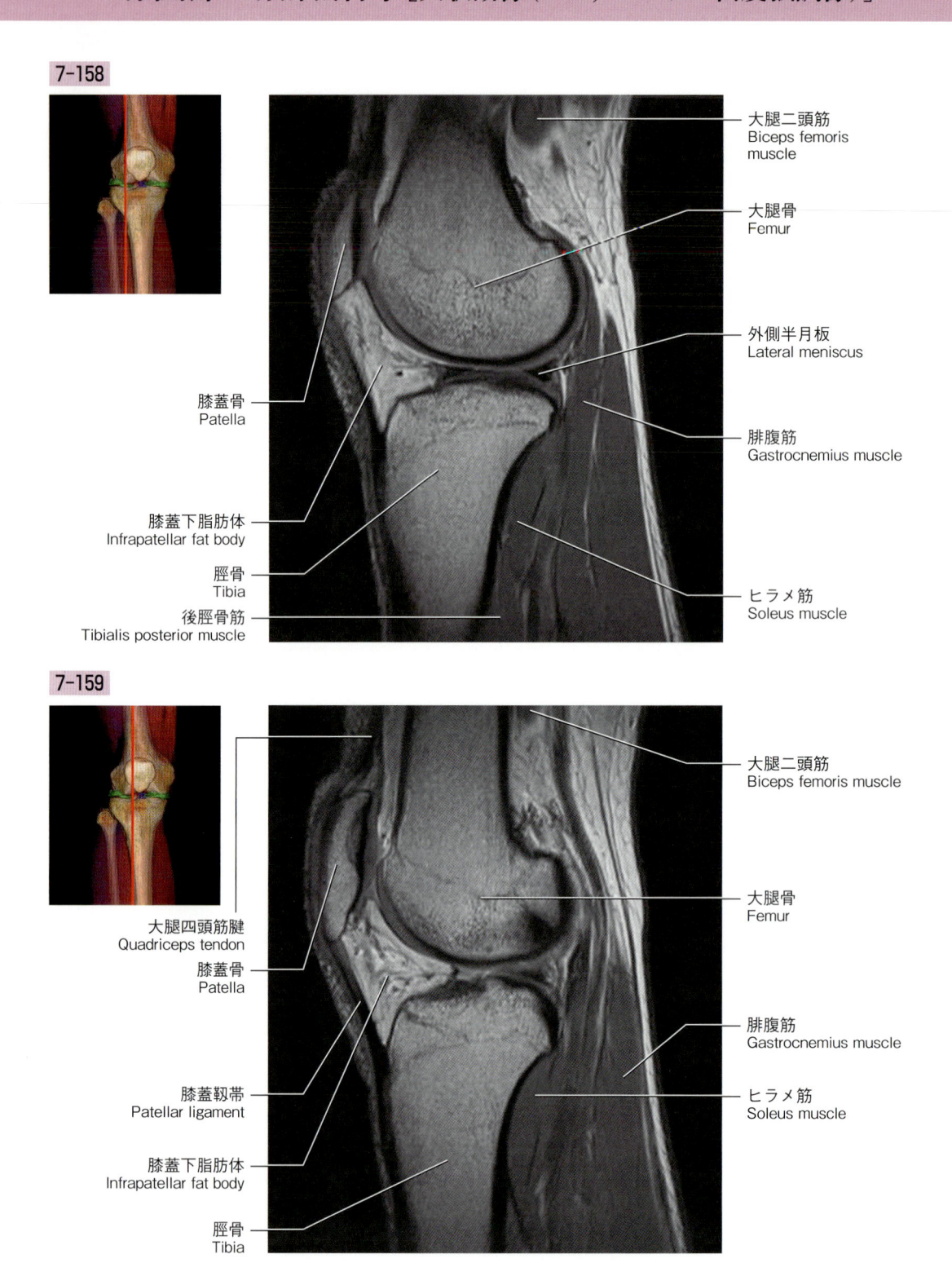

7-159

- 大腿二頭筋 Biceps femoris muscle
- 大腿骨 Femur
- 腓腹筋 Gastrocnemius muscle
- ヒラメ筋 Soleus muscle
- 大腿四頭筋腱 Quadriceps tendon
- 膝蓋骨 Patella
- 膝蓋靱帯 Patellar ligament
- 膝蓋下脂肪体 Infrapatellar fat body
- 脛骨 Tibia

> **NOTE** 大腿動・静脈は遠位部で内転筋管の中を通り，内転筋腱裂孔を抜けて膝窩部に至る．膝窩で大腿動・静脈はそれぞれ膝窩動・静脈となる．膝窩動脈捕捉症候群とは，腓腹筋の付着異常や異常筋・線維束により，膝窩動脈が捕捉あるいは圧排される．捕捉のくり返しにより膝窩動脈の内皮傷害を生じ，最終的に閉塞，下肢の虚血性障害を引き起こす病態である．

膝関節の断層解剖［矢状断像（MRI，プロトン密度強調像）］

7-160

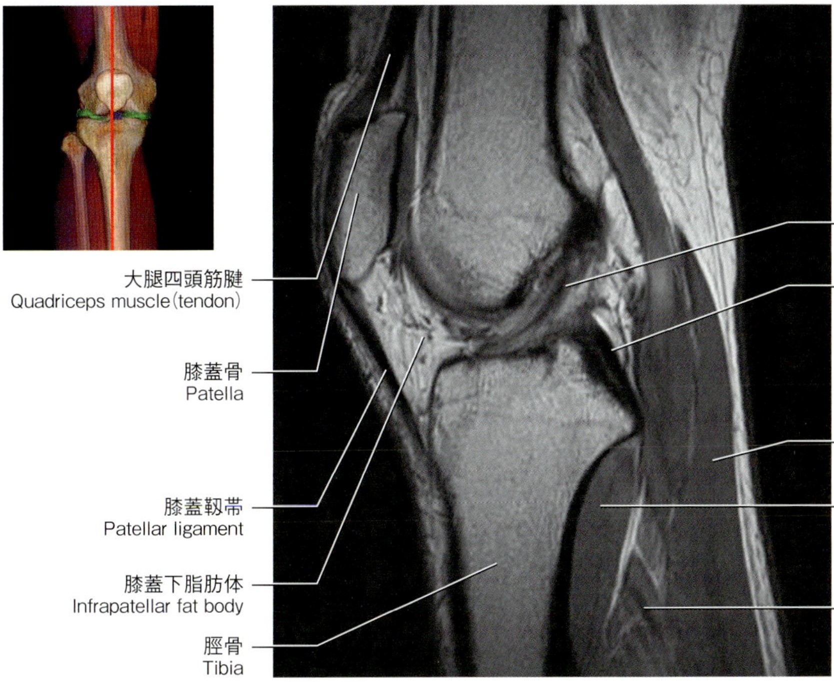

- 大腿四頭筋腱 Quadriceps muscle (tendon)
- 膝蓋骨 Patella
- 膝蓋靱帯 Patellar ligament
- 膝蓋下脂肪体 Infrapatellar fat body
- 脛骨 Tibia
- 前十字靱帯 Anterior cruciate ligament
- 後十字靱帯 Posterior cruciate ligament
- 腓腹筋 Gastrocnemius muscle
- 膝窩筋 Popliteus muscle
- ヒラメ筋 Soleus muscle

7-161

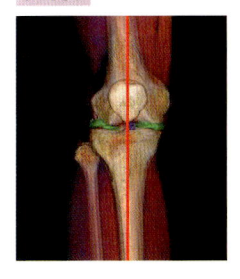

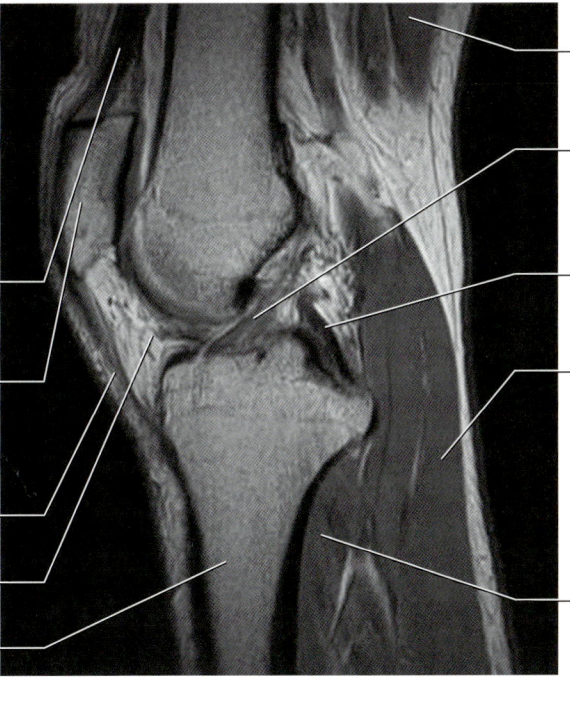

- 大腿四頭筋腱 Quadriceps muscle (tendon)
- 膝蓋骨 Patella
- 膝蓋靱帯 Patellar ligament
- 膝蓋下脂肪体 Infrapatellar fat body
- 脛骨 Tibia
- 半膜様筋 Semimembranosus muscle
- 前十字靱帯 Anterior cruciate ligament
- 後十字靱帯 Posterior cruciate ligament
- 腓腹筋 Gastrocnemius muscle
- 膝窩筋 Popliteus muscle

膝関節の断層解剖 ［矢状断像（MRI，プロトン密度強調像）］

7-162

- 大腿四頭筋腱 Quadriceps muscle (tendon)
- 膝蓋骨 Patella
- 膝蓋下脂肪体 Infrapatellar fat body
- 脛骨 Tibia
- 半膜様筋 Semimembranosus muscle
- 大腿骨 Femur
- 後十字靱帯 Posterior cruciate ligament
- 腓腹筋 Gastrocnemius muscle
- 膝窩筋 Popliteus muscle
- ヒラメ筋 Soleus muscle

7-163

- 内側広筋 Vastus medialis muscle
- 膝蓋下脂肪体 Infrapatellar fat body
- 内側半月板 Medial meniscus
- 脛骨 Tibia
- 半膜様筋 Semimembranosus muscle
- 大腿骨 Femur
- 内側半月板 Medial meniscus
- 腓腹筋 Gastrocnemius muscle

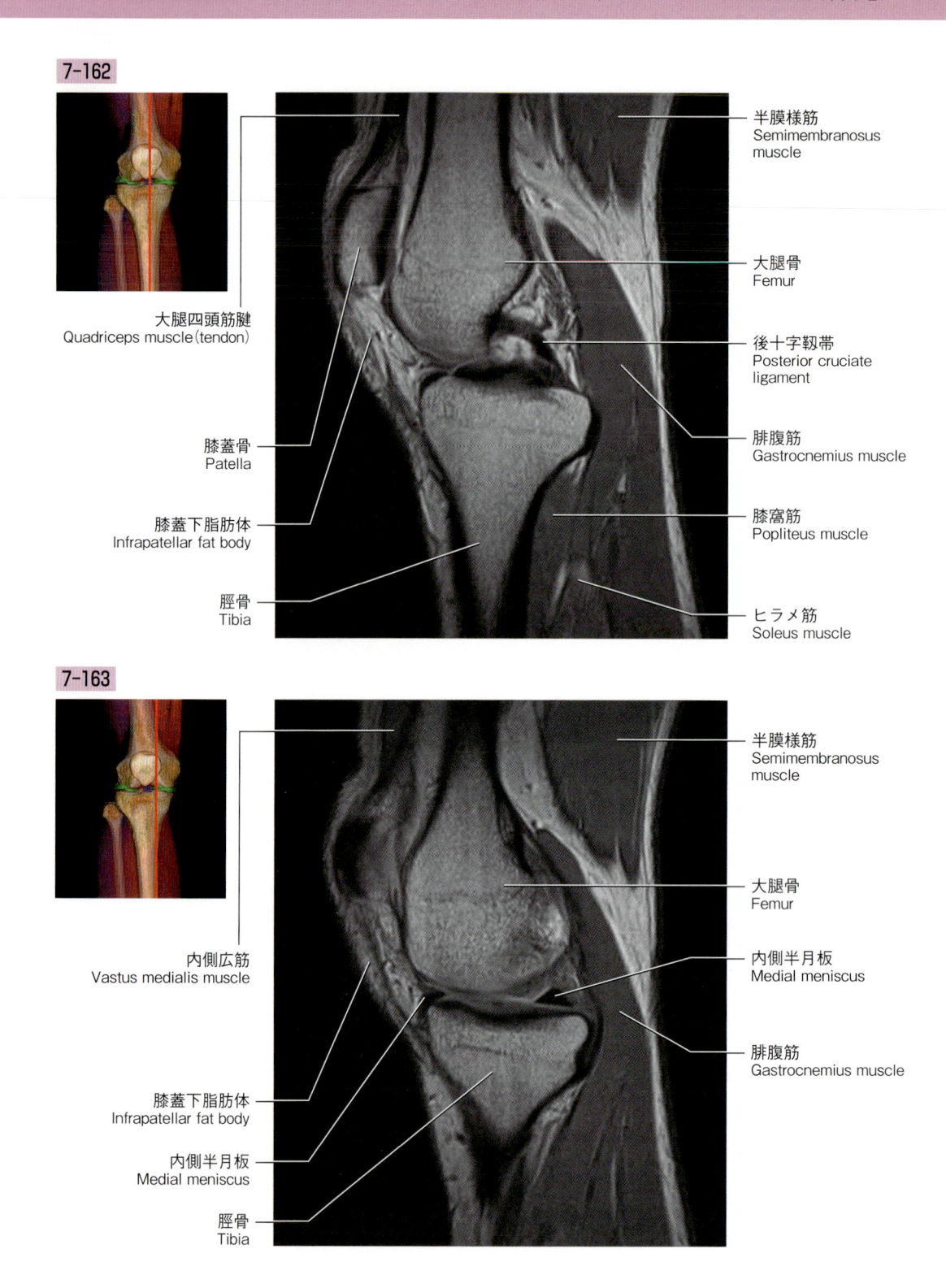

膝関節の断層解剖 ［矢状断像（MRI, プロトン密度強調像）］

7-164

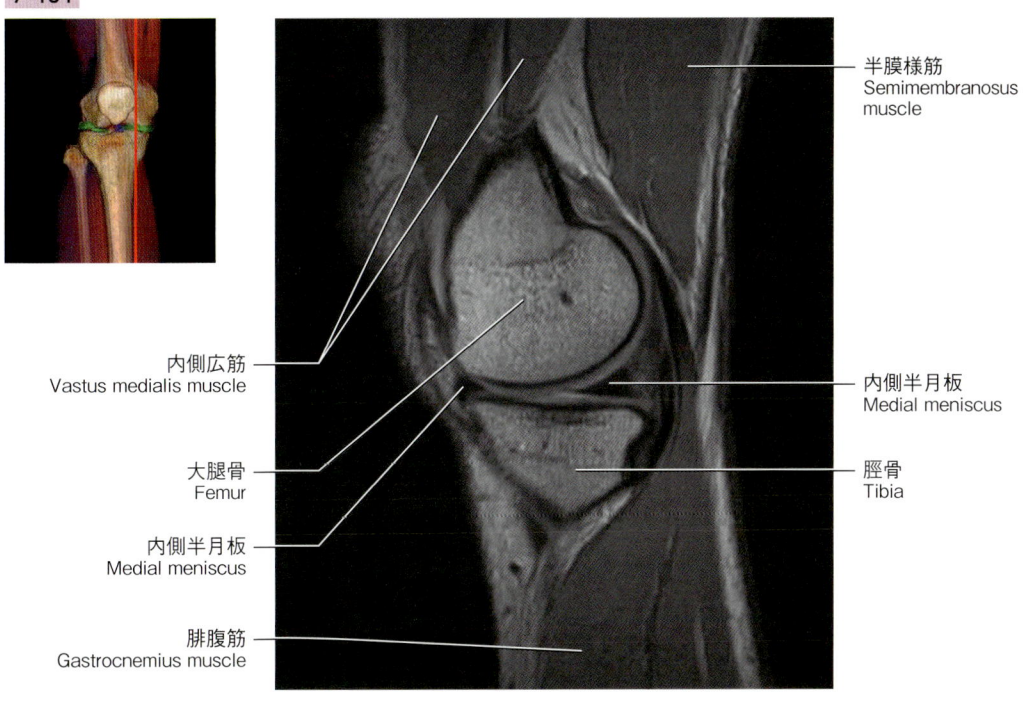

- 半膜様筋 Semimembranosus muscle
- 内側広筋 Vastus medialis muscle
- 大腿骨 Femur
- 内側半月板 Medial meniscus
- 腓腹筋 Gastrocnemius muscle
- 内側半月板 Medial meniscus
- 脛骨 Tibia

7-165

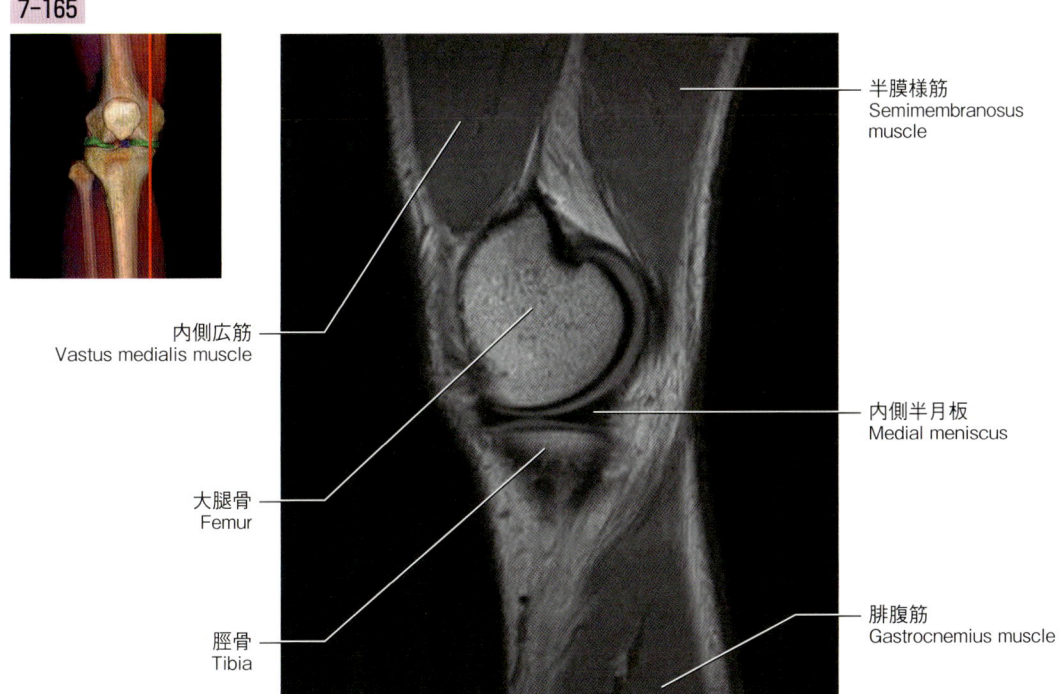

- 半膜様筋 Semimembranosus muscle
- 内側広筋 Vastus medialis muscle
- 大腿骨 Femur
- 内側半月板 Medial meniscus
- 脛骨 Tibia
- 腓腹筋 Gastrocnemius muscle

膝関節の断層解剖 ［矢状断像（MRI，プロトン密度強調像）］

7-166

- 半膜様筋 Semimembranosus muscle
- 内側広筋 Vastus medialis muscle
- 大腿骨 Femur

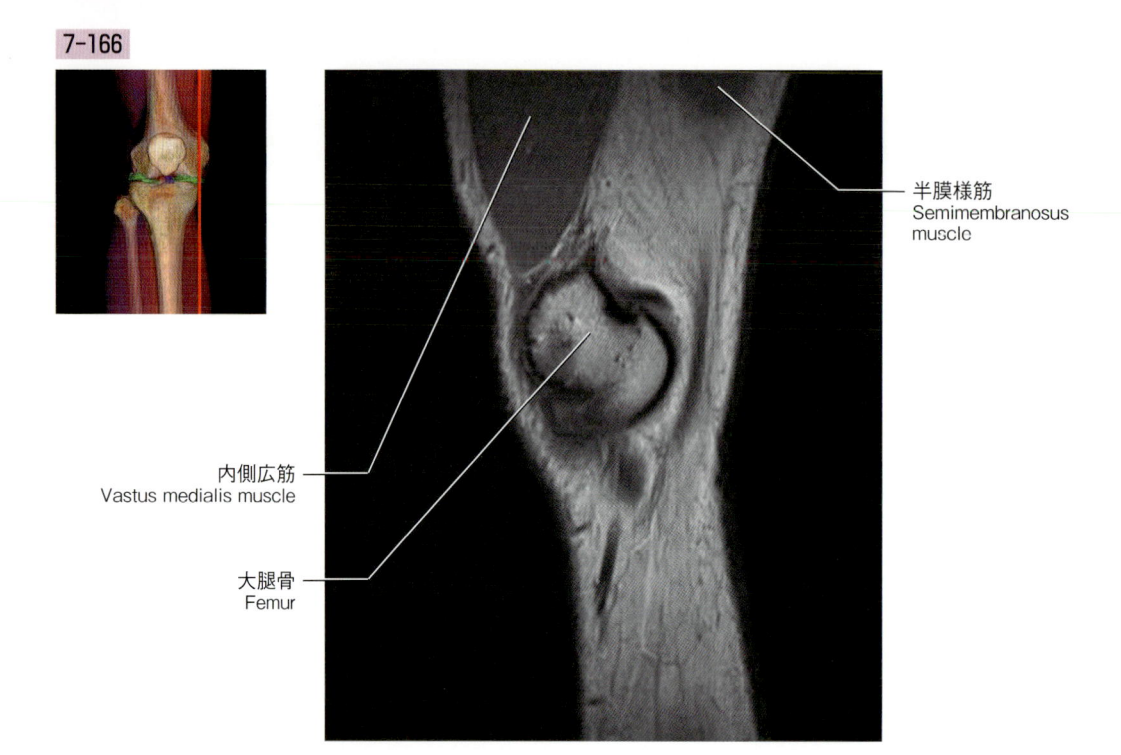

足関節と足 (CT, VR像)

7-167 足関節部の外観（前面）

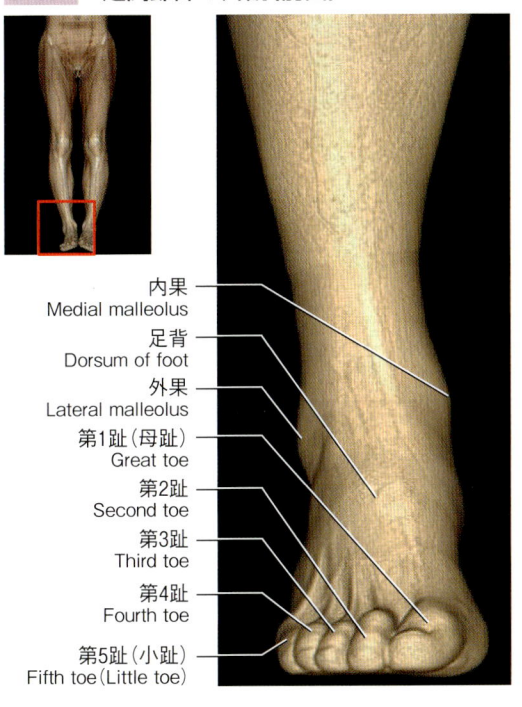

- 内果 Medial malleolus
- 足背 Dorsum of foot
- 外果 Lateral malleolus
- 第1趾（母趾）Great toe
- 第2趾 Second toe
- 第3趾 Third toe
- 第4趾 Fourth toe
- 第5趾（小趾）Fifth toe (Little toe)

7-168 足関節と足の筋・腱（前面）

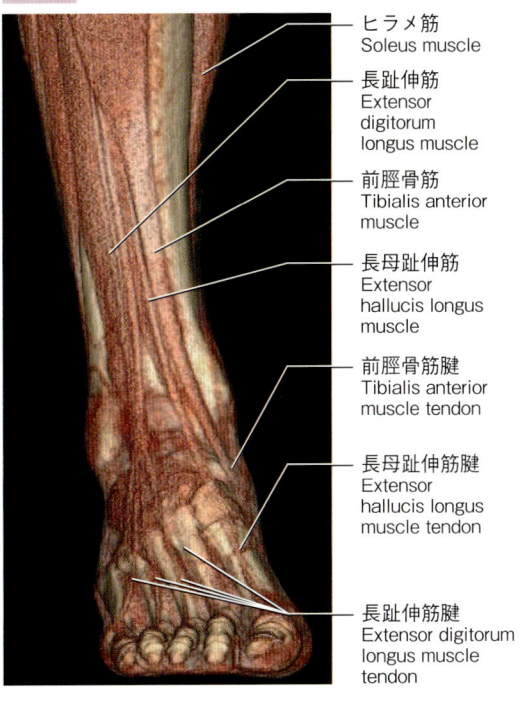

- ヒラメ筋 Soleus muscle
- 長趾伸筋 Extensor digitorum longus muscle
- 前脛骨筋 Tibialis anterior muscle
- 長母趾伸筋 Extensor hallucis longus muscle
- 前脛骨筋腱 Tibialis anterior muscle tendon
- 長母趾伸筋腱 Extensor hallucis longus muscle tendon
- 長趾伸筋腱 Extensor digitorum longus muscle tendon

7-169 足関節と足の筋・腱（内側面）

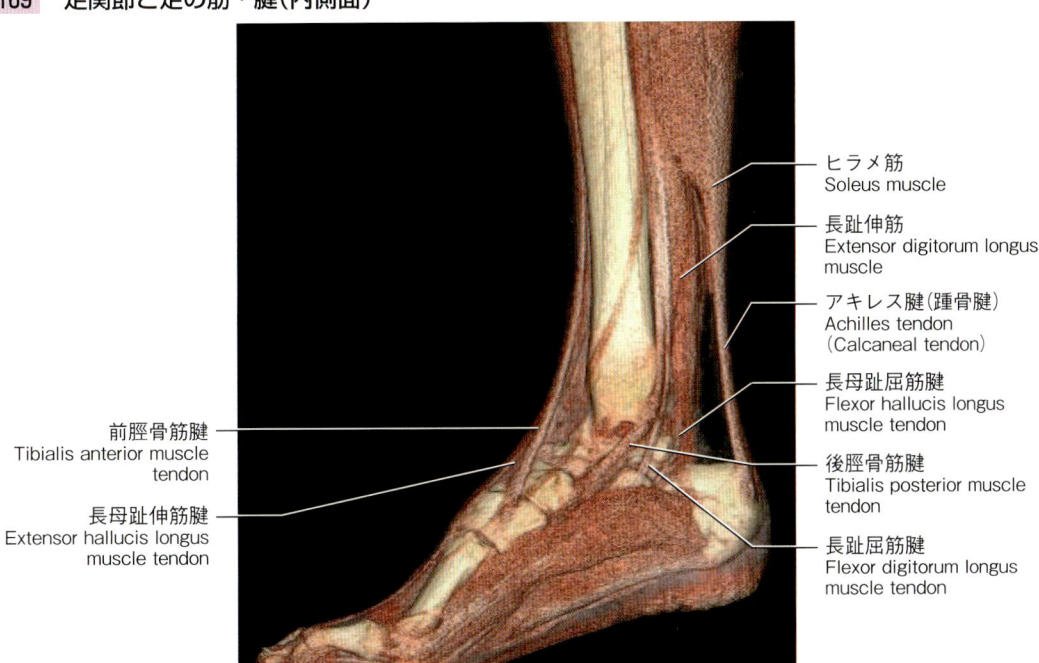

- ヒラメ筋 Soleus muscle
- 長趾伸筋 Extensor digitorum longus muscle
- アキレス腱（踵骨腱）Achilles tendon (Calcaneal tendon)
- 長母趾屈筋腱 Flexor hallucis longus muscle tendon
- 後脛骨筋腱 Tibialis posterior muscle tendon
- 長趾屈筋腱 Flexor digitorum longus muscle tendon
- 前脛骨筋腱 Tibialis anterior muscle tendon
- 長母趾伸筋腱 Extensor hallucis longus muscle tendon

NOTE 足とは，足関節と足部からなる機能的ユニットである．足関節は脛骨下端の関節面と内果・外果の関節面でつくられる果間関節窩と距骨滑車で形成される螺旋関節である．関節窩の天井部分は脛骨天蓋とよばれることがある．外側側副靱帯は外果に起始する３つの靱帯から構成される．

足関節と足（CT, VR像）

7-170　足関節と足の筋・腱（外側面）

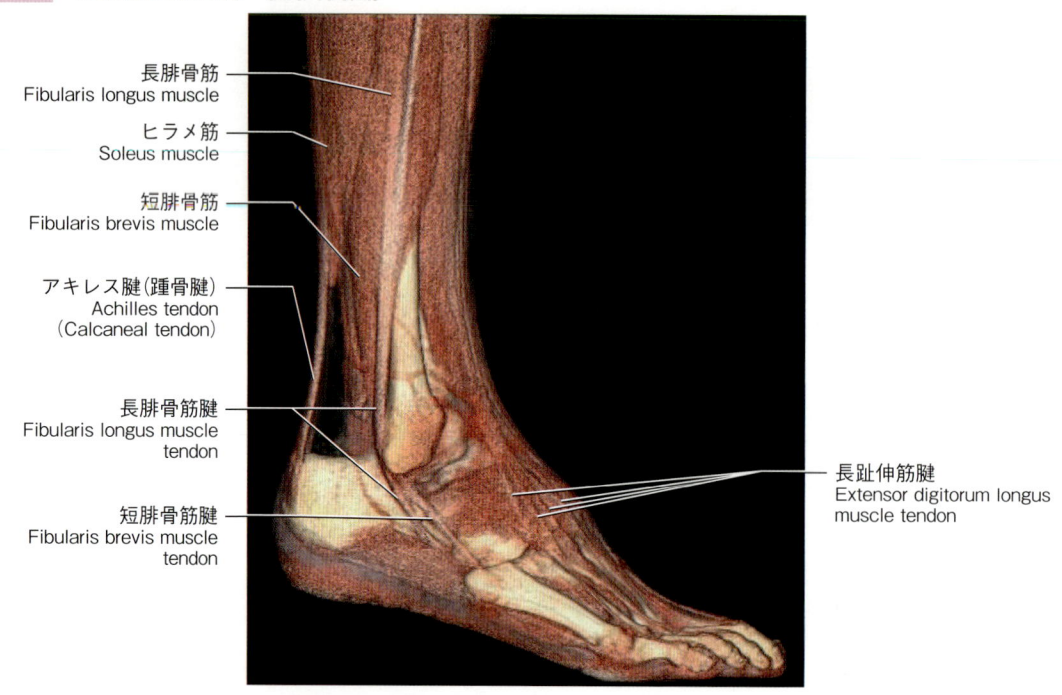

- 長腓骨筋　Fibularis longus muscle
- ヒラメ筋　Soleus muscle
- 短腓骨筋　Fibularis brevis muscle
- アキレス腱（踵骨腱）　Achilles tendon（Calcaneal tendon）
- 長腓骨筋腱　Fibularis longus muscle tendon
- 短腓骨筋腱　Fibularis brevis muscle tendon
- 長趾伸筋腱　Extensor digitorum longus muscle tendon

7-171　足関節と足の骨（前面）

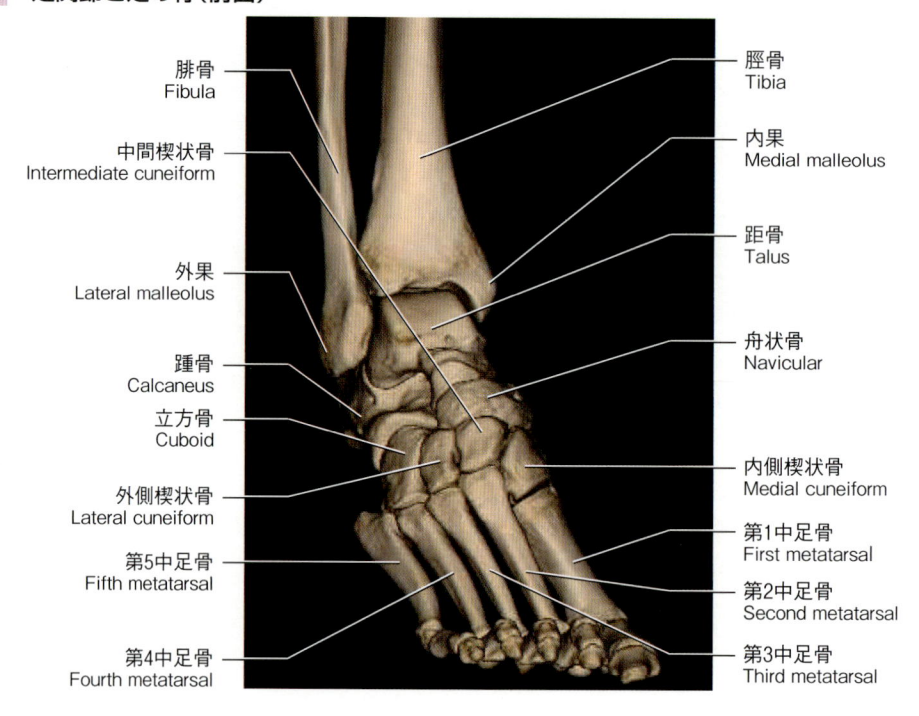

- 腓骨　Fibula
- 中間楔状骨　Intermediate cuneiform
- 外果　Lateral malleolus
- 踵骨　Calcaneus
- 立方骨　Cuboid
- 外側楔状骨　Lateral cuneiform
- 第5中足骨　Fifth metatarsal
- 第4中足骨　Fourth metatarsal
- 脛骨　Tibia
- 内果　Medial malleolus
- 距骨　Talus
- 舟状骨　Navicular
- 内側楔状骨　Medial cuneiform
- 第1中足骨　First metatarsal
- 第2中足骨　Second metatarsal
- 第3中足骨　Third metatarsal

> **NOTE**　内側側副靱帯は内側より足関節の安定をはかる．この靱帯は非常に強靱で，内果に頂点をおいた扇状を形成し，浅層と深層に分けられる．

足関節と足（CT, VR像）

7-172 足関節の骨（内側面）

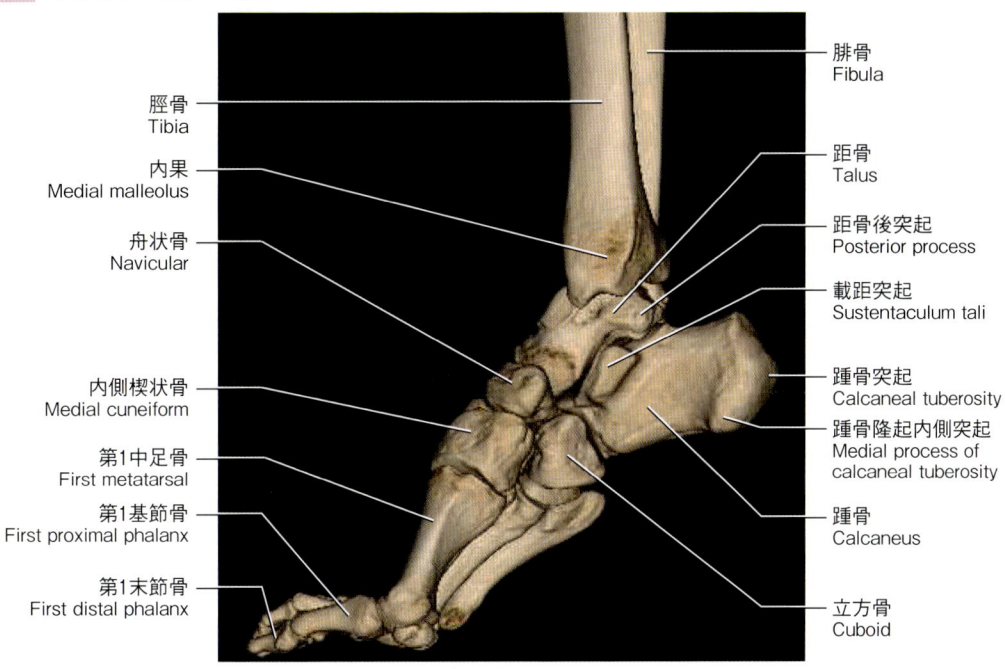

腓骨 Fibula
脛骨 Tibia
内果 Medial malleolus
舟状骨 Navicular
内側楔状骨 Medial cuneiform
第1中足骨 First metatarsal
第1基節骨 First proximal phalanx
第1末節骨 First distal phalanx
距骨 Talus
距骨後突起 Posterior process
載距突起 Sustentaculum tali
踵骨突起 Calcaneal tuberosity
踵骨隆起内側突起 Medial process of calcaneal tuberosity
踵骨 Calcaneus
立方骨 Cuboid

7-173 足関節の骨（外側面）

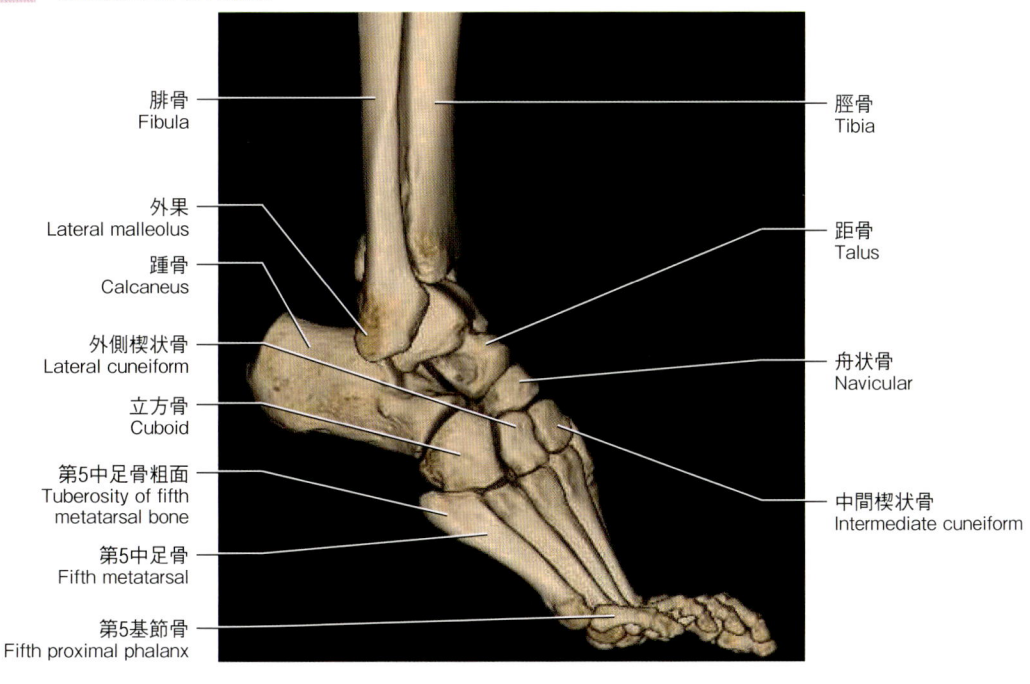

腓骨 Fibula
外果 Lateral malleolus
踵骨 Calcaneus
外側楔状骨 Lateral cuneiform
立方骨 Cuboid
第5中足骨粗面 Tuberosity of fifth metatarsal bone
第5中足骨 Fifth metatarsal
第5基節骨 Fifth proximal phalanx
脛骨 Tibia
距骨 Talus
舟状骨 Navicular
中間楔状骨 Intermediate cuneiform

NOTE 足部は後足部・中足部・前足部に分けられ，後足部は距骨と踵骨，中足部は残りの足根骨，前足部は中足骨と趾節骨で構成される．距骨と踵骨の間に距骨下関節，踵骨と立方骨および距骨と舟状骨の間に横足根関節［Chopart（ショパール）関節］，足根骨と中足骨の間に足根中足関節［Lisfranc（リスフラン）関節］が存在する．

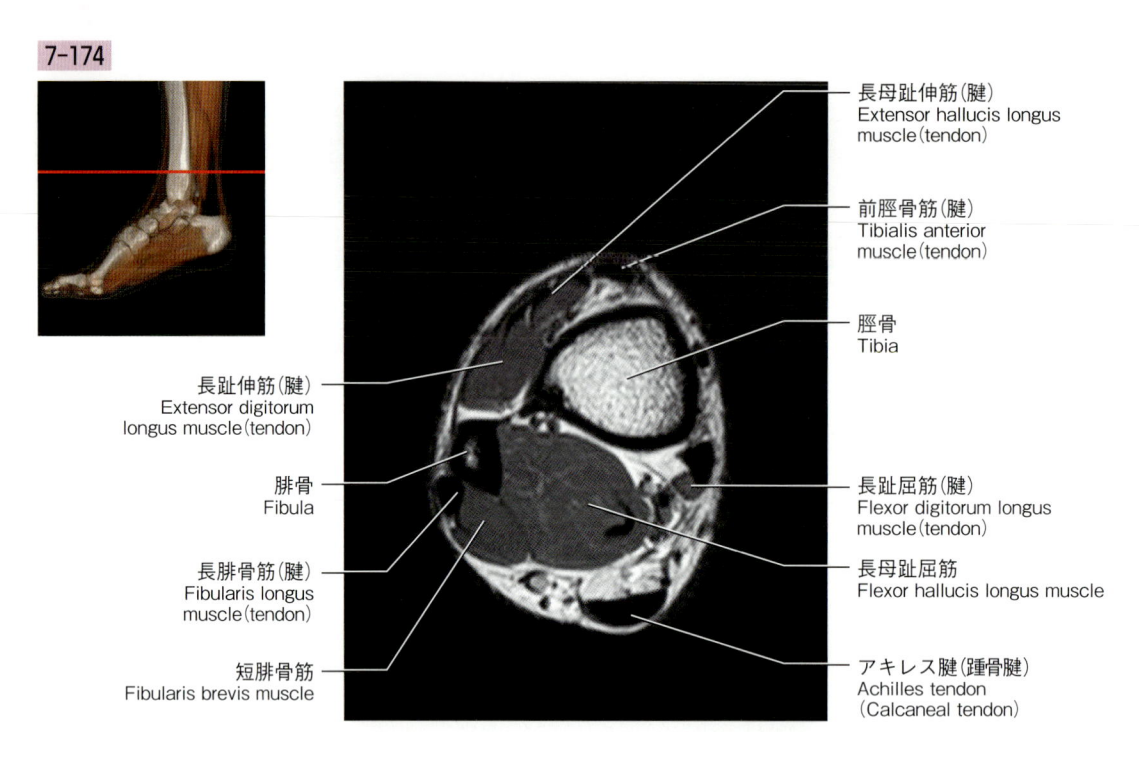

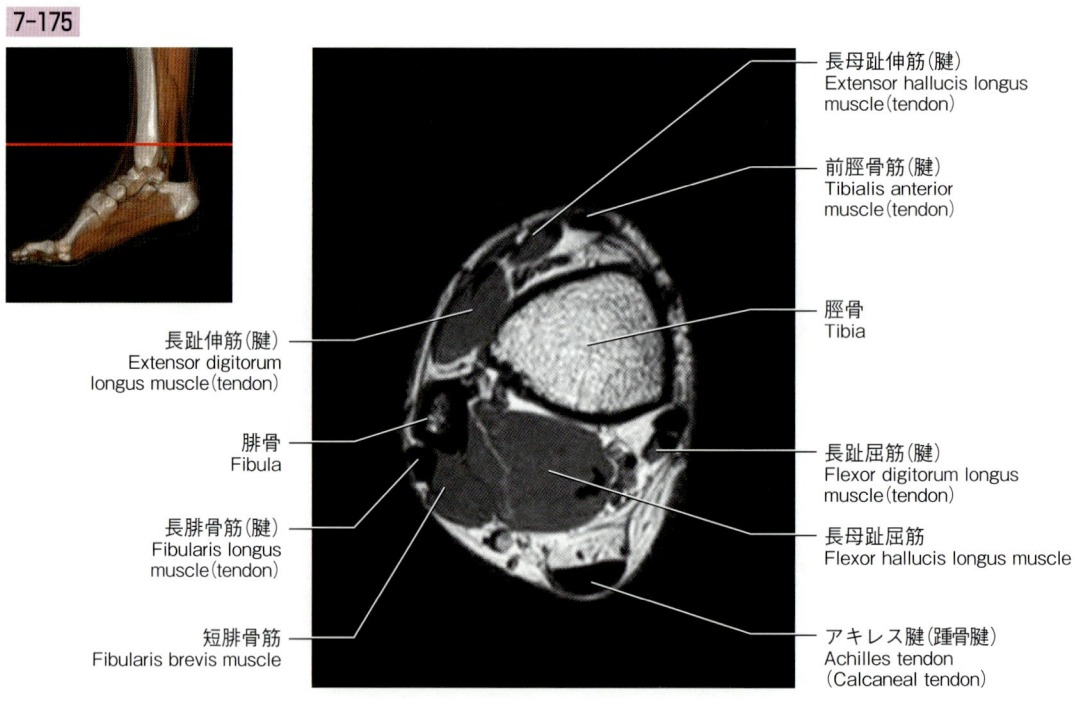

396 足関節と足の断層解剖 ［横断像（MRI，プロトン密度強調像）］

7-174

- 長母趾伸筋（腱） Extensor hallucis longus muscle（tendon）
- 前脛骨筋（腱） Tibialis anterior muscle（tendon）
- 脛骨 Tibia
- 長趾伸筋（腱） Extensor digitorum longus muscle（tendon）
- 腓骨 Fibula
- 長腓骨筋（腱） Fibularis longus muscle（tendon）
- 短腓骨筋 Fibularis brevis muscle
- 長趾屈筋（腱） Flexor digitorum longus muscle（tendon）
- 長母趾屈筋 Flexor hallucis longus muscle
- アキレス腱（踵骨腱） Achilles tendon（Calcaneal tendon）

7-175

- 長母趾伸筋（腱） Extensor hallucis longus muscle（tendon）
- 前脛骨筋（腱） Tibialis anterior muscle（tendon）
- 脛骨 Tibia
- 長趾伸筋（腱） Extensor digitorum longus muscle（tendon）
- 腓骨 Fibula
- 長腓骨筋（腱） Fibularis longus muscle（tendon）
- 短腓骨筋 Fibularis brevis muscle
- 長趾屈筋（腱） Flexor digitorum longus muscle（tendon）
- 長母趾屈筋 Flexor hallucis longus muscle
- アキレス腱（踵骨腱） Achilles tendon（Calcaneal tendon）

NOTE 足関節の腱はその筋腹が下腿に存在するもので構成され，足関節の外側・内側・後方・前方を通る腱に分類される．

足関節と足の断層解剖［横断像（MRI, プロトン密度強調像）］

7-176

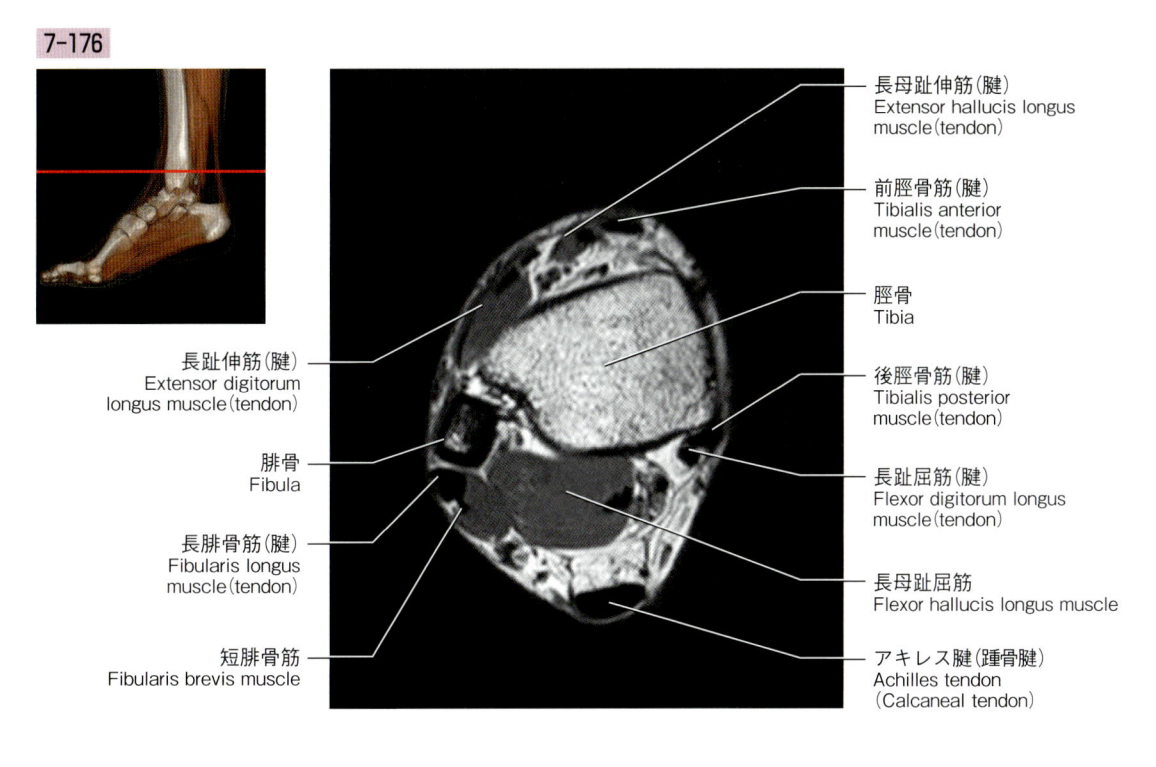

- 長母趾伸筋（腱） Extensor hallucis longus muscle (tendon)
- 前脛骨筋（腱） Tibialis anterior muscle (tendon)
- 脛骨 Tibia
- 後脛骨筋（腱） Tibialis posterior muscle (tendon)
- 長趾屈筋（腱） Flexor digitorum longus muscle (tendon)
- 長母趾屈筋 Flexor hallucis longus muscle
- アキレス腱（踵骨腱） Achilles tendon (Calcaneal tendon)
- 長趾伸筋（腱） Extensor digitorum longus muscle (tendon)
- 腓骨 Fibula
- 長腓骨筋（腱） Fibularis longus muscle (tendon)
- 短腓骨筋 Fibularis brevis muscle

7-177

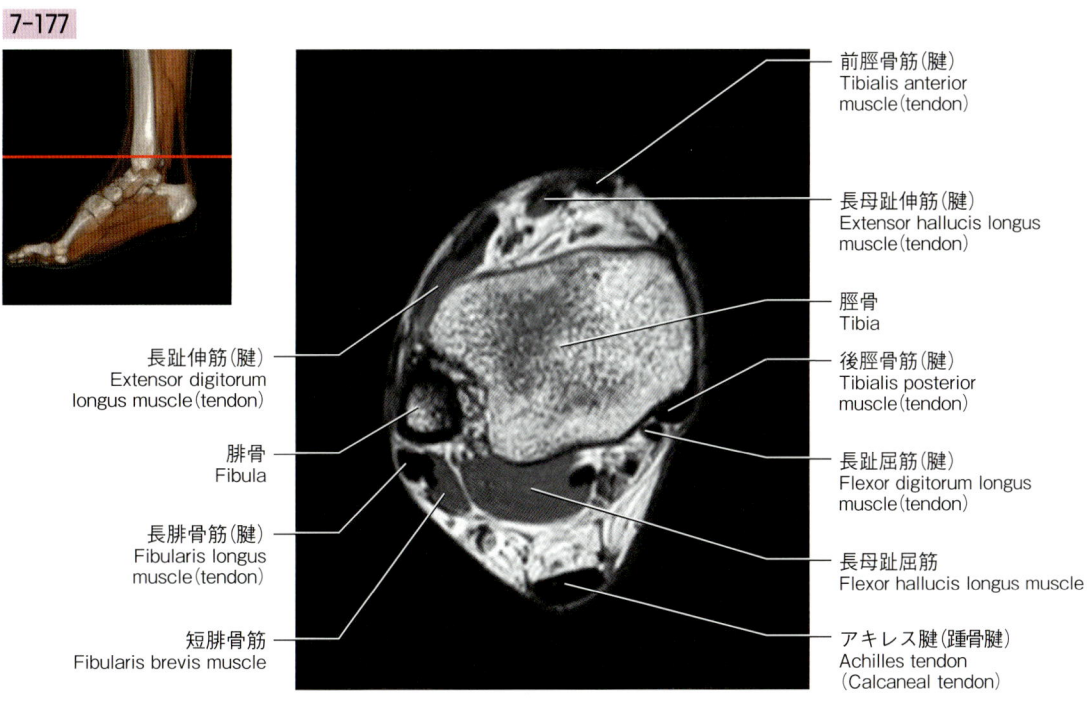

- 前脛骨筋（腱） Tibialis anterior muscle (tendon)
- 長母趾伸筋（腱） Extensor hallucis longus muscle (tendon)
- 脛骨 Tibia
- 後脛骨筋（腱） Tibialis posterior muscle (tendon)
- 長趾屈筋（腱） Flexor digitorum longus muscle (tendon)
- 長母趾屈筋 Flexor hallucis longus muscle
- アキレス腱（踵骨腱） Achilles tendon (Calcaneal tendon)
- 長趾伸筋（腱） Extensor digitorum longus muscle (tendon)
- 腓骨 Fibula
- 長腓骨筋（腱） Fibularis longus muscle (tendon)
- 短腓骨筋 Fibularis brevis muscle

NOTE 外側では長・短腓骨筋腱が外果の後方を走行し，腓骨と踵骨の間にある上腓骨筋支帯と下腓骨筋支帯により，外果後面の腱溝の中を通過するように固定されている．近位部では共通の腱鞘をもつため，MRIで長・短腓骨筋腱が分離不可能なことがある．

足関節と足の断層解剖 ［横断像（MRI, プロトン密度強調像）］

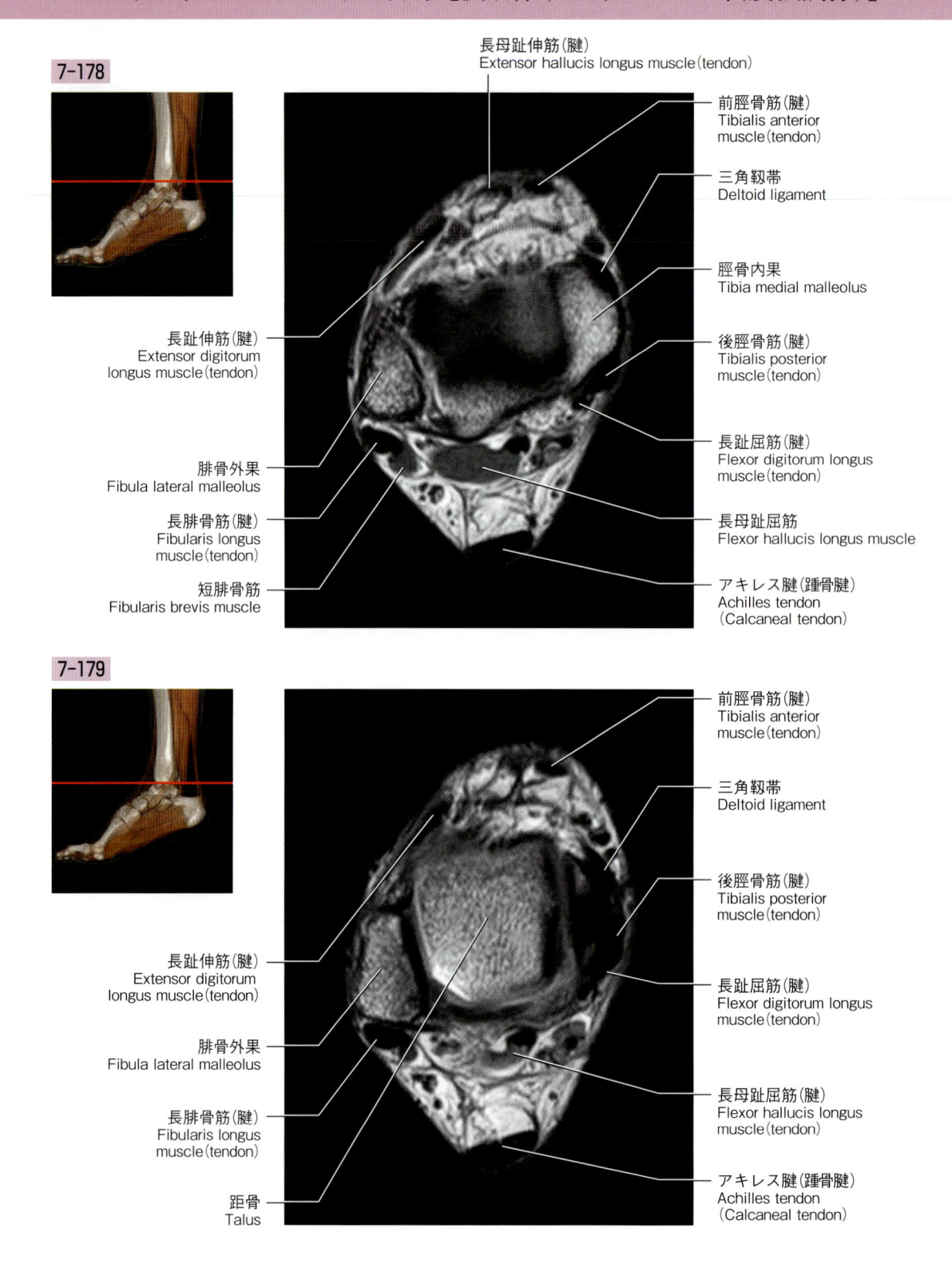

7-178

- 長母趾伸筋（腱） Extensor hallucis longus muscle (tendon)
- 前脛骨筋（腱） Tibialis anterior muscle (tendon)
- 三角靱帯 Deltoid ligament
- 脛骨内果 Tibia medial malleolus
- 後脛骨筋（腱） Tibialis posterior muscle (tendon)
- 長趾屈筋（腱） Flexor digitorum longus muscle (tendon)
- 長母趾屈筋 Flexor hallucis longus muscle
- アキレス腱（踵骨腱） Achilles tendon (Calcaneal tendon)
- 長趾伸筋（腱） Extensor digitorum longus muscle (tendon)
- 腓骨外果 Fibula lateral malleolus
- 長腓骨筋（腱） Fibularis longus muscle (tendon)
- 短腓骨筋 Fibularis brevis muscle

7-179

- 前脛骨筋（腱） Tibialis anterior muscle (tendon)
- 三角靱帯 Deltoid ligament
- 後脛骨筋（腱） Tibialis posterior muscle (tendon)
- 長趾屈筋（腱） Flexor digitorum longus muscle (tendon)
- 長母趾屈筋（腱） Flexor hallucis longus muscle (tendon)
- アキレス腱（踵骨腱） Achilles tendon (Calcaneal tendon)
- 長趾伸筋（腱） Extensor digitorum longus muscle (tendon)
- 腓骨外果 Fibula lateral malleolus
- 長腓骨筋（腱） Fibularis longus muscle (tendon)
- 距骨 Talus

NOTE 内側では前方より後脛骨筋腱，長趾屈筋腱，長母趾屈筋腱が順番に脛骨内果後方の内果溝を下行する．これらの内側の腱は内果，距骨，踵骨，および屈筋支帯で形成される足根管の中を後脛骨動・静脈，脛骨神経とともに通過する．足根管内のガングリオンなどにより起こる脛骨神経の絞扼性神経障害は足根管症候群として知られる．

足関節と足の断層解剖［横断像（MRI，プロトン密度強調像）］

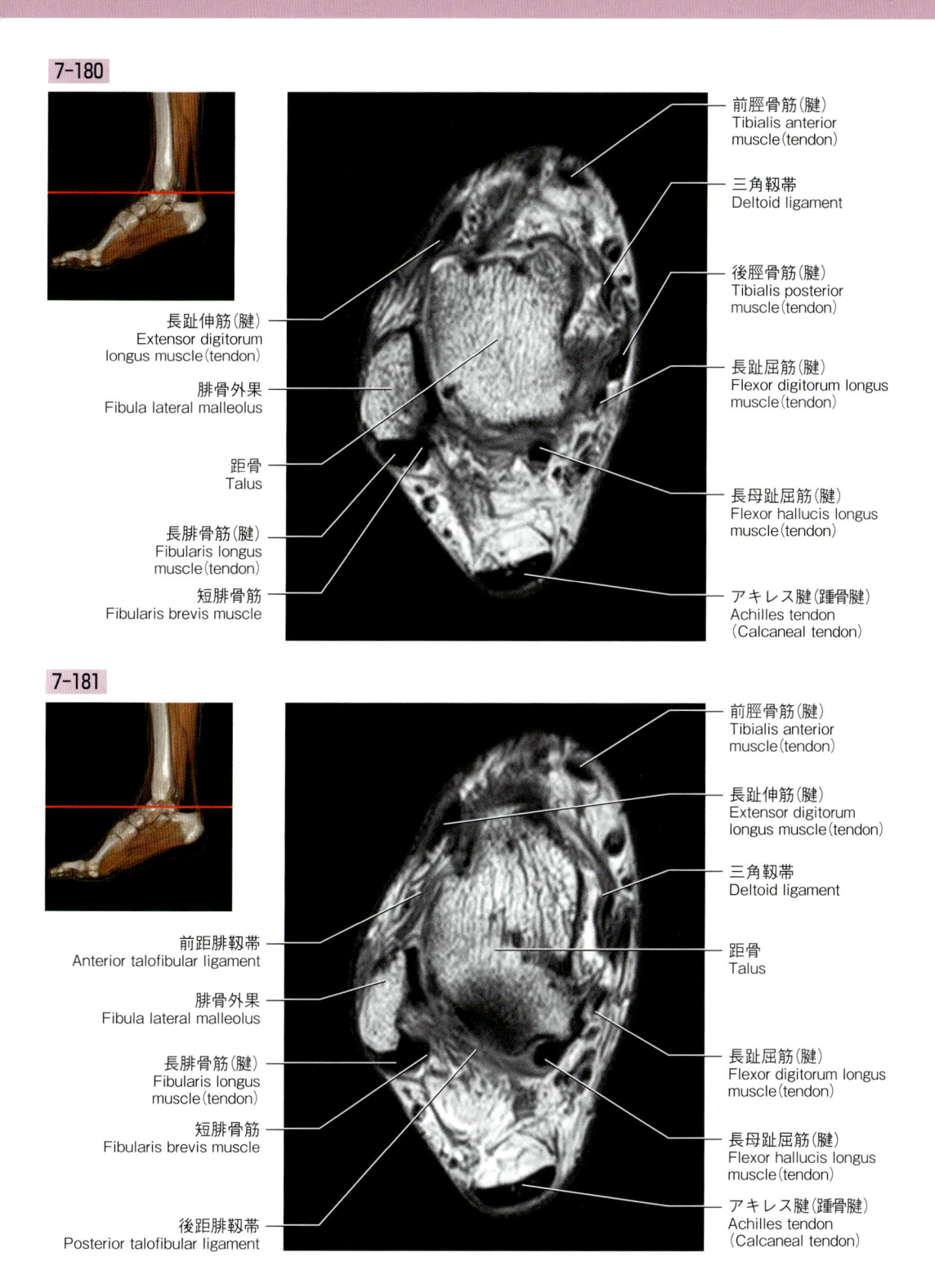

7-180

- 前脛骨筋（腱） Tibialis anterior muscle (tendon)
- 三角靱帯 Deltoid ligament
- 後脛骨筋（腱） Tibialis posterior muscle (tendon)
- 長趾屈筋（腱） Flexor digitorum longus muscle (tendon)
- 長母趾屈筋（腱） Flexor hallucis longus muscle (tendon)
- アキレス腱（踵骨腱） Achilles tendon (Calcaneal tendon)
- 長趾伸筋（腱） Extensor digitorum longus muscle (tendon)
- 腓骨外果 Fibula lateral malleolus
- 距骨 Talus
- 長腓骨筋（腱） Fibularis longus muscle (tendon)
- 短腓骨筋 Fibularis brevis muscle

7-181

- 前脛骨筋（腱） Tibialis anterior muscle (tendon)
- 長趾伸筋（腱） Extensor digitorum longus muscle (tendon)
- 三角靱帯 Deltoid ligament
- 距骨 Talus
- 長趾屈筋（腱） Flexor digitorum longus muscle (tendon)
- 長母趾屈筋（腱） Flexor hallucis longus muscle (tendon)
- アキレス腱（踵骨腱） Achilles tendon (Calcaneal tendon)
- 前距腓靱帯 Anterior talofibular ligament
- 腓骨外果 Fibula lateral malleolus
- 長腓骨筋（腱） Fibularis longus muscle (tendon)
- 短腓骨筋 Fibularis brevis muscle
- 後距腓靱帯 Posterior talofibular ligament

NOTE 後方に存在するアキレス腱は，下腿三頭筋（腓腹筋とヒラメ筋）の腱で，距骨隆起に停止する人体で最大の腱である．アキレス腱の近位部は卵円形であるが，踵骨付着部付近では扁平な形をしている．

足関節と足の断層解剖 ［横断像（MRI，プロトン密度強調像）］

7-182

- 長趾伸筋(腱) Extensor digitorum longus muscle(tendon)
- 前脛骨筋(腱) Tibialis anterior muscle(tendon)
- 距骨 Talus
- 後脛骨筋(腱) Tibialis posterior muscle(tendon)
- 三角靱帯 Deltoid ligament
- 腓骨外果 Fibula lateral malleolus
- 長趾屈筋(腱) Flexor digitorum longus muscle(tendon)
- 長腓骨筋(腱) Fibularis longus muscle(tendon)
- 長母趾屈筋(腱) Flexor hallucis longus muscle(tendon)
- アキレス腱(踵骨腱) Achilles tendon (Calcaneal tendon)

7-183

- 前脛骨筋(腱) Tibialis anterior muscle(tendon)
- 舟状骨 Navicular
- 三角靱帯 Deltoid ligament
- 後脛骨筋(腱) Tibialis posterior muscle(tendon)
- 距骨 Talus
- 長趾伸筋(腱) Extensor digitorum longus muscle(tendon)
- 第3腓骨筋 Fibularis tertius muscle
- 中間楔状骨 Intermediate cuneiform
- 短腓骨筋(腱) Fibularis brevis muscle(tendon)
- 長腓骨筋(腱) Fibularis longus muscle(tendon)
- 長趾屈筋(腱) Flexor digitorum longus muscle(tendon)
- 長母趾屈筋(腱) Flexor hallucis longus muscle(tendon)
- 踵骨 Calcaneus
- アキレス腱(踵骨腱) Achilles tendon (Calcaneal tendon)

NOTE 前方では内側より順に前脛骨筋腱，長母趾伸筋腱，長趾伸筋腱，第3腓骨筋が上・下伸筋支帯の下を通過する．

足関節と足の断層解剖 ［横断像（MRI, プロトン密度強調像）］

7-184

- 内側楔状骨 Medial cuneiform
- 前脛骨筋（腱） Tibialis anterior muscle (tendon)
- 中間楔状骨 Intermediate cuneiform
- 舟状骨 Navicular
- 跳躍靱帯（ばね靱帯） Spring ligament
- 母趾外転筋 Abductor hallucis muscle
- 足底方形筋 Quadratus plantae muscle
- 踵骨 Calcaneus
- 長趾伸筋（腱） Extensor digitorum longus muscle (tendon)
- 第3腓骨筋 Fibularis tertius muscle
- 立方骨 Cuboid
- 短腓骨筋（腱） Fibularis brevis muscle (tendon)
- 長腓骨筋（腱） Fibularis longus muscle (tendon)

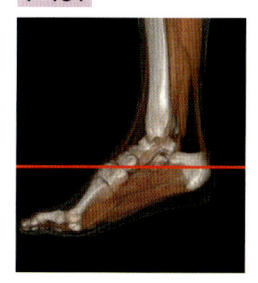

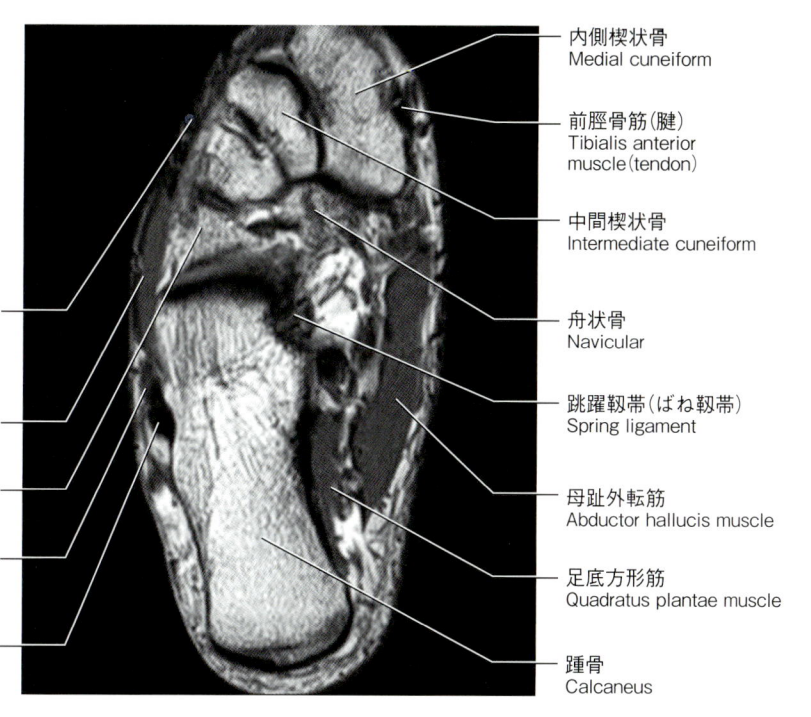

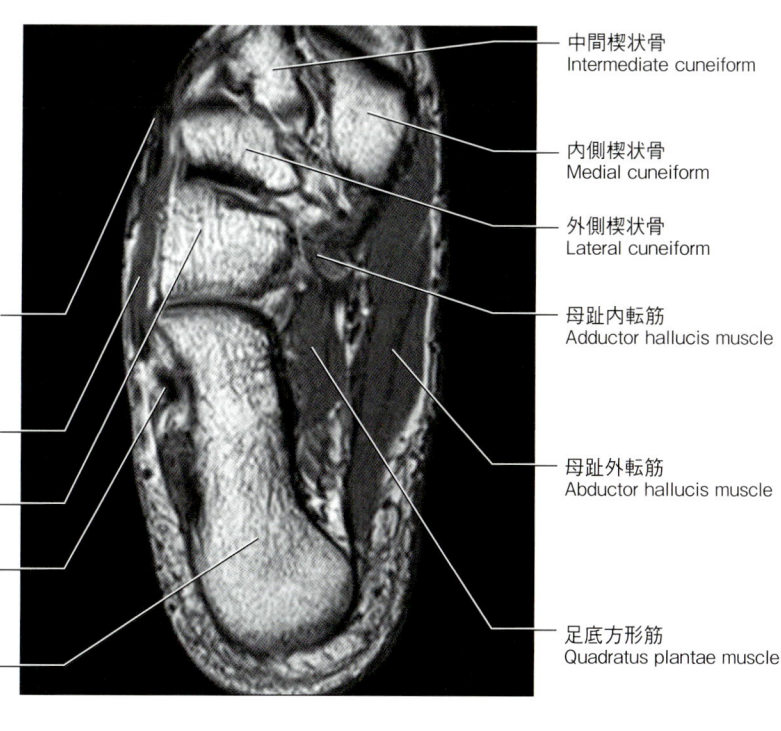

7-185

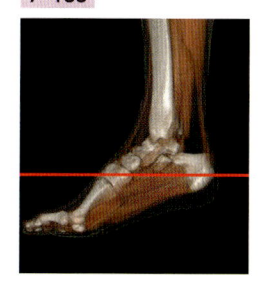

- 中間楔状骨 Intermediate cuneiform
- 内側楔状骨 Medial cuneiform
- 外側楔状骨 Lateral cuneiform
- 母趾内転筋 Adductor hallucis muscle
- 母趾外転筋 Abductor hallucis muscle
- 足底方形筋 Quadratus plantae muscle
- 長趾伸筋（腱） Extensor digitorum longus muscle (tendon)
- 第3腓骨筋 Fibularis tertius muscle
- 立方骨 Cuboid
- 長腓骨筋（腱） Fibularis longus muscle (tendon)
- 踵骨 Calcaneus

足関節と足の断層解剖 [冠状断像（MRI，プロトン密度強調像）]

7-186

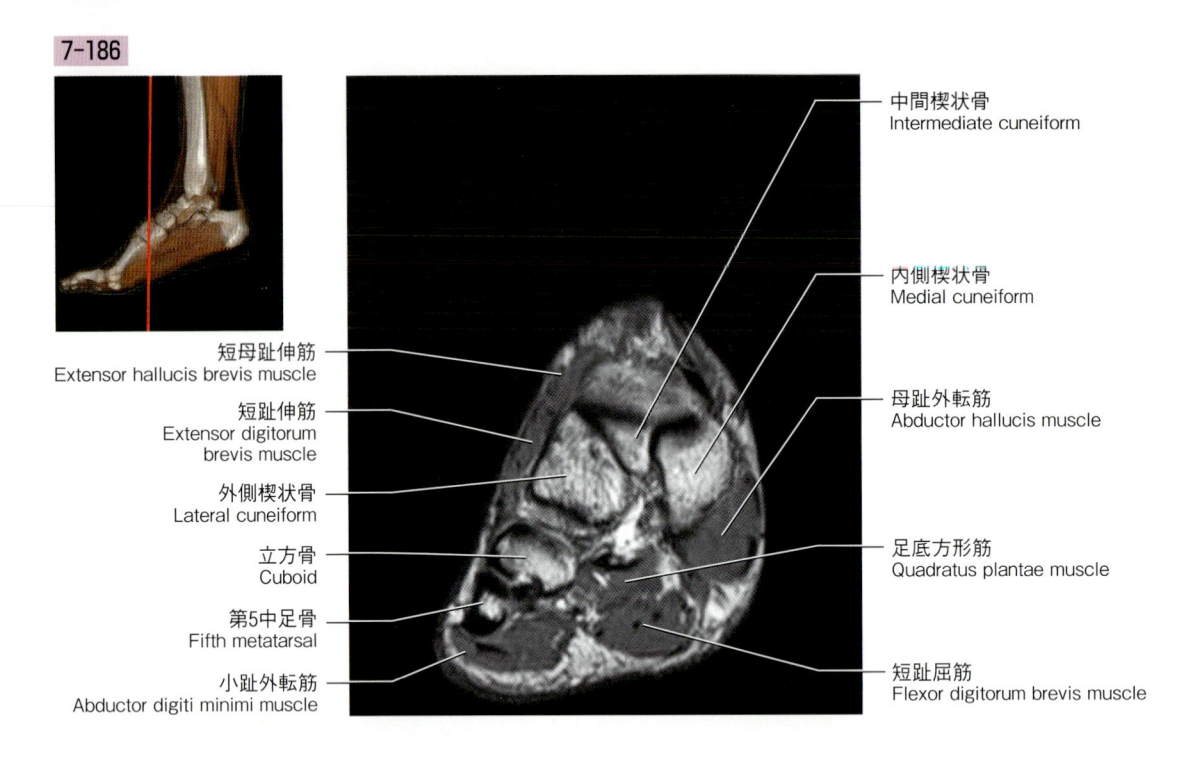

- 中間楔状骨 Intermediate cuneiform
- 内側楔状骨 Medial cuneiform
- 母趾外転筋 Abductor hallucis muscle
- 足底方形筋 Quadratus plantae muscle
- 短趾屈筋 Flexor digitorum brevis muscle
- 短母趾伸筋 Extensor hallucis brevis muscle
- 短趾伸筋 Extensor digitorum brevis muscle
- 外側楔状骨 Lateral cuneiform
- 立方骨 Cuboid
- 第5中足骨 Fifth metatarsal
- 小趾外転筋 Abductor digiti minimi muscle

7-187

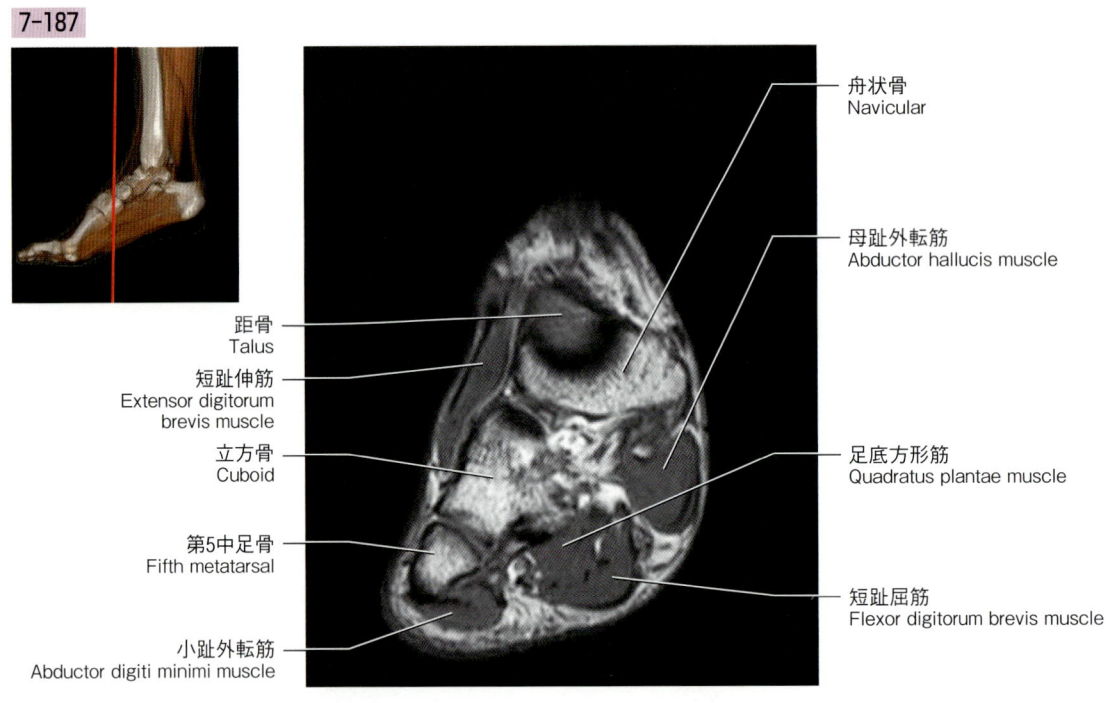

- 舟状骨 Navicular
- 母趾外転筋 Abductor hallucis muscle
- 足底方形筋 Quadratus plantae muscle
- 短趾屈筋 Flexor digitorum brevis muscle
- 距骨 Talus
- 短趾伸筋 Extensor digitorum brevis muscle
- 立方骨 Cuboid
- 第5中足骨 Fifth metatarsal
- 小趾外転筋 Abductor digiti minimi muscle

足関節と足の断層解剖　[冠状断像（MRI, プロトン密度強調像）]

403

7-188

距骨	Talus
底側踵舟靱帯	Plantar calcaneonavicular ligament
後脛骨筋(腱)	Tibialis posterior muscle (tendon)
母趾外転筋	Abductor hallucis muscle
足底方形筋	Quadratus plantae muscle
短趾屈筋	Flexor digitorum brevis muscle
長趾伸筋	Extensor digitorum longus muscle
短趾伸筋	Extensor digitorum brevis muscle
立方骨	Cuboid
第5中足骨	Fifth metatarsal
小趾外転筋	Abductor digiti minimi muscle

7-189

底側踵舟靱帯	Plantar calcaneonavicular ligament
後脛骨筋(腱)	Tibialis posterior muscle (tendon)
母趾外転筋	Abductor hallucis muscle
足底方形筋	Quadratus plantae muscle
短趾屈筋	Flexor digitorum brevis muscle
距骨	Talus
短趾伸筋	Extensor digitorum brevis muscle
立方骨	Cuboid
小趾外転筋	Abductor digiti minimi muscle

VII

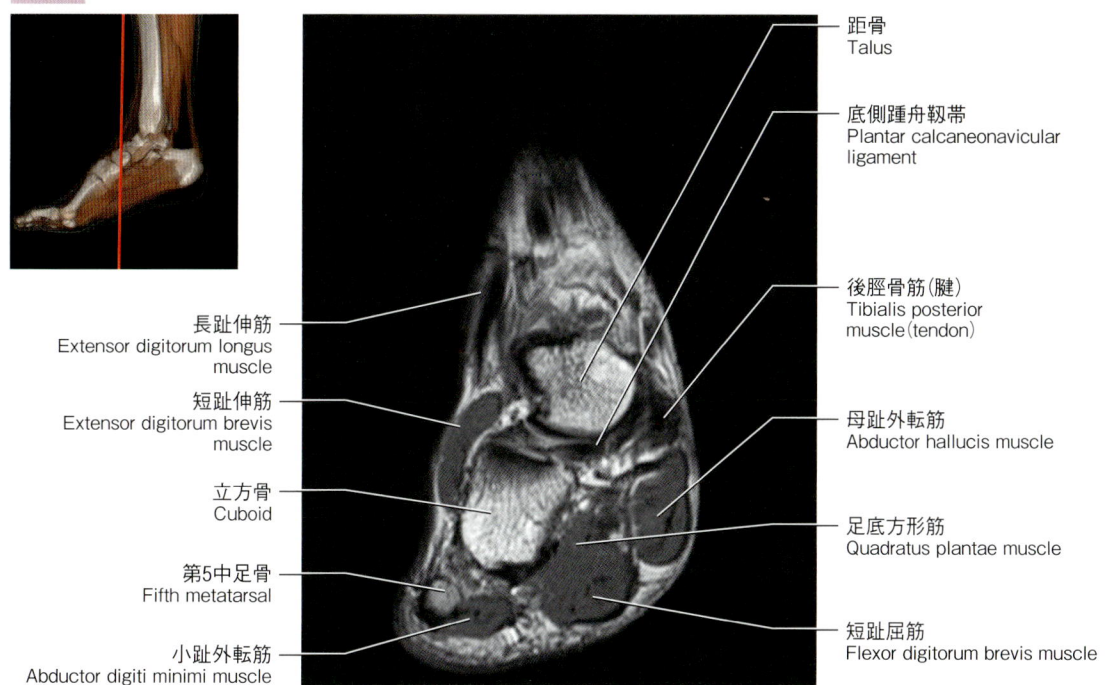

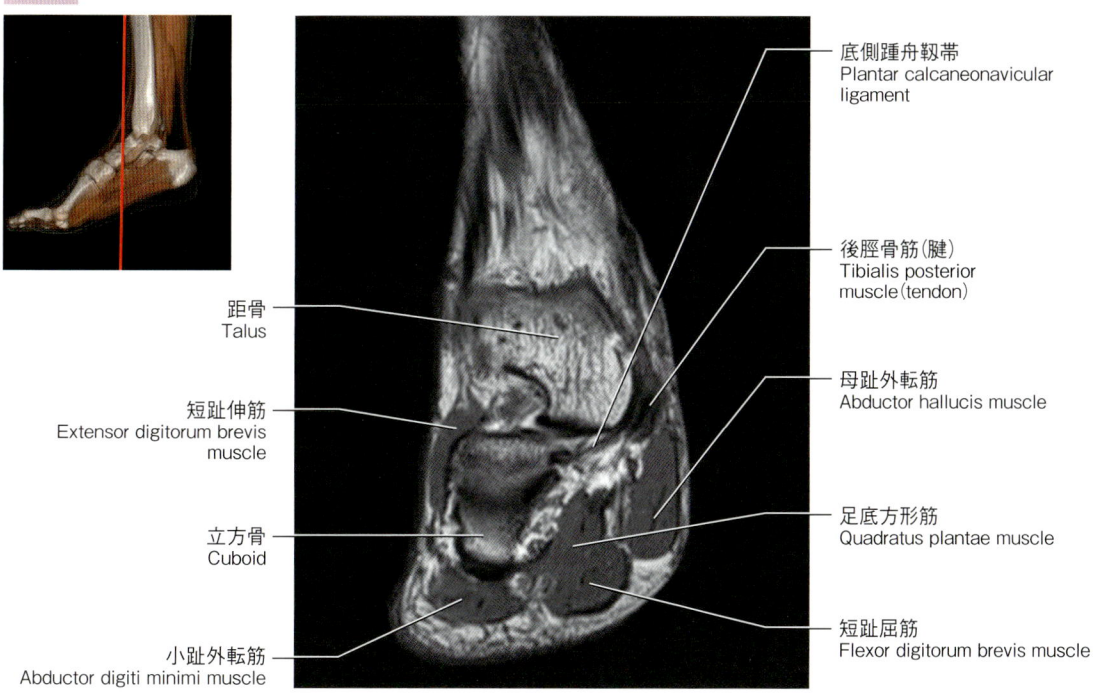

足関節と足の断層解剖 ［冠状断像（MRI, プロトン密度強調像）］

7-190

- 脛骨 Tibia
- 三角靱帯 Deltoid ligament
- 後脛骨筋（腱）Tibialis posterior muscle (tendon)
- 距骨 Talus
- 短趾伸筋 Extensor digitorum brevis muscle
- 母趾外転筋 Abductor hallucis muscle
- 踵骨 Calcaneus
- 足底方形筋 Quadratus plantae muscle
- 長足底靱帯 Long plantar ligament
- 短趾屈筋 Flexor digitorum brevis muscle
- 小趾外転筋 Abductor digiti minimi muscle

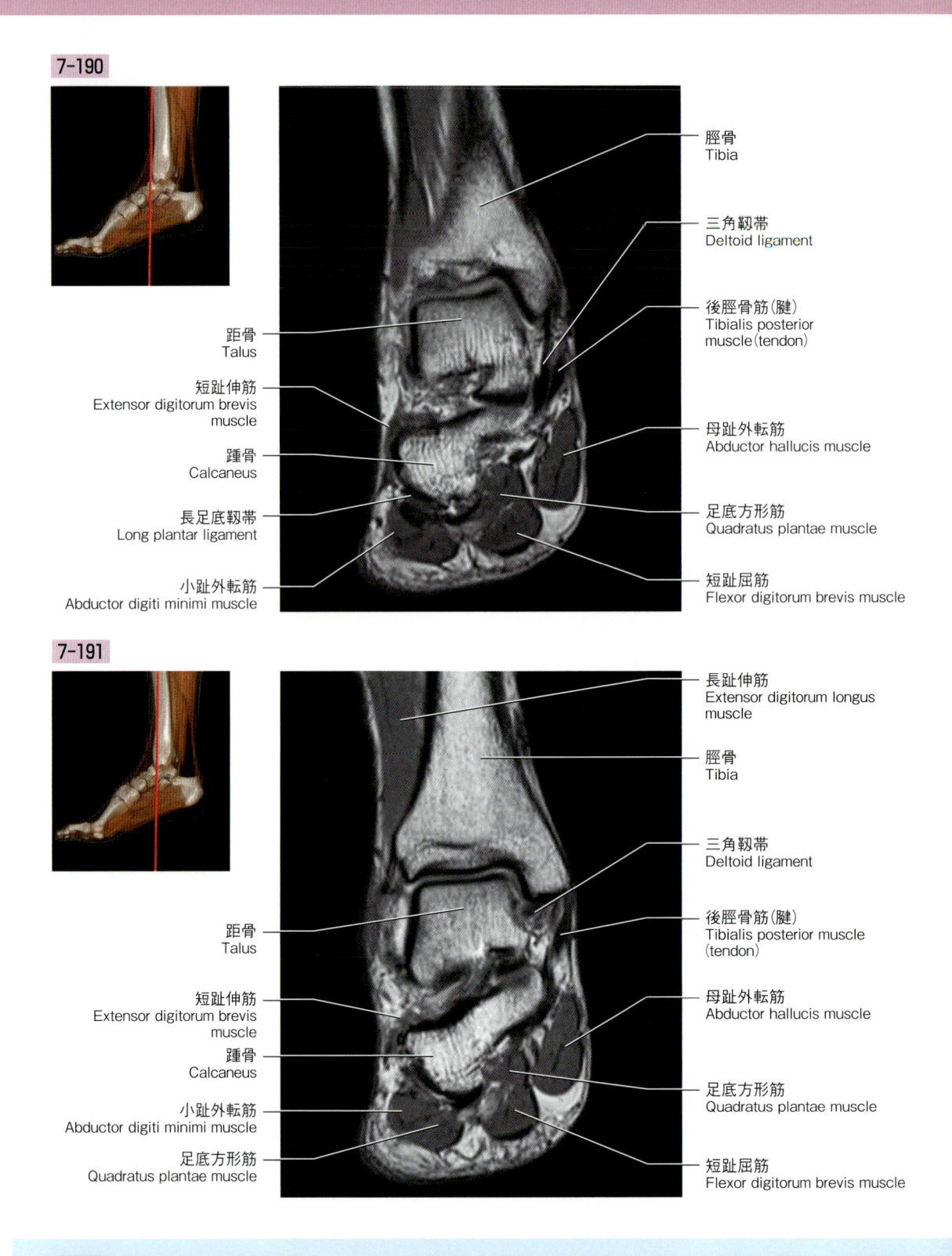

7-191

- 長趾伸筋 Extensor digitorum longus muscle
- 脛骨 Tibia
- 三角靱帯 Deltoid ligament
- 後脛骨筋（腱）Tibialis posterior muscle (tendon)
- 距骨 Talus
- 短趾伸筋 Extensor digitorum brevis muscle
- 母趾外転筋 Abductor hallucis muscle
- 踵骨 Calcaneus
- 足底方形筋 Quadratus plantae muscle
- 小趾外転筋 Abductor digiti minimi muscle
- 短趾屈筋 Flexor digitorum brevis muscle
- 足底方形筋 Quadratus plantae muscle

NOTE 距骨下関節は後距骨下関節と距踵舟状骨関節（右前距骨下関節）に分けられる．これらの間には，距骨溝と踵骨溝で形成される外側前方に開いた漏斗状の非関節腔隙があり，足根洞とよばれる．足根洞には豊富な脂肪組織，後脛骨動脈と腓骨動脈の吻合枝，神経終末枝が存在し，距骨と踵骨の連結を関節包と靱帯が補強する．足根洞の異常に起因した足部外側の疼痛，足根洞部の圧痛，後足部の動揺は足根洞症候群として知られる．

足関節と足の断層解剖 ［冠状断像（MRI, プロトン密度強調像）］

7-192

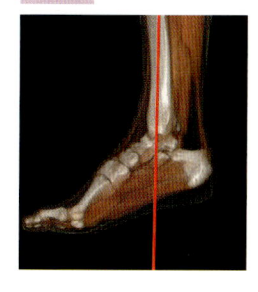

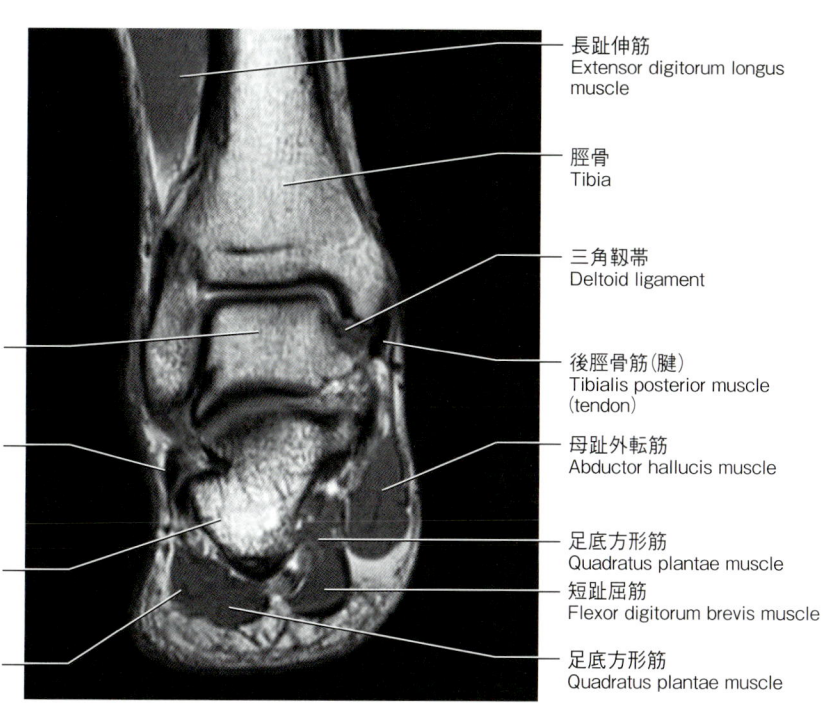

- 長趾伸筋 Extensor digitorum longus muscle
- 脛骨 Tibia
- 三角靱帯 Deltoid ligament
- 距骨 Talus
- 後脛骨筋（腱） Tibialis posterior muscle (tendon)
- 長腓骨筋（腱） Fibularis longus muscle (tendon)
- 母趾外転筋 Abductor hallucis muscle
- 足底方形筋 Quadratus plantae muscle
- 踵骨 Calcaneus
- 短趾屈筋 Flexor digitorum brevis muscle
- 小趾外転筋 Abductor digiti minimi muscle
- 足底方形筋 Quadratus plantae muscle

7-193

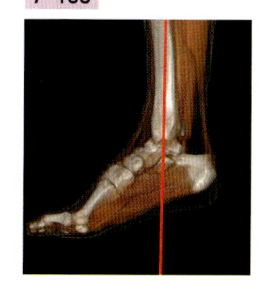

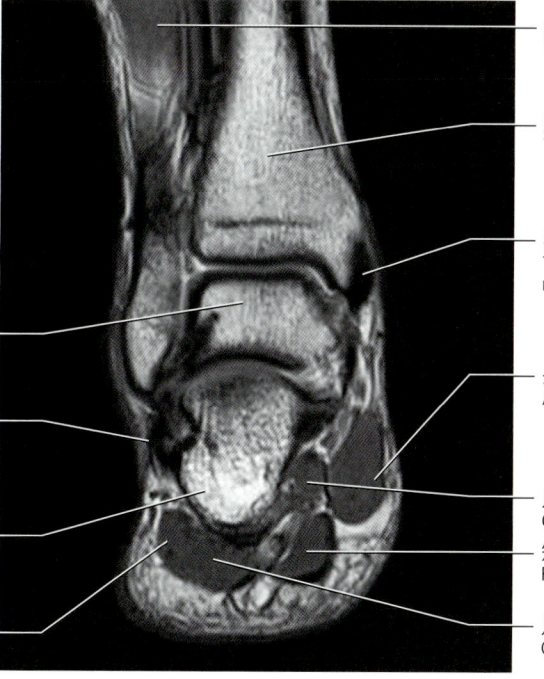

- 長趾伸筋 Extensor digitorum longus muscle
- 脛骨 Tibia
- 後脛骨筋（腱） Tibialis posterior muscle (tendon)
- 距骨 Talus
- 母趾外転筋 Abductor hallucis muscle
- 長腓骨筋（腱） Fibularis longus muscle (tendon)
- 足底方形筋 Quadratus plantae muscle
- 踵骨 Calcaneus
- 短趾屈筋 Flexor digitorum brevis muscle
- 小趾外転筋 Abductor digiti minimi muscle
- 足底方形筋 Quadratus plantae muscle

足関節と足の断層解剖 ［冠状断像（MRI, プロトン密度強調像）］

7-194

- 腓骨 Fibula
- 脛骨 Tibia
- 後脛骨筋（腱） Tibialis posterior muscle (tendon)
- 後距腓靱帯 Posterior talofibular ligament
- 母趾外転筋 Abductor hallucis muscle
- 長腓骨筋（腱） Fibularis longus muscle (tendon)
- 足底方形筋 Quadratus plantae muscle
- 踵骨 Calcaneus
- 短趾屈筋 Flexor digitorum brevis muscle
- 小趾外転筋 Abductor digiti minimi muscle
- 足底方形筋 Quadratus plantae muscle

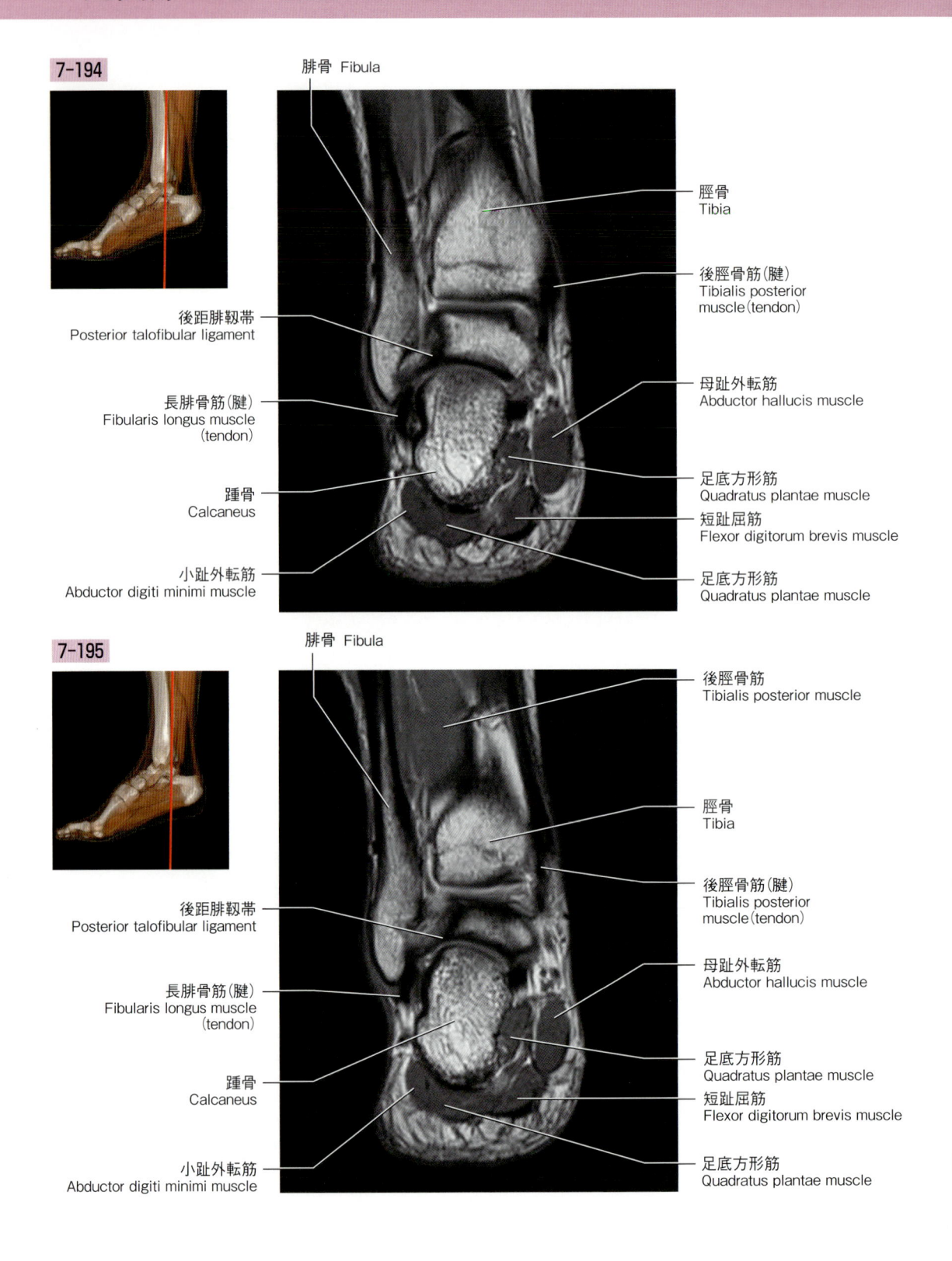

7-195

- 腓骨 Fibula
- 後脛骨筋 Tibialis posterior muscle
- 脛骨 Tibia
- 後脛骨筋（腱） Tibialis posterior muscle (tendon)
- 後距腓靱帯 Posterior talofibular ligament
- 母趾外転筋 Abductor hallucis muscle
- 長腓骨筋（腱） Fibularis longus muscle (tendon)
- 足底方形筋 Quadratus plantae muscle
- 踵骨 Calcaneus
- 短趾屈筋 Flexor digitorum brevis muscle
- 小趾外転筋 Abductor digiti minimi muscle
- 足底方形筋 Quadratus plantae muscle

足関節と足の断層解剖 ［冠状断像（MRI，プロトン密度強調像）］

7-196

- 長母趾屈筋 Flexor hallucis longus muscle
- 脛骨 Tibia
- 足底方形筋 Quadratus plantae muscle
- 母趾外転筋 Abductor hallucis muscle
- 短趾屈筋 Flexor digitorum brevis muscle
- 腓骨 Fibula
- 踵骨 Calcaneus
- 小趾外転筋 Abductor digiti minimi muscle
- 足底方形筋 Quadratus plantae muscle

7-197

- 長趾屈筋 Flexor digitorum longus muscle
- 後脛骨筋 Tibialis posterior muscle
- 長母趾屈筋 Flexor hallucis longus muscle
- 足底方形筋 Quadratus plantae muscle
- 母趾外転筋 Abductor hallucis muscle
- 足底腱膜 Plantar aponeurosis
- 短腓骨筋 Fibularis brevis muscle
- 踵骨 Calcaneus

NOTE 足底筋膜は中央部・内側部・外側部により構成されるが，重要なのは最も強靱な中央部で，これは足底腱膜ともよばれる．足底腱膜は踵骨隆起のやや内側より起始し，MTP関節（Metatarsophalangeal joint：中足趾節関節）レベルで各足趾の中足骨・基節骨・腱鞘などに付着する．足底筋膜炎は長距離ランナーなど足底筋膜への反復性ストレスにより引き起こされる踵骨付着部付近の炎症で，足底筋膜近位部に圧痛を訴える．

足関節と足の断層解剖 ［冠状断像（MRI, プロトン密度強調像）］

7-198

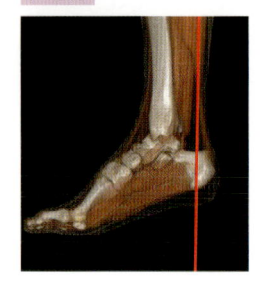

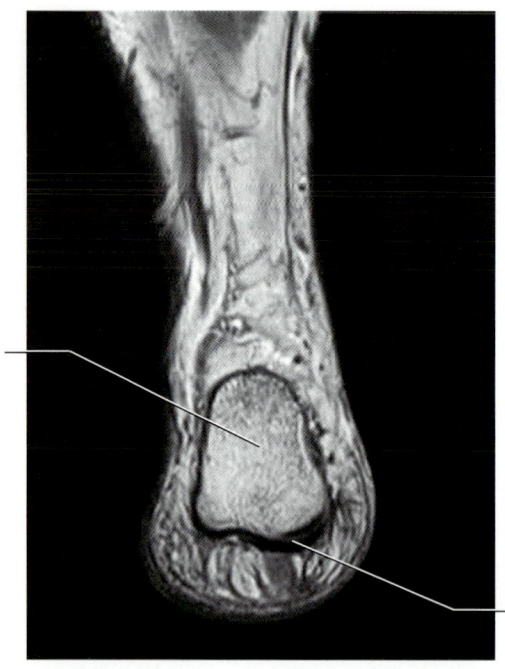

踵骨
Calcaneus

足底腱膜
Plantar aponeurosis

7-199

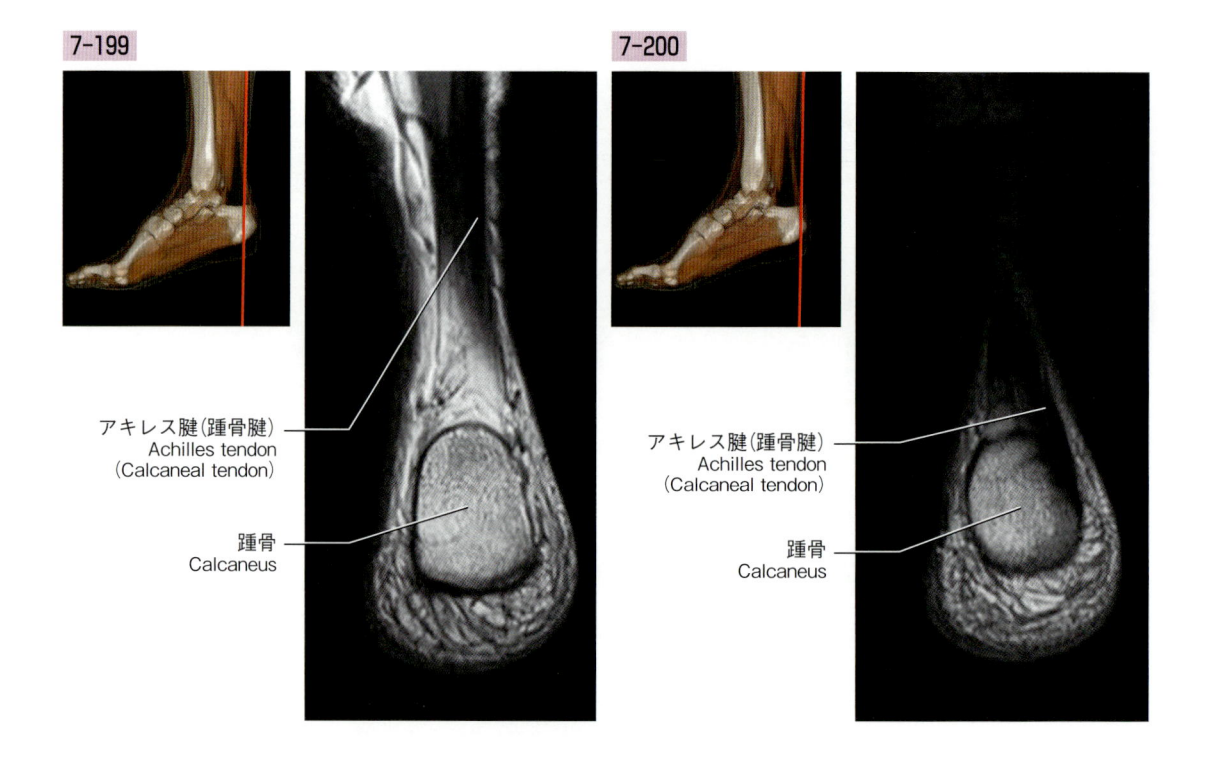

アキレス腱（踵骨腱）
Achilles tendon
(Calcaneal tendon)

踵骨
Calcaneus

7-200

アキレス腱（踵骨腱）
Achilles tendon
(Calcaneal tendon)

踵骨
Calcaneus

足関節と足の断層解剖 [矢状断像（MRI, プロトン密度強調像）]

7-201

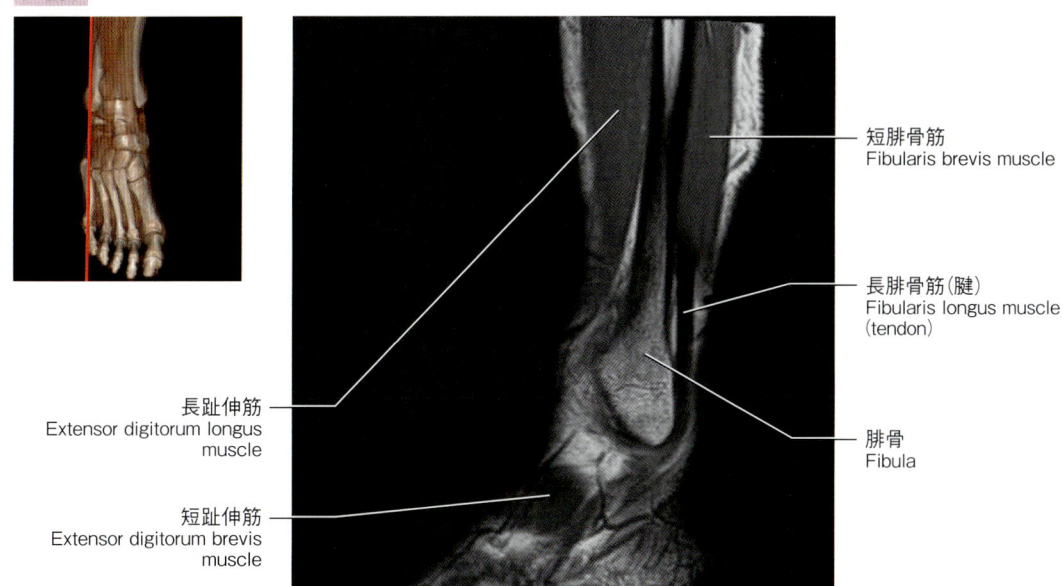

- 長趾伸筋 Extensor digitorum longus muscle
- 短趾伸筋 Extensor digitorum brevis muscle
- 第5中足骨 Fifth metatarsal
- 短腓骨筋 Fibularis brevis muscle
- 長腓骨筋（腱）Fibularis longus muscle (tendon)
- 腓骨 Fibula
- 骨間筋 Interosseous muscle

7-202

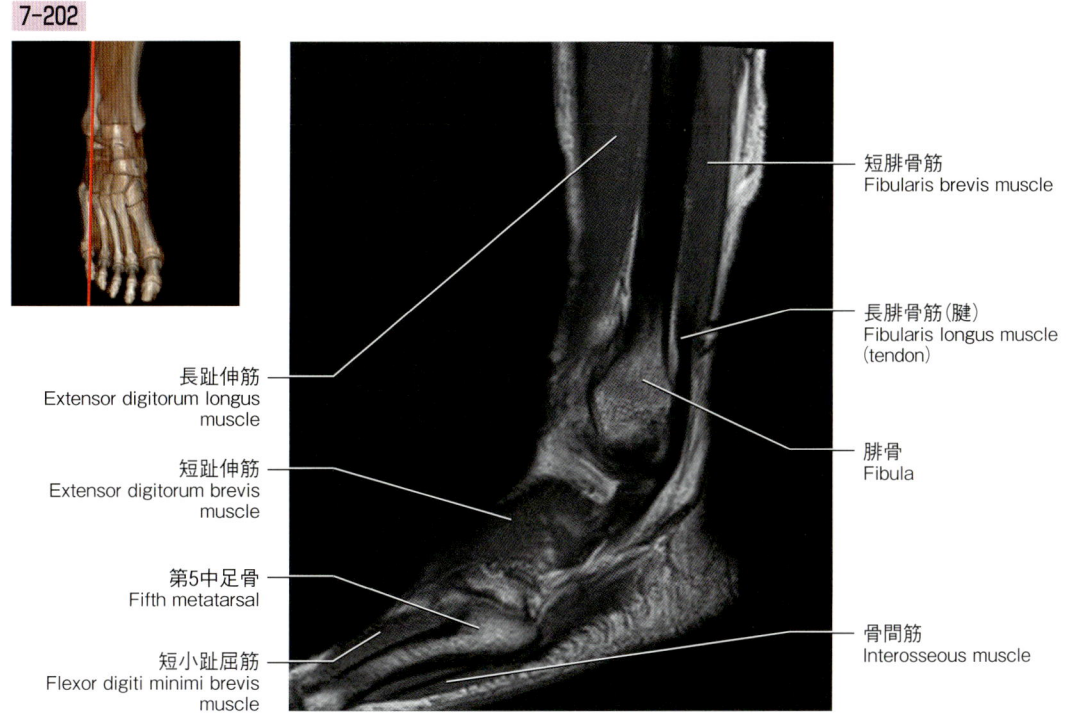

- 長趾伸筋 Extensor digitorum longus muscle
- 短趾伸筋 Extensor digitorum brevis muscle
- 第5中足骨 Fifth metatarsal
- 短小趾屈筋 Flexor digiti minimi brevis muscle
- 短腓骨筋 Fibularis brevis muscle
- 長腓骨筋（腱）Fibularis longus muscle (tendon)
- 腓骨 Fibula
- 骨間筋 Interosseous muscle

足関節と足の断層解剖　[矢状断像（MRI，プロトン密度強調像）]

7-203

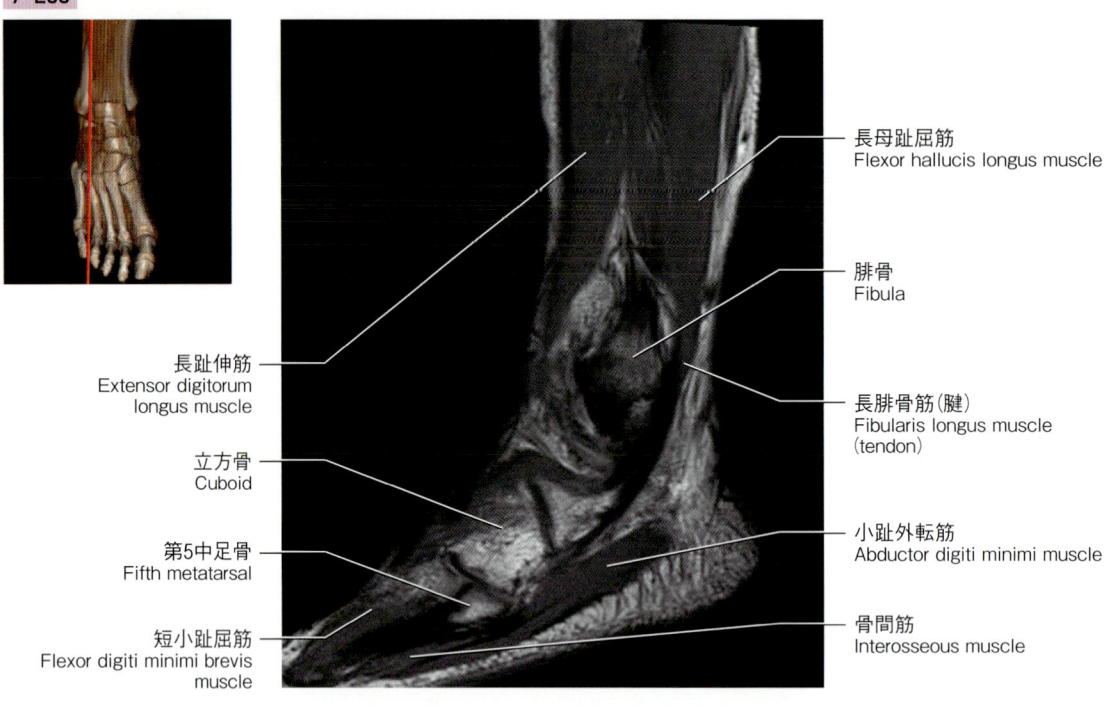

- 長母趾屈筋 Flexor hallucis longus muscle
- 腓骨 Fibula
- 長趾伸筋 Extensor digitorum longus muscle
- 長腓骨筋（腱） Fibularis longus muscle (tendon)
- 立方骨 Cuboid
- 第5中足骨 Fifth metatarsal
- 小趾外転筋 Abductor digiti minimi muscle
- 短小趾屈筋 Flexor digiti minimi brevis muscle
- 骨間筋 Interosseous muscle

7-204

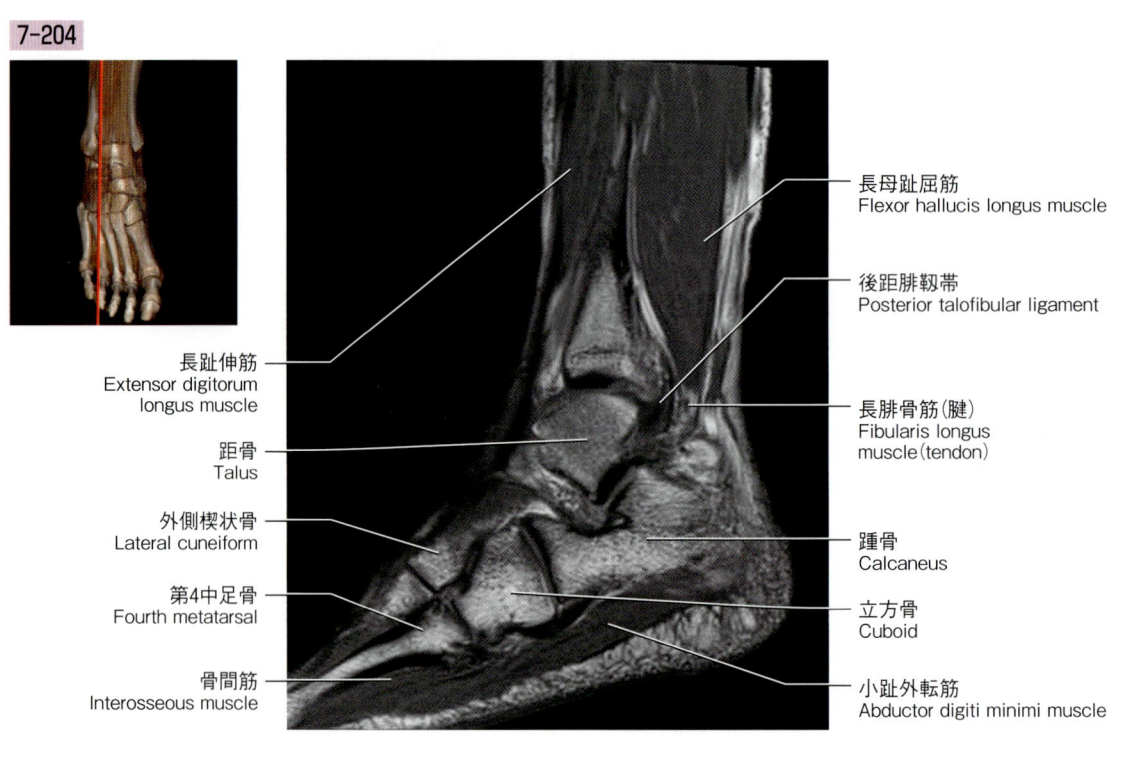

- 長母趾屈筋 Flexor hallucis longus muscle
- 後距腓靱帯 Posterior talofibular ligament
- 長趾伸筋 Extensor digitorum longus muscle
- 長腓骨筋（腱） Fibularis longus muscle (tendon)
- 距骨 Talus
- 外側楔状骨 Lateral cuneiform
- 踵骨 Calcaneus
- 第4中足骨 Fourth metatarsal
- 立方骨 Cuboid
- 骨間筋 Interosseous muscle
- 小趾外転筋 Abductor digiti minimi muscle

足関節と足の断層解剖 ［矢状断像（MRI，プロトン密度強調像）］

7-205

- 脛骨 Tibia
- ヒラメ筋 Soleus muscle
- 長母趾屈筋 Flexor hallucis longus muscle
- 後距腓靱帯 Posterior talofibular ligament
- 距骨 Talus
- アキレス腱（踵骨腱） Achilles tendon (Calcaneal tendon)
- 外側楔状骨 Lateral cuneiform
- 踵骨 Calcaneus
- 第3中足骨 Third metatarsal
- 立方骨 Cuboid
- 骨間筋 Interosseous muscle
- 足底方形筋 Quadratus plantae muscle

7-206

- 脛骨 Tibia
- ヒラメ筋 Soleus muscle
- 長母趾屈筋（腱） Flexor hallucis longus muscle (tendon)
- 距骨 Talus
- 骨間距踵靱帯 Talocalcaneal interosseous ligament
- アキレス腱（踵骨腱） Achilles tendon (Calcaneal tendon)
- 舟状骨 Navicular
- 踵骨 Calcaneus
- 中間楔状骨 Intermediate cuneiform
- 立方骨 Cuboid
- 骨間筋 Interosseous muscle
- 外側楔状骨 Lateral cuneiform
- 第3中足骨 Third metatarsal

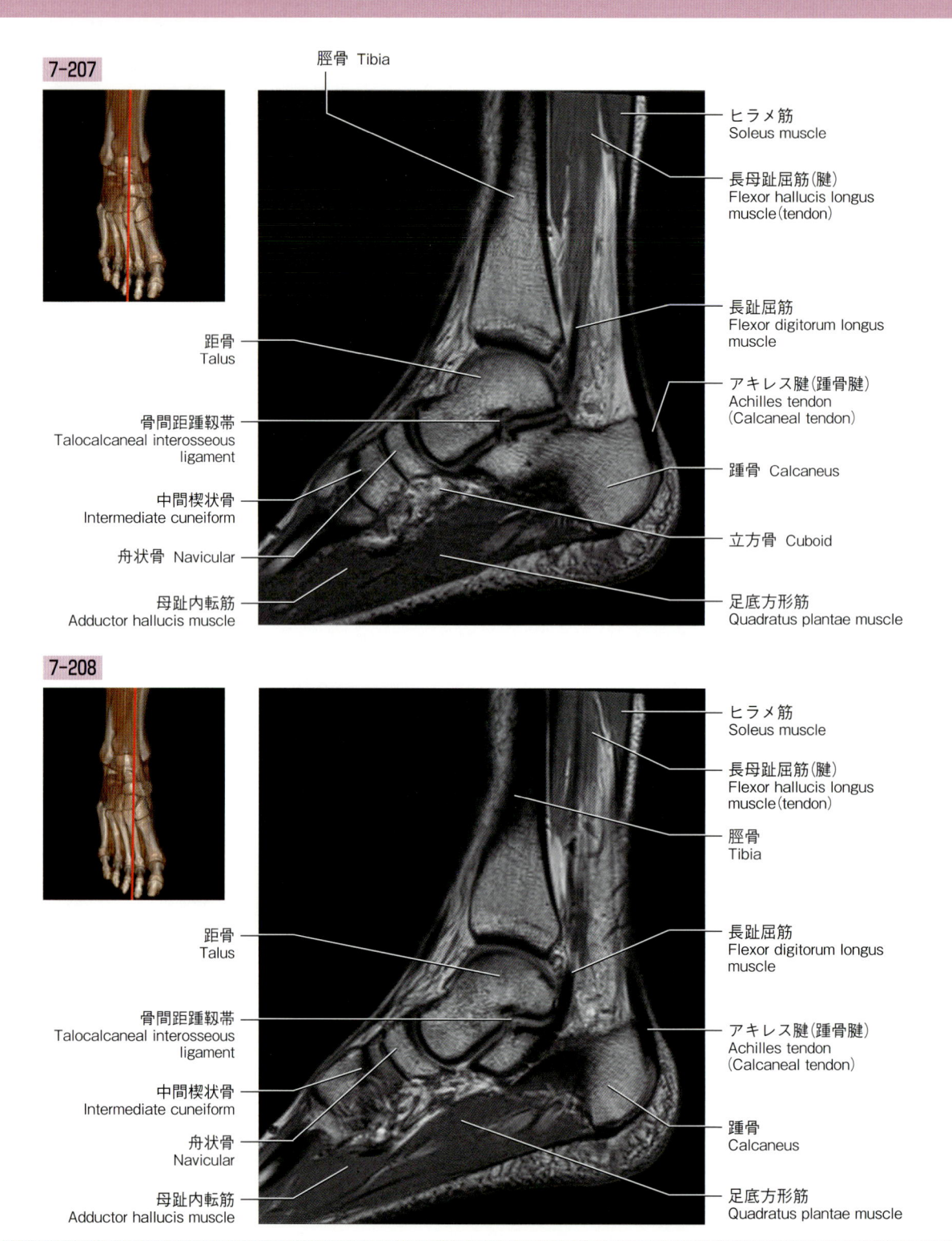

足関節と足の断層解剖 ［矢状断像（MRI, プロトン密度強調像）］

7-207

- 脛骨 Tibia
- ヒラメ筋 Soleus muscle
- 長母趾屈筋（腱） Flexor hallucis longus muscle (tendon)
- 長趾屈筋 Flexor digitorum longus muscle
- アキレス腱（踵骨腱） Achilles tendon (Calcaneal tendon)
- 踵骨 Calcaneus
- 立方骨 Cuboid
- 足底方形筋 Quadratus plantae muscle
- 距骨 Talus
- 骨間距踵靱帯 Talocalcaneal interosseous ligament
- 中間楔状骨 Intermediate cuneiform
- 舟状骨 Navicular
- 母趾内転筋 Adductor hallucis muscle

7-208

- ヒラメ筋 Soleus muscle
- 長母趾屈筋（腱） Flexor hallucis longus muscle (tendon)
- 脛骨 Tibia
- 長趾屈筋 Flexor digitorum longus muscle
- アキレス腱（踵骨腱） Achilles tendon (Calcaneal tendon)
- 踵骨 Calcaneus
- 足底方形筋 Quadratus plantae muscle
- 距骨 Talus
- 骨間距踵靱帯 Talocalcaneal interosseous ligament
- 中間楔状骨 Intermediate cuneiform
- 舟状骨 Navicular
- 母趾内転筋 Adductor hallucis muscle

> **NOTE** アキレス腱 Achilles tendon
> 　Achilles（アキレス）は，ギリシャ神話に登場する英雄で神ではない．桁外れに強いが致命的弱点があり，トロイア戦争でその部位を射られ死にいたった．母親が，生まれたばかりの彼を不死の体にしようと神の川に浸したが，ふくらはぎから踵を掴んでいたため，そこだけ神水の効きめが及ばなかった．解剖名だけではなく「強者の弱点」の意味をもつ．

足関節と足の断層解剖　[矢状断像（MRI，プロトン密度強調像）]

7-209

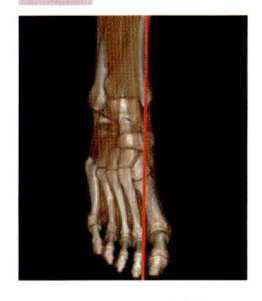

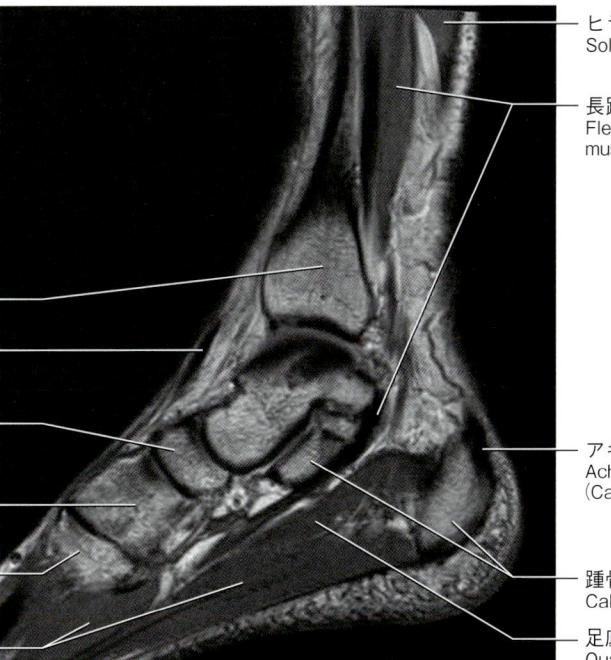

- ヒラメ筋 Soleus muscle
- 長趾屈筋（腱） Flexor digitorum longus muscle（tendon）
- 脛骨 Tibia
- 前脛骨筋（腱） Tibialis anterior muscle（tendon）
- 舟状骨 Navicular
- 内側楔状骨 Medial cuneiform
- 第1中足骨 First metatarsal
- 短母趾屈筋 Flexor hallucis brevis muscle
- アキレス腱（踵骨腱） Achilles tendon（Calcaneal tendon）
- 踵骨 Calcaneus
- 足底方形筋 Quadratus plantae muscle

7-210

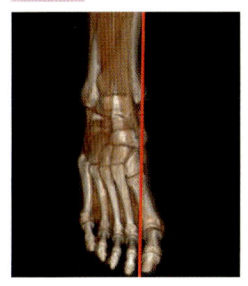

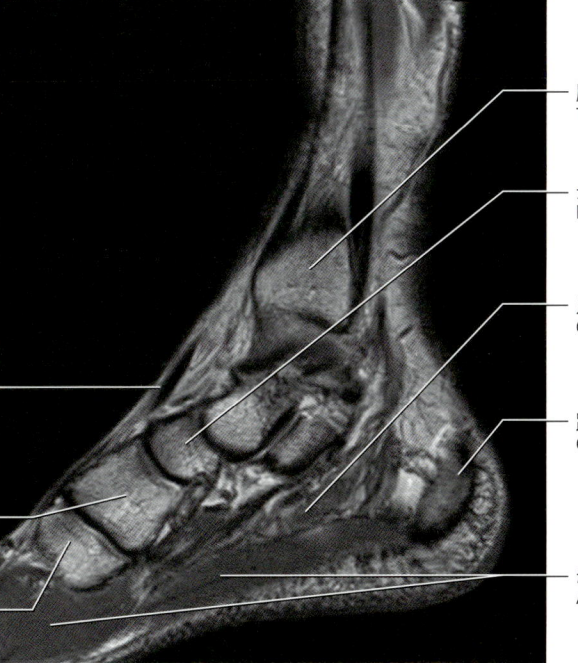

- 脛骨 Tibia
- 舟状骨 Navicular
- 前脛骨筋（腱） Tibialis anterior muscle（tendon）
- 内側楔状骨 Medial cuneiform
- 第1中足骨 First metatarsal
- 足底方形筋 Quadratus plantae muscle
- 踵骨 Calcaneus
- 母趾外転筋 Abductor hallucis muscle

414 足関節と足の断層解剖 ［矢状断像（MRI，プロトン密度強調像）］

7-211

- 脛骨 Tibia
- 長趾屈筋（腱） Flexor digitorum longus muscle（tendon）
- 前脛骨筋（腱） Tibialis anterior muscle（tendon）
- 内側楔状骨 Medial cuneiform
- 距骨 Talus
- 第1中足骨 First metatarsal
- 舟状骨 Navicular
- 短母趾屈筋 Flexor hallucis brevis muscle
- 母趾外転筋 Abductor hallucis muscle

7-212

- 脛骨 Tibia
- 長趾屈筋（腱） Flexor digitorum longus muscle（tendon）
- 前脛骨筋（腱） Tibialis anterior muscle（tendon）
- 内側楔状骨 Medial cuneiform
- 第1中足骨 First metatarsal
- 舟状骨 Navicular
- 母趾外転筋 Abductor hallucis muscle
- 短母趾屈筋 Flexor hallucis brevis muscle

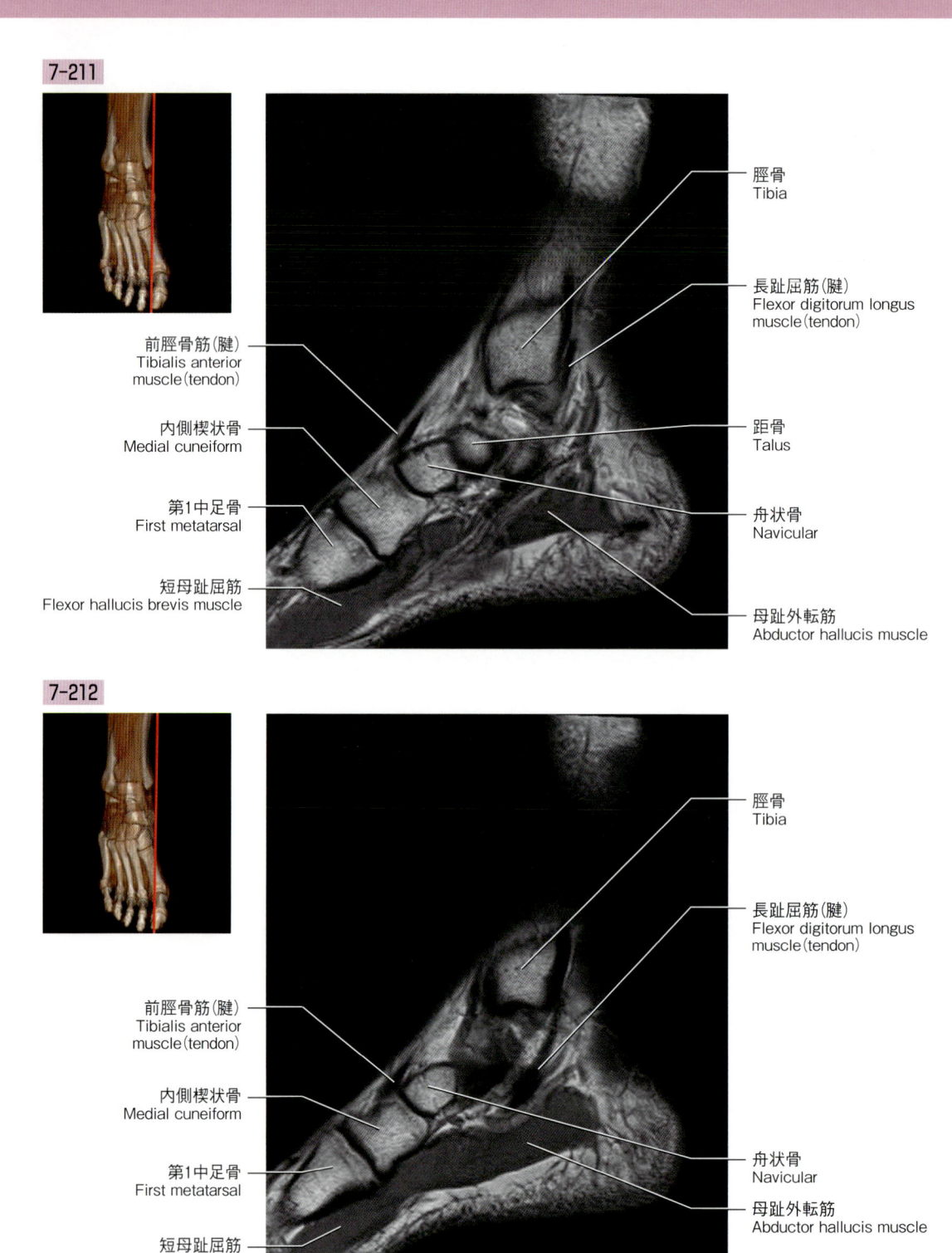

足関節と足の断層解剖　[矢状断像（MRI，プロトン密度強調像）]

7-213

- 脛骨 Tibia
- 長趾屈筋（腱） Flexor digitorum longus muscle（tendon）
- 前脛骨筋（腱） Tibialis anterior muscle（tendon）
- 内側楔状骨 Medial cuneiform
- 第1中足骨 First metatarsal
- 短母趾屈筋 Flexor hallucis brevis muscle
- 舟状骨 Navicular
- 母趾外転筋 Abductor hallucis muscle

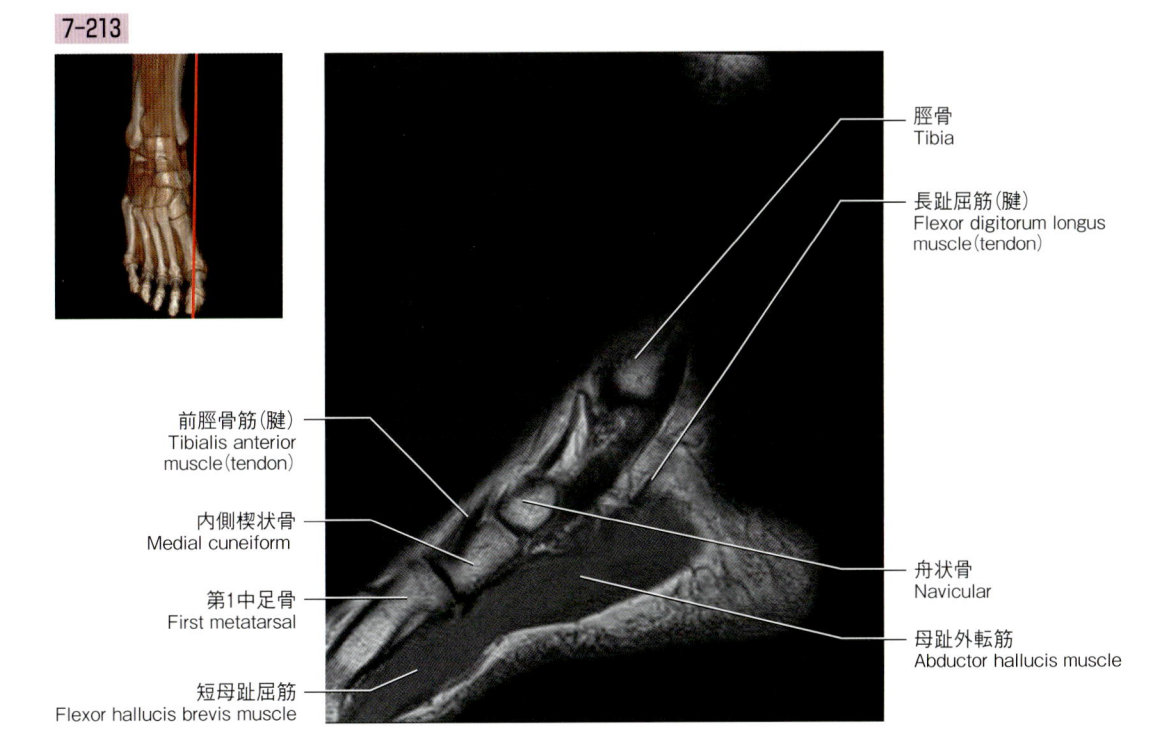

和文索引

あ

アキレス腱(踵骨腱) 393, 394, 396-400, 408, 411-413
足(あし)関節→足(そく)関節
アブミ骨 109, 113, 116
アルツハイマー病 39

い

胃 229, 235-238, 245, 249-251, 254-258, 262-264
胃十二指腸動脈 230, 240, 242, 243, 251, 255
一次運動野 7, 8
一次視覚皮質 21
陰茎海綿体 283-285, 362-364
咽頭 71
咽頭結節 4
咽頭収縮筋 94
陰囊 283
インピンジメント症候群 320

う

ウィリス動脈輪 12
ウェルニッケ野 7
迂回槽 23
烏口肩峰アーチ 320
烏口突起 172-175, 310, 311, 313, 315, 320, 321
烏口腕筋 314, 315, 317, 320, 321
右心耳 213, 214
右心室 182, 187-189, 192-194, 206, 207, 213-222, 224-226
右心房 182, 187, 188, 191, 207, 214-216, 218, 221, 222, 226
運動失語 7
運動前野 7

え

鋭縁部 208
腋窩静脈 307
腋窩動脈 306
腋窩部 308
遠位指節間関節(DIP 関節) 340, 351
円回内筋 326-333, 336, 337, 339
縁上回 7, 20, 21, 43
延髄 24-26, 32, 41, 55-57, 64
　錐体 56

お

横隔膜 194, 249, 254
横隔膜脚 250, 258, 261, 262
横口蓋縫合 4
横行結腸 235, 236, 238, 250-254, 260-265
横後頭溝 6
横静脈洞 13, 42, 43
黄色靱帯 150, 158, 159, 163
横舌筋 97, 98
横側頭回 28, 40
横突起 123-129, 133, 138-140, 143, 144, 147, 151-153
横突孔 123, 126-129
オトガイ 4
オトガイ結節 2
オトガイ孔 2
オトガイ舌筋 81-83, 94, 95, 97-100
オトガイ舌骨筋 82-84, 98-100
オトガイ隆起 2, 3, 5

か

外果 393-395
回外筋 331-333, 335, 336, 338
外頸動脈 76-80
外後頭隆起 2-4
外耳孔 2
外耳道 25, 75, 89, 102, 114, 116, 117
回旋運動 338
外側顆《脛骨》 375
　《大腿骨》 375, 383, 384
外側顆上稜 324
外側環軸関節 125, 129
外側楔状骨 394, 395, 401, 402, 410, 411
外側溝 6
外側広筋 282, 283, 285, 286, 293, 295-297, 355, 362-365, 369-371, 376, 381-383, 386, 387
外側後頭側頭回 43, 61, 65, 66, 68
外側後脈絡動脈(LPChA) 16
外側塊 125-127, 129-131, 134, 135
外側上顆《上腕骨》 324, 326
　《大腿骨》 375
外側仙骨動脈 273
外側仙骨稜 164
外側線条体動脈(LSA) 16

外側側副靱帯
　《膝関節》 371, 383-385
　《肘関節》 336
外側大腿回旋動脈 273, 279
外側中葉枝 183
外側直筋 23, 28, 29, 34, 35, 73, 97
外側肺底枝 183
外側半規管 109, 111, 112, 116, 118, 119
外側翼突筋 76, 77, 90-92, 99-101
回腸 236
外腸骨静脈 280, 281, 285, 286, 291, 292, 295, 296, 354, 360, 361
外腸骨動脈 273, 280, 281, 285, 286, 291, 292, 295, 296, 353, 360, 361
外転神経(CN VI) 44, 47, 55, 66
回内筋 338
回内筋症候群 328
海馬 18, 23, 29, 30, 39, 40, 51, 61, 62, 66, 67
海馬体尾部 62
海馬傍回 23, 39, 51, 62, 65-67
海馬傍回鈎 23, 30, 66
蓋板 32, 63, 64
外腹斜筋 253, 355
外閉鎖筋 282, 285-287, 293, 295-297, 362-364, 366-368
外包 22, 37
解剖頸 311
回盲部 228
下咽頭 83-86
下オリーブ核 41
下顎角 2, 5, 91
下顎管 81, 91, 92, 98-100
下顎頸 76, 77
下顎後静脈 78, 79
下顎骨 5
　関節突起 5
　筋突起 5
下顎枝 2, 5, 77-81, 90, 91, 98-102
下顎体 2, 5, 83, 84, 91-95, 97-99
下顎頭 25, 27, 28, 38, 39, 75, 76, 89, 90, 101
顆間窩 375
下眼窩裂 2, 98
下関節突起 123, 128, 130, 136, 139, 141, 142, 144, 145, 149, 151-153, 155, 156, 158, 159, 162
顆間隆起 375
下丘 63
蝸牛 66, 109, 112, 113, 115, 116, 120

蝸牛岬角　115
角回　7, 20
顎下腺　70, 82, 83, 91, 92, 101, 107
顎関節突起　4
顎舌骨筋　82-84, 93-95, 100
顎二腹筋
　　後腹　91
　　前腹　84, 93, 95, 98-100, 107
下行結腸　235-238, 244, 245, 250-253, 255, 265, 266
下項線　4
下行大動脈　182, 186, 187, 190, 192, 193, 203, 205, 206, 213-219, 225, 226
下後腸骨棘　269
下肢の主な静脈　354
下肢の主な動脈　353
下斜筋　96
下小脳脚　31
下垂体　23, 32, 37, 52, 64, 65
　　後葉　63
　　前葉　63
下垂体柄　38
下舌枝　183
下前腸骨棘　269, 358
下前頭回　7, 28, 35
　　眼窩部　7
　　三角部　7
　　弁蓋部　7
下前頭溝　6
下双子筋　282, 293, 361, 365-368
鵞足　379
下側頭回　7, 28, 29, 37, 61, 65, 66, 68
下側頭溝　6
下腿　355
下大静脈　159, 190, 216, 217, 222, 223, 230, 231, 239, 241, 246, 244, 245, 249-253, 257, 262, 286, 288, 296, 300
肩（かた）関節→肩（けん）関節
下腸間膜静脈　230, 246
下腸間膜動脈　230, 239, 240, 243
下直筋　29, 33, 34, 97
下椎切痕　139, 151, 157
滑車神経（CN IV）　44, 46, 53
下殿動脈　273
下頭斜筋　76-78, 104-106, 131, 135, 136
下頭頂小葉　7
　　縁上回　7
　　角回　7
下鼻甲介　25, 31, 33-35, 77, 96-98
下鼻道　96, 97
下腹部　228

下方関節唇　314
ガレン大静脈　13
下肋骨窩　139
肝円索　246
肝円索裂　250, 251, 254, 261
眼窩回　22, 35
眼窩下管　96
眼窩下孔　2
感覚失語　7
眼窩骨折　96
眼窩脂肪体　73, 75
眼窩上孔　2
眼窩部　7
眼窩吹き抜け骨折　73
肝管　257
眼球　22, 29, 91, 92, 96
肝区域　246-248
寛骨臼　358
寛骨臼蓋　368
環指　340
環軸関節　129, 130
冠状縫合　2, 3
肝静脈　239, 241
冠静脈洞　217
関節窩《肩》　172-175, 310
関節下結節　311
関節唇　313, 316, 317
関節突起　2
関節突起間関節　128, 130
肝臓　217, 229-232, 238, 242-245, 249, 254-264
　　横断面　232
環椎後頭関節　124, 125, 129, 130
環椎十字靱帯　131
冠動脈　208-210
眼動脈　12, 16
冠動脈洞（Valsalva 洞）　207
カントリー線　246
上鼻甲介　98
顔面神経（CN VII）　44, 48, 55, 62, 66
　　鼓室部　112, 116
　　膝神経節　112
　　迷路部　111

● き

ギオン管　345
気管　70, 71, 87, 88, 94, 95, 103, 104, 180, 182-186, 190, 192, 195, 196, 202, 205
気管支　182
気管支異物　183
気管食道溝　87
奇静脈　76, 186, 187, 191

奇静脈弓　190
奇静脈合流部　191
基節骨
　《手》342, 351, 352
　　第2――　346, 349
　　第3――　346, 347
　　第4――　346, 349
　《足》第5――　395
キヌタ骨　109
　　体部　112, 113, 115, 116, 118
　　短脚　113
　　長脚　113, 116
　　豆状突起　119
脚間窩　46
脚間槽　23, 32, 40, 50-52, 66
嗅球　45, 63
嗅溝　22
嗅索　37, 63
弓状線維　23
嗅神経（CN I）　45
橋　23, 24, 31, 32, 39-41, 52-55, 63, 64, 66
胸郭　170-174
　　断層解剖
　　　横断像　175, 176
　　　冠状断像　177, 178
　　　矢状断像　179
頬筋　78-81, 91, 98
胸筋部　308
胸骨　170, 229
頬骨　76, 77, 89-91
頬骨弓　2-4, 75, 76, 97-100
胸骨体　171-173, 176, 177, 179
胸骨柄　171-173, 175, 177, 179
胸鎖関節　172, 175, 178, 310
胸鎖乳突筋　78-88, 90-94, 102-105, 107, 108, 131, 132, 134, 135, 309
橋前槽　32, 63
胸椎　122, 138, 139, 170
　　第2――（T2）　175
　　第3――（T3）　175
　　第10――（T10）　176
　　断層解剖
　　　横断像（CT）　140, 141
　　　横断像（MRI）　146, 147
　　　冠状断像（CT）　142, 143
　　　冠状断像（MRI）　148
　　　矢状断像（CT）　144, 145
　　　矢状断像（MRI）　149, 150
棘突起　179
椎骨　139
椎体　178, 179
胸部の血管　182
棘下窩　311

棘下筋(腱)　175, 313, 314, 318-322
棘間靱帯　136, 137, 150, 162, 163
棘孔　4
棘上窩　311
棘上筋(腱)　175, 312, 316-322
　中心腱　312
棘上靱帯　162, 163
棘突起　123, 126-128, 130, 132, 136-143, 147, 150-153, 155, 156, 158, 159, 162, 163
距骨　394, 395, 398-400, 402-405, 410-412, 414
　後突起　395
季肋部　228
近位指節間関節(PIP関節)　340, 351
筋突起　2

● く

区域気管支　183
クイノー分類　246
空腸　236
くも膜　42, 150
くも膜下腔　146, 147, 160, 161, 163

● け

鶏冠　45
脛骨　369-372, 375, 381-383, 385-391, 394-397, 404-407, 411-415
　外側顆　375
　粗面　369, 375
　内果　398
　内側顆　375
頸最長筋　131
茎状突起　2-4
頸静脈　84
頸静脈孔　4
頸神経叢　134
頸椎　122-126
　第1——(C1)(環椎)　123-126
　　後弓　123, 125, 131
　　前弓　125, 131
　第2——(C2)(軸椎)　123-126
　　棘突起　125
　　椎体　129
　　歯突起　131
　第3——(C3)　123
　第4——(C4)　123
　第5——(C5)　123
　第6——(C6)　123
　第7——(C7)(隆椎)　123, 176
　断層解剖
　　横断像(CT)　127, 128

　　横断像(MRI)　131
　　冠状断像(CT)　129
　　冠状断像(MRI)　134, 135
　　矢状断像(CT)　130
　　矢状断像(MRI)　136, 137
頸動脈　83
頸動脈管　4
茎乳突孔　4
頸半棘筋　80
頸板状筋　79, 80, 91, 92
脛腓関節　375
頸部リンパ節のレベルシステム　107, 108
頸肋　129
結合腱　348
月状骨　342, 344, 349
結石　268, 269
楔前部　19, 20, 43
楔部　20, 43
肩関節　308-311
　断層解剖
　　横断像　312-314
　　冠状断像　315-317
　　矢状断像　318-322
肩甲下窩　310
肩甲下筋　86, 87, 175, 313-317, 320-322
肩甲挙筋　79-87, 91, 105, 106
肩甲棘　174, 311
肩甲頸　310, 311
肩甲骨　86, 170, 171, 175, 176, 178, 179, 309-314, 316, 317, 321, 322
　外側縁　174, 310, 311
　下角　310, 311
　内側縁　174, 310, 311
肩鎖関節　172, 173, 178, 179, 310
腱索　226
犬歯(糸切歯)　5
剣状突起　171-173, 176, 179
腱板疎部　314
肩峰　172-174, 310-312, 316-321

● こ

口蓋骨　4
口蓋扁桃　78, 79, 101
口蓋隆起　98
口角挙筋　80-82
後下行枝(PD)　208, 209, 211, 212
後下小脳動脈(PICA)　10, 14, 67
後弓　124, 126, 127, 130, 136, 137
後距腓靱帯　399, 406, 410, 411
咬筋　76-80, 89, 90, 97-100
後脛骨筋(腱)　383, 384, 387, 388, 393, 397-400, 403-407

後脛骨静脈　354
後脛骨動脈　353
後結節　123-128
硬口蓋　32, 94-98
後交通動脈　12, 52
後交連　32, 63
後骨間神経症候群　329
後根　133
交叉槽　63
後室間溝　208, 209
後斜角筋　92
後十字靱帯　372, 377-379, 382-384, 389, 390
後縦靱帯　163
甲状切痕　71
甲状腺　70, 86-88, 93, 94, 102, 103, 185
鉤状突起
　《頸骨》　123, 124, 128, 129, 134
　《篩骨》　96
　《尺骨》　324
甲状軟骨　70, 84-86, 94, 101-103, 108
　下角　71
　上角　71
　側板　71
後上葉枝　183
項靱帯　136, 137
後仙骨孔　164
後側壁枝(PL)　212
後大脳動脈(PCA)　9-12, 14-16, 46, 51, 52, 65
喉頭　71
後頭蓋　3, 4, 26, 125, 129
後頭回　7
喉頭蓋　71, 82, 95
喉頭蓋谷　82
後頭極　6
後頭骨　2, 4
後頭直筋　131
後頭葉　6
鉤突窩　324, 332, 333
後乳頭筋　206, 216, 220, 224
広背筋　309
後肺底枝　183
後半規管　109-112, 117-120
硬膜　19, 28, 31, 42, 43, 150
硬膜外脂肪　150, 158, 162, 163
硬膜外静脈　162
硬膜静脈洞　13
肛門挙筋　282, 293, 362
口輪筋　91
股関節　355-359
　断層解剖
　　横断像　360-362

冠状断像　363-365
矢状断像　366-368
骨間距踵靱帯　411, 412
骨間筋(腱)　347-349, 351, 352, 409-411
骨盤部
　女性　274, 275-278
　　断層解剖
　　　横断像　291-293
　　　冠状断像　294-298
　　　矢状断像　299-303
　　動脈　279
　男性　268, 269-272
　　断層解剖
　　　横断像　280-283
　　　冠状断像　284-287
　　　矢状断像　288-290
　　動脈　273
骨癒合　357
鼓膜被蓋　116
固有肝静脈　255
固有肝動脈　230, 240, 242, 243, 251

●さ

最外包　22
載距突起　395
最長筋　146, 147, 159
臍部　228
鎖骨　85-93, 100-105, 170, 171, 173, 175, 178, 179, 308-312, 315-317, 320-322
坐骨　268, 283, 356-358, 362, 365, 367, 368
坐骨海綿体筋　365
鎖骨下窩　308
鎖骨下静脈　307
鎖骨下動脈　88, 104, 182, 185, 190, 306
鎖骨胸筋三角　308, 309
坐骨棘　269
坐骨結節　269, 356
坐骨神経　368
坐骨直腸窩　282, 293
坐骨動脈　353
左心耳　213
左心室　182, 187-189, 193, 194, 206, 207, 215-217, 219-226
　短軸像　206
　長軸像　206
左心房　182-184, 187, 189, 190, 192, 206, 207, 213-215, 218, 219, 223-226
三角筋　312-322
　肩甲棘部　309

肩峰部　309
鎖骨部　309
三角筋部　308
三角骨　342, 349
三角靱帯　398-400, 404, 405
三角線維軟骨複合体　349
三角部　7
三腔断像　207
三叉神経(CN V)　24, 44, 47, 54, 66
三尖弁　215, 221, 226
三半規管　55, 56, 109

●し

視覚野　7
耳下腺　40, 41, 70, 78-81, 89, 102-104
耳管　117
耳管開口部　77
耳管隆起　77
四腔断像　207
子宮　274-279, 291, 292, 295, 297, 298
子宮筋層　291, 292, 295, 296, 300, 301
子宮頸部　291, 292, 300-302
四丘体槽　22, 23, 32, 42, 50
子宮体部　300, 302
子宮動脈　279
子宮内膜　291, 292, 295, 296, 300, 301
指屈筋(腱)　346
視交叉　23, 32, 37, 38, 45, 51, 63-65
篩骨洞　70, 71, 73-75, 94-98
篩骨蜂巣　24
視索　31, 38, 39, 45, 50, 65
示指　340
示指伸筋　343, 344
視床　18, 21, 22, 30, 31, 39-41
矢状　144
視床灰白隆起動脈(TTA)　16
視床下部　50
視床間橋　17, 22, 32
耳小骨　109
視床膝状体動脈(TGA)　16
視床穿通動脈(TPA)　16
視床部　8
矢状縫合　3
指伸筋(腱)　341, 347, 348, 351, 352
視神経(CN II)　18, 23, 34-37, 44, 45, 51, 73, 97
歯槽突起　78
膝蓋下脂肪体　378, 379, 388-390
膝蓋骨　369-372, 375-377, 381, 388-390

膝蓋靱帯　370-372, 379, 388, 389
膝窩筋(腱)　380, 382-384, 387, 389, 390
膝窩動脈　353
膝窩動脈捕捉症候群　388
室間孔　17, 21, 32
膝関節　355, 369-372, 375
　断層解剖
　　横断像　376-380
　　冠状断像　381-385
　　矢状断像　386-392
室頂　17
歯突起　124-127, 129, 130, 134, 136, 137
尺側手根屈筋　328, 329, 333-336, 343, 344, 350
尺側手根伸筋(腱)　323, 334, 343-345
尺側皮静脈　307
斜台　25, 63, 64, 75, 76
尺骨　324, 328, 329, 334, 337, 342-344, 349
尺骨神経　326, 327
尺骨頭　340
尺骨動脈　306
縦隔
　断層解剖
　　横断像　185-187
　　冠状断像　188-190
　　矢状断像　191-194
十字靱帯　384
舟状骨
　《足》　394, 395, 400-402, 411-415
　《手》　342, 344, 349-352
縦舌筋　97, 98
十二指腸　235-237, 242, 243, 255, 256, 261
　下行脚　251, 252
　水平脚　252, 253
終板　63
終板槽　63
手関節・手　340-342
　断層解剖
　　横断像　343-346
　　横断像(第3指)　347, 348
　　冠状断像　349, 350
　　冠状断像(第3指)　351, 352
手関節屈筋群　331
手関節伸筋群　331
主気管支　183, 186, 196, 200-203, 205
手根管　345
上咽頭　78
上縁　310
小円筋　314, 320-322

消化管　235, 236
　　冠状断面　238
　　バリエーション　237
上角　311
上顎洞　5, 24-26, 28-30, 33-36, 70, 71, 76, 77, 92, 93, 96, 97
上顎洞自然口　96
松果体　32, 41, 63, 67
上-下葉枝　183
上眼窩裂　2, 98
上眼瞼挙筋　29, 33, 34
小鉗子　20, 21
上眼静脈　97, 98
上関節突起　123, 128, 130, 136, 139, 141, 142, 144-146, 149, 151-153, 155, 156, 158, 159, 162
上関節面　125, 126
上丘　22, 41, 63, 67
小胸筋　175
小結節　310, 311
小結節稜　310
上行結腸　235-237, 238, 244, 252, 253, 255, 257, 260
上項線　3
上行大動脈　182, 186, 187, 189, 192, 205, 207, 213, 214, 218, 219, 221, 222, 226
上後腸骨棘　269
小後頭直筋　91-93
上鼓室　115
踵骨　394, 395, 400, 401, 404-408, 410-413
踵骨腱（アキレス腱）　393, 394, 396-400, 408, 411-413
踵骨突起　395
踵骨隆起内側突起　395
小趾（第5趾）　393
小指　340
小指外転筋　345, 346, 350
小趾外転筋　402-407, 410
小指球　340
上矢状静脈洞　13, 40-43
小指伸筋（腱）　345
硝子体　74, 91
小指対立筋（腱）　345, 346, 350
上肢の静脈　307
上肢の動脈　306
上斜筋　33, 34, 96
上小脳脚　24, 32, 53, 54, 63
上小脳動脈（SCA）　12, 14, 65
小腎杯　268, 269, 286
上舌枝　183
上前腸骨棘　268, 269, 358
上前頭回　7, 19-21
上前頭溝　6

上殿動脈　273
上双子筋　360, 361
掌側骨間筋　346
上側頭回　7, 27, 37, 41, 42, 61
上側頭溝　6
上大静脈　186, 187, 189, 191, 205, 213, 218, 222
小腸　229, 235, 237, 254, 360
上腸間膜静脈　230, 231, 233, 234, 238, 239, 241, 244, 251, 252, 255, 256, 262
上腸間膜動脈　230, 231, 238-240, 242, 243, 251, 252, 255, 256, 263, 295
上腸間膜動脈症候群　251
上直筋　29, 33-35, 72, 96, 97
上椎切痕　139, 151, 157
小殿筋　280-282, 285-287, 291, 292, 296, 297, 360, 361, 363-368
小転子　356, 357, 359, 367
上頭頂小葉　7
小内転筋　365
小脳　6, 23-26, 28-32
小脳脚　8, 66, 67
小脳前葉虫部　22, 42, 50-52
小脳第一裂　32, 64
小脳虫部　24, 43, 51-53, 56, 57, 68
小脳テント　28, 31, 32, 42, 61-64, 66-68
小脳半球　53-59, 61-64
小脳扁桃　26, 55-58, 62-64, 67, 68
紙様板　73, 96
上半規管　109-111, 116, 118-120
上半規管裂隙症候群　119
上腹部の血管系　239
上腹部の静脈　241, 244, 245
上腹部の動脈　240, 242, 243
小葉間裂（水平裂）　180, 181, 195, 197-201
小菱形筋　84-88
小菱形骨　342, 345, 349, 351
上肋骨窩　139
上腕筋　309, 323, 325-332, 335-338
上腕骨　310, 311, 313-320, 324-328, 331, 332, 336, 337
　　外側上顆　324, 326
　　内側上顆　324, 326, 331-333, 338
上腕骨滑車　324, 331, 338
上腕骨小頭　324, 331-333, 335-337
上腕骨頭　175, 310, 311
上腕三頭筋（腱）　309, 314, 317-320, 323, 325, 327, 332-338
上腕三頭筋腱膜　323
上腕静脈　307
上腕動脈　306

上腕二頭筋（腱）　309, 315-317, 319, 320, 323, 325-328, 330-332, 335-337
食道　71, 87, 88, 185-187, 192, 200, 216, 217, 237, 249, 263
食道奇静脈陥凹　200
ショパール関節　395
シルビウス裂　6, 22, 27, 28, 38, 39, 40, 50, 65
腎盂　268, 269, 271, 272, 286, 287
腎盂尿管移行部　252
心窩部　228
神経根　133, 161, 162, 167, 168
心交差　209
深指屈筋（腱）　323, 328, 329, 331-334, 336-339, 341, 343-348, 350-352
心室中隔　187, 206, 207, 215, 216, 220, 222, 224-226
人字縫合（ラムダ縫合）　2, 3
真珠腫，弛緩部型（上鼓室型）　115, 116
腎静脈　230, 239, 241, 244, 251, 256, 257, 263, 264
腎髄質　258
腎錐体　286, 287, 296-298
心切痕　180
心臓　205-207
腎臓　230, 231, 234, 241-245, 250-253, 257-261, 264, 265
　　横断面　234
　　断層解剖　横断像　213-217
心臓
　　断層解剖
　　　　冠状断像　221-223
　　　　左心室短軸像　224, 225
　　　　左心室長軸像　225
　　　　三腔断像　226
　　　　四腔断像　226
　　　　矢状断像　218-220
深大腿動脈　273, 279, 283, 293, 353
腎静脈　230, 231, 234, 239, 241-245, 250-252, 256-261, 263, 264
腎動脈　230, 231, 234, 239, 240, 242, 243, 251, 257, 258, 261-264
腎杯　258, 259
腎皮質　258, 268-272, 277, 278, 285-287, 296

● す

髄核　158, 163
髄核内裂　163
膵管　256, 257
膵鉤部　252

水晶体　23, 29, 74, 91
膵臓　231, 238, 244, 245, 250, 251, 262-265
　横断面　233
膵体部　230, 242, 243, 251, 255
膵胆管合流部　257
膵頭部　230, 242, 243, 251, 252, 255, 256, 262
膵尾部　256
髄膜　42
頭蓋骨　2, 3
頭蓋底　4
頭蓋縫合早期癒合症　2

● せ

正円窓　116
声帯　85
正中環軸関節　124, 125, 127, 130
正中口蓋縫合　4
正中仙骨稜　164, 165, 167
精嚢　269, 272, 280, 281, 287-290
声門　85
声門下腔　86
脊髄　26, 32, 41, 60, 64, 131-133, 135-137, 146-148
脊髄円錐　150, 163
脊柱　122
脊柱管　130, 144, 154, 156
脊柱起立筋　253, 288-290, 299, 300, 302, 303
脊椎　128
セゴン骨折　382
舌　79-81
舌咽神経(CN IX)　44, 48, 56, 57, 67
舌下神経(CN XII)　44, 49, 60
舌骨　70, 71, 83, 94, 95, 100, 101
舌骨下筋群　83, 84
舌骨舌筋　100
切歯窩　4
舌中隔　79, 80, 98-100
舌動脈　97
線維輪　158, 163
前下小脳動脈(AICA)　9, 10, 12, 14
前弓　123, 124, 126, 127, 130, 136, 137
前鋸筋　309, 312, 313, 315
仙棘靱帯　281
前距腓靱帯　399
前脛骨筋(腱)　355, 369-372, 380-382, 386, 387, 393, 396-401, 413-415
前脛骨静脈　354
前脛骨動脈　353
前結節　123-128

前交通動脈(Acom)　12
前交連　22, 32, 85
前鼓室陥凹　113
仙骨　122, 154, 155, 160, 161, 164, 165, 167, 356-358, 360
　岬角　164, 166
　上関節突起　164
仙骨角　164
仙骨管　165, 166
前骨間神経症候群　328
前骨間動脈　306
仙骨孔　165, 168
仙骨尖　164
仙骨翼　164, 165, 167, 168
仙骨裂孔　164
前根　133
浅指屈筋(腱)　328, 329, 331-333, 337-339, 341, 343-347, 350-352
前室間溝　208, 209
前斜角筋　108, 134, 135
前十字靱帯　372, 377, 378, 383, 384, 389
前縦靱帯　162, 163
前障　21, 22, 37
前上行枝　6
線条体　18, 21
　被殻　21
　尾状核　21
前上葉枝　183
前水平枝　6
前正中裂　26, 56-59
前仙骨孔　164
浅大腿動脈　273, 279, 283, 293, 353
前大脳動脈(ACA)　9-12, 14-16, 50, 51, 65, 72
仙腸関節　154, 155, 160, 161, 164, 165, 167, 168, 268
仙椎　122, 164
　断層解剖
　　横断像(CT)　165
　　横断像(MRI)　167
　　冠状断像(CT)　165
　　冠状断像(MRI)　168
　　矢状断像(CT)　166
仙椎椎体　162, 163, 166, 167
穿通枝　16
前庭　109, 111, 112, 116, 119, 120
前庭水管　111, 112
前頭極　6, 21
前頭極枝　10
前頭骨　2, 3
前頭前野　7
前頭洞　21, 29-33, 70-72, 93-96
前頭縫合　3
前頭葉　6

前乳頭筋　206, 215, 220, 222, 224, 226,
前肺底枝　183
前脈絡叢動脈(AChA)　12, 14-16
前立腺　269, 272, 273, 281, 282, 286-290
前立腺肥大症　272
前腕正中皮静脈　307, 323

● そ

総肝管　257
総肝静脈　255
総肝動脈　230, 232, 240, 242, 243, 251, 256, 262
総頚動脈　81-88, 103, 107, 108, 134, 136, 182, 185, 189
総指伸筋　323, 328, 329, 332, 333, 343-346
総大腿動脈　353
総胆管　257, 261
総腸骨静脈　354
総腸骨動脈　257, 273, 279, 285, 353
総鼻道　96, 97
僧帽筋　81-87, 89-93, 106-108, 131, 132, 136, 146, 147, 175, 309, 312, 315-317
僧帽弁　86, 219, 223
　後尖　215, 225, 226
　前尖　215, 225, 226
足関節・足　355, 393-395
　断層解剖
　　横断像　396-401
　　冠状断像　402-408
　　矢状断像　409-415
足根管症候群　398
側切歯　5
足底筋　377-379
足底筋膜炎　407
足底腱膜　407, 408
足底方形筋　401-407, 411-413
側頭極　6, 35, 36
側頭筋　72-77, 90, 91, 97, 99
側頭骨　2, 3
　断層解剖
　　横断像　110
　　冠状断像　115-117
　　矢状断像　118-120
側頭葉　6
側頭連合野　7
側脳室　22, 30-32
　後角　17, 61
　下角　17, 39, 61, 65-67
　前角　17, 36
　体部　17

足背　393
側腹部　228
鼠径部　228

● た

第一頸神経　44
第1趾(母趾)　393
第2〜4趾　393
第5趾(小趾)　393
第一小臼歯　5
第1対角枝(D1)　208, 209, 211-213, 219, 220, 224
第1中隔枝　211
第1背側骨間筋　345
大円筋　175, 317, 320-322
大鉗子　20, 21
大胸筋　175, 314, 320-322
　胸骨部　309
　鎖骨部　309
大結節　310, 311
大結節稜　310
大後頭孔(大孔)　4, 26
大後頭直筋　91-93, 105, 106
第三大臼歯(親しらず)　5
第三脳室　17, 22, 32, 40, 50, 64-66
第3腓骨筋　400, 401
帯状回　18-20, 32, 36-42
帯状溝　31, 32, 37
　縁部　19, 31
帯状束　20
大腎杯　268, 287
体性感覚野　7, 8
大槽　26, 32, 42, 58, 59, 63
大腿　355
大腿筋膜張筋　280-285, 291-295, 355, 361, 362
大腿骨　283, 356-359, 362, 365, 366, 372, 375-377, 381, 382, 387, 388, 390-392
　外側顆　375, 383, 384
　外側上顆　375
　内側顆　375, 383, 384
　内側上顆　375
大腿骨頭　356-361, 363-368
大腿骨頭壊死, 特発性　363
大腿四頭筋(腱)　370-372, 388-390
大腿静脈　282-284, 293, 294, 354, 362
大腿直筋　281-285, 292-294, 355, 361, 362, 366-368
大腿動脈　282-284, 293, 294, 362
大腿動脈穿刺　273
大腿二頭筋(腱)　356, 370, 371, 376-379, 383-388

大大脳静脈　13
大腿方形筋　362, 365-367
大腸　229, 235, 237
大殿筋　160, 161, 280-283, 287, 288, 290-293, 297-299, 302, 303, 356, 360-362, 365-368
大転子　356-359, 361, 364-366
大動脈　146, 147, 159, 241, 263
大動脈弓　186, 189, 190, 192, 205
大動脈洞　189
大動脈弁　187, 189, 192, 215, 219, 222, 226
大内転筋　283, 286-288, 290, 299, 302, 356, 365-368
第二小臼歯　5
大脳外側窩槽　22, 29
大脳鎌　19, 20, 42, 43
大脳脚　8, 22, 23, 40, 50-52, 63, 64, 66
大脳の表面解剖　6, 7
大伏在静脈　354, 370
大葉間裂(斜裂)　180, 181, 195
　左──　196-200, 203, 204
　右──　196-201
大腰筋　158-161, 257-261, 264, 265, 285-287, 290, 296-299, 302, 303
第四脳室　17, 24, 32, 42, 52-55, 63, 64, 67
第四脳室外側口　53
大菱形骨　342, 345, 349
唾液腺　70
多裂筋　106, 146, 147, 159
短趾屈筋　402-407
短趾伸筋　402-404, 409
短小趾屈筋　409, 410
淡蒼球　22, 31, 38
短橈側手根伸筋(腱)　343-345
短内転筋　283, 295, 296, 299, 303, 363-365, 367, 368
胆嚢　230, 231, 233, 238, 242, 245, 251, 255, 257, 260
　横断面　233
胆嚢管　257
短腓骨筋(腱)　384, 394, 396-401, 407, 409
短母指外転筋　345, 351
短母趾屈筋　413-415
短母指屈筋　350
短母趾伸筋　402
短母指伸筋　344

● ち

恥骨　268, 269, 272, 286, 287, 356-358, 362-364

恥骨下枝　283, 358
恥骨筋　281-283, 285, 293-295, 300, 302, 355, 362-364
恥骨結合　268
恥骨結節　356, 358
恥骨上枝　358
腟　274, 275, 278, 292, 293, 296, 300, 301
中咽頭　78-83
肘窩　323
中間気管支幹　183
中間楔状骨　394, 395, 400-402, 411, 412
中間広筋　283, 286, 362-366
中肝静脈　244-246, 249, 250, 255, 256, 261
肘関節　323, 324
　断層解剖
　　横断像　325-329
　　冠状断像　330-334
　　矢状断像　335-339
中間仙骨稜　164, 165
中間肺動脈幹　184
肘筋　323, 326-329, 334-336
中指　340
中斜角筋　92
中手骨　342, 351, 352
　第1──　345, 346, 350
　第2──　345, 346, 349
　第3──　345, 346
　第4──　345, 346, 349
　第5──　345, 394, 395, 402, 403, 409, 410
中手指節関節(MCP関節)　351
中小脳脚　24, 31, 41, 54, 55, 63
中心管　32
中心溝　6, 19-21
中心後回　7, 8, 19, 20
中心後溝　6
中心前回　7, 8, 19, 20
中心前溝　6
中心傍小葉　19
虫垂　253
肘正中皮静脈　307, 323
中節骨《手》　342, 351, 352
　第2──　347, 349
　第3──　347-349
　第4──　349
　第5──　346
中切歯　5
中前頭回　7, 19, 20
中足骨
　第1──　394, 395, 413-415
　第2──　394
　第3──　394, 411

第4—— 394, 410
第5—— 395
中足趾節関節(MTP 関節) 407
中側頭回 27-29, 37, 41, 42, 61
中大脳動脈(MCA) 9, 10, 12, 14-16, 50, 51, 65, 72
中殿筋 280-282, 285-287, 291-293, 295-298, 356, 360, 361, 363-368
肘頭 323, 324, 326, 327, 333, 336, 337, 338
肘頭窩 324
中脳 31, 41
中脳水道 17, 23, 32, 41, 51, 52, 64, 67
中脳被蓋 23, 32, 64
中鼻甲介 24, 25, 31, 33-36, 76, 96-98
中鼻道 96, 97
肘部管症候群 327
虫部小節 42, 64
虫部垂 64, 67, 68
虫部錐体 64
虫部葉 64
聴覚野 7
蝶形骨 2
蝶形骨洞 23, 24, 31, 32, 36-38, 71, 74, 75, 93-95, 99, 100
鳥距溝 42, 43
腸脛靱帯 376-379, 381, 382
腸脛靱帯症候群 378
腸骨 154, 155, 160, 161, 165, 167, 168, 268, 356-358, 360, 361, 363-368
腸骨筋 160, 285-287, 296, 297, 363, 364
腸骨稜 269, 356
蝶篩陥凹 74
長趾屈筋(腱) 393, 396-400, 407, 412-415
長趾伸筋(腱) 355, 381-383, 393, 394, 396-401, 403-405, 409, 410
長掌筋 328, 329, 331-333
長足底靱帯 404
長橈側手根伸筋(腱) 328, 335, 338, 339, 343-345
長内転筋 283, 285, 294, 355
長腓骨筋(腱) 370, 380, 382-384, 394, 396-401, 405, 406, 409, 410
長母指外転筋(腱) 343, 344
長母趾屈筋(腱) 384, 385, 393, 396-400, 407, 410-412
長母指屈筋(腱) 341, 343, 344, 346, 350
長母指伸筋 343

長母趾伸筋(腱) 393, 396-398
跳躍靱帯(ばね靱帯) 401
腸腰筋 280-285, 291-295, 360-364, 366-368
蝶鱗縫合 4
腸肋筋 159
直回 22, 35, 64
直静脈洞 13, 43
直腸 235-238, 360, 361, 365

● つ

椎間関節 123, 128, 130, 136, 141, 142, 144-146, 149, 153, 155, 156, 158, 159, 162
椎間孔 124, 128-130, 132, 138, 140-142, 144, 145, 148, 149, 151, 153, 157, 158, 162
椎間板 128-130, 134, 136, 137, 142, 144-146, 148-150, 153, 154, 156-158, 160-163
椎間板ヘルニア 163
椎弓 127, 128, 139, 147, 152
椎弓根 130, 139, 140, 142, 147-149, 151-154, 157, 159-162
椎弓切除術 147
椎弓板 123, 126, 132, 139, 140-142, 144, 146, 147, 152, 153, 158, 159
椎孔 127, 128, 139, 140, 152, 153, 158, 159
椎骨 135
椎骨動脈(VA) 9, 12, 16, 26, 56-60, 64, 66, 67, 74-87, 131-134
椎骨脳底動脈(VA-BA) 14
椎前筋 131, 132, 134, 136
 頸長筋 79-82, 84-87
 頭長筋 76-78
椎体 123, 124, 127, 128, 130, 133, 134, 136-142, 144-162
使いすぎ症候群 332
ツチ骨 109
 頸部 118
 頭部 112, 113, 115, 118
 柄 113, 114, 116, 118, 119

● て

底側踵舟靱帯 403
テニス肘 332, 333
デュピュイトラン拘縮 346
テンソル解析 8

● と

島 22

洞 29
ドゥ・ケルヴァン病 343
島回 28
動眼神経(CN III) 44, 46, 52
頭頸部 70, 71
 断層解剖
  横断像 72-88
  冠状断像 96-106
  矢状断像 89-95
橈骨 324, 329, 331-337, 342-344, 349, 351, 352
橈骨窩 324
橈骨頸 324
橈側手根伸筋 323
橈骨粗面 324
橈骨頭 324, 328
橈骨動脈 306
頭最長筋 76, 77
頭斜筋 92, 93
豆状骨 342, 350
橈側手根屈筋(腱) 345
橈側手根伸筋 325-331, 333, 335
橈側皮静脈 307, 323
頭頂間溝 6
頭長筋 101
頭頂孔 3
頭頂後頭溝 6, 19, 20, 31, 32
頭頂骨 2, 3
頭頂葉 6
頭頂連合野 7
頭半棘筋 73-80, 90, 91, 93-95, 106, 131, 132
頭板状筋 76-80, 90-92, 105, 106, 131, 132, 136
島皮質 37-40
動脈円錐 192, 193, 213, 219, 221, 222
透明中隔 21, 37-39
島輪状溝 22
鈍縁枝(OM) 212

● な

内果 393-395
内頸静脈 76-88, 91, 92, 102, 103, 107, 108, 131-133, 185
内頸動脈(ICA) 9, 10, 12, 16, 51-55, 73, 75-80, 131-133
 サイフォン部 65
内耳神経(CN VIII) 44, 48, 55, 62, 66
内耳道 61, 109, 111, 112, 115, 116, 120
内側および外側顆間結節 375
内側顆《脛骨》 375

《大腿骨》　375, 383, 384
内側顆上稜　324
内側眼窩回　22
内側楔状骨　394, 395, 401, 402,
　　413-415
内側広筋　355, 369-372, 376, 381,
　　382, 384, 385, 390-392
内側後頭側頭回　30, 42, 43, 65, 66,
　　68
内側後脈絡動脈(MPChA)　10, 16
内側上顆
　　《上腕骨》　324, 326, 331-333, 338
　　《大腿骨》　375
内側線条体動脈(MSA)　16
内側側副靱帯
　　《膝関節》　371, 372, 382
内側中葉枝　183
内側直筋　23, 30, 33, 34, 73, 74, 96,
　　97
内側肺底枝　183
内側毛帯　63
内側翼突筋　78, 91, 92, 100, 101
内腸骨動脈　273, 279, 280, 287, 296,
　　353
内腸骨静脈　354
内腹斜筋　253, 360
内閉鎖筋　280-282, 286-288, 290-
　　293, 296-299, 302, 303, 360-362,
　　364, 365
内包　21, 30, 37, 38
内包前脚　22
ナッツクラッカー症候群　251
軟口蓋　37, 38, 94, 95, 99, 100
軟膜　42, 150

● に

乳頭筋　189
乳頭体　32, 50, 51, 63, 64
乳頭突起　152
乳突洞　112
乳突蜂巣　24, 25, 73-75, 89, 102-
　　104, 110
乳様突起　2-4, 26, 76, 77, 89, 103,
　　104
尿管　230, 231, 257, 268, 269-272,
　　280, 286, 290
尿道　293
尿道海綿体　284, 285

● の

脳
　　断層解剖
　　　　横断像　19-26

　　　　冠状断像　33-43
　　　　矢状断像　27-32
脳回　6, 7
脳幹部
　　断層解剖
　　　　横断像　50-60
　　　　冠状断像　65-68
　　　　矢状断像　61-64
脳弓　32, 38, 39
脳弓柱　22
脳溝　6
脳室　17, 54
脳静脈　13
脳神経　44
　　断層解剖
　　　　横断像　45-49
　　分類　44
脳脊髄液　17, 131, 133, 135-137,
　　150, 162
脳底動脈(BA)　9, 10, 12, 16, 23, 24,
　　52-56, 64-66, 72, 73
脳動脈　9-11
脳動脈支配領域　14, 15
脳動脈瘤　12
脳葉　6
脳梁　8, 20, 31, 32, 41
　　膝　21, 31, 32, 36
　　体部　36-40
脳梁膨大　21, 32

● は

肺
　　断層解剖
　　　　横断像　195-197
　　　　冠状断像　198-200
　　　　矢状断像　201-204
肺区域　180, 181
肺尖後枝　183
肺尖枝　183
肺静脈　183, 184, 186, 187, 192, 193,
　　205, 207, 213-215, 219, 223
背側骨間筋　346
肺動脈　182-184, 186, 189-193,
　　201-203, 211
肺動脈幹　182-184, 186, 188, 189,
　　192, 193, 213
肺動脈弁　187, 192, 213, 219, 221
灰白質　61
薄筋　355, 356, 364, 365, 370
白質　61
白線　253, 280, 284
薄束結節　58
ばね靱帯(跳躍靱帯)　401
馬尾　161

馬尾神経　158, 159, 163
パペッツの回路　18
ハムストリング　362, 366, 370
バルサルバ洞　189, 207, 214
破裂孔　4
半球間槽　34
半月板　373, 374
　　外側——　371, 372, 374, 382 384,
　　387, 388
　　内側——　371, 372, 374, 382-384,
　　390, 391
半腱様筋　370, 376
伴行静脈　88
ハンフリー靱帯　373
半膜様筋　356, 368, 370, 376, 377,
　　389-392
半卵円中心　20

● ひ

鼻咽頭　25, 26, 37, 71, 76-78, 95
被殻　21, 22, 29, 30, 37, 38
皮下脂肪　136, 137
鼻腔　70, 71, 75-77, 96
腓骨　372, 380, 384, 386, 394-397,
　　406, 407, 409, 410
尾骨　122, 162-166, 356-358, 360,
　　361
鼻骨　2, 3, 75
腓骨外果　398-400
腓骨頸　375
腓骨静脈　354
腓骨体　375
腓骨頭　375
腓骨動脈　353
膝(ひざ)関節→膝(しつ)関節
肘(ひじ)関節→肘(ちゅう)関節
皮質　6, 23, 24
脾腫　232
尾状核　18, 21, 22, 30, 31, 37, 38
脾静脈　230, 231, 239, 241, 244, 245,
　　246, 250, 251, 255-257, 263-265
脾臓　230, 231, 232, 241-243, 245,
　　250, 251, 257-259, 265, 266
　　横断面　232
左下肺静脈　183, 184, 187, 193, 205,
　　213, 214, 215, 219, 223
左下葉動脈　190
左肝静脈　244, 245, 246, 249, 255,
　　262
左冠動脈　211, 212
左冠動脈回旋枝(LCX)　205, 208,
　　209, 214-217, 219, 220, 222, 223,
　　225, 226
　　遠位部　212

近位部　212
後下行枝　212
後側壁枝　212
鈍縁枝　212
左冠動脈主幹部（LMT）　208, 209, 211-213, 219, 222
左冠動脈前下行枝（LAD）　205, 208, 209, 213-217, 219-222, 224-226
　遠位部　211, 212
　近位部　211, 212
　中間部　211, 212
左冠動脈洞　214, 219, 222
左季肋部　228
左上肺静脈　183, 184, 186, 205, 213
左側腹部　228
左腸骨部　228
鼻中隔　25, 33, 75-77, 96-98
尾椎　122
脾動脈　230, 232, 240, 242, 243, 250, 256, 257, 263-265
腓腹筋　355, 369-372, 376-380, 383-391
　外側頭　370
　内側頭　370
ヒラメ筋　355, 371, 372, 380, 384, 385, 387-390, 393, 394, 411-413
ヒラメ静脈　354
披裂軟骨　85

● ふ

フォルクマン拘縮　325
腹横筋　253
腹腔動脈　230-232, 234, 239, 240, 242, 243, 250, 251, 255-257, 363
副腎　230, 231, 234, 250, 251, 258, 259
　横断面　234
副神経（CN XI）　44, 49, 57-60, 67
副腎動脈　234
腹直筋　253, 261, 264, 280-282, 284, 288-292, 299-303, 355, 360, 361, 366-368
副突起　152, 153
副鼻腔　70, 71
副鼻腔炎　36
腹部
　血管系（上腹部）　239
　静脈（上腹部）　241, 244, 245
　臓器　228, 229
　臓器（上腹部）　230, 231
　体表解剖　228
　断層解剖
　　横断像　249-253
　　冠状断像　254-259

　　矢状断像　260-266
　　動脈（上腹部）　240, 242, 243
腹部大動脈　230, 231, 239, 240, 242, 243, 249-253, 257, 273, 285, 289, 296, 301
腹部の9領域　228
副葉間裂　195
プルサック腔　115
ブローカ野　7

● へ

ベイカー嚢胞　377
米国心臓協会（AHA）分類　211, 212
閉鎖管　281, 282
閉鎖孔　268, 356-358
閉鎖稜　358
ベツォルド膿瘍　104
弁蓋部　7
片側顔面痙攣　48
扁桃体　23, 29, 38, 39, 51, 65, 66
片葉　56

● ほ

方形回内筋　343, 349, 351, 352
膀胱　268-281, 284-286, 288-290, 292-296, 299-302, 360, 363, 364
縫工筋　280-284, 292-294, 355, 360-362, 366, 367, 372, 376-380, 383-385
縫合骨　3
房室間溝　208, 209
房室結節枝　208, 209, 211
傍脊椎脂肪組織　148
放線冠　21
母趾（第1趾）　393
母指　340
母趾外転筋　401-407, 413-415
母指球　340
母指対立筋　345, 350
母趾内転筋　401, 412
母指内転筋　346
ホムンクルス　8

● ま・み

末節骨
《手》　342, 351
　第1──　346
　第3──　348
《足》　第1──　395

右下肺静脈　182-184, 205, 214, 215, 223

右下葉動脈　190
右肝静脈　244, 245, 246, 249, 250, 261
右冠動脈（RCA）　205, 208, 209, 211, 214-222, 224, 226
　遠位部　211
　近位部　211
　後下行枝　211
　中間部　211
　房室結節枝　211
右冠動脈洞　214, 218, 221, 226
右季肋部　228
右上肺静脈　182-184, 186, 187, 192, 205, 213, 214, 223
右側腹部　228
脈絡叢　21, 30, 41, 42, 62

● む・め

無冠動脈洞　215, 218, 222, 226

迷走神経　44, 48, 57, 58, 67

● も

盲腸　238
門脈　230, 239, 249, 251, 256
　右枝　244-246, 250, 256
　左枝　244-246, 249, 250, 255, 256, 261
　本幹　241, 244-246, 251, 256, 261, 262
モンロー孔（室間孔）　17, 21, 32

● ゆ

有鈎骨　342, 345, 349, 350
有頭骨　342, 345, 349, 351, 352

● よ

腰筋　253
腰椎　122, 151, 152
　第1──（L1）　151, 268
　　椎体　162, 163
　第2──（L2）　151
　第4──（L4）　123, 151, 356-358
　　棘突起　357
　第3──（L3）　151, 152
　第5──（L5）　151, 356
　　横突起　164
　　下関節突起　164
　　棘突起　357
　　椎体　164
　断層解剖

横断像(CT)　153
　　横断像(MRI)　158, 159
　　冠状断像(CT)　154, 155
　　冠状断像(MRI)　160, 161
　　矢状断像(CT)　156, 157
　　矢状断像(MRI)　162, 163
腰方形筋　159, 253
翼状突起
　　外側板　4, 77
　　内側板　4, 77

● ら

ラムダ縫合(人字縫合)　2, 3
卵円孔　4
卵円窓　116
卵巣　274-279, 291, 292, 296, 298, 299, 303

● り

梨状筋　280, 291, 360, 365

梨状筋症候群　368
リスバーグ靱帯　373
リスフラン関節　395
立方骨　394, 395, 401-403, 410-412
菱形筋　175
輪状甲状関節　71, 102
輪状軟骨　70, 85, 86, 94, 95, 102, 103
　　前弓　71
鱗状縫合　2, 3

● る

涙骨　2
涙腺　96
ルシュカ孔　53

● れ

レンズ核　22, 38
　　淡蒼球　22, 38
　　被殻　22, 38

● ろ

漏斗　63
漏斗陥凹　17
漏斗胸　176
ローゼンミューラー窩　77
ローランド溝　6
肋横突関節　140, 143, 144, 147
肋椎関節　140-142, 146, 147
肋軟骨　177
肋間筋　88
肋骨　87, 88, 140-144, 146, 147, 170, 171, 175, 176, 229, 268, 269, 310

● わ

腕橈骨筋　323, 325-332, 335-337
腕頭静脈　185, 205
腕頭動脈　182, 185, 189, 190

欧文索引

A

Abdominal aorta　230, 231, 239, 240, 242, 243, 249-253, 257, 273, 285, 289, 296, 301
Abducens nerve　44, 47, 55, 66
Abductor digiti minimi muscle
　《Foot》　402-407, 410
　《Hand》　345, 346, 350
Abductor hallucis muscle　401-407, 413-415
Abductor pollicis brevis muscle　345, 351
Abductor pollicis longus muscle (tendon)　343, 344
Accessory nerve　44, 49, 57-60, 67
Accessory process　152, 153
Accompanying vein (Companion vein)　88
Acetabular roof　368
Acetabulum　358
Achilles tendon (Calcaneal tendon)　393, 394, 396-400, 408, 411-413
Acromioclavicular joint　172, 173, 178, 179, 310
Acromion　172-174, 310-312, 316-321
Acute margin of the heart　208
Adductor brevis muscle　283, 295, 296, 299, 303, 363-365, 367, 368
Adductor hallucis muscle　401
Adductor longus muscle　283, 285, 294, 355
Adductor magnus muscle　283, 286-288, 290, 299, 302, 356, 365-368
Adductor minimus muscle　365
Adductor pollicis muscle　346
Adrenal gland　230, 231, 250, 251, 258, 259
AHA (American Heart Association) 分類　211, 212
Alveolar process　78
Alzheimer 病　39
Ambient cistern　23
Amygdala　23, 29, 38, 39, 51, 65, 66
Anatomical neck　311
Anatomy　266
Anconeus muscle　323, 326-329, 334-336
Angle of mandible　2, 5, 91
Angular gyrus　7, 20

Anterior arch　123-127, 130, 131, 136, 137
Anterior ascending ramus　6
Anterior basilar segmental bronchus　183
Anterior cerebellar vermis　22, 42, 50-52
Anterior cerebral artery (ACA)　9, 10, 12, 14-16, 72
Anterior choroidal artery (AChA)　14-16
Anterior commissure　22, 32, 85
Anterior communicating artery (Acom)　12
Anterior cruciate ligament　372, 377, 378, 383, 384, 389
Anterior horizontal ramus　6
Anterior inferior cerebellar artery (AICA)　9, 10, 12, 14
Anterior inferior iliac spine　269, 358
Anterior interosseous artery　306
Anterior interosseous nerve syndrome　328
Anterior interventricular sulcus　208, 209
Anterior lobe of the pituitary gland (Adenohypophysis)　63
Anterior longitudinal ligament　162, 163
Anterior nerve root　133
Anterior papillary muscle　206, 215, 220, 222, 224, 226
Anterior sacral foramina　164
Anterior segmental bronchus　183
Anterior superior iliac spine　268, 269, 358
Anterior talofibular ligament　399
Anterior tibial artery　353
Anterior tibial veins　354
Anterior tubercle　123-128
Anulus fibrosus　158, 163
Aorta　146, 147, 159, 241, 263
Aortic arch　186, 189, 190, 192, 205
Aortic valve　187, 189, 192, 215, 219, 222, 226
Apex of the sacrum　164
Apical segmental bronchus　183
Apicoposterior segmental bronchus　183
Aponeurosis of triceps brachii muscle　323

Appendix　253
Aqueduct　17, 23, 32, 41, 51, 52, 64, 67
Arytenoid cartilage　85
Ascending aorta　182, 186, 187, 189, 192, 205, 207, 213, 214, 218, 219, 221, 222, 226
Ascending colon　235-237, 238, 244, 252, 253, 255, 257, 260
Atlanto-axial joint　129, 130
Atlanto-occipital joint　124, 125, 129, 130
Atlas (C1)　123, 124
Atrioventricular branch　208, 209, 211
Auditory area　7
Axillary artery　306
Axillary region　308
Axillary vein　307
Axis (C2)　123
Azygos　76
Azygos arch　190
Azygos vein　186, 187, 191

B

Baker 嚢胞　377
Bankart lesion　319
Basilar artery (BA)　9, 10, 12, 16, 23, 24, 52-56, 64-66, 72, 73
Basilic vein　307
Bezold 膿瘍　104
Biceps brachii muscle (tendon)　309, 315-317, 319, 320, 323, 325-328, 330-332, 335-337
Biceps femoris muscle (tendon)　370, 371, 376-379, 383-388
　Long head　356
Body of fibula　375
Body of lateral ventricle　17
Body of mandible　2, 5, 83, 84, 91-95, 97-99
Body of sternum　171-173, 176, 177, 179
Brachial artery　306
Brachial veins　307
Brachialis muscle (tendon)　309, 323, 325-332, 335-338
Brachiocephalic artery　182, 185, 189, 190
Brachiocephalic vein　185, 205
Brachioradialis muscle　323, 325-

332, 335-337
Broca's area　7
Bronchi　182
Bronchus intermedius　183
Buccinator muscle　78-81, 91, 98

● C

Caecum　238
Calcaneal tendon→Achilles tendon をみよ
Calcaneal tuberosity　395
Calcaneus　394, 395, 400, 401, 404-408, 410-413
Calcarine sulcus　42, 43
Calyx of kidney　258, 259
Cantlie 線　246
Capitate　342, 345, 349, 351, 352
Capitulum of humerus　324, 331-333, 335-337
Carotid artery　83
Carotid canal　4
Carpal tunnel　345
Cauda equina　158, 159, 161, 163
Caudate nucleus　21, 22, 30, 31, 37, 38
Celiac artery　230, 231, 239, 240, 242, 243, 250, 251, 255-257, 263
Central canal　32
Central sulcus　6, 19-21
Cephalic vein　307, 323
Cerebellar hemisphere　53-59, 61-64, 66, 67
Cerebellar peduncle　8
Cerebellar tonsil　26, 55-58, 62-64, 67, 68
Cerebellar vermis　24, 43, 51-53, 56, 57, 68
Cerebellum　6, 23-32
Cerebral peduncle　8, 22, 23, 32, 40, 50-52, 63, 64, 66
Cerebrospinal fluid　131, 133, 135-137, 150, 162
Cervical nerve　44
Cervical plexus　134
Cervical vertebrae　122
　　C1(Atlas)　123, 124
　　C2(Axis)　123
　　C3〜C6　123
　　C7(Vertebra prominens)　123
Chiasmatic cistern　63
Chin　4
Chopart 関節　395
Choroid plexus　21, 30, 41, 42, 62
Cingulate gyrus　18-20, 32, 36-42

Cingulate sulcus　31, 32, 37
Cingulum　20
Circular sulcus of insula　22
Cistern of lateral cerebral fossa　22, 29
Cisterna lamina terminalis　63
Cisterna magna　26, 32, 42, 58, 59, 63
Claustrum　21, 22, 37
Clavicle　85-93, 100-105, 170, 171, 173, 175, 178, 179, 308-312, 315-317, 320-322
Clavipectoral triangle　308, 309
Clivus　25, 63, 64, 75, 76
Coccygeal vertebrae　122
Coccyx　122, 162-165, 356-358, 360, 361
Cochlea　66, 109, 112, 113, 115, 116, 120
Common bile duct　257, 261
Common carotid artery　81-88, 103, 107, 108, 134, 136, 182, 185, 189
Common femoral artery　353
Common hepatic artery　230, 240, 242, 243, 251, 256, 262
Common hepatic vein　255
Common iliac artery　257, 273, 279, 285, 353
Common iliac vein　354
Common liver duct　257
Common nasal meatus　96, 97
Concha bullosa　97
Condylar process　2, 4, 5
Conjoint tendon　348
Conus arteriosus　192, 193, 213, 219, 221, 222
Conus medullaris of spinal cord　150, 163
Coracoacromial arch　320
Coracobrachialis muscle　314, 315, 317, 320, 321
Coracoid process　172-175, 310, 311, 313, 315, 320, 321
Corona radiata　21
Coronal suture　2, 3
Coronary sinus　217
Coronoid fossa　324, 332, 333
Coronoid process《Mandible》　2, 5　　　　《Ulna》324
Corpus callosum　8, 20, 31, 32, 41
　　Body　36-40
　　Genu　21, 31, 32, 36
　　Splenium　21, 32
Corpus cavernosum(penis)　283-

285, 362-364
Corpus cavernosum urethrae　284, 285
Cortex　6, 24
Costal cartilage　177
Costotransverse joint　140, 143, 144, 147
Costovertebral joint　140-142, 146, 147
Couinaud 分類　246
Crest of greater tubercle(Lateral lip)　310
Crest of lesser tubercle(Medial lip)　310
Cricoid cartilage　70, 85, 86, 94, 95, 102, 103
　　Anterior ring　71
Cricothyroid joint　71, 102
Crista galli　45
Cruciate ligament　384
Cruciate ligament of atlas　131
Crus of diaphragm　250, 258, 261, 262
Crux of heart　209
Cubital fossa　323
Cubital tunnel syndrome　327
Cuboid　394, 395, 401-403, 410-412
Cuneus　20, 43

● D

de Quervain 病　343
Deep femoral artery　273, 279, 283, 293, 353
Deltoid ligament　398-400, 404, 405
Deltoid muscle　312-322
　　Acromial part　309
　　Clavicular part　309
　　Spinal part　309
Deltoid region　308
Descending aorta　182, 186, 187, 190, 192, 193, 203, 205, 206, 213-219, 225, 226
Descending colon　235-238, 244, 245, 250-253, 255, 265, 266
Descending part of duodenum　251, 252
Diaphragm　194, 249, 254
Digastric muscle
　　Anterior belly　84, 93, 95, 98, 99, 100, 107
　　Posterior belly　91
DIP 関節(Distal interphalangeal joint)《Hand》340, 351

Distal phalanx《Hand》 342, 351
Dorsal interosseous muscle 346
Dorsum of foot 393
Duodenum 235-237, 242, 243, 255, 256, 261
Dupuytren 拘縮 346
Dura mater 19, 28, 31, 42

● E

Endometrium 291, 292, 295, 296, 300, 301
Epidural fat 150, 158, 162, 163
Epidural vein 162
Epigastric fossa 228
Epiglottic vallecula 82
Epiglottis 71, 82, 95
Epipharynx 78
Epitympanic recess 113
Epitympanum 115
Erector spinae muscle 253, 288-290, 299, 300, 302, 303
Esophagus 71, 87, 88, 185-187, 192, 200, 216, 217, 237, 249, 263
Ethmoidal cells 24
Ethmoidal sinus 70, 71, 73-75, 94-98
Extens 351, 352
Extensor carpi radialis 323
Extensor carpi radialis brevis muscle(tendon) 343-345
Extensor carpi radialis longus muscle(tendon) 328, 335, 338, 339, 343-345
Extensor carpi radialis muscle 325-329, 333, 335
Extensor carpi radialis(Longus and brevis)muscles 330, 331
Extensor carpi ulnaris muscle (tendon) 323, 334, 343-345
Extensor digiti minimi muscle (tendon) 345
Extensor digitorum brevis muscle 402-404, 409
Extensor digitorum longus muscle (tendon) 355, 381-383, 393, 394, 396-401, 403-405, 409, 410
Extensor digitorum muscle (tendon) 323, 328, 329, 332, 333, 341, 343-348
Extensor hallucis brevis muscle 402
Extensor hallucis longus muscle (tendon) 393, 396-398
Extensor indicis muscle 343, 344

Extensor pollicis brevis muscle 344
Extensor pollicis longus muscle 343
External acoustic opening 2
External auditory canal 25, 75, 89, 102, 114, 116, 117
External capsule 22, 37
External carotid artery 76-80
External iliac artery 273, 280, 281, 285, 286, 291, 292, 295, 296, 353, 360
External iliac vein 280, 281, 285, 286, 291, 292, 295, 296, 354, 361
External oblique(muscle) 253, 355
External occipital protuberance 2-4
Extreme capsule 22
Eyeball 22, 29, 91, 92, 96

● F

Facet joint 123, 128, 130, 136, 141, 142, 144-146, 149, 153, 155, 156, 158, 159, 162
Facial nerve 44, 48, 55, 62, 66
　Geniculate ganglion 112
　Labyrinthine segment 111
　Tympanic segment 112, 116
Falx cerebri 19, 20, 42, 43
Fastigium 17
Femoral artery 282-284, 293, 294, 362
Femoral vein 282-284, 293, 294, 354, 362
Femur 283, 356-359, 362, 365, 366, 372, 375-377, 381, 382, 387, 388, 390-392
Fibula 372, 380, 384, 386, 394-397, 406, 407, 409, 410
Fibula lateral malleolus 398-400
Fibular artery(Peroneal artery) 353
Fibular veins(Peroneal veins) 354
Fibularis brevis muscle(tendon) 384, 394, 396-401, 407, 409
Fibularis longus muscle(tendon) 370, 380, 382-384, 394, 396-401, 405, 406, 409, 410
Fibularis tertius muscle 400, 401
Fifth lumbar vertebrae(L5) 356
Fifth metacarpal 345
Fifth metatarsal 394, 395, 402, 403,

409, 410
Fifth middle phalanx 《Hand》 346
Fifth proximal phalanx 《Foot》 395
Fifth toe(Little toe) 393
First diagonal branch(D1) 208, 209, 211-213, 219, 220, 224
First distal phalanx《Foot》 395
　　　　　　　　　《Hand》 346
First dorsal interosseous muscle 345
First major septal branch 211
First metacarpal 345, 346, 350
First metatarsal 394, 395, 413-415
First proximal phalanx 《Foot》 395
First rib 87, 88
Fissura interhemisphaerica 34
Fissura prima cerebelli 32, 64
Fissure of round ligament 250, 251, 254, 261
Flexor carpi radialis brevis muscle (tendon) 345
Flexor carpi ulnaris muscle 328, 329, 333-336, 343, 344, 350
Flexor digiti minimi brevis muscle 409, 410
Flexor digitorum brevis muscle 402-407
Flexor digitorum longus muscle (tendon) 393, 396-400, 407, 412-415
Flexor digitorum muscle(tendon) 346
Flexor digitorum profundus muscle (tendon) 323, 328, 329, 331-334, 336-339, 343, 344, 346-348, 350-352
Flexor digitorum superficialis muscle(tendon) 328, 329, 331-333, 337-339, 343-347, 350-352
Flexor hallucis brevis muscle 413-415
Flexor hallucis longus muscle (tendon) 384, 385, 393, 396-400, 407, 410-412
Flexor pollicis brevis muscle 350
Flexor pollicis longus muscle (tendon) 343, 344, 346, 350
Flocculus 56
Folium of vermis 64, 67
Foramen lacerum 4
Foramen magnum 4, 26
Foramen of Luschka 53
Foramen of Monro 17, 21, 32

Foramen ovale 4
Foramen spinosum 4
Forceps minor 20, 21
Fornix 32, 38, 39
Fornix column 22
Fossa radialis 324
Fourth distal phalanx
　《Hand》 347
Fourth lumbar vertebrae(L4)
　356-358
Fourth metacarpal 345, 346, 349
Fourth metatarsal 394, 410
Fourth middle phalanx
　《Hand》 349
Fourth proximal phalanx
　《Hand》 346, 349
Fourth toe 393
Fourth ventricle 17, 24, 32, 42,
　52-55, 63, 64, 67
Frontal bone 2, 3
Frontal horn 17
Frontal lobe 6
Frontal pole 6, 21
Frontal sinus 21, 29-33, 70-72,
　93-96
Frontopolar branch 10

● G

Galen 大静脈(Great vein of Galen,
　Great cerebral vein) 13
Gallbladder 230, 231, 238, 242, 245,
　251, 255, 257, 260
Gallbladder duct 257
Gastrocnemius muscle 355, 369-
　372, 376-380, 383-391
　Lateral head 370
　Medial head 370
Gastroduodenal artery 230, 240,
　242, 243, 251, 255
Gemellus inferior muscle 282, 293,
　361, 365-368
Gemellus superior muscle 360,
　361
Genioglossus muscle 81-83, 94,
　95, 97-100
Geniohyoid muscle 82-84, 98-100
Glenoid cavity 174, 310
Glenoid labrum 313, 316, 317
Globus pallidus 22, 31, 38
Glossopharyngeal nerve 44, 48,
　56, 57, 67
Glottic space 85
Gluteus maximus muscle 160, 161,
　280-283, 287, 288, 290-293, 297-

299, 302, 303, 356, 360-362, 365-
368
Gluteus medius muscle 280-282,
　285-287, 291-293, 295-298, 356,
　360, 361, 363-368
Gluteus minimus muscle 280-282,
　285-287, 291, 292, 296, 297, 360,
　361, 363-368
Gracile tubercle 58
Gracilis muscle 355, 356, 364, 365,
　370
Great cerebral vein(Great vein of
　Galen) 13
Great saphenous vein(Long
　saphenous vein) 354, 370
Great toe 393
Greater trochanter 356-359, 361,
　364-366
Greater tubercle 310, 311
Grey matter 61
Guyon's canal 345
Gyrus 6

● H

Hamate 342, 345, 349, 350
Hamstring 362, 366
Hard palate 32, 94-98
Head of femur 356-361, 363-368
Head of fibula 375
Head of humerus 310, 311
Head of mandible 25, 27, 28, 38,
　39, 75, 89, 90, 101
Head of radius 324, 328
Hepatic duct 257
Hepatic vein 239, 241, 244, 245,
　249, 250, 255, 261, 262
Hill-Sachs lesion 319
Hippocampus 18, 23, 29, 30, 39, 40,
　51, 61, 62, 66, 67
Hippocampus tail 62
Horizontal part of duodenum 252,
　253
Humerus 310, 311, 313-320, 324-
　328, 331, 332, 336, 337
Humphry 靭帯 373
Hyoglossus muscle 100
Hyoid bone 70, 71, 83, 94, 95, 100,
　101
Hypochondrium 228
Hypoglossal nerve 44, 49, 60
Hypopharynx 83-86
Hypothalamus 50
Hypothenar eminence 340

● I・J

Ileocecum 228
Ileum 236
Iliac crest 269, 356
Iliacus muscle 160, 285-287, 296,
　297, 363, 364
Iliocostalis muscle 159
Iliopsoas muscle 280-285, 291-
　295, 360-364, 366-368
Iliotibial tract(band) 376-379,
　381, 382
Ilium 154, 155, 160, 161, 165, 167,
　168, 268, 356-358, 360, 361, 363-
　368
Incisive fossa 4
Incus 109
　Body 112, 113, 115, 116, 118
　Lenticular process 119
　Long crus 113, 116
　Short crus 113
Inferior angle 310, 311
Inferior articular process 123, 128,
　130, 136, 139, 141, 142, 144, 145,
　149, 151-153, 155, 156, 158, 159,
　162
　L5 164
Inferior cereblellar peduncle 31
Inferior costal facet 139
Inferior frontal gyrus 7, 28, 35
　Opercular part 7
　Orbital part 7
　Triangular part 7
Inferior frontal sulcus 6
Inferior glenoid labrum 314
Inferior gluteal artery 273
Inferior lingular bronchus 183
Inferior mesenteric artery 230,
　239, 240, 243
Inferior mesenteric vein 230
Inferior nasal concha 25, 31, 33-
　35, 77, 96-98
Inferior nasal meatus 96, 97
Inferior nuchal line 4
Inferior oblique muscle 96
Inferior olivary complex 41
Inferior orbital fissure 2, 98
Inferior parietal lobule 7
　Angular gyrus 7
　Supramarginal gyrus 7
Inferior pubic ramus 283, 358
Inferior rectus muscle 29, 33, 34,
　97
Inferior temporal gyrus 7, 28, 29,
　37, 61, 65, 66, 68

Inferior temporal sulcus   6
Inferior vena cava   159, 190, 216, 217, 222, 223, 230, 231, 239, 241, 244, 245, 249-253, 257, 262, 286, 288, 296, 300
Inferior vertebral notch   139, 151, 157
Infraclavicular fossa   308
Infraglenoid tubercle   311
Infraglottic space   86
Infrahyoid muscles   83, 84
Infraorbital canal   96
Infra-orbital foramen   2
Infrapatellar fat body   378, 379, 388-390
Infraspinatus muscle (tendon)   175, 313, 314, 318-322
Infraspinous fossa   311
Infundibular recess   17
Infundibulum of the pituitary gland   63
Inguinal region   228
Insertion of flexor digitorum superficialis muscle   341
Insertion of flexor hallucis longus muscle   341
Insula   22
Insular cortex   37-40
Insular gyri   28
Insular ribbon   22
Intercondylar eminence   375
Intercondylar fossa   375
Intercostal muscle   88
Intermediate cuneiform   394, 395, 400-402, 411, 412
Intermediate sacral crest   164, 165
Internal auditory canal   61, 109, 111, 112, 115, 116, 120
Internal capsule   21, 30, 37, 38
　Anterior limb   22
Internal carotid artery (ICA)   9, 10, 12, 16, 51-55, 73, 75-80, 131-133
　Siphon   65
Internal iliac artery   273, 279, 280, 287, 296, 353
Internal iliac vein   354
Internal jugular vein   76-88, 91, 92, 102, 103, 107, 108, 131-133
Internal oblique muscle   253, 360
Interosseous muscle (tendon)   347-349, 351, 352, 409-411
Interpeduncular cistern   23, 32, 40, 50-52, 66
Interpeduncular fossa   46

Interspinous ligament   136, 137, 150, 162, 163
Interthalamic adhesion   17, 22, 32
Interventricular foramen (Foramen of Monro)   17, 21, 32
Interventricular septum   187, 206, 207, 215, 216, 220, 222, 224-226
Intervertebral disc   128-130, 134, 136, 137, 142, 144-146, 148-150, 153-158, 160-163
Intervertebral foramen   124, 128-130, 132, 138, 140-142, 144, 145, 148, 149, 151, 153, 157, 158
Intranuclear cleft   163
Intraparietal sulcus   6
Ischial spine   269
Ischial tuberosity   269, 356
Ischiocavernosus muscle   365
Ischiorectal fossa   282, 293
Ischium   268, 283, 356-358, 362, 365, 367, 368
IVR (interventional radiology)   279

Jefferson 骨折   126
Jejunum   236
Joints of foot   355
Jugular foramen   4
Jugular vein   84

● K・L

Kidney   230-245, 250-253, 257-261, 264, 265
Knee joint   355

Lacrimal bone   2
Lacrimal gland   96
LAD (Left anterior descending coronary artery)
　Apical   211, 212
　Middle   211, 212
　Proximal   211, 212
Lambdoid suture   2, 3
Lamina   123, 126, 132, 139-142, 144, 146, 147, 152, 153, 158, 159
Lamina papyracea   73, 96
Lamina terminalis   63
Large intestine   229, 235, 237
Larynx   71
Lateral aperture of fourth ventricle   53
Lateral atlanto-axial joint   125, 129
Lateral basilar segmental bronchus   183

Lateral border   174, 310, 311
Lateral circumflex femoral artery   273, 279
Lateral collateral ligament   371, 383-385
Lateral condyle
　《Femur》   375, 383, 384
　《Tibia》   375
Lateral cuneiform   394, 395, 401, 402, 410, 411
Lateral epicondyle
　《Femur》   375
　《Humerus》   324, 326
Lateral malleolus   393-395
Lateral mass   127, 129, 135
　Atlas   125, 126, 129-131, 134
Lateral meniscus   371, 372, 382-384, 387, 388
Lateral occipitotemporal gyrus   43, 61, 65, 66, 68
Lateral posterior choroidal artery (LPChA)   16
Lateral pterygoid muscle   76, 77, 90-92, 99-101
Lateral rectus muscle   23, 28, 29, 34, 35, 73, 97
Lateral region   228
Lateral sacral arteries   273
Lateral sacral crest   164
Lateral segmental bronchus   183
Lateral semicircular canal   109, 111, 112, 116, 118, 119
Lateral striate arteries (LSA)   16
Lateral sulcus   6
Lateral supraepicondylar ridge   324
Lateral ventricle   22, 30-32, 36
Latissimus dorsi   309
LCX [Left circumflex (coronary) artery]   205, 208, 209, 214-217, 219, 220, 222, 223, 225, 226
　Distal   212
　OM (Obtuse marginal branch)   212
　PD (Posterior descending branch)   212
　PL (Posterolateral branch)   212
　Proximal   212
Left anterior descending artery   205, 208, 209, 213-217, 219-222, 224-226
Left aortic sinus   214, 219, 222
Left atrial appendage   213
Left atrioventricular groove   208, 209

Left atrium　182-184, 187, 189, 190, 192, 206, 207, 213-215, 218, 219, 223-226
Left glenoid cavity　172, 173, 175
Left hypochondrium　228
Left iliac region　228
Left inferior lobar artery　190
Left inferior pulmonary vein　183, 184, 187, 193, 205, 213-215, 219, 223
Left internal jugular vein　185
Left internal thoracic artery　182
Left lateral region　228
Left main trunk(LMT)　208, 209, 211-213, 219, 222
Left major fissure　196-200, 203, 204
Left portal vein　244, 245, 249, 250, 255, 256, 261
Left superior pulmonary vein　183, 184, 186, 205, 213
Left ventricle　182, 187-189, 193, 194, 206, 207, 215-217, 219-226
Leg　355
Lens　23, 29, 74, 91
Lentiform nucleus　22, 38
　Globus pallidus　22, 38
　Putamen　22, 38
Lesser trochanter　356, 357, 359, 367
Lesser tubercle　310, 311
Levator anguli oris muscle　80-82
Levator ani muscle　282, 293, 362
Levator palpebrae superioris muscle　29, 33, 34
Levator scapulae muscle　79-87, 91, 105, 106
Linea alba　253, 280, 284
Lingual artery　97
Lingual septum　79, 80, 98-100
Lisfranc 関節　395
Liver　217, 229-231, 238, 242-245, 249, 254-264
Long plantar ligament　404
Long saphenous vein(Great saphenous vein)　354, 370
Longissimus capitis muscle　76, 77
Longissimus cervicis muscle　131
Longissimus muscle　146, 147, 159
Longitudinal muscle of tongue　97, 98
Longus capitis muscle　101
Lumbar vertebrae　122, 151
　L1　151, 268
　L2〜L5　151

Lunate　342, 344, 349
Luschka 孔(Foramen of Luschka)　53

● M

Main bronchus　183, 186, 196, 200-203, 205
Main portal vein　241, 244, 245, 251, 256, 261, 262
Major calyces　268, 287
Major fissure(Oblique fissure)　180, 181
　Left ——　196-200, 203, 204
　Right ——　196-201
Major forceps　20, 21
Malleus　109
　Head　112, 113, 115, 118
　Manubrium　113, 114, 116, 118, 119
　Neck　118
Mamillary body　32, 50, 51, 63, 64
Mammillary process　152
Mandibular canal　81, 91, 92, 98-100
Manubrium of sternum　171-173, 175, 177, 179
Marginal ramus of cingulate sulcus　19, 31
Masseter muscle　76-80, 89, 90, 97-100
Mastoid antrum　112
Mastoid cells　24, 25, 73-75, 89, 102-104, 110
Mastoid process　2-4, 26, 76, 77, 89, 103, 104
Maxillary sinus　5, 24-26, 28-30, 33-36, 70, 71, 76, 77, 92, 93, 96, 97
MCP 関節(Metacarpophalangeal joint)　351
Medial and lateral intercondylar tubercle　375
Medial basilar segmental bronchus　183
Medial border　174, 310, 311
Medial collateral ligament　371, 372, 382
Medial condyle
　《Femur》　375, 383, 384
　《Tibia》　375
Medial cuneiform　394, 395, 401-415
Medial epicondyle
　《Femur》　375
　《Humerus》　324, 326, 331-333, 338
Medial frontral gyrus　22
Medial lemniscus　63
Medial malleolus　393-395
Medial meniscus　371, 372, 382-384, 390, 391
Medial occipitotemporal gyrus　30, 42, 43, 65, 66, 68
Medial posterior choroidal artery (MPChA)　10, 16
Medial process of calcaneal tuberosity　395
Medial pterygoid muscle　78, 91, 92, 100, 101
Medial rectus muscle　23, 30, 33, 34, 73, 74, 96, 97
Medial segmental bronchus　183
Medial striate arteries(MSA)　16
Medial supraepicondylar ridge　324
Median antebrachial vein(Median vein of forearm)　307, 323
Median atlanto-axial joint　124, 125, 127, 130
Median cubital vein　307, 323
Median palatine suture　4
Median sacral crest　164, 165, 167
Medulla oblongata　24-26, 32, 41, 55-57, 64
Medullary pyramid　56
Mental foramen　2
Mental protuberance　2, 3, 5
Mental tubercle　2
Mesopharynx　78-83
Metacarpal　342, 351, 352
Midbrain　31, 41
Middle cerebellar peduncle　24, 31, 41, 54, 55, 63
Middle cerebral artery(MCA)　9, 10, 12, 14-16, 50, 51, 65, 72
Middle frontal gyrus　7, 19, 20
Middle hepatic vein　244, 245, 249, 250, 255, 256, 261
Middle nasal concha　24, 25, 31, 33-36, 76, 96-98
Middle nasal meatus　96, 97
Middle phalanx
　《Hand》　342, 351, 352
Middle temporal gyrus　27-29, 37, 41, 42, 61
Minor calyces　268, 269, 286
Minor fissure(Horizontal fissure)　180, 181, 197-201
Mitral valve　219, 223
Mitral valve anterior leaflet　215,

225, 226
Mitral valve posterior leaflet   215, 225, 226
Monro 孔(Foramen of Monro)   17, 21, 32
MRCP(magnetic resonance cholangiopancreatography)   257
MTP 関節(Metatarsophalangeal joint)《Foot》   407
Multifidus muscle   106, 146, 147, 159
Mylohyoid muscle   82-84, 93-95, 100
Myometrium   291, 292, 295, 296, 300, 301

● N

Nasal bone   2, 3, 75
Nasal cavity   70, 71, 75-77, 96
Nasal septum   25, 33, 75-77, 96-98
Nasopharynx   25, 26, 37, 71, 76-78, 95
Navicular   394, 395, 400-402, 411-415
Neck of fibula   375
Neck of mandible   76, 77
Neck of radius   324
Neck of scapula   310, 311
Nerve root   133, 161, 162, 167, 168
Nine abdominal regions   228
Nodulus   42, 64
Non-coronary sinus   215, 218, 222, 226
Nuchal ligament   136, 137
Nucleus pulposus   158, 163
Nutcracker syndrome   251

● O

Obliquus capitis inferior muscle   76-78, 104-106, 131, 135, 136
Obliquus capitis muscle   92, 93
Obturator canal   281, 282
Obturator crest   358
Obturator externus muscle   282, 285-287, 293, 295-297, 362-364, 366-368
Obturator foramen   268, 356-358
Obturator internus muscle   280-282, 286-288, 290-293, 296-299, 302, 303, 360-362, 364, 365
Occipital bone   2, 4
Occipital condyle   3 ,4, 26, 125, 129
Occipital gyri   7

Occipital horn   17 ,61
Occipital lobe   6
Oculomotor nerve   44, 46, 52
Odontoid process   124-127, 129, 130, 131, 134, 136, 137
Olecranon   323, 324, 326, 327, 333, 336-338
Olecranon fossa   324
Olfactory bulb   45, 63
Olfactory nerve   37, 45, 63
Olfactory sulcus   22
OM(Obtuse marginal branch)   212
Opening of eustachian tube   77
Opening of maxillary sinus   96
Opercular part   7
Ophthalmic artery   12, 16
Opponens digiti minimi muscle (tendon)   345, 346, 350
Opponens pollicis muscle   345, 350
Optic chiasm   23, 32, 37, 38, 45, 51, 63-65
Optic nerve   18, 23, 34-37, 44, 45, 51, 73, 97
Optic tract   31, 38, 39, 45, 50, 65
Orbicularis oris muscle   91
Orbital gyri   22, 35
Orbital part   7
Orifice of azygos vein   191
Oval window   116
Ovary   274-279, 291, 292, 296, 298, 299, 303
Overuse syndrome   332

● P

Palatine bone   4
Palatine tonsil   78, 79, 101
Palmar interosseous muscle   346
Palmaris longus muscle   328, 329, 331-333
Pancreas   231, 238, 244, 245, 250, 251, 262-265
Pancreas body   230, 242, 243, 251, 255
Pancreas head   230, 242, 243, 251, 252, 255, 256, 262
Pancreas tail   256
Pancreatic duct   256, 257
Pancreaticobiliary duct   257
Papez の回路   18
Papillary muscle   189
Paracentral lobule   19
Parahippocampal gyrus   23, 39, 51, 62, 65-67

Paravertebral fat   148
Parietal association area   7
Parietal bone   2, 3
Parietal foramen   3
Parietal lobe   6
Parieto-occipital sulcus   6, 19, 20, 31, 32
Parotid gland   40, 41, 70, 78-81, 89, 102-104
Patella   369-372, 375-377, 381, 388-390
Patellar ligament   370-372, 379, 388, 389
PD(Posterior descending branch)   212
Pectineus muscle   281-283, 285, 293-295, 300, 302, 355, 362-364
Pectoral region   308
Pectoralis major muscle   175, 314, 320-322
　Clavicular part   309
　Sternal part   309
Pectoralis minor muscle   175
Pedicle   130, 139, 140, 142, 147-149, 151-154, 157, 159, 160-162
Peroneal artery(Fibular artery)   353
Pharyngeal constrictor muscles   94
Pharyngeal tubercle   4
Pharynx   71
Pineal body   32, 41, 63, 67
PIP 関節(Proximal interphalangeal joint)《Hand》   340, 351
Piriformis muscle   280, 291, 360, 365
Pisiform   342, 350
Pituitary gland   23, 32, 37, 52, 65
Pituitary stalk   38
PL(Posterolateral branch)   212
Plantar aponeurosis   407, 408
Plantar calcaneonavicular ligament   403
Plantaris muscle   377-379
Pons   23, 24, 31, 32, 39-41, 52-55, 63, 64, 66
Popliteal artery   353
Popliteus muscle(tendon)   380, 382-384, 387, 389, 390
Portal vein   230, 239, 249, 251, 256
Postcentral gyrus   7, 19, 20
Postcentral sulcus   6
Posterior arch   124, 126, 127, 130, 136, 137
　Atlas   123, 125, 131

Posterior basilar segmental bronchus 183
Posterior cerebral artery (PCA) 9, 10, 12, 14-16, 46, 51, 52, 65
Posterior colliculus 63
Posterior commissure 32, 63
Posterior communicating artery (Pcom) 12, 52
Posterior cruciate ligament 372, 377-379, 382-384, 389, 390
Posterior descending branch 208, 209, 211
Posterior fat pad 325
Posterior inferior cerebellar artery (PICA) 10, 14, 67
Posterior inferior iliac spine 269
Posterior interosseous nerve syndrome 329
Posterior interventricular sulcus 208, 209
Posterior lobe of the pituitary gland (Neurohypophysis) 63
Posterior longitudinal ligament 163
Posterior nerve root 133
Posterior papillary muscle 206, 216, 220, 224
Posterior process《Talus》395
Posterior sacral foramen 164
Posterior segmental bronchus 183
Posterior semicircular canal 109-112, 117-120
Posterior superior iliac spine 269
Posterior talofibular ligament 399, 406, 410, 411
Posterior tibial artery 353
Posterior tibial veins 354
Posterior tubercle 123-128
Precentral gyrus 7, 19, 20
Precentral knob 19
Precentral sulcus 6
Precuneus 19, 20, 43
Prefrontal cortex 7
Prepontine cistern 32, 63
Prevertebral muscle 131, 132, 134, 136
　Longus capitis muscle 76-79
　Longus colli muscle 79-82, 84-87
Primary motor area 7
Primary visual cortex 21
Promontory 115
Pronator quadratus muscle 343, 349, 351, 352
Pronator syndrome 328

Pronator teres muscle 326-333, 336, 337, 339
Proper hepatic artery 230, 240, 242, 243, 251
Proper hepatic vein 255
Prostate 269, 272, 273, 281, 282, 286-290
Proximal phalanx
　《Hand》342, 351, 352
Prussak 腔 (Prussak's space) 115
Psoas major muscle 158-161, 257-261, 264, 265, 285-287, 290, 296-299, 302, 303
Psoas muscle 253
Pterygoid process
　Lateral plate 4, 77
　Medial plate 4, 77
Pubic (bone) 268, 269, 272, 286, 287, 356-358, 362-364
Pubic region 228
Pubic symphysis 268
Pubic tubercle 356, 358
Pulmonary artery 182-184, 186, 189-193, 201, 203
Pulmonary trunk 182-184, 186, 188, 189, 192, 193, 213
Pulmonary valve 187, 192, 213, 219, 221
Pulmonary vein 207
Putamen 21, 22, 29, 30, 37, 38
Pyramid of the vermis 64

● Q

Quadratus femoris muscle 362, 365-367
Quadratus lumborum muscle 159, 253
Quadratus plantae muscle 401-407, 411-413
Quadriceps muscle (tendon) 370-372, 388-390
Quadrigeminal cistern 22, 23, 32, 42, 50

● R

Radial artery 306
Radial collateral ligament 336
Radial tuberosity 324
Radius 324, 329, 331-337, 342-344, 349, 351, 352
Ramus of mandible 2, 5, 77-81, 90, 91, 98-102
RCA (Right coronary artery) 205,

208, 209, 214-222, 224, 226
　Atrioventricular branch 208, 209, 211
　Distal 211
　Middle 211
　Posterior descending branch 211
　Proximal 211
Rectum 235-238, 360, 361, 365
Rectus abdominis muscle 253, 261, 264, 280-282, 284, 288-292, 299-303, 355, 360, 361, 366-368
Rectus capitis posterior major muscle 91-93, 105, 106
Rectus capitis posterior minor muscle 91-93
Rectus capitis posterior muscle 131
Rectus femoris muscle 281-285, 292-294, 355, 361, 362, 366-368
Renal artery 230, 231, 239, 240, 242, 243, 251, 257, 258, 261-264
Renal cortex 258, 268-272, 277, 278, 285-287, 296
Renal medulla 258
Renal pelvis 268, 269, 271, 272, 286, 287
Renal pyramids 286, 287, 296-298
Renal vein 230, 239, 241, 244, 251, 256-258, 261-264
Retrobulbar fat 73, 75
Retromandibular vein 78, 79
Rhomboid minor muscle 84-88
Rhomboid muscle 175
Rib 87, 88, 140-144, 146, 147, 170, 171, 175, 176, 229, 310
Right aortic sinus 214, 218, 221, 226
Right atrial appendage 213, 214
Right atrioventricular groove 208, 209
Right atrium 182, 187, 188, 191, 207, 214-216, 218, 221, 222, 226
Right glenoid cavity 172, 173, 175
Right hypochondrium 228
Right inferior lobar artery 190
Right inferior pulmonary vein 182-184, 205, 214, 215, 223
Right lateral region 228
Right major fissure 196-201
Right portal vein 244, 245, 250, 256
Right superior pulmonary vein 182-184, 186, 187, 192, 205, 213, 214, 223

Right ventricle 182, 187-189, 192-194, 206, 207, 213-222, 224-226
Rolando 溝(Rolando's fissure) 6
Rosenmüller 窩(Rosenmüller fossa) 77
Rotator interval 314
Round window 116

● S

Sacral ala 164, 165, 167, 168
Sacral canal 165, 166
Sacral cornu 164
Sacral foramen 165, 168
Sacral hiatus 164
Sacral promontory 164, 166
Sacral vertebrae 122
  S1〜S5 166
Sacroiliac joint 154, 155, 160, 161, 164, 165, 167, 168, 268
Sacrospinous ligament 281
Sacrum 122, 154, 155, 160, 161, 164, 165, 167, 356-358, 360
Sagittal 144
Sagittal suture 3
Sartorius muscle 280-284, 292-294, 355, 360-362, 366, 367, 372, 376-380, 383-385
Scalenus anterior muscle 108, 134, 135
Scalenus medius muscle 92
Scalenus posterior muscle 92
Scaphoid 342, 344, 349-352
Scapula 86, 170, 171, 175, 176, 178, 179, 309-314, 316, 317, 321, 322
Scrotum 283
Scutum 116
Second metacarpal 345, 346, 349
Second metatarsal 394
Second middle phalanx
  《Hand》 347, 349
Second proximal phalanx
  《Hand》 346, 349
Second thoracic vertebrae 175
Second toe 393
Segond 骨折 382
Semicircular canal 55, 56
Semimembranosus muscle 356, 368, 370, 376, 377, 389-392
Seminal vesicle 269, 272, 280, 281, 287-290
Semioval center 20
Semispinalis capitis muscle 73-80, 90, 91, 93-95, 106, 131, 132
Semitendinosus muscle 370, 376

Septum pellucidum 21, 37-39
Serratus anterior muscle 309, 312, 313, 315
Seventh thoracic vertebrae(T7) 176
Sigmoid colon 235-238, 254, 265, 363, 364
Sigmoid sinus 13, 24
Sinus 29
Sinus of aorta 189
SMA syndrome(Superior mesenteric artery syndrome) 251
Small intestine 229, 235, 237, 254, 360
Smaller SMV sign 252
Soft palate 37, 38, 94, 95, 99, 100
Soleus muscle 355, 371, 372, 380, 384, 385, 387-390, 393, 394, 411-413
Somatosensory area 7
Sphenoethmoidal recess 74
Sphenoidal bone 2
Sphenoidal sinus 23, 24, 31, 32, 36-38, 71, 74, 75, 93-95, 99, 100
Sphenosquamous suture 4
Spinal canal 130, 144, 154, 156
Spinal cord 26, 32, 41, 60, 64, 131-133, 135-137, 146-148
Spine 128
Spine of scapula 174, 311
Spinous process 123, 125-128, 130, 132, 136-143, 146, 147, 150-153, 155, 156, 158, 159, 162, 163, 179
  L4, L5 357
Spleen 230, 231, 241-243, 245, 250, 251, 257-259, 265, 266
Splenic artery 230, 240, 242, 243, 250, 256, 257, 263-265
Splenic vein 230, 231, 239, 241, 244, 245, 250, 251, 255-257, 263-265
Splenius capitis muscle 76-80, 90-92, 105, 106, 131, 132, 136
Splenius cervicis muscle 79, 80, 91, 92
Spring ligament 401
Squamous suture 2, 3
Stapes 109, 113, 116
Sternoclavicular joint 172, 175, 178, 310
Sternocleidomastoid muscle 78-88, 90-94, 102-105, 107, 108, 131, 132, 134, 135, 309
Sternum 170, 229

Stomach 229, 235-238, 245, 249-251, 254-258, 262-264
Straight gyrus 22, 35, 64
Straight sinus 13, 43
Striatum 18, 21
  Caudate nucleus 21
  Putamen 21
Styloid process 2-4
Stylomastoid foramen 4
Subarachnoid space 146, 147, 160, 161, 163
Subclavian artery 88, 104, 182, 185, 190, 306
Subclavian vein 307
Subcutaneous fat 136, 137
Submandibular gland 70, 82, 83, 91, 92, 101, 107
Subscapular fossa 310
Subscapularis muscle 86, 87, 175, 313-317, 320-322
Sulcus 6
Superficial femoral artery 273, 279, 283, 293, 353
Superior angle 311
Superior articular facet 125, 126
Superior articular process 123, 128, 130, 136, 139, 141, 142, 144-146, 149, 151-153, 155, 156, 158, 159, 162
Superior articular process
  Sacrum 164
Superior border 310
Superior cerebellar artery(SCA) 12, 14, 65
Superior cerebellar peduncle 24, 32, 53, 54, 63
Superior colliculus 22, 41, 63, 67
Superior costal facet 139
Superior frontal gyrus 7, 19-21
Superior frontal sulcus 6
Superior gluteal artery 273
Superior lingular bronchus 183
Superior mesenteric artery 230, 231, 238-240, 242, 243, 251, 252, 255, 256, 263, 295
Superior mesenteric vein 230, 231, 238, 239, 241, 244, 251, 252, 255, 256, 262
Superior nasal concha 98
Superior nuchal line 3
Superior oblique muscle 33, 34, 96
Superior ophthalmic vein 97, 98
Superior orbital fissure 2, 98
Superior parietal lobule 7
Superior pubic ramus 358

Superior rectus muscle 29, 33-35, 72, 96, 97
Superior sagittal sinus 13, 40-43
Superior segmental bronchus 183
Superior semicircular canal 109-111, 116, 118-120
Superior temporal gyrus 4, 7, 27, 37, 41, 42, 61
Superior temporal sulcus 6
Superior tibiofibular joint 375
Superior vena cava 186, 187, 189, 191, 205, 213, 218, 222
Superior vertebral notch 139, 151, 157
Supinator muscle 331-333, 335, 336
Supra-orbital foramen 2
Supramarginal gyrus 7, 20, 21, 43
Supraspinatus muscle(tendon) 175, 312, 316-322
Supraspinous fossa 311
Supraspinous ligament 162, 163
Surfer's ear 114
Sustentaculum tali 395
Sylvius 裂(Sylvian fissure) 6, 22, 27, 28, 38, 39, 40, 50, 65
S 状結腸(Sigmoid colon) 235-238, 254, 265, 363, 364
S 状結腸過長症 237
S 状静脈洞(Sigmoid sinus) 13, 24

● T

Talocalcaneal interosseous ligament 411, 412
Talus 394, 395, 398-400, 402-405, 410-412, 414
Tectal plate 32, 63, 64
Tegmentum of midbrain 23, 32, 64
Temporal association area 7
Temporal bone 2, 3
Temporal horn 17, 39, 61, 65-67
Temporal lobe 6
Temporal muscle 72-77, 90, 91, 97, 99
Temporal pole 6, 35, 36
Tendinous cord 226
Tennis elbow 332
Tensor fasciae latae muscle 280-285, 291-295, 355, 361, 362
Tenth thoracic vertebrae(T10) 176
Tentorium cerebelli 28, 31, 32, 42, 61-64, 66-68

Teres major muscle 175, 317, 320-322
Teres minor muscle 314, 320-322
Thalamogeniculate arteries(TGA) 16
Thalamoperforate arteries(TPA) 16
Thalamotuberal arteries(TTA) 16
Thalamus 8, 18, 21, 22, 30, 31, 39, 40, 41
Thenar eminence 340
Thigh 355
Third distal phalanx《Hand》 348
Third metacarpal 345, 346
Third metatarsal 394, 411
Third middle phalanx 《Hand》 347-349
Third proximal phalanx 《Hand》 346, 347
Third thoracic vertebrae 175
Third toe 393
Third ventricle 17, 22, 32, 40, 50, 64-66
Thoracic vertebrae 122, 138, 170
Thyroid cartilage 70, 84-86, 94, 101-103, 108
 Inferior horn 71
 Lamina 71
 Superior horn 71
Thyroid gland 70, 86-88, 93, 94, 102, 103, 185
Thyroid notch 71
Tibia 369-372, 375, 381-383, 385-391, 394-397, 404-407, 411-415
Tibia medial malleolus 398
Tibial tuberosity 369, 375
Tibialis anterior muscle(tendon) 355, 369-372, 380-382, 386, 387, 393, 396-401, 413-415
Tibialis posterior muscle(tendon) 383, 384, 387, 388, 393, 397-400, 403-407
Tongue 79-81
Torus tubarius 77
Trachea 70, 71, 87, 88, 94, 95, 103, 104, 180, 182-186, 190, 192, 195, 196, 202, 205
Tracheoesophageal groove 87
Transverse abdominal muscle 253
Transverse colon 235, 236, 238, 250-254, 260-265
Transverse foramen 123, 126-129
Transverse muscle of tongue 97,

98
Transverse occipital sulcus 6
Transverse palatine suture 4
Transverse process 123-129, 133, 138-140, 143, 144, 147, 151-153 L5 164
Transverse sinus 13, 42, 43
Transverse temporal gyrus 28, 40
Trapezium 342, 345, 349
Trapezius muscle 81-87, 89-93, 106-108, 131, 132, 136, 146, 147, 175, 309, 312, 315-317
Trapezoid 342, 345, 349, 351
Triangular fibrocartilage complex 349
Triangular part 7
Triceps brachii muscle(tendon) 309, 314, 317-320, 323, 325, 327, 332-338
Tricuspid valve 215, 221, 226
Trigeminal nerve 24, 44, 47, 54, 66
Triquetrum 342, 349
Trochlea of humerus 324, 331, 338
Trochlear nerve 44, 46, 53
Tuberosity of fifth metatarsal bone 395
Twelfth rib 268, 269

● U

U-fiber 23
Ulna 324, 328, 329, 334, 337, 342-344, 349
Ulnar artery 306
Ulnar head 340
Ulnar nerve 326, 327
Umbilical region 228
Uncinate process 96, 123, 124, 128, 129, 134, 252
Uncus of the parahippocampal gyrus 23, 30, 66
Ureter 230, 231, 257, 268, 269-272, 280, 286, 290
Ureteropelvic junction 252
Urethra 293
Urinary bladder 268-281, 284-286, 288-290, 292-296, 299-302, 360, 363, 364
Uterine artery 279
Uterine body 300, 302
Uterine cervix 291, 292, 300-302
Uterus 274-279, 291, 292, 295, 297, 298
Uvula vermis 64, 67, 68

● V

Vagina 274, 275, 278, 292, 293, 296, 300, 301
Vagus nerve 44, 48, 57, 58, 67
Valsalva 洞 189, 207, 214
Vastus intermedius muscle 283, 286, 362-366
Vastus lateralis muscle 282, 283, 285, 286, 293, 295-297, 355, 362-365, 369-371, 376, 381-383, 386, 387
Vastus medialis muscle 355, 369-372, 376, 381, 382, 384, 385, 390-392
Ventral median fissure 26, 56-59
Ventricle 54
Vertebra prominens(C7) 123
Vertebral arch 127, 128, 139, 147, 152
Vertebral artery(VA) 9, 12, 16, 26, 56-60, 64, 66, 67, 74-87, 131-134
Vertebral body 123, 124, 127, 128, 130, 133, 134, 136-142, 144-154, 156-162, 178, 179
  Axial 129
  L1 162, 163
  L5 164
  S1 162, 163, 166
  Sacrum 167
Vertebral foramen 127, 128, 139, 140, 152, 153, 158, 159
Vertebrobasilar artery(VA-BA) 14
Vestibular aqueduct 111, 112
Vestibule 109, 112, 116, 119, 120
Vestibulocochlear nerve 44, 48, 55, 62, 66
Visual area 7
Vitreous body 74, 91
Vocal cord 85

Volkmann 拘縮 325

● W

Wernicke's area 7
White matter 61
Willis 動脈輪 12
Wrisberg 靱帯 373

● X・Y・Z

Xiphoid process 171-173, 176, 179

Yellow ligament 150, 158, 159, 163

Zygoma 76
Zygomatic arch 2-4, 75, 76, 97-100
Zygomatic bone 77, 89-91

3次元画像から学ぶCT・MRI断層解剖
定価(本体7,000円+税)

2014年3月28日発行　第1版第1刷©

編著者　似鳥　俊明
　　　　にたとり　としあき

発行者　株式会社　メディカル・サイエンス・インターナショナル
　　　　代表取締役　若松　博
　　　　東京都文京区本郷1-28-36
　　　　郵便番号 113-0033　電話(03)5804-6050

印刷：三美印刷／表紙装丁：トライアンス

ISBN 978-4-89592-768-0　C 3047

本書の複製権・翻訳権・上映権・譲渡権・公衆送信権(送信可能化権を含む)は(株)メディカル・サイエンス・インターナショナルが保有します。
本書を無断で複製する行為(複写，スキャン，デジタルデータ化など)は，「私的使用のための複製」など著作権法上の限られた例外を除き禁じられています．大学，病院，診療所，企業などにおいて，業務上使用する目的(診療，研究活動を含む)で上記の行為を行うことは，その使用範囲が内部的であっても，私的使用には該当せず，違法です．また私的使用に該当する場合であっても，代行業者等の第三者に依頼して上記の行為を行うことは違法となります．

JCOPY 〈(社)出版者著作権管理機構 委託出版物〉
本書の無断複写は著作権法上での例外を除き禁じられています．複写される場合は，そのつど事前に，(社)出版者著作権管理機構(電話 03-3513-6969, FAX 03-3513-6979, info@jcopy.or.jp)の許諾を得てください．